Laparoscopic Surgery

Laparoscopic Surgery

GARTH H. BALLANTYNE, M.D., F.A.C.S., F.A.S.C.R.S.
Associate Professor of Surgery
Department of Surgery
Yale University School of Medicine
New Haven, Connecticut
Assistant Chief of Surgical Services
West Haven Veterans Administration Medical Center
West Haven, Connecticut

PATRICK F. LEAHY, M.B., B.Ch., B.A.O., M.Ch., F.R.C.S.I.
Consultant
General Surgeon
Blackrock Clinic
Blackrock
Dublin, Ireland

IRVIN M. MODLIN, M.D., Ph.D., F.R.C.S., F.C.S., F.A.C.S.
Professor of Surgery
Yale University School of Medicine
Chief of Endoscopic Surgery
Yale-New Haven Hospital
New Haven, Connecticut

W.B. SAUNDERS COMPANY
A Division of Harcourt Brace & Company
Philadelphia/London/Toronto/Montreal/Sydney/Tokyo

W.B. SAUNDERS COMPANY

A Division of Harcourt Brace & Company

The Curtis Center
Independence Square West
Philadelphia, PA 19106

Library of Congress Cataloging-in-Publication Data

Laparoscopic surgery / [edited by] Garth H. Ballantyne, Patrick F.
Leahy, Irvin M. Modlin. — 1st ed.
    p.   cm.
    ISBN 0-7216-6648-5
    1. Endoscopic surgery.   2. Laparoscopic surgery.   I. Ballantyne,
Garth H.   II. Leahy, Patrick F.   III. Modlin, Irvin M.
        [DNLM: 1. Laparoscopy—methods.   2. Surgery, Operative—methods.
WO 500 L299 1994]
RD33.53.L37 1994
617'.05—dc20
DNLM/DLC   93-4894

Laparoscopic Surgery   ISBN 0-7216-6648-5

Text copyright © 1994 by W.B. Saunders Company
Illustrations copyright © 1994 by United States Surgical Corporation

All rights reserved. No part of this publication may be reproduced or transmitted in any form or by any means, electronic or mechanical, including photocopy, recording, or any information storage and retrieval system, without permission in writing from the publisher.

Printed in United States of America

Last digit is the print number: 9   8   7   6   5   4   3   2

To my father, Robert Heath Ballantyne, whose efforts in training me during my youth gave me the determination and skills to complete this opus; and to my wife, Helen, whose skills in raising our family and whose love, support and tolerance gave me the time to devote to this project

GHB

To Karen and Ronan

PFL

To my wife, Maria, without whose patience, support and understanding of the future this work could not have been accomplished

IMM

Preface

The practice of surgery has remained remarkably stable over the last five hundred years. Radical changes in the philosophy and technique of surgery were prompted during this time period by only a handful of distinct events. Rapid evolution in surgical thought was ignited by the revelation of true human anatomy by Vesalius with the publication of his *De Humani Corporis Fabrica* in 1543, the introduction of the scientific method into surgical research by John Hunter in the 18th century, the description of an effective and safe suturing technique for the closure of enteric wounds and the construction of anastomoses by Lembert in 1826, the use of nitrous oxide for the extraction of teeth by Wells in 1844 and the administration of ether by Morton at the Massachusetts General Hospital in 1846, and finally the demonstration of the microbial basis of surgical wound infection and the development of antiseptic surgery by Lord Lister in the second half of the 19th century. The summation of these breakthroughs spawned the birth of elective general surgery in the late 19th century. Indeed, the application of these discoveries allowed gifted surgeons such as Bilroth, Halsted, Moynihan, Miles and Mayo to introduce successfully into clinical practice by the close of the 19th century virtually all of the gastrointestinal operations still used today. Whereas surgical technique has evolved throughout the 20th century, it would be fair to say that the gastrointestinal operations we learned during our residencies were 19th century operations using 19th century instruments. The advent of videolaparoscopic cholecystectomy in 1989 has once again ignited an explosive period of growth not only in the practice of gastrointestinal surgery but also, in all branches of surgery. Thus, we are witnessing one of the six most fertile periods of surgical growth in the last five hundred years. What is the basis of this revolution?

The use of the laparoscope in the performance of abdominal operations is not a new idea. Indeed, gynecologists have performed safe and effective laparoscopic procedures for decades. Moreover, a number of "advanced laparoscopic procedures" were accomplished with traditional laparoscopes during the 1980s but these excited little interest at the time. Thus, it was not the application of laparoscopy to cholecystectomy which kindled this revolution in surgical thinking. When Eddie Joe Reddick and William Saye turned a videolaparoscope toward the gallbladder, however, immense excitement was generated and many new ideas about the practice of all fields of surgery burst forth. Attachment of a video camera to a traditional laparoscope breached the isolation that separated gastrointestinal surgery from the rest of society for nearly a century and opened the floodgate of biotechnology transfer from the rest of 20th century civilization into the practice of general surgery. Whereas fields of surgery such as cardiac surgery have long benefitted from modern electronics, videolaparoscopic cholecystectomy was the first insertion of space age technology into gastrointestinal surgery technique. This transfer of 20th century technology has continued to feed the rapid evolution not only of abdominal surgery but also of other vastly divergent areas of surgery.

Laparoscopic Surgery is a snapshot of the philosophy, practice, techniques and results of surgery amidst a period of rapid evolution. The purpose of this book is to disseminate rapidly the advances achieved by the pioneers of this new era of surgical practice. As a result, internationally recognized authorities have been selected to pen each of the sixty-two chapters in this textbook. In particular, contributions were solicited from the master surgeons throughout the United States and Europe who pioneered these new surgical techniques such as Eddie Joe Reddick, Phillip Mouret, Bernard Dallemagne, Namir Katkhouda, Karl Zucker, Dennis Fowler, John Corbitt Jr. and Robert Beart. Just as the five previous major advances of surgical practice were born both in the private practice of surgery such as that of John Hunter and in university departments of surgery such as that of Vesalius, the seminal thinkers and creative forces in our current revolution in surgical practice come from both private practice and university based settings. The contents of this book are directed toward practicing general surgeons and colon and rectal surgeons. Many of the sections, however, should interest gynecologists, urologists and thoracic surgeons. Furthermore, the design is intended to introduce medical students and surgical residents to the basic principles of laparoscopic surgery.

Laparoscopic Surgery is both a textbook and atlas of surgical practice. **Section I. Fundamentals** presents a broad base of information with which all laparoscopic surgeons should be familiar. Technical information on equipment, imaging and electrocautery relevant to laparoscopic surgery is detailed. The tactics of setting up an operating room are considered. Important issues in selection of anesthesia and the pathophysiology of a pneumoperitoneum are explored. Considerations of laparoscopy in pregnant women are summarized. Additionally, an extensive review of complications associated with laparoscopic surgery is compiled.

Section II. General Techniques of Laparoscopic Surgery presents step by step instructions for the accomplishment of techniques, which are applied commonly in a wide variety of laparoscopic procedures. These include trocar insertion, tissue approximation and ligation, techniques of exposure, retraction and dissection and methods of anastomosis. The next four sections present didactic material in an organ system approach.

Section III. Surgery of the Upper Gastrointestinal Tract reviews the pathophysiology of peptic ulcer disease and explores potential applications of laparoscopic surgery in this area. Indications for splenectomy and the technique of laparoscopic splenectomy are outlined. Past results and the future role of laparoscopy in the management of pancreatic diseases are detailed.

Section IV. Surgery of the Biliary System reviews in detail the results of firmly established areas of laparoscopic surgery: the treatment of acute and chronic cholecystitis. In addition, issues about various approaches to the management of common bile duct stones are presented.

Section V. Surgery of the Lower Gastrointestinal Tract reviews the results of treatment of diseases of the appendix and colon. Specifically, the results of laparoscopy in the management of appendicitis are compiled and presented. The pathophysiology of diverticular disease is reviewed and the potential role of laparoscopy in patients afflicted with this malady is explored. The role of laparoscopy in the management of colorectal cancer is one of the most controversial areas of application of this technology. Consequently, an extensive review of previous debates about the merits of various surgical techniques for the treatment of colorectal cancer is provided for reference. Armed with this background the reader will be better prepared to evaluate renewed debate about issues such as high ligation of vessels during the performance of laparoscopic resection for colorectal malignancies. Information about methods of staging colorectal cancers is offered since new technologies may allow improved preoperative and laparoscopic intraoperative staging in the immediate future. Potential roles of laparoscopic surgery in the management of intestinal obstruction, functional disorders of the colon and colonic volvulus are surveyed.

Section VI. Surgery for Other Disorders assembles important information from a wide spectrum of disorders. Results of laparoscopy as a diagnostic modality and in the management of the acute abdomen are detailed. Important considerations and issues in the treatment of inguinofemoral hernias are reviewed. The early experience and technique of thoracoscopic procedures are presented. The early results of laparoscopy in the treatment of genitourinary afflictions are outlined. The appearance of a broad range of obstetric and gynecologic conditions is presented in color so that laparoscopic surgeons will better recognize these conditions when they are unexpectedly encountered. Additionally, the role of laparoscopy in the management of endometriosis is discussed.

Section VII. Techniques of Laparoscopic Surgery is the surgical atlas portion of this book. Nearly all of currently performed laparoscopic operations are addressed. Each chapter discusses patient selection, preoperative evaluation of the patient, equipment required for the procedure, positioning of video equipment, trocar placement and size selection, positioning of the patient, methods of dissection, specific step by step instructions for the operation, techniques of closure, postoperative management of the patient, criteria for patient discharge and specific complications of the procedure. The techniques of the operations are illustrated both by color slides of actual operations and by detailed line drawings. Thomas McCracken has synthesized images from still photographs and videotapes to produce line drawings, which reveal the three dimensional relationships of the instruments and the details of the surgical anatomy. In keeping with an atlas format, each figure illustrates a passage of the text. Consequently, legends have been omitted from this section. A special thank you must be extended to the United States Surgical Corporation, which underwrote much of the cost of the extensive set of figures incorporated into this volume. Many of the instruments depicted herein are tradenames of the U.S. Surgical Corporation and are denoted by an asterisk (*).

The final section of the book, **Section VIII. Postdoctoral Training of Laparoscopic Surgery,** focuses on two areas which are critical during the present period of transition as practicing surgeons learn these new techniques. The requisite components of courses that teach laparoscopic surgery to practicing surgeons are enumerated so that surgeons may better judge the quality of courses in which they may enroll. In the final chapter of *Laparoscopic Surgery*, often-used criteria for the granting of hospital privileges for new laparoscopic procedures are reviewed.

The philosophy, instrumentation, technique and results of laparoscopic surgery have entered a remarkable period of rapid evolution. *Laparoscopic Surgery* attempts to paint a broad picture of surgical practice in late 1993. Thus, the information contained herein can be used by practicing surgeons and surgeons still in training to shape a strategy for inserting and developing this rapidly evolving field in their own clinical practice.

GARTH H. BALLANTYNE, M.D., F.A.C.S., F.A.S.C.R.S.
PATRICK F. LEAHY, M.B., B.CH., B.A.O., M.CH., F.R.C.S.I.
IRVIN M. MODLIN, M.D., PHD., F.R.C.S., F.C.S., F.A.C.S.

Contributors

DAVID N. ARMSTRONG, M.D., M. Chir., F.R.C.S.
Attending Colon and Rectal Surgeon
Georgia Baptiste Hospital
Atlanta, GA

Volvulus of the Colon

M.E. ARREGUI, M.D., F.A.C.S.
Director of Fellowship in Laparoscopy, Endoscopy and Ultrasound
St. Vincent's Hospital and Health Care Center
Indianapolis, IN

Iliopubic Tract Inguinal Hernia Repair with Inlay Buttress of Mesh

ROBERT W. BAILEY, M.D.
Division Head of General Surgery
Department of Surgery
Greater Baltimore Medical Center
Baltimore, MD

Complications
Management of Acute Cholecystitis
Vagotomy

JOHN C. BALDWIN, M.D., F.A.C.S.
Professor of Surgery
Yale University School of Medicine
Chief, Division of Cardiovascular Surgery
Yale-New Haven Hospital
New Haven, CT

Diagnostic and Therapeutic Thoracoscopy

GARTH H. BALLANTYNE, M.D., F.A.C.S., F.A.S.C.R.S.
Associate Professor of Surgery
Department of Surgery
Yale University School of Medicine
Assistant Chief of Surgical Services
West Haven VA Medical Center
West Haven, CT

Physics of Electrosurgery
Colorectal Cancer
Preoperative and Intraoperative Staging of Colorectal Cancer
Volvulus of the Colon
Polypectomy
Right Hemicolectomy with Extracorporeal Anastomosis
Anterior Resection for Rectal Prolapse
Closure of an Ileostomy
Abdominal Perineal Resection

JORIS BANNENBERG, M.D.
Assistant Professor of Surgery
Department of Surgical Research
University of Amsterdam
Academic Medical Center
Amsterdam, Netherlands

Setting Up and Running Courses

ROBERT W. BEART, M.D., F.A.C.S., F.A.S.C.R.S.
Professor of Surgery
Colon & Rectal Surgery
Department of Surgery
University of Southern California
School of Medicine
USC Healthcare Consultation Center
1510 San Pablo Street, Suite 514
Los Angeles, CA

Right Colectomy

BROCK M. BORDELON, M.D.
Department of Surgery
University of Utah School of Medicine
Salt Lake City, UT

Laparoscopy in the Pregnant Patient

GENE D. BRANUM, M.D.
Assistant Professor of Surgery
Department of Surgery
Emory University Medical Center
Atlanta, GA

Modern Treatment of Gallstones: Cholecystectomy

PHILIP F. CAUSHAJ, M.D., F.A.C.S., F.A.S.C.R.S.
Associate Professor of Surgery
University of Massachusetts Medical School
Associate Program Director
University of Massachusetts General Surgery Residency Program
Chair, Department of Surgery
The Medical Center of Central Massachusetts
Worcester, MA

Diagnostic Laparoscopy
Appendectomy

Contributors

WILLIAM G. CHEADLE, M.D.
Assistant Professor of Surgery
University of Louisville
Norton Hospital
University of Louisville
Jewish Hospital
Norton-Children's Hospital
Veterans Administration Medical Center
Appendectomy for Acute Appendicitis

ANTHONY V. COLETTA, M.D., F.A.C.S.
Associate Clinical Professor of Surgery
Medical College of Pennsylvania
Attending Surgeon
Bryn Mawr Hospital
Bryn Mawr, PA
Drainage of a Diverticular Abscess
Closure of a Hartmann's Colostomy

JOHN A. COLLER, M.D., F.A.C.S., F.A.S.C.R.S.
Staff Surgeon
Department of Colon and Rectal Surgery
Lahey Clinic
Burlington, MA
Equipment

JOHN D. CORBITT, JR., M.D., F.A.C.S.
Chairman
Department of Surgery
John F. Kennedy Medical Center
Atlantis, FL
Herniorrhaphy

ANTHONY J. CUNNINGHAM, M.D., F.A.N.Z.C.A., F.F.A.R.C.S.I., F.R.C.P.C.
Professor of Anesthesia
Royal College of Surgeons
St. Stephen's Green
Dublin, Ireland
Anesthesia

BERNARD DALLEMAGNE, M.D.
Service de Chirurgie
Clinique Saint-Joseph
Leige, Belgium
Nissen Fundoplication

DUDLEY SETH DANOFF, M.D., F.A.C.S.
Clinical Faculty
Department of Urology
University of California School of Medicine
Urologic Surgeon
Cedars-Sinai Medical Center and U.C.L.A. Medical Center
Los Angeles, CA
Pelvic Lymphadenectomy

MICHELE D. DAVIS, M.D.
Resident in General Surgery
St. Mary's Hospital
Waterbury, CT
Colorectal Cancer
Preoperative and Intraoperative Staging of Colorectal Cancer

LEON DAYKHOVSKY, M.D.
Assistant Director, Laser Research Center
Cedars-Sinai Medical Center
Clinical Instructor in Surgery
University of California at Los Angeles
Los Angeles, CA
Clinical Instructor in Surgery
Wadsworth Veterans Administration Hospital
Los Angeles, CA
Exploration of the Common Bile Duct

MICHAEL P. DIAMOND, M.D.
Associate Professor,
Department of Obstetrics and Gynecology, Surgery, and Molecular Physiology and Biophysics
Vanderbilt University Medical Center
Nashville, TN
Endometriosis

H.A.F. DUDLEY, M.B., F.R.C.S.
Emeritus Professor of Surgery
London University
London, UK
The Acute Abdomen

TITUS D. DUNCAN, M.D., F.A.C.S.
Assistant Clinical Professor
Department of Surgery
Emory University Medical Center
Atlanta, GA
Director of Minimally Invasive Surgery
Georgia Baptiste Medical Center
Atlanta, GA
Inguinofemoral Hernias

DOUGLAS B. EVANS, M.D.
Assistant Professor of Surgery
M.D. Anderson Cancer Center
Houston, TX
Placement of a Feeding Jejunostomy

ANDREA FERRARA, M.D.
Staff Colon and Rectal Surgeon
Colon and Rectal Clinic of Orlando
Orlando, FL
Functional Disorders of the Colon

STEPHEN J. FERZOCO, M.D.
Resident in General Surgery
Brigham and Women's Hospital
Boston, MA
Splenic Surgery

L. PETER FIELDING, M.B., B.S., F.R.C.S., F.A.C.S.

Clinical Professor of Surgery
Yale University School of Medicine
Chairman, Department of Surgery
St. Mary's Hospital
Waterbury, CT

Intestinal Obstruction

JOHN L. FLOWERS, M.D.

Assistant Professor of Surgery
Department of Surgery
Director
Center for Advances in Videoscopic Surgery
Department of Surgery
University of Maryland School of Medicine
Baltimore, MD

Complications
Management of Acute Cholecystitis
Vagotomy

KENNETH A. FORDE, M.D., F.A.C.S.

Professor of Clinical Surgery
College of Physicians and Surgeons
Columbia University
New York, NY
Attending Surgeon
Presbyterian Hospital
New York, NY

Hospital Credentialing

DENNIS L. FOWLER, M.D., F.A.C.S.

Assistant Clinical Professor of Surgery
University of Missouri
Kansas City, MO

Techniques of Exposure, Retraction, and Dissection
Gastric Resection

THOMAS S. FRENCH, M.D.

Chief Resident in General Surgery
University of Massachusetts Medical Center Coordinated Surgical Residency Program
Worcester, MA

Appendectomy

M.M. GAZAYERLI, M.D., F.R.C.S. (C)

Director, Laparoscopic Laser Surgery Institute, Michigan
Staff Surgeon
Madison Community Hospital
Madison Heights, Michigan
North Oakland Medical Center
Pontiac, MI

Iliopubic Tract Inguinal Hernia Repair with Inlay Buttress of Mesh

CHARLES GELEZ, M.D.

General Surgeon
Lyon, France

Lysis of Adhesions

ALEX GERSHMAN, M.D.

Clinical Instructor, Division of Surgery-Urology
UCLA Medical Center
University of California School of Medicine
Clinical Instructor and Research Scientist
Cedars-Sinai Medical Center
Los Angeles, CA

Pelvic Lymphadenectomy

LEO A. GORDON, M.D., F.A.C.S.

Attending Surgeon
Cedars-Sinai Medical Center
Los Angeles, CA

Exploration of the Common Bile Duct

SCOTT M. GRAHAM, M.D.

Assistant Professor of Surgery
Director of Surgical Endoscopy
University of Maryland Medical School
Attending Surgeon
University of Maryland Medical Center
Baltimore, MD

Laparoendoscopic Management of Common Bile Duct Stones

FREDERICK L. GREENE, M.D., F.A.C.S.

Professor of Surgery
Director of Surgical Oncology and Surgical Endoscopy
University of South Carolina School of Medicine
Columbus, SC

Operating Room Configuration

JAMES HAEBE, M.D.

Assistant Professor
University of Ottawa
Department of Obstetrics and Gynecology
Ottawa General Hospital
Ottawa, Ontario

Obstetric and Gynecologic Disorders

LAWRENCE E. HARRISON, M.D.

Chief Resident in Surgery
University of Massachusetts Medical Center Coordinated Surgical Residency Program
Worcester, MA

Diagnostic Laparoscopy
Appendectomy

H.S. HELMY, M.B., B. CH., M.D.

Lecturer in Surgery
Department of Surgery
Cairo University
Cairo, Egypt

Iliopubic Tract Inguinal Hernia Repair with Inlay Buttress of Mesh

Contributors

JOHN G. HUNTER, M.D.
Associate Professor of Surgery
Emory University School of Medicine
Chief, Gastrointestinal Surgery
Emory University Hospital
Atlanta, GA
Laparoscopy in the Pregnant Patient

D. ALAN JOHNS, M.D.
Director
GYN Laparoscopy Center
Harris-Methodist Hospital
Fort Worth, TX
Endometriosis

NAMIR KATKHOUDA, M.D.
Associate Professor of Surgery
Hospital Saint-Roch
University of Nice
Chief of Endoscopic Surgery
Hospital Saint-Roch
Nice, France
Laparoscopic Treatment of Peptic Ulcer Disease

WILLIAM E. KELLY, JR., M.D., F.A.C.S.
Richmond Surgical Group
Richmond, VA
Left Hemicolectomy

GERALD M. LARSON, M.D., F.A.C.S.
Professor of Surgery
University of Louisville
Louisville, KY
Humana Hospital University of Louisville
Jewish Hospital
Norton-Children's Hospital
Veterans Administration Medical Center
Appendectomy for Acute Appendicitis

STEVEN D. LEACH, M.D.
Fellow in Surgical Oncology
M.D. Anderson Cancer Center
Houston, TX
Approaches to Pancreatic Disease

PATRICK F. LEAHY, M.B., B.Ch., B.A.O., M.Ch., F.R.C.S.I.
Consultant General Surgeon
Blackrock Clinic
Blackrock
Dublin, Ireland
Esophagogastrectomy
Low Anterior Resection

WALTER E. LONGO, M.D.
Assistant Professor of Surgery
Head of Research, Section of Colon and Rectal Surgery
Department of Surgery
Saint Louis University School of Medicine
St. Louis, MO
Treatment of Lower Gastrointestinal Diverticular Disease

ROBERT D. MADOFF, M.D.
Clinical Assistant Professor of Surgery
Director of Research
Division of Colon and Rectal Surgery
Department of Surgery
University of Minnesota Medical School
Minneapolis, MN
Imaging

PAUL F. MANSFIELD, M.D.
Assistant Professor of Surgery
M.D. Anderson Cancer Center
Houston, TX
Placement of a Feeding Jejunostomy

DAN C. MARTIN, M.D., F.A.C.O.G.
Associate Professor
Department of Obstetrics and Gynecology
University of Tennessee
Memphis, TN
Reproductive Surgeon
Baptist Memorial Hospital
Memphis, TN
Obstetric and Gynecologic Disorders

EDWARD M. MASON, M.D., F.A.C.S.
Assistant Clinical Professor
Department of Surgery
University of Georgia School of Medicine
Georgia Baptiste Hospital
Atlanta, GA
Inguinofemoral Hernias

DIRK MEIJER, M.D.
Assistant Professor of Surgery
Department of Surgical Research
University of Amsterdam
Academic Medical Center
Amsterdam, Netherlands
Setting Up and Running Courses

WILLIAM C. MEYERS, M.D., F.A.C.S.
Professor of Surgery
Duke University School of Medicine
Chief, Gastrointestinal Surgery
Duke University Hospital
Durham, NC
Modern Treatment of Gallstones: Cholecystectomy

P. JEFFREY W. MILSOM, M.D., F.A.C.S., F.A.S.C.R.S.
Director of Research
Section of Colon and Rectal Surgery
Cleveland Clinic
Cleveland, OH
Closed and Open Techniques of Trocar Insertion

Contributors

IRVIN M. MODLIN, M.D., Ph.D., F.R.C.S., F.C.S., F.A.C.S.
Professor of Surgery
Yale University School of Medicine
Chief of Endoscopic Surgery
Yale-New Haven Hospital
New Haven, CT
Splenic Surgery
Approaches to Pancreatic Disease

WILLIAM MORGAN, M.D.
Staff Urologist
Medical College of Virginia
Richmond, VA
Urologic Disorders

ANNE C. MOSENTHAL, M.D.
Chief Resident in General Surgery
University of Massachusetts Medical Center Coordinated Surgical Residency Program
Worcester, MA
Diagnostic Laparoscopy

JEAN MOUIEL, M.D.
Professor of Surgery
Hospital Saint-Roch
Chief of General Surgery
Hospital Saint-Roch
Nice, France
Laparoscopic Treatment of Peptic Ulcer Disease

PHILLIPPE MOURET, M.D.
General Surgeon
Lyon, France
Lysis of Adhesions

JOHN J. MURRAY, M.D., F.A.C.S., F.A.S.C.R.S.
Staff Surgeon
Department of Colon and Rectal Surgery
Lahey Clinic
Burlington, MA
Equipment

JUAN J. NOGUERAS, M.D.
Staff Colorectal Surgeon
Department of Colorectal Surgery
Cleveland Clinic Florida
Fort Lauderdale, FL
Anastomosis

MARGRET ODDSDOTTIR, M.D.
Fellow in Laparoscopic Surgery
Emory University Medical Center
Atlanta, GA
Peptic Ulcer Disease

DAVID M. OTA, M.D., F.A.C.S.
Professor of Surgery
University of Missouri School of Medicine
Medical Director
University of Missouri Ellis Fischel Cancer Center
Columbia, MO
Placement of a Feeding Jejunostomy

S. PATERSON-BROWN, M.B., F.R.C.S.
Senior Registrar
Department of Surgery
St. Mary's Hospital
London, UK
The Acute Abdomen

JOHN H. PEMBERTON, M.D., F.A.C.S., F.A.S.C.R.S.
Associate Professor of Surgery
Mayo Medical School
Mayo Clinic,
Rochester, Minnesota
St. Mary's Hospital
Rochester, MN
Functional Disorders of the Colon

HIRAM C. POLK, JR., M.D., F.A.C.S.
Ben A. Reid, Sr. Professor and Chairman
Department of Surgery
University of Louisville School of Medicine
Louisville, KY
Appendectomy for Acute Appendicitis

MICHAEL PONTARI, M.D.
Resident in Urology
Yale University School of Medicine
Yale-New Haven Hospital
New Haven, CT
Urologic Disorders

EDDIE JOE REDDICK, M.D., F.A.C.S.
General Surgeon
Nashville, TN
Cholecystectomy

HARRY REICH, M.D., F.A.C.O.G.
Private Practice
Wyoming Valley GYN Associates
Kingston, PA
Oophorectomy

JUAN A. SANCHEZ, M.D.
Assistant Professor of Clinical Surgery
Division of Thoracic and Cardiovascular Surgery
University of Miami School of Medicine
Miami, FL
Jackson Memorial Hospital
Miami, FL
Diagnostic and Therapeutic Thoracoscopy

Contributors

LAWRENCE A. SAPERSTEIN, M.D.

Resident in Surgery
Department of Surgery
Stanford University Medical School
Stanford, CA

Modern Treatment of Gallstones: Cholecystectomy

THOMAS R. SCOTT, M.D.

Attending Surgeon
York Hospital
York, PA

Laparoendoscopic Management of Common Bile Duct Stones

ANTHONY J. SENAGORE, M.D., M.S.

Associate Professor of Surgery
Michigan State University
East Lansing, Michigan
Ferguson-Bladgett Hospital
Grand Rapids, MI

Tissue Approximation and Ligation Techniques

STEPHEN J. SHAPIRO, M.D., F.A.C.S.

Assistant Clinical Professor of Surgery
UCLA School of Medicine
Los Angeles, CA
Attending Surgeon
Cedars-Sinai Medical Center
Los Angeles, CA

Exploration of the Common Bile Duct

NATHANIEL J. SOPER, M.D.

Associate Professor of Surgery
Department of Surgery
Washington University School of Medicine
St. Louis, MO

Small Bowel Resection

DAVID I. SOYBEL, M.D.

Assistant Professor of Surgery
Harvard Medical School
Brigham and Woman's Hospital
Boston, MA

Peptic Ulcer Disease

JOHN SPENCER, M.S., F.R.C.S.

Reader in Surgery
Royal Postgraduate Medical School
Hammersmith Hospital
London, U.K.
Consultant Surgeon
Hammersmith Hospital,
London, U.K.

Cardiomyotomy

MICHAEL P. SPENCER, M.D.

Clinical Instructor of Surgery
Division of Colon and Rectal Surgery
Department of Surgery
University of Minnesota Medical School
Minneapolis, MN

Imaging

TORGNY SVENBERG, M.D., Ph.D.

Associate Professor of Surgery
Karolinska Institute
Chief, Colon and Rectal Surgery
Karolinska Hospital
Stockholm, Sweden

Pathophysiology of Pneumoperitoneum

NANCY C. TAYLOR, R.N.

Research Assistant
University of South Carolina School of Medicine
Columbus, SC

Operating Room Configuration

JOSEPH F. UDDO, JR., M.D., F.A.C.S.

Clinical Assistant Professor of Surgery
Louisiana State University Medical School
4224 Houma Blvd, Suite 450
Metaire, LA

Antrectomy with Billroth II Anastomosis
Right Hemicolectomy with Intracorporeal Anastomosis

OZURU O. UKOHA

Resident in General Surgery
St. Mary's Hospital
Waterbury, CT

Intestinal Obstruction

ANTHONY M. VERNAVA, III, M.D., F.A.C.S.

Associate Professor of Surgery
Chief, Section of Colon and Rectal Surgery
Department of Surgery
Saint Louis University School of Medicine
St. Louis, MO

Treatment of Lower Gastrointestinal Diverticular Disease

STEPHEN WAISBREN, M.D., Ph.D.

Resident in Surgery
Yale University School of Medicine
Yale-New Haven Hospital
New Haven, CT

Physics of Electrosurgery

STEVEN D. WEXNER, M.D., F.A.C.S.,
F.A.S.C.R.S.

Residency Program Director
Department of Colorectal Surgery
Director
Anorectal Physiology Laboratory
Chairman, Continuing Medical Education
Cleveland Clinic Florida
Fort Lauderdale, FL

Anastomosis

KARL A. ZUCKER, M.D., F.A.C.S.

Professor of Surgery
Department of Surgery
University of New Mexico School of Medicine
Chief, Division of Surgical Endoscopy
University of New Mexico Hospital
Staff Surgeon
Veterans Administration Medical Center
Albuquerque, NM

Complications
Management of Acute Cholecystitis
Vagotomy

Contents

SECTION I FUNDAMENTALS — 1

1. **Equipment** — 3
   John A. Coller & John J. Murray
2. **Imaging** — 15
   Michael P. Spencer & Robert D. Madoff
3. **Physics of Electrosurgery** — 22
   Stephen Waisbren & Garth H. Ballantyne
4. **Operating Room Configuration** — 34
   Frederick L. Greene & Nancy C. Taylor
5. **Anesthesia** — 42
   Anthony J. Cunningham
6. **Pathophysiology of Pneumoperitoneum** — 61
   Torgny Svenberg
7. **Laparoscopy in the Pregnant Patient** — 69
   Brock M. Bordelon & John G. Hunter
8. **Complications** — 77
   John L. Flowers, Karl A. Zucker & Robert W. Bailey

SECTION II GENERAL TECHNIQUES OF LAPAROSCOPIC SURGERY — 95

9. **Closed and Open Techniques of Trocar Insertion** — 97
   P. Jeffrey W. Milsom
10. **Tissue Approximation and Ligation Techniques** — 107
    Anthony J. Senagore
11. **Techniques of Exposure, Retraction, and Dissection** — 114
    Dennis L. Fowler
12. **Anastomosis** — 125
    Steven D. Wexner & Juan J. Nogueras

SECTION III SURGERY OF THE UPPER GASTROINTESTINAL TRACT — 135

13. **Peptic Ulcer Disease** — 137
    Margret Oddsdottir & David I. Soybel
14. **Splenic Surgery** — 154
    Stephen J. Ferzoco & Irvin M. Modlin
15. **Approaches to Pancreatic Disease** — 165
    Steven D. Leach & Irvin M. Modlin

SECTION IV SURGERY OF THE BILIARY SYSTEM — 173

16 Modern Treatment of Gallstones: Cholecystectomy — 175
William C. Meyers, Gene D. Branum & Lawrence A. Saperstein

17 Management of Acute Cholecystitis — 183
Karl A. Zucker, Robert W. Bailey & John L. Flowers

18 Laparoendoscopic Management of Common Bile Duct Stones — 198
Scott M. Graham & Thomas R. Scott

SECTION V SURGERY OF THE LOWER GASTROINTESTINAL TRACT — 213

19 Appendectomy for Acute Appendicitis — 215
Gerald M. Larson, William G. Cheadle & Hiram C. Polk, Jr.

20 Treatment of Lower Gastrointestinal Diverticular Disease — 222
Walter E. Longo & Anthony M. Vernava, III

21 Colorectal Cancer — 233
Michele D. Davis & Garth H. Ballantyne

22 Preoperative and Intraoperative Staging of Colorectal Cancer — 266
Michele D. Davis & Garth H. Ballantyne

23 Intestinal Obstruction — 284
L. Peter Fielding & Ozuru O. Ukoha

24 Functional Disorders of the Colon — 290
John H. Pemberton & Andrea Ferrara

25 Volvulus of the Colon — 301
David N. Armstrong & Garth H. Ballantyne

SECTION VI SURGERY FOR OTHER DISORDERS — 317

26 Diagnostic Laparoscopy — 319
Lawrence E. Harrison, Anne C. Mosenthal & Philip F. Caushaj

27 The Acute Abdomen — 327
S. Paterson-Brown & H.A.F. Dudley

28 Inguinofemoral Hernias — 332
Titus D. Duncan & Edward M. Mason

29 Diagnostic and Therapeutic Thoracoscopy — 345
Juan A. Sanchez & John C. Baldwin

30 Urologic Disorders — 351
Michael Pontari & William Morgan

31 Obstetric and Gynecologic Disorders — 366
James Haebe & Dan C. Martin

32 Endometriosis — 379
Michael P. Diamond & D. Alan Johns

SECTION VII TECHNIQUES OF LAPAROSCOPIC SURGERY 395

33 Esophagogastrectomy 397
Patrick F. Leahy

34 Cardiomyotomy 400
John Spencer

35 Vagotomy 405
Robert W. Bailey, Karl A. Zucker & John L. Flowers

36 Laparoscopic Treatment of Peptic Ulcer Disease 420
Namir Katkhouda & Jean Mouiel

37 Nissen Fundoplication 430
Bernard Dallemagne

38 Gastric Resection 441
Dennis L. Fowler

39 Antrectomy with Billroth II Anastomosis 444
Joseph F. Uddo, Jr.

40 Cholecystectomy 448
Eddie Joe Reddick

41 Exploration of the Common Bile Duct 456
Stephen J. Shapiro, Leo A. Gordon & Leon Daykhovsky

42 Placement of a Feeding Jejunostomy 467
David M. Ota, Douglas B. Evans & Paul F. Mansfield

43 Small Bowel Resection 473
Nathaniel J. Soper

44 Lysis of Adhesions 484
Phillippe Mouret & Charles Gelez

45 Appendectomy 499
Lawrence E. Harrison, Thomas S. French & Philip F. Caushaj

46 Polypectomy 508
Garth H. Ballantyne

47 Right Colectomy 522
Robert W. Beart

48 Right Hemicolectomy with Intracorporeal Anastomosis 526
Joseph F. Uddo, Jr.

49 Right Hemicolectomy with Extracorporeal Anastomosis 536
Garth H. Ballantyne

50 Left Hemicolectomy 547
William E. Kelly, Jr.

51 Anterior Resection for Rectal Prolapse 565
Garth H. Ballantyne

52 Low Anterior Resection 575
Patrick F. Leahy

53 Drainage of a Diverticular Abscess 583
Anthony V. Coletta

54 Closure of an Ileostomy 590
Garth H. Ballantyne

55 Closure of a Hartmann's Colostomy 598
Anthony V. Coletta

56 Abdominal Perineal Resection 605
Garth H. Ballantyne

57 Herniorrhaphy 625
John D. Corbitt Jr.

58 Iliopubic Tract Inguinal Hernia Repair with Inlay Buttress of Mesh 640
M.M. Gazayerli, M.E. Arregui & H.S. Helmy

59 Oophorectomy 650
Harry Reich

60 Pelvic Lymphadenectomy 661
Dudley Seth Danoff & Alex Gershman

SECTION VIII	**POSTDOCTORAL TRAINING FOR LAPAROSCOPIC SURGERY**	**675**
61	**Setting Up and Running Courses** Joris Bannenberg & Dirk Meijer	**677**
62	**Hospital Credentialing** Kenneth A. Forde	**686**
	Index	**691**

Section I
Fundamentals

Chapter 1
Equipment

John A. Coller
John J. Murray

One of the most characteristic aspects of laparoscopic surgery is that it is so technologically intensive. This markedly different approach to operative intervention has created an explosive response to the need for innovative instrumentation. Manufacturers have initiated a vigorous research and development effort in an attempt to solve some of the challenging problems. At the present time, the technological envelope is rapidly expanding. The following description of equipment and instrumentation is intended to provide a sampling of available products. It must be understood that the inclusion of a particular model does not imply superiority just as the failure to mention a product should not be construed as suggesting inferiority.

IMAGING SYSTEM

Laparoscope

The laparoscopic telescope provides the means of acquiring an image of the abdominal cavity. In the 1960s the Hopkins rod-lens system was developed, replacing the less optically efficient simple lens system that had been in use for some time. The Hopkins telescope, which is a series of quartz rod lenses, greatly enhanced image clarity and light transmission. Light is delivered into the abdominal cavity by a fiber bundle surrounding the rod lens. The light exits the scope as a ring at the tip of the instrument. The diameter of the telescope plays a crucial role in the quality of image production. Most procedures are currently being performed with either a 5- or 10-mm instrument. The smaller scope transmits less light into the abdominal cavity and delivers a smaller and less brilliant image to the viewing lens. Consequently, the tip of the scope must be positioned closer to the field of operation. The 10-mm telescope is the most widely used instrument, particularly if operative work is not going to be limited to a focal area. If adhesions are a concern, initial entry with a 5-mm scope at a remote site can facilitate selection of a safe entry point for the larger telescope.

Telescopes are either forward viewing or oblique. The 0-degree instrument provides an image that is directly in front of the scope (Fig. 1-1). Oblique viewing scopes commonly have an angle of 30 degrees to 45 degrees off the center line of the instrument. The oblique viewing scope is helpful in visualizing areas that are not accessible head-on, such as over the dome of the liver. At the proximal end of the telescope, there is an eyepiece. Although one can use this for direct viewing in the traditional fashion, it is now primarily used as an attachment for the camera. The adapter, which joins the camera and the telescope by means of a C-mount, also contains a focusing lens. Some telescopes have been constructed so that the camera is an integral and nondetachable element of the telescope. The telescope is the unheralded low technology member of the imaging system. However, it is very important to understand that the final image on the monitor will be no better than the initial laparoscope view. A poor or damaged telescope is a bad start.

Circon ACMI offers a HydroLaparoscope system that provides distal lens washing as well as an irrigation channel directed toward the operative site (Fig. 1-2). A flexible laparoscope with 90-degree tip deflection that can be passed through an 11-mm cannula is produced by Fujinon Corporation.

Charged Coupled Device (CCD) Camera, the Image Sensor

More than any other single component, it was the development of the current video technology that removed the limitations of traditional laparoscopic procedures and paved the way for multihanded operations. Miniature lightweight cameras are used to deliver the image from the laparoscope to the video monitor. These cameras weigh as little as 40 grams and are getting lighter.

The essential element in the miniature camera is the CCD chip. This is the same digital imaging technology that provides photographs from the space probes. Currently, most camera systems employ a single chip. There are approximately 300,000 light sensitive pixels on the chip surface that measures only about 1/2 inch on the diagonal (Fig. 1-3).

Each pixel responds electrically in proportion to the number of photons to which it is exposed. In order to distinguish color, the surface of the CCD is covered by a matrix filter of the three primary colors—red, green, and blue. Since any color can be produced by a combination of the three primary colors, it takes three adjoining pixels to render the proper color at any one point in the image. The greater the pixel content of a CCD, the higher the resolution of the final image. CCD chip technology is similar to many computer-related components in that development growth is quadrupling about every 3 to 5 years. Therefore, it is anticipated that single chip cameras with more than 1 million pixels will be available in the reasonably near future. It is interesting to note that for astronomical usage, it is anticipated that chips with 100 million pixels will be available by the mid-1990s. As large as this seems, it should be remembered that the human retina has more than 100 million rods and cones.

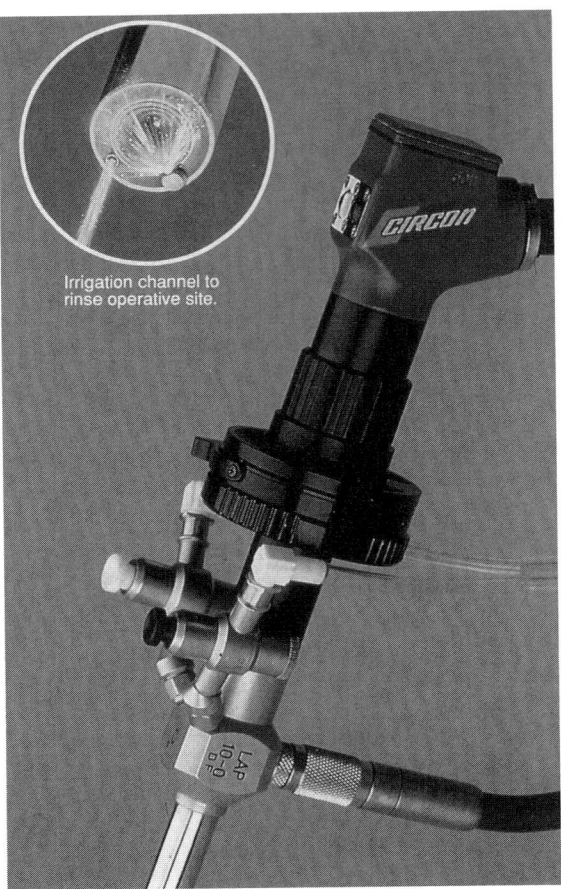

Figure 1-2. Circon ACMI HydroLaparoscope with lens washing and irrigation channel.

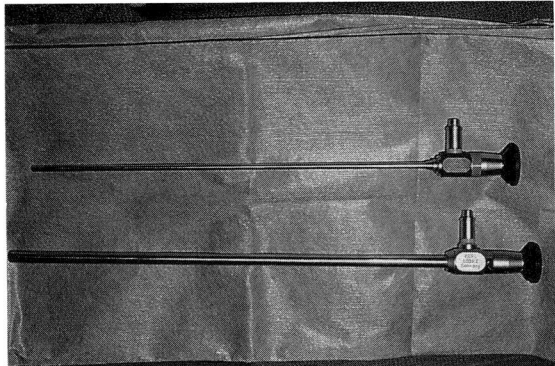

Figure 1-1. Karl Storz 10- and 5-mm 0-degree laparoscope.

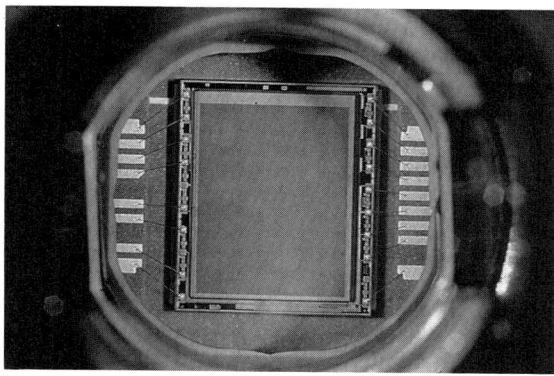

Figure 1-3. CCD chip surface. The center rectangle contains approximately 300,000 pixels.

In an effort to enhance resolution with currently available pixel density, the camera can be made with more than a single chip. Stryker Endoscopy produces a three-chip camera. Each chip is dedicated to one of the three primary colors. The horizontal resolution for this camera is 750 lines. By contrast, most single chip cameras produce between 470 and 560 lines of horizontal resolution. The camera is mounted to the eyepiece of the laparoscope with a C-mount endoscopic coupler (Fig. 1-4A). This permits rapid attachment when switching from one scope to another. The coupler has a focusing knob. Manual focusing may be necessary, particularly at the extremes of distance to the object. Alternatively, the camera and laparoscope may be integrated as a single unit as in the case of the Storz Laparocam. This 10-mm unit minimizes video adjustments and lessens the likelihood of problems with the scope/camera interface (Fig. 1-4B).

The power supply and electronic control for the camera are located away from the operative field and are connected to the camera by cable. Common to nearly all power units is a white balance control. To the human brain, compensation for the type of illumination is automatic. White appears white despite the illumination temperature. On the other hand, a video camera registers a different temperature color depending upon the type of light source being used. If a lower color temperature source is used (e.g., 3700 K tungsten), the video camera registers more orange whereas a high color temperature source (e.g., 5500 K xenon or 6000 K metal halide) would produce a bluer response. Such pictures would provide an unnatural rendering to the human eye. Therefore, the camera is pointed at something that the human eye accepts as being white. When the white balance circuit is activated, it in effect tells the camera what white should look like with the particular type of illumination being used. Once white has been electrically defined, all other colors will then appear appropriately.

Additional camera controls often provide for a manual light intensity boost. This might be located on the control unit, the camera, or the light source. Solos Endoscopy produces a Dual Image camera system. Two separate images can be projected to different video screens, switched between screens, or placed in split screen. This capability is useful for certain complex operations. Simultaneous visualization from inside a viscus, e.g., a common bile duct, or on both sides of a mesentery is often helpful in expediting safe dissection (Fig. 1-5).

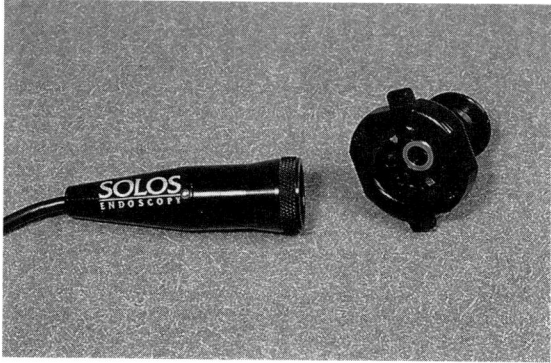

A

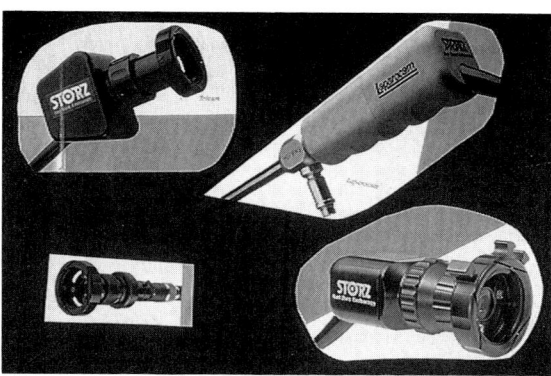

B

Figure 1-4. A, Solos Endoscopy single CCD chip videocamera with detached C-mount and focusing adapter. B, Karl Storz cameras include a three-chip Tricam with 600-line resolution, an integrated camera and scope Laparocam, a diagnostic office camera with 400-line resolution, and a single chip Supercam with 450-line resolution.

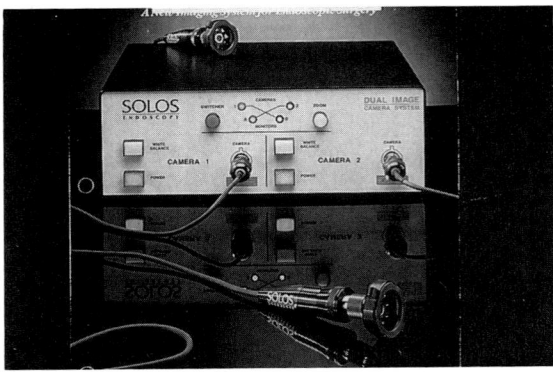

Figure 1-5. Solos Endoscopy Dual Image camera system.

The light sensitivity of a camera is an indication of the amount of light that is required to produce an image. A sensitivity of 5 lux is generally acceptable (1 lux = 0.1 footcandle; 1 footcandle is the light that is provided by 1 candle at a distance of 1 foot).

Light Source

A high intensity light source is a requisite for satisfactory laparoscopic imaging. Although several light sources are used for laparoscopic surgery, the most commonly used units employ either a xenon or metal halide bulb. Both of these sources provide a color temperature that is in the range of daylight (5500 K) or slightly higher. Bulbs have a life expectancy in the 250-hour range. Spare bulbs should always be available. An hours of use meter is a helpful feature. The light is delivered to the laparoscope by fiberoptic cable (Fig. 1-6).

Most light sources either have or can be fitted with adapters that accommodate the light cables for other manufacturers. However, best results are usually obtained when camera and light source are designed to interact. Changes in light level at the camera CCD surface will automatically adjust the illumination intensity. This type of electronic integration will greatly reduce annoying glare and blooming. Manual overrides are available to over- or underilluminate if desired.

Video Monitor and Documentation and Recording

See Chapter 2 for further explanations of these components.

INSUFFLATOR

Exposure of the operative field is a crucial requirement for safe dissection in any surgical procedure. In laparoscopic surgery, exposure is achieved by insufflation of the peritoneal cavity with gas. The distention obtained with pneumoperitoneum permits safe introduction and manipulation of cannulas to accommodate the laparoscopic telescope and laparoscopic instruments. Although a variety of inert gases have been employed for this purpose, carbon dioxide, inexpensive and readily available, is now the sole agent used for laparoscopic surgery. Because of its solubility, relatively large quantities of carbon dioxide can be safely absorbed and excreted by the lungs. Carbon dioxide is also noncombustible, permitting the use of lasers and electrocautery instruments in the operative field. The insufflator regulates the flow of carbon dioxide from a pressurized reservoir and monitors intra-abdominal pressure. The flow of carbon dioxide ceases automatically when a preselected intra-abdominal pressure is achieved. An intra-abdominal distention pressure of 12 to 15 mm Hg will provide adequate exposure for most procedures. When intra-abdominal pressure is sustained at levels greater than 15 mm Hg, the risk for pulmonary and hemodynamic complications increases because of restricted excursion of the diaphragm and decreased venous return.

Commercially available insufflators vary in the range of flow rates they deliver and the format used for display of information. The instrument selected should provide clear and precise display of the level of intra-abdominal pressure, the rate of carbon dioxide insufflation, the volume of gas infused, and the re-

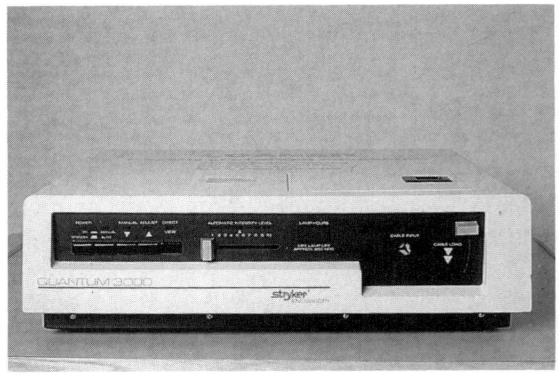

Figure 1-6. Stryker Endoscopy Quantum 3000 has automatic brightness control with constant color temperature.

sidual volume in the carbon dioxide tank. Insufflators are equipped with an alarm to signal an increase in intra-abdominal pressure beyond the maximum pressure previously selected. The alarm may be inadvertently triggered by compression of the abdominal wall, closure of the infusion port on the laparoscopic cannula, kinking of the infusion tubing, or inappropriate placement of the infusion needle or laparoscopic cannula. The rate of carbon dioxide insufflation can be adjusted to provide slow (1 to 2 liters/min) or rapid (6 to 10 liters/min) infusion. The most recently introduced insufflators are capable of providing a peak flow of 10 to 15 liters/min. Insufflation of carbon dioxide should begin at a slow rate. The small caliber of the insufflation needle limits flow to 1 to 2 liters/min. Slow infusion of carbon dioxide will minimize the potential for injury if the insufflation needle or laparoscopic cannula has been incorrectly positioned in a extraperitoneal location or within an abdominal viscus or vessel. Incorrect placement will be indicated by an unexpectedly high pressure, an abnormally low flow rate, or the evident development of subcutaneous emphysema. When pneumoperitoneum has been safely established, the rate of carbon dioxide insufflation should be increased to maintain distention. Advanced laparoscopic procedures require insertion of multiple laparoscopic cannulas. A rapid rate of carbon dioxide insufflation compensates for leakage of gas around the cannulas and for the escape of carbon dioxide that accompanies instrumentation of the cannulas or use of suction equipment in the operative field. Adequate exposure of the operative field is thereby maintained. A recirculating pump that exchanges and filters carbon dioxide to remove smoke and debris while maintaining stable intra-abdominal distention pressure is an attractive feature available in some models. The ability to evacuate smoke may be particularly helpful in patients requiring extensive use of the laser or electrocautery unit (Fig. 1-7).

VERESS NEEDLE

The pneumoperitoneum may be established after insertion of a cannula using an open technique or blunt needle insufflation. The Veress-type insufflation needle is designed to permit blind entry into the abdominal cavity with minimal likelihood of injury to underlying structures. Just the same, the site of puncture should be at a point that is unlikely

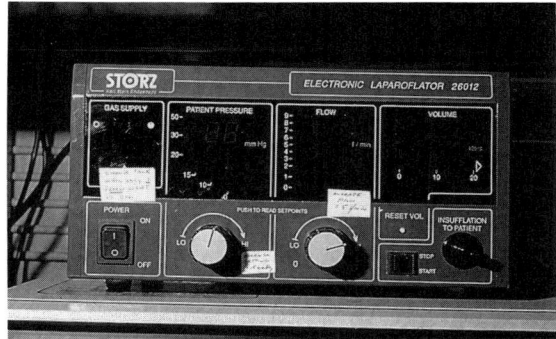

Figure 1-7. Karl Storz Laparoflator provides both digital and analog display of carbon dioxide pressure and flow rates.

to contain adhesions such as the infraumbilical midline. The 2-mm needle has a spring-loaded blunt inner cannula that automatically extends beyond the needle point once the abdominal cavity has been entered (Fig. 1-8A). This blunt cannula has a side hole to permit creation of the pneumoperitoneum. Disposable needles often feature a bead indicator or transparent section for water drop testing to permit visual confirmation of peritoneal cavity entry (Fig. 1-8B).

CANNULA AND TROCAR

The cannula is the conduit by which the laparoscope and various instruments gain access to the abdominal cavity. Versatility is the benchmark for a cannula. It must be easy to insert yet resistive to dislodgment. It must also be able to accept a variety of instruments while maintaining the pneumoperitoneum. With the closed technique, insertion of the first cannula is most critical because this is performed blindly. Subsequent cannulas can be inserted under direct vision. Insertion safety is principally dependent upon the characteristics of the cannula trocar. The trocar tip must offer the most minimal resistance to insertion. The tip and edges must be razor sharp with a narrow angle of attack. If the tip is broad or dull, rather than efficient cutting through the abdominal wall, insertion pressure will result in displacement of the entire wall inwards, closer to or abutting vital tissue or major vessels. If reusable cannulas are used, it is essential that the trocar be regularly inspected, maintained, and replaced if there is any sign of wear or dullness. Recognizing the importance of a consistently sharp trocar has

8   Fundamentals

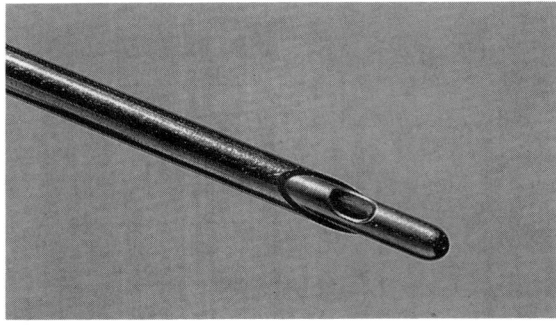

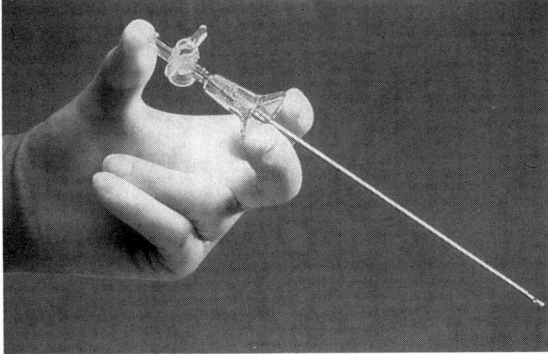

Figure 1-8. A, The tip of a reusable Veress needle. B, A disposable Veress-type needle—the Surgineedle.

led to considerable enthusiasm for one-use disposable cannulas.

These units, such as the USSC* SURGI-PORT* and the Ethicon Endopath, have retractable protective sheaths that cover the trocar tip when not in use. During insertion, the sheath retracts until the trocar tip penetrates the peritoneum at which time the sheath automatically pops back into place to cover the tip and minimize the likelihood of unwanted trauma. Another approach is used by Dexide, Inc. Their Monoscopy brand trocar has a blunt internal spike that pops into place as the beveled trocar tip enters the abdominal cavity. In contrast to the entirely disposable cannula/trocar, some devices combine a reusable cannula with a disposable trocar. This approach is designed to provide a cost savings yet ensure the reliability of a fresh sharp trocar. Wisap provides a disposable trocar in either a conical or pyramidal tip configuration. Core Dynamics produces a stainless steel trocar that is also recyclable (Fig. 1-9).

Once the cannula has been inserted into the abdominal cavity, the trocar is removed. Since the trocar has an airtight fit with the cannula shaft, its withdrawal acts like a plunger. If a loop of bowel or other structure fell against the opening during trocar withdrawal, that tissue could be sucked into the cannula and damaged. Consequently, small holes are placed around the end of the cannula or alternatively, a vent hole may be built into the trocar. An inflation port is generally located along the side of the head of the cannula. Most often this is a stopcock with a luerlock connection. In addition to trocar sharpness, the shaft diameter is an important factor in the ease and safety of abdominal wall penetration. Because a narrow trocar will require less force to create entry into the abdominal cavity, causing less displacement of the wall toward the retroperitoneum, it is often advantageous to use a 5-mm cannula/trocar for the initial placement. A 5-mm laparoscope can then be used to visualize the placement of additional and usually larger ports including one for a 10-mm laparoscope that would generally be used for the operative procedure itself. As more sophisticated instruments have become available, the port diameters have had to become larger. Bowel staplers require cannulas of between 12 and 18 mm in diameter. Larger bore cannulas are available, up to 4 cm and larger, for minimal access purposes such as tissue removal and extracorporeal anastomosis.

A crucial part of an effective cannula is the ability to insert and remove various instruments without loss of pneumoperitoneum. The principal valve in the cannula head that

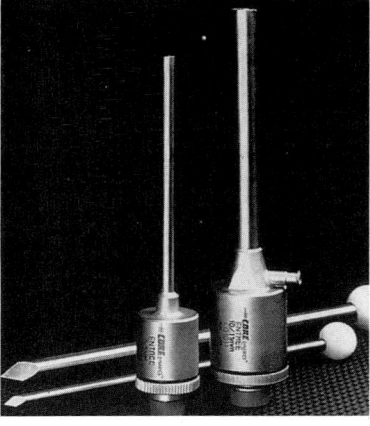

Figure 1-9. Core Dynamics Entree disposable trocar with reusable cannula.

is responsible for preventing gas loss is either a trumpet or flap valve. The trumpet valve must be opened completely prior to the insertion of an instrument, whereas most flap valves can be forced open by the passage of an instrument into the shaft of the cannula. However, using delicate instruments for such mechanical tasks may well interfere with instrument reliability and longevity. When the principal valve is in the open position, the pneumatic seal is actually maintained by a plastic insert or diaphragm that tightly grips the instrument shaft. The insert seal should be able to accommodate all instruments that can be inserted through the cannula or be able to be replaced by a seal that can accommodate smaller sized instruments (Fig. 1-10, A and B).

The shaft of the cannula has to be long enough to permit usage in a thick as well as a thin abdominal wall. However, the farther the cannula slides in toward the operative

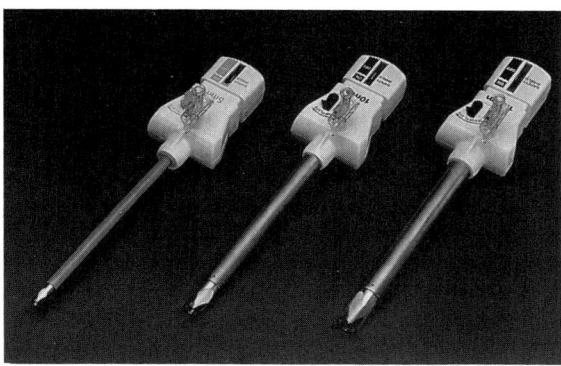

A

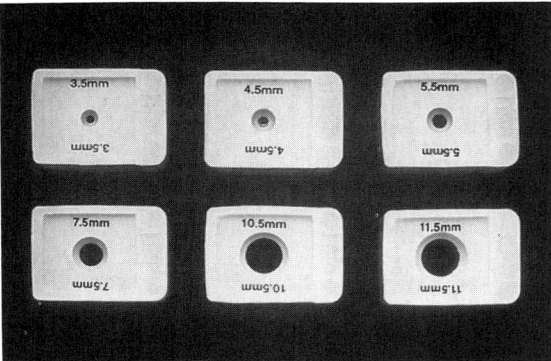

B

Figure 1-10. A, The 5-, 10-, and 12-mm USSC* SURGIPORT* disposable cannula/trocars. B, Reducer inserts adjust the caliber of the cannula for the size of various instruments.

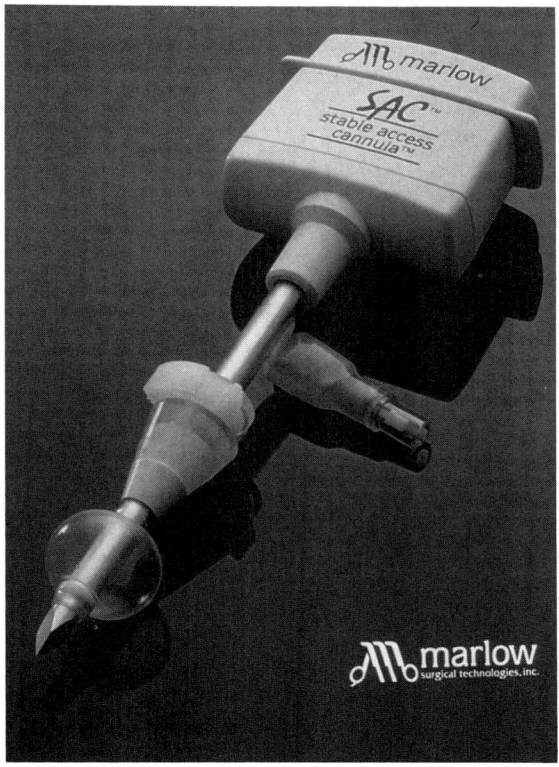

Figure 1-11. Marlow Surgical Technologies, Inc. Cannula with cone and balloon stabilization.

field, the more it encroaches on and interferes with the effector tip of the instrument. An olive may be added to the cannula shaft to limit inward movement of the cannula. The olive also helps to minimize gas leakage should there be a poor seal between the shaft and the abdominal wall (Fig. 1-11). Some shafts are equipped with a spiral ridge that provides resistance to unintentional dislodgment of the cannula. Detachable spiral cannula sheaths can be positioned at various levels of the shaft. Additional approaches that are designed to prevent accidental extrusion of the cannula position include the use of an inflatable balloon or an umbrella-like expansion similar to a Molly fixture (Fig. 1-12).

An open approach can be used for initial entry into the abdominal cavity. In 1971, Hasson[1] described a cannula specifically designed for direct vision placement. This technique offers an extra margin of safety, particularly if numerous adhesions are anticipated. Rather than establishing the pneumoperitoneum with a Veress needle followed by blind entry with a sharp trocar, a mini-incision is

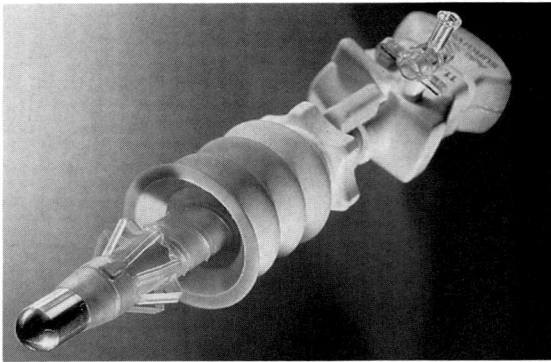

Figure 1-12. This Hasson-type cannula manufactured by USSC is held in place by an umbrella-like expansion unit, which prevents retraction of the unit.

made to facilitate cannula insertion under direct vision. The trocar for the Hasson cannula has an atraumatic rounded tip. Sutures are placed between the fascia and stanchions that are located on the head of the cannula. This fixation prevents the cannula from accidentally being dislodged. An adjustable olive-shaped stopper on the shaft will prevent unintentional inward movement.

The Hasson trocar has occupied a central role in the conventional laparoscopic procedure—the location of the laparoscope throughout the operation. However, as procedures have become more global, extending throughout the abdominal cavity, with multiple entry sites, and with frequent instrument interchange, there is less need for a single predominant Hasson cannula as originally described.

IRRIGATOR

Management of bleeding is a critical issue during laparoscopic procedures. A small pool of blood in the area of dissection can cause a great deal of frustration. A substantial bleeding artery, as might occur in the mesentery, can represent a major challenge if conversion to an open surgical procedure is to be avoided. To handle these events, an efficient high flow irrigator/aspirator unit is required. The basic requirements of this unit include the ability to direct a forceful fluid stream followed by rapid aspiration of clots and fluid. To best accomplish this objective it is necessary to do both jobs through the same tube, alternating the suction and irrigation functions. A single common channel or double channel in a concentric arrangement can be used. In the double channel configuration, irrigation and aspiration can be performed synchronously, which is helpful when trying to break up clots. The outer tube should have side vents for a distance of about 1 cm from the end so that it can function as a pool tip sucker. If side vents extend too high on the suction channel, there will be unnecessary evacuation of pneumoperitoneum during aspiration. A small bore inner cannula will deliver the narrow irrigation stream without appreciable compromise of suction capacity. A thin high pressure stream can be a very helpful tool when used in the procedure of hydrodissection. Many irrigation units can be structured to accept an electrocautery or laser probe without interfering with the irrigation/suction function (Fig. 1-13). The Nezhat-Dorsey hydrodissection pump is a carbon dioxide-powered stand-alone device that provides variable irrigation pressure up to 775 mm Hg.

Operating rooms are universally equipped with nitrogen as a pressure source. The nitrogen-powered Davol Arthro-Flo irrigation system can be used for laparoscopic irrigation. This provides a fluid stream from a 80 psi source and is quite effective in hydrodissection. The disposable diaphragm pump connects to standard irrigation bags.

DISSECTING AND MANIPULATING INSTRUMENTS

The laparoscopic surgeon uses a number of instruments, usually in combination, to per-

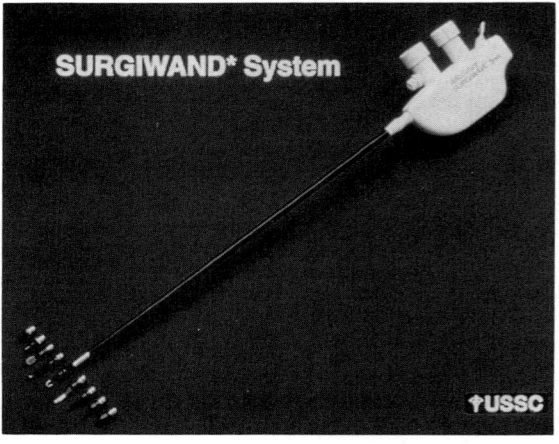

Figure 1-13. The USSC* SURGIWAND* allows for suction, irrigation, and electrocautery with the same instrument. In addition, a central channel permits insertion of laser devices.

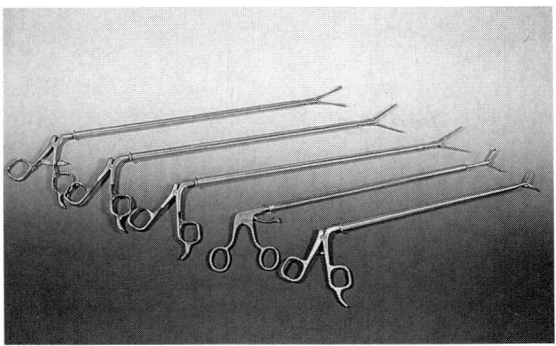

Figure 1-14. Assorted reusable graspers and dissectors with various handle configurations.

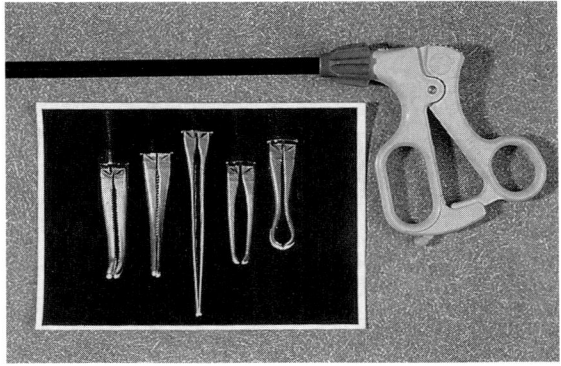

Figure 1-15. Ethicon Endopath bowel instruments include a Babcock and Allis grasper, an occlusive bowel clamp, a Kelly clamp, and a right-angle dissector.

form the tasks of manipulation and dissection. Where appropriate, many instruments have connectors and are insulated for electrocautery. Multipurpose tools have certain advantages from the standpoint of economy of motion. If a single instrument can serve several functions, e.g., retraction, aspiration, irrigation, and electrocautery, instrument exchange time will be minimized and fewer access ports will be required. Virtually any type of effector tip can be placed at the end of an instrument. General purpose graspers and dissectors should have relatively short narrow arms. In contrast to open surgery, one cannot usually dissect as deeply with a single stroke. Some dissection will be performed with teasing, tearing, or stretching maneuvers, which need to be done more discretely than in open surgery. For the most part, in open surgery, bigger mistakes as a result of overaggressive dissection are more easily brought under control. Consequently, bulky dissection instruments are to be avoided when working in close (Fig. 1-14).

Bowel instruments have been adopted along the design of conventional Allis, Babcock, and Kelly clamps. These instruments, because of the requirements for larger effector tips, must be of a bigger diameter, usually 10 mm (Figs. 1-15 and 1-16).

Atraumatic manipulation of tissue along with countertraction can be accomplished with an endoscopic Kittner. This is the laparoscopic equivalent of a sponge stick.

The electrocautery scissors have become the principal dissecting tool for many laparoscopic surgeons. Besides cutting, the tip is used for tearing or scoring, the smooth out-

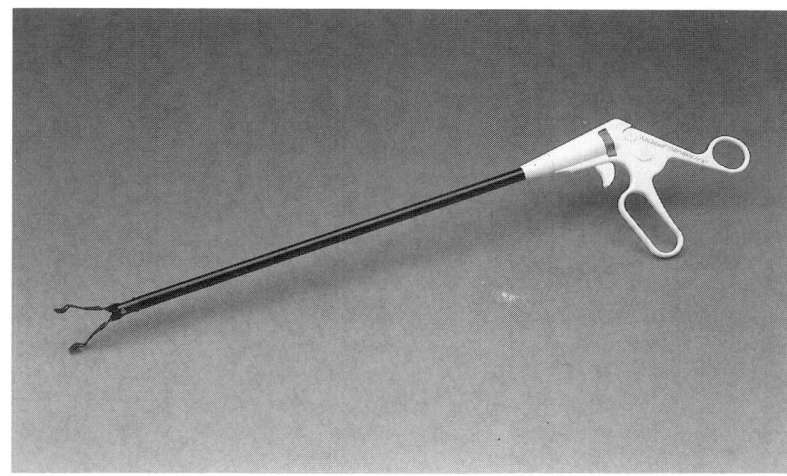

Figure 1-16. ENDO BABCOCK* instrument from USSC features fingertip shaft rotation and a jaw locking mechanism.

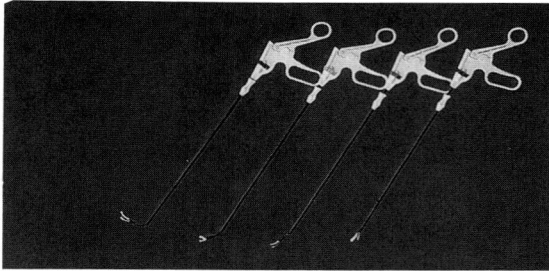

Figure 1-17. Disposable USSC* ROTICULATOR ENDO MINISHEARS* with electrocautery.

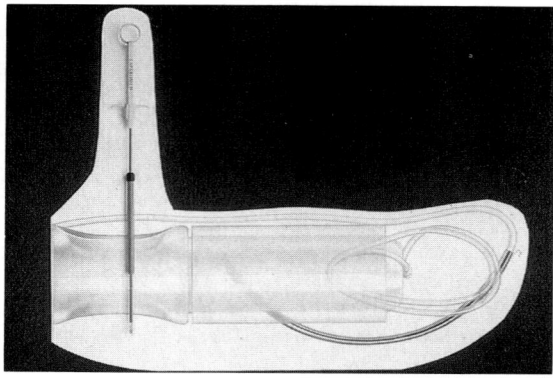

Figure 1-18. Laparomed suture applier provides a suture with a pretied knot.

side surface of the jaws can be used for spreading, and the cautery can handle small vessels. Indeed, if the blades are curved, the scissors can be used to work around a structure, such as a mesenteric vessel. Disposable scissors, such as the 5-mm diameter USSC* ENDO SHEARS* have a 16-mm curved blade that maintains its sharpness throughout long procedures. Finger-controlled shaft rotation permits turning of the blades without abnormal twisting of the wrist. A new ROTICULATOR* version permits articulation of the blades to an angle larger than 90 degrees (Fig. 1-17).

SUTURING AND LIGATION INSTRUMENTS

Intracorporeal suturing and knot tying are among the more advanced operative skills that the laparoscopic surgeon must master. Absorbable and nonabsorbable suture materials with short ski and straight needles are specifically designed for laparoscopic surgery. These long sutures permit either intracorporeal or extracorporeal knot tying. A suture/needle combination may be freestanding or attached to a disposable knot pusher. During the placement of sutures, it is particularly beneficial to have a needle driver that closes with a high mechanical advantage which will allow a firm purchase on the needle. Considerable force must be applied in order to rigidly hold the needle within the small friction area that is provided by most needle jaws. An alternative to the conventional alligator jaw is provided by the Cook surgical curved needle holder. The needle is held in the side slit of a concentric tubular shaft with a central spring-loaded piston-like rod to ensure a firm grasp.

An innovative approach to individual suture placement is offered by Laparomed Corporation with the suture applier. This single use device includes a curved needle with needle driver and pretied knot. Once the suture has been carried through the tissue, the needle is threaded through the final loop of the pretied knot. The knot is then made fast without the need for manual knot tying (Fig. 1-18).

When a free pedicle requires ligation, a pretied suture loop can be applied. This is especially useful for structures that are not suitable for clipping, such as the appendiceal base or larger blood vessels. The ligature is incorporated into its own plastic holder with a preformed loop. With the aid of a protective tube, the loop is carried into the abdominal cavity through a cannula. Once the loop is positioned, it is secured around the structure by simply drawing the loop tight (Fig. 1-19).

Certainly, one of the simplest methods of obtaining hemostasis for vessels not secured with electrocautery or laser is by clipping.

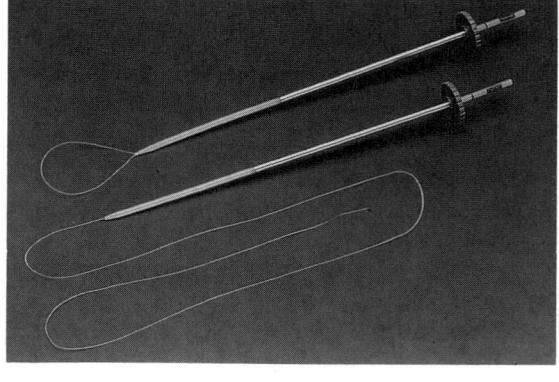

Figure 1-19. USSC* SURGITIE* and SURGIWHIP* provide an easy means of ligating a structure end-on.

Equipment 13

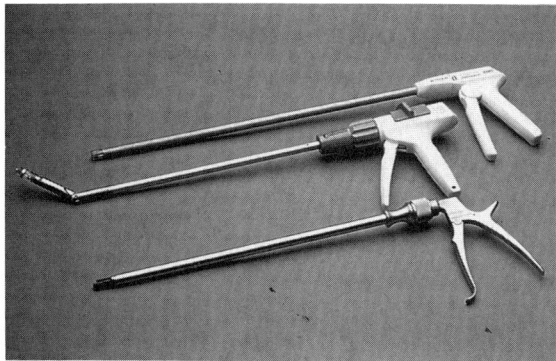

Figure 1-20. Ethicon reusable single clip endoscopic stapler; Ethicon disposable multifeed stapler.

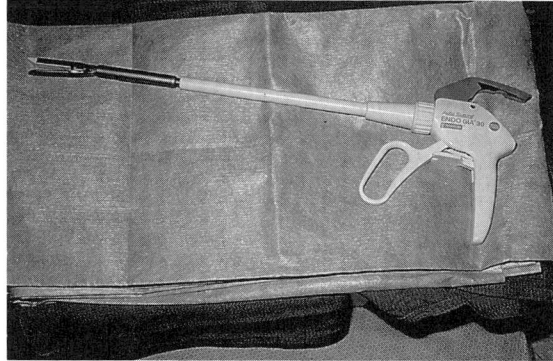

Figure 1-22. USSC ENDO GIA 3-cm linear stapler with knife.

Single load reusable instruments and multiload disposable units are available for application of titanium clips (Fig. 1-20). Disposable units usually contain 20 clips/unit. Since clips are usually placed several at a time, the multiload units considerably increase the speed and efficiency with which a ligature can be accomplished as compared with single clip units (Fig. 1-21, A and B). Clips are most reliable when the blood vessels have been separately and distinctly isolated, as in the case of the cystic artery. If the vascular pedicle is a bit more crowded with surrounding fatty tissue or with communicating vessels as may occur in the mesentery, a USSC* ENDO GIA* with a vascular cartridge may be used. This unit places a 3-cm triple row of staples on both sides of the pedicle division (Fig. 1-22).

STAPLERS AND TACKERS

Instruments are being developed for the mechanical approximation of tissues in an effort to minimize the need for manual suture placement. One of the devices that is show-

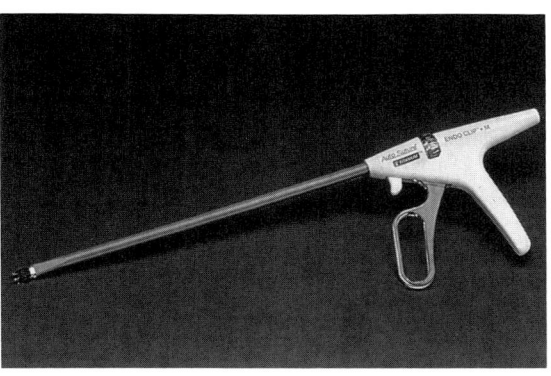

A

B

Figure 1-21. A, The pistol-grip SURGICLIP* applier. B, The palm-grip SURGICLIP* applier.

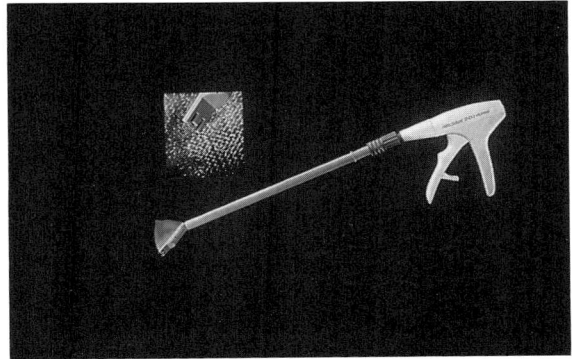

Figure 1-23. USSC* ENDO HERNIA* Stapler with an articulating end facilitates closure of mesenteric defects and hernia repairs.

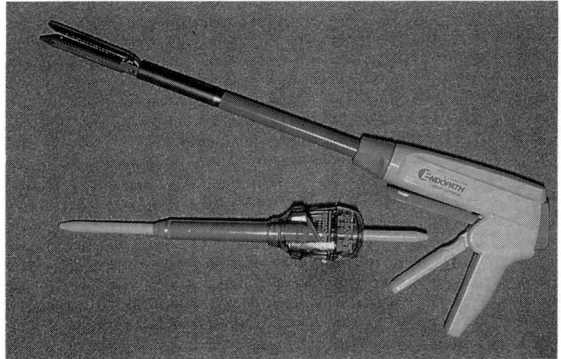

Figure 1-24. Ethicon Endopath 60-mm linear stapler with knife.

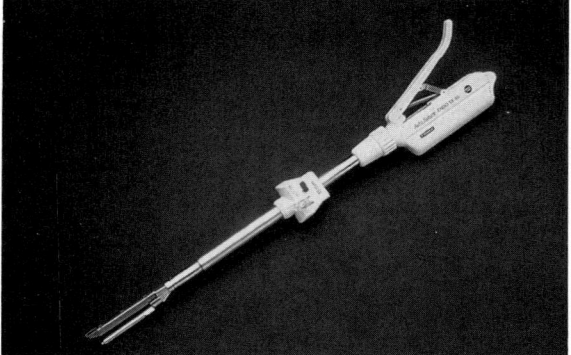

Figure 1-25. USSC ENDO TA* 60-mm gas-powered stapler.

ing promise in tissue approximation is the laparoscopic end-stapler or tacker. This device delivers a large staple end-on in a fashion similar to a skin stapler. On closure, the staple crimps to a box shape, providing a firm but non-necrosing approximation of the tissues. This device is being used for mesenteric closure and for hernia repair with mesh (Fig. 1-23).

Clearly, one of the most impressive applications of mechanical instruments to surgery during the past several decades is that of linear and circular stapling devices. The utility of these devices becomes even more apparent when applied to laparoscopic surgery. In open surgery, the ability to simultaneously occlude and divide a section of bowel is convenient, time saving, and consistently effective. In laparoscopic work, it is, in addition, what makes some of the complex procedures possible. The USSC* ENDO GIA* is a 30-mm linear stapler that is inserted through a 12-mm cannula. A triple row of staples is laid down on both sides of the knife. The standard staple size is suitable for bowel division while a slightly tighter staple cartridge is hemostatic and can be used for vascular ligation. An Ethicon Endopath 60-mm linear stapler places two rows on either side of the knife. An 18-mm cannula is required for its insertion. A 60-mm noncutting linear stapler, the ENDO TA*, is produced by USSC. This unit, which is gas powered, has three rows of staples and passes through a 15-mm cannula (Figs. 1-24 and 1-25).

A broad spectrum of innovative, often very task-specific devices are feverishly being developed to facilitate the demanding challenges of laparoscopic surgery. Many of the new implements will be mere contrivances that fail to contribute to the surgeon's armamentarium. On the other hand, the inventive surgeon cannot help but sense with considerable anticipation the creative approaches, concepts, and tools that will be brought to this new operating environment. Certainly, the biggest changes are yet to come.

REFERENCE

1. Hasson HM. Modified instrument and method for laparoscopy. Am J Obstet Gynecol 1971; 110:886–887.

Chapter 2
Imaging

Michael P. Spencer
Robert D. Madoff

The laparoscopic surgical revolution could not have occurred without technologic advances in laparoscopic imaging. The fundamentals of laparoscopy are not new, and the technique has been employed (albeit sparingly) by gastroenterologists and surgeons since the early 1900s. While Bernheim is credited as the first United States surgeon to utilize the procedure in 1911,[1] much of the pioneering work in the field of laparoscopy has come from Europe. Kalk, a German hepatologist, introduced numerous instruments including a laparscope with an oblique viewing system in the 1920s.[2] This forerunner of today's laparoscopes was essentially a rigid telescope that transmitted an image from the abdominal cavity to the viewer's eye. Not only was the viewing angle narrow, but the majority of light was absorbed by the system, limiting resolution and prohibiting photographic recording.

Laparoscopic surgery was popularized by gynecologists who applied this developing technology to numerous procedures during the 1960s. Semm, a gynecologist and engineer, incorporated the use of fiberoptics, transmitting light through a series of glass rods on the ends of which small lenses are cemented.[3] These fiberoptic cables are composed of an inner core of glass with a relatively high refractive index and a sheathing of low index glass. This system is still relatively inefficient, absorbing 50 per cent or more of the light input. The most advanced systems use fluid-filled cables with quartz ends, markedly diminishing light absorption and providing transmission of the entire color spectrum.

The recent clinical enthusiasm for laparoscopic cholecystectomy and other minimally invasive surgery has propelled and in some cases necessitated the development of new equipment to illuminate, transmit, and record laparoscopic images. Still photography, until recently the principal method of recording images, remains an important medium for documentation. Video technology, however, is now playing a predominant role in this area. Thus, not only have surgeons been required to develop expertise in the expanding field of laparoscopic surgery, they also have had to familiarize themselves with a staggering array of equipment and technology to perform and document their work. This chapter is intended to provide surgeons with a basic understanding of laparoscopic imaging and detail what equipment is available for clinical practice.

DOCUMENTATION

The use of video tape to document laparoscopic procedures is a subject of some debate. There is no doubt as to its usefulness as a teaching aid, both to evaluate surgical techniques and to train others to perform laparoscopic procedures. The video tape is also potentially useful for self-education as it allows the surgeon to review a procedure if postoperative complications arise. However, documenting all procedures to record an operative mishap raises many potential legal questions. Should all surgeons record every procedure? How long should the video be kept? Should the video be filed as part of the medical record? Who (surgical/medical boards or administrative personnel) should dictate these policies? These are questions which confront the practicing surgeon today. At present, it is best to review individual institutional procedures and policies until uniform guidelines are drafted.

BASIC PRINCIPLES OF ENDOSCOPIC IMAGING

Many of the techniques applicable to still photography apply to video recording. In general, the video medium is better adapted to surgical procedures as it eliminates the need to capture a dynamic process with a single or a series of still images. The electronically formed video image is also more sensitive to light than most 35-mm film, making a satisfactory video image easier to obtain.

As with still photography, gross movement of the camera during laparoscopy distorts the image. With video imaging, camera control is crucial not only for recording purposes but also for providing the surgeon with an appropriate visual field. The camera should be moved slowly, attempting to maintain the critical field of vision. The camera operator should be acquainted with the procedure so that he or she can anticipate when magnification is beneficial or when a broader visual field may be required. The laparoscope should be placed at an optimum distance and focused such that the area of interest fills the frame. This is particularly important with laparoscopy, because the viewing field is limited. Frequently, an inexperienced photographer will mentally subtract extraneous objects from view. These distractions, more apparent on review, detour the viewer.

The lens itself can be responsible for distortion and occasionally needs cleaning. The laparoscope may need to be withdrawn and cleansed. Keeping warm water on hand for this purpose will minimize fogging and immersing the tip of the laparoscope in warm water prior to introducing the scope into the abdominal cavity also reduces fogging. Often, simply wiping the scope against the visceral or parietal peritoneum will clear the lens, providing a satisfactory image.

Lighting requirements depend on the ability of the laparoscope to transmit light, the sensitivity of the camera, and the sensitivity of the recording medium. The light source and fiberoptic delivery system are of critical importance. The term "cold light" is utilized when describing the configuration of most lighting systems. The actual light source is separated from the fiberoptic cable by a heat shield to minimize heat transfer to the laparoscope. The principal light sources use halogen or xenon bulbs of approximately 150 or 300 W, respectively. The xenon light source is generally preferred because it is as close to daylight illumination as is currently possible, thus providing optimum color. A comparison of competitive available light sources is presented in Table 2-1.

Fiberoptic transmission is diminished with time, exposure to cleaners, and fractured cables. Periodic replacement is necessary for optimum performance. The longevity of transmission cables will vary, depending on their use and care.

CREATING A LAPAROSCOPIC IMAGE

Following introduction of the laparoscope into the abdominal cavity, illumination is maintained by an external light source connected to the laparoscope. The light is delivered to the tip by multiple fiberoptic cables within the laparoscope. The light is then reflected off an object and travels back through the lens system in the laparoscope to the camera (Fig. 2-1). Video cameras are composed of sensors that emit an electrical signal in response to light; this signal is then transmitted to a monitor and/or video recorder. Sensitivity, the amount of light it takes to make a usable picture, varies between cameras. The greater the sensitivity, the better the camera can see dimly lit scenes. The light sensitivity is specified in lux, which is a subjective determination of the least amount of light needed to discern an image. The greater the lux, the more sensitive the camera.

The sensor is the foundation of the camera. Presently, two types of sensing devices are utilized: solid state chips and vacuum tubes. Solid state technology, however, is the principal format in today's electronic market. Solid state sensors or chips comprise small pieces of silicon whose surfaces contain sensitive areas

Table 2-1. Competitive Light Source Profile

Manufacturer	Model	Lamp Type	Lamp Life (hr)	Universal Cable Input
Cabot	KLI Videolap Light	250 W metal halide	250	Yes
Circon	MV 9082	250 W metal halide	250	No
Dyonics	Autobrite Illuminator II	250 W metal halide	250	No
Medical Dynamics	Insta-Lux 6100	300 W xenon	200	Yes
MP Video	ML-800	250 W metal halide	250	No
Olympus	CLV-U20	300 W xenon	200	No
Solos	ELS-2	175 W xenon	700	Yes
Storz	615C	300 W xenon	250	No
Stryker	Quantum 3000	250 W metal halide	250	No
V. Mueller	LA8000	300 W xenon	500	Yes
Wisap	Endo-Illumination 250	250 W metal halide	250	No
Wolf	5119.00	250 W metal halide	250	Yes

called pixels. Pixels, also known as picture elements, are arranged in a linear format of rows and columns. The total number of pixels in a chip is directly related to resolution; larger chips and smaller pixel size allow increased numbers of pixels and thus higher resolution. The camera's specifications are determined by the chip or chips used and cannot exceed the chip's capacity. The 1/2- and 2/3-inch chip formats currently occupy the majority of the market.

The surface of the sensor is divided into the usable active pixels and black reference pixels. The active pixels create an electronic image when exposed to light. The camera produces a signal by scanning the pixels in a specified fashion. The total information a scanning system collects at any instant produces a frame. A frame is the most basic component that can be perceived by a viewer when the signal is transferred to a monitor. Each frame can be divided into odd and even

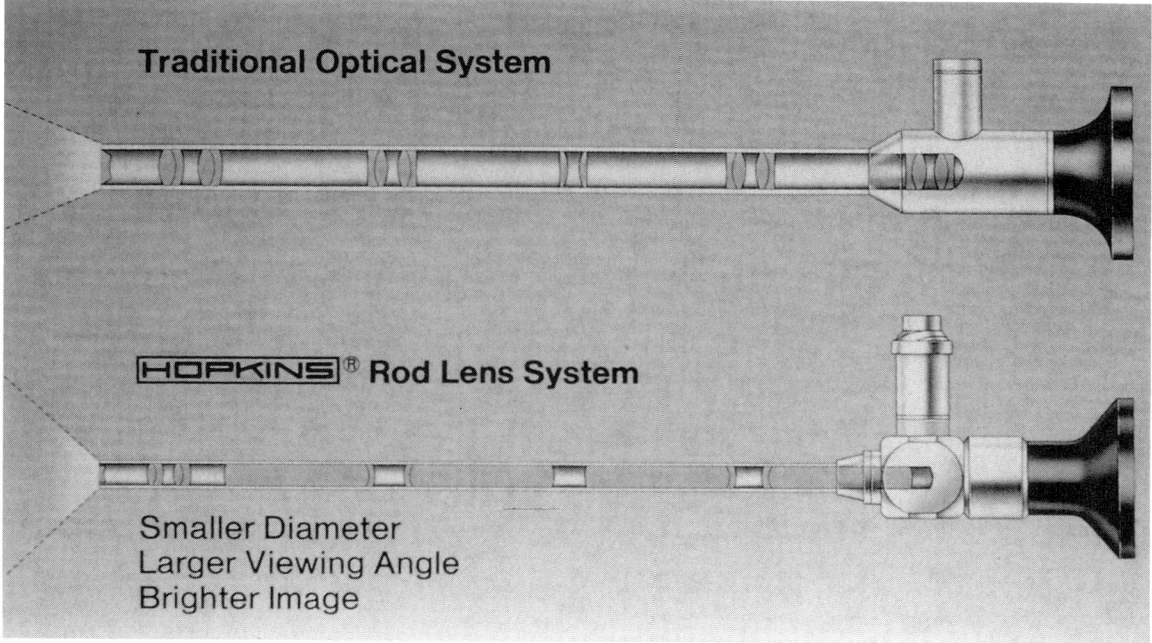

Figure 2-1. Cross-section of traditional and new laparoscope.

fields, which are interlaced by the scanning system. Scanning systems are standardized. The ELARS-170 is used in the United States, Canada, Japan, and South America. This scanning system creates a picture with 525 horizontal lines at a rate of 60 fields or 30 frames/sec (60 Hz). The European CCIR-13 scanning equivalent specifies 625 horizontal lines; this equipment is not compatible with ELARS-170 components.

Color cameras process information based on the primary video colors red, green, and blue (RBG), and white light can be broken down into these components. In order to make the video image appear to the eye as the object would if viewed directly, the camera must be appropriately white-balanced. This is accomplished electronically by pointing the camera at a white object and pushing the "white balance" button. The camera then adjusts its output and processes its signal based on the red, green, and blue components. To create a color image, the camera's sensors are scanned for the primary colors (red, green, and blue) and complementary colors (magenta, yellow, and cyan). Almost any color can be produced by a complex filtering process that varies the primary colors. The camera then processes the output signal based on the primary RGB colors.

The signal output from a camera (based on number of pixels) varies depending on the quality of the camera. Signal output can be one of three types: composite, S-video, and RGB. Composite video, the most common format, is a one-channel signal created by electronically combining all image components. This reduces the signal produced to approximately 330 lines of resolution. S-video comprises two signals: luminance or brightness (Y) and chroma or color (C), the two components of high fidelity recording. S-video produces a superior image with 350 to 425 lines of resolution and improved reproduction capability. The best transmission format available (and also the most expensive) is RBG. This utilizes three channels transmitting all primary components of the color image to the monitor or recorder. The resolution capability of this format exceeds 500 lines of resolution and is superior to the resolution capability of most video recorders and many monitors. The circuitry exists to modify RGB format cameras to S-video and composite systems. This, however, decreases the fidelity of the reproduction and negates the added expense of the RGB camera. Although RGB capability is claimed for some single chip cameras, this is electronically manipulated. Most RGB cameras presently use at least two chips;

Table 2-2. Competitive Camera Profile

Manufacturer	Model	Image Type	Multiple Heads	S-VHS Output	Resolution	Automatic White Balance
Acufex	Auto Shutter HR	2/3 inch	No	Yes	450	Yes
Baxter	AR6500	1/2 inch	No	Yes	450	Yes
Cabot	CCD 3000	1/2 inch	No	No	400	Yes
Circon	Endo Video V	1/2 inch	Yes	Yes	400	Yes
Concept	Intra Vision	1/2 inch	Yes	Yes	420	No
Dyonics	DYOCAM 750	2/3 inch	Yes	Yes	450	Yes
MP Video	MC-800	1/2 inch	Yes	Yes	400	Yes
Medical Dynamics	5960 RGB	1/2 inch	Yes	Yes	430	Yes
Olympus	OTV-S2	1/2 inch	No	No	330	Yes
Solos	VCM-2	1/2 inch	Yes	Yes	500	Yes
Solos	VCM-1	1/2 inch	Yes	No	400	Yes
Solos	Dual Image	1/2 inch × 2	Yes	Yes × 2	500	Yes
Storz	Tri-Cam	3-chip	No	Yes	600	Yes
Storz	Super Cam	1/2 inch	No	Yes	450	Yes
Stryker	777	3-chip	Yes	Yes	750	Yes
Stryker	590	1/2 inch	Yes	Yes	450	Yes
Weck	Colocast	1/2 inch	Yes	Yes	420	Yes
Wisap	Endo View	1/2 inch	No	Yes	450	Yes
Wolf	S5368.10	1/2 inch	Yes	Yes	400	Yes

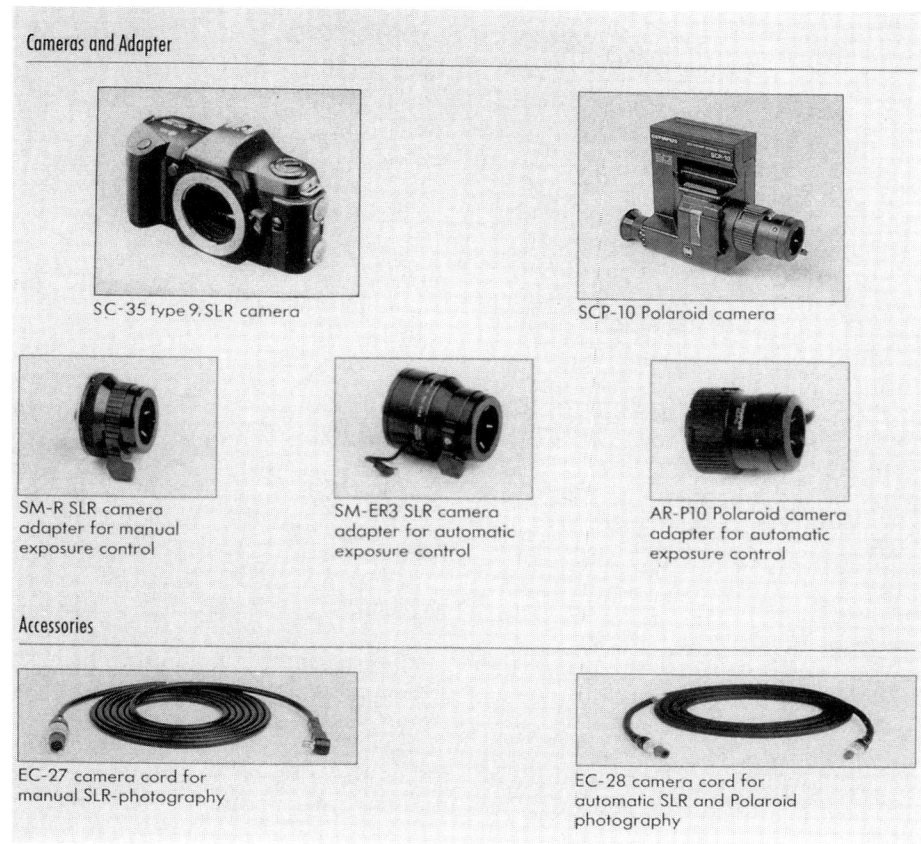

Figure 2-2. Adapters for conventional 35-mm and Polaroid cameras.

single chip cameras lack the resolution capacity of true RGB cameras. Camera profiles are characterized in Table 2-2.

RECORDING MEDIA AND MONITORS

Monitors

Selecting a video monitor has been complicated by the vast array of options and features currently available. The first consideration is the number of monitors needed. Most laparoscopists prefer at least two monitors, allowing the surgeon and assistants to position themselves on either side of the operating table while maintaining visualization of the external operative field and monitor at all times. The second monitor also provides the security of a backup if any technical problems arise. The appropriate screen size is highly operator dependent; careful consideration must be given to the operating room setup and the distance the surgeon will be from the monitor.

Most medical grade monitors provide 400 lines of resolution or more, providing a good match with the resolution capacity of the majority of cameras presently used. If the resolution of the camera exceeds 400 lines, at least one monitor should have equivalent resolution capability. A useful feature to consider is "loop-through." This allows transmission of the signal to several monitors in series, simplifying connections and making transporting equipment between operating suites or elsewhere easier. The multitude of options available for monitors allows a great degree of flexibility; however, component compatibility must be maintained to assure the best image reproduction.

Still Photography

Laparoscopic images can be recorded with traditional still photography or with an increasing number of video modalities. Although less frequently used, still photography maintains a small niche in the field of laparoscopic surgery. Its principal role is to provide photographs or slides for illustration or instructional purposes. Companies such as Olympus and Solos have adapters available for standard 35-mm or Polaroid photography (Fig. 2-2). The adapter splits the laparoscopic image, sending it to both cameras, thus diminishing slightly the quality of the video image. Still photographs obtained in this manner are generally superior to the quality of images transferred from VHS recorders to 35-mm formats. The resolution with still photography, however, is inferior to that produced on the video monitor or with a video printer because of the limitations of the laparoscope. Provided a xenon light source is utilized, no special flash is needed. Generally, a high resolution 200 ASA film will provide the best reproduction.

Video Recorders

Video technology continues to expand rapidly, making it difficult to keep current in the field. The most common video recording format at this time is VHS. The VHS or composite video is popular because it is relatively inexpensive and readily available and permits ideal recording times of an hour or longer. The VHS format is limited, however, in that the resolution capacity is 330 lines or less. The recording, therefore, is frequently inferior to the image produced on the monitor when the procedure is being performed.

S-video, while more expensive, provides a superior match for the majority of components utilized in laparoscopic surgery. While the recording time is similar to that of VHS, definition is superior with up to 425 lines of resolution. The improved reproduction produces an image very close to the resolution capacity of many laparoscopic camera and monitors in use. The S-video uses higher quality recording tape than VHS. Standard VHS tape is compatible with S-video but leads to diminished resolution.

Video tape recorders do not lend themselves well to editing. This is a major drawback to those who are creating recordings for instructional purposes. It is also difficult to transfer the video image to other formats such as 35-mm film without jeopardizing the quality of the reproduction.

Alternative Recording Media

Until recently, the resolution capability of RGB cameras and high resolution monitors (more than 500 lines) exceeded the reproduction quality of most recording formats. For those interested in producing photographic prints, video printers have been introduced (Fig. 2-3). The video printer produces prints directly from the electronic image, bypassing the loss of resolution that occurs when the video format is transferred to 35-mm film. Because the video image is more light sensitive, the electronically produced print also has better contrast at low light levels. Video printers are available in both black and white and color. High resolution printers, with reso-

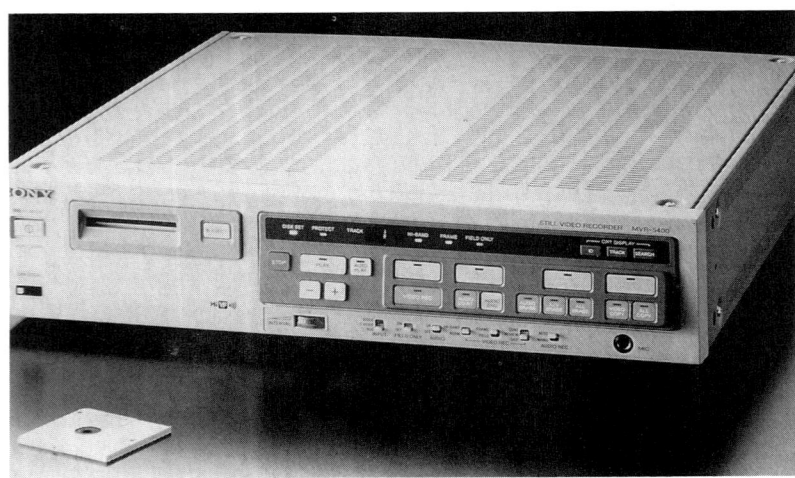

Figure 2-3. The Sony Mavigraph is an example of a currently available video printer.

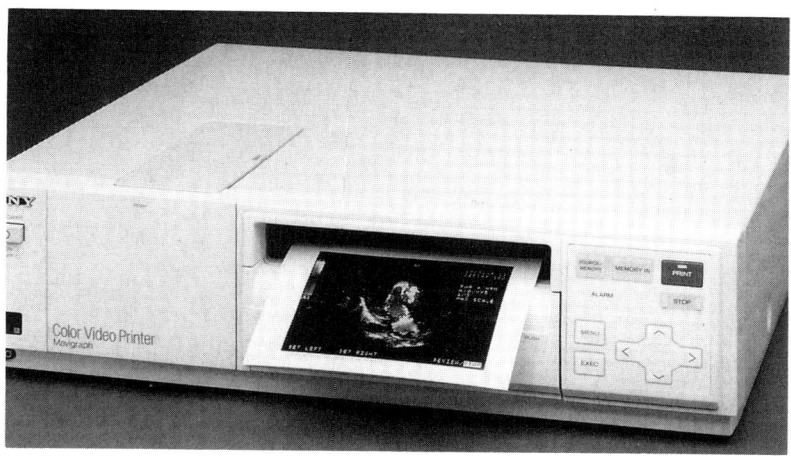

Figure 2-4. Sony MVR-5400 high resolution magnetic disc recorder.

lution exceeding 500 lines, are also now available.

The latest high resolution recorders marketed in 1992 use laser disc and magnetic disc formats. The Sony MVR-5400 (Fig. 2-4) still video recorder has the ability to record video images on a 2-inch floppy disc and reproduce an image with over 500 lines of resolution. The laser disc should also have comparable recording capacity and offer far superior editing capability and increased reliability with extended use. While not all advances are applicable to general practice, the disc format offers exciting possibilities when linked to office or personal computers. When coupled with RGB cameras and high resolution monitors, the laser and magnetic disc offer the cleanest recorded image available and is a tool for electronic photography, publishing, and presentation applications.

REFERENCES

1. Bernheim BM. Organoscopy; cystoscopy of the abdominal cavity. Ann Surg 1911; 53:764–767.
2. Kalk H. Erfahrunzen mit der laparoskopic. Z Klin Med 1929; 111:303–348.
3. Semm K. Advances in pelviscopic surgery. Curr Probl Obstet Gynecol 1982; Vol. 5.

BIBLIOGRAPHY

Classen N, Phillip J. Electronic endoscopy of the gastrointestinal tract. Endoscopy 1984; 16:167–169.
Gadacz TR, Talamin MA, Lillemoele D, et al. Laparoscopic cholecystectomy. Surg Clin North Am 1990; 70:1249–1262.
Hirschowitz B. Photography through the fiber gastroscope. Am J Dig Dis 1963; 8:389–395.
Sivak MV. Gastroenterologic Endoscopy. Philadelphia, W.B. Saunders Company, 1987.
Soper NJ. Laparoscopic cholecystectomy. Curr Probl Surg 1991; 28:585–655.

Chapter 3
Physics of Electrosurgery

Stephen Waisbren
Garth H. Ballantyne

Although the techniques of electrosurgery are relatively new, surgeons have treated vascular, metastatic, and infectious lesions with other methods of cauterization for millennia. The Egyptian Edwin Smith Surgical Papyrus recommended that tumors of the breast be burned with the "fire stick."[1] In Roman times, Celsus prescribed cautery for severe hemorrhage: "When circumstances do not even admit [ligature], the blood vessels can be burnt with a red-hot iron."[2] This same method was utilized in the seventh century. Paulus Aegineta resorted to "cautery with fire . . . when the bleeding proceeds from vessels being corroded by mortification."[3] This therapy continued to be espoused four hundred years later in Arabia by Avicenna (980–1037). He described the best technique for achieving hemostasis with cautery: "For arresting hemorrhage, great heat is required, with vigorous cauterization, so that a firm thick eschar is produced which will not readily come off. It is this crust forming under the eschar which stops the blood-flow. . . ."[4] Even sixteenth century surgical practice remained much the same. Peter Lowe would "cauterize the [veins and arteries] with hot irons" when other techniques failed to stop hemorrhage.[5] By the end of the eighteenth century and throughout the nineteenth century hot iron cautery began to lose favor.[6] The 2000-year-old technique of ligature was revitalized, and cauterization techniques were rarely described.[7]

Renewed interest in the techniques of cauterization began at the turn of this century with the introduction of electrosurgery. In the 1890s, D'Arsonval and Oudin studied the physiologic effects of alternating currents.[8] D'Arsonval demonstrated in 1891 in Paris that high frequency currents above 10,000 Hz could pass through human tissue without causing pain or neuromuscular stimulation. These currents, however, produced heat. Twenty years later Pozzi introduced the term "fulguration." By using high frequency and high voltage from the end of his resonator, he was able to report cures of "deep seated" cancers.[8] In France, Doyen improved the circuitry and added a return electrode. The work of Doyen led to standardization of early electrocautery units in Europe. Meanwhile in America, William Clark, ignorant of the work of his European colleagues, developed a cautery apparatus that used a single spark that was shorter and hotter than that of the previous multiple spark models. After observing the changes in cellular morphology caused by his electrosurgical unit, he termed his technique "desiccation" because it resulted in cell shrinkage.[9] Despite the successes of these pioneering surgeons, electrocautery was slow to gain widespread acceptance. It was still regarded as unscientific, not suitable for a proper surgeon.

The surgeon who was willing to risk his considerable reputation on the new electrosurgical technique was Harvey Cushing (1869–1939). In 1926, at the age of 57, he initiated the modern era of electrocautery.

Part of his success was due to chance. The other part could only be attributed to his open and insightful mind. At the American Surgical Association meeting in June 1925, he happened to come across a demonstration of a cutting diathermy machine incising a large chunk of beef. Instead of just dismissing the new technique with ridicule, as some of his residents had anticipated, he was rather intrigued. Soon thereafter he experimented with the "electrified needle" on the brain, but found little advantage over conventional techniques.[10] However, the next year he discovered William T. Bovie's electrified loop and the modern era of electrosurgery was born.

Bovie (1882–1958) was not a doctor (Fig. 3-1). Although his Ph.D. thesis was in the area of plant physiology, his first appointment at Harvard was as an instructor in bacteriology. There he received a gift of a high frequency generator, but was forbidden to bring the apparatus into his laboratory. Bovie was advised by his director that his work with electrosurgery was a "waste of time" and would bring him "nothing but discredit."[10] Thus, it was not until 3 years later, when he was promoted to a position as a physicist with the Harvard Cancer Commission, that he had an opportunity to experiment with electrosurgery.

The City of Boston enlisted his help to develop a diathermy machine to treat young women for gonorrhea. Since the commercially available techniques were inadequate for these experiments, he found it necessary to build his own high frequency generator. Simultaneously with his new task, enthusiasm for radiation therapy for cancer began to wane with the physicians in his own department. Up until that time, radiation therapy was viewed as the next great hope for treatment of solid tumors. In addition, a few articles had appeared in the English literature on electrosurgery and a number of the new interns became interested in surgery as a treatment for cancer. Hence, a few of the younger residents experimented on minor surgical procedures with Bovie's electrosurgical apparatus. Thus, the stage was set for Harvey Cushing.

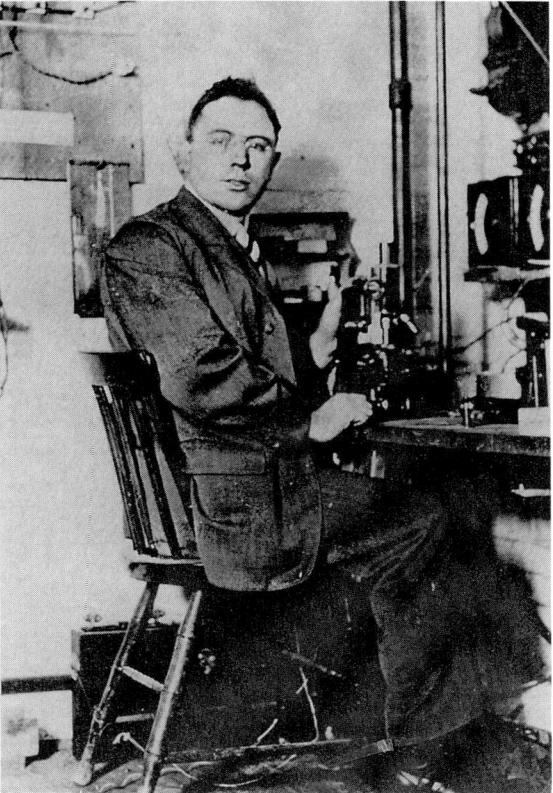

Figure 3-1. William Bovie working at his alternating current switchboard. (Reprinted from Goldwyn RM. Bovie: The man and the machine. Ann Plast Surg 1979; 2:135–153.)

Cushing turned to the Bovie apparatus (Figs. 3-2 and 3-3) only after conventional techniques failed him. In an attempt to remove a painless, slowly enlarging cranial mass of unknown etiology, Cushing was met with an impossibly bloody field. Pondering his predicament, he turned to the new Bovie apparatus. The operation, Cushing wrote, "was a perfect circus—many ringed." After the operating room was rewired, Cushing was initially unable to find any competent assistance because the New England Surgical Association was meeting in Boston at the same time. Instead, he had "four or five coughing Frenchmen with colds in their head" and a medical student blood donor who fainted and fell to the floor. Despite these difficulties, the operation was a complete success. Bleeding was negligible even though the tumor proved to be a vascular myeloma.[10]

Cushing was so impressed with the success of the electrosurgical unit that he called back

24 Fundamentals

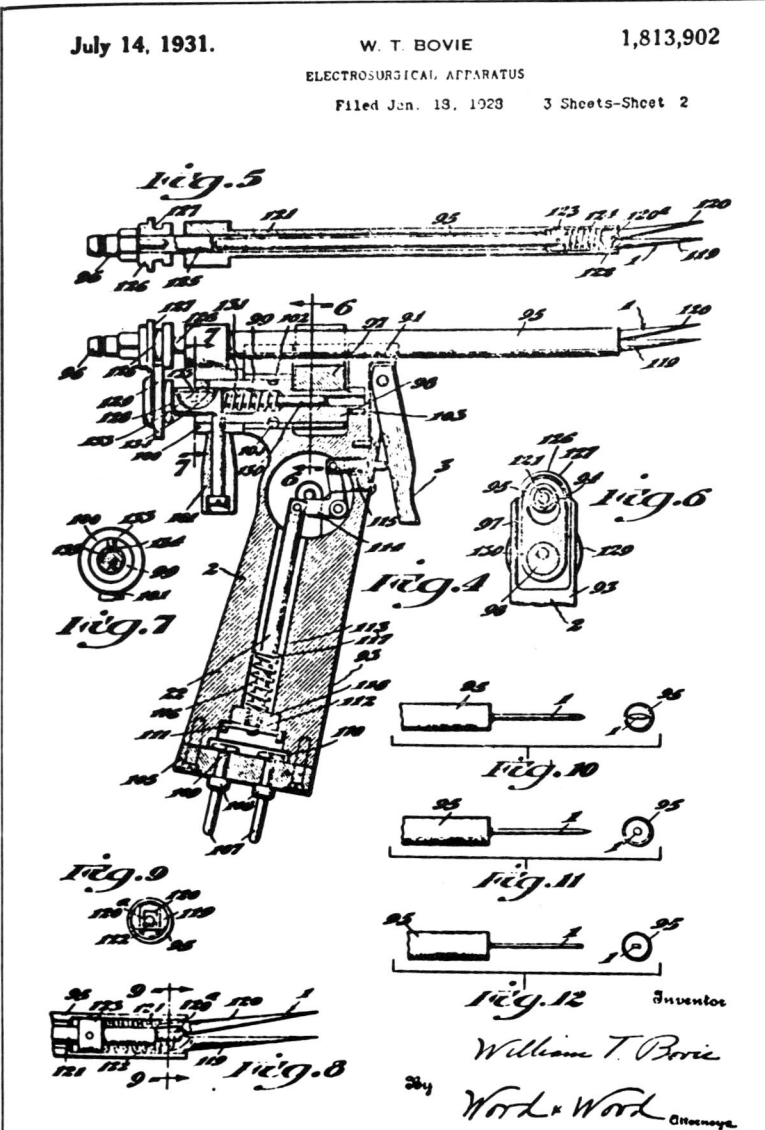

Figure 3-2. The pistol style electrosurgical unit diagrammed for Bovie's patent application filed in 1928. (Reprinted from Goldwyn RM. Bovie: The man and the machine. Ann Plast Surg 1979; 2:135–153.)

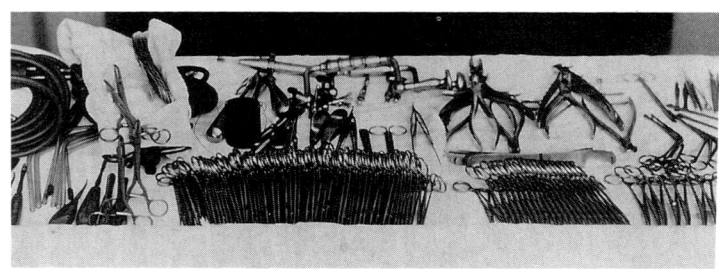

Figure 3-3. Harvey Cushing's surgical instruments. On the left, alongside the classical surgical tools, is the Bovie apparatus. (From the Historical Library at the Yale University School of Medicine.)

a number of his patients whose tumors he had previously deemed "inoperable." As Cushing became more familiar with the apparatus, he made a number of changes in his operative technique. These included substituting rectal administration of ether for inhalation to avoid possible explosions. In addition, he recognized the importance of grounding of the electrosurgical unit after his assistants received a number of strong electric shocks.

One early convert to Bovie's machine was the physiologist Ivan P. Pavlov. John Fulton, in his 1946 biography of Cushing, recalled how Pavlov was to become interested in electrosurgery. Pavlov, having saved enough of his Nobel Prize to pay for a trip to America, visited Harvey Cushing during the International Physiologic Congress (Fig. 3-4). It was an eventful trip. On the New Haven train line Pavlov "was promptly and deftly separated, at the point of a revolver, from his pocketbook containing what was left of his prize money."[11] Despite the difficulties, this 80-year-old survivor of the Russian Revolution, now penniless, proved to be an eager and untiring guest. Cushing treated Pavlov to a demonstration of the electrosurgical apparatus. "Pavlov was so much interested that he all but put his prominent whiskers into the operative field. After the operation was completed, he made enquiries about the electrosurgical knife, whereupon H.C. produced a large slab of beef and had Pavlov inscribe his name with the cutting current"[11] (Fig. 3-5).

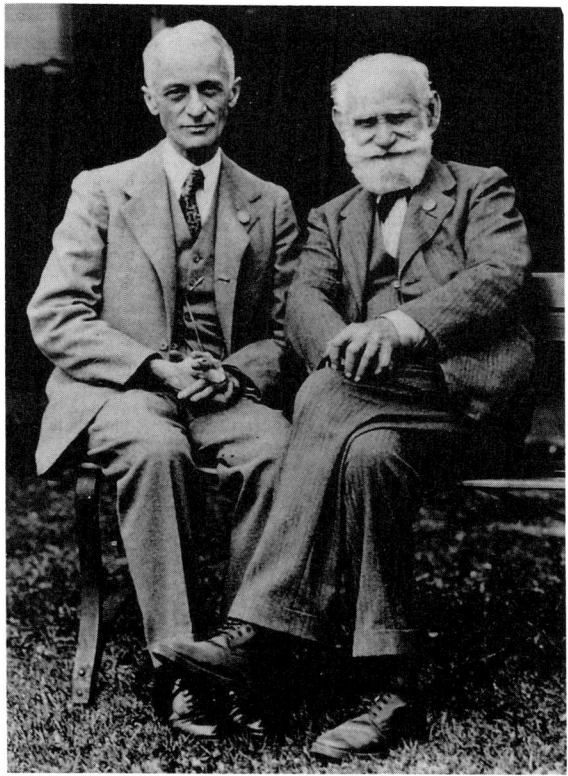

Figure 3-4. Harvey Cushing and Ivan Pavlov photographed in 1929. Pavlov, at the age of 80, amazed his hosts with his energy, inquisitiveness, and enthusiasm. (From the Historical Library at the Yale University School of Medicine.)

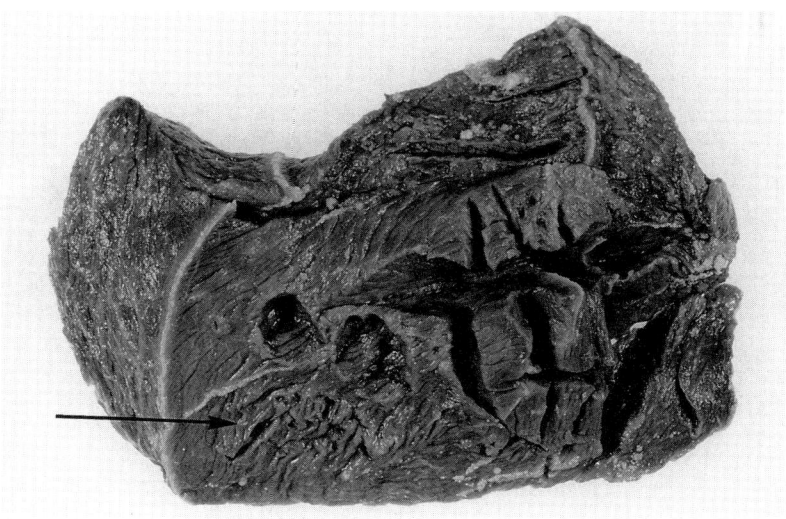

Figure 3-5. A piece of steak in which Pavlov used the Bovie apparatus to sign his name. His signature is discernible on the lower half of the meat. At the arrow a "P" is most visible. The beef has been preserved and is displayed with pride in the office of the chief librarian at the Yale University School of Medicine Historical Library. (From the Historical Library at the Yale University School of Medicine.)

Despite the enthusiastic support of the group from Boston[12] and from physiologists from around the world, many surgeons continued to view electrocautery as primitive. Stevenson and Reid, for example, wrote in 1941 that "in spite of our intense dislike for electrocoagulation, there are moments when it may be used for selected purposes."[13] Thirty-seven years later Glover, Bendick, and Link wrote that "many academic surgeons oppose all use of [the Bovie], especially by their house officers in training."[8] Despite these reservations, the "Bovie" remains standard equipment in just about every operating room.

Despite the eventual success of his apparatus, Bovie, the man, never garnered any rewards, financial or academic, for his work on the electrosurgical unit. He sold his patent rights for the machine to the Liebel-Flarsheim Company for one dollar. Additionally, his academic career at Harvard suffered because of his interest in electrosurgery. Since he spent so much time in the operating room testing each improvement on his apparatus, he was unable to complete the tasks for which he was hired. Thus, when his grant ran out and his application for tenure was denied, he left his position at Harvard for a professorship in Biophysics at Northwestern University.

Despite his "failure" at Harvard, his achievements were recognized nationally. He was elected to many prestigious societies and received a number of awards. He was in great demand throughout the United States as a lecturer. Still, after his years at Harvard, he rarely published the results of any of his experiments. Bovie remained at Northwestern for only 2 years until he moved to Maine to continue his research. In Maine, his career as an academic faltered. Despite his popularity as a lecturer at local colleges, his research was undisciplined and, apparently, unproductive. When he died in 1958 at age 75 his estate was so poor that money had to be raised from neighbors to pay for his burial.

ELECTROCAUTERY IN ENDOSCOPIC SURGERY

Whereas electrocautery has been begrudgingly applied in abdominal surgery, fulguration and endotherm snare extraction rapidly became standard treatment for polypoid lesions of the rectum and distal sigmoid colon accessible with rigid endoscopes. In 1948 Scarborough and Klein[14] reported the treatment by electrodesiccation of 211 polyps in 112 patients. Similarly, Castro and colleagues[15] successfully coagulated 105 adenomas in 95 patients. Furthermore, several groups applied fulguration to the treatment of early colorectal cancers. Jackes[16] successfully treated with fulguration seven of eight patients with malignant polyps. Between 1949 and 1950, 214 polypoid carcinomas of the rectum were treated by fulguration at the Mayo Clinic.[17] Treatment was unsuccessful in only five patients. Consequently, by the dawn of the era of flexible endoscopy, electrocautery was well established as standard therapy for polypoid lesions accessible with endoscopes.

In the early 1970s, Wolff and Shinya reported the efficacy and safety of colonoscopic polypectomy. In February 1973, they described in *The New England Journal of Medicine* the successful removal of 303 polyps in 218 patients using a "wire loop threaded through the polyethylene tube and introduced via the biopsy channel of the colonoscope."[18] In September 1973, they reported on the removal of an additional 499 polyps from 350 patients.[19] Following these reports, electrocautery has become an essential part of flexible sigmoidoscopy and electrocautery.

It was the experience with colonoscopy that familiarized general surgeons with endoscopic electrosurgery. When the pioneers of laparoscopic general surgery performed operations that had traditionally been completed with open techniques, they were already adept at electrocautery through an endoscope. Using this familiar technique in previously unfamiliar settings made the transition from open to closed techniques possible.

PHYSICS

Frequency

The frequency of the current used in electrocautery must be within a range that does not stimulate neuromuscular tissue. As all high school biology students know, stimulating a frog muscle with a battery will cause the muscle to contract. However, if the current placed across the neuromuscular junction is an alternating current, the depolarization will quickly be reversed. This will result in muscle tetany. At alternating current frequencies greater than 100,000 Hz, insufficient time is available for ionic current to flow and cause a depolarization. Instead, the ions move only short distances. Because this kinetic energy is dissipated as heat, a cell that is stimulated with alternating current greater than 100,000 Hz will become hot.[20] In practice, most generators operate at currents with a frequency of 250,000 to 350,000. Diathermy units are based upon a high frequency current administered across a large surface area. This unfocused current heats the patient but does not injure tissue (Fig. 3-6).

Electrocautery Cutting

Electrocautery cutting of tissue is accomplished by concentrating the density of the current, by increasing the power (voltage), and by altering the waveform. The electrosurgical knife, which has a small surface area, serves as the active electrode (Fig. 3-7). A passive electrode with a large surface area is attached to the patient (often incorrectly referred as the "grounding plate"). This discrepancy of surface area between the two electrodes results in a dense current at the tip of the electrosurgical knife and a dispersed current at the passive electrode. The relatively high density of current at the tip of the electrosurgical knife enables the electricity to cut tissue. Empirical experience has demonstrated that an undamped continuous sinusoidal waveform effectively incises tissue (Fig. 3-8).[8] Such a current, however, produces virtually no coagulation. During cutting, a thin layer of tissue surrounding the knife evaporates.

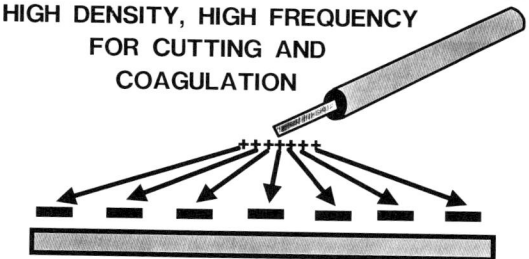

Figure 3-7. Electrocautery cutting is produced by focusing a current with a high frequency at the tip of the electrocautery device. The tissue at the tip of the monopolar electrocautery instrument is vaporized. The large surface area of the passive electrode ("grounding plate") rapidly disperses the intensity of the current.

Coagulation

Coagulation is accomplished by much the same means as cutting but with a different current wave pattern. Empirical experience has revealed that a damped sinusoidal waveform achieves the best coagulation with little cutting of tissues (Fig. 3-9). To provide coagulation the current is interrupted with "off times" which range from 50 to 150 μseconds. The ratio of on time:off time determines the level of coagulation. Usually, a ratio of 1:5 to 1:10 produces the best results.[20]

Electrocautery coagulation does not actually cause clot formation. Instead, electrocautery coagulation is achieved by desiccation of cells.

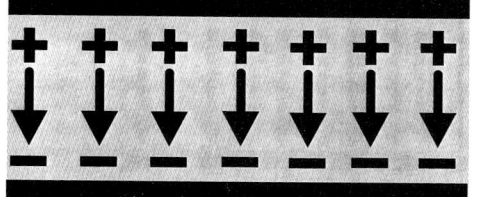

Figure 3-6. Diathermy, a system for warming patients, is achieved with a current of high frequency applied over a large surface area. The unfocused current heats the tissue but does not have sufficient energy to injure the tissue.

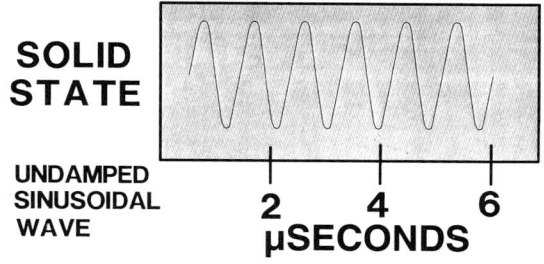

Figure 3-8. A current with an undamped sinusoidal waveform at a high frequency produces electrocautery cutting of tissue.

The heat generated by the current boils out the water in the tissue, which produces a zone of desiccated cells. This barrier of dehydrated cells attains the hemostatic effect.

Blended Currents

To achieve cutting with hemostasis it is necessary to combine the features of both cutting and coagulation currents. These blended currents with a combination of pure waveform and pulsed waveform with various on times and off times provide an intermediate level of cutting with adequate coagulation (Fig. 3-10).[8,20] It should be noted that the tip of the electrocautery instruments affects the characteristics of the current. A fine needle-like electrotrode increases the cutting properties of the current and minimizes the coagulation effect.

Fulguration

Fulguration refers specifically to tissue destruction caused by "spark gapping." In this technique the active electrode is held several millimeters from the tissue. The current must be of sufficient magnitude that it will jump the gap between electrode and tissue. The cross-sectional area of the resulting "sparks" is very small and as a result the density of the current upon tissue contact is extremely high. This produces deep tissue penetration and a large zone of tissue desiccation and injury. Furthermore, the sparks tend to

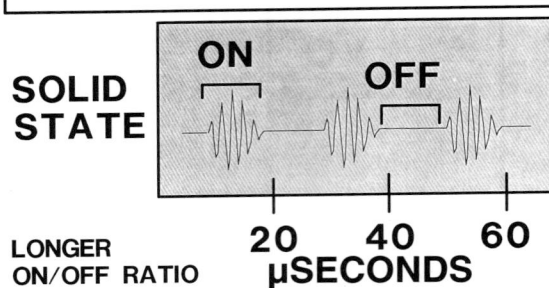

Figure 3-10. Blended currents which both cut tissues and coagulate are achieved by altering the on:off ratio of the pulsed waveform.

wander around a relatively large area of contact, which also contributes to the large zone of injury. A high voltage current facilitates fulguration by ionizing the gas in the gap between the active electrode and the tissue.

Differences in Solid State and Vacuum Tube Generated Currents

Modern electronics have greatly improved electrocautery. The current generated by the classic spark-gap and vacuum tube circuits decayed over time. Consequently, the initial current of the pulse was much greater than that after a few seconds of use. The gradual decay in current resulted in greater penetration of the current into surrounding tissue, resulting in a larger zone of coagulation and tissue injury.

The nature of cutting currents generated by solid state circuits differs somewhat from classical spark-gap and vacuum tube circuits. Classical circuits generate a current output which oscillates every 1/120 second.[20] The sinusoidal pattern of the waveform remains intact, but the magnitude of each wave varies with time. This oscillation causes some coagulation and injury to surrounding tissue. In contrast, the output of current from modern solid state circuits is more stable, and the magnitude of each sinusoidal waveform remains more constant over time. Schroeder and colleagues[21] found that a Valley Lab electrocautery unit on a setting of 3 produced tissue damage in rat colons for a depth of 0.38 ± 0.21 mm. As a result, solid state circuitry produces a more "pure cutting" current that causes little coagulation and produces a very limited zone of tissue injury.

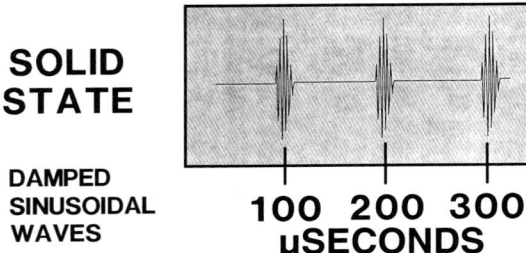

Figure 3-9. A current with a damped sinusoidal waveform, which is interrupted for periods of 50 to 150 μseconds causes coagulation. The ratio of the on time to the off time determines the level of coagulation.

Surprisingly, classical spark-gap and vacuum tube circuits are superior to solid state circuits for fulguration. This is probably due to the higher initial pulse of current and the higher voltage produced by the classical circuits (Fig. 3-11).[20]

Monopolar and Bipolar

Solid state electrocautery units permit either monopolar or bipolar operation. Described previously is the monopolar electrocautery in which the current passes from the active electrode to the passive electrode ("grounding plate") attached to the patient. In bipolar operation, the electrocautery instrument (e.g., forceps) contains both the active and passive electrodes (Fig. 3-12). The current flows from one tip of the forceps, through the grasped tissue, to the other tip. Unlike monopolar coagulation, there is little dissipation of current. Bipolar coagulation results in better control because cellular damage is limited to the tissue held by the forceps.

APPLICATIONS OF ELECTROCAUTERY TO LAPAROSCOPIC SURGERY

During open abdominal procedures, surgeons can maintain or reestablish hemostasis with several techniques that have been perfected over the last century. During open procedures, large amounts of blood and clots can be quickly removed from the operative

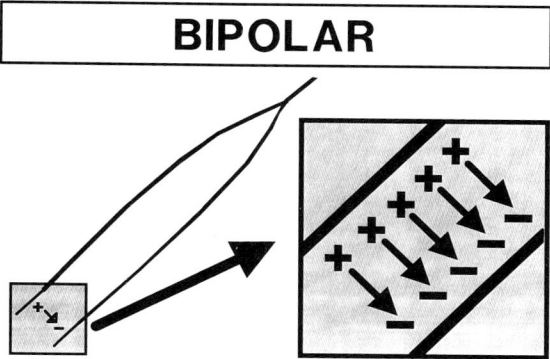

Figure 3-12. A bipolar electrocautery device contains both the active and passive electrodes. Thus, the current passes only through the tissue grasped by the instrument.

field with suction or sponge-like laparotomy pads. Sites of hemorrhage can be clamped with multiple clamps of various types and then tied with sutures. Alternatively, the bleeding vessels can be ligated rapidly with sutures. Whereas these methods remain dramatically effective during open abdominal operations, implementation of these techniques during laparoscopic procedures is difficult, and the results are unreliable.

Application of traditional techniques of hemostasis during laparoscopic procedures is tedious at best and often impossible. The currently available suction devices for use during laparoscopic procedures are limited in their ability to remove clots and large volumes of blood by their narrow diameter. Even small clots rapidly clog these devices. The use of suction devices with larger calibers is impractical because high rates of suction exceed the flow rates of the carbon dioxide insufflators and deflate the pneumoperitoneum, which obscures the view through the laparoscope. Application of clamps is limited by the number of available trochars. Tying knots on sutures is slow regardless of the technique. Placement of suture ligatures is encumbered by the two-dimensional telecast of the procedure and the limitation of movement of the needle imposed by the laparoscopic needle holder and the trochar. Finally, jets of blood streaming from points of hemorrhage may coat the lens of the telescope and result in limited visibility.

Meticulous hemostasis must be maintained throughout laparoscopic procedures. Even small amounts of blood stain the tissues and obscure the tissue planes. During laparoscopic

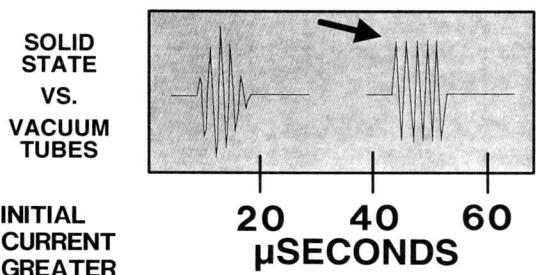

Figure 3-11. Solid state (transitors) equipment produces a damped sinusoidal waveform (*left*). In contrast, older vacuum tube circuitry produces a higher initial current (*right*). As a result, the older circuitry penetrated tissue to a greater depth.

procedures, orientation within the abdomen is almost entirely dependent upon visual clues. Unfortunately, hemorrhage, even after it has been well controlled, may lead to disorientation because of obfuscation of these visual clues and subsequent deviation from planned paths of dissection. Thus, successful laparoscopic surgery requires not only meticulous hemostasis but also a virtually bloodless operative field. Electrocautery meets these demands of laparoscopic surgery.

ADAPTATION OF ELECTROCAUTERY DEVICES FOR LAPAROSCOPY

Dissection with electrocautery is an effective technique for the performance of laparoscopic procedures. Many traditional surgical instruments have been adapted for use in laparoscopic operations. Karl Zucker, for example, developed an instrument for dissection of Kalot's triangle called the Maryland Dissector. This instrument has a working end much like a small curved clamp and is wired for monopolar electrocautery. This allows careful dissection of small structures with the magnified image of the video laparoscope and meticulous hemostasis. Similarly, various types of scissors have been adapted for laparoscopic use. In most cases, these instruments are wired as a monopolar electrocautery device. This setup permits use of the scissors as both a scissors and an electrocautery knife. Thus, tissues can be transected with a sequence of cauterization and sharp cutting or by simultaneous use of cutting and cautery. This integration of two types of instruments into one greatly facilitates laparoscopic procedures since it reduces the number of times instruments must be withdrawn from the abdomen and reintroduced through trochars.

New electrocautery instruments have also been developed for laparoscopic procedures. The angle of attack and the limitations of movement dictated by operating through trochars requires novel methods of dissection. The SURGIWAND* Tip system (Fig. 3-13), for example, provides nine different tips for this electrocautery dissection instrument. Each tip incorporates a different combination of shapes and surface areas to promote a variety of mixtures of hook, blunt, sharp, and electrocautery dissection. The tips with needle-like ends have small surface areas and, consequently, focus the energy of the electrocautery and promote the cutting properties of the cautery device. The blunt tips with large surface areas diffuse the current when ap-

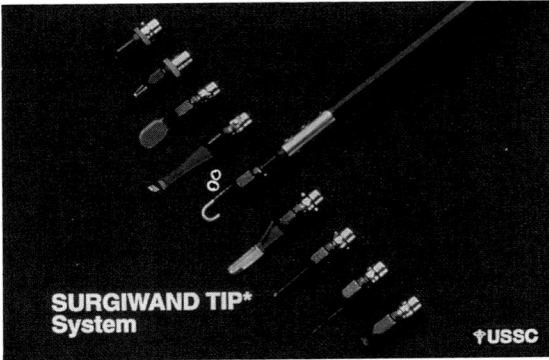

Figure 3-13. The SURGIWAND* Tip system allows a wide variety of tips for different combinations of electrocautery and blunt dissection.

plied en face but can still focus the current when applied along their narrow edge. As a result, these instruments can be used for both blunt dissection as well as an electrocautery knife. The hook tips allow simultaneous retraction and cauterization of the tissue. These instruments illustrate the modern trend in the design of laparoscopic surgical instruments: the marriage of at least two functions into one instrument.

SPECIAL CONSIDERATIONS FOR AN OPERATING LAPAROSCOPE

Use of a monopolar electrocautery device through an operating laparoscope induces a magnetic field around the long axis of the cautery instrument.[22] This in turn induces an electric charge in the metal casing of the laparoscope. Indeed, the induction of the magnetic field may sap as much as 50–70 per cent of force of the electrocautery current. If the laparoscope is not grounded, it becomes a capacitor and stores the charge. As a result, the federal Food and Drug Administration has dictated that any laparoscope greater than 7 mm in diameter must be encased in a metal sleeve. This allows discharge of the induced charge over a large surface area with little risk of injury.

SAFETY OF ELECTROCAUTERY

Karl Semm has raised concerns about the use of electrocautery during laparoscopic procedures. He writes in his textbook *Endoscopic Abdominal Surgery* that "there is compelling biophysical and medical considerations why the therapeutic use of high-frequency current can no longer be considered safe in the closed abdominal cavity."[23] Semm points out that the course of the current to the grounding plate is unpredictable and consequently the possibility of injury is unpredictable. He cites anecdotal case reports of injury to distal organs such as the colon and changes in menstrual function. Bowel injuries have been reported by others.[24] Deaths have also been reported after use of unipolar electrocautery for laparoscopic sterilization procedures.[25] Despite the theoretical concerns raised by Semm, many experimental as well as clinical studies attest to the safety of the use of electrocautery devices during laparoscopic procedures.

EXPERIMENTAL STUDIES

The recent application of laparoscopic techniques to general surgery procedures has once again focused attention on the safety of unipolar electrocautery devices. Saye and colleagues[26] performed experiments to address specifically the possibility of secondary sparking during the use of electrocautery and also distal burns caused by an increase in electrical resistance in distal organs. They found that secondary sparking is unlikely to occur and that the sparks jump less than 2 to 3 mm. Additionally, it was pointed out that the humidification of air increases the voltage required for sparking and, furthermore, that the dielectric constant of carbon dioxide is 5 per cent greater than that of air. Thus, the conditions found within a carbon dioxide pneumoperitoneum actually decrease the probability that spontaneous sparking will occur. It was pointed out, however, that smoke from electrocautery increases the chances of sparking. If smoke begins to accumulate, it should be allowed to dissipate before further cauterization is undertaken. In sharp contrast, the second set of experiments indicated that secondary burns from electrocautery were likely to occur under certain conditions. Saye and collegues warned that extreme caution should be used when applying unipolar electrocautery to appendix- and duct-like structures. Application of electrocautery to the omentum should be limited to short durations.

ELECTROCAUTERY IN LAPAROSCOPIC CHOLECYSTECTOMY

The safety of electrocautery during laparoscopic cholecystectomy has been studied in both experimental models and clinical trials. Soper and colleagues[27] studied the effects of electrocautery on surrounding tissues during laparoscopic cholecystectomy in pigs. There was no histologic evidence of injury to bile ducts, liver, or intestines in five animals sacrificed immediately after the operation. Similarly, there were no alterations in liver function tests and no histologic evidence of ongoing hepatocyte injury in the gallbladder bed or cholestasis when the animals were sacrificed at 1 month after the operation.

The clinical safety of unipolar electrocautery in laparoscopic cholecystectomy has been confirmed in many clinical trials. Corbitt,[28] for example, directly compared the morbidity and mortality of laparoscopic cholecystectomy using a laser with the use of unipolar electrocautery and found both equally safe. Similarly, the Southern Surgical Club[29] reported about an equal percentage of complications in patients who underwent laser laparoscopic cholecystectomy and those treated with electrocautery. In a series of 1,339 laparoscopic cholecystectomies using electrocautery dissection, Larson and colleagues[30] reported two complications directly attributable to the electrocautery: a small cautery burn of the common bile duct that required repair and a cautery perforation of the duodenum. Similarly, in a focused review of 12 biliary duct injuries that occurred during laparoscopic cholecystectomies, Meyers and colleagues[31] attributed one late biliary stricture to excessive use of electrocautery during the dissection of the cystic duct. This injury may indeed illustrate the admonition offered by Saye's group against cauterization of duct-like structures. Arguing from a somewhat different perspective, Voyles and colleagues[32] contend that electrocautery is better than lasers for laparoscopic cholecystectomy because of the equal safety but cheaper cost of electrocautery instruments. Many other large clinical trials have also supported the safety of monopolar electrocautery for laparoscopic cholecystectomy.[33,34]

ELECTROCAUTERY FOR ADVANCED GASTROINTESTINAL LAPAROSCOPIC PROCEDURES

Laparoscopic techniques are being applied to the full spectrum of gastrointestinal diseases. At present, however, only limited and often anecdotal experience with these procedures has been reported. Consequently, the safety of the use of electrocautery in various advanced gastrointestinal laparoscopic procedures is not yet established. Nonetheless, early experience supports the use of electrocautery in these operations. Bailey and colleagues[35] have performed laparoscopic selective vagotomy with the use of electrocautery dissection. Similarly, Bastug and colleagues[36] have reported successful laparoscopic lysis of adhesions with electrocautery for small bowel obstruction. German surgeons have reported much experience with bipolar electrocautery in laparoscopic appendectomies.[37] Early experience with laparoscopic-assisted colon resections also suggests that electrocautery can be safely used in these more difficult and lengthy procedures.[38,39] Although careful assessment of large clinical series is warranted, preliminary information indicates that monopolar or bipolar electrocautery can be used safely in the full spectrum of laparoscopic procedures.

CAUTIONS ON TECHNIQUE

Electrocautery can be safely used during laparoscopic procedures. Nonetheless, as with any type of surgical intervention, injury is possible. The following guidelines may help to diminish the risk of inadvertent injury of surrounding tissues or distant organs.

1. Insufflate the peritoneum with carbon dioxide whenever possible.
2. Make sure there is good contact between the patient and the grounding pad.
3. Make sure the entire conductive surface of the electrocautery device is visible whenever electrocautery is applied. The two-dimensional appearance of the video image may not warn you that the back side of the cautery device is in contact with adjacent tissues.
4. Avoid transecting appendix-like or duct-like structures with electrocautery. Flow of current down these tube-like structures may lead to tissue injury at distant sites. These structures are better ligated with clips or stapling devices and then sharply divided.
5. Do not allow smoke from electrocautery to accumulate since smoke promotes spontaneous sparking.

Summary

The techniques of cauterization have progressed greatly over the past six millennia. Although bleeding is no longer controlled with the application of hot irons, cautery remains a well proven tool for the general surgeon. As laparoscopic surgical techniques are used more frequently, electrosurgical procedures may replace the scalpel and ligature as the primary tools of the general surgeon. Harvey Cushing and William Bovie would be very surprised to find how their work has made the modern laparoscopic revolution possible.

The greatest advantage of electrocautery for the novice laparoscopic surgeon is previous experience with this technique during the performance of standard open abdominal procedures. The use of this familiar technique of dissection will facilitate the transition to the performance of laparoscopic procedures. Laparoscopic surgery requires meticulous hemostasis since even small amounts of hemorrhage stain tissues and obscure tissue planes. Loss of these visual clues may lead to disorientation of the surgeon during laparoscopic procedures. Electrocautery dissection admirably meets these rigorous demands.

REFERENCES

1. Breasted JH. The Edwin Smith Surgical Papyrus. Published in facsimile and hieroglyphic transliteration with translation and commentary in two volumes. Chicago, The University of Chicago Press, 1930, pp 365–366.
2. Celsus (Spencer WG, trans). De Medicina. Cambridge, MA, Harvard University Press, Vol II, p 81.
3. Adams F, trans. The Seven Books of Paulus Aegineta. Translated from the Greek with a commentary embracing a complete view of the knowledge possessed by the Greeks, Romans, and Arabians on all subjects connected with medicine and surgery. London, The Sydenham Society, 1846, Book IV, p 129.
4. Gruner OC. A Treatise on the Canon of Medicine of Avicenna Incorporating a Translation of the First Book. London, Luzac & Co, 1930, No. 1072, pp 525–526.
5. Lowe P. The Whole Course of Chirurgie, Wherein Is Briefly Set Downe the Causes, Signes, Prognostications & Curations of All Sorts of Tumors, Wounds, Ulcers, Fractures, Dislocations & all other Diseases. London, Thomas Purfoot, 1597, Sixth Treatise, Chap VI.
6. Hunter J. A Treatise on the Blood, Inflammation, and Gun-Shot Wounds. London, George Nicol, 1794, p 535.
7. Cooper A. In Tyrrell F, ed. The Lectures of Sir Astley Cooper, Bart, F.R.S., Surgeon to the King, etc., on the Principles and Practice of Surgery, 5th American ed. Philadelphia, Haswell, Barrington, and Haswell, 1839, pp 424–453.
8. Glover JL, Bendick PJ, Link WJ. The use of thermal knives in surgery: Electrosurgery, lasers, plasma scalpel. Curr Probl Surg 1978; 15:1–78.

9. Kelly HA, Ward GE. Electrosurgery. Philadelphia, WB Saunders, 1932.
10. Goldwyn RM. Bovie: The man and the machine. Ann Plast Surg 1979; 2:135–153.
11. Fulton JF. Harvey Cushing: A Biography. Springfield, IL, Charles C Thomas, 1946, pp 578 and 671.
12. Cushing H, Bovie WT. Electrosurgery as an aid to the removal of intracranial tumors. Surg Gynecol Obstet 1928; 47:751.
13. Stevenson JM, Reid MR. The fundamental principles of surgical technic. In Bancroft FW, ed. Operative Surgery. New York, Appleton-Century Company, 1941, p 262.
14. Scarborough RA, Klein RR. Polypoid lesions of the colon and rectum. Am J Surg 1948; 76:723–727.
15. Castro AF, Ault GW, Smith RS. Adenomatous polyps of the colon and rectum. Surg Gynecol Obstet 1951; 92:1264–1271.
16. Jackes H. Fulguration of malignant lesions of the rectum. Treat Serv Bull 1952; 7:157.
17. Lochridge EP, Jackman RJ. Evaluation of conservative management of certain polypoid lesions of the lower part of the large intestine. Dis Colon Rectum 1958; 1:101–109.
18. Wolff WI, Shinya H. Polypectomy via the fiberoptic colonoscope. N Engl J Med 1973; 288:329–332.
19. Wolff WI, Shinya H. A new approach to colonic polyps. Ann Surg 1973; 178:367–378.
20. Sittner WR, Fitzgerald JK. High-frequency electrosurgery. In Berci G, ed. Endoscopy. New York, Appleton-Century-Crofts, 1976, pp 214–220.
21. Schroeder T, Brackett K, Joffe SN. An experimental study of the effects of electrocautery and various lasers on gastrointestinal tissue. Surgery 1987; 101:691–697.
22. Hulka JF. Textbook of Laparoscopy. New York, Grune & Stratton, Inc, 1985, p 26.
23. Semm K (Friedrich ER, trans). Operative Manual for Endoscopic Abdominal Surgery. Chicago, Year Book Medical Publishers, Inc, 1987, pp 81–91.
24. Levy BS, Soderstrom RM, Dail DH. Bowel injuries during laparoscopy: Gross anatomy and histology. J Reprod Med 1985; 30:168–179.
25. Peterson HB, Ory HW, Greenspan JR, et al. Deaths associated with laparoscopic sterilization by unipolar electrocoagulation devices, 1978 and 1979. Am J Obstet Gynecol 1981; 139:141.
26. Saye WB, Miller W, Hertzmann P. Electrosurgery thermal injury: Myth or misconception? Surg Laparosc Endosc 1991; 1:223–228.
27. Soper NS, Barteau JA, Clayman RV, Becich MJ. Safety and efficacy of laparoscopic cholecystectomy using monopolar electrocautery in the porcine model. Surg Laparosc Endosc 1991; 1:17–22.
28. Corbitt JD Jr. Laparoscopic cholecystectomy: Laser versus electrosurgery. Surg Laparosc Endosc 1991; 1:85–88.
29. Meyers WC, Branum GD, Farouk M, et al. A prospective analysis of 1518 laparoscopic cholecystectomies: The Southern Surgeons Club. N Engl J Med 1991; 324:1073–1078.
30. Larson GM, Vitale GC, Casey J, et al. Multipractice analysis of laparoscopic cholecystectomy in 1,983 patients. Am J Surg 1992; 163:221–226.
31. Davidoff AM, Pappas TN, Murray EA, et al. Mechanisms of major biliary injury during laparoscopic cholecystectomy. Ann Surg 1992; 215:196–202.
32. Voyles CR, Meena AL, Petro AB, et al. Electrocautery is superior to laser for laparoscopic cholecystectomy. Am J Surg 1990; 160:457.
33. Peters JH, Ellison EC, Innes JT, et al. Safety and efficacy of laparoscopic cholecystectomy: A prospective analysis of 100 initial patients. Ann Surg 1991; 213:3–12.
34. Zucker KA, Bailey RW, Gadacz TR, Imbembo AL. Laparoscopic guided cholecystectomy. Am J Surg 1991; 161:36–44.
35. Bailey RW, Flowers JL, Graham SM, Zucker KA. Combined laparoscopic cholecystectomy and selective vagotomy. Surg Laparosc Endosc 1991; 1:45–49.
36. Bastug DF, Trammell SW, Boland JP, et al. Laparoscopic adhesiolysis for small bowel obstruction. Surg Laparosc Endosc 1991; 1:259–262.
37. Pier A, Götz F, Bacher C. Laparoscopic appendectomy in 625 cases: from innovation to routine. Surg Laparosc Endosc 1991; 1:8–13.
38. Monson JR, Darzi A, Carey PD, Guillou PJ. Prospective evaluation of Laparoscopic-assisted colectomy in an unselected group of patients. Lancet 1992; 340:831–833.
39. Phillips EH, Franklin M, Carroll BJ, Fallas MJ, Ramos R, Rosenthal D. Laparoscopic Colectomy. Ann Surg 1992; 216:703–707.

Chapter 4
Operating Room Configuration

Frederick L. Greene
Nancy C. Taylor

The surgeon who embarks upon minimally invasive surgery using laparoscopic intervention must have a keen understanding, not only of equipment, but also of the specific needs that must be met by the operating room and its personnel. Since most hospitals are not currently configured for the performance of this type of surgical procedure, standard operating suites must be utilized and configured to allow laparoscopic surgical procedures to be done efficiently and safely.

The initial requirement is to have an operating suite that is large enough to contain the increased number of instruments and technical equipment needed for these types of procedures. Whether one is using laparoscopy primarily for biliary tract surgery or performing thoracoscopy for pulmonary resection, the size requirement is virtually the same. Operating rooms that are traditionally set aside for major abdominal or thoracic surgery are quite suitable for laparoscopic surgical procedures. It is not appropriate to perform these procedures in smaller rooms traditionally used by the ophthalmologists or ear, nose, and throat surgeons or to use "procedure rooms" designed for endoscopic procedures or changing of casts.

Standard operating rooms generally include appropriate electrical outlets, but it is important to remember that the electrical support of monitors and electrocautery, laser, and additional equipment may place a burden on the electrical supply of a conventional operating suite. The electrical supply and appropriate grounding in an operating room must be surveyed and the engineering staff of the hospital must be involved in determining appropriate operating room support as well as in monitoring ongoing electrical needs.

Laparoscopic surgery is performed on a standard operating room table, but the importance of adaptation to fluoroscopy must be kept in mind. Since the use of the C-arm fluoroscopic units for biliary tract intervention will expand in the future, the operating room table should be adaptable for total fluoroscopic support. In addition, the operating room table should rotate into multiple positions, including Trendelenburg, reverse Trendelenburg, right and left angulation, and standard flexion and lithotomy positions. The performance of laparoscopic surgery will require various positions depending upon the procedure performed and the anatomical requirements of the individual technique. Indeed, exposure for many of the gastrointestinal procedures is almost exclusively obtained through position changes of the patient. The operating room table should allow for the placement of a foot rest to protect the patient from sliding while also having additional supports to maintain the patient in angled positions if needed. By having an appropriate, electronically manipulated operating room table, it is easier to place the patient into position and potential intraoperative problems are reduced. The patient's arms may be placed in an abducted position on arm boards or at the patient's side, depending on the monitoring needs. Regardless of the arm position used, appropriate padding of the ulnar nerve and avoidance of hyperabduction at the shoulder are important to avoid neurologic injury.

Lighting in the operating room, although important for laparoscopic surgery, is less of an issue because of the need to reduce overall lighting when monitors are used. It is important, however, to have appropriate operating room lights that can be dimmed and moved out of position easily while video monitors are in use. Mobility of the ceiling-mounted operating room lights is especially important since the monitors frequently need to be placed in areas occupied by these mounted lights. Appropriate tracks for light movement are needed to position the monitors without interference from ceiling-mounted lights.

It is important to have needed equipment placed in the operating room prior to entrance of the patient for induction of anesthesia. This is not the time to continue searching for needed instrumentation since this will interfere with the induction of anesthesia and reduce the patient's confidence in the planned surgical procedure because of unnecessary disruption. Instrument cards or laminated wall mountings should be developed to help nursing personnel and technicians set up the room appropriately and to recognize the instrument requirements of the surgeon involved. Operating rooms designated for laparoscopic surgery are beneficial since equipment can be stored in these rooms, thus reducing the need for transportation of instrumentation.

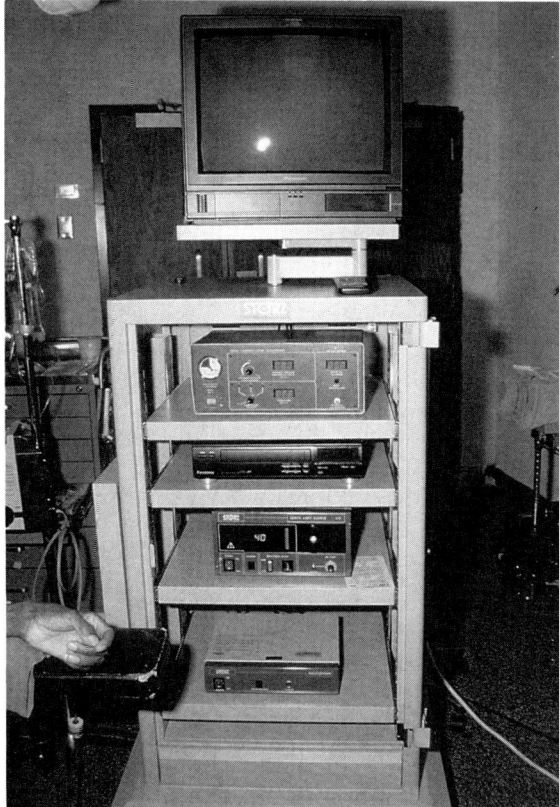

Figure 4-2. Placement of monitors to facilitate change of position in the operating room. The insufflator and light source are stored as a unit.

Basic laparoscopic surgical equipment includes one or two television monitors that can be mounted on a cart at least 5 to 6 feet in height or ceiling-mounted to allow for the best viewing by the surgical team (Fig. 4-1). If the same room will be used for a variety of laparoscopic procedures, it is appropriate to have cabinet-mounted monitors to allow for these to be moved into appropriate locations depending on the operation performed (Fig. 4-2). High resolution television monitors are mandatory and should be purchased to interface appropriately with the laparoscopic instrumentation that is used.

Additional equipment needed for laparoscopic procedures, regardless of the type of operation performed, are insufflators for carbon dioxide and the electrocautery or laser units used for dissection. These units will become more compact in the future, but still require additional space on each side of the

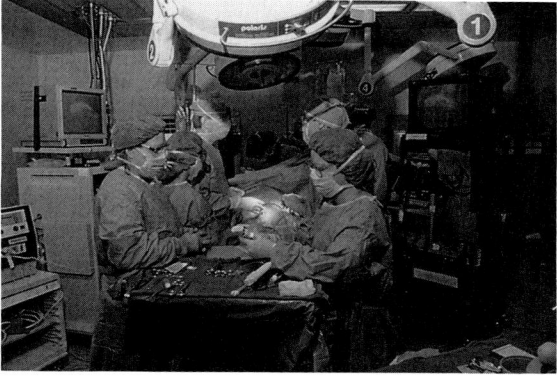

Figure 4-1. Positioning of monitors for laparoscopic surgery to allow optimum viewing.

operating room table. It is important to have backup equipment available since these devices are mandatory for safe and efficient laparoscopic procedures. One important consideration is to properly arrange the many electric cords and cables that are placed in the sterile field. Generally, tubing from the carbon dioxide insufflator, the light cable for the laparoscope, and the grounding cable from the patient to the electrocautery unit can be led directly from the operating table to these units placed behind the operative team. Cables or fibers connecting the electrocautery or laser units, respectively, are best positioned to allow for full mobility in the hands of the operating surgeon.

In addition, operating room tables and Mayo stands should be available to display instrumentation for open procedures, if needed, as well as to contain the specific laparoscopic instrumentation necessary to perform the procedure (Fig. 4-3). Since the patient may be placed in a steep reverse Trendelenburg position, especially for laparoscopic biliary tract procedures, it is appropriate to apply compression balloons or to wrap the patient's legs to avoid venous stasis. If pneumatic compression balloons are used, the electrical pumping device for these should be placed at the foot of the table and out of the way of the operating team and instrument tables. When the patient is positioned on the table in a supine position, it is important to place the foot board to meet the patient's feet at a right angle and to ensure that the foot of the patient is not everted or inverted when placed in a steep reverse Trendelenburg position. This will avoid potential neurologic injury or pressure injury during a lengthy procedure.

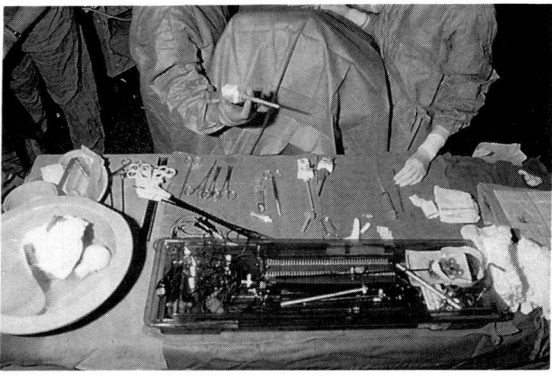

Figure 4-3. Laparoscopic instruments placed on a suitable table adjacent to the scrub nurse.

LAPAROSCOPIC CHOLECYSTECTOMY

The operating room configuration and placement of instrumentation for laparoscopic cholecystectomy depend upon the choice of patient position. In the United States, laparoscopic cholecystectomy is usually performed with the patient in a full supine position.[1] The surgeon generally stands to the left side of the patient with the assistant on the patient's right side (Fig. 4-4). Two television monitors are used and positioned at the head of the table to allow the surgeon's first assistant and camera operator to have an unencumbered view at all times. It is important to place these monitors at a height that allows clear vision, and this may require movement of anesthesia machines as well as rotation of the operating room table into a different floor position, depending on the layout of the room. As in standard open abdominal procedures, the scrub nurse will generally stand opposite the surgeon and to the right side of the first assistant. This will also allow the nurse to have full access not only to instruments needed for the laparoscopic procedure, but also for the instruments that have been prepared for open cholecystectomy if needed. This equipment should be displayed on a large back table and available for use at all times.

If the lithotomy position is chosen for biliary tract intervention, monitors should be similarly placed at the head of the table, but the surgeon is generally stationed between the patient's legs, which are positioned in stirrups. The assistant will continue to be on the patient's right side and the camera operator along the left side of the operating table. This configuration is used primarily in European countries,[2] but may become more common as additional laparoscopic procedures are introduced.

LAPAROSCOPIC APPENDECTOMY

Although laparoscopic appendectomy was described approximately 10 years ago by Semm in Germany,[3] the surgeon embarking on minimally invasive surgery is generally more familiar with laparoscopic biliary tract procedures rather than appendiceal resection. The configuration of the operating table as well as the instrument tables is generally the same as that for laparoscopic biliary tract procedures. The major difference is in the positioning of the operating team as well as

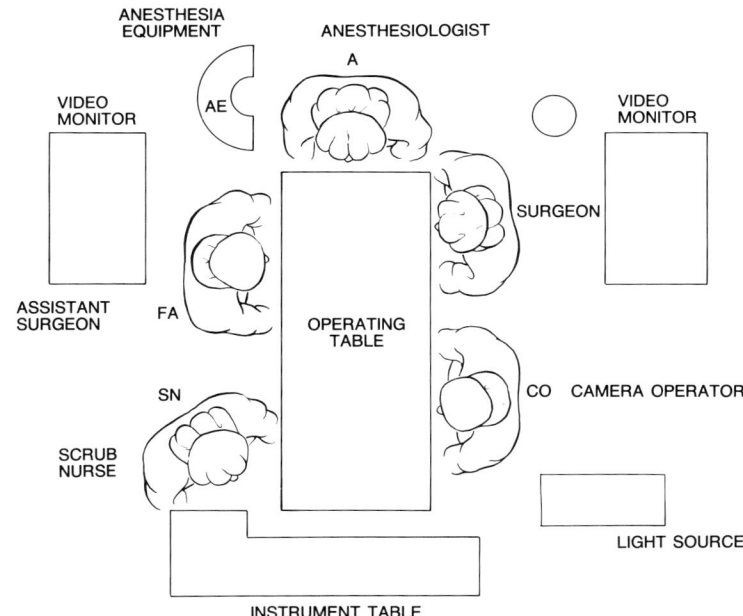

Figure 4-4. Diagram showing position of operating team and equipment for laparoscopic cholecystectomy.

the monitors. The surgeon will generally stand on the patient's left side and requires a monitor to be positioned near the foot of the bed for best viewing[4] (Fig. 4-5). The table is positioned in the Trendelenburg position for laparoscopic appendectomy to help mobilize the small bowel from the pelvis during the procedure. The table will also be angled into a left lateral position to allow free access to the region of the cecum and appendix. As noted previously for biliary tract procedures, the European approach involves placing the patient into the lithotomy position. The scrub nurse is positioned on the surgeon's left, and the assistant stands across from the surgeon on the opposite side of the operating table. If one monitor is used, it can generally be placed at the foot of the table between the patient's legs or positioned across from the operating surgeon, but within view of other

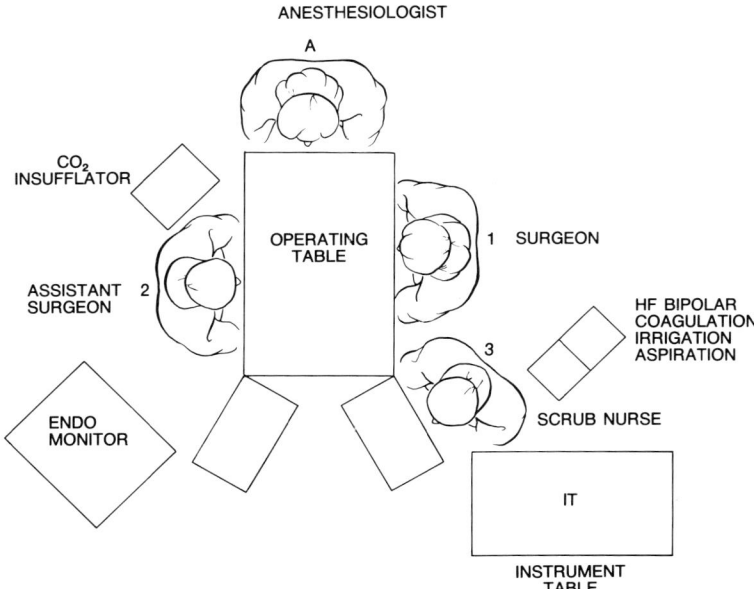

Figure 4-5. Positions for operating team and instruments for laparoscopic appendectomy.

members of the team. The insufflator for carbon dioxide may be placed near the head of the table, and the electrocautery or laser unit may be placed opposite the insufflator and out of the way of the operating team.

LAPAROSCOPIC HERNIORRHAPHY

For laparoscopic herniorrhaphy the patient generally will be placed in the supine position.[5] Standard equipment for a laparoscopic approach is used, and placement of the insufflator, electrocautery or laser unit, and instrument tables will be similar to that described earlier for laparoscopic cholecystectomy. The monitors should be placed near the foot of the operating table because the surgeon and assistant will be facing the pelvic region. Since several different techniques for hernia repair have been advocated, positioning of the surgeon and operating team will be dictated by the innovations that develop in this operative approach and the surgeon's preference.

LAPAROSCOPIC SMALL BOWEL RESECTION

The positioning of the patient and video monitors for both small bowel and large bowel resection will be dictated by the specific portions of bowel resected and the methods used for removal of resected bowel from the abdominal cavity. Placement of the patient in the supine position will be satisfactory for all procedures involving the small intestine and the configuration of the monitors and operative equipment will generally correspond to that used in biliary tract procedures.

LAPAROSCOPIC COLON RESECTION

Techniques for performing laparoscopic colon resections remain in a period of evolution. In general, the surgeon should approach these procedures in a manner similar to the way these operations are performed using traditional open techniques. If the sigmoid colon is normally mobilized from the left side of the patient during open procedures, the same should be done during laparoscopic procedures. The monitors and other equipment are then distributed around the patient based on these position preferences of the surgeon. Performance of major intestinal resection using laparoscopic techniques will continue to dictate that appropriate instruments be available throughout the procedure to allow the surgeon to convert to an open celiotomy when necessary.

Exposure during colonic resections is principally achieved by changes of position of the patient. The cecum, sigmoid colon, and rectum are exposed by dropping the patient into deep Trendelenburg position. The transverse colon and flexures become visible when the patient is placed in the reverse Trendelenburg position. Rotation up of the right or left side of the patient displays the right and left gutters, respectively.

In the performance of laparoscopic resections of the left colon and rectum, the patient is placed in lithotomy position[6] (Fig. 4-6). This allows access to the perineum for several important tasks. (1) In operations for neoplastic disease, the lesion is generally not visible through the laparoscope but is located by passing a rigid proctosigmoidoscope or flexible endoscope through the anus and advancing it up to the distal edge of the lesion. The light of the endoscope becomes visible through the laparoscope when the light intensity of the laparoscope is turned down. The lesion as well as the distal point of resection is then marked by the laparoscopic surgeon with sutures or clips. (2) The lithotomy position allows removal of the specimen transanally. (3) In this position, an end-to-end anastomosis can be constructed with a circular stapling device introduced through the anus. (4) In women, exposure of the distal rectum is improved by retraction of the uterus with a uterine elevator, which is inserted through the vagina. The primary monitor is positioned between the legs of the patient. A second monitor is put near the left arm or shoulder of the patient. The second monitor is useful for mobilization of the descending colon and splenic flexure. The endoscopy light source and monitor are placed by the knee of one of the patient's legs. This permits observation of the luminal image through the endoscope by both the endoscopist and laparoscopic surgeon.

Distribution of equipment for laparoscopic resections of the right colon is similar to that for laparoscopic cholecystectomy. The primary monitor is put near the right shoulder of the patient. A secondary monitor placed near the left shoulder may be helpful when an assistant is on the right side of the patient. The patient can be placed in a supine position

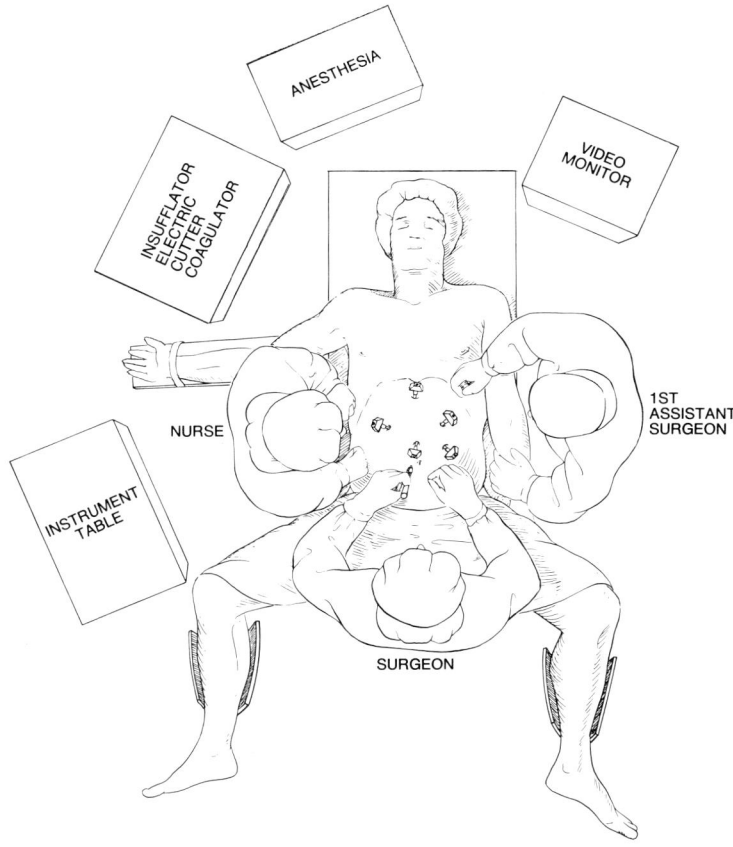

Figure 4-6. Positions for operating team and instruments for laparoscopic resections of the left colon and rectum.

if the location of the lesion is known for certain. Otherwise the patient is placed in lithotomy position so that the lesion can be localized by intraoperative colonoscopy. In addition, some surgeons prefer to stand between the legs of the patient during mobilization of the right colon.

LAPAROSCOPIC VAGOTOMY AND ANTIREFLUX PROCEDURES

The management of peptic ulcer disease laparoscopically, using posterior truncal vagotomy and anterior seromyotomy, continues to open vistas for future management of this entity using minimally invasive procedures. Reports by Mouiel and Katkhouda[7] describe placing the patient in the lithotomy position with the legs spread apart. The operating surgeon stands between the patient's legs with the first and second assistant on the patient's left and right, respectively.[6] The videoendoscopic system, including irrigation and suction, is placed on the patient's left. A second monitor in addition to electrocautery or laser is placed on the right. The operating surgeon may stand between the patient's legs or on the left side of the patient, which is the current position for laparoscopic cholecystectomy. If either of these positions is used, monitors should be placed near the head of the operating table and again elevated to a position that is convenient for all members of the surgical team. Instrumentation for open celiotomy must be available and placed on a back table convenient to the scrub nurse. In addition to vagotomy, laparoscopic approaches for esophageal reflux are possible and may convert traditional open procedures to those that are performed laparoscopically.

Dallemagne and colleagues in Belgium[8] reported laparoscopic Nissen fundoplication using a lithotomy position for facilitation of the procedure. The surgeon is positioned between the patient's legs with the assistants on the right and left sides of the operating table. The reverse Trendelenburg position is used, which allows the abdominal viscera to fall away from the upper abdominal region. This positioning requires the video monitor to be stationed at the head of the operating table.

The scrub nurse may be positioned to the right side of the patient with the instrument table in easy reach. If the lithotomy position is chosen for laparoscopic surgical procedures such as laparoscopic Nissen fundoplication or vagotomy, the patient's feet and lower calves must be positioned properly in the leg supports. These supports are preferable to the more limited "candy cane" stirrups that are at times used for gynecologic procedures. Absolute care and attention must be given to patient positioning for these procedures to assure that no pressure injuries or neurologic deficits occur during a potentially long operative procedure.

OPERATIVE THORACOSCOPY

For traditional intrapleural procedures that use a formal thoracotomy, thoracoscopic approaches may be possible. These include subtotal or total lobar resections of lung or truncal vagotomy.[9] Diagnostic thoracoscopy has been performed for many years and usually requires general anesthesia and a formal operating room environment.

Operating room and equipment needs for thoracoscopic surgery will generally be similar to those required for abdominal operations. The major difference will be in patient position, because a full right or left lateral decubitus position as used for traditional thoracotomy is required. It is imperative that appropriate padding be placed under areas of potential pressure and that the patient be carefully secured to the operating table. An insufflator will not be necessary since establishment of a pneumothorax and use of a double lumen endotracheal tube will assure adequate exposure of the lung, pleura, or mediastinum on the operative side.

The surgeon will usually be positioned facing the patient's back as is traditional in open thoracotomy. Monitors should be placed at the head of the operating table and across from the operating surgeon. A second monitor for the assistant should be available and placed also at the patient's head. The scrub nurse should be positioned opposite the surgeon and should have instruments available for thoracotomy if this becomes necessary.

DIAGNOSTIC AND STAGING LAPAROSCOPY

Traditionally, laparoscopy or peritoneoscopy was advocated for intra-abdominal inspection and biopsy to resolve diagnostic dilemmas in patients with abdominal pain, masses, or unexplained ascites. In response to the current interest in therapeutic laparoscopy, diagnostic evaluations, especially for biopsy of liver or lymph nodes, have again become popular, especially in preoperative staging of malignancy.[10] Operating room and instrument needs are identical to those described for therapeutic maneuvers such as cholecystectomy.

Since diagnostic laparoscopy may be directed by previously performed imaging studies, adequate viewing areas should be available in the operating room to facilitate the display and utilization of these studies. X-ray view boxes should not be hidden behind doors or the anesthesia equipment.

Although diagnostic laparoscopy may be performed in an outpatient setting using local or sedation anesthesia, a suitable operating room must be used to ensure the safety of the procedure and to provide a facility for conversion to open techniques, if this becomes necessary. Standard insufflators and electrocautery or laser techniques must be available to control bleeding and to assist in lymph node dissection if this is planned.

Conclusion

As new procedures and techniques for laparoscopic surgery become popular, additional equipment needs and variations in operating room configuration will be necessary. It is anticipated that the popularity of minimally invasive surgical procedures will dictate the development and construction of dedicated facilities in existing operating room suites or construction of free-standing units for laparoscopic surgery. It is important for surgeons to remain involved in the planning of these facilities and to take a leadership role in working with health care administrators in the design and construction of efficient operating environments.

REFERENCES

1. Berci G, Sackier J. Laparoscopic cholecystectomy. Prob Gen Surg 1991; 8:284–319.
2. Dubois F, Icard P, Berthelot G, Levard H. Coeliscopic cholecystectomy: Preliminary report of 36 cases. Ann Surg 1991; 211:60–62.
3. Semm K. Die endoskopische appendektomie. Gynäkolog Prax 1983; 7:26.
4. Pier A, Gotz F, Bacher C. Laparoscopic appendec-

tomy in 625 cases: From innovation to routine. Surg Laparosc Endosc 1991; 1:8–13.
5. Corbitt JD. Laparoscopic herniorrhaphy. Surg Laparosc Endosc 1991; 1:23–25.
6. Fowler D, White S. Laparoscopy-assisted sigmoid resection. Surg Laparosc Endosc 1991; 1:183–188.
7. Mouiel J, Katkhouda N. Laparoscopic vagotomy in the treatment of chronic duodenal ulcer disease. Prob Gen Surg 1991; 8:358–365.
8. Dallemagne B, Weerts JM, Jehaes C, et al. Laparoscopic Nissen fundoplication: Preliminary report. Surg Laparosc Endosc 1991; 1:138–143.
9. Dubois F. Laparoscopic vagotomies. Prob Gen Surg 1991; 8:348–357.
10. Warshaw AL, Gu Z-Y. Laparoscopy for preoperative staging of malignant tumors of the foregut. Prob Gen Surg 1990; 7:65–74.

Chapter 5
Anesthesia

Anthony J. Cunningham

The advent of laparoscopic cholecystectomy was the catalyst that aroused the interest of general surgeons worldwide in laparoscopy and closed abdominal surgery.

The historical milestones in the evolution of laparoscopic surgery have been detailed by Gastin et al.[1] in a recent comprehensive review. Laparoscopy and laparoscopic surgery are not new; as far back as 1910, Jacobeus in Stockholm discussed the application of endoscopy and pneumoperitoneum to inspect the pleura and peritoneum. For the most part, gynecologists developed the instrumentation, operative principles, and techniques of laparoscopic surgery. The lack of attention given by general surgeons to laparoscopy until recent times may be attributed to its perceived role as a diagnostic rather than a therapeutic tool. However, the frontiers and horizons of laparoscopic surgery may not be limited to cholecystectomy but may extend to appendendectomy, inguinal hernia repair, peptic ulcer disease, laparoscopic nephrectomy, and splenectomy.[2-4]

The publication by Steptoe[5] in 1967 of the widely adopted technique of laparoscopy in gynecologic practice was followed by several reviews outlining the anesthetic considerations for these procedures.[6,7] The creation of a pneumoperitoneum by insufflation of the abdominal cavity with carbon dioxide (CO_2) and the assumption of the lithotomy position with a steep head-down (Trendelenburg) position had several potential hemodynamic and respiratory consequences. However, these gynecologic procedures were generally of short duration and were performed on young, otherwise healthy, female patients. Changes in hemodynamic and respiratory function associated with intraperitoneal CO_2 insufflation during these short procedures were extensively investigated and found to be relatively insignificant.

New intra-abdominal laparoscopic surgical techniques have been developed, performed, and advocated for older patients who may have coexisting cardiac and/or pulmonary disease.[8] These general surgical laparoscopic procedures involve a position change for the patient from Trendelenburg to reverse Trendelenburg and longer periods of intraperitoneal CO_2 insufflation compared with gynecologic procedures.

This chapter will incorporate data on the physiologic consequences of pneumoperitoneum creation derived from early studies involving gynecologic procedures and will focus on the unique anesthetic considerations involved in laparoscopic cholecystectomy.

LAPAROSCOPIC CHOLECYSTECTOMY—COMPARISON WITH TRADITIONAL OPEN CHOLECYSTECTOMY

There are approximately 500,000 cholecystectomies performed annually in the United States.[9] For decades, these procedures were performed through a right upper quadrant incision, which proved to be a safe and efficient means of managing cholelithiasis. Although the overall reported mortality for open cholecystectomy in some series was less than 0.1 per cent, surgery for complications of gallstones in the elderly may be associated with mortality of up to 10 per cent.[10] Most patients experience significant postoperative impairment of pulmonary function, pain, discomfort, ileus, and prolonged convalescence.

The major source of complications in the open cholecystectomy procedure is the abdominal incision. Medicare data summarized by the Office of Research and Demonstrations, Health Care Financing Administration, on 94,056 patients who underwent open cholecystectomy in 1986 classified adverse complications during the index stay into five groups: death, complications related to the bile duct, other gastrointestinal complications related to surgery, general surgical complications, and "other" events.[11] The overall adverse event rate was 22.4 per cent and the in-hospital mortality rate was 1.95 per cent. Infectious complications related to surgery were reported in 11.8 per cent of cases and general surgical complications in 5.4 per cent. Wound dehiscence was another potential complication of the open procedure (Table 5-1).

Upper abdominal procedures, including open cholecystectomy, produce significant impairment of pulmonary mechanics, ventilation, and defense mechanisms independent of the effects of general anesthesia. The adverse effects of upper abdominal procedures on pulmonary function were outlined in two comprehensive reviews.[12,13] Vital capacity, which is critical for effective coughing, is reduced in the hours after surgery by as much as 40 to 50 per cent of preoperative values.

Table 5-1. Open Cholecystectomy 1986–The Gold Standard

Adverse Event Rate 22.4%
  Mortality
  Bile duct injuries
  Gastrointestinal injuries
  General surgical complications
  Wound dehiscence
  Wound infection
  Pulmonary infections

Data from 94,056 patients, Medicare Office of Research and Demonstrations, Health and Financing Administration.

Gradual restoration of vital capacity over the next 5 to 7 days is usual.

Functional residual capacity, the lung volume at which a balance occurs between the natural tendency of the lung to retract and the rib cage to expand, is reduced soon after upper abdominal surgery to 70 to 80 per cent of preoperative values. Gradual restoration of lung function begins on the second or third postoperative day. Full recovery takes a few days longer, even after resumption of gastrointestinal function.

The reductions in functional residual capacity and vital capacity after upper abdominal surgery are principally caused by incisional pain and reflex diaphragmatic dysfunction.[14] Following upper abdominal surgery, breathing is restricted with rapid shallow breaths. Two particular aspects of pulmonary defense mechanisms, coughing and removal of particulate matter, are adversely affected by these changes in breathing patterns. Other factors include the absence of spontaneous sighs, impaired mucociliary activity, and mechanical disruption of the abdomen. Local irritation, surgical influences (packs or retractors), and bowel distention are potent inhibitors of diaphragmatic function and contribute to the reduction in FRC and the 10 to 20 per cent incidence of atelectasis reported with open cholecystectomy.[15]

The past decade witnessed the evolution of alternative methods for the management of cholelithiasis, including gallstone dissolution therapy,[16] endoscopic and percutaneous techniques of stone extraction,[17] biliary lithotripsy,[18] and the technique of gallstone removal via "minilaparotomy."[19] Drug therapy for gallstones may be appropriate for only a fraction of patients, and the most optimistic data indicate that in only 20 to 40 per cent of carefully selected patients is stone dissolution seen within 2 years.[15] Likewise, in a German study, only 19 per cent of 5824 patients were considered eligible for lithotripsy, and dissolution was incomplete in most patients with more than one stone.[20] Thus, most of these new techniques were not universally adopted because their application was limited by stone content, location, size, and number. In addition, these techniques left intact a gallbladder already known to harbor lithogenic bile. The recent advent of a minimally invasive laparoscopic technique which, in most cases, safely removes the diseased gallbladder as well as its contained stones, soon became so widely accepted and adopted that a prospective randomized control trial of laparoscopic cholecystectomy became almost impossible to undertake because of patient demand and ethical considerations.[21]

Laparoscopic cholecystectomy has rapidly emerged as a popular alternative to traditional laparotomy and cholecystectomy in the management of cholelithiasis.[22] The technique was first described in France by Phillipe Mouret in 1988 (personal communication), was first reported in the literature by Perissat et al.,[23] and was refined and popularized in the United States by Reddick and Olsen.[24] Laparoscopic cholecystectomy retains the benefit of completely removing the gallbladder with the advantages of shorter hospital stay, more rapid return to normal activities, less pain associated with the small, limited incisions, and less postoperative ileus compared to the open laparotomy technique[25-27] (Table 5-2).

The major benefits claimed for laparoscopic cholecystectomy are thought to result from elimination of the abdominal incision. Holohan[15] claimed that the overall adverse event rate of 22.4 per cent with open cholecystectomy was more than 6 times the rate of complications calculated from summary data of laparoscopic cholecystectomy compiled from 11 studies involving 3225 patients.[15] The most comprehensive assessment to date of laparoscopic cholecystectomy has been undertaken by Meyers et al.[28] under the auspices of The Southern Surgeons Club in a prospective study of 1518 patients distributed equally between academic and community hospitals. The 5.1 per cent complication rate included seven patients with bile duct injuries. The most common complication was superficial infection at the site of insertion of the umbilical trocar. The judgment of experienced surgeons in this study on the risk/benefit ratio of laparoscopic compared with open cholecystectomy was highlighted by the fact that during the study period, the 59 participating surgeons performed only 12 per cent of cholecystectomies by the traditional open technique.

There never have been, and there may never be, any prospective randomized studies directly comparing laparoscopic with open cholecystectomy. Frazee et al.,[29] in a prospective nonrandomized study of 16 patients undergoing open cholecystectomy and 20 patients undergoing laparoscopic cholecystectomy, reported postoperative forced vital capacity (FVC) measured 52 per cent, forced expiratory volume in 1 second (FEV_1) 53 per cent, and forced expiratory flow (FEF) 53 per cent of baseline values for open cholecystectomies compared with FVC, FEV_1 and FEF of 73, 72, and 81 per cent, respectively, for laparoscopic cholecystectomy. The location and type of abdominal incision have been shown repeatedly to influence the extent of postoperative pulmonary impairment.[30] Frazee et al.[29] claimed that the 20 to 25 per cent better FEV_1, FVC, and FEF values in patients undergoing laparoscopic cholecystectomy were a result of minimal muscle disruption and less postoperative pain. This improvement in pulmonary function may translate into a lower incidence of respiratory complications. The differences in pulmonary function were present despite longer anesthetic and operating times in the laparoscopic group.

SPECIAL CONSIDERATIONS

Surgical Technique

The operative technique involves the intraperitoneal insufflation of carbon dioxide through a Veress needle inserted into a small infraumbilical incision, with the patient in a 15- to 20-degree Trendelenburg position.[15] The electronic variable flow insufflator terminates flow when a preset intra-abdominal pressure of 12 to 15 mm Hg has been reached. A cannula is inserted in place of the needle to provide and maintain insufflation adequate for surgery. A video laparoscope is inserted through the cannula and the operative field is visualized by high resolution television camera-monitor systems.

The diseased gallbladder is removed by means of instruments introduced through cannulas via three additional small (5 to 11 mm) skin incisions. These cannulas or tro-

Table 5-2. Laparoscopic Cholecystectomy —Comparison with Traditional Open Cholecystectomy

Characteristics
    Eliminates the abdominal incision
    Preserves diaphragmatic function
Potential benefits
    Reduced adverse events
    Pulmonary function preserved
    Less postoperative ileus
    Early ambulation
    Economic
        Shorter hospital stay
        Earlier return to work and normal activities

cars are inserted under direct vision for placement and control of the instruments required to dissect the gallbladder. The sites of trocar/cannula insertion may vary, but they usually include one to the right of the midline to avoid the falciform ligament and two right upper quadrant sites.

The patient's position is then changed to steep reverse Trendelenburg, with left lateral tilt, to facilitate retraction of the gallbladder fundus and to minimize the diaphragmatic dysfunction associated with the induced pneumoperitoneum. The cystic duct and cystic artery are identified and clamped. Laser dissection was commonly used initially to remove the gallbladder from the hepatic bed but, with experience and familiarity with laparoscopic techniques, electrocautery became the norm.[28] The video laparoscope is removed to an upper midline abdominal position to allow visualization of gallbladder removal through the periumbilical cannula by means of claw forceps or extractor.

Indications/Contraindications

Indications for laparoscopic cholecystectomy are the same as for the open procedure, i.e., symptomatic cholelithiasis and chronic cholecystitis. Early contraindications to the laparoscopic technique in the surgical literature included the presence of large stones, evidence of acute inflammation, common bile duct stones, pregnancy, or a history of previous abdominal surgery.[31] Morbid obesity and the possibility of adhesions associated with previous intra-abdominal surgery were considered relative contraindications (Table 5-3).

The indications for the laparoscopic technique have become more liberal recently after case reports confirmed its efficacy and safety in patients with acute cholecystitis[32] and during pregnancy.[33] The technique has rapidly emerged as a cost-effective treatment for symptomatic gallbladder disease with low morbidity. Laparoscopic cholecystectomy has become the routine method of cholecystectomy, not only in teaching centers, but also in community hospitals where most cholecystectomies take place.[34] Dubois et al.[8] claim that laparoscopic surgery causes minimum trauma and stress and is the procedure of choice for high operative risk patients, especially those with cardiac and respiratory disease. The low morbidity rate associated with laparoscopic surgery in some patients older than 80 years has been advanced as a claim that it is the technique of choice for the elderly. Phillips et al.[35] suggested that common bile duct injury, the most serious surgical complication, could be reduced by cholangiography.

The presence of preexisting lung disease has not been considered a relative contraindication to laparoscopic cholecystectomy. Recent case reports[36] and studies,[37] documenting profound intraoperative hypoxemia and respiratory acidosis in patients with preexisting chronic obstructive and restrictive lung disease, suggest that preoperative arterial blood gas analysis and pulmonary function tests are appropriate in patients with cardiopulmonary disease undergoing laparoscopic cholecystectomy. In this era of cost containment, these patients may not be suitable for admission on the morning of surgery if such preoperative investigations are not available at the preoperative screening clinic. Restrictive or obstructive lung disease may be relative contraindications to a laparoscopic cholecystectomy technique. Conversion to open cholecystectomy may be indicated if problems of high airway pressures, hypercarbia, or refractory hypoxemia are encountered during anesthesia.

Conversion to Open Cholecystectomy

The evolving role of laparoscopic cholecystectomy in the management of gallbladder disease has been the subject of extensive recent editorial comment.[38-40] Continuing controversies regarding the technique include the role of preoperative cholangiography, the strategy for dealing with choledocholithiasis, the management of the acutely inflamed gallbladder, and the arguments for and against the use of lasers in the cystic duct dissection. Despite the widespread acceptance of the

Table 5-3. Indications and Contraindications for Laparoscopic Cholecystectomy

Established indications
  Cholelithiasis
  Chronic Cholecystitis
Controversial indications/contraindications
  Acute cholecystitis
  Pregnancy
  Previous abdominal surgery
  Morbid obesity
  Cardiorespiratory disease

Table 5-4. Reported Indications for Conversion from Laparoscopic to Open Cholecystectomy

Authors	Study Period	Study Design	Location	Institution	Patients	Conversion to Open Cholecystectomy
Spangenberger et al. (1990)[41]	1989–90	Retrospective	Cologne, Germany	Teaching	100	1 (1%) 1 Bile duct leak
Peters et al. (1991)[42]	1989–90	Prospective	Columbus, Ohio	Community	100	4 (4%) 1 CBD Injury 1 uncertain anatomy 2 acute inflammation
Nathanson et al. (1991)[43]	?	Retrospective	Dundee, Scotland	Teaching	61	1 (2%) 1 Dilated CBD with stones
Graves et al. (1991)[44]	1989–90	Retrospective	Nashville, Tennessee	Community	304	21 (6.9%) 6 acute cholecystitis 6 chronic scarring 2 Rule Out CBD injury 1 CBD injury 1 obesity 1 benign liver tumor 1 small intestine injury
Cuschieri et al. (1991)[45]	1989–90	Retrospective	European Multi-center	Mixed Teaching Community	1236	45 (3.6) 33 technical difficulties 8 uncontrolled bleeding 2 CBD injury 1 rupture empyema 1 instrument failure

CBD, common bile duct.
Cunningham AJ, Schlanger M. Intraoperative hypoxemia complicating laparoscopic cholecystectomy in a patient with sickle hemoglobinopathy. Anesth Analg 1992; 75:838–843.

technique, early series suggest that some complications are more commonly associated with laparoscopic cholecystectomy compared to traditional open cholecystectomy.

Table 5-4 details the indications for conversion from laparoscopic to open cholecystectomy in five recent published series.[41-45] The conversion rates varied from 1.0 to 6.9 per cent. Experience from several institutions suggests that the incidence of common bile duct injuries may be higher with this procedure, and conversion to open cholecystectomy was usually caused by difficulty in identifying and mobilizing the cystic duct, suspected or confirmed common bile duct injury, uncontrolled bleeding from the cystic artery, acute inflammatory changes, and stones present in the common bile duct.

The absence of data concerning anesthesia-related complications of laparoscopic cholecystectomy in the anesthesia literature is conspicuous apart from isolated case reports and letters describing the uneventful anesthetic management of such cases.[46-48] Greville et al.[49] reported a case of nonfatal intraoperative pulmonary air embolism following inadvertent puncture of the liver by the sapphire tip of the neodymium-yttrium-garnet laser, which was cooled by air flowing from ports proximal to the tip. We reported the first case of profound and sustained intraoperative hypoxemia associated with high peak airway pressures, which necessitated the conversion from laparoscopic to traditional open cholecystectomy.[36]

COMPLICATIONS OF LAPAROSCOPIC CHOLECYSTECTOMY

Many data have been accumulated regarding the complications of laparoscopy. The complications unique to laparoscopic cholecystectomy were recently reviewed by Ponsky[50] (Table 5-5).

Table 5-5. Complications of and Adverse Physiologic Changes with Laparoscopic Cholecystectomy

Trocar insertion
Trendelenburg position
Pneumoperitoneum creation
Exogenous CO_2
Reverse Trendelenburg and Lateral Tilt

Table 5-6. Laparoscopic Cholecystectomy Trocar Insertion

Bleeding
  Abdominal wall vessels
  Intra-abdominal vessels
    Aorta
    Iliac arteries
    Inferior vena cava
  Hepatic/splenic tears
Gastrointestinal trauma
  Perforation
  Avulsion of adhesions
  Omental disruption
Herniation

Trocar Insertion

Injuries have been reported to occur as the trocar is blindly introduced prior to insertion of the laparoscope. Such injuries have included bleeding from abdominal wall vessels, gastrointestinal tract perforations, hepatic and splenic tears, major vascular trauma, avulsion of adhesions, omental disruption, and hernia at the trocar insertion site (Table 5-6).

The most frequent complications are associated with creation of the initial pneumoperitoneum. These include pneumomentum, subcutaneous emphysema, mediastinal emphysema, pneumothorax, hypoxemia, hypotension, cardiovascular collapse, carbon dioxide embolism, and cardiac dysrhythmias. Complications associated with the cholecystectomy, i.e., hemorrhage, bile duct injury, common bile duct stones, perihepatic collections, and infection, are similar to those that may occur with traditional open cholecystectomy, although the frequency may differ. Perforation of the gallbladder itself, although not usually significant during the performance of open cholecystectomy, may preclude successful completion of the laparoscopic approach.

Laparoscopy itself introduces four potential major physiologic alterations in the anesthetized patient—the initial Trendelenburg position, creation of the pneumoperitoneum, introduction of exogenous CO_2, and the reverse Trendelenburg position.

Trendelenburg Position

In the 1860s, Friedrich Trendelenburg, a German urologic surgeon, popularized the high pelvic posture that still bears his name.[51]

In gynecologic and laparoscopic cholecystectomy procedures, the patient is normally placed in a 10- to 20-degree Trendelenburg position to keep small bowel and colon out of the pelvis and to minimize complications associated with blind trocar insertion. The physiologic effects of the head-down Trendelenburg position in normal and hypovolemic patients have been recently reviewed by Wilcox and Vandam[52] and are highlighted in Table 5-7.

Cardiovascular Effects

Conventional wisdom suggests that postures with the head lowered are more favorable to the circulation; postures with the head raised are more favorable to respiration.[53] The cardiovascular changes associated with the Trendelenburg position may be influenced by the extent of the head-down tilt, the patient's age, intravascular volume status, associated cardiac disease, anesthetic drugs, and ventilation techniques. Bivins et al.,[54] in a noninvasive study of healthy normovolemic subjects placed in a 15-degree headdown position, showed only a 1.8 per cent (median) central displacement of blood volume. This small volume shift was not enough to cause significant hemodynamic changes. Pricolo et al.,[55] in a recent study of 13 normotensive patients in a 10-degree head-down position, reported a small but significant (10 per cent) increase in cardiac index, without elevation of central venous pressure, pulmonary capillary wedge pressure, heart rate, or systemic vascular resistance. In contrast, central venous pressure and pulmonary capillary wedge pressure significantly increased, and cardiac index decreased with head-down positioning of normotensive patients with coronary artery disease. In healthy normotensive patients, the baroreceptor reflex may be responsible for the stable cardiovascular status with the head-down position. However, in patients with coronary artery disease, the autotransfusion associated with steep head-dependent positioning may produce cerebral congestion and potentially harmful baroreceptor reflex changes.

RESPIRATORY EFFECTS

Pulmonary function changes associated with the head-down position will depend on the patient's age and preoperative lung function, the degree of head-down tilt, body size, anesthetic agents, and ventilatory techniques. The Trendelenburg position has been reported to reduce vital capacity because of the increased weight of the abdominal viscera on the diaphragm.[56] These changes may be more marked in obese, elderly, or debilitated patients and may be enhanced by placement of surgical packs and retractors in the upper abdomen. Studies of healthy anesthetized spontaneously ventilating volunteers in a 20-degree head-down tilt showed vital capacities 86 per cent of values in the sitting position.[57] A change to a 35-degree head-down tilt showed no changes in minute volume or pH, although the work of breathing was increased. At a 45-degree head-down position, decreased functional residual capacity, total lung volume, and pulmonary compliance were demonstrated. Scott and Slawson,[58] in a study of 26 healthy anesthetized spontaneously ventilating volunteers in a 30-degree head-down position for 1 hour, reported that the observed changes in lung volumes did not result in major changes in gas exchange. A compensatory increase in respiratory rate and occasional deep sighs maintained adequate arterial oxygenation and CO_2 excretion.

ENDOBRONCHIAL INTUBATION

The potential for inadvertent right mainstem bronchus intubation with resultant hypoxemia associated with Trendelenburg posi-

Table 5-7. Physiological Effects of the Trendelenburg Position in Laparoscopic Cholecystectomy

Cardiovascular changes
  Patient
    Age
    Tilt
    Intravascular volume
    Associated disease
    Anesthetic agents
    Ventilatory techniques
  Cardiac output
  Preload: cardiac filling pressure
  Contractility: neural/humeral
  Afterload
Respiratory changes
  Lung volumes
  Minute ventilation
  Work of breathing
Mainstem bronchus intubation

tioning was highlighted by Wilcox and Vandam.[52] The endotracheal tube, firmly secured at its proximal end, does not always move cephalad with the trachea as the diaphragm presses upwards and displaces the lung and carina.[59]

Pneumoperitoneum Creation

Pneumoperitoneum creation involves the intraperitoneal insufflation of CO_2 through a Veress needle with the patient in 15- to 20-degree Trendelenburg position. The potential difficulties that may be encountered with pneumoperitoneum creation are outlined in Table 5-8.

TECHNICAL DIFFICULTIES

Technical difficulties may be encountered with pneumoperitoneum creation. Lew et al.[60] reported extensive surgical emphysema that involved the neck, chest, and abdomen and extended down to the groin. The mechanism postulated in this case report was subcutaneous insufflation of CO_2 from a poorly stabilized Veress insufflation needle.

CARDIOVASCULAR EFFECTS

In the early days of gynecologic laparoscopy, intra-abdominal pressures (IAP) up to 40 mm Hg were created. Laparoscopic cholecystectomy technology includes an electronic variable flow insufflator, which terminates flow when a preset IAP of 12 to 15 mm Hg has been reached. The volume of gas insufflated may exceed 50 liters because intra-abdominal gas may quickly escape through the multiple trocar/cannula puncture sites.

The cardiovascular and respiratory changes associated with pneumoperitoneum creation have been studied extensively in experimental and clinical investigations. The extent of these changes will depend on the IAP attained, the volume of CO_2 absorbed, intravascular volume, ventilatory technique, surgical conditions, and anesthetic agents.

Marshall et al.[61] reported no significant changes in cardiac output in a series of anesthetized, spontaneously ventilating patients in whom IAPs were in the range of 15 to 20 cm H_2O. Smith et al.[62] studied the cardiovascular effects of stepwise increases of IAP up to a maximum of 25 cm H_2O in anesthetized, mechanically ventilated patients. At 25 cm H_2O IAP, increased airway pressure, intrathoracic pressure (ITP), central venous pressure (CVP), and femoral venous pressure were accompanied by hypertension, tachycardia, and increased end-tidal carbon dioxide tensions. Based on data obtained from a study of the effects of progressive increasing W in horizontal and tilted, anesthetized, mechanically ventilated patients, Kelman et al.[63] claimed that moderate increases of IAP (up to 25 cm H_2O) may be accompanied by an increased effective cardiac filling pressure (CVP − ITP) and therefore (by Starling's law) an increased cardiac output. When IAP was further raised to 40 cm H_2O, tachycardia, hypotension, and reduced CVP and cardiac output were observed. These changes were most marked in the horizontal compared with the head-down tilt position. The authors speculated that increased IAP has two opposite effects on the cardiovascular system: it forces blood out of the abdominal organs and inferior vena cava into the central venous reservoir; at the same time it dams blood back in the legs and thus tends to decrease the central blood volume.

The relative roles of the factors that contribute to cardiac output changes may be difficult to separate, but the increased cardiac output at lower IAP may result from increased cardiac filling pressures, caused partly by mechanical factors and partly by sympathetically mediated constriction of capacitance vessels and a hypercarbia-induced effect on cardiac efferent sympathetic activity.[64] Ivankovich et al.[65] reported a reduction of more than 60 per cent in inferior vena caval blood flow and cardiac output in an experimental dog study when the IAP exceeded 40 mm Hg.

The effects of general anesthetic agents and intravascular volume on hemodynamic func-

Table 5-8. Potential Complications of Pneumoperitoneum Creation in Laparoscopic Cholecystectomy

Technical difficulties
Cardiac output changes
   Preload: cardiac filling pressure
   Contractility: neural/humeral
   Afterload
Respiratory function
   Hypercarbia
   Hypoxemia
Pneumothorax
Regurgitation of gastric contents

tion associated with pneumoperitoneum creation has been investigated. Diamant et al.[66] reported a 35 per cent reduction in inferior vena caval blood flow and cardiac output when intraperitoneal insufflation of nitrogen, nitrous oxide, and CO_2 produced an IAP of 40 mm Hg under basal pentobarbital anesthesia. The addition of 1 minimal alveolar concentration halothane in combination with hypovolemia (15 per cent blood volume loss) depressed the preinduction cardiac output more than the addition of halothane anesthesia alone or induction of hypovolemia alone. Johannsen et al.[67] compared the hemodynamic effects of 2 kPa intra-abdominal pressure and 30-degree Trendelenburg tilt in a prospective study of 16 mechanically ventilated patients randomly selected to receive either halothane anesthesia or balanced anesthesia with pethidine and thiopental. In both groups, similar reductions in cardiac index were accompanied by significant elevations in systemic vascular resistance.

In summary, studies in gynecologic patients have consistently shown only minor hemodynamic changes during laparoscopic procedures with CO_2 insufflation when IAP did not exceed 25 mm Hg. However, these short duration studies were performed in young, relatively healthy, women in the Trendelenburg position. Considering the widespread adoption of laparoscopic cholecystectomy, there is a remarkable paucity of data concerning the hemodynamic and respiratory function changes in normal patients and in those with cardiorespiratory disorders associated with prolonged CO_2-induced pneumoperitoneum in a steep head-up position. This lack of critical experimental and clinical assessment of the physiologic changes associated with laparoscopic cholecystectomy is in marked contrast to the systematic evaluation of diagnostic laparoscopy in the late 1960s and early 1970s. This situation may have arisen because of the fulsome welcome given to laparoscopic cholecystectomy by general surgeons, health care providers, and the medical/lay press. However, recent disquiet has been expressed concerning the seeming uncritical acclaim given to this new procedure.[68]

RESPIRATORY FUNCTION

The limited available data concerning laparoscopic cholecystectomy suggest that the hemodynamic and respiratory function changes may differ from those reported with gynecologic laparoscopic procedures. Liu et al.,[69] in a prospective observational study of 16 otherwise healthy patients (mean age 40.2 ± 3.5 years, operating time 137 ± 13 minutes) noted no significant cardiac output changes, despite an increased mean arterial pressure ($PaCO_2$) and end-tidal CO_2 with CO_2 pneumoperitoneum. Wittgen et al.[37] compared the hemodynamic and ventilatory effects of laparoscopic cholecystectomy in 20 patients with normal cardiopulmonary status [ASA (American Society of Anesthesiologists) physical status I] and 10 patients with documented cardiac and pulmonary disease (ASA II-III). The patients without cardiopulmonary disease had increased end-tidal CO_2 and $PaCO_2$ and decreased pH values following CO_2 insufflation, but the changes were not statistically significant. During CO_2 insufflation, no significant change occurred in minute volume and peak inspiratory pressure. In contrast, significant decreases in arterial pH values and increases in $PaCO_2$ were observed in patients with cardiopulmonary disease following CO_2 insufflation. These patients had significantly increased minute ventilation and peak inspiratory pressures when values before CO_2 insufflation were compared with values obtained after CO_2 insufflation.

Early reports of anesthesia for laparoscopy using halothane emphasized the dangers of hypercarbia if patients were allowed to breathe spontaneously. Seed et al.[70] reported an increased CO_2 output (from 135.4 ± 2.5 to 150.9 ± 6.9 ml/min) after the start of insufflation. This increased CO_2 output was associated with increased end-tidal CO_2 concentrations from 4.7 to 5.4 per cent. Desmond and Gordon[71] observed tachypnea, increased minute ventilation, and respiratory acidosis in a study of 10 patients spontaneously breathing nitrous oxide/oxygen and 0.5 to 1.0 per cent halothane. The authors considered the hypoventilation secondary to the steep Trendelenburg position and the pneumoperitoneum-induced splinting of the diaphragm to be potentially hazardous, especially in combination with halothane.

In addition to the potential for pneumoperitoneum-induced hypoventilation and respiratory acidosis, hypoxemia may also be encountered, especially in the context of preexisting lung disease. The possible factors that might contribute to the development of intraoperative hypoxemia are listed in Table 5-9. Intraoperative hypoxemia may be caused by a reduction in alveolar oxygen tension (PAO_2), an increased alveolar/arterial O_2 ten-

Table 5-9. Intraoperative Hypoxemia during Laparoscopic Cholecystectomy—Differential Diagnosis

Preexisting conditions
   Cardiopulmonary disease
   Morbid obesity
Hypoventilation
   Patient position
   Pneumoperitoneum
   Endotracheal tube obstruction
   Inadequate ventilation: spontaneous/controlled
Intrapulmonary shunting
   Reduced functional residual capacity (pneumoperitoneum-induced)
   Endobronchial intubation
   Pneumothorax
   Emphysema: mediastinum/subcutaneous
   Bowel distention: nitrous oxide-induced
   Pulmonary aspiration of gastric contents
Reduced cardiac output
   Hemorrhage: trochar injury
   Inferior vena caval compression
   Impaired venous return: pneumoperitoneum
   Dysrhythmias: hypercarbia/volatile anesthetic agents
   Myocardial depression: drug-induced/acidosis
   CO_2 venous embolism

sion difference, or a reduction in cardiac output, singly or in combination. A reduction in PAO_2 may be caused by reduced or absent inspired oxygen concentration and decreased alveolar ventilation. Kinking of the endotracheal tube, blockade with secretions, and a herniated or ruptured cuff are potential causes of intraoperative hypoxemia not confined to laparoscopic cholecystectomy. An increased alveolar/arterial O_2 tension difference may also lead to intraoperative hypoxemia. This will be most commonly associated with increased intrapulmonary shunting and decreased mixed venous oxygen tension. Inadvertent endobronchial intubation caused by frequent positional changes from Trendelenburg position to reverse Trendelenburg and left lateral tilt position are potential consequences of the procedure.

A tension pneumothorax has been reported as a complication during laparoscopic cholecystectomy following trocar insertion and intraperitoneal carbon dioxide insufflation.[72] A congenital defect of the diaphragm (patent pleuroperitoneal canal) through which the insufflated gas passes into the thoracic cavity has been suggested as the underlying mechanism.[7] Gastric regurgitation has been reported during gynecologic laparoscopic procedures. Duffy[73] reported gastric regurgitation in 2 of 93 fasting patients undergoing elective gynecologic laparoscopic procedures. During laparoscopic cholecystectomy there are several factors that increase IAP and predispose patients to regurgitation, including the initial steep head-down tilt, insufflation of intraperitoneal gas, and pressure exerted on the abdomen by the surgical team.

A reduction in functional residual capacity relative to closing volume may be associated with the development of intraoperative atelectasis and intrapulmonary shunting. These changes may be associated with general anesthesia because of the cephalad shift of the diaphragm associated with the supine position,[12] the loss of inspiratory muscle tone, the appearance of end-expiratory tone in the abdominal expiratory muscles, changes in intrathoracic blood volume associated with induction of anesthesia,[74] and the influence of muscle relaxants on diaphragmatic exclusion.[75] The reduction in functional residual capacity associated with general anesthesia may be compounded by the CO_2-induced pneumoperitoneum during laparoscopic cholecystectomy. A reduced cardiac output secondary to pneumoperitoneum-induced reduction in venous return or drug-induced myocardial depression may reduce mixed venous O_2 tension. The larger the intrapulmonary shunt and the greater the reduction in mixed venous O_2 tensions, the greater the reduction in arterial oxygen tension.

Exogenous CO_2

Historically a number of gases have been used to facilitate laparoscopic surgery. Peritoneal gas insufflation is essential to enable exposure, visualization, and manipulation of intra-abdominal contents. The ideal insufflation gas would be colorless, physiologically inert, inexplosive in the presence of electrocautery and laser coagulation, and capable of pulmonary excretion. Although nitrous oxide and room air have been used for diagnostic gynecologic procedures, they are unsuitable when electrocautery is required. For these reasons and because of its ready availability, low cost, and proven efficacy, carbon dioxide has evolved as the insufflation gas of choice for laparoscopic surgery.[69]

A highly diffusable gas, CO_2 is absorbed across the peritoneal surface and is ultimately carried by the systemic and portal venous systems to the right heart and pulmonary circulation. According to Henry's law of solubility, CO_2 concentration in solution will equal CO_2 partial pressure (PCO_2) times solubility coefficient.[76] Although the volume of CO_2 carried in solution is small, most of the CO_2 enters and leaves the blood as CO_2 itself. The greater part of the CO_2 diffuses into the erythrocytes where hydration to carbonic acid occurs rapidly in the presence of carbonic anhydrase, and the subsequent ionization is promoted by the buffeting capacity of hemoglobin for the hydrogen ion. In this way considerable quantities of bicarbonate ion are formed, and these diffuse into the plasma in exchange for chloride ion which diffuses in the opposite direction. Lesser quantities of CO_2 are transported by hemoglobin as carbamino compounds. The ability of the body to store CO_2 varies with its metabolic production and exogenous CO_2 load, mixed venous CO_2 tension, cardiac output, alveolar ventilation, and the respiratory gas exchange quotient. The CO_2 stores of the body can be considered as two compartments, namely, the alveolar-arterial stores, equilibrated as alveolar PCO_2, and peripheral stores, which are equilibrated with mixed venous PCO_2.

The interactions of exogenous CO_2 load, volatile anesthetic agents, and ventilatory techniques have been the subject of extensive clinical investigation in the past two decades.

Early reports of anesthesia for gynecologic laparoscopy using halothane emphasized the hazards of hypercarbia if patients were allowed to breathe spontaneously.[6,7] Several factors may contribute to the hypercarbia reported with halothane anesthesia and spontaneous ventilation—respiratory center depression by premedicant and anesthetic drugs, absorption of carbon dioxide from the peritoneal cavity, and impairment of ventilation by mechanical factors such as abdominal distention and the use of a steep Trendelenburg position. Hodgson et al.[77] emphasized the importance of keeping the intra-abdominal pressure less than 25 mm Hg in spontaneously ventilating patients, thus avoiding any unnecessary restriction of diaphragmatic movement.

Desmond and Gordon[71] reported increased arterial carbon dioxide tensions and arrhythmias in 10 spontaneously breathing patients anesthetized with halothane and concluded that controlled ventilation was indicated for these procedures. Lewis et al.[78] observed that the $PaCO_2$ may be highest after the completion of the surgical procedure, once the intra-abdominal pressure has been released and suggested that these patients may be at most risk for cardiac arrhythmias after completion of the procedure, independent of the technique of ventilation used. Scott[79] reported incidences of arrhythmias (mostly unifocal or multifocal premature ventricular contractions) in up to 27 per cent of patients undergoing laparoscopy with halothane anesthesia and spontaneous ventilation. If nitrous oxide replaced carbon dioxide as the insufflation gas, the incidence of arrythmias decreased to 5 per cent, despite the use of halothane and a spontaneous ventilation technique.[80] However, carbon dioxide is the preferred insufflation gas, despite the increased postoperative discomfort associated with its use. Its greater solubility should minimize complications if inadvertent vascular injury occurred.[81]

The cardiopulmonary responses to CO_2 insufflation were prospectively evaluated by Lie et al.[69] in a study of 16 otherwise healthy patients undergoing laparoscopic cholecystectomy. All patients were paralyzed and controlled ventilation was used. End-tidal CO_2 tension and $PaCO_2$ increased from 31.4 ± 0.7 to 42.1 ± 1.6 mm Hg and from 33.3 ± 0.7 to 43.7 ± 1.2 mm Hg, respectively, during the course of the procedure. Arterial pH decreased from 7.43 ± 0.01 to 7.34 ± 0.01, while bicarbonate concentration remained constant. Thirteen of the 16 patients required increased minute ventilation to correct hypercarbia detected by capnography. Blood pressure increased from 78 ± 2 mm Hg (mean) at the start to 98 ± 2 mm Hg. This increase was coincidental with the maximal $PaCO_2$. Wittgen et al.[37] reported significant increases in arterial carbon dioxide tensions and decreases in pH during carbon dioxide insufflation in a group of 10 patients with previously documented cardiac and respiratory disease compared with patients without underlying disease.

The hemodynamic consequences of intraoperative hypercarbia were addressed by Rasmussen et al.[64] in a study of 12 patients with ischemic heart disease in whom $PaCO_2$ levels reached 55 to 65 mm Hg. In this situation, significant increases in systolic blood pressure, heart rate and cardiac output were reported, while shortening of the pre-ejection period, left ventricular ejection time, and the decrease in pre-ejection period/left ventricular ejection time ratio suggested increased mechanical cardiac activity. Hypercarbia caused sympathetic nervous system stimulation as demonstrated by 2- to 3-fold increases in plasma catecholamine concentrations.

A number of case reports have described acute hypotension, hypoxemia, and cardiovascular collapse associated with laparoscopy.[6,82] Postulated causes included: hypercarbia caused by hypoventilation or absorption of carbon dioxide from the peritoneal surface inducing dysrhythmias, especially if the myocardium is sensitized by volatile anesthetic agents, reflex increase of vagal tone caused by excessive stretching of the peritoneum, compression of the inferior vena cava leading to decreased cardiac output, and hemorrhage and venous gas embolism. A number of case reports have described the clinical conditions associated with venous CO_2 embolism during laparoscopy.[83,84] Venous CO_2 embolism in these cases was associated with profound hypotension, cyanosis, and asystole after pneumoperitoneum creation. The authors suggested that CO_2 could enter a tributary of the portal system during attempts to establish the pneumoperitoneum.

Reverse Trendelenburg Position

Laparoscopic cholecystectomy is unique in that a change in body position from Trendelenburg when establishing pneumoperitoneum to reverse Trendelenburg during dissection of the gallbladder is necessary to avoid inadvertent bowel injury and to provide optimum exposure. Additional changes in position are undertaken when the patient is placed supine for an intraoperative cholangiogram. The conventional wisdom is that the change to reverse Trendelenburg should be accompanied by respiratory advantages and cardiovascular disadvantages.[52] The limited data available suggest that, in otherwise healthy patients, these cardiac output changes are insignificant.[69] However, these changes may not be so benign in patients with established cardiorespiratory disease.

GUIDELINES FOR ANESTHETIC MANAGEMENT

Choice of Anesthetic Technique

The choice of anesthetic technique for laparoscopic cholecystectomy is mostly limited to general anesthesia because of patient discomfort associated with pneumoperitoneum creation and the extent of position changes associated with the procedure.[85] Controlled ventilation is recommended because several factors may induce hypercarbia, including depression of ventilation by anesthetic agents, absorption of carbon dioxide from the peritoneal cavity, and mechanical impairment of ventilation by the pneumoperitoneum and the initial steep Trendelenburg position.[46]

High intra-abdominal pressures during laparoscopic cholecystectomy may increase the risk of passive regurgitation of gastric contents.[73] Outpatients presenting for laparoscopic cholecystectomy may have higher volumes of gastric contents at lower pH, increasing the potential risk of acid aspiration.[86] Cuffed endotracheal tube placement should minimize the risk of acid aspiration should reflux occur. Following induction of anesthesia, a urinary bladder catheter and nasogastric tube are placed. Bladder catheterization is undertaken to avoid trauma to intra-abdominal contents at the time of trocar insertion. Intraoperative gastric decompression may reduce the risk of visceral puncture at the time of pneumoperitoneum creation and may improve laparoscopic visualization and ease retraction of the right upper quadrant structures.[46]

Local anesthesia, in combination with 2 μg/kg of fentanyl, has been used for ambulatory laparoscopic gynecologic procedures.[85] This technique has been associated with occasional vagal reflexes, manifested by hypotension, bradycardia, and nausea precipitated by uterine manipulation, acute respiratory alkalosis, and less than optimal surgical conditions. A combination of abdominal and tubal insufflation with a local anesthetic, paracervical block, and 100 μg of fentanyl was advocated by Penfield[87] as a suitable technique for ambulatory laparoscopic tubal ligation.

Epidural anesthesia has been suggested as a suitable alternative to general anesthesia for outpatient laparoscopy. The effects of epidural anesthesia on control of ventilation have been investigated in healthy unpremedicated subjects.[88] The administration of 5 mg/kg of lidocaine increased the slope of the ventilatory response to CO_2 significantly from its control values. Epidural lidocaine may have a stimulating effect on ventilatory control mechanisms arising from systemic effects of the drug. High levels of sympathetic denervation (extending from C4 to T7) induced by epidural block with 1.5 per cent lidocaine did not impair circulatory and ventilatory responses to carbon dioxide in awake healthy humans.[89] In a study of the respiratory effects of epidural anesthesia in seven healthy female patients undergoing laparoscopic tubal ligation, no significant changes in ventilatory variables were observed in the Trendelenburg position.[90] In contrast, CO_2 insufflation significantly increased minute ventilation (from 9.1 ± 1.0 to 11.8 ± 2.6 liters/min) and respiratory rate (from 16.9 ± 1.9 to 23.1 ± 3.3 breaths/min), whereas $PaCO_2$ remained constant throughout the study.

To date, local or regional anesthetic techniques, with the exception of correspondence concerning continuous epidural anesthesia in patients with cystic fibrosis,[91] have not been advocated for laparoscopic cholecystectomy. The high level of sympathetic denervation required, the patient position changes, and the mandatory pneumoperitoneum may be associated with adverse ventilatory and circulatory responses in the older and potentially sicker patients undergoing laparoscopic cholecystectomy. Conversion to general anesthesia would be required if surgical conditions necessitated a change from laparoscopic to open cholecystectomy.

Anesthetic Agents

PREMEDICATION

A suggested outline for the anesthetic management of patients undergoing laparoscopic cholecystectomy is presented in Table 5-10. Limited data are available concerning the impact of anesthetic management on postoperative outcome following laparoscopic cholecystectomy. Stanton[48] reported an initial high 42 per cent incidence of nausea and vomiting in the postoperative period. A change in anesthetic technique, including the addition of an antiemetic agent and substitution of intramuscular diclofenac for intravenous opioids, was associated with a reduction of postoperative nausea and vomiting in that particular center. Parris and Lee[92] speculated on the etiology of nausea and vomiting following laparoscopic cholecystectomy. Neurogenic effects secondary to traction on the celiac axis, peritoneal distention with carbon dioxide, and splanchnic manipulation were all implicated. The authors claimed that administration of the nonsteroidal anti-inflammatory agent ketorolac (60 mg intramusculary following induction), intraoperative metoclopramide (10–20 mg) intravenously, and prophylactic droperidol (0.625 mg) before the end of surgery essentially eliminated this problem in their patient population.

Table 5-10. Guidelines for Anesthetic Management in Laparoscopic Cholecystectomy

Premedication
  Benzodiazepines
  Nonsteroidal anti-inflammatory agents
  Antiemetic agents
Anesthesia
  General
  Intubation
  Controlled ventilation
Induction agents
  Barbiturates
  Propofol
  Etomidate
Relaxants
  Depolarizing
  Non-depolarizing
Monitoring
  Electrocardiogram (leads II and V5)
  Blood pressure
  Temperature
  Esophageal stethoscope
  End-tidal CO_2
  Oximetry
  Fractional inspired oxygen concentration
  Airway pressure
Maintenance
  N_2O/O_2/isoflurane or Air/O_2/isoflurane

PERIOPERATIVE NARCOTIC ADMINISTRATION

During laparoscopic cholecystectomy, intraoperative cholangiography may be crucial for the diagnosis of unsuspected common bile duct stones. The actions of certain drugs, such as cholinergic agents or narcotic agents used before surgery for preanesthetic medication and during surgery as part of a balanced anesthetic technique, have been reported to cause spasm of the choledochoduodenal sphincter (sphincter of Oddi).[93] Spasm of the sphincter may give rise to cholangiographic findings indistinguishable from those produced by a stone impacted in the common bile duct. Narcotic-induced sphincter spasm may cause unnecessary conversion to open cholecystectomy for exploration of the common bile duct, with its accompanying morbidity. However, several studies have shown that narcotic-induced spasm of the sphincter of Oddi may be antagonized by several drugs including naloxone,[94] glucagon,[95] and nalbuphine.[96]

Fentanyl, a potent narcotic analgesic noted for its rapid onset of action, relative cardiovascular stability, and negligible histamine release,[97] is widely used as a supplement in balanced anesthetic techniques. There are, however, conflicting reports on its effects on intrabiliary pressure (IBP). Arguelles et al.,[98] in an experimental study, noted a significant increase in IBP with all narcotics except pentazocine. IBP increases ranged from 85.7 per cent for meperidine to 143.4 per cent for fentanyl. No significant changes in IBP were noted during halothane and enflurane anesthesia. In a human study comparing the effects of equianalgesic doses of intravenous fentanyl, morphine, meperidine, and pentazocine on common bile buct pressures, Radnay et al.[99] demonstrated increases of 99.5, 52.7, 61.3, and 15.1 per cent, respectively. The effects of both morphine and fentanyl peaked at 10 minutes, meperidine at 8 minutes, and pentazocine at 6 minutes.

The potential difficulties associated with fentanyl-supplemented anesthesia seem overstated. Jones et al.[95] prospectively assessed the incidence of choledochoduodenal sphincter spasm during biliary tract surgery in 100 patients who received fentanyl in doses up to 10 μ/kg as part of a balanced anesthetic technique. The incidence of failure of passage of the contrast material into the duodenum was 3 per cent. In each of the three patients with cholangiographic evidence of sphincter spasm, contrast material flowed freely into the duodenum after the administration of 2 mg of glucagon. The advent of perioperative non-steroidal anti-inflammatory agents and the tendency for less postoperative pain associated with the laparoscopic approach may obviate the need for perioperative narcotic administration. However, if such narcotic administration is deemed necessary, it would appear that sphincter of Oddi spasm is uncommon during fentanyl-supplemented anesthesia, and this method of anesthesia may be appropiate for this type of biliary tract surgery.

THE NITROUS OXIDE CONTROVERSY

The use of nitrous oxide (N_2O) during laparoscopic cholecystectomy is controversial because of concerns regarding its ability to produce bowel distention during surgery and to increase postoperative emetic sequelae. N_2O is about 30 times more soluble than nitrogen. Thus, a closed air-containing space may accumulate N_2O more rapidly than it can eliminate nitrogen. Eger and Saidman[100] observed an increase of more than 200 per cent in intestinal lumen after 4 hours of N_2O breathing. Lonie and Harper[101] reported a reduction in postoperative vomiting from 49 to 17 per cent when N_2O was omitted in a prospective randomized study of 87 patients undergoing gynecologic laparoscopic procedures. Scheinin et al.[102] reported significantly less intraoperative bowel distention, earlier return of postoperative bowel function, and a shorter postoperative hospital stay in a group of patients randomly selected to receive air compared with those receiving N_2O during elective colonic surgery.

In contrast, Muir et al.,[103] in an extensive randomized and blinded study involving 780 patients, found no association between the use of N_2O and the subsequent development of postoperative nausea and vomiting. Interestingly, female gender, younger age, and a previous history of postoperative nausea and vomiting were found to be factors associated with postoperative nausea and vomiting. The safety and efficacy of N_2O specifically during laparoscopic cholecystectomy was investigated by Taylor et al.[104] There was no significant difference between the groups receiving air and N_2O with respect to operating conditions or bowel distention. More importantly, there were no time-related changes in either variable during the course of surgery. Finally, the incidence of postoperative nausea and vomiting was similar in both treatment groups.

In summary, there is no conclusive evidence to date that demonstrates a clinically significant effect of N_2O on surgical conditions during laparoscopic cholecystectomy or on the incidence of postoperative emesis. N_2O, therefore, may still be a useful adjuvant during general anesthesia for this procedure.

MONITORING

Suggested monitoring guidelines for laparoscopic cholecystectomy are included in Table 5-10. Standard intraoperative monitoring should include continuous electrocardiogram (leads II and V5), pulse oximetry, end-tidal capnography, neuromuscular function, inspired oxygen fraction, peak airway pressure, esophageal temperature, and urinary output. Urinary bladder catheter and nasogastric tubes are placed to avoid injury to intraabdominal contents during trocar insertion.

The most controversial issue involved in the appropriate monitoring of patients during laparoscopy involves the issue of whether radial arterial cannulation should be undertaken to assess the effectiveness of oxygenation and ventilation after pneumoperitoneum creation. The end-tidal carbon dioxide tension ($PetCO_2$) is most commonly used as a noninvasive substitute for $PaCO_2$ ($PaCO_2$ OVER) in evaluating the adequacy of ventilation during laparoscopic cholecystectomy. However, $PetCO_2$ may differ considerably from $PaCO_2$ because of ventilation-perfusion (Va/Q) mismatching, and erroneous clinical decisions may be reached if the two values are assumed to be equal, to change proportionally, or even to change in the same direction.[105] In a study of otherwise healthy, mechanically ventilated patients undergoing laparoscopic cholecystectomy, equal and proportional increases in $PetCO_2$ and $PaCO_2$ were observed following CO_2 insufflation.[69] In this patient population, end-tidal CO_2 monitoring should suffice. In contrast, patients with preoperative cardiopulmonary disease demonstrated significant increases in $PaCO_2$ OVER and decreases in pH after CO_2 insufflation, which was not reflected by comparable increases in $PetCO_2$ OVER.[37] The difference between $PaCO_2$ and $PetCO_2$ OVER (P[a − et]CO_2) will increase if there is a greater contribution of ventilation from high Va/Q regions. Therefore, radial artery cannulation for continuous blood pressure recording and frequent arterial blood gas analysis is appropriate in patients with preoperative cardiorespiratory disease and in situations in which intraoperative hypoxemia, high airway pressures, or elevated $PetCO_2$ are encountered.

Summary

Laparoscopic cholecystectomy is a relatively new surgical procedure, enjoying ever increasing popularity and presenting new anesthetic challenges. The advantages of shorter hospital stay and more rapid return to normal activities are combined with less pain associated with the small limited incisions and less postoperative ileus compared with the traditional open cholecystectomy. The major benefits claimed for laparoscopic cholecystectomy are thought to result from elimination of the abdominal incision. Prospective nonrandomized studies have reported 20 to 25 per cent improvement in FEV_1 and FVC, attributable to minimal muscle disruption and less postoperative pain following laparoscopic cholecystectomy compared with open cholecystectomy. The laparoscopic technique was so quickly adopted and so widely accepted that prospective randomized studies became almost impossible to undertake because of patient demand and ethical considerations.

The early laparoscopic cholecystectomy series were confined to relatively healthy patients with symptomatic cholelithiasis and chronic cholecystitis. Indications for the procedure soon became more liberal after case reports confirmed its efficacy in patients with acute cholecystitis, in the elderly, and in association with obesity, pregnancy, and previous abdominal surgery. Recent case reports and studies documenting intraoperative hypoxemia and respiratory acidosis in patients with preexisting chronic obstructive and restrictive lung disease suggest there may be some patients who will poorly tolerate the procedure. The conversion rate from laparoscopic to open cholecystectomy varies from 1 to 6 per cent in some series. Conversion is most commonly required for technical difficulties—identification of the cystic duct, common bile duct injuries, cystic artery bleeding, and common bile duct stones.

Complications associated with the procedure relate to traumatic injuries sustained during blind trocar insertion and physiologic changes associated with the initial Trendelenburg position, creation of the pneumoperitoneum, introduction of exogenous CO_2, and reverse Trendelenburg position. Trocar insertion injuries include bleeding from abdominal wall vessels, gastrointestinal tract perforation, hepatic and splenic tears, and major vascular trauma.

The physiologic changes during diagnostic laparoscopy associated with the Trendelenburg position and pneumoperitoneum creation were systematically investigated in the late 1960s and early 1970s. These studies showed only minor hemodynamic and ventilatory changes when the IAP did not exceed 25 mm Hg. However, these short duration procedures were performed in young, relatively healthy women in the Trendelenburg position. Considering the widespread adoption of laparoscopic cholecystectomy, there is a remarkable paucity of data concerning the hemodynamic and respiratory function changes in normal patients and in patients with cardiopulmonary diseases following prolonged CO_2-induced pneumoperitoneum in a steep head-up position. The limited available data, in otherwise healthy patients, suggest that these interventions may be associated with negligible cardiac output changes, despite increases in mean arterial pressure and end-tidal CO_2. In contrast, hypercarbia, respiratory acidosis, increased peak airway pressures, and minute ventilation requirements may be manifest in patients with preexisting cardiopulmonary disease. Intraoperative hypoxemia (attributed to tension pneumothorax, aspiration, inferior vena caval compression, and CO_2 embolism) have been reported during laparoscopic procedures.

The choice of anesthetic technique for laparoscopic cholecystectomy is mostly limited to general anesthesia. A continuous epidural technique was reported in patients with cystic fibrosis. However, the high sympathetic denervation required, the patient position changes, and the mandatory pneumoperitoneum may be associated with patient discomfort and adverse ventilatory and circulatory responses in the older and potentially sicker patients undergoing laparoscopic cholecystectomy. Cuffed endotracheal tube placement and controlled ventilation are recommended to minimize the risk of acid aspiration and to avoid hypercarbia secondary to depression of ventilation by anesthetic agents, absorption of carbon dioxide from the peritoneal cavity, and mechanical impairment of ventilation by the pneumoperitoneum and the initial steep Trendelenburg position.

Postoperative nausea and vomiting have been frequently noted after laparoscopic cholecystectomy. An anesthetic technique incorporating metoclopramide to promote gastric emptying, droperidol as a prophylactic antiemetic agent, and substitution of the nonsteroidal inflammatory agent ketorolac for intravenous opioids has been reported to significantly reduce these unpleasant sequelae.

Narcotic-induced sphincter of Oddi spasm may cause unnecessary conversion to open cholecystectomy for exploration of the common bile duct, with its accompanying morbidity. The potential difficulties associated with fentanyl-supplemented anesthesia seem overstated. The advent of perioperative nonsteroidal anti-inflammatory agents and the tendency for less postoperative pain associated with the laparoscopic approach may obviate the need for perioperative narcotic administration. The use of N_2O during laparoscopic cholecystectomy is controversial because of concerns regarding its ability to produce bowel distention during surgery and to increase postoperative emetic sequelae. However, there is no conclusive evidence to date that demonstrates a clinically significant effect of N_2O on surgical conditions during laparoscopic cholecystectomy or on the incidence of postoperative emesis.

Standard intraoperative monitoring should include continuous electrocardiogram (leads II and V5), pulse oximetry, end-tidal capnography, neuromuscular function, inspired oxygen fraction, peak airway pressure, esophageal temperature, and urinary output. Urinary bladder catheter and nasogastric tubes are placed to avoid injury to intra-abdominal contents during trocar insertion. The end-tidal carbon dioxide tension is most commonly used as a noninvasive substitute for $PaCO_2$ in evaluating the adequacy of ventilation during laparoscopic cholecystectomy. However, $PetCO_2$ may differ considerably from $PaCO_2$ because of ventilation-perfusion mismatching. Therefore, radial artery cannulation for continuous blood pressure recording and frequent arterial blood gas analysis are appropriate in patients with preoperative cardiorespiratory disease and in situations where intraoperative hypoxemia, high airway pressures, or elevated $PetCO_2$ are encountered.

Laparoscopic cholecystectomy is a major advance in the management of patients with symptomatic gallbladder disease. Initial uncritical enthusiasm for and acceptance of the procedure have been tempered by recent cautionary reports of unique associated complications. Until more clinical experience is obtained and until more extensive evaluations of the hemodynamic and ventilatory changes associated with the procedure are done, anesthesiologists should adopt a critical and cautious approach. Because of its perceived safety, in this era of cost containment, older and sicker patients may present for this procedure on the day of surgery without adequate preoperative evaluation. Finally, anesthesiologists should not hesitate to recommend conversion to an open procedure if hemodynamic, oxygenation, or ventilation difficulties arise during the procedure.

REFERENCES

1. Gaskin TA, Isobe JH, Mathews JL, et al. Laparoscopy and the general surgeon. Surg Clin North Am 1991; 71:1085–1097.
2. McKiernan J, Saye W. Laparoscopic general surgery. J Med Assoc Ga 1990; 79:148.
3. Semm K. Endoscopic appendectomy. Endoscopy 1983; 15:59–64.
4. Whitworth C, Whitworth P, Sanfillipo J. Value of diagnostic laparoscopy in young women with possible appendicitis. Surg Gynecol Obstet 1988; 167:187–190.
5. Steptoe PC. In: Laparoscopy in Gynaecology. Edinburgh, ES Livingstone Ltd, 1967, p 1.
6. Alexander GD, Noe FE, Brown EM. Anesthesia for pelvic laparoscopy. Anesth Analg 1969; 48:14–18.
7. Calverley RK, Jenkins LC. The anaesthetic management of pelvic laparoscopy. Can Anaesth Soc J 1973; 20:679–686.
8. Dubois F, Berthelot G, Levard H. Laparoscopic cholecystectomy: Historical perspective and personal experience. Surg Laparosc Endosc 1991; 1:52–57.
9. McSherry CK. Cholecystectomy: The gold standard. Am J Surg 1989; 158:174–178.
10. Luna CK, Heimbach DM, Olson H, Hanson J. Hospital stay following biliary tract surgery: A comparison of two community hospitals. Arch Surg 1986; 121:693–696.
11. Health Care Financing Special Report. Health Care Financing Administration, Office of Research and Demonstrations, June 1990, Vol 3.
12. Craig DB. Postoperative recovery of pulmonary function. Anesth Analg 1981; 60:46–52.
13. Wahba RWM. Perioperative functional residual capacity. Can J Anaesth 1991; 38:384–400.
14. Ford GT, Whitelaw WA, Rosenal TW. Diaphragm function after upper abdominal surgery in humans. Am Rev Respir Dis 1983; 127:431–436.
15. Holohan TV. Laparoscopic cholecystectomy. Lancet 1991; 338:801–803.
16. Pitt HA, McFadden DW, Gadacz TR. Agents for gallstone dissolution. Am J Surg 1987; 153:233–246.
17. Martin DF, Tweedle DEF. Endoscopic management of common duct stones without cholecystectomy. Br J Surg 1987; 74:209–211.
18. Sackmann M, Delius M, Sauerbrunch T. Shock wave lithotripsy of gallbladder stones: The first 175 patients. N Engl J Med 1988; 318:393–397.
19. Burhenne HJ, Stoller JL. Minicholecystectomy and radiologic stone extraction in high risk cholelithiasis patients: Preliminary experience. Am J Surg 1985; 149:632–635.
20. Sackmann M, Pauletzki J, Sauerbruch T. The effect of ursodiol on the efficacy and safety of extracorporeal shock-wave lithotripsy of gallstones: Results of the first five years with 711 patients. Ann Intern Med 1991; 114:290–296.
21. Neuebauer E, Troidl H, Spangenberger W, et al. Conventional versus laparoscopic cholecystectomy and the randomized controlled trial. Br J Surg 1991; 78:150–154.
22. Way LW. Changing therapy for gallstone disease. N Engl J Med 1990; 323:1273–1274.
23. Perissat J, Collet DR, Belliard R. Gallstones: Laparoscopic treatment, intracorporeal lithotripsy followed by cholecystectomy or cholecystectomy—A personal technique. Endoscopy 1989; 21:373–374.
24. Reddick EJ, Olsen DO. Laparoscopic laser cholecystectomy: A comparison with mini-lap cholecystectomy. Surg Endosc 1989; 3:131–134.
25. Du Bois F, Icard P, Berthelot G, Levard H. Coelioscopic cholecystectomy: Preliminary report of 36 cases. Ann Surg 1990; 211:60–62.
26. Grace PA, Quereshi A, Coleman J, et al. Reduced postoperative hospitalization after laparoscopic cholecystectomy. Br J Surg 1991; 78:160–162.
27. Jones RM, Fletcher DR, McLellan DG, et al. Laparoscopic cholecystectomy: Initial experience. Aust N-Z J Surg 1991; 61:261–266.
28. Meyers WC, The Southern Surgeons Club. A prospective analysis of 1518 laparoscopic cholecystectomies. N Engl J Med 1991; 324:1073–1078.
29. Frazee RC, Roberts JW, Okeson GC, et al. Open versus laparoscopic cholecystectomy: A comparison of postoperative pulmonary function. Ann Surg 1991; 213:651–653.
30. Johnson WC. Postoperative ventilatory performance: Dependence on surgical incision. Am Surg 1975; 41:615–619.
31. Gadacz TR, Talamini MA. Traditional versus laparoscopic cholecystectomy. Am J Surg 1991; 161:336–338.
32. Flowers JL, Bailey RW, Scovill WA, Zucker KA. The Baltimore experience with laparoscopic management of acute cholecystitis. Am J Surg 1991; 161:388–392.
33. Pucci RO, Seed RW. Case report of laparoscopic cholecystectomy in the third trimester of pregnancy. Am J Obstet Gynecol 1991; 165:401–402.
34. Wilson P, Leese T, Morgan WP, et al. Elective laparoscopic cholecystectomy for "all-comers." Lancet 1991; 338:795–797.
35. Phillips EH, Berci G, Carroll B. The importance of intraoperative cholangiography during laparoscopic cholecystectomy. Am Surg 1990; 56:256–261.
36. Cunningham AJ, Schlanger M. Intraoperative hypoxemia complicating laparoscopic cholecystectomy in a patient with sickle hemoglobinopathy. Anesth Analg 1992; 75:838–843.
37. Wittgen CM, Andrus CH, Fitzgerald SD, et al. Analysis of the hemodynamic and ventilatory effects of laparoscopic cholecystectomy. Arch Surg 1991; 126:997–1001.
38. Paterson-Brown S, Garden OJ, Carter DC. Laparoscopic cholecystectomy. Br J Surg 1991; 78:131–132.
39. Cameron JL, Gadacz TR. Laparoscopic cholecystectomy. Ann Surg 1991; 213:1–2.
40. Perissat J, Vitale GC. Laparoscopic cholecystectomy: Gateway to the future. Am J Surg 1991; 161:408.
41. Spangenberger W, Klein J, Troidl H. Laparosko-

41. (cont.) pische cholezystektomie—Erste erfahrungen und ergenbrisse. Langenbecks Arch Chir 1990; Suppl 11:1361–1368.
42. Peters JH, Ellison C, Innes JT, et al. Safety and efficacy of laparoscopic cholecystectomy. A prospective analysis of 100 patients. Ann Surg 1991; 213:3–12.
43. Nathanson LK, Shimi S, Cushieri A. Laparoscopic cholecystectomy: The Dundee technique. Br J Surg 1991; 78:155–159.
44. Graves HA, Ballinger JF, Anderson WJ. Appraisal of laparoscopic cholecystectomy. Ann Surg 1991; 213:655–663.
45. Cuschieri A, Du Bois F, Mouiel J, et al. The European experience with laparoscopic cholecystectomy. Am J Surg 1991; 161:385–387.
46. Marco AP, Yeo CJ, Rock P. Anesthesia for a patient undergoing laparoscopic cholecystectomy. Anesthesiology 1990; 73:1268–1270.
47. Greville AC, Clements EAF. Anaesthesia for laparoscopic cholecystectomy using the Nd:Yag laser. The implications for a district general hospital. Anaesthesia 1990; 45:944–945.
48. Stanton JM. Anaesthesia for laparoscopic cholecystectomy. Anaesthesia 1991; 46:317.
49. Greville AC, Clements EAF, Erwin DC, et al. Pulmonary air embolism during laparoscopic laser cholecystectomy. Anaesthesia 1991; 46:113–114.
50. Ponsky JL. Complications of laparoscopic cholecystectomy. Am J Surg 1991; 161:393–395.
51. Editorial: Friedrich Trendelenburg (1844–1924). Trendelenburg's position. JAMA 1969; 207:1143–1144.
52. Wilcox SW, Vandam LD. Alas, poor Trendelenburg and his position! A critique of its uses and effectiveness. Anesth Analg 1988; 67:574–578.
53. Miller AH. Surgical posture with symbols for its record on the anesthetist's chart. Anesthesiology 1940; 1:241–245.
54. Bivins HG, Knopp R, dos Santos PAL. Blood volume distribution in the Trendelenburg position. Ann Emerg Med 1885; 14:641–643.
55. Pricolo VE, Bruchard KW, Gann DS. Trendelenburg versus PASG application hemodynamic response in man. J Trauma 1986; 26:718–726.
56. Case EH, Stiles JA. The effect of various surgical positions on vital capacity. Anesthesiology 1946; 7:29–31.
57. Schiller WR. The Trendelenburg position. Surgical requirements. In Martin JT, ed. Positioning in anesthesia and surgical requirements. Philadelphia, WB Saunders, 1987, pp 89–97.
58. Scott DB, Slawson KB. Circulatory effects of prolonged Trendelenburg position. Br J Anaesth 1968; 40:103–107.
59. Heinonen J, Takki S, Tammisto T. Effect of the Trendelenburg tilt and other procedures on the position of endotracheal tubes. Lancet 1969; 1:850–853.
60. Lew JKL, Gin T, Oh TE. Anaesthetic problems during laparoscopic cholecystectomy. Anaesth Intensive Care 1992; 20:91–92.
61. Marshall RL, Jebson PJR, Davie IT, Scott DB. Circulatory effects of carbon dioxide insufflation of the peritoneal cavity for laparoscopy. Br J Anaesth 1972; 44:680–684.
62. Smith I, Benzie RJ, Gordon NLM, et al. Cardiovascular effects of peritoneal insufflation of carbon dioxide for laparoscopy. Br Med J 1971; 3:410–411.
63. Kelman GR, Swapp GH, Smith I, et al. Cardiac output and arterial blood-gas tension during laparoscopy. Br J Anaesth 1972; 44:1155–1162.
64. Rasmussen JP, Dauchot PJ, De Palma RG, et al. Cardiac function and hypercarbia. Arch Surg 1978; 113:1196–1200.
65. Ivankovich AD, Miletich DJ, Albrecht RF, et al. Cardiovascular effects of intraperitoneal insufflation with carbon dioxide and nitrous oxide in the dog. Anesthesiology 1975; 42:281–287.
66. Diamant M, Benumof JL, Saidman LJ. Hemodynamics of increased intra-abdominal pressure: Interaction with hypovolemia and halothane anethesia. Anesthesiology 1978; 48:23–27.
67. Johannsen G, Andersen M, Juhl B. The effect of general anesthesia on the haemodynamic events during laparoscopy with CO_2-insufflation. Acta Anaesthesiol Scand 1989; 33:132–136.
68. Lennon F. Laparoscopic cholecystectomy: A cautionary note. Br J Surg 1991; 78:1400.
69. Liu SY, Leighton T, Davis I, et al. Prospective analysis of cardiopulmonary responses to laparoscopic cholecystectomy. J Laparoendosc Surg 1991; 1:241–246.
70. Seed RF, Shakespear TF, Muldoon MJ. Carbon dioxide homeostasis during anesthesia for laparoscopy. Anesthesia 1970; 25:223–231.
71. Desmond J, Gordon RA. Ventilation in patients anaesthetized for laparoscopy. Can Anaesth Soc J 1970; 17:378–387.
72. Whiston RJ, Eggers KA, Morris RW, Stamatakis JD. Tension pneumothorax during laparoscopic cholecystectomy. Br J Surg 1991; 78:1325.
73. Duffy BL. Regurgitation during pelvic laparoscopy. Br J Anaesth 1979; 51:1089–1090.
74. Slocum HC, Hoeflich EA, Allen CR. Circulatory and respiratory distress from extreme positions on the operating table. Surg Gynecol Obstet 1947; 84:1065–1068.
75. Froese AB, Bryan CA. Effects of anesthesia and paralysis on diaphragmatic mechanics in man. Anesthesiology 1974; 41:242–248.
76. Nunn JF. Carbon dioxide. In Nunn JF, ed. Applied Respiratory Physiology, 3rd ed. London, Butterworth & Co, 1987, pp 207–234.
77. Hodgson C, McClelland RMA, Newton JR. Some effects of peritoneal insufflation of carbon dioxide at laparoscopy. Anaesthesia 1970; 25:382–385.
78. Lewis DG, Ryder W, Burn N, et al. Laparoscopy—An investigation during spontaneous ventilation with halothane. Br J Anaesth 1972; 44:685–691.
79. Scott DB. Some effects of peritoneal insufflation of carbon dioxide at laparoscopy. Anaesthesia 1970; 25:590–594,.
80. Scott DB, Julian DG. Observations on cardiac arrhythmias during laparoscopy. Br Med J 1972; 1:411–413.
81. Sharp J, Pierson W, Brady C. Comparison of CO_2 and N_2O induced discomfort during peritoneoscopy under local anesthesia. Gastroenterology 1982; 82:453–456.
82. Lee CM. Acute hypotension during laparoscopy: A case report. Anesth Analg 1975; 54:142–143.
83. Clarke CC, Weeks DB, Gusdon JP. Venous carbon dioxide embolism during anesthesia. Anesth Analg 1977; 56:650–652.
84. Root B, Levy MN, Pollack S, et al. Gas embolism death after laparoscopy delayed by "trapping" in the portal circulation. Anesth Analg 1978; 57:232–237.
85. Brown DR, Fishburne JI, Roberson VO, Hulka JF.

86. Cunningham AJ. Acid aspiration: Mendelson's syndrome. Ann R Coll Phys Surg Can 1987; 20:335–340.
    Ventilatory and blood gas changes during laparoscopy with local anesthesia. Am J Obstet Gynecol 1976; 124:741–745.
87. Penfield AJ. Laparoscopic sterilization under local anesthesia. 1200 cases. Obstet Gynecol 1977; 49:725–727.
88. Labille T, Clergue F, Samii K, et al. Ventilatory response to CO_2 following intravenous and epidural lidocaine. Anesthesiology 1985; 63:179–183.
89. Dohi S, Takeshima R, Naito H. Ventilatory and circulatory responses to carbon dioxide and high level sympathectomy induced by epidural blockade in awake humans. Anesth Analg 1986; 65:9–14.
90. Ciofolo MJ, Clergue F, Seebacher J, et al. Ventilatory effects of laparoscopy under epidural anesthesia. Anesth Analg 1990; 70:357–361.
91. Edelman DS. Laparoscopic cholecystectomy under continuous epidural anesthesia in patients with cystic fibrosis. Am J Dis Child 1991; 145:723–724.
92. Parris WCV, Lee EM. Anesthesia for laparoscopic cholecystectomy. Anaesthesia 1991; 46:997.
93. Chessick KC, Black S, Hoye SJ. Spasm and operative cholangiography. Arch Surg 1975; 110:53–57.
94. McCammon RL, Viegas OJ, Stoelting RK, Dryden GE. Naloxone reversal of choledochoduodenal sphincter spasm associated with narcotic administration. Anesthesiology 1978; 48:437.
95. Jones RM, Detmer M, Hill AB, et al. Incidence of choledochoduodenal sphincter spasm during fentanyl supplemented anesthesia. Anesth Analg 1981; 60:638–640.
96. Humphrey HK, Fleming NW. Opioid-induced spasm of the sphincter of Oddi apparently reversed by nalbuphine. Anesth Analg 1992; 74:308–310.
97. Bovill JG. Opioid analgesics in anesthesia: With special reference to their use in cardiovascular anesthesia. Anesthesiology 1984; 61:731–755.
98. Arguelles JE, Franatovic Y, Romo-Salas F, Aldrete JA. Intrabiliary pressure changes produced by narcotic drugs and inhalation anesthetics in guinea pigs. Anesth Analg 1979; 58:120–123.
99. Radnay PA, Brodman E, Manikikar D, Duncalf D. The effect of equi-analgesic doses of fentanyl, morphine, meperidine and pentazocine on common bile duct pressure. Anaesthetist 1980; 29:26–29.
100. Eger EI II, Saidman LJ. Hazards of nitrous oxide anesthesia in bowel obstruction and pneumothorax. Anesthesiology 1963; 26:61–66.
101. Lonie DS, Harper NJN. Nitrous oxide and anaesthesia: The effect of nitrous oxide anaesthesia on the incidence of vomiting following gynaecological laparoscopy. Anaesthesia 1986; 41:703–707.
102. Scheinin B, Lindgren L, Scheinin TM. Peroperative nitrous oxide delays bowel function after colonic surgery. Br J Anaesth 1990; 64:154–158.
103. Muir JJ, Warner MA, Offord KP, et al. Role of nitrous oxide and other factors in postoperative nausea and vomiting. A randomized and blinded prospective study. Anesthesiology 1987; 66:513–518.
104. Taylor E, Feinstein R, White PF, Soper N. Anesthesia for laparoscopic cholecystectomy: Is nitrous oxide contraindicated? Anesthesiology 1992; 76:541–543.
105. Yamanaka MK, Sue DY. Comparison of arterial-end-tidal PCO_2 difference and dead space/tidal volume ratio in respiratory failure. Chest 1987; 92:832–835.

Chapter 6
Pathophysiology of Pneumoperitoneum

Torgny Svenberg

Pneumoperitoneum is used during laparoscopy and laparoscopic surgery to enable visualization of abdominal structures. A pressure within the abdomen of approximately 15 to 20 mm Hg is required, which is maintained by means of automatic gas insufflation. Approximately 5 liters of gas are needed to increase the intra-abdominal pressure to 15 mm Hg,[1] depending on the weight and muscle strength of the anterior abdominal wall. Figure 6-1 illustrates this pneumoperitoneum prior to laparoscopic cholecystectomy in a female patient. Most studies on the effects of pneumoperitoneum on circulation and ventilation have been carried out during brief gynecologic laparoscopic procedures in young women without concomitant cardiopulmonary or other systemic disease. However, with recent technologic developments, this method is now suggested for a wide variety of surgical procedures. Sections II through VII of this book focus on a number of abdominal operations now being performed through the laparoscope. Many of these will probably become standard surgical teaching within a few years. These procedures, although considered less traumatic than their conventional counterparts, however, will last longer and in general will be performed on older and less fit patients than the gynecologic operations referred to previously. Therefore, the specific problems with laparoscopic surgery, i.e., those related to new surgical instruments, to pneumoperitoneum, and to unusual postures of the patient during surgery, should be well known by the surgeon. He or she should also know how to best monitor the patient during surgery and how to detect and treat sudden dangerous complications.

This chapter will review current knowledge on the pathophysiology of pneumoperitoneum and also discuss its possible consequences during longer procedures in old patients. To start off, it must be reemphasized that the reviewed data, with few exceptions, were obtained from animal studies or from brief laparoscopic procedures performed on young women. Hence, the extrapolation of these results to longer operations on patients with concomitant heart and lung problems must be made with caution.

Insight into the pathophysiology of pneumoperitoneum has largely emerged from gynecologic laparoscopy, performed on a large scale since the 1960s. This knowledge will be reviewed, together with appropriate animal data, as follows: first, considerations leading to the present use of carbon dioxide as the gas of choice will be given; second, the effects of pneumoperitoneum on respiration and circulation will be presented; and third, other effects of increased intra-abdominal pressure and some further matters of surgical interest in relation to pneumoperitoneum will be listed.

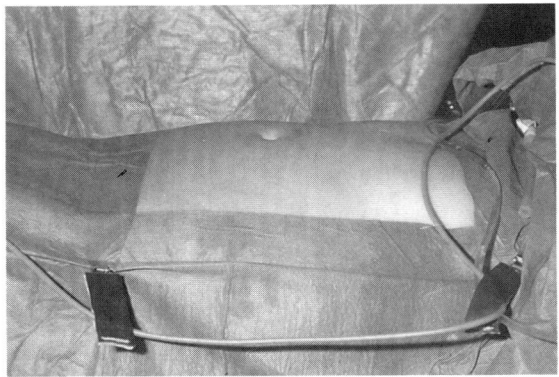 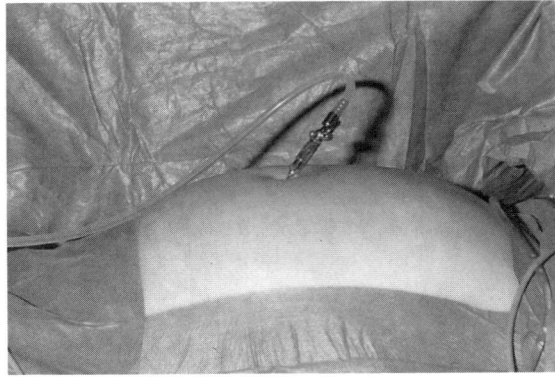

Figure 6-1. Pneumoperitoneum, prior to laparoscopic cholecystectomy in a 45-year multiparous female. The pictures were taken before (*left*) and after (*right*) carbon dioxide insufflation to an intra-abdominal pressure of 13 mm Hg.

HISTORICAL NOTES

Pneumoperitoneum has been used clinically in a few situations apart from laparoscopy. Earlier in this century, insufflation of air in the abdomen was used in the treatment of pulmonary tuberculosis as a way to collapse diseased lower parts of the lungs.[2] Peritoneal insufflation of air has also been used prior to surgical treatment of large ventral abdominal hernias. The abdominal wall was distended to facilitate repositioning of abdominal organs away from the hernia sac. A few reviews describe the method of daily air insufflations for 7 to 10 days before hernia repair.[3-5] The most common among reported adverse effects is perforation of the bowel by the needle used for abdominal puncture. Finally, pneumoperitoneum has been used in the radiologic diagnosis of inguinal hernias, particularly in children.[6]

CHOICE OF GAS FOR PNEUMOPERITONEUM

The ideal gas for pneumoperitoneum should be nontoxic, colorless, readily soluble in blood, easily ventilated through the lungs, noninflammable, and cheap. Room air, oxygen, and nitrous oxide have been abandoned because of the risk of combustion caused by the necessary use of diathermy or laser during laparoscopic surgery. There is no such risk with carbon dioxide. It is cheap, colorless, highly soluble in blood with a solubility coefficient of 0.49 at 37°C as compared to 0.013 for nitrogen,[7] and readily expired via the lungs. These properties have popularized the use of carbon dioxide for the induction of pneumoperitoneum. Its high solubility in blood allows rapid absorption and elimination after surgery and has also been suggested to increase the margin of safety, should the gas be injected into the circulation by mistake. Animal experiments have shown carbon dioxide to be less lethal than both room air and oxygen when used to induce gas embolism.[8,9] Recently, helium has been suggested to be more suitable than carbon dioxide[10] because it causes less acidosis (discussed later). Helium is, however, poorly soluble in blood, with a solubility coefficient of 0.0098 in human blood at 37°C,[11] compared to 0.49 for carbon dioxide.[7] Therefore, helium appears not to be an ideal gas for pneumoperitoneum since it poses a much greater threat than carbon dioxide in the case of accidental gas embolism.

GAS EMBOLISM

Gas embolism is a rare but dangerous complication of pneumoperitoneum. Many instances of gas embolism have been reported,[12-14] some with lethal outcome.[15,16] Embolism results from the injection of gas into the circulation. This usually occurs at the beginning of a laparoscopic operation, as a result of faulty positioning of the needle used for gas insufflation. The commonly used pumps for insufflation of gas give a flow of several liters of gas per minute. This by far exceeds the rate known to induce lethal gas embolism in animals.[17] It is therefore important to test that the Veress needle is correctly placed within free peritoneal cavity before gas insufflation is started and to inject the gas slowly at first. Circulatory collapse usually develops within seconds after gas injection into systemic veins or, rarely, after a delay of 30 minutes following insufflation into the portal venous system.[18] Gas trapped in the pulmonary artery will have a number of acute effects on central hemodynamics.[19] Pulmonary artery obstruction will cause right ventricular dilatation and failure. Increased pressure in the right ventricle may cause gas embolism into the left ventricle through a patent foramen intraventriculare, which has been reported to be present in 20 per cent of the population.[20] Further, markedly decreased left ventricular output will result in diminished coronary circulation and a decrease in arterial blood pressure. At the same time, the impaired pulmonary circulation rapidly causes hypoxia and anoxia. Unless gas embolism is quickly detected and proper measures are taken to stop further gas insufflation, the series of events described earlier rapidly kills the patient.

Early during gas embolism, a typical "mill wheel" murmur can be heard over the heart. Thus, an ordinary precordial stethoscope should be used during gas insufflation.[21] Doppler ultrasonography may also be used. A decrease in end-tidal carbon dioxide pressure is another early signal of gas embolism in the pulmonary artery caused by increased physiologic dead space. Electrocardiographic changes typical of gas embolism should also be looked for during gas insufflation. These are widening of QRS interval and ventricular tachycardia.[21] There are several relatively simple means of reducing the dangers of gas embolism. External cardiac massage breaks up large gas bubbles into smaller ones that can be circulated into the peripheral pulmonary vessels. Placing the patient in the left lateral decubitus position with a sharp head-down tilt helps to move gas from the outflow tract of the right ventricle toward the apex of the heart. Intracardiac aspiration of gas could be undertaken through a central venous catheter. These techniques have been compared in animal experiments and were found to be equally effective in preventing death from gas embolism.[19] Finally, treatment with hyperbaric oxygen may be instituted, particularly with embolism from gases other than carbon dioxide.[7,22]

VENTILATORY EFFECTS OF PNEUMOPERITONEUM

A number of studies have documented the fact that peritoneal gas insufflation may interfere with lung function. An investigation of patients during gynecologic laparoscopy using local anesthesia revealed a significant decrease of vital capacity and a compensatory increase in ventilatory rate during carbon dioxide pneumoperitoneum with intraperitoneal pressure of 12 to 18 mm Hg. No significant effects on ventilatory parameters by a 20-degree Trendelenburg tilt were observed in this study.[23] Similarly, no adverse effects on carbon dioxide exchange or different oxygenation parameters were found to be caused by the position of the patient or by pneumoperitoneum. The authors noted more abdominal discomfort for several hours after carbon dioxide pneumoperitoneum compared with nitrous oxide. This may be explained by the creation of carbonic acid from carbon dioxide. Thus, a decrease in peritoneal pH to 6.9 after 15 minutes of pneumoperitoneum using 100 per cent carbon dioxide compared with pH 7.35 using 5 per cent carbon dioxide in air has been reported.[24]

In studying similar patients but with epidural anesthesia, another group found increased minute ventilation and respiratory rate during carbon dioxide pneumoperitoneum.[25] No significant changes in ventilatory variables were observed to result from positioning the patients in the Trendelenburg position. Although the Trendelenburg position is known to decrease functional residual capacity, total lung volume, and lung compliance,[26,27] these studies[25] demonstrate that pneumoperitoneum has more dramatic effects on ventilation than head-down tilt of the patient. These data have all been obtained from young women with ASA (American Society of Anesthesiologists) physical status I.

Several studies have documented the fact that carbon dioxide pneumoperitoneum causes increased arterial carbon dioxide tension ($PaCO_2$), hypercapnia, and a decrease in arterial pH.[23,28–32] In patients with normal lung function, hypercarbia is easily compensated for by increased ventilation. During laparoscopic cholecystectomy on 16 patients (ASA classes I and II), an increase in $PaCO_2$ from 31.4 ± 0.7 to 42.1 ± 1.7 mm Hg (mean $\pm$ SEM) and a concomitant decrease in arterial pH from 7.43 ± 0.01 to 7.34 ± 0.01 was recorded.[33] These changes were readily compensated for by increased ventilation. In another recent study on laparoscopic cholecystectomy, 10 patients of ASA classes II and III were included and compared with 20 patients of ASA class I. Significantly greater increases in $PaCO_2$ (31.9 ± 8.4 [mean $\pm$ SD] to 46.0 ± 9.2 versus 30.7 ± 2.9 to $36.6 \pm$

5.1 mm Hg) and decreases in pH (7.45 ± 0.08 to 7.33 ± 0.06 versus 7.47 ± 0.03 to 7.40 ± 0.05) were seen in ASA classes II and III patients compared with ASA class I patients. In one ASA class II patient, acidosis could not be controlled with hyperventilation. Therefore, carbon dioxide pneumoperitoneum had to be terminated and the operation completed as a formal open cholecystectomy.[34]

Taken together, these investigations clearly reveal a potential disadvantage with carbon dioxide for inducing pneumoperitoneum, at least in patients with concomitant lung problems, in that hypercarbia and respiratory acidosis are induced. A recent publication proposes helium to be a more appropriate medium in this respect.[10] No problems with hypercarbia or acidosis were encountered in this animal investigation. The possible merits and drawbacks (see before under "Gas Embolism") with the use of helium for pneumoperitoneum await further study.

CIRCULATORY EFFECTS OF PNEUMOPERITONEUM

Several publications describe untoward circulatory effects caused by pneumoperitoneum. These range from sudden vasovagal reflexes easily managed by atropine administration,[23,29,35,36] to circulatory collapse caused by high pressure tension pneumoperitoneum requiring immediate laparotomy or abdominal puncture.[37-39] One study reported a 97 per cent incidence of cardiac arrhythmias during laparoscopy, pneumoperitoneum, and anesthesia.[40] Premedication with a β-receptor antagonist significantly reduced the incidence of supraventricular tachycardia, ventricular ectopic beats, and atrioventricular dissociation. Another report drew attention to the importance of not using cardiostimulatory anesthetic drugs such as halothane or bolus doses of succinylcholine to avoid cardiac arrhythmias during pneumoperitoneum.[41]

In young women during laparoscopy, carbon dioxide pneumoperitoneum with moderate elevations of intra-abdominal pressure to 20 mm Hg caused increased arterial and central venous pressures and tachycardia.[29] A further increase of intra-abdominal pressure to 30 mm Hg reversed these effects and caused decreased arterial and central venous pressures, suggesting impairment of venous return from the lower part of the body. The authors concluded that pressure within the abdominal cavity should be kept below 20 mm Hg during laparoscopy. These findings were explored in a series of dog experiments.[42] At abdominal pressures of 40 mm Hg, both cardiac output and inferior vena caval flow were reduced by more than 60 per cent. A comparison between carbon dioxide and nitrous oxide pneumoperitoneum[42] showed that both gases had similar effects except for the expected hypercarbia and slight acidosis induced by carbon dioxide.

All human investigations found in the literature prior to the writing of this chapter showed increases in arterial and central venous pressure during pneumoperitoneum with moderate intra-abdominal pressures of 15 to 20 mm Hg. This would be expected to cause increased cardiac output by increasing blood flow to the heart, further augmented by the Trendelenburg position. Several studies during gynecologic laparoscopy[30,43] accordingly demonstrate increased cardiac output, as revealed by dye dilution techniques, at intra-abdominal pressures of 15 to 20 mm Hg. Some investigations, using impedance cardiography, showed either decreased[44,45] or slightly increased cardiac output[31] during pneumoperitoneum of 15 to 20 mm Hg. Thus, the question of the influence on cardiac output by pneumoperitoneum, of longer duration in particular, has not yet been answered. Further studies using more sensitive techniques for measuring cardiac output are needed to evaluate the risks related to pneumoperitoneum and different body postures on patients with compromised heart function.

RELEASE OF VASOPRESSIN BY PNEUMOPERITONEUM

The release of arginine vasopressin (AVP) has long been known to occur in relation to abdominal surgery.[46,47] Animal data suggest that increased intra-abdominal pressure, not stress by itself, releases AVP via a reflex involving visceral pain receptors and the posterior spinal nerve roots.[48,49] Release of AVP, measured with radioimmunoassay, was later reported to occur during pneumoperitoneum in man.[50] This finding was confirmed in a larger study by others.[51] A 5-fold increase in plasma AVP was recorded in 50 per cent of the patients, using carbon dioxide pneumoperitoneum with intra-abdominal pressures of only 6 to 10 mm Hg. This increase in plasma AVP was not associated with changes in cardiopulmonary function, except for a significant increase in central venous and right atrial pressures. Several research groups suggested that intrathoracic pressure receptors mediate AVP release during pneumoperitoneum.[52–55]

Vasopressin regulates urine flow and therefore much of the body's water balance.[56] A normal adult human kidney is capable of producing urine concentrated to 1200 mosMol/kg of water at a flow of 0.5 ml/min. In the absence of AVP, as in diabetes insipidus, the kidney is unable to concentrate the urine, which flows at a rate of 15 to 20 ml/min with a concentration of only 30 mosMol/kg of water. AVP is currently considered to regulate certain channels in the plasma membrane of the kidney's convoluted tubules and collecting ducts.[56] Following reaction with specific AVP receptors on the "blood" side of the cell, cyclic adenosine monophosphate is generated, which activates a protein kinase that phosphorylates a membrane protein on the "luminal" side of the cell. This protein renders the membrane more water permeable. Plasma osmolality is considered to be the most important determinant of AVP release under physiologic conditions.[57]

AVP has long been known to reduce blood flow in the splanchnic circulation.[58] This property of the peptide has made it useful in the treatment of bleeding esophageal varices. AVP is believed to exert its effect by constriction of splanchnic arteries.[59] The peptide has also been demonstrated to cause relaxation of isolated portal veins,[60] which may contribute to the reduction in portal venous pressure induced by AVP.

POSSIBLE HAZARDS WITH PNEUMOPERITONEUM: AREAS FOR FUTURE RESEARCH

There is a potential risk of functional impairment for three organs within the abdominal cavity, i.e., the liver, the kidneys, and the gut, during increased intra-abdominal pressure, particularly with a concomitant release of AVP. These organs are briefly discussed to suggest some areas where research efforts should be directed to fully evaluate the risks associated with pneumoperitoneum.

Kidney

Animal experiments have demonstrated that increasing intra-abdominal pressure to 15 mm Hg induces oliguria while intra-abdominal pressure of 30 mm Hg is associated with anuria.[61,62] Tension ascites caused by liver disease is known to adversely affect kidney function[63–65] and has been proposed to be the pathophysiologic cause of hepatorenal syndrome.[63,66] Following laparocentesis that lowered intra-abdominal pressure from 35 to 15 mm Hg, glomerular filtration rate, renal plasma flow, and urine production increased dramatically.[63] Long-term improvement of kidney function was obtained by means of LeVeen peritoneovenous shunts in six patients in the same study. In a small sample of trauma patients with hemorrhage within the abdominal cavity, polyuria and restoration of kidney function were obtained by surgical decompression of the abdomen.[62] Whether the impairments of renal function described previously were caused by increased intra-abdominal pressure restricting renal vein blood flow, by an increase in circulating AVP with maximal antidiuretic stimulus, or by the combination of these events remains to be investigated.

Liver and Intestines

Several hours of elevated intra-abdominal pressure, associated with increased plasma levels of AVP, as can occur during long laparoscopic sessions, probably reduce hepatic and intestinal oxygenation because of constriction of the splanchnic arteries. This reduces portal blood flow, which is normally around 1000 to 1200 ml/min in the adult liver, contributing 70 per cent of the oxygen supply to the liver.[67] Portal vein pressure, normally about 7 mm Hg,[67] is at least doubled during pneumoperitoneum, a feature that further impairs portal blood flow. These possible adverse effects of pneumoperitoneum on hepatic parenchymal oxygenation deserve further investigation. Similarly, the combined effects of elevated intra-abdominal pressure and increased AVP levels may be hazardous for the intestinal circulation, at least in subjects with occlusive atherosclerotic lesions of the main intestinal arteries.

OTHER FACTORS OF SURGICAL INTEREST

Venous Return

Venous return from the lower extremities is compromised by pneumoperitoneum, although counteracted by a steep Trendelenburg tilt. With laparoscopic procedures in the upper part of the abdomen, however, a reverse Trendelenburg position is preferred. Thus, reduced venous return from the lower extremities may render the patient susceptible to development of deep vein thrombosis in the lower leg. Whether or not prophylactic measures against thromboembolism should be undertaken has not been stated in a number of recent articles on laparoscopic surgery.[1,68,69]

Postoperative Ileus

Postoperative ileus is a common and sometimes troublesome problem following conventional abdominal surgery. This type of bowel paralysis, mainly affecting the large bowel, is thought to result from sympathetic inhibition by peritoneal pain reflexes.[70] It has been claimed that ileus is less of a problem after laparoscopic procedures.[71] Less peritoneal trauma may be expected to cause a decreased neural response, resulting in less gut motility inhibition. However, a number of studies, both in animals and man, reveal that postoperative ileus is independent of the degree of bowel manipulation and of the duration of surgery.[72-76] Further studies are clearly required to document the influence of different laparoscopic surgical procedures on postoperative gut motility.

Peritoneal Inflammation

A few publications deal with the problem of pain after laparoscopic procedures.[77,78] Since nonsteroidal anti-inflammatory drugs are effective in controlling pain following laparoscopy, the authors speculate that peritoneal inflammation is an important cause of postoperative pain. Peritoneal biopsies 2 to 3 days after laparoscopy with carbon dioxide pneumoperitoneum showed vascular and neural damage with bleeding and neuromata formation. This could, in theory, predispose to the formation of peritoneal adhesions. However, in a recent study patients who had conventional and laparoscopic appendectomies underwent laparoscopy again after 3 months. Significantly fewer peritoneal adhesions were seen in patients who had laparoscopic surgery.[79]

Summary and Conclusions

Pneumoperitoneum at intra-abdominal pressures of 15 to 20 mm Hg has a number of well defined effects on respiration and circulation. A pressure increase within the abdominal cavity, particularly in combination with the Trendelenburg position, reduces functional residual capacity, total lung volume, and lung compliance. Pneumoperitoneum increases arterial and central venous pressures by squeezing blood out of the abdominal viscera, presumably resulting in increased cardiac output, again further reinforced by the head-down tilt position of the patient. The use of carbon dioxide for pneumoperitoneum results in hypercapnia and acidosis. This is easily compensated for by increased ventilation. In patients with impaired lung function, however, this may not be possible. In a recently reported case this problem necessitated the conversion of a laparoscopic cholecystectomy to a conventional laparotomy. Thus, the ideal gas or gas mixture for pneumoperitoneum is still not at hand. Helium is probably not the solution due to its poor blood solubility and high cost.

Pneumoperitoneum, at relatively low intra-abdominal pressures of 6 to 10 mm Hg, is associated with the release of vasopressin into the circulation. The main function of this posterior pituitary hormone is to regulate the body's water balance by concentrating urine. Furthermore, it reduces splanchnic blood flow by constricting splanchnic arteries. Raised plasma levels of vasopressin, in combination with possible mechanical effects of elevated intra-abdominal pressure, may therefore adversely affect kidney function and put the liver and gut at risk for reduced oxygenation.

These effects of pneumoperitoneum should be taken into consideration when selecting laparoscopic surgery of longer duration for older or otherwise physically compromised patients. Close cooperation between the surgeon and anesthesiologist is mandatory; together they should master the diagnosis and treatment of sudden complications, particularly gas embolism.

REFERENCES

1. Grace PA, Quereshi A, Coleman J, et al. Reduced postoperative hospitalization after laparoscopic cholecystectomy. Br J Surg 1991; 78:160–162.
2. Veress J. Neues instrument zur ausfuhrung von brust- und bauchpunktionen. Dtsch Med Wochenschr 1938; 41:1480–1481.

3. Johnson WC. Preoperative progressive pneumoperitoneum in preparation for repair of large hernias of the abdominal wall. Am J Surg 1972; 124:63–68.
4. Raynor RW, DelGuerico LRM. Update on the use of preoperative pneumo-peritoneum prior to the repair of large hernias of the abdominal wall. Surg Gynecol Obstet 1985; 161:367–371.
5. Coopwood RW, Smith RJ. Treatment of large ventral and scrotal hernias using preoperative pneumoperitoneum. J Natl Med Assoc 1989; 81:402–404.
6. Timberlake GA, Ochsner MG, Powell RW. Diagnostic pneumoperitoneum in the pediatric patient with a unilateral inguinal hernia. Arch Surg 1989; 124:721–723.
7. Etches RC. Hyperbaric oxygen and CO_2 embolism. Can J Anaesth 1989; 36:270–271.
8. Graff TD, Arbegast NR, Phillips OC, et al. Gas embolism: A comparative study of air and carbon dioxide as embolic agents in the systemic venous system. Am J Obstet Gynecol 1959; 78:259–265.
9. Kunkler A, King H. Comparison of air, oxygen and carbon dioxide embolization. Ann Surg 1959; 149:95–99.
10. Leighton TA, Bongard FS, Liu S-Y, et al. Comparative cardiopulmonary effects of helium and carbon dioxide pneumoperitoneum. Surg Forum 1991; 42:485–487.
11. McDonald and Wann, eds. In: Physiological Aspects of Anesthetics and Inert Gases, London, Academic Press, 1978, p 254.
12. Chamberlain G, Carron Brown J. Gynecological Laparoscopy. The Report of the Working Party of the Confidential Enquiry into Gynecological Laparoscopy. London, Royal College of Gynecologists, 1978.
13. Bruhl W. Comparisons of laparoscopy and liver biopsy under vision, the results of a survey. Germ Med Monthly 1967; 12:31–32.
14. DePlater RMH, Jones ISC. Non-fatal carbon dioxide embolism during laparoscopy. Anesth Intensive Care 1989; 17:359–361.
15. Gottlieb JD, Ericsson JA, Sweet RB. Venous air embolism, a review. Anesth Analg 1965; 44:773–779.
16. Whitby JD. Early cases of air embolism. Anesthesia 1964; 19:579–584.
17. Adornato DC, Gildenberg PL, Ferrario CM. Pathophysiology of intravenous air embolism in dogs. Anesthesiology 1978; 49:120–127.
18. Root B, Levy M, Pollack S, et al. Gas embolism death after laparoscopy delayed by trapping in portal circulation. Anaesth Analg 1978; 57:232–237.
19. Alvaran SB, Toung JK, Graff TE, et al. Venous air embolism: Comparative merits of external cardiac massage, intracardiac aspiration and left lateral decubitus position. Anesth Analg 1978; 57:166–170.
20. Edwards JE. Congenital malformations of the heart and great vessels: Malformations of the atrial septal complex. In Gould SE, ed. Pathology of the Heart. Springfield, IL, Charles C Thomas, 1968, p 262.
21. Östman PL, Pantle-Fisher FH, Faure EA, et al. Circulatory collapse during laparoscopy. J Clin Anesth 1990; 2:129–132.
22. McGrath BJ, Zimmerman JE, Williams JF, et al. Carbon dioxide embolism treated with hyperbaric oxygen. Can J Anaesth 1989; 36:586–589.
23. Brown DR, Fishburne JI, Robertson VO, et al. Ventilatory and blood gas changes during laparoscopy with local anesthesia. Am J Obstet Gynecol 1976; 124:741–745.
24. Khan I, Devroey P, Van den Berg M, et al. The effect of pneumoperitoneum gases on fertilization, cleavage and pregnancy in human in-vitro fertilization and gamete intra-Fallopian transfer. Hum Reprod 1989; 4:323–326.
25. Ciofolo MJ, Clergue F, Seebacher J, et al. Ventilatory effects of laparoscopy under epidural anesthesia. Anesth Analg 1990; 70:357–361.
26. Nunn JF. Applied Respiratory Physiology, 2nd ed. London, Butterworths, 1977, pp 63–93.
27. Wilcox S, Vandam LD. Alas, poor Trendelenburg and his position! A critique of its uses and effectiveness. Anesth Analg 1988; 67:574–578.
28. Hodgson C, McClelland RMA, Newton JR. Some effects of the peritoneal insufflation of carbon dioxide at laparoscopy. Anesthesia 1970; 25:382–390.
29. Motew M, Ivankovich AD, Bieniarz J, et al. Cardiovascular effects and acid-base and blood gas changes during laparoscopy. Am J Obstet Gynecol 1973; 115:1002–1012.
30. Marshall RL, Jebson PJR, Davie IT, et al. Circulatory effects of carbon dioxide insufflation of the peritoneal cavity for laparoscopy. Br J Anaesth 1972; 44:680–684.
31. Versichelen L, Serreyn R, Rolly G, et al. Physiopathologic changes during anesthesia administration for gynecologic laparoscopy. J Reprod Med 1984; 29:697–700.
32. Brampton WJ, Watson RJ. Arterial to end-tidal carbon dioxide tension difference during laparoscopy. Anesthesia 1990; 45:210–214.
33. Liu S-Y, Leighton T, Davis I, et al. Prospective analysis of cardiopulmonary responses to laparoscopic cholecystectomy. J Laparoendosc Surg 1991; 1:241–246.
34. Wittgen CM, Andrus CH, Fitzgerald SD, et al. Analysis of the hemodynamic and ventilatory effects of laparoscopic cholecystectomy. Arch Surg 1991; 126:997–1001.
35. Doyle DJ, Mark PWS. Laparoscopy and vagal arrest. Anesthesia 1989; 44:448.
36. Harris MNE, Plantevin OM, Crowther A. Cardiac arrhythmias during anesthesia for laparoscopy. Br J Anaesth 1984; 56:1213–1217.
37. Cameron PA, Rosengarten PL, Johnson WR, et al. Tension pneumoperitoneum after cardiopulmonary resuscitation. Med J Aust 1991; 155:44–47.
38. Ralston C, Clutton-Brock TH, Hutton P. Tension pneumoperitoneum. Intensive Care Med 1989; 15:532–533.
39. Yip A, Lau WY, Wong KK. Tension pneumoperitoneum: An unusual urological cause. Br J Urol 1989; 64:199–200.
40. Burns JMA, Hart DM, Hughes RL, et al. Effects of nalodol on arrhythmias during laparoscopy performed under general anesthesia. Br J Anaesth 1988; 61:345–346.
41. Lip H, Delhaas E. Cardiovascular collapse during laparoscopy. Am J Obstet Gynecol 1990; 162:873.
42. Ivankovich AD, Miletich DJ, Albrecht RF, et al. Cardiovascular effects of intraperitoneal insufflation with carbon dioxide and nitrous oxide in the dog. Anesthesiology 1975; 42:281–287.
43. Kelman GR, Swapp GH, Smith I, et al. Cardiac output and arterial blood-gas tension during laparoscopy. Br J Anaesth 1972; 44:1155–1162.
44. Siekmann U, Dimler H. Veränderungen hämodynamisher Kenngrössen in den verschiedenen Phasen der Pelviskopie. Zentralbl Gynäkol 1989; 111:99–109.
45. Johannsen G, Andersen M, Juhl B. The effect of general anesthesia on the hemodynamic events during laparoscopy with CO_2-insufflation. Acta Anesthesiol Scand 1989; 33:132–136.
46. Moran WH, Miltenberger FW, Shuayb WA, et al. The

relationship of antidiuretic hormone secretion to surgical stress. Surgery 1964; 56:99–107.
47. Moran WH, Zimmermann B. Mechanisms of antidiuretic hormone (ADH) control of importance to the surgical patient. Surgery 1967; 62:639–644.
48. Husain MK, Manger WM, Rock TW, et al. Vasopressin release due to manual restraint in the rat: Role of body compression and comparison with other stressful stimuli. Endocrinology 1979; 104:641–644.
49. Ukai M, Moran WH, Zimmermann B. The role of visceral afferent pathways on vasopressin secretion and urinary excretory patterns during surgical stress. Ann Surg 1968; 168:16–28.
50. Punnonen R, Viinamäki O. Vasopressin release during laparoscopy: Role of increased intra-abdominal pressure. Lancet 1982; 1:175–176.
51. Herruzo SJA, Castellano G, Larrodera L, et al. Plasma arginine vasopressin concentration during laparoscopy. Hepatogastroenterology 1989; 36:499–503.
52. Douglas JE, Noon N. Pericardial tamponade and excessive secretion of antidiuretic hormone. South Med J 1983; 76:1327–1328.
53. Gauer OH, Henry JP, Sieker HO, et al. The effect of negative pressure breathing on urine flow. J Clin Invest 1954; 33:287–296.
54. Ledsome JR, Ngsee J, Wilson N. Plasma vasopressin concentration in the anesthetized dog before, during and after atrial distension. J Physiol 1983; 338:413–421.
55. Schulz HD, Fater DC, Sundet WD, et al. Reflexes elicited by acute stretch of atrial vs pulmonary receptors in conscious dogs. Am J Physiol 1982; 242:H1065-H1076.
56. Ramsay DJ. Posterior pituitary gland. *In* Greenspan FS, Forsham PH, eds. Basic and Clinical Endocrinology, 2nd ed. Los Altos, CA, Lange Medical Publishers, 1986, pp 132–134.
57. Hammer M, Ladefoged J, Olgaard K. Relationship between plasma osmolality and plasma vasopressin in human subjects. Am J Physiol 1980; 238:E313-E317.
58. Richardson PDI, Withrington PD. Liver blood flow. II. Effect of drugs and hormones on liver blood flow. Gastroenterology 1981; 81:356–375.
59. Granger DN, Richardson PDI, Kvietys PR, et al. Intestinal blood flow. Gastroenterology 1980; 78:837–863.
60. Hughes J, Vane JR. An analysis of the response of the isolated portal vein of the rabbit to electrical stimulation and to drugs. Br J Pharmacol 1967; 30:46–66.
61. Thorington JM, Schmidt CF. A study of urinary output and blood-pressure changes resulting in experimental ascites. Am J Med Sci 1923; 165:880–886.
62. Richards WO, Scowill W, Shin B, et al. Acute renal failure associated with increased intra-abdominal pressure. Ann Surg 1983; 197:183–87.
63. Cade R, Wagemaker H, Vogel S, et al. Hepatorenal syndrome. Studies of the effect of vascular volume and intraperitoneal pressure on renal and hepatic function. Am J Med 1987; 82:427–438.
64. Hecker R, Sherlock S. Electrolyte and circulatory changes in terminal liver failure. Lancet 1956; 2:1121–1125.
65. Papper S, Belsky JL, Bleifer KH. Renal failure in Laënnec's cirrhosis of the liver. I. Description of clinical and laboratory features. Ann Intern Med 1959; 51:759–773.
66. Mullane JF, Gliedman ML. Elevation of the pressure in the abdominal inferior vena cava as a cause of hepato-renal syndrome in cirrhosis. Surgery 1969; 59:1135–1146.
67. Sherlock S. *In* Diseases of the Liver and Biliary System, 7th ed. New York, Blackwell Scientific Publications, 1985, pp 135–136.
68. The Southern Surgeons Club. A prospective analysis of 1518 laparoscopic cholecystectomies. N Engl J Med 1991; 324:1073–1078.
69. Nathanson LK, Shimi S, Cuschieri A. Laparoscopic cholecystectomy: The Dundee technique. Br J Surg 1991; 78:155–159.
70. Livingston EH, Passaro EP. Postoperative ileus, a review. Dig Dis Sci 1990; 35:121–132.
71. Perissat J, Collet D, Belliard R, et al. Traitement laparoscopique par litotripsie intra-corporelle suivie de cholecystostomie ou cholecystectomie. Chirurgie 1990; 116:243–247.
72. Graber JN, Schulte WJ, Condon RE. The duration of postoperative ileus related to the extent and site of operative dissection. Surg Forum 1980; 31:141–144.
73. Rimback G, Cassuto J, Faxen A, et al. Effect of intra-abdominal bupivicaine instillation on postoperative colonic motility. Gut 1986; 27:170–175.
74. Condon RE, Covles VE, Schulte WJ, et al. Resolution of postoperative ileus in humans. Ann Surg 1986; 203:574–581.
75. Kewenter J, Kock NG. Studies on intestinal motility the first few days after partial gastrectomy and after cholecystectomy. Acta Chir Scand 1963; 125:248–253.
76. Noer T. Roentgenological transit time through the small intestine in the immediate postoperative period. Acta Chir Scand 1968; 124:557–580.
77. Gillberg LE, Harsten AS, Ståhl LB. The effect of diclofenac sodium on post laparoscopy pain. Anesthesiology 1991; 75:A21.
78. Comyn DJ. Minimising pain after laparoscopy. Presented at the 9th World Congress of Anesthesiologists, Washington DC, May 1988, A0004.
79. De Wilde RL. Good-bye to late bowel obstruction after appendectomy. Lancet 1991; 2:1012.

Chapter 7
Laparoscopy in the Pregnant Patient

Brock M. Bordelon
John G. Hunter

Since Hancock reported the first drainage of an appendiceal abscess in the puerperal period,[1] much discussion has taken place regarding the proper evaluation and care of disease requiring surgery in the pregnant patient. Recent advances in laparoscopic techniques, in particular the advent of laparoscopic cholecystectomy and appendectomy, add a new dimension to this dialogue.[2,3] However, enthusiasm for laparoscopic procedures in this population must be tempered by the scarcity of meaningful data regarding the safety and efficacy of laparoscopy in the pregnant patient. While technical limitations imposed by the gravid uterus can usually be overcome by an inventive laparoscopist, solid understanding of the physiologic effects of the pneumoperitoneum upon the uterus and fetus is still lacking. Nevertheless, diagnostic and therapeutic laparoscopy during pregnancy is being performed in carefully selected patients.[4,5] Before we endorse laparoscopic access to all pathologic conditions that require surgery in the pregnant patient, we must be aware of several technical and safety considerations regarding laparoscopy during pregnancy.

SAFETY AND TECHNICAL CONSIDERATIONS

Three issues central to a discussion of laparoscopy during pregnancy are: (1) How should one attain laparoscopic access without endangering the uterus or its blood supply during Veress needle or primary trocar placement? (2) What modifications in trocar placement must be made to allow smooth conduction of the procedure in the presence of an enlarged uterus? (3) What are the possible adverse effects of a sustained carbon dioxide (CO_2) pneumoperitoneum upon fetal physiology and blood flow?

Veress needle and primary trocar placement in the pregnant patient require careful consideration of the position of the uterus at various stages of pregnancy. During the first trimester, the gravid uterus lies in the pelvis and is unlikely to be injured by a needle or trocar placed near the umbilicus. By the beginning of the second trimester, the fundus of the uterus has risen above the pelvic brim to lie halfway between the symphysis pubis and umbilicus (Fig. 7-1). By the end of the second trimester, the uterine fundus lies well above

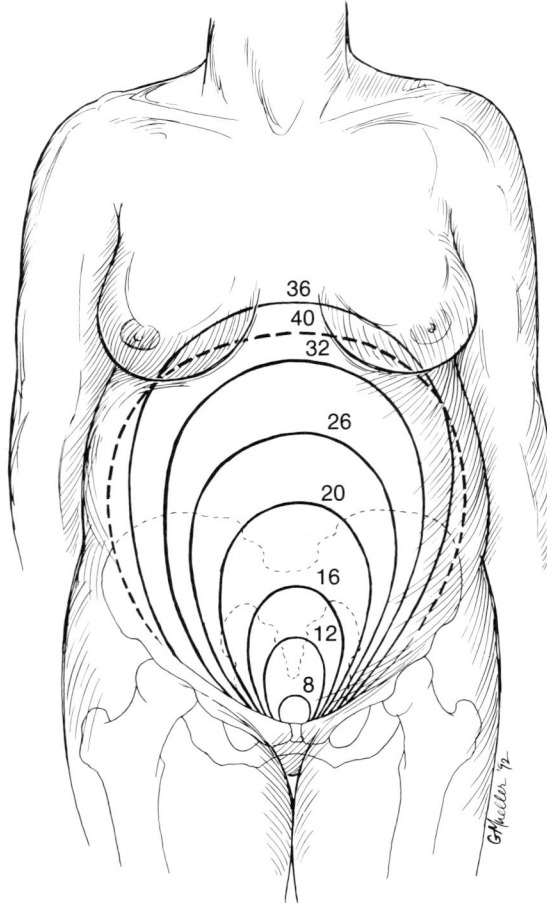

Figure 7-1. Enlargement of the uterus during pregnancy from the 8th week of gestation to term.

general, ports should be placed higher on the abdominal wall, with the cephalad displacement dictated by uterine size. For laparoscopic cholecystectomy, this requires positioning the right anterior axillary trocar, as well as the telescope trocar in some situations, above the level of the umbilicus (Fig. 7-2). Placement of accessory trocars during laparoscopic appendectomy is dictated by uterine size as well as by the position of the appendix. Similar to the situation faced during laparoscopic cholecystectomy, this entails cephalad displacement of the accessory ports (Fig. 7-3). Localization of the appendix prior to accessory trocar placement facilitates their proper positioning.

A more complex problem is whether a CO_2 pneumoperitoneum of 15 mm Hg will impair blood delivery to the fetus or blood return from the fetus or alter the carbon dioxide tension in the fetus independent of maternal

the umbilicus. The Veress needle may therefore be safely placed through the umbilicus until about 16 to 18 weeks of gestation, but must be directed toward either axilla, rather than toward the pelvis. The primary trocar should then be placed well above the crest of the fundus, followed by placement of the remaining trocars under direct visualization. Alternatively, open laparoscopy with a blunt-tipped trocar can be performed at the umbilicus. Beyond approximately 20 weeks of gestation, the gravid uterus would prevent adequate visualization of the gallbladder or appendix in most patients.

Proper trocar placement is essential in any laparoscopic procedure to facilitate removal of the diseased organ. An enlarged uterus restricts the area available for trocar placement, and careful consideration must be given to precise trocar positioning in this setting. In

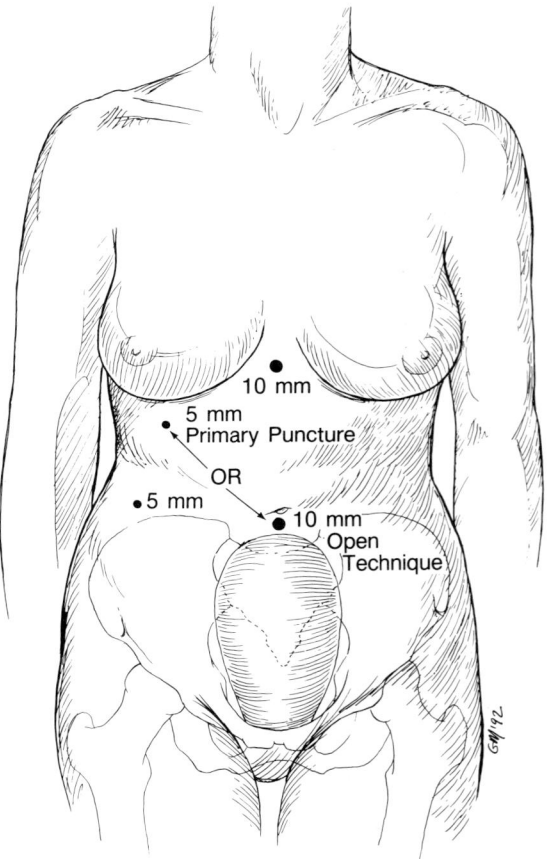

Figure 7-2. Trocar positioning for laparoscopic cholecystectomy during the second trimester of pregnancy.

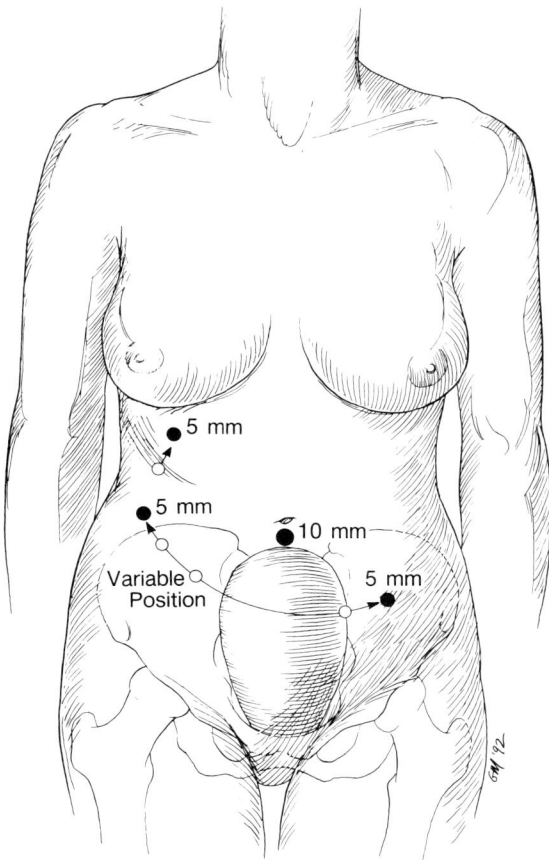

Figure 7-3. Trocar positioning for laparoscopic appendectomy during the second trimester of pregnancy. Position of the inferior trocar is dependent upon uterine size and appendiceal location.

carbon dioxide tension. The answers to these questions are currently unknown and will probably never be known for the human fetus. The safety of a CO_2 pneumoperitoneum in healthy adults has been evaluated extensively, with no adverse effects on cardiac output or acid-base status reported.[6,7] However, these early studies were performed on healthy young persons subjected to brief laparoscopic procedures. Careful monitoring of acid-base status and carbon dioxide tension (PCO_2) has been shown to be extremely important in less healthy individuals subjected to a prolonged CO_2 pneumoperitoneum.[8] Translation of these data to a pregnant woman undergoing a 2-hour laparoscopic cholecystectomy is difficult.

Brief elevation of intra-abdominal pressure to less than or equal to 15 mm Hg should not have significant deleterious effects upon maternal or fetal blood flow. The Valsalva maneuver, coughing, and straining all increase intra-abdominal pressure and are not correlated with fetal distress. However, prolonged maintenance of a pneumoperitoneum may aggravate impaired venous return resulting from the gravid uterus compressing the inferior vena cava with the patient in the recumbent position. Conscientious monitoring of maternal blood pressure during induction of the pneumoperitoneum and maintaining insufflation pressure between 10 to 12 mm Hg can help avoid serious consequences, and elevation of the right hip 30 degrees can alleviate uterine compression of the vena cava.[9]

Maternal hypercarbia and acidosis resulting from a prolonged CO_2 pneumoperitoneum may have significant detrimental effects upon the fetus. Alterations in maternal acid-base status are reflected across the placenta, but the rate at which this occurs is unclear. Removal of fetal CO_2 by the placenta is rapid, and under normal conditions umbilical venous PCO_2 is 3 to 4 mm Hg higher than uterine venous PCO_2.[10] Nevertheless, it is conceivable that CO_2 absorption during a lengthy laparoscopic procedure could generate fetal acidosis. To avoid this possibility, compulsive monitoring of maternal end-tidal CO_2 is prudent in this setting. Because it has been shown that end-tidal CO_2 values may not accurately reflect PCO_2 and acid-base changes, monitoring of arterial blood gases may be warranted during longer procedures.[8]

Fetal heart rate has been shown to correlate with fetal distress during the perinatal period and may be of value to assess fetal well-being perioperatively, although this is unproven. We have therefore used fetal heart rate monitoring during induction of anesthesia and periodically throughout laparoscopic procedures as the only available method to detect fetal distress.[11] Bradycardia or tachycardia during or after peritoneal insufflation should prompt immediate evacuation of the pneumoperitoneum. If such heart rate alterations are reproduced with repeated insufflation, the laparoscopic procedure should be terminated.

With careful consideration, we feel that laparoscopic surgery can be safely undertaken during pregnancy with certain caveats. Laparoscopy is unlikely to be technically feasible past the 20th week of gestation because the uterus will obscure the operative field and prevent the creation of an adequate pneumoperitoneum. Insufflation pressure should be kept less than or equal to 12 mm Hg to prevent significant alterations in maternal or placental blood flow. Careful end-tidal CO_2 and, in certain circumstances, arterial blood gas monitoring is essential. Finally, fetal heart rate monitoring is helpful as the only noninvasive means to assess fetal well-being.

We have gathered some preliminary data regarding the effects of a CO_2 pneumoperitoneum upon the fetus in studies performed upon pregnant sheep. At 100 days of gestation, fetal sheep have reached the end of the second trimester and weigh between 1000 and 1500 g; their physiology and size are similar to the human fetus of a similar gestational age. Prior to pneumoperitoneum creation, arterial and central venous pressure lines were placed in both the fetus and ewe, and continuous end-tidal CO_2 monitoring was performed upon the ewe. Two abdominal trocars were placed in the ewe, one connected to an insufflator and the other to a pressure transducer. Fetal and maternal arterial blood gases and heart rate were monitored during induction and maintenance of both a CO_2 and a nitrous oxide (N_2O) pneumoperitoneum (Table 7-1).

Several interesting observations were made with this experimental model. No fetal hypoxia was noted, and fetal pH and PCO_2 closely followed maternal parameters; direct absorption of CO_2 by the fetus was minimal. Use of N_2O produced less prominent maternal and fetal acid-base disturbances. No hyper- or hypotension was seen with a pneumoperitoneum created with either agent. However, fetal tachycardia was seen with a CO_2 pneumoperitoneum of greater than 10 mm Hg, while no tachycardia was experienced in the presence of a N_2O pneumoperitoneum. When the same experiments were performed upon a stressed fetus, induction of a CO_2 pneumoperitoneum precipitated reversible bradycardia upon initial insufflation. Upon reinsufflation, an irreversible bradycardia was experienced, followed by fetal demise. Based upon these preliminary investigations, we have concluded that limited, yet demonstrable, alterations in the physiology of the normal fetus are seen with the creation of a pneumoperitoneum, and these alterations are less prominent when nitrous oxide is used as the insufflation agent. Additionally, monitoring for fetal decelerations appears to be important, because the pneumoperitoneum may contribute to the demise of a stressed fetus.

Several critical questions regarding the safety of laparoscopic surgery during pregnancy remain unanswered. Animal studies are needed that focus on carbon dioxide absorption and elimination as well as alterations in maternal and fetal blood flow in the presence of a CO_2 pneumoperitoneum. In addition, the optimal method of perioperative fetal monitoring has yet to be identified. Until these problems are resolved satisfactorily, pregnant patients must be informed that the effects of the pneumoperitoneum upon the fetus are unknown.

SPECIFIC PROCEDURES

Currently, there are three frequent indications for laparoscopy in the pregnant patient: diagnosis and management of ectopic pregnancy, evaluation of right lower quadrant pain, and cholecystectomy. The vast majority of experience with laparoscopy during pregnancy has been gained with the diagnosis, and more recently treatment, of ectopic pregnancy. Before applying laparoscopic techniques to biliary tract and appendiceal disease in pregnancy, the general surgeon must be familiar with the gynecologic literature.

ECTOPIC PREGNANCY

For several years, gynecologists have been using laparoscopy as an aid in the diagnosis

Table 7-1. Effects of the Pneumoperitoneum upon Fetal and Maternal Physiology in a Pregnant Sheep Model

Intra-Abdominal Pressure and Ventilator Settings	Ewe		Fetus	
	pH	PCO_2	pH	PCO_2
0, TV-750, RR-8	7.40	34	7.35	44
15 mm Hg CO_2, TV-750, RR-8	7.33	44	7.27	54
15 mm Hg CO_2, TV-1000, RR-10	7.43	30	7.35	44
15 mm Hg N_2O, TV-750, RR-8	7.39	36	7.37	41

of suspected extrauterine pregnancy.[12] Laparoscopic evaluation of suspected ectopic pregnancy is highly accurate and has drastically reduced the rate of incorrect diagnosis at laparotomy since its introduction.[13]

When extrauterine pregnancy is encountered at laparoscopy, therapy can be undertaken in most cases without resorting to laparotomy. The first laparoscopic evacuation of a tubal pregnancy was reported by Shapiro and Adler in 1973,[14] and many large series have since been published confirming the safety of this approach.[15,16] Magos and co-workers[17] successfully treated 24 of 25 ectopic pregnancies, including several that had ruptured, with laparoscopic salpingotomy, salpingectomy, or salpingooophorectomy. Successful laparoscopic management of ruptured ectopic pregnancy requires hemodynamic stability, a hemoperitoneum that does not impair visualization, and proficiency with endoscopic suturing techniques.

APPENDICITIS

Appendicitis is the most common nongynecological cause of acute abdomen during pregnancy, with an estimated frequency of 1 case of acute appendicitis per 1500 pregnancies.[18] Significant complications of appendicitis in pregnancy was recognized early in this century by Babler,[19] who reported maternal and fetal mortality rates of 24 and 40 per cent, respectively, in a review of more than 200 cases. Early operative intervention is paramount, as the risk of fetal loss is dramatically higher in the presence of perforation.[9,20,21]

Accurate preoperative diagnosis of appendicitis during pregnancy is notoriously difficult for several reasons. As was demonstrated by Baer in 1932, the appendix is displaced cephalad and laterally and its tip rotates counterclockwise as the uterus enlarges.[22] By the 8th month of gestation, the appendix lies well above the iliac crest in 93 per cent of patients (Fig. 7-4). Additionally, the gravid uterus lifts the abdominal wall away from the abdominal viscera, and findings associated with inflammation of the parietal peritoneum may be absent.[20] The difficulty encountered in this setting is reflected by an incorrect diagnosis at laparotomy rate that ranged from 20 to greater than 40 per cent.[9,23]

Laparoscopy has been proposed as a method to increase diagnostic accuracy in the pregnant patient with right lower quadrant pain. Much success has already been found with laparoscopy as an aid in the diagnosis of appendicitis in young women of reproductive age, a group in whom diagnosis is notoriously inaccurate.[24,25] Proponents of diagnostic laparoscopy in this setting note that when the diagnosis is found to be incorrect at laparotomy and a normal appendix is removed, a complication rate approaching 15 per cent may be expected.[26,27] Although the rate of fetal loss resulting from incorrect diagnosis at laparotomy in the pregnant patient is disputed, it remains an important consideration.[25,28] Diagnostic laparoscopy can potentially prevent unnecessary appendectomy in the pregnant patient, as well as prevent a delay in diagnosis of appendicitis, both of which increase the rate of fetal loss.

Spirtos et al.,[29] reported on the use of laparoscopy as an aid in the diagnosis of appendicitis in 13 pregnant women. All patients were in the first trimester of pregnancy, and all had successful laparoscopic visualization

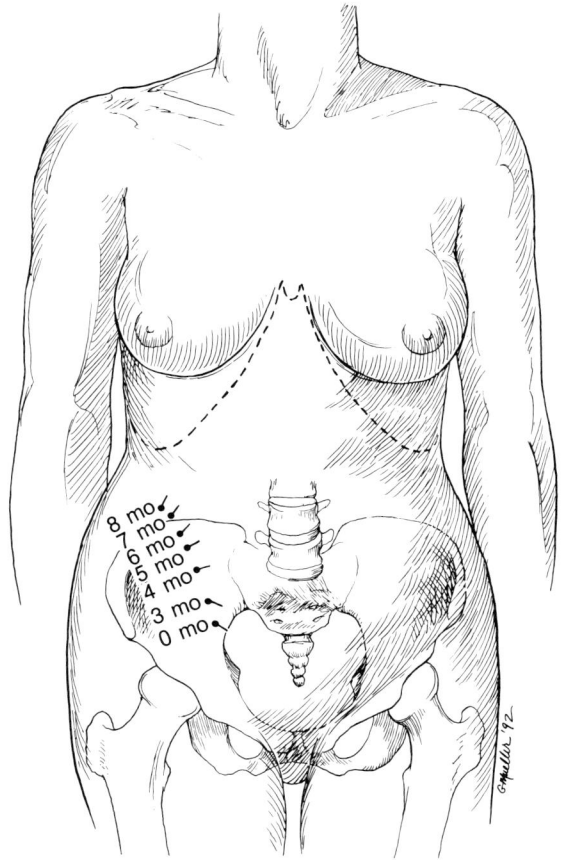

Figure 7-4. Positional changes of the appendix during pregnancy.

of the appendix. Twelve patients had appendicitis confirmed by laparoscopy and underwent open appendectomy, and one patient with a normal appearing appendix recovered without further intervention. No maternal complications and no fetal losses occurred in this group. The authors point out that diagnostic laparoscopy is technically feasible even in the advanced stages of gestation with the use of open laparoscopy. In the latter stages of pregnancy, diagnostic laparoscopy may also be helpful in localizing the optimal incision site for removal of an inflamed appendix.

Laparoscopic appendectomy, first performed in 1982,[3] is technically possible in the pregnant patient, at least in the early stages of pregnancy before the uterus rises out of the pelvis. In 1990, Tamir et al.[25] reported a single case of laparoscopic appendectomy during the first trimester, although no follow-up data were given. In the same year, Schriber[30] reported laparoscopic appendectomy in six pregnant women without maternal or fetal complications. These anecdotal reports support the notion that laparoscopic appendectomy is possible during pregnancy. Timely diagnosis may be an even more important advantage of diagnostic evaluation of the pregnant patient, as "the mortality of appendicitis complicating pregnancy is the mortality of delay."[19]

Technical Considerations in Laparoscopic Appendectomy

Optimal visualization of the appendix is difficult at times even during standard open exploration in the pregnant patient, as the uterus intrudes upon the operative field and the incision is frequently misplaced. Optimal trocar positioning is aided by locating the appendix with the telescope prior to inserting the accessory trocars; in general, the accessory ports will be placed more cephalad during the second trimester to avoid injury to the gravid uterus (see Fig. 7-3). Elevation of the right flank 30 degrees is helpful in appendiceal exposure during the open procedure and may be similarly beneficial during a laparoscopic procedure.[9,31] If an acutely inflamed appendix is discovered, rapid removal can be facilitated with the use of new laparoscopic linear stapling devices. With laparoscopic exploration, there is no obligation to remove a normal appendix. The appropriate course of action will depend upon the circumstances of the individual patient.

CHOLECYSTECTOMY

Biliary tract disease is relatively frequent in pregnancy, possibly reflecting the decreased gallbladder emptying and increased bile saturation with cholesterol seen with pregnancy. Conservative management of biliary colic or acute cholecystitis is generally espoused, though intractable symptoms or complications necessitate cholecystectomy between 1 and 6 times per 10,000 pregnancies.[32,33]

An aggressive surgical approach has been recommended by Dixon et al.,[34] who found a higher rate of fetal loss in patients treated nonoperatively than in those undergoing elective cholecystectomy. In the Mayo Clinic series of 20 pregnant patients undergoing cholecystectomy, only one spontaneous abortion occurred 42 days following a first trimester operation.[33] A similar experience was reported by Printen and Ott,[35] who performed cholecystectomy in four patients during the second trimester without fetal loss. Friley and Douglas[36] reviewed eight pregnant patients with biliary tract disease who were managed operatively; six delivered viable infants, while two were lost to follow-up. Despite their successes, all of the authors mentioned above recommend conservative, nonoperative management as first line therapy.

The acceptance of laparoscopic cholecystectomy as a safe, effective, and superior alternative to traditional open cholecystectomy in nonpregnant patients has been overwhelming.[37] Pregnancy, however, is considered by some authors to be an absolute contraindication to laparoscopic cholecystectomy.[2,38] The possible adverse effects of a sustained CO_2 pneumoperitoneum on fetal physiology are poorly understood. As the uterus rises above the level of the umbilicus after the 20th week of gestation, trocar positioning and optimal visualization become difficult. In addition, there is at least a theoretical concern that maintaining intra-abdominal pressure in the range of 10 to 15 mm Hg could have an adverse effect upon placental blood flow.

Despite these concerns, case reports and small series of laparoscopic cholecystectomy in pregnant patients are beginning to appear in the literature. Swedish investigators recently published a report of a successful laparoscopic cholecystectomy during the 22nd week of gestation, subsequently followed by the delivery of a healthy term infant.[5] The largest series to date was reported by Soper et al.,[11] who successfully performed laparoscopic cholecystectomy in five women, all in the second trimester of pregnancy, without maternal or fetal morbidity.

Most authors agree that when elective cholecystectomy is necessary during pregnancy the optimal time to operate is during the second trimester.[11,33] By that stage, the peak period of spontaneous abortion has passed, organogenesis is complete, the induction of premature labor may be less likely, and the uterus is not sufficiently large to encroach upon the operative field.[33,39] Liberal use of therapeutic tocolysis has yielded significant success in controlling premature labor in these patients, although the usefulness of prophylactic tocolytic therapy is debatable.[40,41] Certainly, the same considerations should be applied to laparoscopic cholecystectomy in the pregnant patient.

Technical Considerations in Laparoscopic Cholecystectomy

In trocar positioning, illustrated in Figure 7-2, one must take into consideration the distance between the uterus and the planned operative field. By late in the second trimester of gestation, the uterus lies well above the umbilicus. At that point, the uterus would restrict telescope maneuverability and sufficiently increase intra-abdominal pressure to prevent the creation of an adequate pneumoperitoneum. Cholangiography should either be omitted from the procedure or performed with shielding to prevent fetal exposure to ionizing radiation. Laparoscopic ultrasound is another alternative for imaging the bile duct without risking ionizing radiation.

PROSPECTS FOR THE FUTURE

As was alluded to earlier, much basic scientific investigation needs to be completed before laparoscopic cholecystectomy or appendectomy is recommended for all pregnant patients. As more experience is gained, however, it is likely that laparoscopic surgery will be safely performed during the first two trimesters of gestation. Diagnostic laparoscopy, already used in the diagnosis of potential ectopic pregnancy, may be useful in the evaluation of the pregnant trauma patient in order to avoid unnecessary laparotomy or abdominal computed tomographic scanning. Laparoscopic gynecologic procedures during pregnancy have also been reported.[4] However, beyond the more common procedures of cholecystectomy and appendectomy, elective laparoscopic surgery, like all elective operations during pregnancy, should be limited in the pregnant patient.

REFERENCES

1. Hancock H. Disease of the appendix coeci cured by operation. Lancet 1848; 2:380–382.
2. Zucker KA, Bailey RW, Gadacz TR, Imbembo AL. Laparoscopic guided cholecystectomy. Am J Surg 1991; 161:36–44.
3. Semm K. Endoscopic appendectomy. Endoscopy 1983; 15:59–64.
4. Nezhat F, Nezhat C, Silfen SL, Fehnel SH. Laparoscopic ovarian cystectomy during pregnancy. J Laparoendosc Surg 1991; 1:161–164.
5. Arvidsson D, Gerdin E. Laparoscopic cholecystectomy during pregnancy. Surg Laparosc Endosc 1991; 1:193–194.
6. Marshall RL, Jebson PJR, Davie IT, Scott DB. Circulatory effects of carbon dioxide insufflation of the peritoneal cavity for laparoscopy. Br J Anaesth 1972; 44:680–684.
7. Motew M, Ivankovich AD, Bienarz J, et al. Cardiovascular effects and acid-base and blood gas changes during laparoscopy. Am J Obstet Gynecol 1973; 115:1002–1012.
8. Wittgen CM, Andrus CH, Fitzgerald SD, et al. Analysis of the hemodynamic and ventilatory effects of laparoscopic cholecystectomy. Arch Surg 1991; 126:997–1001.
9. Horowitz MD, Gomez GA, Santiesteban R, et al. Acute appendicitis during pregnancy: Diagnosis and management. Arch Surg 1985; 120:1362–1367.
10. Battaglia FC, Meschia G. Fetal respiratory physiology. In Battaglia FC, Meschia G, eds. An Introduction to Fetal Physiology. Orlando, FL, Academic Press, Inc, 1986; pp 175–195.
11. Soper NJ, Hunter JG, Petrie RH. Laparoscopic cholecystectomy during pregnancy. Surg Endosc 1992; 6:115–117.
12. Esposito JM. The laparoscope: An aid in the diagnosis of intact ectopic gestation. J Reprod Med 1972; 9:158–160.
13. Reich H, Freifeld ML, McGlynn F, Reich E. Laparoscopic treatment of ectopic pregnancy. Obstet Gynecol 1987; 69:275–279.
14. Shapiro HI, Adler DH. Excision of an ectopic pregnancy through the laparoscope. Am J Obstet Gynecol 1973; 117:290–291.
15. Pouly JL, Manhes H, Mage H, et al. Conservative laparoscopic treatment of 321 ectopic pregnancies. Fertil Steril 1986; 46:1093–1097.
16. DeCherney AH, Diamond MP. Laparoscopic salpingostomy for ectopic pregnancy. Obstet Gynecol 1987; 70:948–950.
17. Magos AL, Baumann R, Turnbull AC. Managing gynaecological emergencies with laparoscopy. Br Med J 1989; 299:371–374.

18. Babaknia A, Parsa H, Woodruff JD. Appendicitis during pregnancy. Obstet Gynecol 1977; 50:40–44.
19. Babler EA. Perforative appendicitis complicating pregnancy. JAMA 1908; 51:1310–1313.
20. Cunningham FG, McCubbin JH. Appendicitis complicating pregnancy. Obstet Gynecol 1975; 45:415–420.
21. Gomez A, Wood M. Acute appendicitis during pregnancy. Am J Surg 1979; 137:180–183.
22. Baer JL, Reis RA, Arens RA. Appendicitis in pregnancy with changes in position and axis of normal appendix. JAMA 1932; 98:1359–1364.
23. Saranson EL, Bauman S. Acute appendicitis in pregnancy. Difficulties in diagnosis. Obstet Gynecol 1963; 22:382–386.
24. Whitworth CM, Whitworth PW, Sanfillipo J, Polk HC. Value of diagnostic laparoscopy in young women with possible appendicitis. Surg Gynecol Obstet 1988; 167:187–190.
25. Tamir IL, Bongard FS, Klein SR. Acute appendicitis in the pregnant patient. Am J Surg 1990; 160:571–576.
26. Chang FC, Hogle HH, Welling DR. The fate of the negative appendix. Am J Surg 1973; 126:752–754.
27. Dunn EL, Moore EE, Elerding SE, et al. The unnecessary laparotomy for appendicitis—Can it be decreased? Am Surg 1982; 48:320–323.
28. Saunders P, Milton PJD. Laparotomy during pregnancy: An assessment of diagnostic accuracy and fetal wastage. Br Med J 1973; 3:165–167.
29. Spirtos NM, Eisenkop SM, Spirtos TW, et al. Laparoscopy—A diagnostic aid in cases of suspected appendicitis. Its use in women of reproductive age. Am J Obstet Gynecol 1987; 156:90–94.
30. Schriber JH. Laparoscopic appendectomy in pregnancy. Surg Endosc 1990; 4:100–102.
31. Weingold AB. Appendicitis in pregnancy. Clin Obstet Gynecol 1983; 26:801–809.
32. Landers D, Carmona R, Crombleholme W, Lim R. Acute cholecystitis in pregnancy. Obstet Gynecol 1987; 69:131–133.
33. Hill NM, Johnson CE, Lee RA. Cholecystectomy in pregnancy. Obstet Gynecol 1975; 46:291–295.
34. Dixon NP, Faddis DM, Silberman H. Aggressive management of cholecystitis during pregnancy. Am J Surg 1987; 154:292–294.
35. Printen KJ, Ott RA. Cholecystectomy during pregnancy. Am Surg 1978; 44:432–434.
36. Friley MD, Douglas G. Acute cholecystitis in pregnancy and the puerperium. Am Surg 1972; 38:314–317.
37. Peters JH, Ellison EC, Innes JT, et al. Safety and efficacy of laparoscopic cholecystectomy. A prospective analysis of 100 initial patients. Ann Surg 1991; 213:3–12.
38. Gadacz TR, Talamini MA, Lillemoe KD, Yeo CJ. Laparoscopic cholecystectomy. Surg Clin North Am 1990; 70:1249–1262.
39. Simon JA. Biliary tract disease and related surgical disorders during pregnancy. Clin Obstet Gynecol 1983; 26:810–821.
40. Allen JR, Helling TS, Langenfeld M. Intra-abdominal surgery during pregnancy. Am J Surg 1989; 158:567–569.
41. Hopkins MP, Duchol MA. Adnexal surgery in pregnancy. J Reprod Med 1986; 31:1035–1037.

Chapter 8
Complications

John L. Flowers
Karl A. Zucker
Robert W. Bailey

This chapter focuses on complications of laparoscopy and their management. The discussion is organized into two sections. The first section reviews the pertinent literature from the disciplines of gynecology and gastroenterology and discusses complications related to the general performance of laparoscopy. The second section concentrates on complications arising from the laparoscopic performance of specific general surgical procedures such as cholecystectomy, appendectomy, herniorrhaphy, and others. The available current literature is discussed and suggestions for management of particular complications are offered.

GENERAL MORBIDITY AND MORTALITY

Since the widespread adoption of operative laparoscopy by gynecologists in the late 1960s and early 1970s, a large volume of literature has been generated citing the safety and efficacy of the technique.

The information on laparoscopic morbidity and mortality arises from three main sources. The first of these are retrospective surveys taken by professional organizations, most notably the American Association of Gynecological Laparoscopists (AAGL). Annual surveys by this group have been conducted since 1973.[1] The second group of sources are several large literature reviews from both the United States and Europe.[2-5] Finally, there are impressive personal series compiled by several authors, which are widely quoted.[6,7] Table 8-1 is a summary of some of the largest series and their respective morbidity and mortality rates. Operative morbidity and mortality figures are well established, in the range of 4 per cent and less than 0.1 per cent, respectively.[8,10]

Despite the sheer volume of these data, several caveats are in order before the results can be extrapolated to general surgical procedures performed under laparoscopic guidance. Most data regarding laparoscopic complications arise from retrospective analyses and are therefore likely to underestimate the true incidence of complications. A 1984 prospective study of gastroenterologists in Dallas showed higher than usual major and minor morbidity rates of 2.3 and 5.1 per cent, respectively, with a 0.5 per cent mortality.[11] Poor response rates (often 20 to 40 per cent) from data such as the AAGL surveys may even further exaggerate the inherent inaccuracy of such studies.[10,12,13]

The majority of gynecologic laparoscopic procedures are performed on otherwise healthy young women.[8] Many general surgical procedures, on the other hand, are performed in a relatively older patient population who frequently have significant comorbid disease. In addition, longer and more

Table 8-1. Review of Large Laparoscopic Surveys

Series	Number of Cases	Major Complications (%)	Total Complications (%)	Death Rate (per 100,000 Cases)
Reidel et al.[3]	292,462	0.19	0.19	5.1
Phillips et al.[9] (1975 National Survey)	298,029	0.46 (D) 0.37 (S)	0.41	5.2 (D) 2.5 (S)
Phillips et al.[12] (1975 AAGL Survey)	117,705	0.31 (D) 0.28 (S)	0.29	4.2 (T)
Loffler and Pent[2]	32,719		2.40	
Henning[4]	36,207	0.18	0.87	66.0
	94,382			64.0
RCOG Inquiry[5]	50,247		3.50	8.0
Phillips et al.[13] (1982 AAGL Survey)	125,560	0.14 (S)	0.14	
Peterson et al.[10] (1988 AAGL Survey)	36,928	1.5	0.15	5.4

D, diagnostic; S, sterilization; T, total.

complex procedures have been made possible over the last 5 years by the development of video laparoscopy and more sophisticated instrumentation. The degree of surgical dissection and subsequent physiologic alteration encountered with current laparoscopic procedures is therefore quite different from that which occurred during diagnostic laparoscopy or laparoscopic sterilization 20 years ago. It is anticipated that the types and frequency of complications will differ accordingly.

Interpretation of the existing data on laparoscopic complications presents other difficulties. Diagnostic and therapeutic procedures with different inherent morbidity are frequently grouped together. The definition of "major" and "minor" complications is often not specified or rates are not given. Furthermore, data from different centers around the world may not be applicable to American practice patterns; indications and operator experience sometimes differ markedly.[3,4,11] In spite of these drawbacks, the existing body of laparoscopic morbidity and mortality data provides a useful starting point for the evaluation of newer general surgical laparoscopic procedures. The most common complications of laparoscopy and their approximate frequency are listed in Table 8-2. Many of these specific complications will be discussed in the next sections.

ANESTHESIA-RELATED COMPLICATIONS

Local and regional anesthetic techniques have been used for more than 20 years with great success in gynecologic laparoscopic surgery. However, the duration and complexity of newer therapeutic laparoscopic procedures have made general anesthesia with endotracheal intubation the anesthesia of choice in most laparoscopic general surgical procedures. For this reason, the discussion will be limited to complications encountered during general anesthesia. A classification of anesthesia-related complications is given in Table 8-3.

Knowledge of the physiologic effects of carbon dioxide pneumoperitoneum is helpful in understanding the pathogenesis of potential complications, which may be broadly divided into cardiovascular and respiratory effects.

Cardiovascular effects are the sum of a va-

Table 8-2. Laparoscopic Complication Rate

Complication	Per Cent
Pneumoperitoneum complications	0.7
Bleeding	0.6
Perforation injuries	0.3
Electrical complications	0.2
Infection	0.1
Bowel burns	<0.1
Cardiac arrest	<0.1
Laparotomy rate	0.6

Modified from Phillips JM. Complications in laparoscopy. Int J Gynaecol Obstet 1977; 15:157–162.

Table 8-3. Anesthesia-Related Complications

Cardiovascular
   Electrocardiographic changes
   Arrhythmia
   Hypotension
   Cardiac Arrest

Pulmonary
   Aspiration of gastric contents
   Endobronchial intubation
   Pneumothorax/Pneumomediastinum
   Pulmonary edema
   Hypercarbia

---

riety of complex influences, which may vary during the course of a normal case. The usual effects are an increase in cardiac output, increased systolic and diastolic blood pressure, and a decrease in peripheral vascular resistance.[14]

Respiratory changes include a decrease in tidal volume and functional residual capacity from diaphragmatic elevation. Hypercarbia [increased arterial carbon dioxide tension ($PaCO_2$)] and resultant mild respiratory acidosis may also occur because of transperitoneal absorption of carbon dioxide.[15,16] These changes are seldom of clinical significance in healthy adults but may be potentially dangerous in patients with preexisting cardiopulmonary disease.[17]

Cardiovascular complications related to anesthesia include electrocardiographic changes, cardiac arrhythmia, hypotension, and cardiac arrest. Common electrocardiographic changes include left axis deviation, increased R-wave amplitude, and T-wave inversion. They are usually promptly reversed with evacuation of pneumoperitoneum and are believed to be caused by benign positional changes resulting from abdominal distention and diaphragm elevation.[18]

Cardiac arrhythmias are common during laparoscopy, occurring in up to 17 per cent of cases.[19] Frequently observed rhythms include premature supraventricular contractions, aberrant QRS conduction, and sinus tachycardia. Premature ventricular contractions, bigeminy, and fusion beats may also be seen. These latter rhythms may be early indications of hypoxia and should be observed carefully.

The exact mechanism of arrhythmia during laparoscopy is unclear. Contributing factors may include hypercarbia from carbon dioxide insufflation, inhalation anesthetics, and sympathetic stimulation from hypercarbia. Some data show a higher incidence of arrhythmia with carbon dioxide than with nitrous oxide.[19–21] Hypoxia, vagal stimulation, positional changes, and type of inhalation agent are also implicated as possible factors contributing to the occurrence of arrhythmias. Enflurane and isoflurane are less arrhythmogenic than halothane, which may increase the level of circulating catecholamines and precipitate abnormal cardiac rhythm.[22] Careful regulation of $PaCO_2$ with appropriate ventilation will prevent significant hypercarbia and usually control intraoperative cardiac arrhythmia.

Acute hypotension may occur during laparoscopy. The differential diagnosis includes arrhythmia caused by hypercarbia, vagal reflex, hemorrhage, gas embolism, and inferior vena cava compression caused by elevated intra-abdominal pressure.[20] Careful attention to intra-abdominal pressure and maintenance of adequate ventilation and intravascular volume will help to prevent this complication. Management of acute hypotension from the surgeon's perspective includes a rapid check of the abdomen for hemoperitoneum, immediate removal of all instruments and evacuation of the pneumoperitoneum, return of the patient to a neutral position, and a search for other causes.

Fortunately, cardiac arrest is a rare complication of laparoscopy. It occurs in approximately 0.03 per cent of cases.[8] Possible explanations include increased $PaCO_2$, catecholamine stimulation, gas embolism, and cardiac arrhythmia, especially with halothane sensitization of the myocardium.[23] Although rare, the occurrence of unexplained circulatory collapse in otherwise healthy individuals underscores the importance of appropriate patient monitoring during laparoscopy.

Potential pulmonary complications related to anesthesia include aspiration of gastric contents, endobronchial intubation, pneumothorax, and acute pulmonary edema. Aspiration occurs most frequently during induction, intubation, and extubation. Reflux of gastric contents and subsequent aspiration are much greater concerns during laparoscopy performed under local or regional anesthesia. Estimates of the incidence of clinically significant gastric reflux range from 0.002 to 0.2 per cent during elective procedures to as high as 20 per cent during emergency gynecologic laparoscopic procedures.[5,24,25] There is some evidence that this concern is more theoretical than real.[26] With the widespread use of general anesthesia and endotracheal intubation, the risk is minimized, although it is recognized that aspiration may occur in the presence of a cuffed endotracheal tube. Routine evacuation of stomach contents will decrease the likelihood of gross aspiration. Endobronchial intubation may lead to sudden intraoperative arterial oxygen desaturation. Upward displacement of the diaphragm, combined with steep Trendelenberg positioning, has been shown to alter the position of endotracheal tubes during laparoscopy.[27] This potentially serious complication may be avoided by awareness and a high index of suspicion. Some authors recommend taping the endotracheal tube at 19 to 20 cm (women) or 21 to 22 cm (men) from the angle of the mouth or using a shorter endotracheal tube.[14]

Pneumothorax and pneumomediastinum may occur during laparoscopy, but most cited references are case reports; a good estimate of the actual frequency does not exist.[28,29] In the absence of direct diaphragmatic trauma, the etiology of these conditions is unclear. Several potential explanations have been proposed. The most popular is that carbon dioxide, which gains access to the retroperitoneum, dissects cephalad into the thorax. Congenital defects or pores in the diaphragm that have not completely closed are also implicated. Pneumothorax may be observed, aspirated, or treated with tube thoracostomy, depending on the patient's symptoms. Pneumomediastinum is generally observed unless the patient is symptomatic. Parenteral administration of antibiotics is recommended until the carbon dioxide is reabsorbed, which usually occurs at 24 to 48 hours.[30]

Acute pulmonary edema, although infrequent, may occur during laparoscopic surgery. Underlying cardiopulmonary disease such as congestive heart failure, chronic obstructive pulmonary disease, or arrhythmia may be exacerbated during anesthesia and laparoscopy. Increased central venous pressure, the Trendelenberg position, fluid overload, transient hypoxia, and administration of narcotics may increase the chances for pulmonary edema. One should also be aware that sudden appearance of pulmonary edema may be the first sign of carbon dioxide gas embolism.[19]

FACTORS INFLUENCING THE INCIDENCE OF LAPAROSCOPIC COMPLICATIONS

A variety of factors combine to dramatically alter the surgeon's perception during laparoscopic surgery. First and most obvious is transposition of the operative view to a two-dimensional television monitor. Images are magnified and depth of field is reduced. This arrangement brings with it a loss of three-dimensional depth perception and other visual cues upon which the surgeon has come to rely. The surgeon is at the mercy of a complex chain of technology including a fiberoptic laparoscope, solid state video camera chip, light source, television monitor, and ancillary equipment such as videocassette recorders and thermal printers. Any of the links of this chain may malfunction at a critical moment and jeopardize a surgical procedure.

A second potential source of complications arises from laparoscopic instrumentation. Most laparoscopic instruments are unfamiliar to practicing general surgeons. They tend to be longer and more unwieldy and transmit less grasping strength than traditional instruments. The typical working distance from the operative field is approximately 18 inches, and fine movements of the instrument tips are greatly magnified by the laparoscope and video camera. Smaller incisions used for minimally invasive surgery deny access to the surgeon's hand and virtually eliminate tactile sensation and the valuable information it provides.

In addition, surgeons have had to work with instrumentation that was not designed for laparoscopic general surgical procedures. Procedure-specific instrumentation is expensive and is just now becoming widely available. Laparoscopic cholecystectomy was originally performed with gynecologic laparoscopic instruments, and it was quickly realized these instruments were insufficient for the task. Development of new instrumentation is proceeding rapidly, but a new set of problems is arising. The quality of laparoscopic trocars and instruments may vary widely among manufacturers, and standardization of operating port and instrument sizes has not yet occurred. These issues serve to further confuse the novice laparoscopic surgeon.

Coordination between surgeon and camera operator is also essential to the success of the procedure. Instruments must always be inserted into the peritoneal cavity under direct vision; "blind" insertion of instruments may lead to inadvertent visceral injury (Fig. 8-1). When video laparoscopic procedures are performed as a team, operative times and morale are likely to improve and the potential for complications is likely to decrease.

Patient selection is another issue that may

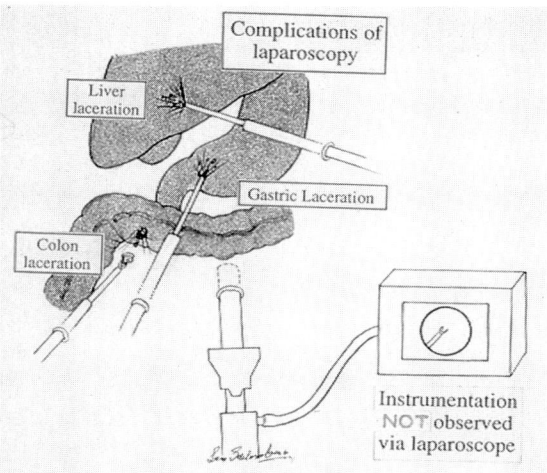

Figure 8-1. Potential complications that may occur with "blind" insertion of instruments into the peritoneal cavity.

have an impact on the incidence of complications during laparoscopy. As new laparoscopic procedures are rapidly developed, the practicing surgeon must acquire the necessary operative skills without the luxury of prolonged supervised training offered during surgical residency. One way to minimize the occurrence of complications is to avoid performing procedures on patients with absolute contraindications to laparoscopy and carefully consider those patients with relative contraindications. Absolute and relative contraindications to laparoscopy are listed in Table 8-4.

The issue of training is central to the discussion of complications of laparoscopy. Phillips[8] notes that operator experience is the primary determinant of the incidence of laparoscopic complications. His data show an inverse correlation between number of laparoscopic procedures performed and the incidence of complications, with significant decrements in the incidence of complications after performance of 50 and 100 laparoscopic procedures. An additional sharp decline in both the incidence of failed attempts at laparoscopy and the number of procedures requiring laparotomy was observed after performance of 250 procedures. A 1975 national survey corroborates these data; a significant progressive decline in complication rates was seen for surgeons performing 40 to 60 laparoscopic procedures, and an additional improvement was seen for those physicians performing 61 to 80 procedures.[9] Mintz[31] notes a similar trend correlating experience and fewer complications in a 1977 review of 99,204 laparoscopies performed in France.

COMPLICATIONS OF PNEUMOPERITONEUM

Choice of Insufflation Agent

Room air, oxygen, nitrous oxide, and carbon dioxide have all been used as agents for peritoneal insufflation during laparoscopy. Selection of an insufflating gas should take into account respiratory and cardiovascular side effects, ability to support combustion, cost, availability, and degree of peritoneal irritation.

Carbon dioxide has emerged as the agent of choice for general surgical and gynecologic laparoscopic procedures. It is readily available and inexpensive, suppresses combustion, and has a high solubility coefficient in blood, which may lessen the severity of gas embolization. Disadvantages of carbon dioxide include greater peritoneal irritation and subsequent postoperative discomfort than with nitrous oxide and a higher incidence of cardiac arrhythmia.[19]

The use of nitrous oxide is essentially limited to diagnostic laparoscopy under local anesthesia. Its advantages as an insufflating agent include a lower incidence of cardiac arrhythmia and an analgesic effect, which allows improved tolerance of pneumoperitoneum in the awake patient. Disadvantages of nitrous oxide include lower solubility in blood than carbon dioxide, which is theoretically worse in the event of gas embolism, and the ability to support combustion. This latter property contraindicates its use in the presence of electrocautery and laser energy, thereby all but eliminating its use in general surgical laparoscopic procedures.

Table 8-4. Contraindications to Laparoscopy

Absolute contraindications
    Generalized peritonitis
    Uncorrectable coagulopathy
Relative contraindications
    Inability to tolerate general anesthesia
    Prior abdominal surgery
    Carcinomatosis
    Minor bleeding disorders
    Pregnancy
    Morbid obesity

Extraperitoneal Insufflation

This complication includes subcutaneous emphysema and insufflation of the preperitoneal space, omentum, or mesentery (Fig. 8-2). Subcutaneous emphysema is relatively common during laparoscopy. It may occur anywhere along the abdomen or spread along any contiguous fascial planes, including the head and neck, thorax, back, and scrotum. Rarely, it may occur in conjunction with pneumothorax or pneumomediastinum.[32] Most cases are caused by improper positioning of the insufflation needle, but the condition may occur from leakage around a trocar site, especially if the trocar has been repeatedly dislodged and the area is traumatized. It has also been described in patients in whom intra-abdominal pressure is grossly elevated either intentionally or from insufflator malfunction. Leaning against the patient's abdomen during the procedure may also elevate intra-abdominal pressure. Despite its disconcerting appearance, subcutaneous emphysema is usually painless and resolves spontaneously. Some authors advocate aspiration of the gas pocket if symptoms occur, but this is usually unnecessary.[20]

Preperitoneal insufflation is a complication that may be difficult to detect (Fig. 8-3). Insufflation pressures may not be abnormally high and abdominal percussion may be sym-

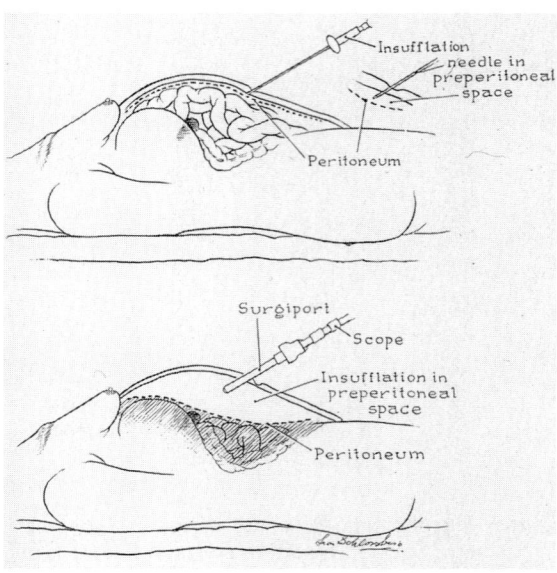

Figure 8-3. Illustration of the mechanism of preperitoneal insufflation. The tip of the Veress needle is accidentally placed in the preperitoneal space (*top*), and a large amount of gas is trapped in the preperitoneal space, which goes unrecognized until insertion of the laparoscope (*bottom*).

metric and tympanitic. The best means of identifying erroneous needle placement is instillation and subsequent recovery of saline injected through the Veress needle. The condition is generally diagnosed upon insertion of the laparoscope at which time the intact parietal peritoneum is seen. It must be recognized that the dislodged parietal peritoneum is quite close to underlying bowel, and the layer must be opened with care. The condition may be managed with aspiration of the gas pocket and reinsertion of the needle at another location. Alternatively, the peritoneal layer may be opened under direct vision with a laparoscopic scissors, or an open laparoscopy may be performed. Evacuation of the gas pocket by manual pressure on the abdominal wall is discouraged; it may exacerbate dissection of the gas into the retroperitoneum and distort retroperitoneal structures such as the ureters.

Omental and mesenteric insufflation also results from malposition of the insufflation needle or primary trocar. The condition is generally well tolerated as long as hemorrhage does not occur; however, there may be visual impairment of the operative field. Omental insufflation may be managed by dissection into the gas pocket under direct

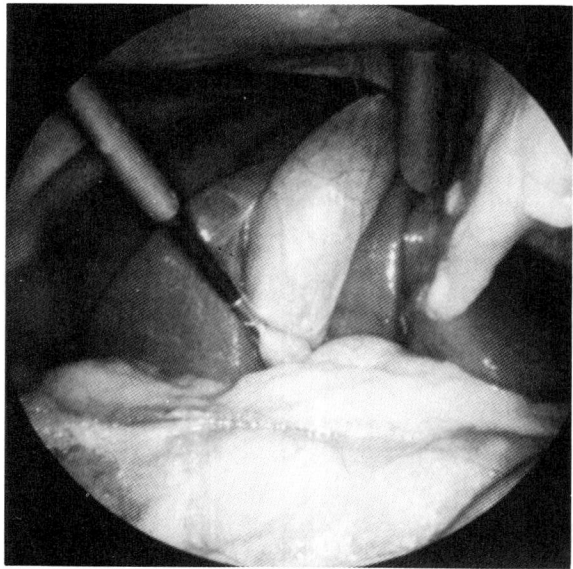

Figure 8-2. Inadvertent omental insufflation by a Veress needle during laparoscopic cholecystectomy.

vision to create a vent into the peritoneal cavity.

Needle and Trocar Injuries

Insertion of the Veress needle and trocars is responsible for a significant number of injuries during laparoscopy. Injuries to most portions of the gastrointestinal tract, genitourinary tract, and major vessels have been reported. The severity of these injuries ranges from inconsequential needle punctures to fatalities from hemorrhage and unrecognized bowel perforation.[33-36] Estimates of the combined incidence of Veress needle and trocar injuries are approximately 0.2 to 0.3 per cent.[2] A recent study from Germany reviewing laparoscopic data from 1983 through 1985 revealed that needle and trocar accidents to the gastrointestinal tract accounted for 38 per cent of all complications, which required repeated laparotomy or laparoscopy. Major vessel injury by the same mechanism was responsible for 23 per cent of repeated procedures.[37]

Some insight into these injuries was gained with a recent survey of Canadian gynecologists, reviewing 136,997 laparoscopies from 1985 through 1987.[38] A total of 274 injuries caused by needle and trocar insertion were reported. The true frequency of injury could not be determined from the survey data. Injuries to blood vessels were most common, followed in decreasing frequency by injuries to bowel, uterus, and abdominal wall. Of these injuries, 39.8 per cent were caused by the Veress needle, 37.9 per cent were caused by insertion of the primary trocar, and 22.2 per cent were caused by the secondary trocar. More injuries occurred with the group of surgeons who had not received laparoscopic training during residency and in situations in which difficulty was encountered during trocar insertion.

This data shows that 22.2 per cent of injuries in the series were caused by insertion of the secondary trocar. Complications caused by secondary trocar insertion should theoretically approach 0 since the trocar should always be inserted under direct vision. These and other data suggest that at least some insufflation needle and trocar injuries are preventable.[31,38]

A variety of methods have been suggested to minimize the occurrence of Veress needle and trocar insertion complications. Elevation of the abdominal wall with the surgeon's hand or towel clips provides resistance to needle and trocar insertion, but has never been shown to decrease the incidence of complications.[38] The patient should be placed in the Trendelenberg position to displace bowel from the pelvis. The insufflation needle should be inserted in the midline and directed caudally at an angle toward the hollow of the sacrum. The most important step is verification of an intraperitoneal location of the Veress needle.

Several manuevers are available to help ensure the proper location of the needle tip. Injection of saline with aspiration through the Veress needle is the single most reliable test. Intra-abdominal pressure should be monitored constantly during insufflation. Initial entry pressure should be less than or equal to 6 mm Hg. Gas insufflation should begin at 1 liter/min and intra-abdominal pressures should increase slowly to the desired level (10 to 15 mm Hg). High flow insufflation should not be used until an adequate pneumoperitoneum is established. Abdominal distention should be symmetric; asymmetric percussion tympany may indicate insufflation of bowel or the preperitoneal space. Loss of percussion dullness over the liver should occur as gas enters the peritoneal cavity. None of these methods is foolproof, however, and any irregularity should prompt a thorough reassessment of Veress needle placement.

Other steps may be taken during laparoscopy to prevent and detect needle and trocar injuries. Reusable operating trocars should be kept sharp, and undue force should never be used during insertion. Disposable trocars have recently been marketed in an effort to improve the safety of these devices. The potential advantages of the disposable instruments include a retractable safety shield to cover the trocar tip after the abdominal wall is penetrated and the fact that single use instruments do not have the opportunity to dull. No data exist at the present time to confirm these advantages. It should also be recognized that the safety shield offers no protection to fixed structures such as bowel which may adhere to the posterior aspect of the abdominal wall.

A thorough search for injuries should be undertaken during exploratory laparoscopy, including inspection of the posterior aspect of the abdominal wall and the bowel underlying the insertion site. In patients at risk for underlying adhesions to the abdominal wall or in whom abdominal entry may be otherwise difficult there are other options available for the establishment of pneumoperitoneum. The

Veress needle may be inserted into the abdominal cavity at an alternate site such as in the right upper quadrant, transuterine, or through the rectouterine space.[39] Preoperative real-time abdominal ultrasound has been reported to "map" the location of adhesions to the abdominal wall prior to needle insertion.[40] Finally, open laparoscopy should be considered in patients in whom the potential for injury during creation of the pneumoperitoneum exists.

Open Laparoscopy

The modern technique of open laparoscopy was popularized by Hasson in 1974.[41] The primary advantage of this technique is that access to the peritoneal cavity is gained under direct vision; therefore, bowel and vascular injuries should be virtually nonexistent. Despite the theoretic advantages of this method, the vast majority of laparoscopies are still performed using a closed method. Only 4 per cent of procedures in the 1982 AAGL survey were open.[13]

Data regarding the complication rate for open laparoscopy are scarce. A 1985 survey of 10,840 open laparoscopies reported 19 wound infections and 6 bowel lacerations for a complication rate of 0.2 per cent.[42] Fitzgibbons et al.[43] recently reported 350 laparoscopic cholecystectomies performed by open laparoscopy. Two cases of umbilical cellulitis were attributed to the technique (0.6 per cent). A single bowel injury was also noted, but the etiology of this injury is unclear. As noted earlier, the complication rate for Veress needle and trocar insertion during closed laparoscopy is approximately 0.2 to 0.3 per cent. Therefore, the complication rates for the two approaches are apparently similar at the present time, although the potential for major vascular injury is less with open laparoscopy. It would seem prudent for surgeons to be facile with both methods so that open laparoscopy may be used in patients in whom risk of bowel or vascular injury is high.

Abdominal Wall Injuries

Abdominal wall complications during laparoscopy may be classified as early or late. Early complications include hemorrhage and infection. Hemorrhage is by far the more common occurrence. The most benign form of hemorrhage is periumbilical ecchymosis, which occurs from a combination of damage to the delicate periumbilical venous plexus and excessive traction on the abdominal wall during establishment of pneumoperitoneum.

Another frequent type of abdominal wall hemorrhage stems from damage to the superficial epigastric, inferior epigastric, or unnamed muscular abdominal wall vessels. Injuries to vessels of the abdominal wall are a frequent source of morbidity, occurring in 0.25 to 6.0 per cent of cases.[2,44] Incidence of this type of injury may increase as more complex procedures use increasing numbers and larger sizes of trocars.

Hemorrhage from abdominal wall vessels is usually manifest by troublesome oozing around the trocar, either internally or externally. However, a large hematoma may occasionally develop without signs of shed blood. Continued bleeding should not be tolerated because a significant extraperitoneal hematoma may develop (Fig. 8-4). Initial methods of management include use of the trocar as a lever to apply pressure to the posterior aspect of the anterior abdominal wall. If this is unsuccessful after several minutes, the trocar may be removed and a Foley catheter placed through the opening. Inflation of the balloon and upward traction may tamponade the bleeding site.[45] An alternative method is transabdominal laparoscopic suture ligation of the bleeding point. If all these methods fail, exploration of the wound with hematoma evacuation and suture ligature of the bleeding vessel should be performed. Injuries to abdominal wall vessels may be avoided in thin patients by transillumination and inspection of the abdominal wall prior to trocar insertion.

The low incidence of superficial wound infection is one of the advantages of laparoscopy. The exact reason for the apparent decrease in wound infection is not clear;

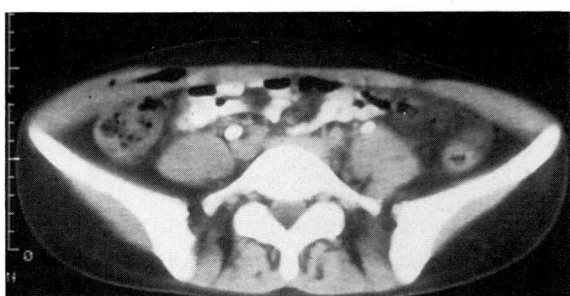

Figure 8-4. Unrecognized abdominal wall hematoma arising from a trocar insertion site.

commonly quoted rates are approximately 0.8 to 1.3 per cent.[5,46] Pathogens from laparoscopic sterilization procedures are usually skin flora such as *Staphylococcus epidermidis* or *β-hemolytic Streptococcus*. Management is identical to that of traditional wound infections. Although most instances of wound infection are relatively benign, it should be noted that necrotizing fasciitis of the abdominal wall has been reported after diagnostic laparoscopy.[47] Good surgical technique, proper cleaning and sterilization of laparoscopic equipment, and antibiotic prophylaxis when indicated will help minimize the incidence of wound infection.

The primary late abdominal wall complication following laparoscopic surgery is hernia formation. Herniation through laparoscopic entry sites is uncommon, with an incidence of less than 0.1 per cent.[7] When it occurs, hernia formation is usually the result of infection rather than improper fascial closure.[48] Routine closure of all fascial defects greater than 5 mm is advocated to minimize this complication. In patients with preexisting umbilical hernias simultaneous umbilical herniorrhaphy may be performed with their laparoscopic procedure. Open laparoscopy should be used in these cases to avoid inadvertent injury to contents of the hernia sac.

Postoperative Pain

A complication unique to laparoscopic surgery is the occurrence of postoperative shoulder pain. Most discomfort associated with laparoscopy is mild incisional pain that is easily controlled with nonsteroidal anti-inflammatory agents or oral narcotics. As many as one third of patients may experience significant transient discomfort in one or both shoulders following laparoscopic surgery. Severe pain, however, occurs in less than 5 per cent of cases.[31] It is usually described as an arthralgia-like ache and resolves spontaneously in 24 to 48 hours. In a recent series of 375 laparoscopic cholecystectomies, shoulder pain was noted in 11 per cent of patients and resolved within 24 hours in all cases.[49]

The etiology of this referred shoulder pain is believed to be either stretching of the diaphragm caused by pneumoperitoneum or direct irritation of the diaphragm by CO_2. Slow initial insufflation (1.0 to 1.5 liters/min) and complete removal of CO_2 at the end of the procedure may help to minimize this complication.

COMPLICATIONS RELATED TO INSTRUMENTATION

Equipment Failures and Electrical Injury

All surgeons who have performed endoscopic and laparoscopic procedures are familiar with the frustration experienced during the learning phase of new surgical procedures. Acclimation to new technology such as video laparoscopy compounds this feeling, especially when equipment failures occur. It behooves the surgeon to master the operation and troubleshooting of all hardware and instrumentation upon which he or she is dependent. A designated operating room nursing staff committed to laparoscopic surgery is valuable in the transition to this new technology.

We hope that electrical injuries are only of historical significance at this point. All laparoscopic surgeons should be aware that electrocution and cutaneous burns of numerous body parts of both the surgeon and patient have been reported.[50,51] The development of solid state electrosurgical generators and implementation of strict nursing practice and biomedical engineering standards have drastically reduced the occurrence of these incidents.

Gastrointestinal Injury

The complication of gastrointestinal injury is second only to hemorrhage in frequency. The incidence in large series ranged from 0.06 to 0.4 per cent.[3,4,7,10,35,52,53] A broad range of injuries were reported, from simple recognized Veress needle perforations and minor trocar lacerations to major unrecognized intestinal burns resulting in fatal sepsis. Injuries to the stomach, small bowel, colon, liver, and spleen have been described.[52-59] Causes of intestinal injury are difficult to determine in many reports. Many series did not list visceral injuries according to mechanism. The primary causes were instrumental perforation and thermal burn, but the relative frequency was unclear and existing data were conflicting. Forty-two percent of visceral injuries reported by Yuzpe[38] were caused by Veress needle or trocar insertion. Mintz' review[31] of 123 major visceral injuries revealed that 79 per cent of bowel injuries were caused by instrumental perforation and 21 per cent by thermal burn. However, Loffer and Pent's review[2] of 56,106 laparoscopies noted 43 bowel burns and only 20 bowel perforations. A 5-year review of 3600 laparoscopic sterilization procedures at Johns Hopkins Hospital revealed 11 gastrointestinal injuries, 10 of which were attributed to thermal burn.[33] An article by Levy et al.[58] suggested that 5 of those injuries may have actually been perforations.

Management of bowel injury depends on the mechanism and severity of the insult, although all laparoscopic injuries may be managed by the same basic principles. Determination of the presence of an injury must occur, the extent and severity of the injury must be determined, and the appropriate method of repair must be chosen. Recognized puncture of the small bowel during Veress needle insertion is often inconsequential and was formerly managed expectantly. As laparoscopic skills have increased, many surgeons would perform suture repair of inadvertent enterotomies just as in open cases. Larger punctures or lacerations such as those created with instruments or large trocars should be repaired with primary closure or resection as appropriate. Laparoscopic repair may be attempted by the experienced surgeon, recognizing that conversion to laparotomy should ensue if the injury cannot be properly assessed or treated through the laparoscope. Whenever the gastrointestinal tract is violated with an insufflation needle, a new needle should always be used for reinsertion.

Thermal injury to the small bowel is a different case. The zone of injury surrounding a bowel burn is essentially a full thickness injury and includes a significantly greater area than that which is readily visible. Resection of the involved segment is generally indicated. It should be remembered that electrocautery and laser are not the only mechanisms of thermal injury. The tip of the laparoscope can burn intra-abdominal organs if left in contact with them for any length of time, as may occur during prolonged loss of pneumoperitoneum.

The issue of thermal injury to bowel has recently resurfaced with the use of monopolar electrocautery during laparoscopic cholecystectomy. Significant concern over the safety of monopolar cautery during sterilization procedures arose as a result of a Centers for Disease Control report in 1981 describing three deaths attributed to monopolar cautery. The AAGL issued a statement in 1981 suggesting that alternatives to monopolar cautery be used during laparoscopic sterilization. In a subsequent histologic review of cases of suspected bowel burns and original animal experiments, Levy et al.,[58,59] concluded that the majority of injuries ascribed to bowel burns were actually more consistent with traumatic laceration or puncture. Based on these results, the AAGL has withdrawn their previous position statement. Review of the early experience with laparoscopic cholecystectomy does not reveal an increased incidence of bowel injury with the use of monopolar electrocautery.

Vascular Injury

The incidence of vascular injury (defined as "bleeding" or "hemorrhage") during laparoscopy is approximately 0.1 to 0.6 per cent.[2,60] Major vascular injuries occur in about 0.03 to 0.06 per cent of cases.[3,31] Injury to a major vessel is the second most common cause of death during laparoscopy, following anesthesia.[20] Just as with gastrointestinal injuries, the true incidence of specific injuries is difficult to determine, probably owing to underreporting and inconsistent classification from large reviews.

A 1989 review of case reports of major vascular injuries during gynecologic laparoscopy reported 16 cases. The aorta alone was injured in 10 patients, the aorta and another vessel in 2 patients, the common iliac artery and vein in 3 patients, and the iliac artery alone in 1 patient.[34] Delayed diagnosis is common in fatalities. The mechanism of injury is the Veress needle in approximately two thirds of cases and insertion of the primary trocar in one third of cases.

The best management of major vascular injury is prevention. Proper technique of Veress needle insertion and verification of an intraperitoneal location are the two most important steps. If major hemorrhage is verified by aspiration of bright red blood, the Veress needle should be left in place and immediate laparotomy for vascular control should ensue. Waiting until hemodynamic decompensation or shock occurs will greatly increase the morbidity and mortality associated with these injuries.[44]

A unique type of complication related to vascular injury is gas embolism. Fortunately, gas embolism is rare; the approximate incidence during laparoscopy is 0.002 to 0.016 per cent.[61] The presumed etiology is entry of carbon dioxide into the venous circulation from surgical injury.[62,63] Accordingly, analysis of cases of gas embolism show an increased incidence of hemorrhage and high insufflation pressures. Clinical signs of gas embolism include a sudden significant drop in blood pressure, an abrupt increase in end-tidal carbon dioxide concentration, and the appearance of a noisy, gurgling cardiac murmur ("mill wheel" murmur). Cyanosis, arrhythmia, and pulmonary edema may also be present. Diagnosis is facilitated by continuous monitoring of blood pressure, heart sounds, and end-tidal carbon dioxide concentration. Precordial Doppler probe monitoring has also been reported to be useful.[61]

Treatment of suspected gas embolism involves placement of the patient in the Durant position (left lateral decubitus position combined with Trendelenberg position), cardiopulmonary resuscitation if necessary, immediate desufflation and hyperventilation, and insertion of a central venous catheter to attempt aspiration of the gas embolus. Other sources of cardiovascular collapse should also be excluded.

Genitourinary Injury

The literature describing genitourinary injury during laparoscopy consists essentially of case reports; insufficient detail exists in large series to even estimate the true incidence of injury. The bladder and ureter are the most commonly injured genitourinary tract organs during laparoscopic surgery. The etiologies of bladder and ureteral injury are different. Bladder injury almost uniformly occurs as a consequence of perforation of a distended organ during insertion of the Veress needle.[36,64] However, newer procedures such as pelvic lymphadenectomy may be associated with bladder injury during operative dissection.[68] Ureteral injury generally occurs as a result of thermal burn during gynecologic sterilization and the usual site is near the uterosacral ligament.[35] Injuries to urachal sinus remnants have also been reported.[66]

Suspected intraperitoneal bladder injuries may be diagnosed intraoperatively by the sudden appearance of air in the urine-collecting system or by the extravasation of methylene blue dye. Unsuspected bladder injuries are usually diagnosed postoperatively and are based on clinical suspicion. The diagnosis is confirmed by performance of a retrograde cystogram. Ureteral injury is usually diagnosed postoperatively. The patient commonly exhibits abdominal or flank pain, abdominal distention, leukocytosis, and fever. Diagnosis is confirmed with an intravenous pyelogram or retrograde ureterogram.

Small bladder punctures may be managed expectantly or repaired primarily, with bladder decompression and administration of antibiotics for 4 to 5 days being recommended in either case. Injuries larger than 5 mm should be approached by direct suture repair via the laparoscope or open technique as experience permits.[65] The primary risk factor for bladder injury is distention. Routine bladder evacuation is recommended with an indwelling catheter. Some authors advocate preoperative voiding or no bladder emptying,[67,68] but longer procedures and extensive dissection in the pelvis would seem to make routine catheter decompression prudent.

Suspected ureteral injuries should be explored and treated immediately. Treatment options include ureteroureterostomy, stenting and laparoscopic repair, and ureteroneocystostomy.[69] Some authors advocate the technique of hydrodissection to prevent ureteral injury during retroperitoneal gynecologic surgery.[70]

COMPLICATIONS OF SPECIFIC LAPAROSCOPIC PROCEDURES

Laparoscopic Cholecystectomy

The explosion of laparoscopic cholecystectomy into widespread clinical practice is reflected in the surgical literature. As of November 1991, more than 10,000 cases of laparoscopic cholecystectomy have been published. Several recent series have provided detailed information on the incidence and management of complications. A representative sample of these articles is included in Table 8-5.[43,49,71-75]

The mortality of laparoscopic cholecystectomy in these collected series ranged from 0 to 0.9 per cent and morbidity from 3 to 12 per cent. Overall morbidity in most series was 3 to 6 per cent. Biliary injury ranged from 0 to 1.5 per cent. These data included cystic duct injuries and leaks as well as more serious common bile duct injuries. Hemorrhage, as defined in Table 8-4, included hematoma formation and all reported episodes of postoperative bleeding, regardless of transfusion requirement or need for laparotomy. No episodes of major vessel injury occurred in these reports. The incidence of significant hemorrhage was 0 to 0.9 per cent. Bowel injuries occurred slighty less often, from 0 to 0.5 per

Table 8-5. Complications of Laparoscopic Cholecystectomy

Series	No. of Patients	Mortality (%)	Major Morbidity (%)	Total Morbidity (%)	Injuries (%) Biliary[a]	Bowel	Bleeding[b]	Wound Infection (%)
Southern Surgeons[71]	1518	0.07		5.1	0.5	0.3	0.2	1.0
Wolfe et al.[72]	381	0.9	2.4	6	1.3	0.5	0.3	0.5
Bailey et al.[49]	375	0.3	0.6	3.5	1.5	0	0.9	0
Fitzgibbons et al.[43]	350	0		6	0	0.3	0.9	0.6
Graves et al.[73]	304	0		3	0.4	0.3	0	0
Peters et al.[74]	283	0	2.1	5.3	1.4	0	0	1.1
Schirmer et al.[75]	152	0	4	12	0.7	0	0	3.2

[a] Includes bile leaks, cystic duct injury, and common bile duct injury.
[b] Includes hematoma and postoperative bleeding.

cent. Wound infection was somewhat more frequent, occurring in 0 to 3.2 per cent of cases. These results compare favorably with existing data on open cholecystectomy and other laparoscopic procedures. A recent review of 671 open cholecystectomies performed between 1982 and 1987 quoted 0 mortality and 4.2 per cent total morbidity.[76] The incidence of common bile duct injury for open cholecystectomy is 0.1 to 0.5 per cent.[77,78] In spite of the fact that cystic duct injuries are included with the laparoscopic data, the results are generally comparable, and analysis of individual series do not reveal an increased rate of common bile duct injuries. The incidence of other complications from the series in Table 8-4 also compares favorably with existing data from the gynecologic and gastroenterology literature. Bowel injuries and hemorrhagic events during laparoscopic cholecystectomy averaged 0.2 and 0.3 per cent, respectively. Wound infections occurred in an average of 0.9 per cent of cases, as opposed to 1.3 per cent for open cholecystectomies.[76]

However, these data may represent state-of-the-art results. There is some evidence that many practicing surgeons may be experiencing different complication rates. Several tertiary referral centers are beginning to receive patients who sustained bile duct injury during laparoscopic cholecystectomy.[72,74] Data from the Puget Sound, Washington, area reveal a 2.8 per cent bile leak rate in 597 laparoscopic cholecystectomies collected from the surrounding communities.[79] Additional analysis of five of these biliary injuries reveals that each injury occurred during the first 30 cases of the surgeon's experience.[80] Analysis of the series in Table 8-4 reveals that the majority of biliary injuries occurred during the first 100 cases in each series. Longitudinal data from a variety of academic and community practices are necessary before the true incidence of biliary injury and late stricture formation is known.

Management of most complications of laparoscopic cholecystectomy is similar to that with open cholecystectomy. The importance of proper training, meticulous operative dissection, liberal use of operative cholangiography, and the willingness to convert to an open procedure cannot be overstated.[81–83]

The management of biliary leaks deserves special mention. Recognized intraoperative biliary leaks may be treated by laparoscopic repair of the injured duct, laparoscopic common duct drainage, or laparotomy with bile duct repair, drainage, or diversion. The choice depends on the severity of the injury and the expertise of the surgeon.

The management of unrecognized postoperative bile leaks is more complex. Central to the early postoperative diagnosis of biliary injury is a high index of suspicion. Unusual abdominal discomfort, significant hyperbilirubinemia, or signs of cholangitis should prompt concern. A useful screening test is the radionuclide hepatobiliary scan (Fig. 8-5).[84] Extravasation of tracer or obstruction of flow into the duodenum is investigated further by endoscopic retrograde cholangiopancreatography or urgent surgery if necessary. Endoscopic cholangiography will delineate an obstruction or leakage and allow for placement of a stent if conservative management is elected. This approach has proven useful in the management of cystic duct leaks, thus avoiding laparotomy.[74,80] Computed tomographic scanning of the abdomen should be considered in these cases to exclude the presence of a significant fluid collection, which

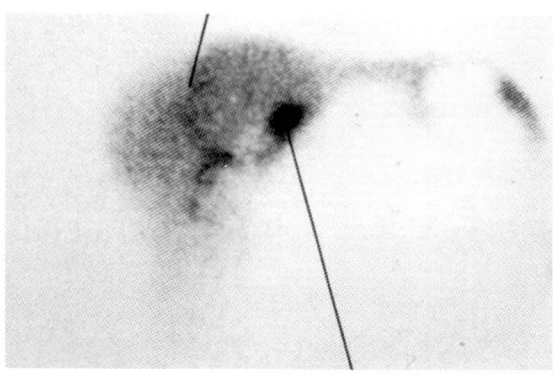

Figure 8-5. Postoperative radionuclide biliary scan in a patient with a cystic duct bile leak.

may be drained percutaneously if present. If surgical exploration is necessary, some surgeons prefer to perform another laparoscopy instead of laparotomy.

Early data suggest that laparoscopic cholecystectomy is safe and effective in experienced hands. Complication rates are similar between published series and consistent with existing gynecologic literature regarding complications of laparoscopy. A definite learning curve exists although it cannot be accurately quantified from currently available data. The incidence of biliary injury appears to be higher during the surgeon's early experience.

Laparoscopic Appendectomy

Potential complications of laparoscopic appendectomy include hemorrhage, wound infection, intra-abdominal infection or abscess, appendiceal stump leakage, fistula formation, and complications related to laparoscopy. Initial reports describe the performance of laparoscopic appendectomy for a variety of indications such as acute and chronic appendicitis, involvement of the appendix with endometriosis, and incidental appendectomy.[85–88] Complication rates are not discussed in detail in these initial studies.

Four significant series evaluating the laparoscopic approach to acute appendicitis have been published to date.[45,89–91] The results are listed in Table 8-6. No mortality is reported in these series and total morbidity ranges from 1.4 to 3.0 per cent. Acute inflammation was present in a majority of cases. Superficial wound infection occurred in 0 to 2.2 per cent and intra-abdominal abscess formation in 0 to 1.4 per cent. Conversion to traditional appendectomy was required in 0 to 4.3 per cent cases, either because of an inability to visualize the appendix or difficulty during operative dissection. Rate of removal of normal appendices varied from 0 to 14 per cent.

Overall morbidity and mortality rates from these early series are quite low and compare favorably with data from open appendectomy. Traditional appendectomy is accompanied by 0.1 to 0.2 per cent mortality and morbidity ranging from less than 5 per cent in uncomplicated appendicitis to greater than 20 per cent in complicated appendicitis.[92] Wound infection and intra-abdominal abscess rates for laparoscopic appendectomy are also impressively low. Early data suggest that laparoscopic appendectomy is safe and effective in the treatment of acute appendicitis, with acceptable complication rates.

However, the role of laparoscopic appendectomy in the treatment of complicated appendicitis is unclear from these data. Rates of perforation and gangrenous appendicitis as well as antibiotic usage are not clear in all series. Treatment of perforated appendicitis was not handled in a consistent manner between series; peritoneal contamination was treated laparoscopically in some cases and in others the procedure was converted to laparotomy.

The rate of removal of normal appendices during laparoscopic appendectomy also remains unclear. The data from Pier and coau-

Table 8-6. Laparoscopic Appendectomy for Acute Appendicitis

Series	No. of Patients	Acute Inflammation (%)	Normal Appendices (%)	Wound Infection (%)	Abscess (%)	Conversion Open (%)	Total Morbidity (%)
Pier et al.[89]	625	85	14	2.2	0.5	2.2	2.7
Valla et al.[90]	465	93	7	0	0.6	1.0	3.0
Schreiber[91]	70	25–75	?	0	1.4	4.3	1.4
Nowzaradan et al.[45]	35	100	0	0	0	0	2.9

thors[89] showed a normal appendectomy rate of 14 per cent during procedures performed with a presumptive diagnosis of acute appendicitis, which is not a substantial improvement over the 10 to 15 per cent rate during open appendectomy. Valla et al.[90] removed normal appendices in 7 per cent of cases. Conversely, Nowzaradan et al.[45] did not remove appendices that were normal in appearance during diagnostic laparoscopy. More prospective data are necessary to answer these remaining questions. A prospective trial comparing open and laparoscopic appendectomy in the United States is now under way.

Laparoscopic Herniorraphy

Data regarding laparoscopic herniorraphy are even more scarce than those available for appendectomy. It is apparent that a large number of general surgeons are performing a variety of laparoscopic hernia repairs, nearly all of which involve preperitoneal or intraperitoneal placement of prosthetic material such as Marlex or Gore-Tex.[92-95] Several surgeons have personal series near or exceeding 100 patients but have not yet published their results[96] (J. Pietrafitta, personal communication, 1991). Indications, contraindications, optimal prosthetic material, optimal surgical technique, recurrence rate and other morbidity, and mortality are all unresolved issues. Available data are insufficient to draw conclusions or make recommendations regarding this technique. Prospective trials designed to answer some of these questions are currently in progress.

Laparoscopic Urologic Procedures

Laparoscopy for the visualization of nonpalpable testes has been reported since the early 1980s[97-98] (M. Gazayerli, personal communication, 1991). The procedures are usually successful with failure to discover the undescended testicle occurring in only 5 to 12.3 per cent of cases. The technology is now being extended to perform orchiectomy in cases of atrophic testes.[99]

More advanced laparoscopic procedures are now being performed such as pelvic lymphadenectomy, nephrectomy, and varicocele ligation. The role of pelvic lymphadenectomy for the staging and treatment of prostate and bladder cancer is undergoing evaluation at a number of centers[68,100] (J. Choe, unpublished

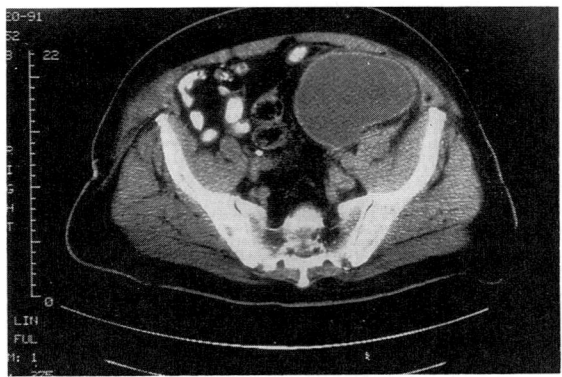

Figure 8-6. Pelvic computed tomographic scan of a patient with fever and leukocytosis 11 days after laparoscopic pelvic lymphadenectomy.

data). Thus far minimal data regarding complications have been reported. Flowers et al.[65] reported an intraoperative bladder laceration and infected pelvic hematoma (Fig. 8-6) in their first 12 patients, for a complication rate of 17 per cent. Figure 8-7 is a postoperative retrograde cystogram demonstrating a recognized intraoperative bladder laceration during laparoscopic lymphadenectomy, which was successfully treated by bladder decompression for 5 days. Vancaillie and Scheussler[101] reported 4 complications (1 bowel injury and 3

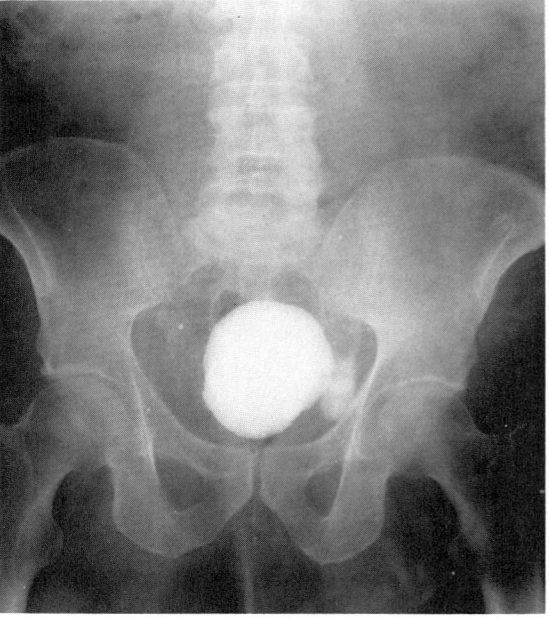

Figure 8-7. Postoperative retrograde cystogram in a patient with a recognized bladder laceration during laparoscopic pelvic lymphadenectomy.

minor complications) in their first 36 patients (11 per cent). Winfield et al.[100] reported 15 cases anecdotally but did not report complication data. Laparoscopic nephrectomy has been successfully performed, but significant data are not yet available.

Laparoscopic Gastrointestinal Surgery

This is another field of laparoscopic surgery still in its infancy. Initial reports of vagotomy, Nissen fundoplication, and colectomy have recently been published.[102-108] Complication data are presented with the realization that existing data merely serve to illustrate the feasibility of the surgical techniques but do not provide definitive information regarding morbidity and mortality rates.

Laparoscopic vagotomy has been performed in both the United States and Europe.[102,103] Indications have been primarily elective, for intractable duodenal ulcer, although the procedure has been performed for perforated duodenal ulcer.[104] Katkhouda and Mouiel[102] reported 10 patients undergoing posterior truncal vagotomy and anterior seromyotomy without complication. The University of Maryland group, in conjunction with other centers, has performed 19 posterior truncal and anterior highly selective vagotomies, with one recurrence and no intraoperative complications, although follow-up is incomplete (unpublished data). Longer follow-up is necessary to determine the true incidence of postvagotomy diarrhea, delayed gastric emptying, and recurrence rates.

Nissen fundoplication has been reported by Dallemagne et al.[105] The procedure was successful in 9 of 12 patients, with 3 patients requiring conversion to an open procedure—two for injury to the gastric fundus and a third for malfunction of video equipment. Postoperative pneumonia occurred in 1 patient (8.3 per cent). No other morbidity or mortality was reported.

Jacobs et al.[106] reported a series of 20 laparoscopic colectomies for a variety of indications. Right hemicolectomy, sigmoid colectomy, Hartmann's procedure, low anterior resection, and abdominoperineal resection were included. There was no operative mortality. Three complications occurred (15 per cent)—postoperative hemorrhage, anastomotic edema requiring tube decompression, and a mechanical small bowel obstruction requiring laparotomy.

Summary

A large body of information has accumulated regarding the general nature of complications of laparoscopic surgery during the past 20 years. It is apparent that laparoscopy is a safe and effective technique. The exact rates of some types of complications remain unclear, primarily owing to the inherent limitations of retrospective data collection. The possibility exists that the incidence of some complications may have been underreported for the same reason. These concerns underscore the need for prospective data collection with new laparoscopic procedures.

Early data suggest that a laparoscopic approach may be applicable for many traditional general surgical procedures. Sufficient data exist for both laparoscopic cholecystectomy and laparoscopic appendectomy to state that morbidity and mortality rates appear to be similar to those of standard cholecystectomy and appendectomy. Insufficient information is available to make the same statements regarding the remainder of laparoscopic general surgical procedures at this time.

REFERENCES

1. Hulka JF, Soderstrom RM, Corson SL, Brooks PG. Complications Committee of the American Association of Gynecological Laparoscopists: First annual report. J Reprod Med 1973; 10:301–306.
2. Loffler FD, Pent D. Indications, contraindications, and complications of laparoscopy. Obstet Gynecol Surv 1975; 30:407–427.
3. Riedel HH, Lehmann-Willenbrock E, Conrad P, Semm K. German pelviscopic statistics for the years 1978–1982. Endoscopy 1986; 18:219–222.
4. Henning H. The Dallas report on laparoscopic complications. Gastrointest Endosc 1985; 31:104–105.
5. Chamberlain G, Carron-Brown J. Gynaecological Laparoscopy: The Report of the Working Party of the Confidential Enquiry into Gynaecological Laparoscopy. London, Royal College of Obstetrics and Gynecology, 1978.
6. Corson SL, Bolognese RJ. Laparoscopy: An overview and results of a large series. J Reprod Med 1972; 9:148–157.
7. Kleppinger RK. Laparoscopy at a community hospital: An analysis of 4300 cases. J Reprod Med 1977; 19:353–363.
8. Phillips JM. Complications in laparoscopy. Int J Gynaecol Obstet 1977; 15:157–162.
9. Phillips J, Hulka J, Keith D, et al. Laparoscopic procedures: A national survey for 1975. J Reprod Med 1977; 18:219–226.
10. Peterson HB, Hulka J, Phillips JM. American Association of Gynecologic Laparoscopists' 1988 membership survey on operative laparoscopy. J Reprod Med 1990; 35:587–589.

11. Kane MJ, Krejs GJ. Complications of laparoscopy in Dallas: A 7 year prospective study. Gastrointest Endosc 1984; 30:237–240.
12. Phillips JM, Hulka B, Hulka J, et al. Laparoscopic procedures: The American Association of Gynecologic Laparoscopists' membership survey for 1975. J Reprod Med 1977; 18:227–232.
13. Phillips JM, Hulka JF, Peterson HB. American Association of Gynecologic Laparoscopists' 1982 membership survey. J Reprod Med 1984; 29:592–594.
14. Shantha TR, Harden J. Laparoscopic cholecystectomy: Anesthesia-related complications and guidelines. Surg Laparosc Endo 1991; 3:173–178.
15. Bongard F, Liu SY. Cardiopulmonary pathophysiology of laparoscopy and pneumoperitoneum. In White RA, Klein SR, eds. Endoscopic Surgery. St. Louis, Mosby-Year Book Inc, 1991, pp 159–171.
16. Liu SY, Leighton T, Davis I, et al. Prospective analysis of cardiopulmonary responses to laparoscopic cholecystectomy. J Laparoendosc Surg 1991; 1:241–246.
17. Wittgen CM, Andrus CH, Fitzgerald SD, et al. Analysis of hemodynamic and ventilatory effects of laparoscopic cholecystectomy. Arch Surg 1991; 126:997–1001.
18. El-Minawi MF, Wahbi O, El-Bagouri IS, et al. Physiologic changes during CO_2 and N_2O pneumoperitoneum in diagnostic laparoscopy: A comparative study. J Reprod Med 1981; 26:338–346.
19. Scott DB, Julian DG. Observations on cardiac arrhythmias during laparoscopic surgery. Br Med J 1972; 1:411–413.
20. Borten M. Laparoscopic Complications. Prevention and Management. Toronto, BC Decker, Inc, 1986, pp 185–195, 253–263, 265–284, 297–361.
21. Harris MNE, Plantevin OM, Crowther A. Cardiac arrhythmia during anesthesia for laparoscopy. Br J Anaesth 1984; 56:1213–1217.
22. Hodgson C, McLelland RMA, Newton JR. Some effects of the peritoneal insufflation of carbon dioxide at laparoscopy. Anaesthesia 1970; 25:382–389.
23. McKenzie R, Wadhwa RK, Bedger RC. Noninvasive measurement of cardiac output during laparoscopy. J Reprod Med 1980; 24:247–250.
24. Duffy BL. Regurgitation during pelvic laparoscopy. Br J Anaesth 1979; 51:1089–1090.
25. Carlsson C, Islander G. Silent gastropharyngeal regurgitation during anaesthesia. Anesth Analg 1981; 60:655–657.
26. Roberts CJ, Goodman NW. Gastro-oesophageal reflux during elective laparoscopy. Anaesthesia 1990; 45:1009–1011.
27. Heinonen J, Takki S, Tammisto T. Effect of Trendelenberg tilt and other procedures on the position of endotracheal tubes. Lancet 1969; 1:850–853.
28. Batra MS, Driscoll JJ, Coburn WA, et al. Evanescent nitrous oxide pneumothorax after laparoscopy. Anesth Analg 1983; 62:1121–1123.
29. Murray DP, Rankin RA, Lackey C. Bilateral pneumothoraces complicating peritoneoscopy. Gastrointest Endosc 1984; 30:45–46.
30. Bailey RW. Complications of laparoscopic general surgery. In Zucker KA, Bailey RW, Reddick EJ, eds. Surgical Laparoscopy. St. Louis, Quality Medical Publishing, Inc, 1991, pp 311–342.
31. Mintz M. Risks and prophylaxis in laparoscopy: A survey of 100,000 cases. J Reprod Med 1977; 18:269–272.
32. Pascual JB, Baranda MM, Taerrero MT, et al. Subcutaneous emphysema, pneumomediastinum, bilateral pneumothorax, and pneumopericardium after laparoscopy. Endoscopy 1990; 22:59.
33. Thompson BH, Wheeless CR. Gastrointestinal complications of laparoscopic sterilization. Obstet Gynecol 1973; 5:669–676.
34. Baadsgaard SE, Bille S, Egeblad K. Major vascular injury during gynecologic laparoscopy. Report of a case and review of published cases. Acta Obstet Gynecol Scand 1989; 68:283–285.
35. Grainger DA, Soderstrom RM, Schiff SF, et al. Ureteral injuries at laparoscopy: Insight into diagnosis, management, and prevention. Obstet Gynecol 1990; 75:839–843.
36. Georgy FM, Fetterman HH, Chefetz MD. Complication of laparoscopy: Two cases of perforated urinary bladder. Am J Obstet Gynecol 1974; 120:1121–1122.
37. Fitzgibbons RJ, Salerno GM, Filipi CJ. Open laparoscopy. In Zucker KA, Bailey RW, Reddick EJ, eds. Surgical Laparoscopy. St. Louis, Quality Medical Publishing, Inc, 1991, pp 87–97.
38. Yuzpe AA. Pneumoperitoneum needle and trocar injuries in laparoscopy: A survey on possible contributing factors and prevention. J Reprod Med 1990; 35:485–490.
39. Wolfe WM, Pasic R. Transuterine insertion of Veress needle in laparoscopy. Obstet Gynecol 1990; 75:456–457.
40. Marin G, Bergamo S, Miola E, et al. Prelaparoscopic echography used to detect abdominal adhesions. Endoscopy 1987; 19:147–149.
41. Hasson HM. Open laparoscopy: A report of 150 cases. J Reprod Med 1974; 12:234–238.
42. Penfield Aj. How to prevent complications of open laparoscopy. J Reprod Med 1985; 30:660–663.
43. Fitzgibbons RJ, Schmid S, Santoscoy R, et al. Open laparoscopy for laparoscopic cholecystectomy. Surg Laparosc Endosc 1991; 1:216–222.
44. McDonald PT, Rich NM, Collins GJ, et al. Vascular trauma secondary to diagnostic and therapeutic procedures: Laparoscopy. Am J Surg 1978; 135:651–655.
45. Nowzaradan Y, Westmoreland J, McCarver CT, Harris RJ. Laparoscopic appendectomy for acute appendicitis: Indications and current use. J Laparoendosc Surg 1991; 1:247–257.
46. Brenner WE, Edelman DA, Black JK. Laparoscopic sterilization with electrocautery, spring-loaded clips, and Silastic bands: Technical problems and early complications. Fertil Steril 1976; 27:256–266.
47. Sotrel G, Hirsch E, Edelin KC. Necrotizing fasciitis following diagnostic laparoscopy. Obstet Gynecol 1983; 62(Suppl):67–69.
48. Fischer JD, Turner FW. Abdominal incisional hernias: A ten year review. Can J Surg 1974; 17:202–204.
49. Bailey RW, Zucker KA, Flowers JL, et al. Laparoscopic cholecystectomy: Experience with 375 patients. Ann Surg 1991; 214:531–541.
50. Neufeld GR. Principles and hazards of electrosurgery including laparoscopy. Surg Gynecol Obstet 1978; 147:705–710.
51. Esposito JM. The laparoscopist and electrosurgery. Am J Obstet Gynecol 1976; 126:633–637.
52. Krebs HB. Intestinal injury in gynecologic surgery: A ten year experience. Am J Obstet Gynecol 1986; 155:509–514.
53. Ilter T, Bolukoglu MA, Musoglu A. Complication rates of diagnostic laparoscopy. Gastrointest Endosc 1986; 32:126.

54. Dancygier H, Jacob RA. Splenic rupture during laparoscopy. Gastrointest Endosc 1983; 29:63.
55. Phillips RS, Reddy R, Jeffers LJ, Schiff ER. Experience with diagnostic laparoscopy in a hepatology training program. Gastrointest Endosc 1987; 33:417–420.
56. Endler GC, Moghissi KS. Gastric perforation during pelvic laparoscopy. Obstet Gynecol 1976; 47(Suppl):40–42.
57. Birns MT. Inadvertent instrumental perforation of the colon during laparoscopy: Nonsurgical repair. Gastrointest Endosc 1989; 35:54–56.
58. Levy BS, Soderstrom RM, Dail DH. Bowel injuries during laparoscopy: Gross anatomy and histology. J Reprod Med 1985; 30:168–172.
59. Soderstrom RM, Levy BS. Bowel injuries during laparoscopy: Causes and medicolegal questions. Contemp Ob/Gyn 1986; March:41–45.
60. Bergqvist D, Bergqvist A. Vascular injuries during gynecologic surgery. Acta Obstet Gynecol Scand 1987; 66:19–23.
61. DePlater RHM, Jones ISC. Non-fatal carbon dioxide embolism during laparoscopy. Anaesth Intensive Care 1989; 17:359–361.
62. Shulman D, Aronson HB. Capnography in the early diagnosis of carbon dioxide embolism during laparoscopy. Can Anaesth Soc J 1984; 31:455–459.
63. Yacoub OF, Cardona I, Coveler, et al. Carbon dioxide embolism during laparoscopy. Anesthesiology 1982; 57:533–535.
64. Deshmukh AS. Laparoscopic bladder injury. Urology 1982; 19:306–307.
65. Flowers JL, Feldman J, Jacobs SC. Laparoscopic pelvic lymphadenectomy. Surg Laparosc Endo 1991; 1:62–70.
66. McLucas B, March C. Urachal sinus perforation during laparoscopy. J Reprod Med 1982; 27:573–574.
67. Akhtar MS, Beere DM, Wright JT, MacRae KD. Is bladder catheterization really necessary before laparoscopy? Br J Obstet Gynaecol 1985; 92:1176–1178.
68. Cooperman AM. Laparoscopic cholecystectomy: Results of an early experience. Am J Gastroenterol 1991; 86:694–696.
69. Gomel V, James C. Intraoperative management of ureteral injury during operative laparoscopy. Fertil Steril 1991; 55:416–419.
70. Nezhat C, Nezhat FR. Safe laser endoscopic excision or vaporization of peritoneal endometriosis. Fertil Steril 1989; 52:149–151.
71. The Southern Surgeons Club. A prospective analysis of 1518 laparoscopic cholecystectomies. N Engl J Med 1991; 324:1073–1078.
72. Wolfe BM, Gardiner BN, Leary BF, Frey CF. Endoscopic cholecystectomy: An analysis of complications. Arch Surg 1991; 126:1192–1198.
73. Graves HA, Ballinger JF, Anderson WJ. Appraisal of laparoscopic cholecystectomy. Ann Surg 1991; 213:655–664.
74. Peters JH, Gibbons GD, Innes JT, et al. Complications of laparoscopic cholecystectomy. Surgery 1991; 110:769–778.
75. Schirmer BD, Edge SB, Dix J, et al. Laparoscopic cholecystectomy: Treatment of choice for symptomatic cholelithiasis. Ann Surg 1991; 213:665–677.
76. Gilliland TM, Traverso LW. Modern standards for comparison of cholecystectomy with alternative treatments for symptomatic cholelithiasis with emphasis on long term relief of symptoms. Surg Gynecol Obstet 1990; 170:39–44.
77. Andren-Sandberg A, Alinder F, Bengmark S. Accidental lesions of the common bile duct at cholecystectomy. Ann Surg 1985; 201:328–332.
78. Madsen CM, Sorensen HR, Truelsen F. The frequency of operative bile duct injuries, illustrated by a Danish County Survey. Acta Chir Scand 1960; 119:92–107.
79. Traverso LW. Laparoscopic cholecystectomy. Pract Gastroenterol 1991; 15:16–27.
80. Ball TJ. Laparoscopic cholecystectomy: Complications call for caution. Pract Gastroenterol 1991; 15:31–45.
81. Hunter JG. Avoidance of bile duct injury during laparoscopic cholecystectomy. Am J Surg 1991; 162:71–75.
82. Stockmann PT, Soper NJ. Early results of laparoscopic cholecystectomy at a teaching institution. In Levine BA, ed. Perspectives in General Surgery. St. Louis; Quality Medical Publishing, 1991, Vol 2, pp 1–24.
83. Flowers JL, Zucker KA, Graham SM, et al. Laparoscopic cholangiography: Results and indications. Ann Surg 1992; 215:209–216.
84. Gelman R, Alexander MS, Zucker KA, Bailey RW. The use of radionuclide imaging in the evaluation of suspected biliary damage during laparoscopic cholecystectomy. Gastrointest Radiol 1991; 16:201–204.
85. Saye WB, Rives DA, Cochran EB. Laparoscopic appendectomy: Three year's experience. Surg Laparosc Endosc 1991; 1:109–115.
86. McKernan JB, Saye WB. Laparoscopic techniques in appendectomy with argon laser. South Med J 1990; 83:1019–1020.
87. Gangal HT, Gangal MH. Laparoscopic appendectomy. Endoscopy 1987; 19:127–129.
88. Semm K. Endoscopic appendectomy. Endoscopy 1983; 15:59–64.
89. Pier A, Gotz F, Bacher C. Laparoscopic appendectomy in 625 cases: From innovation to routine. Surg Laparosc Endosc 1991; 1:8–13.
90. Valla JS, Limonne B, Valla V, et al. Laparoscopic appendectomy in children: Report of 465 cases. Surg Laparosc Endosc 1991; 1:166–172.
91. Schrieber JH. Early experience with laparoscopic appendectomy in women. Surg Endosc 1987; 1:211–216.
92. Condon RE, Telford GL. Appendicitis. In Sabiston D, ed. Textbook of Surgery: The Biological Basis of Modern Surgical Practice, 14th ed. Philadelphia, WB Saunders, 1991, pp 884–898.
93. Corbitt JD. Laparoscopic herniorrhaphy. Surg Laparosc Endo 1991; 1:23–25.
94. Schultz LS, Graber JN, Pietrafitta JJ, Hickok DF. Laser laparoscopic herniorrhaphy: Preliminary results of a clinical trial. J Laparoendosc Surg 1991; 1:41–45.
95. Toy FK, Smoot RT. Toy-Smoot laparoscopic hernioplasty. Surg Laparosc Endo 1991; 1:151–155.
96. Ger R. The laparoscopic management of groin hernias. Contemp Surg 1991; 39:15–19.
97. Scott JES. Laparoscopy as an aid in the diagnosis and management of the impalpable testis. J Pediatr Surg 1982; 17:14–16.
98. Lowe DH, Brock WA, Kaplan GW. Laparoscopy for localization of nonpalpable testes. J Urol 1984; 131:728–729.
99. Castilho LN. Laparoscopy for the nonpalpable testis: How to interpret the endoscopic findings. J Urol 1990; 144:1215–1218.

100. Winfield HN, Donovan JF, See WA, et al. Urological laparoscopic surgery. J Urol 1991; 146:941–948.
101. Vancaillie TG, Schuessler WW. Laparoscopic pelvic lymphadenectomy. In Zucker KA, Bailey RW, Reddick EJ, eds. Surgical Laparoscopy. St. Louis, Quality Medical Publishing, 1991, pp 241–261.
102. Katkhouda N, Mouiel J. A new technique of surgical treatment of chronic duodenal ulcer without laparotomy by videocoelioscopy. Am J Surg 1991; 161:361–364.
103. Bailey RW, Flowers JL, Graham SM, Zucker KA. Combined laparoscopic cholecystectomy and selective vagotomy. Surg Laparosc Endo 1991; 1:45–49.
104. Mouret P, Francois Y, Vignal J, et al. Laparoscopic treatment of perforated peptic ulcer. Br J Surg 1990; 77:1006.
105. Dallemagne B, Weerts JM, Jehaes C, et al. Laparoscopic Nissen fundoplication: Preliminary report. Surg Laparosc Endo 1991; 3:138–143.
106. Jacobs M, Verdeja JC, Goldstein HS. Minimally invasive colon resection (laparoscopic colectomy). Surg Laparosc Endo 1991; 1:144–150.
107. Schlinkert RT. Laparoscopic-assisted right hemicolectomy. Dis Colon Rectum 1991; 34:1030–1031.
108. Fowler DL, White SA. Laparoscopy-assisted sigmoid resection. Surg Laparosc Endosc 1991; 3:183–188.

Section II
General Techniques of Laparoscopic Surgery

Chapter 9
Closed and Open Techniques of Trocar Insertion

P. Jeffrey W. Milsom

Safe entry into the potential space of the peritoneal cavity is the first essential skill the budding laparoscopic surgeon must master. This endeavor may be a rapid and rather uneventful prelude to a laparoscopic operative procedure, but success requires careful adherence to a variety of concepts that ensure maximal safety to the patient as well as optimal exposure.

This chapter will focus on a step by step approach to the techniques available for safe placement of transabdominal trocars and on how to avoid the pitfalls that may ensue subsequent to trocar placement. It is hoped that this chapter will allow the surgeon and the patient maximal opportunity to reap the benefits of the laparoscopic endeavor.

HISTORICAL BACKGROUND

The earliest described laparoscopic procedures were diagnostic maneuvers performed transvaginally in humans in the early twentieth century by Ott[1] of Petrograd. Kelling[2] of Dresden introduced the concept of inducing a preliminary pneumoperitoneum in dogs using a regular type of hypodermic needle, then visualized the peritoneal cavity with a Nitze cystoscope. Jacobeus[3] of Stockholm coined the term laparoscopy and used the technique in humans. Bernheim, an American, reported a method of entry into the peritoneal cavity using a rigid proctoscope, perhaps originating the open technique of instrument insertion.[4] In 1937 Ruddock,[5] also of the United States, reported on 500 procedures accomplished without mortality. Veress,[6] in 1938, described a small bore spring-loaded needle (Fig. 9-1) passed through the abdominal wall to establish a pneumoperitoneum more safely than with conventional needles.

A German gastroenterologist, Kalk,[7] developed a dual trocar technique for performing diagnostic laparoscopy and, in 1951, reported on 2000 procedures completed under local anesthesia without mortality.

Innovation regarding trocars largely developed in the field of gynecology over the ensuing 25 years. Hasson[8] of Chicago described the trocars that bear his name in 1978 (Fig. 9-2), applying them to an open technique of trocar insertion, which he felt lowered the complication rate of trocar insertion in certain patients. The open technique will be described later.

Since 1989, with the rapid increase in interest in general surgical procedures using lap-

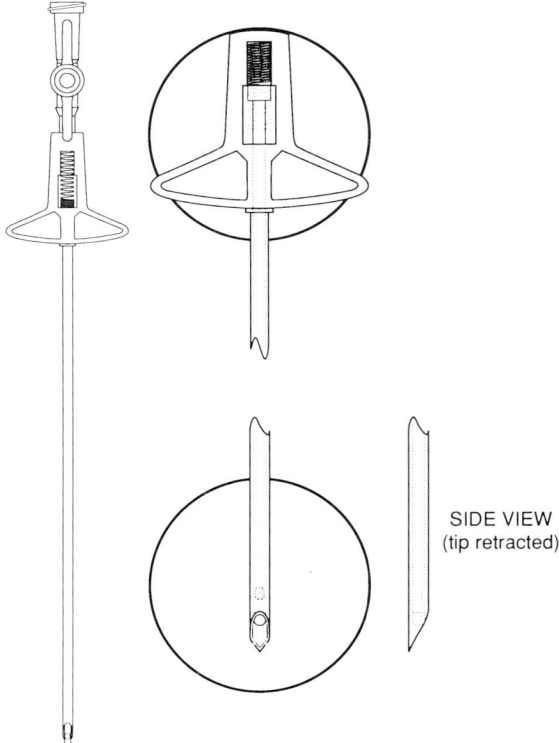

Figure 9-1. SURGINEEDLE* pneumoneedle for initial entry into the peritoneal cavity. The blunt tip retracts as the abdominal wall is traversed, then springs past the sharp tip when the peritoneal cavity is entered.

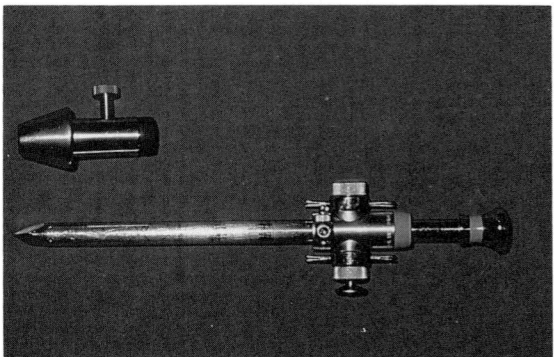

Figure 9-2. Hasson trocar (*bottom*) with notches on either side for attaching fascial sutures. The funnel-shaped adaptor (*top*) fits over the trocar and occludes the fascial opening to prevent leakage of intraperitoneal gas.

aroscopic techniques, a variety of trocars have now become available in both nondisposable and disposable models. The nondisposable types offer the advantage of reliable sharpness and are probably the most popular currently in use (Fig. 9-3).

Future changes in design are envisioned to make laparoscopic entry into the peritoneum even safer. Fiberoptic visualization into the peritoneal cavity through the Veress needle using a mini-telescope, low profile trocars for easier manipulation, and self-adjusting (iris-type) port sizes for universal use (regardless of instrument diameter) are some of the future developments in trocar technology.

DETAILED TECHNIQUE OF TROCAR INSERTION

In this section several techniques (open and closed) for safe entry into the peritoneal cavity will be described, with a step by step description of the procedure. The following section will address common pitfalls and what to do if a complication occurs.

Step One: Creating the Pneumoperitoneum

Prior to surgery, a good history should be obtained and physical examination should be carried out to evaluate the patient's suitability for a laparoscopic procedure. Contraindications to laparoscopy may include pregnancy, coagulation disorders, portal hypertension, or severe lung disease. Other conditions such as hiatal hernia, inguinal hernia, obesity, or multiple previous laparotomies may present hazards to the creation of a pneumoperito-

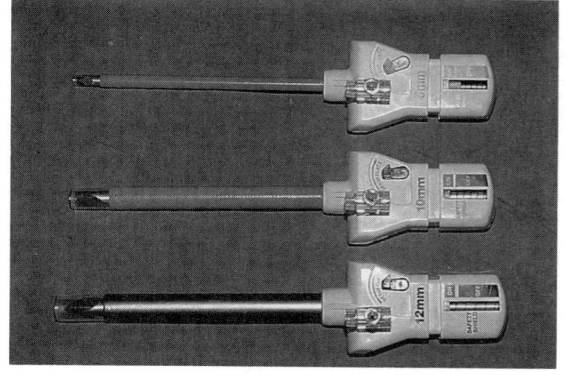

Figure 9-3. Disposable SURGIPORT* trocars come in a variety of diameters, are equipped with safety shields at their tips, and are reliably sharp.

neum. In a patient with an inguinal hernia a truss should be placed over the hernia at surgery if he or she is deemed a suitable candidate.

After induction of general anesthesia and placement of a nasogastric tube and Foley urinary catheter (to deflate the stomach and bladder to their fullest extent), the abdomen is inspected for potential sites of entry. If previous surgical scars are present near the midline or in the lower abdomen, it is wise to consider an open technique. For the vast majority of patients, a site either just above or below the umbilicus is chosen for initial entry using a small bore specialized needle (Veress), which has a spring-loaded blunt tip, allowing for safer entry into the abdomen (see Fig. 9-1). A scalpel and basic surgical instruments are readied on the operating setup, in case any problem during trocar insertion requires an immediate laparotomy.

CLOSED TECHNIQUE

Initial Entry into the Peritoneal Cavity. A 10- to 12-mm curvilinear incision is made just below the umbilicus into the subcutaneous tissue. The anterior abdominal fascia is then cleared of subcutaneous tissue using a tonsil clamp. The patient is placed in the Trendelenburg position (25 to 35 degrees). The Veress needle is inserted into the peritoneal cavity by gentle, steady pressure, stabilizing the ulnar aspect of the hand on the abdominal wall and grasping the needle at midshaft so as to not allow plunging of the needle. Simultaneously, two towel clips placed on opposite edges of the incision are elevated anteriorly to raise the abdominal wall away from the viscera, and the needle is directed toward the pelvis, away from the intestine and great vessels (Fig. 9-4). Two distinct "pops" are generally perceived: one as the needle pierces the fascia, and the second as the needle pierces the peritoneum.

Testing Needle Position. Once the needle is felt to be into the peritoneal cavity, a number of tests are rapidly performed to verify position. None should be considered foolproof.

1. Aspiration/Injection: The Veress needle is loaded with a 10-ml syringe filled with 5 ml of saline solution. Aspiration and injection are performed twice, injecting 2 ml at a time. Aspiration should yield no gas or fluid, and the saline should freely pass out of the syringe.
2. Hanging Drop Test: After the above step reveals no abnormalities, a drop of saline is placed on the top of the opening in the needle, and then the abdominal wall is raised with towel clips or by grasping manually. The drop should easily run into the peritoneal cavity. Alternatively, a half-filled syringe without the plunger can be placed on the needle and the saline should freely run into the abdomen.

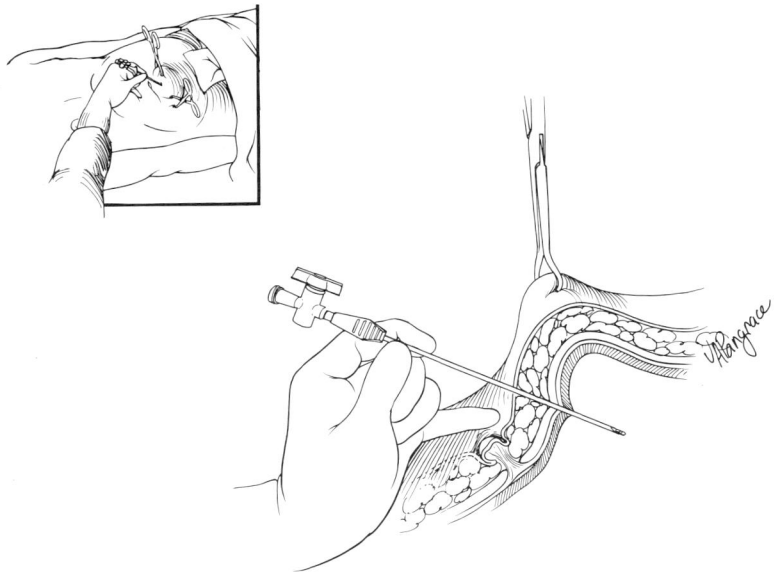

Figure 9-4. Safe entry into the peritoneal cavity with the Veress needle. The patient should be in 25- to 35-degree Trendelenburg position and the needle directed toward the pelvis.

3. **Gentle Movement of the Needle ("Probing")**: The tip of the Veress needle may then be gently moved back and forth (not in and out) to verify free movement of the tip. If it feels fixed, then incorrect placement should be considered, and the needle should be readjusted or removed and the preceding steps repeated.

Insufflation. Once correct needle placement is attained, the carbon dioxide tubing should then be attached to the needle, and the insufflation started at a very low flow rate (1.5 liters/min). If the needle is correctly placed, one should see low pressure (less than 5 to 6 mm Hg) at the outset. If pressures are high, one should initially perform some simple maneuvers: (1) raise the abdominal wall or incision with the towel clips; (2) rotate the needle circumferentially; or (3) alter the needle's position slightly, but do not advance it.

If there is any question about placement, stop the insufflation and start over. Some of the other pressure patterns one may see on insufflation are outlined in Table 9-1. Insufflation is carried out until the abdominal pressure reaches 12 to 15 mm Hg. At this point, the Veress needle is removed, and a trocar is readied for insertion.

The maximum flow rate achievable through the Veress needle is approximately 2.5 liters/min, but it is probably safer to insufflate at 1.5 liters/min to minimize the chance for any cardiorespiratory compromise that may occur with establishment of the pneumoperitoneum. The pneumoperitoneum takes longer to establish initially, but the added safety measure is well worth this time.

OPEN TECHNIQUE

Although some experienced laparoscopists decry the needle method for preliminary pneumoperitoneum before trocar insertion, I believe the only time trocars should be inserted directly into the peritoneal cavity is using the open technique. This entails a direct cut down into the peritoneal cavity, generally in the midline just below the umbilicus, a technique originally described by Hasson of Chicago.[8] At this site, a 1- to 2-cm incision is made in the fascia and either a purse-string suture or two heavy sutures are placed into the fascia, then tied to the special Hasson trocars fitted with a funnel-shaped adapter to occlude the fascial opening (see Fig. 9-2). Alternatively, SURGIGRIP* disposable sleeve available for use with United States Surgical Corporation (Norwalk, CT) trocars may be anchored in place to the fascia with a purse-string suture after placement of the trocar into the peritoneum under direct vision.

This technique is indicated whenever the Veress needle position is uncertain with the closed technique or when multiple adhesions are suspected.

CHOICE OF GAS FOR INSUFFLATION

Although a variety of gases have been utilized for establishment of the pneumoperitoneum, carbon dioxide is almost universally used owing to rapid absorption, low cost, and no combustible properties. It does cause vasodilation, which may rarely cause hypotension in an elderly or dehydrated patient. Ab-

Table 9-1. Aberrant Pressure Patterns during Insufflation

Pressure Pattern	Likely Problem	Solution(s)
Starts high, drops, then rises rapidly	Preperitoneal space	Remove needle, retry or convert to open technique
Starts high and stays high	Needle or tubing obstructed Needle jammed in tissue or against	Check lines Rotate needle, lift abdominal wall anteriorly
Starts low and stays low	Leak in system Needle in bowel or bladder Inguinal or hiatal hernia In vascular system	Check for leaks Caution anesthesia Pressure on inguinal hernia Recheck needle position Abort procedure, release pneumoperitoneum rapidly

sorption can lead to a significant arterial pH decrease and increase in carbon dioxide tension. Thus, the anesthesiologist must observe patients carefully, especially those with chronic obstructive pulmonary disease, in the immediate postoperative period.

Step Two: Insertion of the First Trocar

Once the abdomen has been safely insufflated, the initial trocar is placed at the site of Veress needle insertion. Again, safety is paramount, and this begins with the surgeon taking the trocar (usually 10 or 12 mm diameter) and personally inspecting that it and all subsequent trocars function properly. The trocar valve is closed, the safety shield is tested, and the anterior fascia is engaged with the trocar tip in a perpendicular fashion (Fig. 9-5A). The barrel of the trocar is stabilized with one hand to avoid plunging while the other hand supplies the driving force in a twisting-boring fashion (Fig. 9-5B). To keep danger of vascular-visceral injury to a minimum, the trocar tip is pointed toward the pelvis as the abdominal wall is traversed (Fig. 9-5C). Despite safety shields being present on most disposable trocars, injury may still occur, and the peritoneal entry must be a steady and controlled maneuver. The sharpness of the trocar is a critical part of the control and the major advantage of the disposable models.

Once the initial trocar is placed, the carbon dioxide insufflation line is reattached, and a steady state pressure is maintained at 12 to 15 mm Hg. The tenseness of the abdomen seen at 15 mm Hg pressure may be valuable in inserting further trocars; then the pressure on the abdomen may be lowered to 10 to 12 mm Hg for the duration of the procedure to lower the likelihood of adverse sequelae of the pneumoperitoneum.

Step Three: Insertion of Additional Trocars

The precise placement of additional trocars may now be done under direct vision of the laparoscope, since the initial one is used for visualization of the entire peritoneal cavity. Strategy will vary according to procedure, but generally the further away trocars are from each other, the better.

General rules for trocar placement are:

1. Avoid the rectus sheath if possible.
2. Transilluminate the abdominal wall prior to choosing a site to visualize and avoid blood vessels (Fig. 9-6).
3. Use a clamp to depress the chosen site and inspect the posterior abdominal wall (peritoneal aspect) by laparoscope to be sure the area is free of vessels, ligaments, or adhesions.

Once a site is chosen, especially if you are just beginning laparoscopic endeavors, use larger trocar sizes (10 or 12 mm) since they may be universally used with a convertor/adaptor for almost any instrument.

The insertion procedure is then as follows:

1. Make a skin incision along Langer's lines.
2. Spread subcutaneous tissues with a tonsil clamp to the anterior fascia.
3. Depress the abdominal wall again with a clamp to verify safety of the site with the laparoscope.
4. Check the trocar as previously described, place a fascia-grasping (e.g., SURGIGRIP*) device on the trocar, then place the point perpendicular to fascia and, using a two-hand technique, steadily twist it into the peritoneum under direct laparoscopic guidance.
5. Angle the trocar as soon as its point pierces the peritoneum so it travels horizontally and away from abdominal viscera until it fully enters the abdomen (Fig. 9-7, A and B).
6. Pull back on the trocar tip so it is just inside the abdominal cavity. If the trocar sleeve (e.g., SURGIGRIP*) is used, twist this into the abdominal wall so a portion of the thread is visible, then adjust the trocar shaft so it is just beneath this (Fig. 9-8).

Pitfalls of Trocar Insertion and Their Management

Although the vast majority of trocar insertions performed properly will result in no complications, the expert in any endeavor will know how to expeditiously manage problems if they arise. Specific problems and their management will be enumerated here. Problems with air insufflation have been touched upon earlier.

GAS LEAK AT TROCAR SITE

This may occur during insertion of the initial trocar or when any subsequent trocar is placed. If the leak is only a minor one and

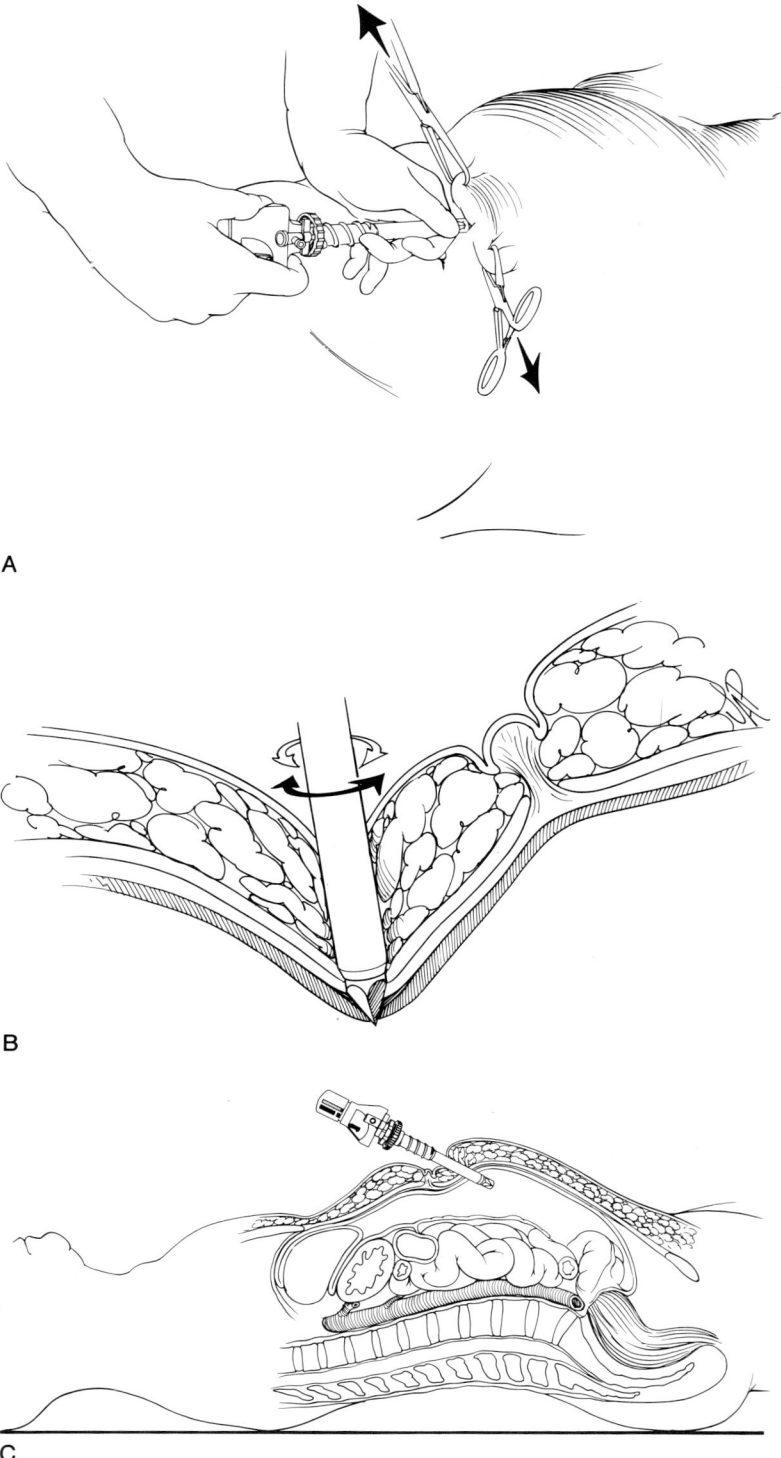

Figure 9-5. A, The initial trocar is placed into the peritoneal cavity using two hands to stabilize the trocar. B, A twisting-boring action is applied to the trocar shaft to gain steady, reliable entry into the peritoneal cavity. C, Always pointing toward the pelvis may minimize the chance for accidental visceral or vessel injury.

Closed and Open Techniques of Trochar Insertion 103

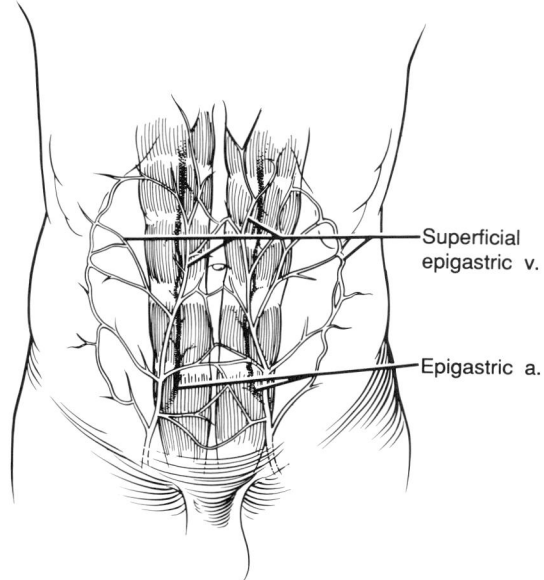

Figure 9-6. Transillumination may help to avoid trocar injury to abdominal wall vessels.

pneumoperitoneum is adequate, this problem may be ignored. Most of the time, the problem requires some correction, and may be remedied simply by (1) verifying that all valves are closed and tubing connections are tight; and (2) scrutinizing the precise leakage site. If the leak is emanating from the fascial edge remove the trocar/fascial gripper, insert an absorbable pursestring suture around the fascial edge, replace the trocar and gripper, and tighten the pursestring suture around the gripper. If the leak is coming from the trocar or equipment, tighten the joints or consider replacing the trocar.

HEMORRHAGE FROM TROCAR SITE

If significant bleeding is noted (usually characterized by spurting or dripping of blood from around a trocar site), attempt to: (1) tighten the surgical gripper into the abdominal wall or (2) replace the trocar with a larger size, then complete the surgery if hemostasis is attained.

If the bleeding continues, or when the trocar is removed at the conclusion of the procedure, the area must be well visualized by a direct surgical approach, enlarging the incision as needed. The bleeding vessel is then suture-ligated. Preventive measures include avoidance of the rectus sheath and other areas that contain large blood vessels and preliminary transillumination of the abdominal wall before trocar placement (Fig. 9-8).

TROCAR WILL NOT ENTER THE PERITONEAL CAVITY

The trocar will not enter the peritoneal cavity because it is hung up in the preperitoneal space (Fig. 9-9A). If this occurs with the initial trocar insertion, the simplest and most rapid solution is to remove the trocar and perform an open insertion. Diagnosis is made by a characteristic pressure pattern on carbon dioxide insufflation (Table 9-1) or if after insertion of the trocar and laparoscopic optical system, no viscera are seen and the foamy yellowish preperitoneal space is seen.

If a secondary trocar is being inserted and will not go through the peritoneum (Fig. 9-9B) check to be sure the safety shield is

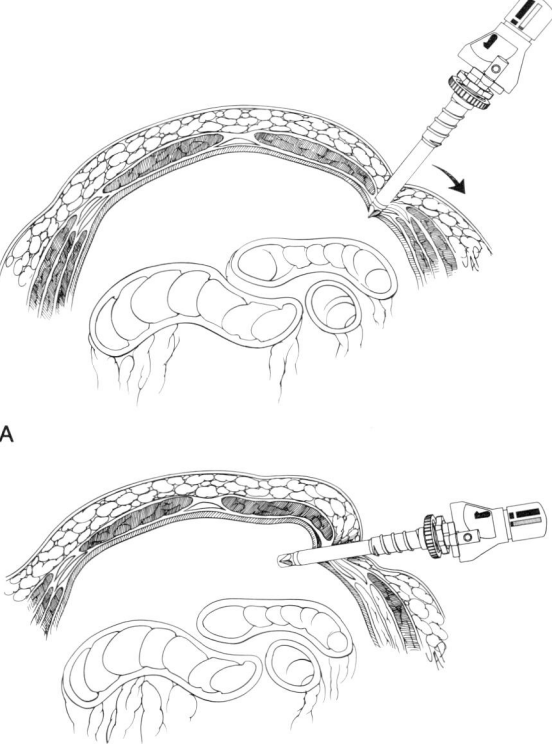

Figure 9-7. A Insert additional trocars under direct visualization starting at right angles to the abdominal wall until the trocar point just pierces the peritoneum and B then angle the trocar so it travels as horizontally as possible, to avoid any potential for visceral injury.

104 General Techniques of Laparoscopic Surgery

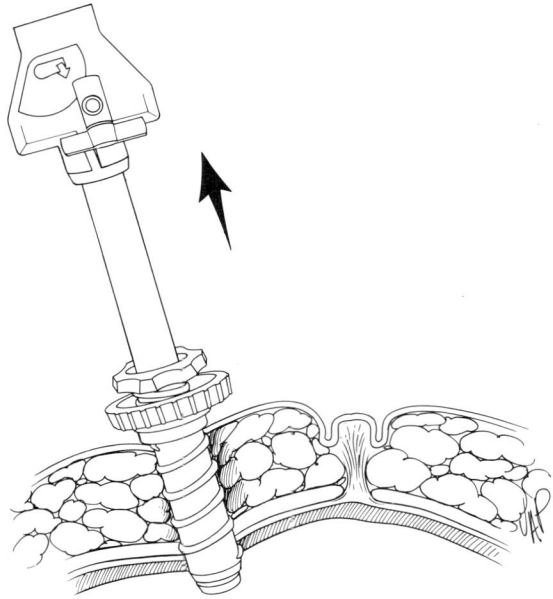

Figure 9-8. The trocar shaft should be adjusted so the abdominal wall gripper is just showing one thread inside the peritoneal cavity and the trocar protrudes just beneath this.

retracting. If it is, advance the trocar tip, tenting the peritoneum into the barrel of the initial trocar under direct vision. Then advance the trocar with a twisting motion and the tip will usually advance through the peritoneum (Fig. 9-9C).

POSSIBILITY OF PERFORATED VISCUS (INTESTINE)

This probably occurs with blind insertion of the Veress needle or the initial trocar owing to improper direction of the trocar (Fig. 9-10). If there is any question of this occurrence, the safest course to follow is to (1) leave the instrument in place as a marker and (2) perform immediate laparotomy and evaluate the intestine thoroughly. Remember that through and through and multiple loop injuries can occur and that concomitant vascular injuries may also occur. The entire gastrointestinal tract needs to be inspected, as does the retroperitoneum in the vicinity. These injuries are handled in a routine open surgical fashion.

Prevention is the key; hints that occult injury to a viscus has occurred include (1) bilious or fecal staining on instrument tips or visualized in the abdomen; (2) intestinal odor at any point in the procedure; or (3) gradual

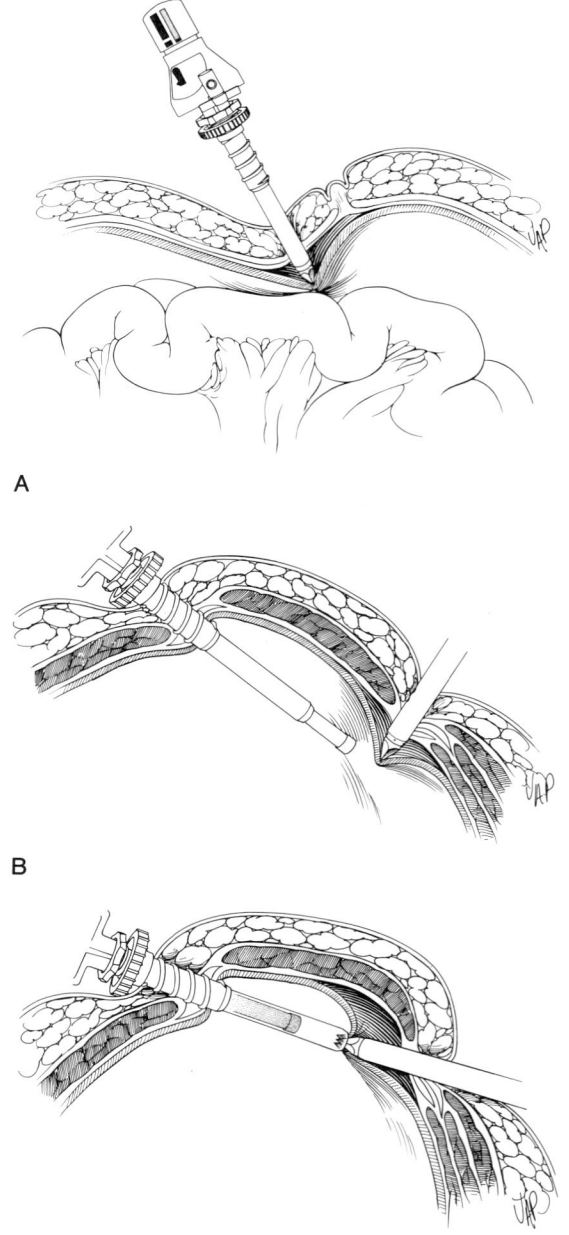

Figure 9-9. A, The trocar is hung up in the preperitoneal space. If the primary trocar will not safely enter the peritoneal cavity, use an open technique for insertion. B, Check that the safety shield is retracted. If the secondary trocar tip will not safely pierce the abdominal wall peritoneum, withdraw the optical system into the primary trocar shaft. C, then advance the secondary trocar tip into the shaft of the primary one. This will usually allow safe entry into the peritoneum.

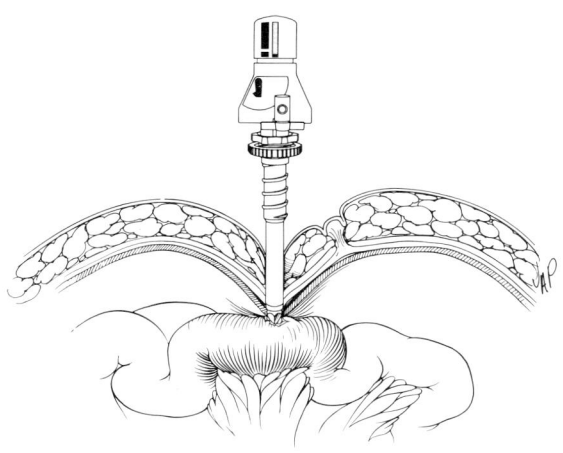

Figure 9-10. Faulty direction of the trocar tip during advancement may lead to visceral injury. Leave the trocar in place as a marker while performing a laparotomy to remedy the situation.

dilation of the intestine during the operation (from pneumoperitoneal air entering the bowel lumen).

SUBCUTANEOUS EMPHYSEMA

Most of the time emphysema is a self-limiting problem. If it is just noted around the trocar sites or anterior abdominal wall, the surgeon should lower the pressure limit on the carbon dioxide insufflator to approximately 10 mm Hg and keep working. If a leak at the fascial level is noted, placement of a fascial purse-string suture may help.

Occasionally, this problem may spread to involve the entire trunk, thighs, and even face and neck. If the emphysema is increasing rapidly, one should consider aborting the procedure for an open technique, primarily so the patient is not alarmed when he or she awakes. The gas is nearly always innocuous and is reabsorbed within 6 to 8 hours.

MAJOR VASCULAR INJURY

If blood rapidly returns after insertion of the trocar or needle or if a major hemorrhage is noted after insertion, the instrument is left in place, a laparotomy is quickly performed, and hemostasis is attained by direct occlusion (Fig. 9-11).

After the patient's condition stabilizes, proximal and distal control of the vessel is attained. The surgeon must remember the possibility of through and through and multi-visceral injury.

Direct open repair is carried out and consideration should be given to aborting the primary surgical indication. A thorough investigation of the entire gastrointestinal tract and retroperitoneum is performed.

POSSIBLE GAS EMBOLISM

One of the rarest but most feared complications, gas embolism may occur with cannulation of a vessel during trocar insertion, or during surgery if a large vein is opened.

Slow insufflation through the Veress needle at the outset of the procedure is an important part of minimizing the risk for gas embolism.

This syndrome may be heralded by arrhythmias, which then are followed by sudden hypotension. A characteristic "mill wheel" murmur may be heard at the left heart border.

If gas embolism is suspected, the pneumoperitoneum is immediately released, and the patient is placed in a steep Trendelenburg in the left lateral decubitus position. A right heart catheter is placed by the anesthesiologist and an attempt to aspirate air from the right heart is made. Special fenestrated central lines exist to better aspirate air from the right heart.

The procedure should be terminated rapidly, and the patient allowed to recover with monitoring of electrocardiograms and myocardial enzyme levels. A careful neurologic examination is also performed to rule out the possibility of air embolism to the systemic circulation through a patent foramen ovale.

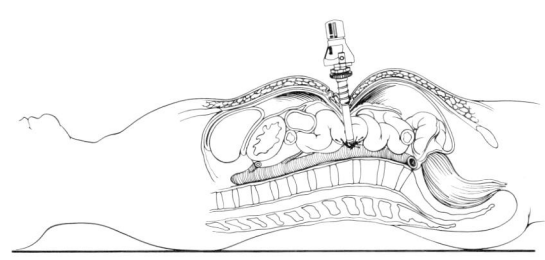

Figure 9-11. Major vascular injury, from faulty direction of the trocar or an inadvertent plunging maneuver, requires immediate laparotomy and evaluation for multiple injuries.

Concluding the Operation: Trocar Removal

Once the laparoscopic procedure has been completed, the trocars should be removed sequentially, plugging the fascial opening with an assistant's digit to maintain pneumoperitoneum while bleeding sites are searched for in the abdominal wall. After removal of all trocars except the laparoscope insertion site, this area is carefully surveyed by withdrawing the trocar to skin level and then slowly drawing the laparoscope and trocar back through the fascia.

Bleeding sites are identified and suture ligated. The entry sites are then irrigated and, if 10 mm or greater, a size 2-0 or 0 absorbable suture is used to close the fascial opening; then the skin is closed with a subcuticular absorbable suture.

Summary

Trocar insertion is the key that will expeditiously and safely unlock the peritoneal cavity to the aspiring laparoscopic surgeon. Armed with the appropriate skills and fundamental tenets regarding trocar insertion, the surgeon will be empowered to perform laparoscopic procedures that maximize patient safety and allow concentration on obliteration of the pathologic process.

REFERENCES

1. Ott DO. Ventroscopic illumination of the abdominal cavity in pregnancy. Z Akus: Zhensk Bolez 1901; 15:7.
2. Kelling G. Uber die Moglichkeit, die Zystoskopie bei Untersuchungen Serosen Hohlungen Anzuwenden Bernierkung zu dem Artikel von Jacobeus. Muench Med Wochenschr 1910; 57:2358.
3. Jacobeus HC. Ueber die Moglichkeit die Zystoskopie bei Untersuchung seroser Hohlung Anzuwenden. Muench Med Wochenschr 1910; 57:2090.
4. Bernheim BM. Organoscopy: Cystoscopy of the abdominal cavity. Ann Surg 1911; 53:764.
5. Ruddock JC. Peritoneoscopy. Surg Gynecol Obstet 1937; 65:623.
6. Veress J. Ein Neues instrument zur Ausführung von Brust- oder Bauchpunktionen und Pneumothoraxbehandlung. Dtsch Med Wochenschr 1938; 41:1480.
7. Kalk H, Bruhl W, Sieke E. Die Gezielte Leberpunktion. Dtsch Med Wochenschr 1943; 69:693.
8. Hasson HM. Open laparoscopy versus closed laparoscopy: A comparison of complication rates. Adv Plann Parent 1978; 13:41-43.

Chapter 10
Tissue Approximation and Ligation Techniques

Anthony J. Senagore

Essential components of any surgical procedure are accurate ligation of bleeding points and reapproximation of any tissue defects created during the surgical dissection. These techniques are second nature to most surgeons, although with the advent of laparoscopic procedures many new instruments and techniques will be required in the surgeon's armamentarium. Many of these techniques are new to the general surgeon, but these skills can be rapidly gained with practice using a closed cardboard box and the laparoscope and camera.

DIFFERENCES BETWEEN LAPAROSCOPIC AND OPEN SURGERY

One of the first differences that immediately becomes obvious to the beginning laparoscopic surgeon is the absence of depth perception. This requires that the surgeon think three dimensionally while looking at a two-dimensional image on the video screen. Typically, orientation is gained rapidly once the surgeon has accurately located the instrument tips in the operating field. However, if the surgeon becomes disoriented, the use of small circular motions with the instruments will allow recognition of the instrument location and its relationship to the adjacent viscera. It is also helpful if the surgeon learns to concentrate on the image on the video screen rather than attempting to watch the hands for guidance. A quick view of the position and angle of trocars as they enter the peritoneal cavity can also give information about the probable position of the instruments. Finally, optimal appreciation of instrument location and motion is best obtained by working ahead of the camera. Working toward the camera yields a reversed image on the screen, which requires an extra step in using the video image to produce appropriate hand motions.

Another difference for the surgeon to overcome when performing laparoscopic procedures is appreciation of the limitations of the instrument motion. Apart from the restrictions placed on the surgeon by the length of the instrument, the field of access is described by a cone with the apex of the cone being the trocar at the fascial level. Therefore, accurate placement of the trocars is required to facilitate the performance of tissue approximation and/or ligation. The locations for optimal trocar placements for suturing are best selected after placement of the central trocar for the laparoscope. This will allow accurate visualization of the proposed operative field so that two needle holders can be placed to allow operation in planes at a 90-degree angle from each other. If the trocars are placed too close to each other or at an incorrect angle, the result will either be an interesting "sword fight" or an inability to accurately secure the knot. The author has found it helpful to use the corkscrew grips for the trocars through which dissection and suturing instruments are placed so that the trocar can be withdrawn as much as possible toward the fascia, thereby maximizing the mobility of the instruments. These grip devices add the security of decreasing the possibility of trocar loss during particularly difficult dissection or suturing.

A factor that is often unappreciated is the advantage gained by accurate patient positioning. Allowing the patient to be placed on the operating table in an appropriate partial decubitus position rather than supine allows gravity to retract the small intestine away from the intended operative field. This frees a trocar from retraction duties, allowing it to be used for temporary tissue approximation during suturing. It also allows the assistant to help in the operative field rather than be relegated to maintaining the small bowel away from the operative sight.

When selecting accurate sights of placement for the trocars, the surgeon must be careful to place the appropriate size trocar for the required instruments. Needle holders, dissectors, and tissue graspers can be placed through a 5-mm port without difficulty. However, larger ligating instruments such as clip appliers or vascular staplers require either the 10- or 12-mm trocars, respectively. Although these trocars can be replaced, it is far easier and less disruptive to the operative procedure to place the appropriate trocar initially. If a larger trocar is placed, it can be down-sized by diaphragm adaptors so that smaller instruments can be placed through the trocar without loss of the pneumoperitoneum.

LAPAROSCOPIC SUTURING

There are a wide variety of needle holders and several needle types available for laparoscopic suturing techniques. The surgeon should be familiar with the different instruments as well as their limitations before beginning clinical suturing. Again, most of these skills can be gained using one of the training boxes or even a simple cardboard box. Generally, one of three needle types is used: an atraumatic straight needle, the ski needle, and the standard semicircular curved needle (Fig. 10-1). For needle passage to be optimal, the use of two needle holders and a relatively short length of suture material (less than 10 cm) is required. One of the needle holders (active) is used to initially grasp the needle near the swaged end while the second needle holder (passive) can be used to manipulate tissue for accurate needle placement. The needle is then driven across the defect to be sutured and is grasped on the other side with the passive needle holder. The suture is accurately secured using one of the knotting techniques to be described later. Either a simple stitch, simple running, or running/locking technique may be used as determined by the surgeon. If a running technique is used, the assistant can use a grasper to maintain tension on the suture line, although slippage can be minimized by using a running/locking technique. Currently laparoscopic suturing limitations are primarily the result of limitations of the instruments. Many of the needle holders do not provide a sufficient grip on the needle, resulting in swiveling and difficulty maintaining accurate direction of needle passage. This is particularly true when the semicurved needle is used. The straight needle also offers some increased tissue resistance on its passage through the tissue, but much of this problem has been alleviated by the introduction of ski needles, which are available with a number of different suture materials. The laparoscopic surgeon should become familiar with all available needle

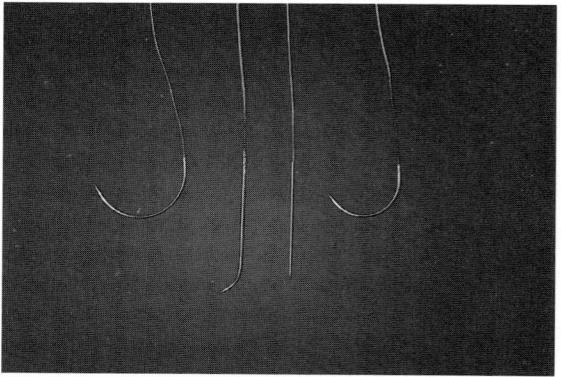

Figure 10-1. Needle types available for laparoscopic suturing include the standard round needle, the straight needle, and the ski needle.

holders, their uses, and their limitations before performing advanced laparoscopic procedures.

KNOT TYING

As was mentioned earlier, accurate, secure knot formation is essential to any operative procedure. Laparoscopic surgery requires learning several new techniques for knot tying, a process that has become second nature for most surgeons. Knot tying can be divided into two general approaches, extracorporeal (throws placed outside the abdominal cavity and then brought down to the operative field by a knot pusher) and intracorporeal (throws of the knot placed directly at the operative site using laparoscopic instrumentation). Generally both techniques are safe and accurate. Extracorporeal knotting does take a bit longer to perform and requires frequent insertion and removal of the knot passer, resulting in a temporary decrease in the degree of pneumoperitoneum. Extracorporeal knotting is performed by placing the suture material under laparoscopic direction and then bringing both ends of the suture out through the same trocar. A single throw or a surgeon's knot is placed extracorporeally and passed down through the trocar to the operative site under laparoscopic visualization to assure accurate ligation. The passer is used to push the knot into place while tension is maintained on both ends of the suture by the surgeon's hand. This process is repeated for two to three more throws as indicated for accurate square knot formation. A variety of knot passers are available including simple rod pushers, ring pushers, one-piece needle/suture and passer systems (Endoknot, Ethicon Inc., Somerville, NJ; SURGIWHIP*, United States Surgical Corp., Norwalk, CT), and specially cut needle holders with slits at the end of the jaws to function as a knot pusher.

The technique for extracorporeal knotting can also be performed using the Roeder external slip knot (Fig. 10-2). This technique is best performed using dry catgut (plain or chromic) or silk suture, which offers the advantage of swelling with hydration, making the knot more secure. For this technique, placement of the suture ligature is performed under laparoscopic guidance with retrieval of the free end and needle through the same trocar. The pneumoperitoneum can be maintained by finger occlusion of the partially open channel. The needle is removed and a single hitch is placed leaving approximately 8 to 10 cm of free suture on one end. This free end is then used to make three complete revolutions around both suture strands while maintaining the single hitch by pinching with the left finger and thumb. After the three revolutions are performed, the tail of the suture is brought through the large loop between the trocar and the surgeon's left finger and thumb. Finally, the end of the suture is brought through the small loop between the initial single hitch and the twists. This free end is clipped approximately 4 mm from the knot. The remaining long free end is then secured, and the knot is brought down through the trocar for accurate laparoscopically guided placement using a knot passer.

Although extracorporeal knotting techniques are useful, they do have several drawbacks. First, success in passing the knot to its eventual location depends on the friction of the suture. Obviously, this technique works best for monofilament or one of the coated sutures. This technique may be more difficult with silk or catgut suture material, which tend to hang up during attempts at passing the knot. In addition, constant tension must be maintained on the free ends of the suture while the pusher is used to accurately place the knot. Failure to do so can result in too loose a knot or worse yet, tangling the knot passer in the suture, which might result in a tear at the site of ligation. Intracorporeal knotting is a skill that requires considerable practice. There are basically three techniques for the formation of secure intracorporeal knots including the standard microsurgical square knot, the internal twist knot, and the Dundee internal knot. The technique used by the individual surgeon will depend on the clinical situation and familiarity with each of the techniques.

The standard microsurgical knot is performed in a fashion similar to instrument tying techniques used by most general surgeons (Fig. 10-3). Again, when laparoscopic suturing and knot tying are performed, the suture should not be longer than approximately 10 cm. If the suture material is too long, it can be very difficult to control the knot-tying process, and the potential for losing the needle and creating iatrogenic injuries greatly increases. In addition, the tail must be kept short so that it can be easily retrieved with limited motion of the needle holder. It is a far easier practice to grasp the needle close to the swaged end and wind the suture around a passive needle holder. It is helpful

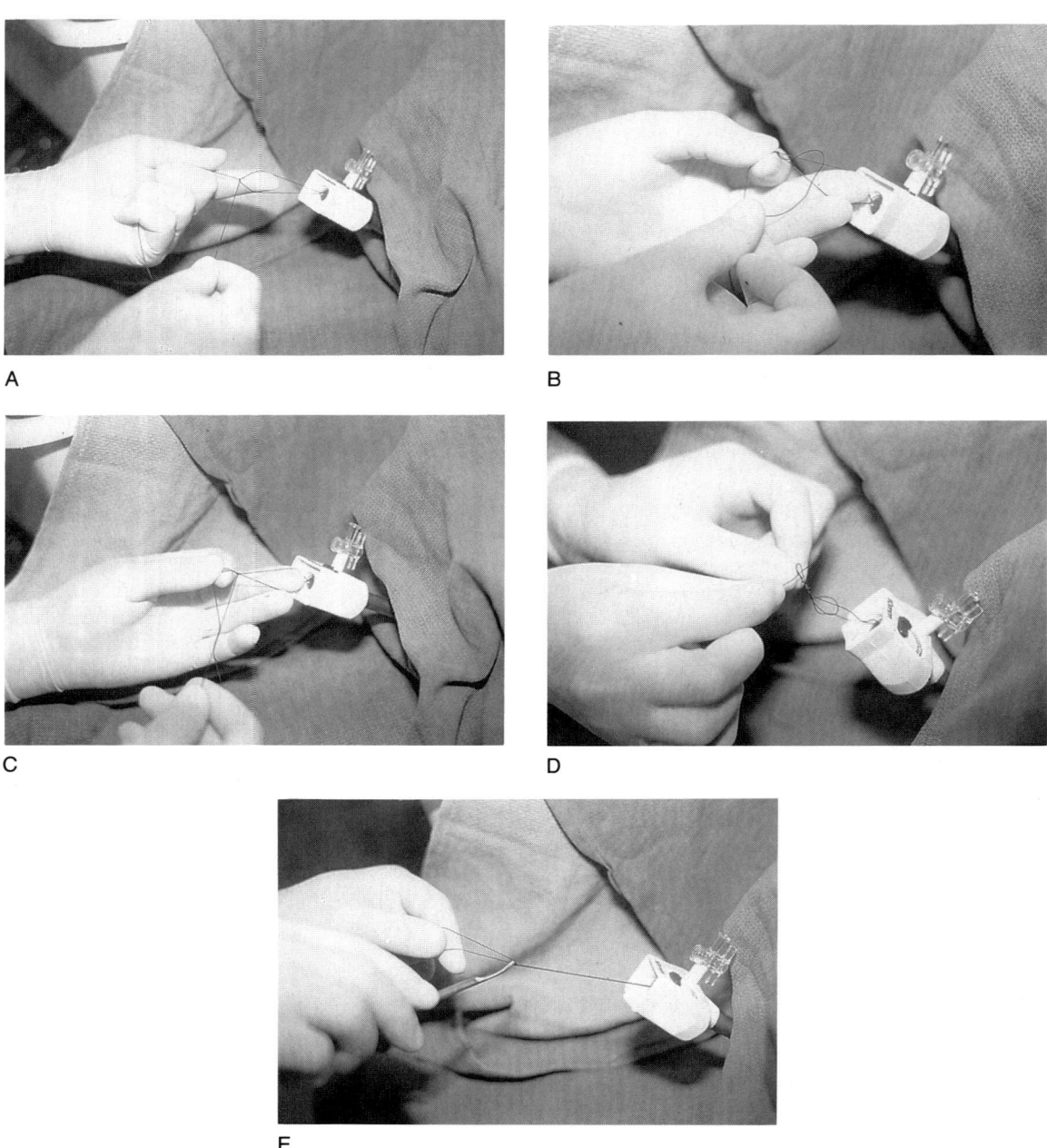

Figure 10-2. Demonstration of the formation of the Roeder slip knot: A, a single hitch is formed, which is then pinched with the index and forefinger of the left hand; B, the free end of the suture is wrapped around both limbs of the suture for three revolutions; C, the free end of the suture is placed through the large loop; D, the free end is brought through the small loop located between the wrap and the initial hitch; and E, the slip knot is cinched down and brought into the operating field by a knot pusher.

Tissue Approximation and Ligation Techniques 111

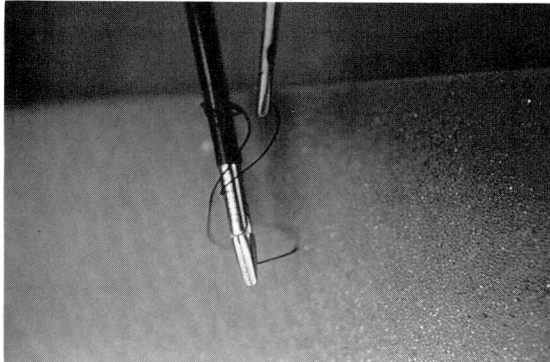

Figure 10-4. Twist knot formation performed by grasping the free end of the suture near the exit point from the structure being ligated and performing four revolutions of the needle holder. The suture is released and the needle holder is used to grasp the needle and pull it through the loop, forming the knot. This can be repeated two to three times to secure the knot.

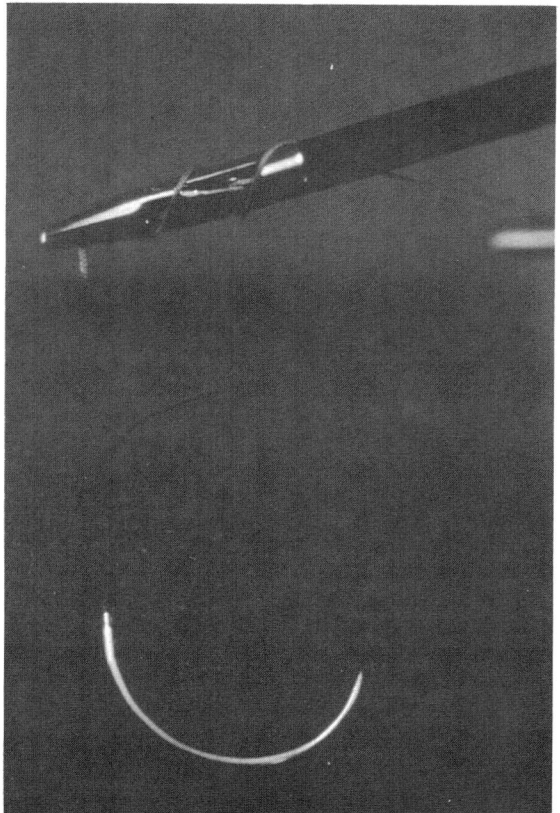

Figure 10-3. The standard microsurgical square knot formed by placing two revolutions of suture around the passive needle holder, which is then used to grasp the free end of the suture. Pulling on both limbs of the suture secures the knot.

to use a double throw initially, forming a surgeon's knot so that appropriate tension can be placed on the initial attempt. This makes subsequent winding and knot tying less likely to loosen the knot, resulting in an insecure closure. The surgeon must also remember to alternate the direction of the wind from clockwise to counterclockwise with subsequent throws to ensure square knot formation. One way to ease the suture off the needle holder is to allow the winds around the passive needle holder to loosen up before pulling through the free end of the suture. This avoids catching of the suture material in the jaws of the needle holder. The winding technique of knot formation can be done in two ways. Once the suture is placed in the tissue, the needle holder on the side closest to the free end of the suture is used to grasp the short free end (Fig. 10-4). This needle holder is then rotated four times forming three com-

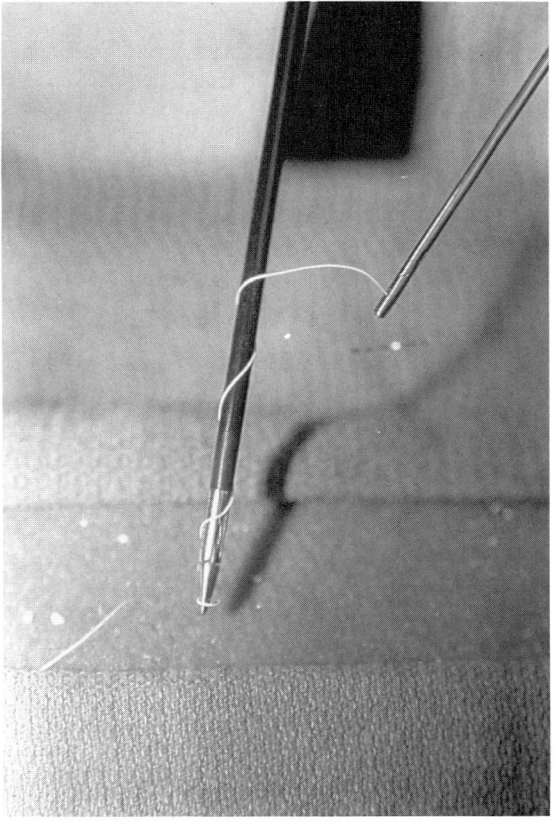

Figure 10-5. Twist knot formation by using the needle limb of the suture to form the four revolutions. The free end of the suture is pulled through these loops forming the knot.

plete loops around the tip of the needle holder. The free end is released and that instrument is used to grasp the other end of the suture. This is best done by removing the needle from the opposite end. The second needle holder is used to grasp the initial end of the suture used to form the twist. The end of the suture is then pulled through the twisted loops, forming the initial throw of the knot. To complete the square knot process, the revolutions around the needle holder are reversed, initially clockwise and subsequently counterclockwise.

An alternative method of tying this knot, if one wishes to perform a running suture and therefore preserve the needle on the end of the suture material, is to use the needle limb for twisting (Fig. 10-5). This is done by grasping the needle in one needle holder to maintain traction on this limb of the suture. A second needle holder (active) is then used to grasp the suture close to the intended sight of ligation. Again, the active needle holder is twisted four times to form three complete loops. The suture is released, and the active needle holder is used to grasp the free end of the suture and pull it through the loops. The passive needle holder is used to maintain tension on the needled limb to secure the knot. Again, this is repeated three to four times depending on the suture material and the structure being ligated to complete the square knot process.

A final technique for internal knot tying is the Dundee internal knot. This knot consists of four components: (1) an external jamming slip loop knot; (2) reversal of the needle through the loop; (3) sliding of the loop from the tail and locking; and (4) a restraining hitch.

The external jamming loop is formed near the free end of the suture extracorporeally (Fig. 10-6). This is then brought down into the operative field through one of the trocars. The suture is then placed into the tissue at the sight of ligation using the attached needle and is pulled through so that the jamming slip loop is brought into apposition with the tissue. Tension is maintained on the suture while the needle is reversed and passed through the loop and pulled through all the way. The suture is then grasped close to the loop and the tail is pulled in the opposite direction to slide the loop down on the suture. This allows the knot to be jammed by pulling on the suture while applying countertraction on the knot with the needle holder. One or two extra hitches are usually required to secure knot formation.

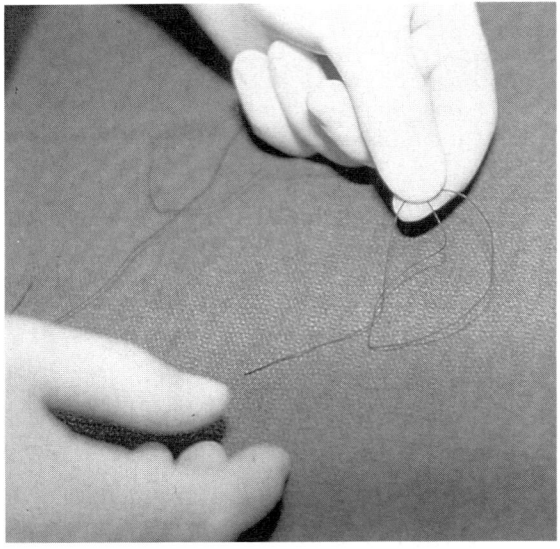

A

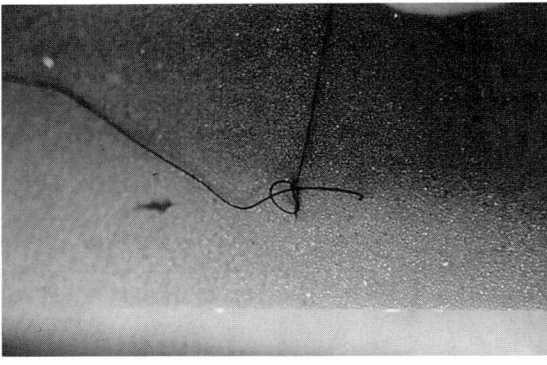

B

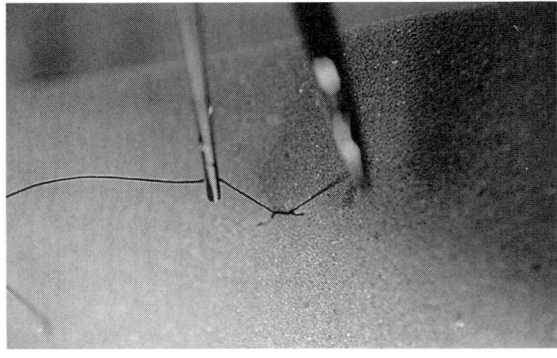

C

Figure 10-6. A demonstration of the Dundee slip knot: A, formation of the external jamming slip loop knot; B, placement of the jamming knot at the ligation site with reversal of the free end of the suture through the loop; and C, pulling of the suture limbs to close the slip loop and form the knot. Several more simple hitches are required to make this knot secure.

A technique not recommended is the use of any metal clips to secure one end of the suture rather than some fashion of knot tying. These clips are small and do not provide appropriate friction to maintain a secure attachment to the suture material, resulting in potential slippage of the suture and possibly complete disruption of the suture line. Knot tying can be quickly mastered with a little bit of practice. The surgeon should accept nothing less for safe, secure closure or ligation.

An alternative to knot-tying techniques is use of one of the commercially available preformed loop/knot instruments. SURGITIE* ligating loop is available with SURGIGUT* SURGIDIAL* and POLYSORB* suture. Although they may save a little time, the same effect can be obtained with a little patience and practice at forming this knot yourself. In this era of cost containment, surgeons must remember to use the most cost-effective technique.

Chapter 11
Techniques of Exposure, Retraction, and Dissection

Dennis L. Fowler

To the extent possible, laparoscopic procedures should be carried out with the same surgical principles that have withstood the scrutiny of surgeons for decades. The basic principles of acquiring exposure, creating traction and countertraction, and providing retraction remain valid during laparoscopy. However, the methods of effecting these principles are somewhat different than for laparotomy. On the other hand, techniques of dissection are more nearly like those used at the time of laparotomy. Blunt dissection, sharp scissor dissection. and cautery or laser dissection are easily performed in a fashion very similar to open surgery once adequate exposure is established. Control of blood vessels can be accomplished laparoscopically with a combination of open surgical techniques and new technclogy such as vascular staplers.

There are two major differences in how the laparoscopic surgeon perceives intra-abdominal structures compared with the surgeon performing laparotomy: The laparoscopic surgeon views the surgical field in two dimensions rather than three, and the laparoscopic surgeon does not have the use of palpation of intra-abdominal structures. With experience, there is essentially no loss of perception of the surgical site with two dimensions. The laparoscope can be moved intermittently to the left or right to provide the equivalent of binocular vision, and hence some semblance of depth perception. Although the laparoscopic surgeon can use tactile sensation through instruments to some extent, it is not nearly as useful as palpation through a laparotomy incision. There are, however, other ways to obtain much the same information, and the use of Doppler probes, ultrasound probes, and nuclear scanning probes via the surgical ports at laparoscopy can potentially provide this information.

EXPOSURE

As in open surgery, unless there is adequate exposure, the procedure cannot be completed precisely, safely, or expeditiously.

Exposure in laparoscopic surgery is dependent upon the following five factors: (1) adequate laparoscope and video equipment, (2) adequate pneumoperitoneum, (3) optimal port placement, (4) position of the patient, and (5) appropriate techniques for use of graspers and retractors.

Laparoscope and Video Equipment

For most laparoscopic procedures, a 5- or 10-mm rigid 0-degree laparoscope is the instrument of choice. An adequate light source and light-carrying cable are essential. Most current generation 5-mm scopes can carry enough light to visualize the field adequately, but a 10-mm scope can deliver more light into the abdomen. In some cases, a rigid laparoscope with a 30- or 45-degree angle tip can provide better visualization of the field. An angled laparoscope can be particularly helpful when an inguinal hernia is being repaired laparoscopically, or when the gallbladder of a morbidly obese patient is removed. In the latter situation, the angled laparoscope can greatly enhance the exposure of the triangle of Calot when the very large omentum and viscera obscure a direct view from the umbilicus. The use of the flexible laparoscope may obviate the need for the angled rigid laparoscope. Although not yet generally available, it would seem to offer a great deal of potential for visualizing the "hard to get to" areas of the abdominal cavity.

To complete the setup for videolaparoscopy, the rigid laparoscope must be coupled with a video camera. Newer high resolution cameras greatly enhance the exposure obtained by improving the video image. Forthcoming technology such as HDTV (High Density Television) will further improve intra-abdominal visualization. The flexible laparoscope does not require a separate camera, for this laparoscope has the chip that initiates the video image built into the end of the laparoscope. Either the newer high resolution camera with the rigid laparoscope or the flexible laparoscope can provide excellent visualization.

Pneumoperitoneum

Without a space in which to work, laparoscopy would not be possible. That space is provided by the inflation of a gas (carbon dioxide) under pressure into the abdominal cavity. Since numerous ports are used and instruments are frequently passed in and out through them, significant amounts of gas are often lost. An essential part of the equipment of surgical laparoscopy is an adequate insufflator. The insufflator should provide at least 6 liters/min flow, and rates of up to 10 liters/min are even more desirable. The most common cause of poor or lost exposure is loss of adequate pneumoperitoneum. Ports with adequate seals and a high volume insufflator are essential to maintain adequate pneumoperitoneum.

Port Placement

Although there is no one way that ports must be placed to provide adequate exposure, satisfactory positioning of ports is critical to the successful completion of the operation. For most gastrointestinal operations, four ports will be adequate, and most of the time, each port will provide access for instruments carrying out a single function. Less commonly, ports will be used for different functions during the same operation. Obviously, one port will be used for the laparoscope. Another port is used as the operating port, and most of the dissection can be done through this port. The remaining two ports of the typical four will be used for graspers or retractors, including one that can be used for forceps by the surgeon when operating with both hands.

Situations occur in which five ports need to be routinely used and also when three can be routinely used. Five ports are used when an organ other than the one that is the focus of the operation needs to be retracted. An example of this is vagotomy, in which the liver must be retracted, yet four ports are needed to do the vagotomy apart from retracting the liver. Three ports are used when there is no need for retraction, e.g., for inguinal herniorrhaphy and appendectomy. In each case, one port is used for the scope, a second is used as the operating port, and the third is used for holding or providing traction. An additional situation in which three ports might be adequate is with the use of an operating laparoscope through which instruments could be passed.

Placement of the port for the laparoscope is very important. For many operations the laparoscope should be placed through the umbilicus, but it is not necessary to restrict the laparoscope to that locale. The laparoscope should be positioned where the best visualization is obtained. It must be placed far enough away from the target organ that a "panorama" view of the area can be obtained and that there is room to work in front of the scope. Yet it must be close enough that the laparoscope can reach into the field for fine, meticulous portions of the operation. This port must also be placed in a location where there is an appropriate angle for visualization of all necessary aspects of the target organ. Finally, the port for the laparoscope must be placed so that it can be manipulated externally with a comfortable reach by the person assigned to do that.

To meet these criteria, the laparoscope is usually best positioned in the umbilicus for cholecystectomy. However, in a patient with extensive upper abdominal adhesions, it might be better to place it in the right mid-abdomen. For right colectomy, the scope can be placed in the left mid-abdomen, and for sigmoid resection it can be placed either at the umbilicus or higher through the abdominal wall.

Satisfactory placement of the operating port is as or more important than placement of the port for the laparoscope. The operating port must be placed in relationship to the laparoscope so that the surgeon can have an angle that is comfortable and familiar to him or her. Although the experienced laparoscopist can operate from any angle in relation to the laparoscope, it is much more difficult to operate from some angles than others. It is particularly difficult to operate from a "straight on" position in which the operating instrument is pointed directly at the laparoscope. When operating port positions on the left or right of the laparoscope are different from what the surgeon is most accustomed to, the movements will seem backward to the surgeon. This will require a period of acclimation before movements become automatic and comfortable. Sometimes this is unavoidable, and with experience, all positions can be effectively utilized.

The second important aspect of operating port placement involves the relationship of this port to the target organ. For the use of blunt dissectors, scissors, clips, or forceps it may not be so critical, but if the use of a stapler is contemplated, the port must be placed in a position to allow the organ to be introduced between the jaws of the stapler. For example, the use of the stapler for dividing the colon at the rectosigmoid junction at the time of sigmoid resection requires that the stapler come across the bowel transversely. The port for the stapler must be low enough on the abdominal wall for the stapler to fit transversely across the distal line of resection and divide it. Additionally the size of this port must be adequate to accommodate any instruments that might be needed to complete the operation.

The remaining ports are for graspers and retractors. These must be positioned with a variety of factors in mind, all having to do with optimal exposure. The ports must be placed not only so that the instruments passed through them can reach and grasp the target organ, but also so that there is room between the port and the target organ to move and place tension on the organ. If the port is too close to the target organ, there is no room to move the organ to place traction on it. Also the two ports must be placed in relation to each other so that the actions through them complement each other, rather than duplicate the same function. In the case of cholecystectomy it is acceptable for these two ports to come toward the gallbladder from the same direction because they are both retracting against a fixed point (the attachment to the liver). Other procedures such as sigmoid resection require that retracting ports be placed on opposite sides of the target organ. For this operation, these ports should be placed in the left mid-abdomen and the suprapubic midline.

The ports for retraction must also be placed so that externally they can be used comfortably by the appropriate person. If the surgeon is using a two-handed technique for the operation (Fig. 11-1), one of these retraction ports must be placed in relation to the operating port so that the surgeon can comfortably use both the operating port and this retraction port from his or her side of the table. For example, to do laparoscopic herniorrhaphy, the surgeon should be using an umbilical port and a lateral port so that he or she can stand on the side of the lateral port and have the two ports immediately in front. If an assistant is to use both retracting ports, they must be placed so that the assistant can comfortably use them for the duration of the operation. In the case of cholecystectomy, the assistant can use the midclavicular and anterior axillary line ports while standing on the patient's right side.

Likewise, if the surgeon is operating the laparoscope with one hand (to move the camera to better simulate depth of field perception) and using the other hand for the

Techniques of Exposure, Retraction, and Dissection   117

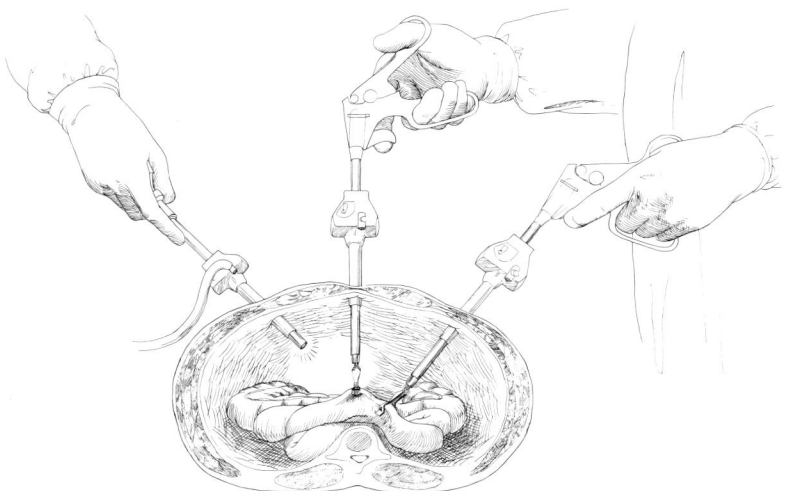

Figure 11-1. The surgeon is operating with both hands, and both ports are positioned comfortably on one side of the patient.

operating port, these two ports must be placed in a relationship which would allow the surgeon to utilize these two ports comfortably from his or her side of the table. During cholecystectomy, placing the laparoscope through an umbilical port and placing the operating port in the upper midline creates an arrangement where the surgeon can manage both comfortably. Finally, any port used for retraction must not only be placed in a position where it can provide the retraction and be managed externally by the person assigned to do so, but it must also be placed so that it does not interfere with the use of the other ports. By placing ports at least a few centimeters apart and never in a direct line toward the target organ, interference between ports can be minimized.

Position of the Patient

For essentially all laparoscopic procedures the patient can be placed in the supine or lithotomy position. However, the exposure of various areas of the peritoneal cavity can be enhanced by changing the angle of the operating table.

For operations in the pelvis, the Trendelenburg position will allow the omentum and small intestine to fall cephalad and lie in the upper portion of the abdominal cavity. The pneumoperitoneum facilitates this by increasing the space available in the upper abdomen. It is almost never necessary to actually hold the small intestine out of the pelvis. For operations in the upper abdomen, placing the patient in the reverse Trendelenburg position may be equally helpful. Specifically, in operations on the gallbladder and biliary tree or at the gastroesophageal junction, the reverse Trendelenburg position may allow the omentum and other viscera to fall toward the pelvis, enhancing exposure.

A small but sometimes significant amount of additional exposure can be obtained by tilting the table right or left. Examples of procedures in which this might help include cholecystectomy, appendectomy (particularly for a retrocecal appendix), and mobilization of the splenic flexure.

Techniques for Retractors and Graspers

Retractors can be placed into the abdominal cavity, and in the case of the uterus, they can be placed in the uterine cavity. A Cohen manipulator is invaluable in holding the uterus and adnexae anteriorly to better expose the pouch of Douglas. This eliminates the need for an intra-abdominal method of retracting the uterus. For intra-abdominal retraction of an organ that cannot be easily grasped (solid organs such as liver or spleen), an expandable retractor which fits through a port and then expands in the abdominal cavity is most effective (Fig. 11-2). The instrument must be blunt and have no sharp or pinching angles that could injure the intra-abdominal structures. An instrument that does not expand to create a broader surface area is much more likely to pierce the liver.

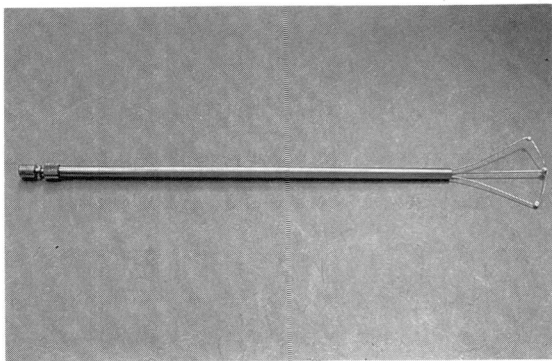

Figure 11-2. This expanded retractor can be collapsed for passage in and out of a 5-mm port.

For retracting or moving the stomach and intestinal tract, atraumatic grasping instruments are most effective (Fig. 11-3). Not only are they adequate for holding the intestine in the desired position, but they also can be moved from one position on the intestine to another as the need for change in exposure dictates. These graspers grip the intestine sufficiently to allow placement of traction on the mesenteric and peritoneal attachments of the intestine, but should release the grip before tearing or injuring the bowel. At the beginning of a sigmoid resection or right colectomy, the bowel can be grasped and retracted medially to put tension on the lateral peritoneal attachments of the mesocolon. As the dissection progresses, the mobilized portion of the intestine can be moved away from the area of dissection allowing better visualization for replacing the grasper in a position to apply traction. The use of retractors or graspers that are held in a fixed position limits the progress of the operation and their use is discouraged.

In summary, good exposure is dependent upon adequate videolaparoscopic equipment, stable pneumoperitoneum, optimal port placement, the patient's position, and skillful use of the appropriate retracting devices. A breakdown in any one of these parts of the operation can result in inadequate exposure. Excellent exposure remains the dominant prerequisite for safe and expeditious surgery.

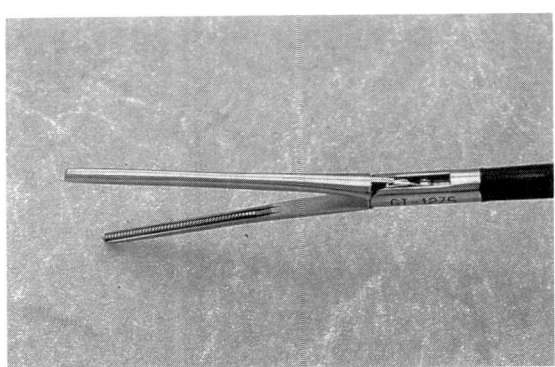
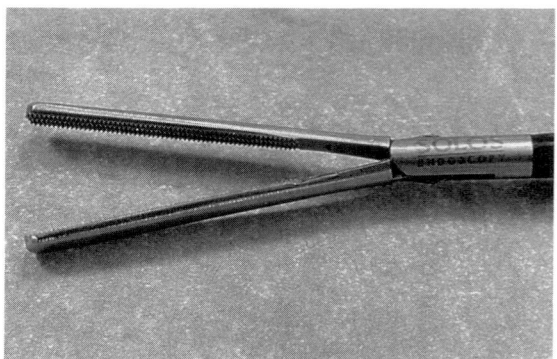
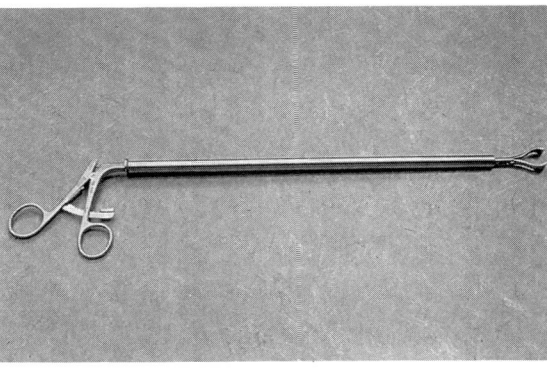
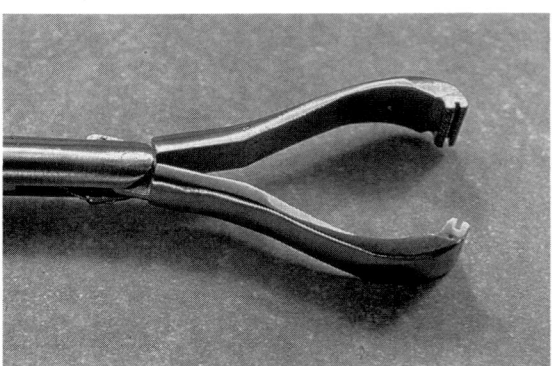

Figure 11-3. The top two photographs show different views of a bowel grasper. The bottom two photographs show a large endoscopic Allis clamp.

DISSECTION TECHNIQUES

The actual techniques of laparoscopic dissection do not differ substantially from those for an open procedure, but this dissection is perhaps even more dependent on adequate exposure than during an open procedure. With the exception of inguinal herniorrhaphy, most laparoscopic procedures can be performed similarly if not actually identically to an open procedure. The method of dissection and the type of instrument used need not be appreciably different.

There are several methods of dissection. Blunt dissection can be effectively used when there are no troublesome small vessels within the tissue. It is particularly effective in the dissection of the triangle of Calot during cholecystectomy. A right angle clamp (Fig. 11-4) can be used to strip the peritoneum from the underlying duct and artery. It can also be effectively used in skeletonizing larger vessels such as the cystic artery or arteries in the mesentery by inserting it right beside the artery and opening the clamp. At any location where it is used, the blunt dissection technique is dependent upon adequate exposure and adequate traction with countertraction.

Sharp dissection can most effectively be done laparoscopically with scissors. A variety of scissors are available. Some are straight, some are curved, some have hook blades, and each of these shapes may or may not be used with electrocautery (Fig. 11-5). Again, some tension on the tissue to be divided facilitates cutting with the scissors. When one is cutting through tissue that bleeds, the use of the coagulating current before mechanically cutting with the scissors can minimize bleeding.

As for open surgery, both electrocautery and laser can be used to dissect. The obvious

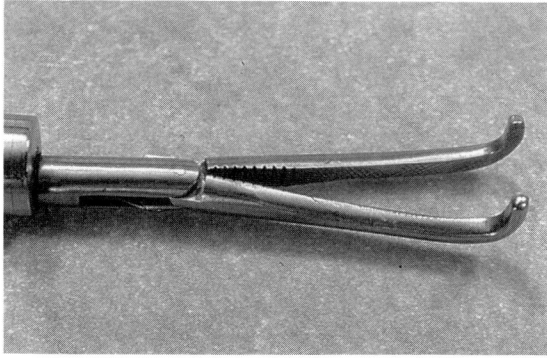

Figure 11-4. This laparoscopic Mixter can be used for blunt dissection.

advantage of these methods is the potential to coagulate blood vessels at the time they are cut. Each of these energy sources has the potential to minimize bleeding, but electrocautery technology is usually much less expensive than laser. Although monopolar cautery is more familiar to American surgeons, bipolar cautery has been used extensively around the world to control bleeding sites during laparoscopy. Bipolar cautery can effectively control arteries as large as the cystic artery. Laser has been less commonly used, but has been shown to be effective for cholecystectomy, herniorrhaphy, and appendectomy, although there is no evidence that it functions better than electrocautery. Dissection techniques using either electrocautery or laser are very dependent upon traction and countertraction.

The laser energy is usually delivered through a small fiber placed in a larger cannula. Irrigation and suction can both be ac-

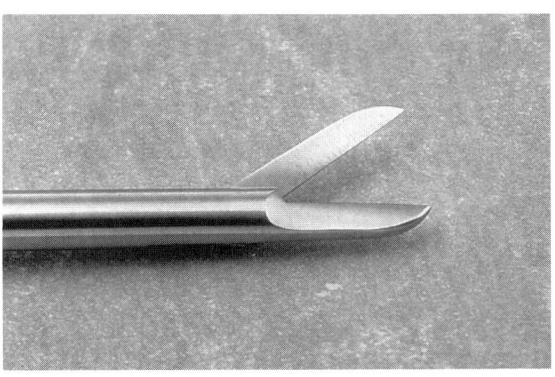 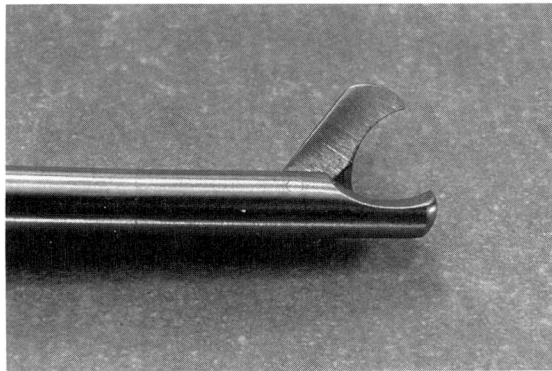

Figure 11-5. These are examples of straight (*left*) and hook (*right*) laparoscopic scissors.

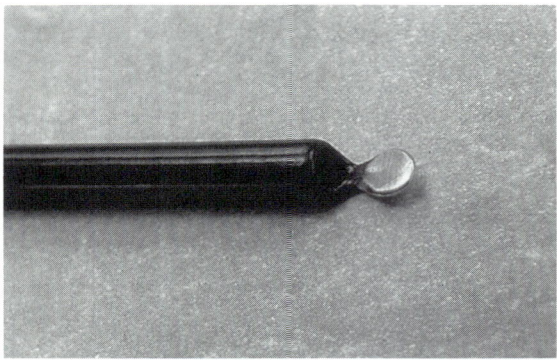 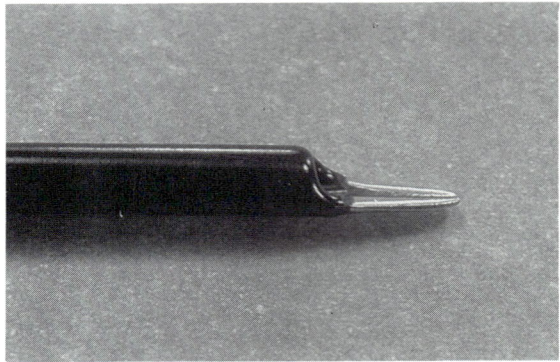

Figure 11-6. On the *left* s a spatula cautery tip and on the *right* is a point cautery tip.

complished through this larger cannula, although not at the same time. However, a great number of electrocautery tips are available. The two most commonly used types of cautery tips are the spatula tip and the hook tip. Although some mechanical blunt dissection can be performed with the hook tip, when tissue is caught in the hook and pulled away from the surrounding tissue, the application of the cautery energy is less effective because of the relatively broad area of contact between the tissue and the tip. The most effective delivery of electrocautery energy is with a very small area of contact between the tip and the tissue. For this, the spatula or a point tip usually functions best (Fig. 11-6). These electrocautery tips must also have irrigation and suction capability. This ability to irrigate or suction provides an additional advantage when the surgeon uses electrocautery or laser.

The most important technique in laparoscopic dissection is to provide traction and countertraction. Whether dissecting bluntly, with the scissors, or with electrocautery or laser, tension on the dissection plane is crucial. This requires the use of effective grasping instruments that can be repositioned as the dissection progresses. Whether the procedure is cholecystectomy, appendectomy, or sigmoid resection, the graspers must be able to pull against a fixed point to provide this tension.

In the case of cholecystectomy, the fixed point will usually be the attachment to the liver. In mesenteric dissection during colectomy, the fixed point will usually be provided by a second grasper. The graspers must initially both be placed on the bowel a few centimeters apart and then pulled in opposite directions to place the bowel and mesentery on tension (Fig. 11-7). Once a portion of the mesentery is dissected and there is an opening in the mesentery, the bowel grasper should be placed on the edge of the mesentery itself to lift it and provide continued traction. Countertraction can be provided with another bowel grasper placed appropriately farther down the bowel. As the dissection progresses a few centimeters, the tension will be lost, and the grasper must be repositioned closer to the point of dissection.

The effective implementation of traction and countertraction techniques during laparoscopic surgery is dependent upon grasping devices appropriate for the organ being dissected. Instruments used to grasp the gallbladder need not be atraumatic, since the gallbladder will be removed, but they must

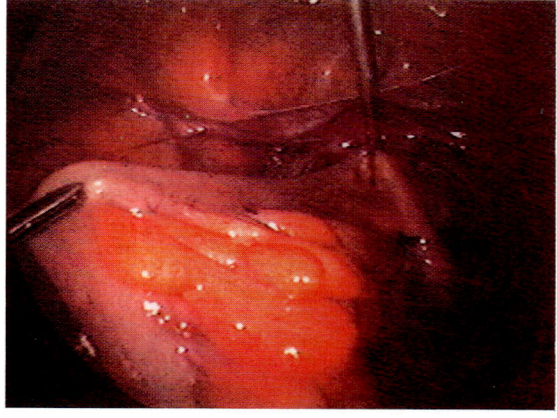

Figure 11-7. Bowel graspers are seen holding the sigmoid colon in two places to provide traction on the mesentery for dissection.

not be so traumatic as to perforate the gallbladder. These graspers grip the gallbladder tightly enough to injure it, but will usually pull off before actually tearing it. Instruments for grasping the stomach or intestine must be atraumatic. During laparoscopic bowel surgery, it is usually necessary to grasp portions of the intestine that are not to be removed. Therefore, these graspers grip much less tightly and either have no teeth or very fine teeth, which will not themselves injure the bowel wall. These instruments must also be easy to move and reposition so that as the dissection progresses, they may be reapplied to continually provide adequate tension on the dissection plane.

Most of the time, the choice of instrument with which to dissect is a matter of personal preference for the surgeon. However, there are certain instances in which one instrument generally works better than another. When a vessel is divided between clips, scissors are preferred because the cut can be placed precisely between the clips. Blunt dissection is most effective for stripping peritoneum from an organ or from vessels. If sharp or cautery dissection is used, there is a risk of injuring the underlying organ or vessel. When the dissection proceeds along a well defined plane, particularly one with some vascularity, electrocautery or laser is very effective for separating tissue along that plane, while at the same time it coagulates small vessels. Examples would include the plane between the gallbladder and the gallbladder fossa and the plane between the greater omentum and the transverse colon.

A technique that has occasional application but has not been fully evaluated is hydrodissection. A small, high pressure stream of saline can be instilled into a poorly defined plane resulting in a thickened, better defined plane. This allows the dissection to proceed more quickly and with less chance of injuring the tissue on either side. It is a particularly helpful technique for dissecting the gallbladder from its fossa when the dissection is difficult. The instillation of saline into the tissue plane reduces the conductivity of the tissue; hence, electrocautery will not work as well, and sharp dissection may be necessary.

New technology will inevitably be developed that will provide further improvements in the surgeon's ability to dissect safely and quickly. The argon beam coagulator and different wavelength lasers, and the ultrasonically activated scalpel are potential additions to the tools available for coagulation and dissection. For now, blunt dissection, sharp scissor dissection, and electrocautery dissection are adequate for essentially all the laparoscopic procedures presently being performed.

CONTROL OF VESSELS

During the initial development of laparoscopic surgical techniques, one of the greatest obstacles was the fear of intractable bleeding. This fear has been eliminated with the development of both techniques and technology to adequately control blood vessels. Obviously, smaller arteries can be controlled with electrocautery, and that is the technique of choice when it is adequate. But many intra-abdominal organs have an arterial supply that is too big to control with electrocautery. There are three basic alternative techniques for controlling the blood supply to an organ being resected: ligatures, clips, and staples. But before these methods can be used, the artery must be located.

Since it is not possible during laparoscopy to palpate the mesentery to localize the arteries, another method of identifying them is desirable. Blind dissection of the mesentery until an artery is encountered can be used, but this can result in an injury to the artery before it is controlled. A Doppler probe (Fig. 11-8) placed through one of the laparoscopic ports can identify all the arteries with sizable pulsatile flow in a very short time and allow a more precise dissection of each artery. Although this technique was initially developed for intestinal surgery, it can also be of help in cholecystecomy when the cystic artery is not easily identified (Fig. 11-9).

The laparoscopic application of a ligature is an effective means of controlling arteries. However, it is best accomplished with the artery still in continuity, and this is time consuming. The cystic artery during cholecystectomy, the superior sigmoid artery during sigmoidectomy, and the ileocolic artery during right colectomy are all examples of arteries that can be effectively ligated laparoscopically. After skeletonizing the vessel, the ligature to be used is passed around the vessel and then it is tied. It can be tied intracorporeally, or both ends can be brought out through a port and it can be tied extracorporeally. Intracorporeal knots are tied with a simple instrument tie under laparoscopic visualization. Extracorporeal knots can be tied either with a Roeder knot or standard surgical

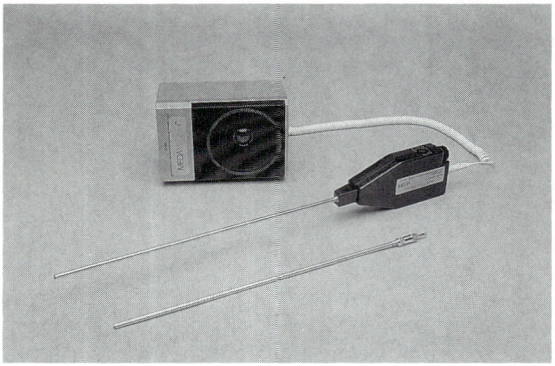

Figure 11-8. This laparoscopic Doppler probe is shown attached to the speaker box. The power supply and all switches are located in the handle. During laparoscopic use, the handle and cord are covered with a sterile drape. The actual probe is detachable and can be sterilized.

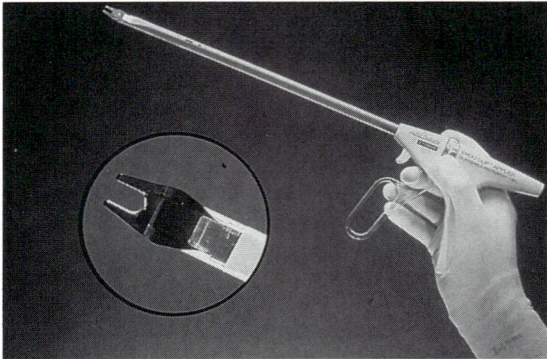

Figure 11-10. The USSC* ENDO CLIP* applier automatically reloads.

knot, each of which can be tightened with a pusher.

If a major vessel is divided without previous control, it can be grasped with a laparoscopic clamp to stop the bleeding, and an adequate ligature can still be applied. However, ligation is much easier while the artery is in continuity and is not bleeding significantly.

A faster and easier way to control substantial arteries is with metal clips. Most arteries encountered during gastrointestinal tract surgery are small enough that they can be safely controlled with a clip. Much the same as when using a ligature, the artery should be skeletonized with blunt dissection, and then one or more clips can be securely placed on the artery with good visualization before it is divided. Automatically loading clip appliers are commercially available (Fig. 11-10). The cystic artery, branches from the gastric and gastroepiploic arteries, and many arteries in the mesentery can be quickly and safely controlled with clips (Fig. 11-11).

The newest technology to be of help in controlling large vessels during gastrointestinal tract surgery is an endoscopic stapler with 2.5-mm staples (Fig. 11-12). The stapler applies three rows of staples on each side of the tissue and then divides the tissue between these rows of staples with a knife. This provides quick and hemostatically secure control of even larger vascular pedicles. It is particularly helpful for the primary vascular pedicles during laparoscopic colectomy (Figs. 11-13 and 11-14) and for controlling both the infundibulopelvic ligament and uterine vessels during hysterectomy.

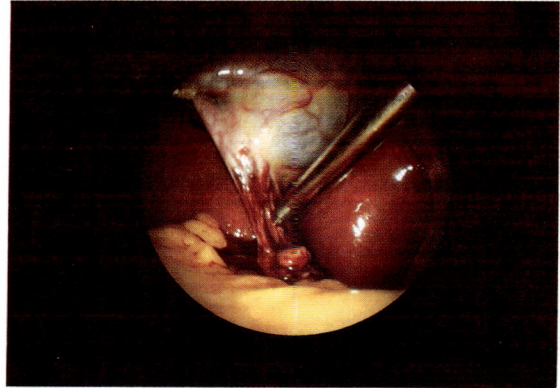

Figure 11-9. The Doppler probe is against the cystic artery, and its signal indicates pulsatile flow.

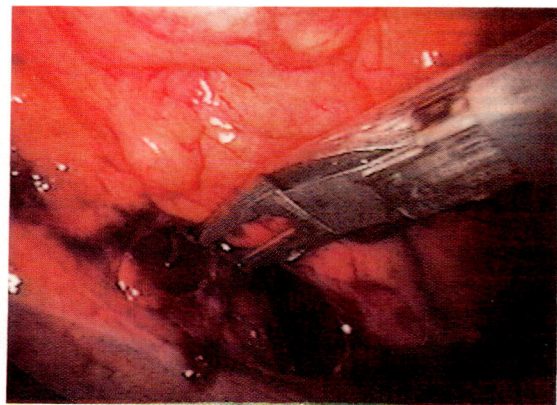

Figure 11-11. The clip applier is positioned to clip the exposed vessel.

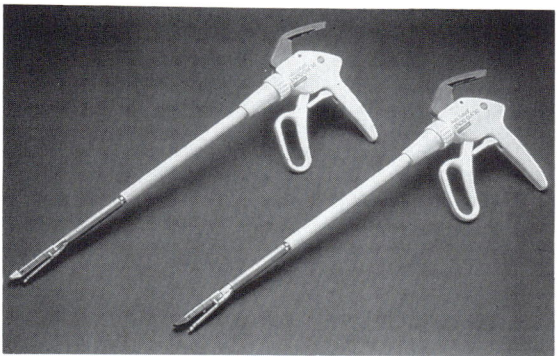

Figure 11-12. These two USSC* ENDO GIA* staplers apply two sets of three rows of staples and cut between these. The cartridge on the lower stapler contains 3.5-mm staples for use on the intestine, and the cartridge on the upper stapler contains 2.5-mm staples for vascular structures.

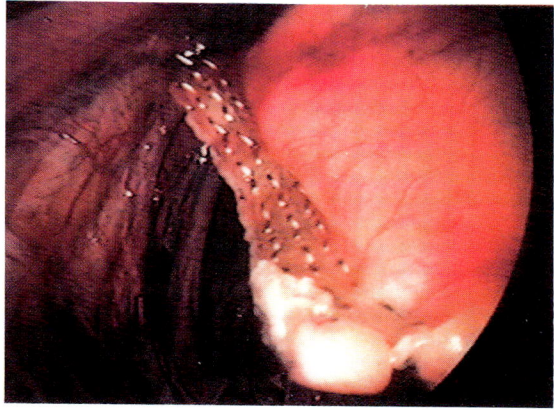

Figure 11-14. These three rows of staples are on the superior sigmoid artery.

As in the case of open surgery, there are many methods for controlling large arteries during laparoscopic surgery. The size of the vessels, the availability of instruments, and the experience of the surgeon will dictate the technique used.

THE FUTURE

The future of laparoscopic surgery will almost certainly include new technology or new applications of old technology to enhance the surgeon's ability to evaluate intra-abdominal disease. Almost certainly on the horizon will be ultrasound probes for laparoscopic use and perhaps even radioactivity-sensing probes for detecting localization of radioactive labeled antibodies. The basis for our ability to operate laparoscopically is our ability to obtain information about the anatomy and pathology of the abdominal cavity. Although laparoscopy provides adequate visualization, it limits the use of our other senses. Technology is now giving us tools to obtain that information formerly acquired by our senses. In some cases it may provide information that we could not have perceived even with our senses at laparotomy. We are limited only by our imagination in the development of newer technology that will further our ability to obtain information from within the abdominal cavity at the time of laparoscopy. With that information, more effective therapy can perhaps be provided.

ACKNOWLEDGMENTS

The author would like to acknowledge the assistance of Sharon A. White, R.N., in the writing of this chapter. In addition to proofreading and making suggestions, she participated in the development of the techniques of exposure and dissection that are discussed here.

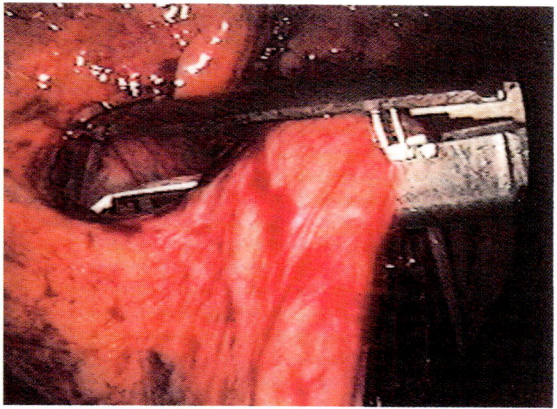

Figure 11-13. The endoscopic stapler is around the superior sigmoid artery during sigmoid resection.

BIBLIOGRAPHY

Bailey RW, Flowers JL, Graham SM, Zucker KA. Combined laparoscopic cholecystectomy and selective vagotomy. Surg Laparosc Endosc 1991; 1:45–49.

Cooperman AM, Katz V, Zimmon D, Botero G. Laparoscopic colon resection: A case report. J Laparosc Surg 1991; 1:221–224.

Fowler DL, White SA. Laparoscopic resection of a submucosal gastric lipoma: A case report. J Laparoendosc Surg 1991; 1:303–306.

Fowler DL, White SA. Laparoscopy-assisted sigmoid resection. Surg Laparosc Endosc 1991; 1:183–188.

Pier A, Gotz F, Bacher C. Laparoscopic appendectomy in 625 cases: From innovation to routine. Surg Laparosc Endosc 1991; 1:8–13.

Zucker KA. Laparoscopic guided cholecystectomy. *In* Zucker KA, ed. Surgical Laparoscopy. St. Louis, Quality Medical Publishing, Inc, 1991.

Chapter 12
Anastomosis

Steven D. Wexner
Juan J. Nogueras

Regardless of which operation is performed on the gastrointestinal tract, basic surgical principles must be followed to achieve a successful outcome. There must be excellent exposure of the operative field, allowing the surgeon adequate visualization of all vital structures. Often this means that retraction of one form or another is required. If resection is planned, the target organ must be mobilized by dividing its attachments to other viscera and retroperitoneal structures and interrupting its vascular supply. At resection, there should be no spillage of enteric contents in the peritoneal cavity. The specimen must be retrieved intact to obtain a complete pathologic analysis. The anastomosis must be circumferentially intact, tension free, and well vascularized. These tenets have held true over the decades of evolving technology and are of paramount importance regardless of the anastomotic technique employed. The excitement associated with the availability of new "minimal access" surgical techniques must not defocus these surgical axioms. Compromise cannot be accepted to facilitate technique, but rather technical advances must keep pace with the rigors of sound surgery. With these thoughts in mind, this chapter reviews the available options for laparoscopic and laparoscopically assisted intestinal anastomoses.

INSTRUMENTATION

The range of available instrumentation is constantly increasing. Initial products were small and were designed for laparoscopic cholecystectomy. Present enthusiasm regarding the potential colorectal applications of laparoscopy, however, have led to the development of instruments more appropriate for intestinal surgery. Some of the bowel clamps now available are illustrated in Figure 12-1.

Resection and Anastomosis

Patients scheduled for elective laparoscopic colonic resection undergo a preoperative mechanical cathartic bowel preparation the day prior to surgery. In addition, both oral and broad spectrum parenteral antibiotics are administered. At least two video monitors should be utilized; these should be positioned at the feet of the stretcher at 45-degree angles toward the operating team. Alternatively, these monitors can be suspended from the ceiling. If four monitors are available, the two additional monitors should be positioned at the head of the stretcher. Figure 12-2 illustrates the arrangement of the patient, the operating room personnel, and the monitors.

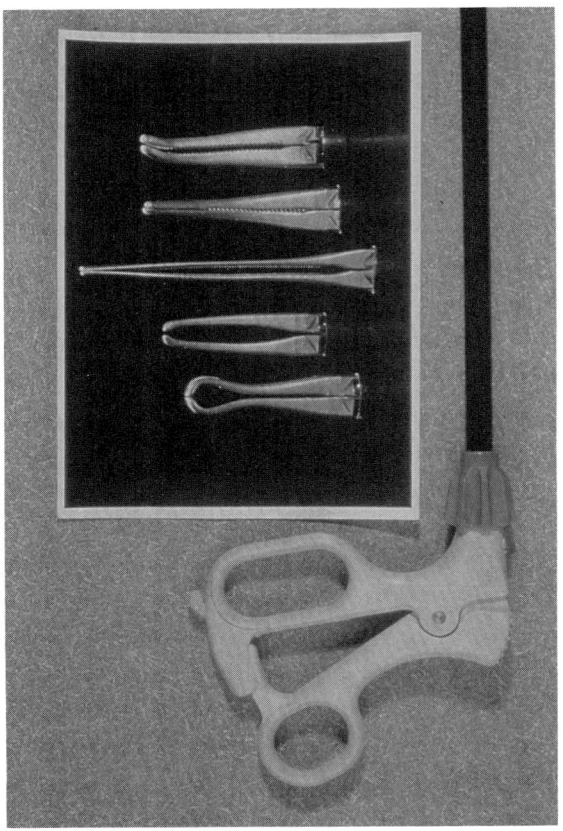

Figure 12-1. Some of the currently available bowel clamps include adaptations of traditional Mixter, Kelly, Dennis, Alis and Babcock clamps.

The patient is placed either in the supine or the supine modified lithotomy position under general anesthesia. A Foley catheter and a nasogastric tube are inserted to minimize the risks of trocar injury to the bladder or stomach, respectively. The abdomen is prepared in the standard fashion and draped to provide a wide exposure. A site is selected for insertion of the insufflator needle. If the patient has had no previous abdominal surgery, we prefer to introduce the Veress needle in the infraumbilical position. In the patient with a prior history of abdominal surgery, the open technique of insertion may be utilized. After a pneumoperitoneum of 15 to 16 mm Hg is established, a large (either 10/11 mm or 12 mm) trocar is inserted in the place of the insufflating needle. The camera is then introduced into this port, and all subsequent port insertions are accomplished under direct visualization.

The selection of port sites depends upon the proposed operation. In general, it is important that ports be close enough to one another so that instruments can reach the operative field with ease, yet not so close that there is ongoing intracorporeal clashing of instruments, so called "sword-fighting." In addition, only ports of a minimum size of 10 mm are used. This allows maximum flexibility for repositioning of the camera, bowel clamps, staplers, and other instruments. This issue highlights an important difference between gallbladder surgery and bowel surgery. In order to significantly decrease the size of a Kocher cholecystectomy incision, the ports utilized for laparoscopic cholecystectomy must be as few in number and as small in diameter as possible. This is crucial since a Kocher incision is often only 8 to 10 cm in length. However, an appreciable reduction from a standard 25 to 30 cm midline celiotomy incision can be realized even after introduction of five 12-mm ports. The right colon is best mobilized after insertion of additional large ports in the right suprapubic position and the right midclavicular line in the right upper quadrant (Fig. 12-3). Similarly, for operations on the left colon, additional large ports are inserted in the left suprapubic position and left midclavicular line in the upper quadrant (Fig. 12-4).

Table positioning can facilitate the retraction of loops of bowel from the operative field. For example, when the sigmoid colon is mobilized, placing the patient in the Trendelenburg position with the table tilted to the right can help keep the loops of small bowel out and away from the pelvis. Similarly, when the hepatic flexure is mobilized, a reverse Trendelenburg position and a table tilt to the left can be helpful. If further retraction is needed, an assistant can insert a laparoscopic retractor through one of the ports. Figure 12-5 illustrates a laparoscopic retractor.

Mobilization of the colon from the retroperitoneum is accomplished by grasping the colon with specially designed noncrushing intestinal clamps (see Fig. 12-1) and retracting in a medial direction, thereby exposing the line of Toldt. This avascular plane is then divided with a combination of blunt and sharp dissection; electrocautery is used for both dissection and hemostasis. Larger vessels located at the flexures are ligated with either surgical clips or endoloops. Once full mobilization has been accomplished, the mesenteric vascular supply is divided. If an extracorporeal anastomosis is planned, this vascular ligation can also be done in an extracorporeal fashion. However, intracorporeal vascular di-

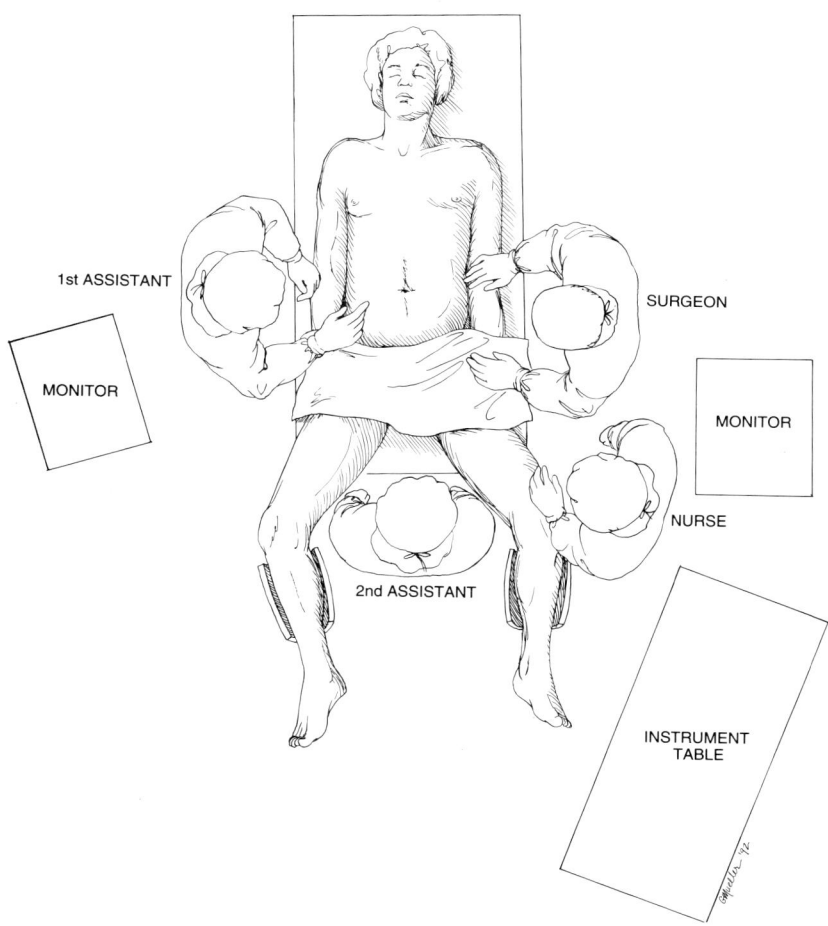

Figure 12-2. Patient positioning.

vision is mandatory if an intracorporeal anastomosis is planned and can also be performed prior to exteriorization for an extracorporeal anastomosis. Vascular division is best facilitated by skeletonization of the vessels and ligation with either clips or suture material. Most vessels are either doubly ligated or doubly clipped. Alternatively, the endoscopic gastrointestinal anastomosis (ENDO GIA*) instruments with the 30-mm vascular cartridge can be used for mesenteric division (Fig. 12-6A). Once the mesentery is divided and the lines of resection are free of vessels, the bowel is ready for transection.

Intracorporeal Anastomosis

In practical terms, although an intracorporeal anastomosis is possible, it is a tedious and expensive procedure. Some of the expense incurred is not only from the mechanical (stapling) devices, but also from the increased time required in surgery to manipulate the bowel in that fashion. Moreover, issues such as bacterial contamination and tumor spillage have not yet been resolved. Nonetheless, for the sake of completeness, the intracorporeal anastomosis technique is discussed.

The technique used in dividing the bowel is an important step in the subsequent anastomosis of the two bowel ends. The ENDO GIA* stapling instrument creates two stapled ends of bowel, thereby minimizing spillage of intraluminal contents. This is preferred to the potential spillage that can easily occur if the bowel is transected and left opened within the peritoneal cavity. Despite diligent preoperative bowel preparation and the use of atraumatic occlusive clamps, fecal contamination is possible and its sequelae are potentially disastrous. Furthermore, if both the

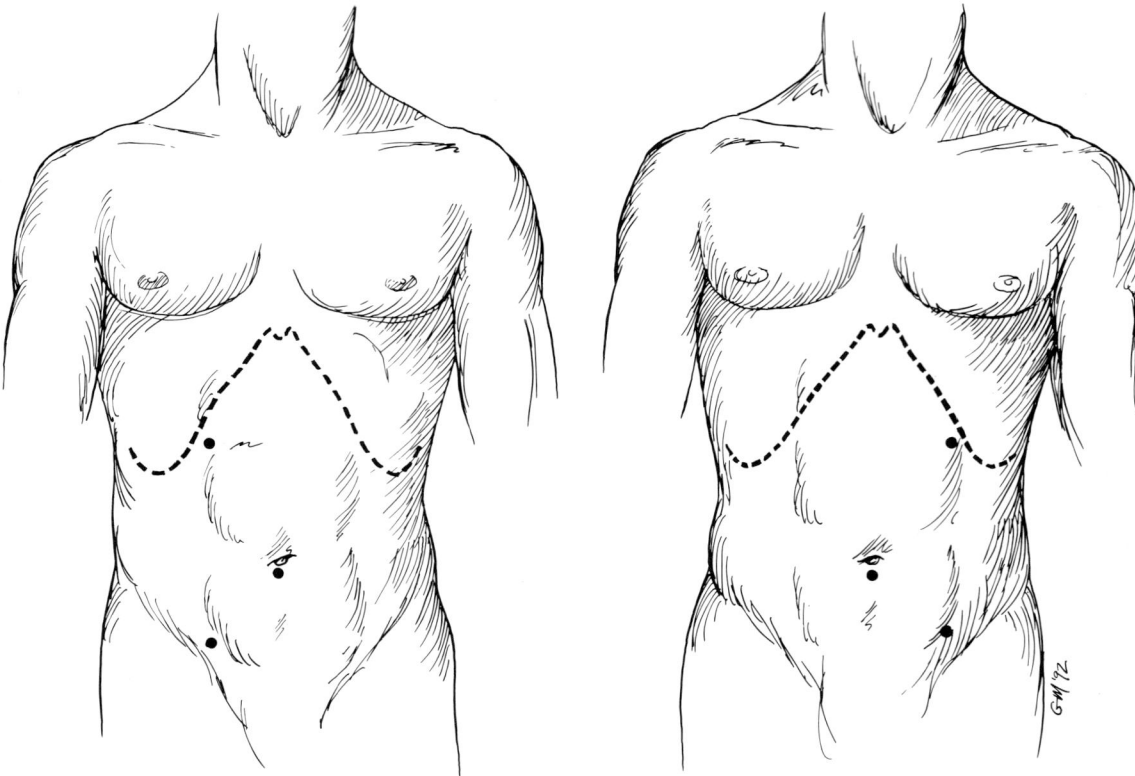

Figure 12-3. Port placement for a right hemicolectomy.

Figure 12-4. Port placement for a left hemicolectomy.

proximal and distal limbs of the bowel are occluded with clamps, two fewer ports are available for subsequent manipulation and anastomosis. Therefore, the ENDO GIA* is a very valuable instrument not only for anastomotic construction but also for preliminary bowel transection. Although the routine use of the original ENDO GIA* instruments was precluded because of their short length (30-mm staple line; Fig. 12-6A), the newer instruments are valuable assets; these instruments are shown in Figure 6B, C, and D. After each end of the bowel is divided (Fig. 12-7A), the bowel ends are grasped with Babcock clamps and the antimesenteric corners of each staple line are excised (Fig. 12-7B). A side-to-side (functional end-to-end) anastomosis is then created with a third application of the ENDO GIA* stapler (Fig. 12-7B Inset). The cut edges of the bowel are then grasped with Babcock clamps and the anastomosis is inspected for hemostasis. The lumen can be irrigated with saline, povidone-iodine, or both. The opposing cut edges of the bowel are held with Babcock clamps, and the enterotomy is closed with an ENDO GIA* stapler (Fig. 12-7C). The excess excised bowel is then removed through one of the large ports. The mesenteric defect can either be closed with a suture or with a series of clips.

Retrieval of the resected specimen can pose a dilemma. There are those who believe that in some situations transanal extraction of the

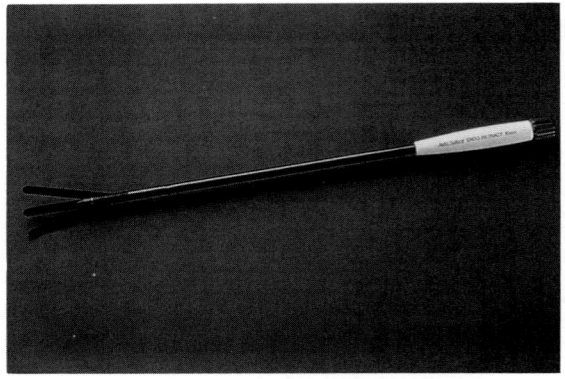

Figure 12-5. A laparoscopic bowel retractor.

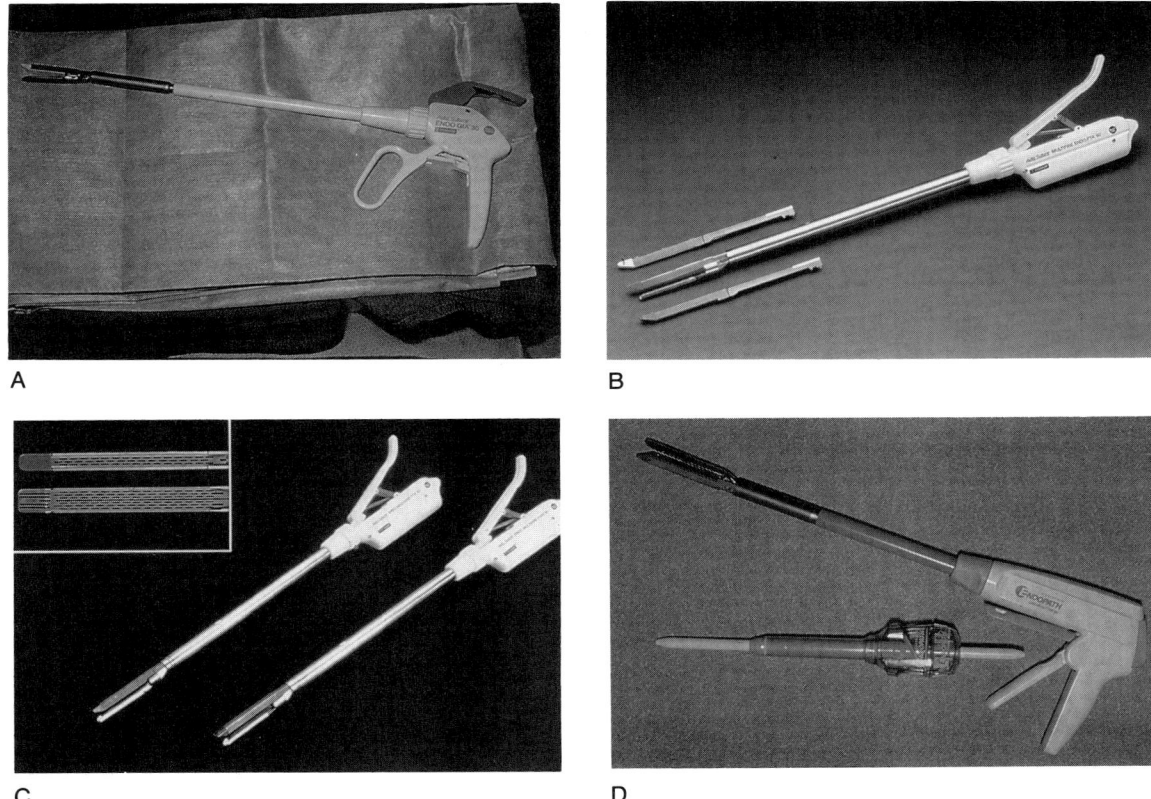

Figure 12-6. Several laparoscopic gastrointestinal stapling instruments are available: A, the ENDO GIA* 30 stapling device; B, the ENDO GIA* 60 stapling device which has both a vascular type cartridge (white) and a second cartridge generally used for bowel (blue); C, the ENDO TA* 60 stapling device which places three rows of staples instead of six and does not have a scalpel blade; D, the endopath stapling device.

resected colon can be performed. However, for the bulky lesion or for a specimen with carcinoma, this option is clearly contraindicated, because of the unphysiologic anal sphincter dilation required to deliver the left colon and its attendant mesentery out of the anus. Moreover, tumor seeding throughout the rectum is certainly a possibility. Clearly, however, the bulky colon does not readily pass through standard size ports. Until larger ports are developed, in most situations the surgeon will need to enlarge one of the port sites in order to retrieve the specimen. Moreover, if a neoplasm has been resected, the specimen may be placed in a plastic bag prior to transabdominal extraction.

If the decision is made to retrieve the specimen through an abdominal incision, consideration should be given to extracorporeal anastomosis. After full intracorporeal mobilization, a small incision is made in the abdominal wall, usually by enlarging one of the laparoscopic ports, through which the mobilized colon is then delivered. The bowel is divided, and either a hand-sewn or a stapled anastomosis is created. This technique takes advantage of the ability to mobilize laparoscopically the colon, thereby permitting a reduction in the size of the incision required to remove the specimen and create the anastomosis.

At the Cleveland Clinic Florida, we have initiated a Laparoscopic Colon Surgery Registry. Our initial experiences with seventy-three patients are based on the application of this combined intracorporeal/extracorporeal approach. The indications for surgery and the operations performed are listed in Table 12-1. Such a combined approach provides a reasonable point from which to initiate a laparoscopic colorectal surgical program by utilizing the advantages of both techniques. The mo-

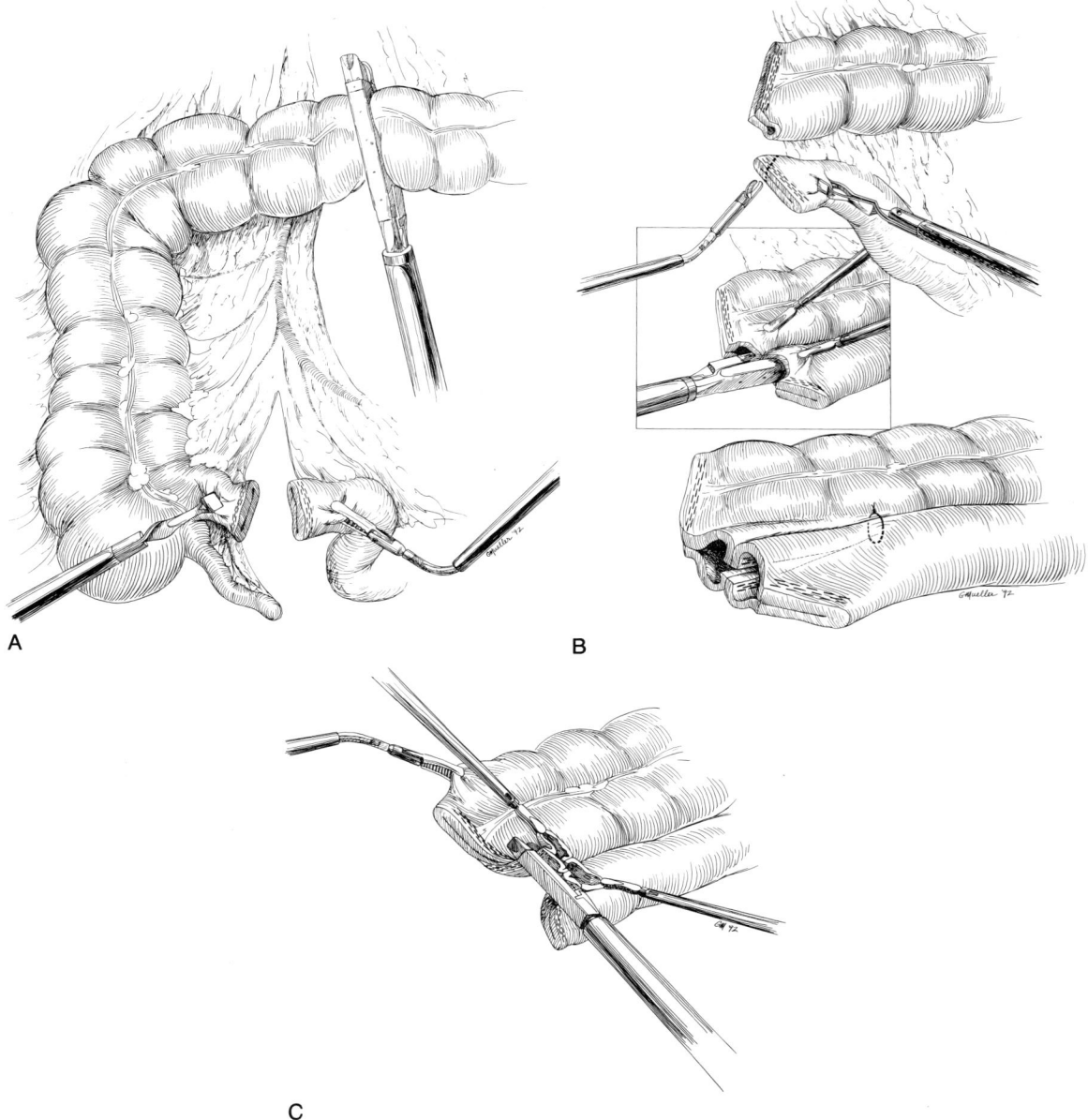

Figure 12-7. Creation of a side-to-side (functional end-to-end) anastomosis: A, bowel division; B, anastomotic creation; C, enterotomy closure.

bilization of the colon can be performed with excellent visualization, while the resection and anastomosis can be accomplished in the more familiar standard fashion. In addition, performance of an extracorporeal anastomosis allows for suture reinforcement of any nonhemostatic portions of the staple line. Furthermore, imbrication of the closed apical enterotomy and placement of a stitch to remove tension from the end of the staple line can be undertaken.

Given infinite patience and time, it is conceivable that an intraperitoneal hand-sewn anastomosis could be constructed. At least two ports would be required for stabilization of both ends of the bowel. The operator would then need two ports for handling the grasper and the needle holder. A continuous running one-layer technique would proceed more quickly than either an interrupted one-layer or a two-layer technique. Suture knot tying can be performed either intracorporeally

Table 12-1. Laparoscopic Colon Surgery, Cleveland Clinic Florida

Indications	
Mucosal ulcerative colitis	19
Cancer	12
Crohn's disease	7
Diverticular disease	8
Familial polyposis	6
Polyps	5
Incontinence	5
Colonic inertia	4
Other	7
Total	73
Procedures	
Total abdominal colectomy	31
with ileoanal reservoir	23
with ileorectal anastomosis	6
with ileostomy	2
Segmental resections	32
Stoma creations	10

or extracorporeally. A disadvantage of this intracorporeal hand-sewn anastomosis is the significant learning curve required to achieve sufficient dexterity with the instruments to complete the operation in a timely fashion. A stapled intracorporeal anastomosis is more appealing because of the avoidance of the tedious suturing demanded to effect a hand-sewn anastomosis. The technique of intracorporeal anastomosis that has the most immediate application is the colorectal anastomosis. Transanal circular stapler introduction is a procedure already familiar to most surgeons. After laparoscopic mobilization of the sigmoid colon, its vascular supply is interrupted. There are a variety of options available to create the end-to-end anastomosis.

HAND-SEWN PURSE-STRING SUTURE

This technique is particularly useful for a Hartmann's closure. After rectal transection, a distal hand-sewn purse-string suture is applied. When this suture is pulled taut, spillage is minimized. The specimen can then be delivered through an enlarged port site. As the proximal end is transected, a purse-string suture is created in the proximal end, and the proximal detachable head of the circular stapler is inserted and secured into the proximal colon. The colon is returned to the abdominal cavity and the port site is closed with either sutures or a series of clamps. Pneumoperitoneum is then reestablished, and the shaft of the stapling instrument is transanally introduced. The rod is then opened once it is properly positioned at the purse-string. Lastly, the purse-string suture is secured around the instrument. The cartridge on the proximal colon is then snapped into position into the distal shaft and the instrument is closed and fired. The anastomosis is then checked for air integrity by filling the pelvis with saline. The technique of laparoscopic circular stapled anastomosis is illustrated in Fig. 12-8.

DOUBLE-STAPLED TECHNIQUE

The advantage of the double-stapled technique is avoidance of the hand-sewn distal purse-string suture, a process that is exceedingly tedious given the current technologic limitations. The rectum is transected with a linear stapling device, closing it off with a row of staples. This technique markedly reduces the risk of spillage. The sigmoid colon is then delivered through an enlarged port site, a proximal purse-string suture is created, and the detachable instrument head is secured in position. The colon is returned to the peritoneal cavity and pneumoperitoneum is reestablished. The instrument is then inserted transanally, and once it is positioned at the level of the staple line, the rod is opened to position the spike through the center of the staple line. The spike is removed through one of the ports, and the two ends of the bowel are connected as described earlier. The technique is shown in Figure 12-8B.

TRIPLE-STAPLING TECHNIQUE

Another potential technique is the triple-stapling technique. In this variation, the detachable head of the circular stapler, under colonoscopic guidance, is transanally inserted to a level proximal to the proximal line of resection. The bowel is transected at proximal and distal ends with a linear stapling instrument. The shaft of the proximal cartridge is then delivered through the linear staple line. The stapling instrument is then transanally introduced, and an anastomosis is performed in the same fashion as described above for the double-stapled technique. This triple-stapled anastomosis has the advantage of obviating the need for a proximal or distal

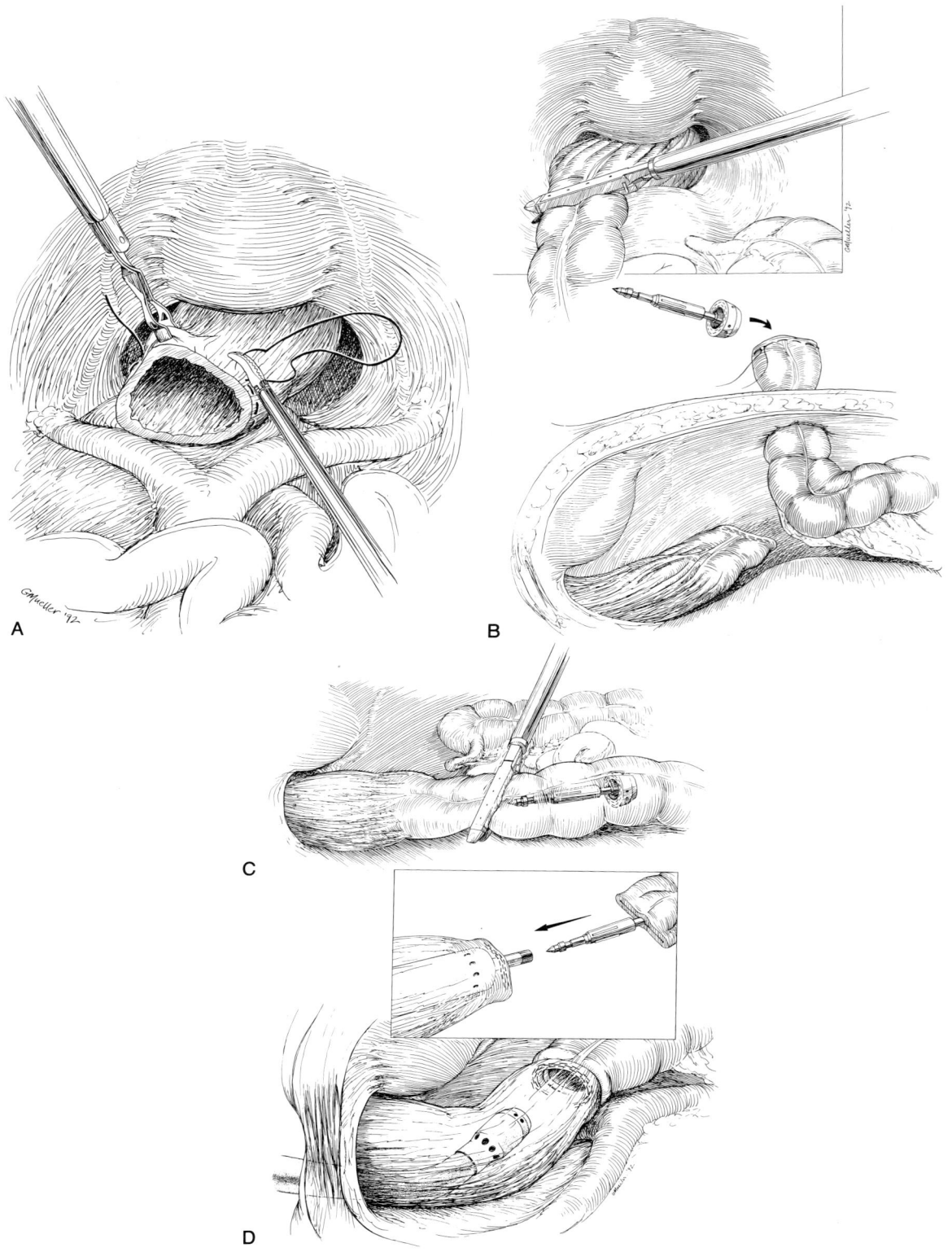

Figure 12-8. A transanal end-to-end circular stapled anastomosis: A, application of the distal purse-string suture; B, stapling the distal segment shut for the double-stapling technique and insertion of the anvil-shaft assembly of the Premium CEEA* into the proximal colon; C, stapling the proximal segment shut for the triple-stapling technique; D, docking of the anvil-shaft assembly with the center rod of the circular stapling device (inset) and retrieval of the anvil after construction of the circular stapled anastomosis.

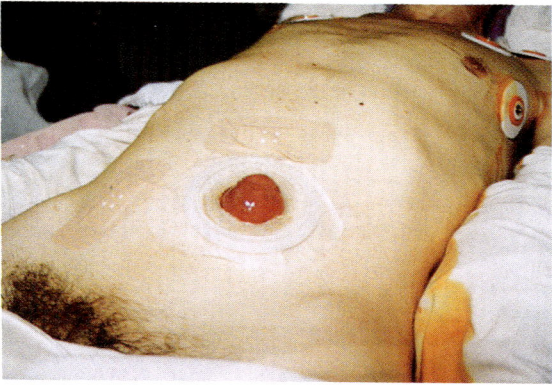

Figure 12-9. A laparoscopically constructed end sigmoid colostomy.

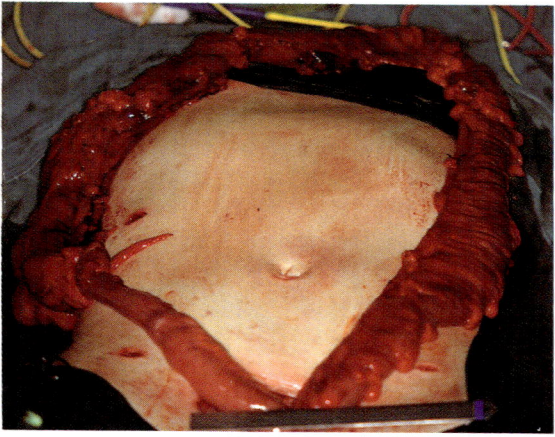

Figure 12-11. A laparoscopic-assisted total abdominal colectomy through a Pfannenstiel incision.

purse-string suture, but the disadvantage of technical difficulties in positioning the cartridge above the line and delivering the shaft through the staple line. This technique is illustrated in Figure 12-8, *C* and *D*.

Conclusions

Throughout the preliminary developmental phases of laparoscopic colorectal surgery, enthusiasm must be tempered with reality. The true morbidity, mortality, and long-term sequelae of the technology remain unknown. Qualified surgeons must, therefore, continue to assess these parameters in a meaningful, prospective fashion to perform the necessary statistical evaluations needed to decide what role laparoscopic colonic surgery will have in the surgical armamentarium.

Given current technical constraints, we perform stoma creations, Hartmann's closures, and palliative abdominoperineal resections as completely laparoscopic procedures (Figs. 12-9 and 12-10). We perform segmental and total colectomies as laparoscopically-assisted procedures utilizing the incision required for specimen removal to also perform vascular ligation, bowel transection, and anastomosis (Figs. 12-11 and 12-12). We perform resec-

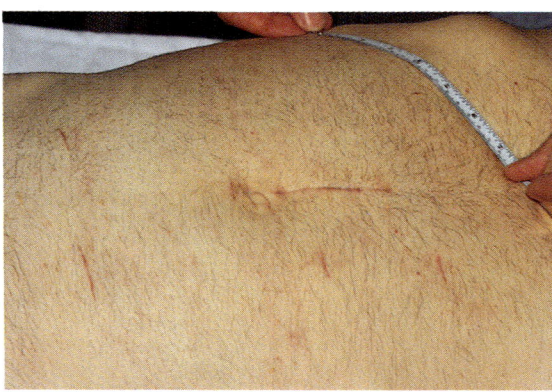

Figure 12-10. This incision after a laparoscopic-assisted right hemicolectomy measures 4.5 cm. The tape measure shows the patient's prior 21 cm subcostal cholecystectomy incision.

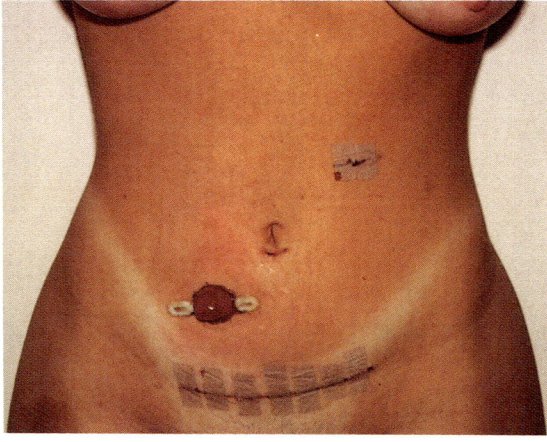

Figure 12-12. The incision after a laparoscopically-assisted ileal pouch anal anastomosis with loop ileostomy.

tions only for benign disease; patients with preoperatively identified carcinomas are offered the option of a laparoscopic or laparoscopically-assisted procedure only within the confines of a prospective randomized trial. However several reports of early port site recurrences after curative resection for malignancy are very worrisome.[1-3] Such responsible conservativism will hopefully insure the longevity of laparoscopic colorectal surgery.

REFERENCES

1. Stitz R. Laparoscopic colectomy. Presented at the American Society of Colon and Rectal Surgeons. Chicago May 2-7, 1993.
2. Guillou P. Laparoscopic colectomy. Presented at the Association of Coloproctology of Great Britain and Ireland. Glasgow May 20-21, 1993.
3. Alexander RJT, Jacques BC, Mitchell KG. Laparoscopically assisted colectomy and wound recurrence. Lancet 1993; 341:249-50.

Section III
Surgery of the Upper Gastrointestinal Tract

Chapter 13
Peptic Ulcer Disease

Margret Oddsdottir
David I. Soybel

The introduction of effective medical therapy for ulcer disease has changed the patterns of surgical management of peptic ulcer disease. Once common, elective procedures for intractable symptoms are now rare. Nevertheless, the incidence of complications requiring emergency surgery has not fallen. In the 15 years that H_2-receptor antagonists and other inhibitors of gastric acid secretion have been available, there has been no reduction in the ulcer-related mortality rate.[1-6]

Recent developments in laparoscopically assisted surgery offer the advantages of an open procedure while promising minimal postoperative discomfort and early return to daily activity. This approach may be advantageous in the management of acute, life-threatening complications of ulcer disease, including those occurring in patients at high risk for surgical complications. For the elective management of peptic ulcer disease, the laparoscopic approach may provide an alternative to protracted courses of medical therapy in carefully selected patients.

To evaluate whether laparoscopically assisted procedures can provide safe and better alternatives to present patterns of medical and surgical management, a number of issues must be addressed. First, we must reevaluate our understanding of how ulcers come into being, why they cause symptoms, and why they fail to heal or recur. It has been widely taught that the presence of luminal acid is a primary factor in the process that causes ulcers to persist and then recur. One alternative hypothesis, currently under active investigation, is that many duodenal ulcers develop and persist because of mucosal inflammatory responses to infestation by a bacterium, *Helicobacter pylori*. In this setting, acid is necessary, but secondary, in the pathogenesis of mucosal injury. Another evolving hypothesis suggests that hydrogen ions (H^+) contribute to nonhealing of duodenal and gastric ulcers, not so much by direct toxic effects on mucosal and submucosal tissue, but by destabilization of endogenous factors that promote mucosal growth, repair, and angiogenesis. If these hypotheses are proved, then development of effective antibacterial regimens and acid-stable growth factor analogues may accelerate healing and reduce recurrence rates in a high proportion of patients. Such developments could significantly alter patterns of ulcer persistence and recurrence. Conventional medical regimens or surgical interventions, which are based on a notion of suppressing gastric acid secretion, may ultimately come to play a much more limited role in management of these diseases.

Second, we must critically examine our understanding of the long term outcomes of patients with acute complications of gastric and duodenal ulcers. In evaluating the natural history of these complications, we should distinguish between those patients having ulcer complications that must be managed surgically (free ulcer perforations or unreversible gastric outlet obstruction) and complications that might be managed expectantly or endoscopically with surgical backup (bleeding ulcers or partial obstructions). The primary objective in all such patients, however, will be to treat the acute complication safely and prevent its early recurrence. The use of laparoscopically assisted approaches should become important in pursuing this primary goal, in conjunction with the development of demonstrably safe techniques for managing bleeding, perforation, and obstruction. The secondary objective of management in such patients will be to reduce the long term incidence of recurrence or other complications. As noted earlier, pursuit of this secondary goal will depend on our evolving understanding of how often and why these ulcers recur in the long term.

Third, we must appreciate the long term complications and costs of current forms of medical therapy and those of emergency and elective surgery, with its potentially low recurrence rates. At a more abstract level, we must at least consider how much it might cost to prove the feasibility of laparoscopically assisted procedures as compared to conventional medical and surgical approaches.

This chapter is divided into four parts. In the first part, we discuss central concepts related to classification, pathogenesis, and natural history of gastric and duodenal ulcers. In the second part, we briefly review the rationale and results of conventional approaches to acute and long term complications of gastric and duodenal ulcers. In the third part, we examine potential costs of medical and surgical approaches to patients with complications of ulcer disease. In the final part, we attempt to identify questions, as yet unanswered, regarding the feasibility and indications for combined laparoscopic/endoscopic approaches to complications of peptic ulcer disease.

PEPTIC ULCER DISEASE: CLINICAL COURSE

Epidemiology and Classification

Peptic ulcer disease is one of the most prevalent gastrointestinal disorders, affecting about 10 per cent of the population at some point in their lives.[7,8] Once much more common in men, the incidence in women, especially elderly women, is rising.[7,8] Overall, in the Western hemisphere, the incidence in the elderly is rising, and the duodenal/gastric ulcer ratio is decreasing.[9,10] It has been postulated that this change might be a result of the aging of the population and the increased use of nonsteroidal anti-inflammatory agents (NSAIDS) in the elderly population.[11,12]

Duodenal ulcers usually are seen in younger patients than gastric ulcers.[12] They typically occur in the first portion of the duodenum, within 1 to 2 cm of the pyloric sphincter and are rarely malignant.[13] When duodenal ulcers occur beyond the first portion of the duodenum, atypical causes of ulceration such as Zollinger-Ellison syndrome, malignancy, or drug-induced ulcers may be suspected.[14]

Gastric ulcers are frequently divided into three types, depending on their location and characteristics.[15] Type I includes the typical benign gastric ulcer, located on the lesser curvature at or proximal to the incisura angularis. In 1959, Oi et al.[16] observed that such lesions are found most frequently in the transition zone between the fundic and antral mucosa (Fig. 13-1). The fact that this junctional zone can occur quite proximally on the lesser curvature, especially in older patients, may account for ulcers that occur near the esophagogastric junction. Such high lying ulcers are sometimes classified as Type IV.[17] Type I gastric ulcers are associated with low to normal acid secretion and account for about 60 per cent of gastric ulcers.[18] Type II ulcers account for approximately 20 per cent of gastric ulcers and are those associated with active duodenal ulcers. Type III account for approximately 20 per cent of gastric ulcers and include those found in the prepyloric region or in the pyloric channel.[15] Both Types II and III gastric ulcers are generally associated with acid hypersecretion and behave like duodenal ulcers.[18] As many as 5 to 10 per cent of benign-appearing gastric ulcers may ultimately prove to be malignant.[19,20] Thus, endoscopic evaluation is mandatory for all gastric ulcers, and circumferential biopsies[8-12] of ulcer margins should be performed. Multiplicity of gastric ulcerations does not exclude the possibility of malignancy.

Pathogenesis and Pathophysiology

A number of authors have conceptualized the pathogenesis of both gastric ulcers (GUs) and duodenal ulcers (DUs) to be interactions

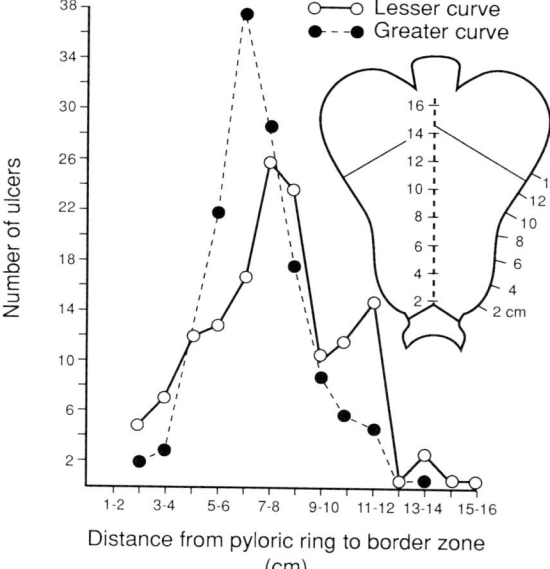

Figure 13-1. Data from Oi and co-workers, showing the distance of gastric ulcers from the pyloric ring to the transitional zone. The transitional zone between the antral-corporal mucosa tends to lie more proximal on the lesser curvature than the greater. (Reproduced with permission from Fromm D. Ulceration of the stomach and duodenum. In Fromm D, ed. Gastrointestinal Surgery. New York, Churchill Livingstone, 1985, p 261.)

of aggressive and defensive factors.[20-23] Patients with duodenal ulcers often are observed to have high basal levels of gastric acid secretion (Fig. 13-2). Such patients also exhibit exaggerated acid secretion to a meal or to stimulation by infusions of gastrin or histamine analogues.[22] An increased parietal cell mass is found in these patients as well. The mechanisms underlying hypertrophy of the parietal cell mass have not been elucidated.[21,24] It is important to note that many patients with DUs exhibit normal levels of basal and stimulated acid secretion (Fig. 13-2). It is generally accepted that high levels of acid secretion, especially at night, are a primary cause of most DUs. The prevailing explanation for the development of DUs has suggested that mucosal defenses are intact, but overwhelmed by the high levels of acid secretion.[21,22,24] However, investigators have only recently begun to evaluate possible alterations in defensive factors (such as duodenal mucus/bicarbonate ion (HCO_3^-) secretion, barrier properties, or mucosal blood flow) in the pathogenesis of DUs.

Patients with Type I GUs generally are found to have low to normal levels of acid secretion. Acid secretion and pepsin activity appear to be necessary for the formation of gastric ulcers, because ulcer healing is accelerated and recurrence rates are reduced when acid secretion is inhibited. However, there appears to be functional susceptibility of gastric mucosa, which leads to ulcerations in the region of the antral-corporal junction.

The reasons for decreased resistance in this region of the gastric mucosa (the locus minoris resistentiae) have not been identified, despite intensive investigation of gastric barrier properties. With regard to these barrier properties, it is known that the surface epithelial cells of gastroduodenal mucosa secret mucus and HCO_3^-, which maintains a neutral pH

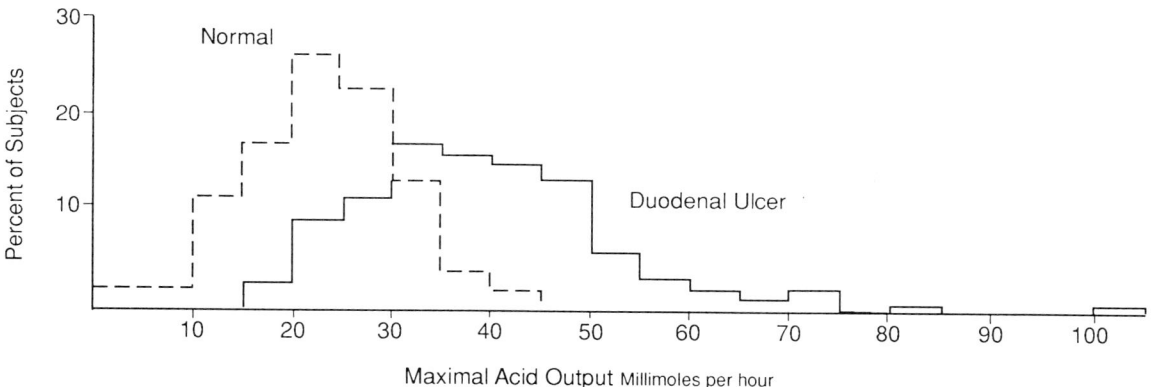

Figure 13-2. Maximal acid response to intravenous infusion of histamine in healthy control subjects and in patients with duodenal ulcers. The median value is significantly greater for duodenal ulcer patients, but more than half of them fall within the normal range. (Reproduced with permission from Grossman MI. Peptic Ulcer: A Guide to the Practicing Physician. Chicago, Year Book Medical Publishers, Inc., 1981.)

near the surface of the mucosa, despite highly acidic conditions in the lumen.[21,22,24] In addition, blood flow to gastric mucosa plays an important role in delivering HCO_3^- and washing out back-diffusing luminal H^+. Disturbances of mucosal perfusion and the mucus-HCO_3^- gel have been demonstrated in experimentally induced gastric injury[23] but have not been systematically explored in more chronic models of injury. Another important protective property involves the ability of the gastric epithelium to be rapidly reconstituted after it has been disrupted. Under normal conditions, surface cells continually slough, and the gaps are resealed by adjacent cells. Following injury by exposure to hypertonic solutions or other topical agents of injury, this process allows rapid migration of epithelial cells to cover the defects. This process depends on a microenvironment which maintains neutral pH, calcium ions, and intact microtubule and microfilament assembly processes.[25] Finally, prostaglandins enhance several of the mechanisms involved in mucosal resistance to injury. Abnormal prostaglandin production has not been verified in patients with peptic ulcer disease.[21]

Whether and how such "barrier" properties might be impaired in patients with Type I GUs remain subjects of speculation. There is evidence of an abnormally high reflux of duodenal contents (containing bile) into the stomachs of patients with Type I GUs.[23] It is not uniformly accepted that such reflux accounts for breakdown of barrier properties in the majority of patients with Type I GUs.

Two clinically relevant factors have been identified that are capable of disrupting mucosal resistance to injury by luminal acid and pepsin: (1) mucosal infestation by the bacterium H. pylori and (2) ingestion of NSAIDs such as aspirin, indomethacin, and ibuprofen.[24,26,27] H. pylori-induced gastritis is found in 95 to 100 per cent of patients with DUs and about 75 to 85 per cent of patients with GUs.[24,26] H. pylori is commonly found in the gastric mucosa of individuals without peptic ulcer disease. However, several reports have suggested that, apart from some atypical ulcers and NSAID-induced ulcers, no "conventional" ulcers exist without H. pylori infection.[21,26] There are several mechanisms by which H. pylori may be involved in ulcer formation: H. pylori infection is associated with impaired duodenal HCO_3^- secretion, decreased hydrophobicity of the mucus, hypergastrinemia, and dense inflammatory reaction. When H. pylori is eradicated from patients who have chronic duodenal ulcers, recurrences may be reduced.[27,28] The evidence supporting a major role for H. pylori in the pathogenesis of ulcer disease is substantial. However, the reason why the majority of persons who have H. pylori infection never develop ulcers is not clear.

Topical exposure of gastric mucosa to NSAIDs can elicit acute superficial erosions and prolonged ingestion may lead to chronic ulceration with bleeding or perforation.[22,24] NSAIDs can exacerbate underlying ulcer disease as well as cause ulcers *de novo*. NSAID-related ulcers have a high risk of complications, occurring equally in the stomach and duodenum.[29,30] Administration of prostaglandin E_2 analogues provides effective prophylaxis against complications of ulcers that occur in patients who require chronic use of NSAIDs.[31,32] These findings have suggested that the ulcerogenic effects of NSAIDs might be largely attributable to their inhibition of prostaglandin synthesis.

Until recently, it seemed reasonable to suggest that factors which caused the ulcer to develop were those which caused the ulcer to persist and recur. This simplified view has been called into question by recent investigation of the role of mucosal growth and angiogenic factors in ulcer healing. Epidermal growth factor is normally found in saliva; it reduces gastric acid secretion and accelerates healing of experimental gastroduodenal ulcers. Transforming growth factor α is found in the acid-secreting region of the stomach; it inhibits acid secretion, stimulates angiogenesis, and may also facilitate healing of mucosal injury. Wright et al.[33] found that cell lineages that express epidermal growth factor immunoreactivity are observed in mucosal crypts adjacent to areas of mucosal injury in a variety of inflammatory conditions of the gut. Such lineages are not observed in normal mucosa. Recent work also has shown that basic fibroblast growth factor is a very potent stimulant of angiogenesis, which is destabilized in the presence of acid and expressed in gastroduodenal mucosa.[34] Based on these preliminary observations, it has been suggested that the progression to chronic ulceration and complications could reflect alterations in mucosal repair processes owing to changes in expression or activity of endogenous growth and angiogenesis factors. If so, it might be predicted that agents that enhance mucosal repair and epithelial reconstitution would be effective in accelerating ulcer healing, even if acid secretion is not suppressed. In this regard, Folkman et al.[34,35] have shown that a form of basic fibroblast growth factor, which is stable in acid, can accelerate healing of experimentally induced duodenal injury more potently than cimetidine. Preliminary work by this group offers the possibility that the drug sucralfate binds endogenous basic fibroblast growth factor, protecting it from destabilization in acid and concentrating it near the areas of mucosal injury.

It might also be predicted that some behaviors would specifically influence ulcer healing and recurrence without necessarily increasing the incidence of ulcer occurrence. At least one risk factor, cigarette smoking, has been implicated in delayed healing of gastroduodenal ulcers but could not be shown to influence the risk of developing an ulcer *per se*. In addition, ingestion of alcohol can cause gastritis and duodenitis and may delay healing, despite the lack of evidence that alcohol is a risk factor for the development of chronic ulceration.[26,36-38]

In summary, it is clear that the pathogenesis of Type I GUs differs from that of DUs and Types II and III GUs. Until recently, clinically relevant information on the origins of these lesions could be summarized by pointing out that Type I GUs require acid to persist and cause complications, but originate in a region of gastric mucosa that has an intrinsic susceptibility to injury by luminal acid and pepsin. Duodenal ulcers and Types II and III GUs originate in the setting of high levels of basal and stimulated acid/pepsin secretion, perhaps abetted by abnormally rapid emptying of acid into the duodenum. This simplified outlook will certainly change. For the present, the surgeon who is involved in the care of patients with ulcer disease must follow closely the development of the newer lines of experimental and clinical investigation. Such inquiries may radically alter our understanding of the events that favor healing of these lesions, thus changing or eliminating current strategies for surgical management of the complications of these lesions.

Natural History of Symptomatic Disease

Peptic ulcers give rise to chronic syndromes, with activity waxing and waning over several years.[8,21] It is important to recognize that the reported "natural histories" of peptic ulcer syndromes are those of medically treated disease, rather than true reflections of the untreated illnesses. Reports of natural history are thus influenced by available medications, patterns of patient compliance, and length of therapy. In addition, the patterns of recurrence and complications may depend on the incidence of relevant behaviors, such as cigarette smoking and NSAID use, as well as the presence of underlying diseases in the population under study.

The outlook for patients with symptoms (mainly pain) caused by duodenal ulcer may be considered for the short term (less than 2 years) and over prolonged follow-up, up to 25 years after the onset of symptoms. Current regimens of sucralfate or antisecretory therapy are capable of healing up to 95 per cent of typical DUs within 12 weeks after therapy is started. Specific cases that are refractory to such management have been attributed to: (1) noncompliance with the regimen; (2) Zollinger-Ellison syndrome and failure to control gastric acid production; (3) persistent *H. pylori* infestation; (4) continued use of NSAIDs or cigarette smoking; (5) large size of the ulcer (greater than 2 cm diameter); and (6) stressful life events (although this remains controversial).

Following conventional medical management, however, recurrence rates in the short term are high. Typical figures suggest that, when therapy is stopped, relapse rates approach 55 per cent at 3 months, 75 per cent at 6 months, and 80 per cent at 12 months (Fig. 13-3).[39-42] "Maintenance" therapy, which follows the initial course of therapy to heal the ulcer, usually involves doses of antisecretory medications given to reduce night-

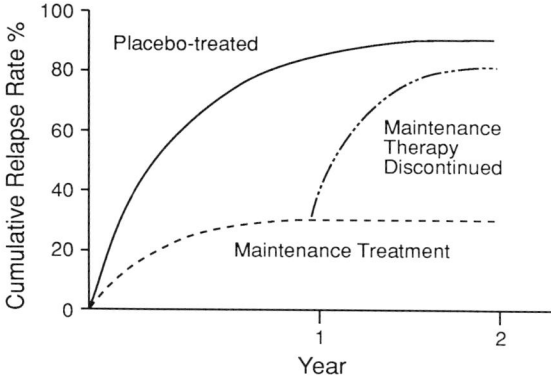

Figure 13-3. Cumulative relapse rate for duodenal ulcer with and without maintenance therapy. When maintenance therapy is discontinued, the ulcer recurrence rate approaches that of no treatment.

time acidity. Such low dose, maintenance regimens can lower recurrence rates to 15 to 20 per cent at 12 months, 20 to 25 per cent at 24 months, and 25 to 30 per cent at 36 months, following initial healing of the ulcer.[41,42] Recurrences during maintenance therapy are unlikely after 3 years. If medication is discontinued, recurrences of symptomatic DUs may continue to appear, even after 25 years of follow-up. At present, it appears that current forms of medical therapy control symptoms of DUs, but the disease may not necessarily be eliminated in all or most patients. It is not yet clear how to quantify the risk that any given patient with a DU might be consigned to a lifetime of therapy. In addition, studies are underway to determine if therapies directed at eradicating *H. pylori* will alter the risk of recurrence.

The long term course of gastric ulcers is not as well defined, since most patients undergo surgery because of the fear of malignancy and negligible recurrence rates following gastric resection. In short term studies of medical management, it appears that antisecretory therapy or sucralfate can heal 90 to 95 per cent of GUs within 12 weeks. Rates of healing are inversely correlated to size of the ulcer.[40-42] If therapy is discontinued after healing, relapse rates may approach 70 to 80 per cent at 2-year follow-up. Most recurrences are diagnosed within the first 6 months after therapy is discontinued. Maintenance therapy with antisecretory agents can reduce these 2-year recurrence rates to 15 per cent, and with sucralfate to approximately 40 per cent.[17,43] In one study, it was suggested that Type I gastric ulcers not associated with specific risk factors such as NSAID use, may "burn out" after 12 to 15 years.[43] The level of disability caused by such symptoms has not been fully explored in the more recent large scale trials of medical therapy for gastric ulcer disease.[42]

PEPTIC ULCER DISEASES: CURRENT MANAGEMENT STRATEGIES

Medical Management of Ulcer Pain

In treating peptic ulcer disease, the physician aims to alleviate symptoms, promote healing, prevent recurrences, and prevent complications. Medical treatment of peptic ulcer disease is very effective in healing ulcers and alleviating symptoms.[19] Recurrences are reduced with maintenance therapy. It is controversial whether the incidence of acute complications can be altered by maintenance therapy.[19,39,42] The natural history and management of acute complications will be discussed later in greater detail.

Patients with chronic symptoms caused by peptic ulcer disease are candidates for initial medical therapy. At present, the most widely used medical treatments for gastric and duodenal ulcers rely on inhibition or neutralization of acid. It should be emphasized that as many as 5 to 10 per cent of Type I benign-appearing gastric ulcers are malignant and malignant ulcers can appear to heal when patients are given antisecretory therapy.[19,20] Therefore, all gastric ulcers require endoscopy with biopsies of the ulcer at the beginning of therapy and at follow-up. Nonhealing after 12 weeks of therapy, rapidly recurring gastric ulcers, or any suspicion of malignancy is an accepted indication for operative treatment.

Different classes of medications available today provide the clinician with tools to decrease intragastric acidity, suppress acid production, and enhance the protective and restorative properties of the mucosa. H_2-receptor antagonists are the agents most widely used to promote ulcer healing, but sucralfate and antacids seem equally effective.[40,44-46] Omeprezole suppresses acid secretion by blocking hydrogen-potassium adenosine triphosphatase, which is the direct mediator of H^+ secretion across the apical membrane of the parietal cell. Omeprazole may be slightly more effective in accelerating rates of ulcer healing and the percentage of ulcers healed than H_2-recestor antagonists.[39,44] Based on considerations noted earlier, omeprazole therapy is not likely to provide substantially more protection against recurrence of DU or GU, once the ulcer has healed.

Agents that promote mucosal healing, without requiring a reduction in gastric acidity, include sucralfate and prostaglandin analogues. The prostaglandin E analogues effectively prevent appearance and complications of NSAID-induced ulcers. It is of interest that prostaglandins are less effective in promoting healing of such ulcers.[29,45] Bismuth compounds suppress *H. pylori* and appear to reduce the rate of early recurrences of healed duodenal ulcers.[19] Sucralfate enhances a number of reparative and protective properties of gastric mucosa.[46] As noted earlier, it may also enhance stability and availability of growth and angiogenesis factors to the injured mucosa.

Surgical Management of Ulcer Pain

Patterns of surgical treatment of peptic ulcer disease have changed over the past 20 years. Previously, approximately 85 per cent of ulcer surgery was performed electively because of intractable pain. At present, given the efficacy of medical management in relieving and preventing recurrence of symptoms, surgery is rarely performed for intractable pain or refractory ulcer healing. The rare indications for elective surgery today include frequent recurrences, history of bleeding and nonhealing, noncompliance with therapy, and the inability to rule out malignancy in a gastric ulcer.

DUODENAL ULCER

The goals of operative ulcer therapy are: (1) effective reduction of acid secretion and (2) management of the specific local complications such as bleeding diathesis, deformity of the pylorus or duodenum with impending obstruction, or penetration into adjacent structures (e.g., pancreatic bed, biliary tract, or colon). All surgical procedures, used presently to manage intractable symptoms of duodenal ulcer, are based on the strategy of suppressing gastric acid secretion.[21,24] Surgery can address the main components that regulate basal and stimulated gastric acid secretion. These components are: (1) cholinergic vagal innervation; (2) antral gastrin secretion; and (3) the parietal cell mass itself. Vagotomy plays a central role in the treatment of duodenal ulcer disease, as the disruption of efferent vagal fibers to the parietal cells directly reduces acid secretion. Additionally, vagal denervation reduces the responsiveness of the parietal cells to circulating endogenous secretagogues such as gastrin.[14] Resting, cephalic, and gastric phases of secretion are affected by vagal section. Antrectomy removes the gastrin-secreting cells and greatly diminishes the gastric phase of acid secretion. Although rarely performed at present, subtotal gastrectomy decreases the parietal cell mass in addition to removing the antrum. This operation has been as effective as vagotomy and antrectomy in controlling recurrences of ulcer disease.[14]

The standard operations used to manage duodenal ulcers include truncal vagotomy with drainage, truncal vagotomy with antrectomy, highly selective vagotomy, or modifications of these procedures. These procedures all can be performed safely in good risk patients under favorable operative conditions. However, in comparisons of the results of these operations, important differences in ulcer recurrence and postoperative complications emerge (Table 13-1).[2,14,47,48]

Highly selective vagotomy has the advantage of leaving antral motility intact, and thus a drainage procedure is unnecessary. This minimizes the incidence and severity of long term postoperative sequelae. The recurrence rate, however, is similar to that of truncal or selective vagotomies, between 5 and 15 per cent over 10 years.[4,47,49,52] Truncal vagotomy and antrectomy have been associated with recurrence rates less than or equal to 2 per cent.[2,47,48] Long term complications of this procedure are not infrequent and can be highly disabling in 1 to 2 per cent of patients. Truncal vagotomy and pyloroplasty carry the same recurrence rate as highly selective vagotomy and postoperative sequelae similar to truncal vagotomy. Except in unusual circumstances, this operation is not recommended for management of intractable ulcer symptoms.

Table 13-1. Recurrence and Mortality and Postoperative Sequelae Following Standard Operations for Duodenal Ulcer

Procedure	Recurrence (%)	Mortality (%)	Mild Symptoms (%)	Severe Symptoms (%)
Truncal vagotomy and drainage	10–15	1	20	1–5
Truncal vagotomy and antrectomy	0–2	1–2	20	1
Parietal cell vagotomy	10–15	<0.5	1–2	<1
Gastric resection (no vagotomy)	2–5	1–2	40–50	>10

Estimates derived from a variety of reports from North American and European centers.

GASTRIC ULCERS

The standard operation for Type I gastric ulcer is partial gastrectomy and Billroth I reconstruction. Current operative mortality rates are 1 to 2 per cent, and recurrence rates are less than 4 per cent. Recurrence rates following vagotomy and drainage approach 20 per cent at 10- to 15-year follow-up.[17,49,50] Regardless of the type of procedure performed, an important principle of management is to excise the ulcer. This will diagnose most unsuspected early gastric cancers as well as remove the postulated locus of least resistance. Vagotomy need not be added when distal resection is used to excise the Type I gastric ulcer.[53] For Type II and III gastric ulcers, vagotomy is required to prevent high recurrence rates, since these ulcers behave similarly to duodenal ulcers.

Management of the Type IV gastric ulcer can be challenging and is tailored to specific circumstances. The method of surgical treatment depends on the size, location, and degree of surrounding inflammation. Pauchet's procedure resects the lesser curvature as high as needed to include the high lying ulcer with the distal gastrectomy specimen. If the risk of narrowing the gastroesophagal junction is too great, then the Csendes procedure, closure of the lesser curvature with Roux-en-Y gastrojejunostomy, may be appropriate.[18,54] If the ulcer cannot safely be included in the resection, then antrectomy without vagotomy has been advocated (Kelling and Madlener) with good results.[18,54]

Based on observations that reduction of acid secretion can lead to healing of most benign gastric ulcers, some authors have advocated highly selective vagotomy with ulcer excision for the treatment of benign gastric ulcers.[17,49,51] Follow-up for 5 years has revealed a 15 per cent recurrence rate for patients with Type I gastric ulcers. For Types II and III gastric ulcers, highly selective vagotomy carries an unacceptably high recurrence rate of 20 to 35 per cent over a 5-year follow-up.[49,55] Completion of a highly selective vagotomy in a patient with a gastric ulcer can be more difficult than when performed for duodenal ulcer, owing to inflammation along the lesser curvature.[49]

Management of Acute Complications of Ulcer Disease

Since the introduction of H_2-receptor antagonists, there has been a general reluctance to refer patients for elective ulcer surgery.[19] Nevertheless, there is no evidence that the incidence of acute complications of ulcer disease has been significantly altered. The incidence of emergency surgery for ulcer complications in the general population has not fallen.[3,56] About 20 per cent of patients with chronic peptic ulcerations will, during their lifetime, develop a complication of their disease.[19] Hemorrhage is the most common complication, followed by perforation and obstruction. The annual complication rate is about 2-fold for patients who have had a previous complication. To date, there are no effective criteria for determining which ulcer in which location will have a tendency for serious complications.

It is well recognized that the first presentation of ulcer disease may involve life-threatening complications.[57,58] Acute, life-threatening complications can occur, without warning, in the elderly, who may tolerate or are unable to verbalize their ulcer complaints. Complications of ulcers tend to have a painless presentation in elderly patients more commonly than in younger patients.[44,58] In addition, life-threatening complications in the absence of previous history are more common in patients taking NSAIDs than in other subgroups of patients with pelvic ulcer disease. Use of NSAIDs is also common in the elderly, which increases their risk of an acute ulcer complication in general.[59,60] Moreover, patients with known pelvic ulcer disease, now receiving maintenance doses of antisecretory therapy, are not immune from sudden development of bleeding, perforation, or obstruction.[24,57,58]

HEMORRHAGE

Bleeding is a common complication of peptic ulcers and carries an overall mortality rate of 10 per cent.[61,62] About 25 per cent of patients seen with a bleeding peptic ulcer have no previous history of an ulcer. The majority of bleeding peptic ulcers stop bleeding spontaneously. About 20 to 30 per cent will continue to bleed or are at high risk of rebleeding.[63] Clinical and endoscopic features of patients at high risk for persistent or recurrent bleeding ulcers are listed in Table 13-2.[60,63–65] Elderly, chronically ill patients do not tolerate repeated bouts with hypovolemia and have statistically increased mortality from bleeding ulcers. In general, the majority of such patients will be better served by early and definitive intervention to stop the bleeding.[20,62,65]

Table 13-2. Clinical Risk Factors for and Endoscopic Features Predicting Recurrent Bleeding from Peptic Ulcer

Risk Factors	Endoscopic Features		
	Stigmata	Prevalence (%)	Further Bleeding (%)
Persistent hypotension	Active arterial bleeding	10	90
Coagulopathy	Nonbleeding visible vessel	25	50
Age greater than 60 years	Adherent clot	10	25
Concurrent illness	Oozing without visible vessel	5	<20
	Flat spot	15	<10
	Clean base	35	<5

Reproduced with permission from Freeman ML. The current endoscopic diagnosis and intensive care unit management of severe ulcer and other nonvariceal upper gastrointestinal hemorrhage. Gastrointest Endosc Clinics North Am 1991; 1:209–239.

The initial management for bleeding peptic ulcers requires endoscopy. At endoscopy the bleeding site is localized and may be effectively treated in up to 90 per cent of patients.[63,66] Of the various techniques available the ones commonly used are heater probe, bipolar coagulation, or injection therapy with epinephrine followed by sclerosing agent; all seem equally effective.[64,66,68]

A close examination of recent reports suggests that expert and expeditious use of endoscopic techniques do, in fact, diminish transfusion requirements, reduce rates of rebleeding, and avert emergency surgery in many patients with ulcers at high risk for rebleeding.[66] In considering different reports of the efficacy of endoscopic hemostatic techniques, however, it is important to note the level of transfusions given and the actual requirement for surgical intervention in the control groups. Most of these reports suggest that, in the groups treated by "sham therapy," the transfusion requirement averages no more than 3 to 4 units, even when the incidence of emergency surgery approaches 30 to 40 per cent. The reduction in transfusion requirements in the treatment is 50 per cent, and the requirement for urgent surgery may be reduced by two-thirds.[64,66] It seems clear that early endoscopy and expeditious referral for surgery, if hemostasis is not rapidly achieved, are responsible for these benefits.

When emergency operation is required, the first operative priority is control of the bleeding site. In the stable patient, it has generally been advocated that a procedure that suppresses acid secretion should be performed. Previously, it has been suggested that patients who do not receive such definitive procedure may be at a significant risk for rebleeding, with high mortality.[62] The most common surgical procedures performed in conjunction with ligation of the bleeding duodenal ulcer include (1) truncal vagotomy combined with pyloroplasty and suture ligation of bleeding vessels and (2) truncal vagotomy combined with antrectomy that either includes the ulcer or involves suture ligation of the bleeding vessel.[49] Truncal vagotomy and antrectomy may be considered an alternative procedure in younger patients who are not in shock and who have a long history of disabling symptoms or previous acute complications. In the unstable and high risk patient, oversewing of the ulcer and/or the feeding vessel is acceptable because it is expedient.[2,69] When surgery is performed semielectively, after successful endoscopic treatment of the bleeding ulcer, highly selective vagotomy may be considered for the duodenal ulcer patient.[59,67,70]

A bleeding gastric ulcer is generally accepted as a more dangerous lesion than a bleeding duodenal ulcer, since it tends to be more persistent and the patients are usually older with multiple medical problems.[2] The procedure of choice is gastric resection that includes the bleeding ulcer. Vagotomy and drainage with excision of the ulcer are alternatives if gastrectomy is not safe or feasible. Simple oversewing of the ulcer is appropriate only for the most unstable patients.[71]

PERFORATION

Perforation of a duodenal ulcer is an indication for emergency operation, except in rare cases when the perforation has closed spontaneously and peritonitis is minimal. Candidates for nonoperative treatment should be less than 70 years of age, have a proven ulcer with evidence of sealed perforation (by Gastrografin study), and have minimal evidence of peritonitis. In some cases, patients may not be operated on because their conditions are clearly beyond salvage owing to multiple system organ failure or the latest stages of peritonitis.[2,14,49]

Simple closure of an ulcer with an omental (Graham) patch is preferred by many surgeons.[56] Others have argued that simple closure is appropriate for the acute ulcer whereas definitive treatment would benefit the patient with a prior history of duodenal ulcer or findings indicating chronic ulcer at the time of the operation.[49,56,72,73] This latter view has been challenged.[49] It may be difficult to obtain an accurate history from these patients, and an intraoperative distinction between chronic and acute ulcer also may be difficult. A number of prospective studies have shown that ulcer symptoms occurred in 60 to 70 per cent of patients after simple closure.[70,73,74,75] As many as 20 to 35 per cent of such patients have required subsequent ulcer surgery.[76,77,78]

Controversy remains over the choice of the operation that will best facilitate ulcer healing and reduce recurrences. Truncal vagotomy with drainage and truncal vagotomy with antrectomy are both associated with significant postoperative gastric sequelae (see above). Since about 30 per cent of patients with perforated ulcers may not experience symptoms of ulcer disease again, it is difficult to recommend a procedure with such significant postoperative side effects. Thus, recent attention has focused on highly selective vagotomy, which has a minimal complication risk and which provides protection against recurrent ulcer equivalent to that of the truncal vagotomy. Several reports have recommended that HSV with patch of the ulcer should be the preferred definitive procedure for perforated duodenal ulcers.[2,49,74]

Perioperative mortality in patients with perforated duodenal ulcers is related to preoperative shock, severe current medical illness, longstanding perforation (more than 24 hours) and age over 60[56,72] (Fig. 13-4). If all risk factors are present, mortality rates approach 100 per cent. If any of the above risk factors are present, simple closure should be performed. In the absence of risk factors, simple closure and definitive surgery carry the same mortality rate.

Perforated gastric ulcers tend to occur in older patients with associated medical illness. Overall, they carry a higher mortality rate

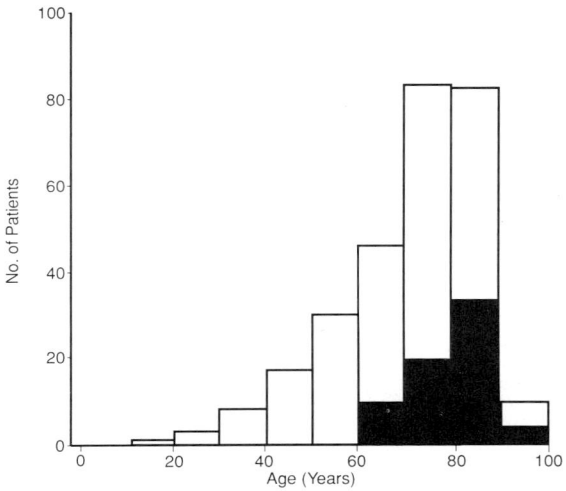

Figure 13-4. Age of patients presenting with perforated peptic ulcers and associated mortality rate. *Shaded areas* represent deaths. (Reproduced with permission from Irvin TT. Mortality and perforated peptic ulcer: A case for risk stratification in elderly patients. Br J Surg 1989; 76:215–218.)

than duodenal ulcers (10 to 40 per cent versus 0 to 10 per cent).[69] Although perforated gastric ulcers most commonly are benign and occur on the anterior wall of the distal stomach, they can perforate posteriorly into the lesser sac and may be associated with gastric cancer. The treatment of choice is partial gastrectomy, including the ulcer.[69] Vagotomy is not necessary for Type I gastric ulcers, but is included for prepyloric ulcers (Type III) or those associated with a duodenal ulcer (Type II). In high risk or unstable patients, simple closure of the ulcer with an omental patch and biopsy or excision of the ulcer may be the most expedient and safest option.[2,17]

OBSTRUCTION

Patients exhibiting gastric outlet obstruction are initially treated nonoperatively using gastric decompression, H_2-receptor antagonist treatment, and intravenous fluid and electrolyte replacement. Endoscopy is used to confirm the mechanical nature of the obstruction, rule out the presence of malignancy, and document coexisting pathologic conditions.[14] In many cases, a component of the obstruction may be acute and will reverse within a few days of gastric decompression.

Gastric outlet obstruction that fails to resolve with short-term conservative therapy, generally represents injury by chronic prepyloric, pyloric, or duodenal ulcer. In such cases, the goal of surgery is to relieve the gastric outlet obstruction and treat the ulcer diathesis.[2,49] Truncal vagotomy combined with antrectomy provides the optimal surgical intervention. It has very low recurrence rates and allows for resection of the scarred pyloroduodenal tissue. A second choice would be truncal vagotomy with gastrojejunostomy. This can be considered for the older patient and for the patient in whom inflammation and excess scarring in the pyloroduodenal region prevent a safe antrectomy and management of the duodenal remnant.

COMPLICATIONS AND COSTS OF MEDICAL AND SURGICAL THERAPIES

Complications and Side Effects

The medical complications of therapies for peptic ulcer disease can be divided into three categories: first, the potential long term side effects of suppression of acid secretion, including the potential for development of gastric carcinoma; second, the pharmacologic side effects of specific medical agents such as H_2-receptor blockers, omeprazole, and sucralfate; and third, physiologic disturbances arising from surgical section of the vagal branches and from disruption or bypass of the pyloric sphincter mechanism.

The implications of profound and sustained suppression of acid secretion are of increasing concern.[40,79] Long term suppression with drugs such as omeprazole causes increases in gastric floral counts and can lead to proliferation of bacterial species not normally found in the mouth or upper gastrointestinal tract. Suppression of acid secretion is also associated with varying elevations of circulating levels of gastrin, which has trophic effects on gut mucosa. Following truncal or highly selective vagotomy, proliferation of epithelial cells has been observed. In addition, with disruption or bypass of the pylorus by pyloroplasty or gastrojejunostomy, bile (a known co-mutagen) is given access to the neutral gastric lumen, gastritis is observed, and luminal concentrations of other mutagens, such as nitrites and nitrosamines, are increased.

One major source of concern regarding the use of antisecretory therapies has been the long term risk of neoplasia in the gastric mucosa. Shortly after cimetidine was introduced, several reports suggested a surge in the incidence of such malignancies in patients given the drug.[79] There is evidence in laboratory animals to suggest that intensive and suprapharmacologic regimens of different forms of H_2-blockers or omeprazole may cause abnormal proliferation of epithelial or endocrine cell elements. However, there is no clinical evidence to suggest that agents currently in use are carcinogenic, either in themselves or because of their ability to suppress gastric acid secretion. It should be noted that long term studies are not yet available to fully establish the absence of such a risk in patients who are taking the most recently introduced agent, omeprazole, or more powerful forms of nonsuppressible and unreversible H_2-blockers.

The major side effects of long term administration of H_2-blockers, omeprazole, or sucralfate are well characterized. Most such side effects are little more than a nuisance and cause no disability. The more serious side effects, such as thrombocytopenia (cimetidine) or asthenia (omeprazole), are generally reversible when the medications are discontinued.

Physiologic disturbances caused by truncal vagal section and disruption or bypass of the pyloric sphincter are also well characterized and need not be catalogued here. However, it is important to recognize the importance of objectively evaluating the disability that may be associated with such syndromes. In this regard, grading of such disabilities was introduced in 1946 by Visick[76] to evaluate patient satisfaction after gastric surgery. In the traditional Visick system any recurrence of peptic ulcer is classified permanently as a failure of treatment with maximal disability. At that time, this may have been appropriate, since recurrence after gastric resection and vagotomy generally implied marginal ulceration, a highly disabling complication that was difficult to treat. Recurrence of peptic ulcer following gastrectomy (with or without vagotomy) or vagotomy and drainage, may be associated with significant or disabling symptoms (Visick III or IV) in up to 20 to 25 per cent of patients. Recently, Busman et al.[77,80] introduced a "dynamic" Visick grading scale that allows for a change in grading as well as evaluating the degree of disability of either the recurrence and/or postoperative sequelae. With this scale, the overall proportion of patients (90 to 95 per cent) with HSV have a Visick Grade I or II in any given year. This is consistent with the benign course of many recurrences after HSV, which often have occurred only once and have been easily treated.

Costs

How do we assess the costs of different treatments for the different forms of peptic ulcer disease? An initial approach might distinguish two categories of patients: those seen with chronic symptoms, mainly pain, and those seen with an acute, life-threatening complication requiring endoscopic and/or surgical intervention. For those seen with pain caused by a DU, for example, we should calculate the cost of 8 to 12 weeks of medication. To this initial expense is added the cost of maintenance therapy for several years. This raises a problem: Should the patient receive continuous maintenance therapy or simply be treated, intermittently, for recurrences and complications as they arise? This question has been addressed by a number of authors[39,41] who compared the costs of continuous maintenance therapies, with lower recurrence rates, to the costs of treating symptomatic recurrences and acute complications as they arose. In addition to the costs of therapy and intervention, absenteeism, loss of work productivity, and changes in overall quality of life should be included in calculating the costs of each recurrence or complication. These approaches have suggested that maintenance therapy with standard H_2-blockers may, in the long run, be cheaper than treating recurrences and complications as they arise.[39]

Jensen,[81] Sonnenberg,[82] and others have compared the cost of chronic maintenance therapy with ranitidine to that of surgery. Jensen's analysis suggested that the costs of elective surgery and ongoing medical therapy might equalize if the patient were to require 8 years of such ongoing therapy. Sonnenberg's analysis demonstrates that adjustment of incidences of recurrences/complications and their costs could lead to the conclusion that elective performance of a highly selective vagotomy is more cost-effective than maintenance schedules in some European health care systems, but not necessarily in the U.S. system as presently organized. Such thought experiments illustrate the potential sensitivity of the cost analysis to changes in: (1) expense of medications; (2) changes in recurrence or complication rates of newer medical therapies; or (3) expense, length of stay, duration, and intensity of postoperative disability following elective surgical procedures such as HSV. Thus, under certain conditions, elective laparoscopically assisted approaches to ulcer disease might be feasible and cost-effective.

For patients seen with acute complications of peptic ulcer disease, the analysis of costs would begin with the recognition that such complications are life-threatening and can lead to significant morbidity. Although actuarial and life insurance companies are in the business of estimating the potential costs of the loss of life, it is not so clear whether and when such estimates should enter into therapeutic decisions. At present, it seems best to continue to evaluate the "costs" of different therapeutic approaches primarily in terms of the reduction of mortality and early and late morbidity. Other considerations such as length and expense of hospital stay and expense of different therapeutic modalities may be included in comparisons of different therapeutic approaches if the risks to life and well-being are balanced.

In the acute circumstance, the analysis of cost would recognize that the primary goal of therapy is to treat the specific complication, prevent early recurrences and other acute complications, and minimize morbidity and disability. The secondary goals would include, but not be limited to, prevention of symptomatic recurrences in the long term. In some settings, such as free perforation, early surgical intervention would remain the mainstay of treatment. In other cases, such as the bleeding ulcer, open surgery to ligate the bleeding vessel would be reserved for patients in whom endoscopic management fails. Laparoscopic approaches can be expected to replace open approaches when they are shown to be equally safe and efficacious in addressing the complication that requires urgent surgery. Whether such patients should, in addition, undergo vagotomy or more radical procedures will depend on the evolution of medications that specifically lower long term incidence of complications and ulcer recurrence.

LAPAROSCOPIC APPROACHES TO PEPTIC ULCER DISEASES

A videoscopic approach to peptic ulcer disease was first investigated by Dubois, at the University of Paris in 1988.[83] He performed bilateral truncal vagotomies through left chest thoracoscopy, combined with endoscopic balloon dilatation of the pylorus. In 1991, Mouiel and Katkhouda, reported their results on laparoscopic posterior truncal vagotomy and anterior seromyotomy.[83,84] Subsequently Bailey et al. have described laparoscopic posterior truncal vagotomy and anterior highly selective vagotomy.[85] The laparoscopic approach to peptic ulcer disease has most of the advantages of traditional surgery, but may eliminate the disadvantages of laparotomy, including prolonged hospital stay and postoperative discomfort. The following briefly summarizes the features of laparoscopically assisted procedures that may be useful in the management of different peptic ulcer diseases. More detailed descriptions of each procedure can be found in the ensuing chapters.

Truncal Vagotomy

Truncal vagotomy consists of dividing the main vagal trunks as they emerge through the esophagal hiatus (Fig. 13-5A). This not only denervates the entire stomach but deprives the entire abdomen of parasympathetic innervation derived from the vagus (vagectomy). Truncal vagotomy is done with relative ease videoscopically, either transthoracically or transabdominally.[83,86] Truncal vagotomy requires a complementary drainage procedure or has to be combined with antrectomy. If the patient has not had a previous drainage procedure or resection, balloon dilation of the pylorus has been performed with fairly good short term success.[47] Gastrojejunostomy has been performed via the laparoscope with newly developed stapling devices

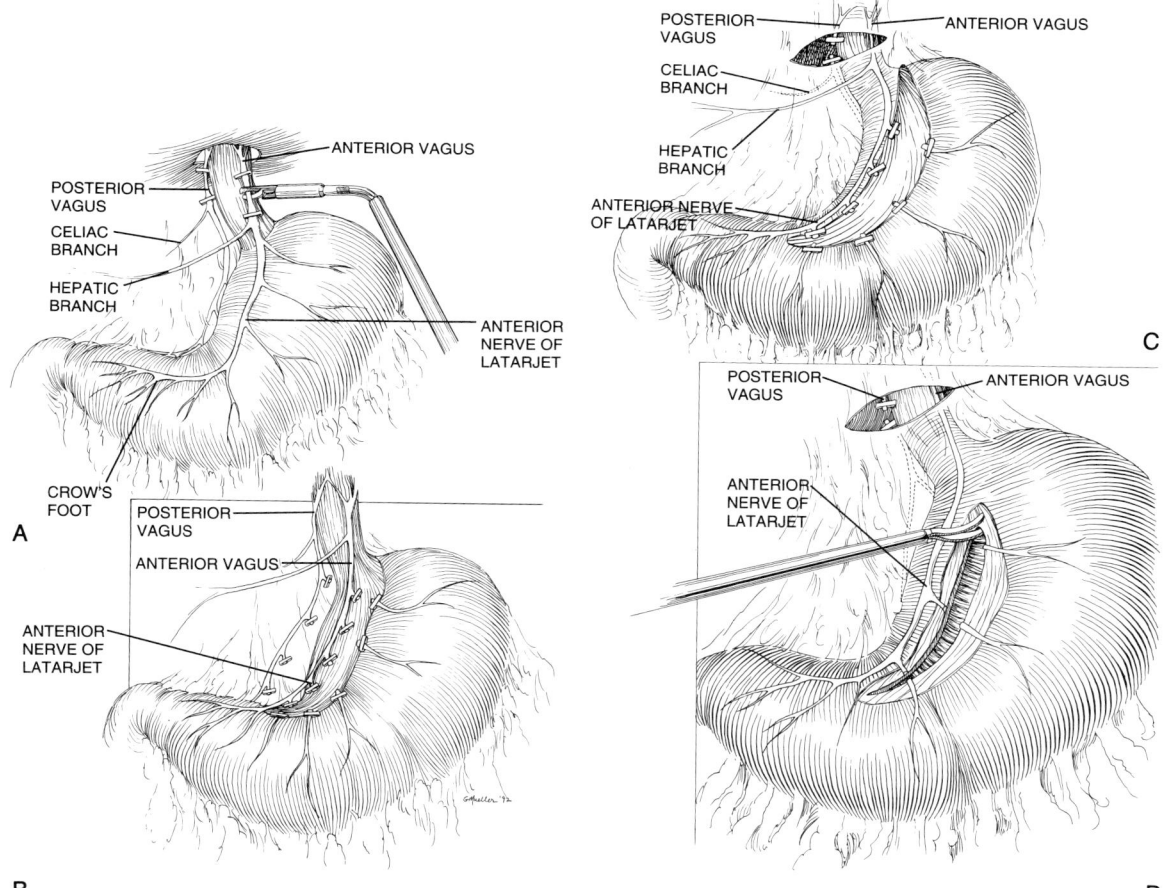

Figure 13-5. Currently established laparoscopically assisted vagotomies: A, truncal vagotomy; B, highly selective vagotomy; C, posterior truncal vagotomy and anterior highly selective vagotomy; D, posterior truncal vagotomy and anterior seromyotomy.

in the laboratory setting. Recently, a laparoscopically assisted pyloromyotomy has been performed, using the neodymium-yttrium-garnet laser, in conjunction with truncal vagotomy.[87]

Highly Selective Vagotomy

Also known as the proximal gastric vagotomy or parietal cell vagotomy, the highly selective vagotomy (HSV) was popularized 20 years ago as an operation that provides gastric vagal denervation, permitting preservation of the pylorus to minimize dumping and diarrhea.[47,49,51] The traditional HSV denervates only the acid-secreting parietal cell portion of the stomach, by dividing all the neurovascular bundles between the anterior and posterior vagus nerves and the lesser curve (Fig. 13-5B). Performed through the laparoscope, HSV can be technically difficult and time-consuming. Modifications are easier to perform laparoscopically and therefore are preferred by most surgeons.[88,89]

Modifications of Selective Vagotomy

ANTERIOR LESSER CURVE SEROMYOTOMY AND POSTERIOR TRUNCAL VAGOTOMY

Described by Taylor in 1979 as a simplified technique for denervating the parietal cell mass, this procedure includes a posterior truncal vagotomy (TV). A seromyotomy is carried out on the anterior gastric wall, along the lesser curvature (Fig. 13-5D). No drainage procedure is required.[90–93] Katkhouda and Mouiel of France reported their initial results of laparoscopic posterior truncal vagotomy and anterior seromyotomy. They recently reported a series of 62 patients with chronic duodenal ulcers. All had excellent results at 2-month follow-up. In 2 years the recurrence rate was 5.6 per cent.[83,84,94] Shapiro et al.[89] compared laparoscopic HSV, posterior TV and anterior seromyotomy, and posterior TV and anterior HSV. They found that the posterior TV and anterior seromyotomy provided the optimal combination of antiulcer prophylaxis and adaptivity to the laparoscopic approach.

POSTERIOR TRUNCAL VAGOTOMY AND ANTERIOR HIGHLY SELECTIVE VAGOTOMY

This procedure was initially described by Hill and Barker[95] as a simple, open technique for denervating the parietal cell mass. They reported results comparable to those for HSV. Although this modification never gained widespread use as an open procedure, it has become a popular approach using the laparoscope (Fig. 13-5C). Bailey et al.[85] first described using posterior TV and anterior HSV done via the laparoscope for duodenal ulcer disease. In their report on the results of 25 patients, there were recurrences in 2 patients, both of whom had prepyloric ulcers. All patients returned to normal activity in 1 week.[96]

GASTRIC RESECTIONS

The antrum constitutes the distal 30 to 40 per cent of the stomach and has a tongue that extends orad along the lesser curvature. Distal gastrectomy removes the antrum, ablates the gastric phase of gastric secretion, and decreases the parietal cell mass. When partial gastrectomy is performed for gastric ulcer, every attempt must be made to excise the ulcer with the gastrectomy specimen. There have been occasional reports on successful antrectomies done via the laparoscope in the laboratory setting. Laparoscopically assisted gastric resection is not yet an established procedure, but will probably be so within a short time with refined techniques and instrumentation.

Summary and Conclusions

In reflecting upon the feasibility and potential usefulness of newer approaches to the management of ulcer disease, it should be emphasized that the indications for surgery in ulcer disease may not necessarily change with the introduction of the laparoscope. Where applicable, laparoscopically assisted surgery may offer advantages in overall patient care, with diminished postoperative discomfort, rapid recovery, and return to normal activity as well as decreased hospital stay. At present, the indications for elective surgery for peptic ulcer disease are few. Semielective procedures are recommended for patients who may be at high risk for developing complications, who have significant or total gastric outlet obstruction, or who may not tolerate or comply with long term medical therapy. At present, the analysis of costs might permit a conclusion that surgery is more cost-effective than long-term maintenance therapies to prevent symptomatic recurrence and acute complications. In particular, with lower recurrence rates and a reduction in postoperative recovery and disability now available with laparoscopic approaches, the stage has been set to debate the relative advantages of laparoscopically assisted approaches over long term therapies. In addition, the feasibility of endoscopic approaches to interruption of vagal inputs or obliteration of the gastrin-secreting G cells in the antrum is under evaluation in the laboratory. These developments could alter our current views about the risks and benefits of medical or invasive interventions in managing the chronic symptoms of this disease.

In the acute setting, laparoscopically assisted closure of acute duodenal perforations has been reported.[97,98] For the high risk patient, simple closure via a minimal approach seems ideal. A simultaneous definitive ulcer operation has not to this date been reported, but will probably be part of the management in the appropriate situation. For duodenal ulcer without obstruction, the procedure of choice is HSV or a modification thereof. Laparoscopically assisted variations of the HSV are clearly feasible.[83–85,88] Despite an expected 10 per cent recurrence rate, the disability caused by the surgery is low. For the perforated gastric ulcer, cancer must be excluded. If simple closure with an omental patch is performed using the laparoscope, adequate biopsy of the ulcer must be ensured. Preferably the ulcer should be excised or included in a partial gastrectomy.

At the present time, a sensible laparoscopic approach has not been worked out for patients whose ulcers are actively bleeding at the time of surgery. When bleeding has been controlled by other measures, semielective surgery via the laparoscope should be considered for patients who may have a high risk of rebleeding or who have required transfusions of many units of blood. The procedure of choice for duodenal ulcer may be HSV or one of its modifications. For gastric ulcer, either gastric resection including the ulcer or HSV with excision of the ulcer are accepted procedures. Type II and III gastric ulcers have an unacceptable high recurrence rate after HSV. Truncal vagotomy with antrectomy is the procedure of choice for these ulcers. With improved techniques, it may become feasible to address these more challenging problems with laparoscopically assisted procedures.

The field of laparoscopically assisted surgery has been developing at an explosive rate. Laparoscopic approaches have changed our approach to biliary colic and cholecystitis. In the field of gastrointestinal surgery, combined use of the endoscope and the laparoscope will certainly offer the patient procedures that are minimally invasive. At the same time, it remains the surgeon's responsibility to ensure that the quality of care provided by such technologies is comparable to that which has now been achieved with conventional surgical approaches.

REFERENCES

1. Bloom BS. Cross-national changes in the effects of peptic ulcer disease. Ann Intern Med 1991; 114:558–562.
2. Sachdeva AK, Zaren HA, Sigel B. Surgical treatment of peptic ulcer disease. Med Clin North Am 1991; 75:999–1012.
3. McConnell DB, Baba GC, Deveney CW. Changes in surgical treatment of peptic ulcer disease within a veterans hospital in the 1970s and the 1980s. Arch Surg 1989; 124:1164–1167.
4. Malangoni MA, Mullins RJ. Proximal gastric vagotomy for duodenal ulcer disease. South Med J 1989; 82:733–735.
5. Gustavsson S, Nyren O. Time trends in peptic ulcer surgery, 1956 to 1986. Ann Surg 1989; 210:704–709.
6. Paimela H, Tuompo PK, Perakyla T, et al. Peptic ulcer surgery during the H_2-receptor antagonist era: A population-based epidemiological study of ulcer surgery in Helsinki from 1972 to 1987. Br J Surg 1991; 78:28–31.
7. Kurata JH, Haile BM. Epidemiology of peptic ulcer disease. J Clin Gastroenterol 1984; 13:289–307.
8. Katz J. The course of peptic ulcer disease. Med Clin North Am 1991; 75:831–840.
9. Bloom BS, Fendrick AM, Ramsey SD. Changes in peptic ulcer and gastritis/duodenitis in Great Britain, 1970–1985. J Clin Gastroenterol 1990; 12:100–108.
10. Bernersen B, Johnsen R, Straume B, et al. Towards a true prevalence of peptic ulcer: The Sörreisa gastrointestinal disorder study. Gut 1990; 31:989–992.
11. Kurata JL. An assessment of nonsteroidal anti-inflammatory drugs as a risk factor in ulcer disease. In Soll AH, moderator. Nonsteroidal Anti-inflammatory Drugs and Peptic Ulcer Disease. Ann Intern Med 1991; 114:311–315.
12. Kurata JL, Honda GD, Frankl H. Hospitalization and mortality rates for peptic ulcers: A comparison of a large HMO and US Data. Gastroenterology 1982; 1008–1016.
13. Oi M, Sakurai Y. The location of duodenal ulcer. Gastroenterology 1959; 36:60–64.
14. Yeo CJ, Zinner MJ. Duodenal ulcer. In Zuidema GD, Ritchie WP Jr, eds. Shackleford's Surgery of the Alimentary Tract, Philadelphia, WB Saunders, 1991, Vol II.

15. Johnson HD. Gastric ulcer: Clarification, bloodgroups, characteristics, secretion patterns and pathogenesis. Ann Surg 1965; 162:996–1002.
16. Oi M, Oshida K, Sugimura S. The location of gastric ulcer. Gastroenterology 1959; 36:45–56.
17. Jordan PH Jr. Gastric ulcer. *In* Scott HW Jr, Sawyers JL, eds. Surgery of the Stomach, Duodenum, and Small Intestine, 2nd ed. Boston, Blackwell Scientific Publications, 1992.
18. Herrington JL Jr, Sawyers JL. Gastric ulcer. Curr Probl Surg 1987; 24:759–865.
19. Rubin W. Medical treatment of peptic ulcer disease. Med Clin North Am 1991; 75:981–998.
20. Barquist E, Zinner M. Peptic ulcer disease. *In* Cameron JL, ed. Current Surgical Therapy, 4th ed. St. Louis, Mosby-Year Book, Inc.
21. Mertz HR, Walsh JH. Peptic ulcer pathophysiology. Med Clin North Am 1991; 75:799–814.
22. Soll AH. Peptic ulcer diseases. J Clin Gastroenterol 1989; 1(Suppl 1):S1–S5.
23. Cheung LY, Ashley SW. The pathogenesis of acid-peptic disease. *In* Moody FG, ed. Surgical Treatment of Digestive Diseases. Chicago, Yearbook Medical Publishers, 1990, pp 155–173.
24. Soll AH. Pathogenesis of peptic ulcer and implications for therapy. N Engl J Med 1990; 322:909–916.
25. Silen, W. Experimental models of gastric ulceration and injury. Am J Physiol 1988; 255:G395–G402.
26. Martin DF, Montgomery E, Dobek AS, et al. *Campylobacter pylori*, NSAIDS, and smoking: Risk factors for peptic ulcer disease. Am J Gastroenterol 1989; 84:1268–1272.
27. Graham DY. *Campylobacter pylori* and peptic ulcer disease. Gastroenterology 1989; 96:615–625.
28. Clearfield HR. *Helicobacter pylori*: Aggressor or innocent bystander? Med Clin North Am 1991; 71:815–829.
29. Weinstein WM. Differentiation of nonsteroidal anti-inflammatory drug-associated and "ordinary" peptic ulcers, pp 309–311. *In* Soll AH, moderator. Nonsteroidal Anti-inflammatory Drugs and Peptic Ulcer Disease. Ann Intern Med 1991; 114:307–319.
30. Bliss DW, Stabile BE. The impact of ulcerogenic drugs on surgery for the treatment of peptic ulcer disease. Arch Surg 1991; 126:609–612.
31. Jones MP, Schubert ML. What do you recommend for prophylaxis in an elderly woman with arthritis requiring NSAIDs for control? Am J Gastroenterol 1991; 86:264–266.
32. Agrawal N. Risk factors for gastrointestinal ulcers caused by nonsteroidal anti-inflammatory drugs (NSAIDs). J Fam Pract 1991; 32:619–624.
33. Wright NA, Pike C, Elia G. Induction of a novel epidermal growth factor-secreting cell lineage by mucosal ulceration in human gastrointestinal stem cells. Nature 1990; 343:82–85.
34. Folkman J, Szabo S, Stovroff M, et al. Duodenal ulcer. Discovery of a new mechanism and development of Angiogenic therapy that accelerates healing. Ann Surg 1991; 214:414–427.
35. Thirlby, RC. Selected summary: A new look at the mechanisms of healing of peptic ulcers by Folkman J, Szabo S, Stovroff M, et al. in Ann Surg 1991; 214:414–427. Gastroenterology 1992; 102:1816–1817.
36. Freston JW. Mechanisms of relapse in peptic ulcer disease. J Clin Gastroenterol 1989; 11(Suppl 1):S34–S38.
37. Anda RF, Williamson DF, Escobedo LG, et al. Smoking and the risk of peptic ulcer disease among women in the United States. Arch Intern Med 1990; 150:1437–1441.
38. Chiverton SG, Hunt RH. Smoking and duodenal ulcer disease. J Clin Gastroenterol 1989; 11(Suppl 1):S29–S33.
39. Earnest DL. Maintenance therapy in peptic ulcer disease. Med Clin North Am 1991; 75:1013–1038.
40. Hixson LJ, Kelley CL, Jones WN, et al. Current trends in pharmacotherapy for peptic ulcer disease. Arch Intern Med 1992; 152:726–732.
41. Wormsley KG. Maintenance treatment with H_2-receptor antagonists in patients with peptic ulcer disease: Reduces morbidity in a significant minority of patients. Br Med J 1988; 297:1392–1394.
42. Howden CW. Maintenance treatment with H_2-receptor antagonists in patients with peptic ulcer disease: Rarely justified in terms of cost or patient benefit. Br Med J 1988; 297:1393–1394.
43. Fry J. Peptic ulcer: A profile. Br Med J 1964; 2:809–812.
44. Arakawa T, Higuchi K, Fukuda T, et al. H_2-receptor antagonist-refractory ulcer: Its pathophysiology and treatment. J Clin Gastroenterol 1991; 13(Suppl 1):S129–S133.
45. Howden CW, Holt S. Acid suppression as treatment for NSAID-related peptic ulcers. Am J Gastroenterol 1991; 86:1720–1722.
46. Szabo S. The mode of action of sucralfate: The $1 \times 1 \times 1$ mechanism of action. Scand J Gastroenterol 1991; 26(Suppl 185):7–12.
47. Johnston D, Blackett RL. A new look at selective vagotomies. Am J Surg 1988; 156:416–427.
48. Hoffmann J, Jensen H-E, Christiansen J, et al. Prospective controlled vagotomy trial for duodenal ulcer. Ann Surg 1989; 209:40–45.
49. Jordan PH Jr. Surgery for peptic ulcer disease. Curr Probl Surg 1991; 28:267–330.
50. Jordan GL Jr, DeBakey ME, Duncan JM Jr. Surgical management of perforated peptic ulcer. Ann Surg 1974; 179:628–633.
51. Schirmer BD. Current status of proximal gastric vagotomy. Ann Surg 1989; 209:131–148.
52. Soper NJ, Kelly KA, van Heerden JA, Ilstrup DM. Long term clinical results after proximal gastric vagotomy. Surg Gynecol Obstet 1989; 169:488–494.
53. Arends TW, Nahrwold DL. Gastric resection and reconstruction. *In* Zuidema GD, Ritchie WP Jr, eds. Shackleford's Surgery of the Alimentary Tract. Philadelphia, WB Saunders, 1991, Vol II.
54. Dulchavsky SA, Fromm D. Benign gastric ulcer. *In* Cameron JL, ed. Current Surgical Therapy, 4th ed., St. Louis, Mosby Year Book, 1992.
55. Sawyers JL. Vagotomy and pyloroplasty. *In* Zuidema GD, Ritchie WP Jr, eds. Shackleford's Surgery of the Alimentary Tract. Philadelphia, WB Saunders, 1991, pp 136–148.
56. Irvin TT. Mortality and perforated peptic ulcer: A case for risk stratification in elderly patients. Br J Surg 1989; 76:215–218.
57. Corinaldesi R, De Giorgio R, Paternico A, et al. Leading article: Asymptomatic peptic ulcer disease. Is it worth looking for? Drugs 1991; 41:821–824.
58. Pounder R. Silent peptic ulceration: Deadly silence or golden silence? Gastroenterology 1989; 96:626–31.
59. Shallcross TM, Heatley RV. Effect of non-steroidal anti-inflammatory drugs on dyspeptic symptoms. Br Med J 1990; 300:368–369.
60. Matthewson K, Pugh S, Northfield TC. Which peptic ulcer patients bleed? Gut 1988; 29:70–74.
61. Greiser WB, Bruner BW, Shamoun JM, et al. Factors affecting mortality in patients operated upon for complications of peptic ulcer disease. Am Surg 1989; 55:7–11

62. Poxon VA, Keighley MRB, Dykes PW, et al. Comparison of minimal and conventional surgery in patients with bleeding peptic ulcer: A multicentre trial. Br J Surg 1991; 78:1344–1345.
63. Starlinger M, Becker HD. Upper gastrointestinal bleeding—Indications and results in surgery. Hepato-Gastroenterology 1988; 38:216–219.
64. NIH consensus development conference. Therapeutic endoscopy and bleeding ulcers. JAMA 1989; 262:1369–1372.
65. Rutgeerts P. Approach to upper gastrointestinal bleeding—When to treat? Can J Gastroenterol 1990; 4:647–649.
66. Morissey JF, Reichelderfer M. Gastrointestinal endoscopy (first of two parts). N Engl J Med 1991; 325:1142–1149.
67. Waring JP, Sanowski RA, Sawyer RL, et al. A randomized comparison of multipolar electrocoagulation and injection sclerosis for the treatment of bleeding peptic ulcer. Gastrointest Endosc 1991; 37:295–298.
68. Hui WM, Ng MMT, Lok ASF, et al. A randomized comparative study of laser photocoagulation, heater probe, and bipolar electrocoagulation in the treatment of actively bleeding ulcers. Gastrointest Endosc 1991; 37:299–304.
69. Dempsey DT, Ritchie WP Jr. Gastric ulcer. In Zuidema GD, Ritchie WP Jr, eds. Shackleford's Surgery of the Alimentary Tract. Philadelphia, WB Saunders, 1991, Vol II.
70. Boey J, Lee NW, Koo J, et al. Immediate definitive surgery for perforated duodenal ulcers. A prospective controlled trial. Ann Surg 1982; 196:338–344.
71. Gorey TF, Lennon F, Heffernan SJ. Highly selective vagotomy in duodenal ulceration and its complications. Ann Surg 1984; 191:181–184.
72. Boey J, Choi SKY, Alagaratnam TT, et al. Risk stratification in perforated duodenal ulcers. A prospective validation of predictive factors. Ann Surg 1987; 205:22–26.
73. Boey J, Lee NW, Wong J, et al. Perforation in acute duodenal ulcers. Surg Gynecol Obstet 1982; 155:193–196.
74. Boey J, Branicki FJ, Alagaratnam TT, et al. Proximal gastric vagotomy: The preferred operation for perforations in acute duodenal ulcer. Ann Surg 1988; 208:169–173.
75. Tanphiphat C, Tanprayoon TN, Thalang A. Surgical treatment of perforated duodenal ulcer: A prospective trial between simple closure and definitive surgery. Br J Surg 1985; 75:370–372.
76. Visick AH. A study of the failures after gastrectomy. Ann R Coll Surg Engl 1948; 3:266.
77. Busman DC, Munting JDK. Dynamic Visick grading after highly selective vagotomy. World J Surg 1988; 12:224–228.
78. Donahue PE. Letter to the editor. Am J Surg 1989; 158:79–80.
79. Soybel DI, Modlin IM. Implications of sustained suppression of gastric acid secretion. Am J Surg 1992; 163:613–622.
80. Busman DC, Volovics A, Munting JDK. Recurrence rate after highly selective vagotomy. World J Surg 1988; 12:217–223.
81. Jensen DM. Economic and health aspects of peptic ulcer disease and H_2-receptor antagonists. Am J Med 1986; 81(Suppl 4B):42–48.
82. Sonnenberg A. Costs of medical and surgical treatment of duodenal ulcer. Gastroenterology 1989; 96:1445–1452.
83. Mouiel J, Katkhouda N. Laparoscopic truncal and selective vagotomy. In Zucker KA, ed. Surgical Laparoscopy. St. Louis, Quality Medical Publishing, 1991.
84. Katkhouda N, Mouiel J. A new technique of surgical treatment of chronic duodenal ulcer without laparotomy by videocoelioscopy. Am J Surg 1991; 161:361–364.
85. Bailey RW, Flowers JL, Graham SM, Zucker KA. Combined laparoscopic cholecystectomy and selective vagotomy. Surg Laparosc Endosc 1991; 1:45–49.
86. Laws HL, Naughton MJ, McKernan JB. Thoracoscopic vagectomy for recurrent peptic ulcer disease. Surg Laparosc Endosc 1992; 2:77–81.
87. Pietraffita JJ, Schultz LS, Graber JN, et al. Laser laparoscopic vagotomy and pyloromyotomy. Gastrointest Endosc 1991; 37:338–343.
88. Legrand M, Detroz B, Honore P, Jacquet N. Laparoscopic highly selective vagotomy. Presented at the SAGES Scientific Session, April 10–12, 1992.
89. Shapiro S, Gordon L, Dayhkovsky L, et al. Development of laparoscopic anterior seromyotomy and right posterior truncal vagotomy for ulcer prophylaxis. J Laparosc Surg 1991; 1:279–286.
90. Taylor TV, Lythgoe JP, McFarland JB, et al. Anterior lesser curve seromyotomy and posterior truncal vagotomy versus truncal vagotomy and pyloroplasty in the treatment of chronic duodenal ulcer. Br J Surg 1990; 77:1007–1009.
91. Taylor TV, Gunn AA, MacLeod DAD, et al. Mortality and morbidity after anterior lesser curve seromyotomy with posterior truncal vagotomy for duodenal ulcer. Br J Surg 1985; 72:950–951.
92. Taylor TV, Gunn AA, MacLeod DAD, et al. Anterior lesser curve seromyotomy and posterior truncal vagotomy in the treatment of chronic duodenal ulcer. Lancet 1982; 1:846–849.
93. Oostvogel HJM, van Vroonhoven TJMV. Anterior lesser curve seromyotomy with posterior truncal vagotomy versus proximal gastric vagotomy. Br J Surg 1988; 75:121–124.
94. Katkhouda N. Laparoscopic vagotomy for chronic duodenal ulcer disease. Presented at the SAGES Postgraduate Course, April 10–12, 1992.
95. Hill GL, Barker CJ. Anterior highly selective vagotomy with posterior truncal vagotomy: A simple technique for denervating the parietal cell mass. Br J Surg 1978; 65:702–705.
96. Zucker KA. Laparoscopic management of peptic ulcer disease. Presented at the SAGES Postgraduate Course, April 10–12, 1992.
97. Mouret P, Francois Y, Vignal J, et al. Laparoscopic treatment of perforated peptic ulcer. Br J Surg 1990; 70:1006.
98. Costalat G, Dravet F, Alquier Y, et al. Treatment of perforated peptic ulcer using the round ligament under celioscopy. J Chir 1991; 128:91–93.

Chapter 14
Splenic Surgery

Stephen J. Ferzoco
Irvin M. Modlin

The spleen is an organ of mesodermal origin. In the adult, it weighs between 75 and 100 grams and is situated in the left upper quadrant, superiorly and posteriorly to the cardia of the stomach where protection is afforded by the ninth, tenth, and eleventh ribs. The spleen is regarded as possessing four distinct physiologic functions which include filtration, storage, hematopoiesis, and immunologic protection.[1] Its principal role is that of filtration since approximately 2 liters of blood per minute pass through the organ.

HISTORIC REVIEW OF SPLENECTOMY

The first reported therapeutic splenectomy was performed by Spencer Wells in 1887 for the disease hereditary spherocytosis.[2] Historical treatises of the sixteenth, seventeenth, and eighteenth centuries report instances of what may have been splenic surgery for trauma. Riegner, in 1883,[3] is credited with ushering in the modern era of splenic surgery based upon his report of a total splenectomy performed on a 14-year-old child who fell from a height and landed on his abdomen.

Thereafter, splenectomy was used for both hematologic disorders as well as splenic injury. Initially, total splenectomy was the operation of choice; however, the recognition that patients with no spleen have an increased risk of developing early and late postoperative infections[4-7] led to a reconsideration of the extent of the procedure. In particular, encapsulated organisms appear to be a major cause of postoperative septic complications. In order to minimize this problem, the technique of partial splenectomy or splenic salvage evolved. Modern methods for avoiding total splenectomy include suture repair, partial resection, splenic reimplantation, microwave coagulation, polyglycolic acid mesh, and the application of hemostatic agents made of collagen, gelatin, cellulose, or fibrin glue.[8-12]

HEMOLYTIC ANEMIAS

Hemolytic anemias are characterized by accelerated destruction of mature red blood cells and are subdivided into congenital or acquired groups. In the congenital disorder, there is an intrinsic abnormality within the erythrocyte whereas acquired hemolytic anemias exhibit an extrinsic factor, which results in the development of an abnormality in an otherwise intrinsically normal cell.[2]

Hereditary Spherocytosis

Hereditary spherocytosis is one of the most investigated of all hereditary anemias. Formerly known as acholuric jaundice, the disease is characterized by small, round red blood cells on the peripheral smear. The primary responsible defect is in spectrin synthesis and results in the development of a more rigid and hence less compliant cell membrane. This rigidity engenders red cell entrapment within the splenic sinusoids and subsequent destruction.

The disease is inherited by the typical Mendelian pattern although 20 per cent of cases arise sporadically.[13] It is predominant in individuals of European origin and usually presents between the ages of 4 and 11 years with anemia, jaundice, and splenomegaly. Treatment for the disease is splenectomy. More conservative approaches have included treatment with steroids, iron and vitamin B_{12} but these have met with little success. Management of patients by elective splenectomy has yielded promising results with resolution of anemia as well as hemolysis.[2]

Hereditary Elliptocytosis

First recognized in 1904 by Dresbach,[14] this disorder is asymptomatic in the majority of patients throughout their lives. On peripheral blood smear, the cells appear elliptical in shape. As in hereditary spherocytosis, the underlying cause of the disease is a defect in the red cell membrane, which results in splenic entrapment of the red blood cell. Splenectomy is recommended for those with hemolysis or massive splenomegaly. In studies in which splenectomy has been the chief treatment modality, there have been reports of long lasting decreased hemolysis and resolution of anemia.[15,16]

Thalassemia

Thomas Cooley first elucidated the clinical picture in 1925 when he reported a series of children with splenomegaly, anemia, and bone changes.[17] The primary defect lies in the synthesis of either the α- or β-globin chain in hemoglobin. Thalassemias are the most common single-gene disorders in the world population.[18] The trait is inherited as an autosomal dominant trait. Homozygous individuals are characterized as having thalassemia major, which is often a fatal disease in childhood. Thalassemia intermedia occurs in individuals who are heterozygous for the trait and clinically exhibit anemia, jaundice, and splenomegaly. The group with thalassemia minor may experience either mild symptoms owing to chronic anemia and occasionally have splenomegaly.

Surgical therapy for patients with thalassemia is reserved for those with either the major or intermedia form, and splenectomy was first proposed in thalassemic patients as a method of slowing the hemolytic process of the spleen. Reemtsma and Elliot[19] reported reduced transfusion requirements in a series of 13 patients who underwent splenectomy. Politis[20] reported a 5-year follow-up in thalassemia major patients treated either with partial splenic embolization or total splenectomy. The partial splenectomy group exhibited fewer postoperative infections and decreased transfusion requirements.

Sickle Cell Disease

First recognized by Herrick in 1910,[21] this disorder of β-chains in hemoglobin leads to an elongated or sickle-shaped red blood cell under conditions of reduced oxygen tension. The sickled cells then become trapped in small blood vessels leading to minute infarcts in various organs.

The first report of splenectomy for children affected with sickle cell disease was in 1927.[22] Studies have addressed the use of splenectomy in increasing erythrocyte life span as well as decreasing the transfusion requirements.[23-25] The best results have been observed in young children who exhibit splenomegaly.[26]

Idiopathic Autoimmune Hemolytic Anemia

This disorder is one of the most common types of acquired hemolytic anemia. Initially described by Chauffard and Troisier in 1908,[27] the disease is characterized by antibodies produced against the individual's own cells. Women are twice as likely to be affected as men, and the presentations include anemia as well as jaundice and splenomegaly, usually after the fifth decade.

Indications for splenectomy are as follows: (1) failure of steroid therapy after a 4- to 6-week trial, (2) the need for excessive doses of steroids to maintain a remission, (3) evidence of toxic manifestations, and (4) contraindication for steroids.[2]

In a number of studies utilizing splenectomy as treatment, 50 to 80 per cent of the patients reported a favorable response.[28-30]

PURPURA

Idiopathic Thrombocytopenic Purpura

Idiopathic thrombocytopenic purpura is the most common immune thrombocytopenia.[13] As the name implies, no clear etiology has been implicated in this disorder although thrombocytopenia associated with antibody production to platelets has been reported.[31] A role for viral infection, drug sensitivity, infectious mononucleosis, or systemic lupus erythematosus as a causative agent in the disease has been suggested. Women are more than twice as likely to have idiopathic thrombocytopenic purpura than men. Platelet counts are low, typically less than 50,000/mm^3,[13] and individuals exhibit bleeding, petechiae, and ecchymosis.

In children afflicted with this disorder the platelet counts generally return to normal without any need for medical treatment. However, spontaneous remissions in adults do not occur with the same high frequency. Steroid treatment and splenectomy are therefore indicated in such patients.

The need for splenectomy in adult patients is suggested by the theory that the spleen may act as either a source of antibody production or a sequestration site of the platelets themselves.[2,31] Previous studies have indicated better results in patients who underwent splenectomy as opposed to a trial course of steroids.[30] Indeed, studies in which splenectomy has been utilized as treatment report success rates as high as 85 per cent.[32,33]

Thrombocytopenic purpura has also been reported in patients infected with the human immunodeficiency virus.[34] Indeed, it appears that nearly 11 per cent of such patients have platelet counts less than 100,000/mm^3.[35] Conflicting reports exist concerning the use of splenectomy in these patients. Thus, Tyler et al.[36] commented that splenectomy should be reserved for medically refractory human immunodeficiency virus-associated thrombocytopenia whereas others report the use of splenectomy as safe and effective therapy.[37–39]

Thrombotic Thrombocytopenic Purpura

Initially described in 1925 by Moschcowitz,[40] thrombotic thrombocytopenia purpura is primarily a disease of arterioles and capillaries. The disorder is of unknown etiology and primarily affects young women although it has been reported in both sexes as well as in all age groups.

The clinical features include fever, purpura, hemolytic anemia, neurologic symptoms, and evidence of renal involvement[2,41] and reflect the formation of microemboli within capillaries and arterioles of many organs.[13] Formerly, the disease was fatal in the majority of patients; however, the use of glucocorticoids and antiplatelet drugs as well as splenectomy and plasmapheresis has resulted in improved survival.[13,42] Thus, in 1980 Cuttner reported that the use of medium molecular weight dextran, steroids, and splenectomy resulted in a remission rate of 87 per cent.[43]

HYPERSPLENISM

Primary Hypersplenism

In 1955 Dameshek provided the classic definition of hypersplenism.[44] The four criteria include: (1) cytopenias of one or more peripheral cell lines, (2) bone marrow hyperplasia, (3) splenomegaly, and (4) correction of the cytopenia following splenectomy.[45,46]

Although the etiology is unclear, Doan proposed that excessive phagocytosis of granulocytes, platelets, and red blood cells by the spleen led to the hematologic changes.[47] Treatment for primary hypersplenism is splenectomy. Studies by Doan et al.[28] and Schwartz et al.[2] have shown excellent results (higher than 90 per cent) with sustained hematologic improvement.

Secondary Hypersplenism

A wide range of diseases may be associated with secondary hypersplenism. Such pathologic conditions usually involve the red pulp of the spleen with subsequent sequestration and destruction of the abnormal erythrocytes. Splenomegaly is the most common finding in patients with portal hypertension secondary to thrombosis of the extrahepatic portal vein and is a frequent physical finding in patients with portal hypertension secondary to cirrhosis.[2]

The primary therapy for this disease has been directed at the reduction of portal hypertension. Indeed, reports of portacaval shunt surgery reveal an improvement of hematologic status.[48,49] The use of the splenectomy is thus somewhat controversial.[50,51] A summary of current opinion suggests that in the rare circumstances in which splenectomy is required, it should be used in conjunction with a splenorenal shunt to decompress the portal circulation.[52]

NEOPLASTIC CONDITIONS

Myeloid Metaplasia

Both agnogenic myeloid metaplasia (AMM) and postpolycythemic myeloid metaplasia (PPMM) are chronic myeloproliferative disorders characterized by splenomegaly, immature granulocytes, distorted and teardrop-shaped erythrocytes, erythroblasts in peripheral blood, and bone marrow fibrosis.[53] Although the etiology of AMM is unknown, PPMM develops in approximately 10 per cent of patients with previous polycythemia vera.[54]

Survival rates for patients with these two disorders differ significantly. Thus, the 5-year survival for patients afflicted with AMM is 60 per cent,[55] whereas PPMM shows a more progressive course with a reported median survival of 2 years.[56]

The use of splenectomy as a treatment for patients with AMM or PPMM remains controversial. Mulder et al.[57] proposed splenectomy for all patients immediately after the diagnosis of AMM while others[58-60] have suggested that splenectomy should be reserved for selected patients. A number of reports state that splenectomy should be used only in rare instances.[2,61,62] Thus, the reported indications for splenectomy in patients with AMM include painful splenomegaly, refractory hemolytic anemia, marked thrombocytopenia, and associated portal hypertension.[58]

A recent review suggested that splenectomy improved the quality of life in most patients with AMM and in many patients with PPMM, although survival was not affected.[60]

Hodgkin's Disease, Lymphomas, and Leukemias

Bryant and Billroth are credited with performing the first splenectomies in the treatment of leukemia and lymphoma.[2] Since then, there have been numerous reports regarding the indications for splenectomy.[63-67] Although the primary therapy for these disorders includes the use of chemotherapy and radiotherapy, splenectomy may be indicated for major splenomegaly, increased transfusion requirements, or cytopenia that precludes systemic therapy.[52]

Adler et al.,[68] in a study of 50 patients with lymphocytic lymphoma and leukemia, reported that splenectomy was worthwhile in lymphoproliferative disease complicated by hematologic depression regardless of marrow findings or the results of other diagnostic studies. Indeed, a number of studies have reported the benefit of splenectomy in patients with Hodgkin's disease.[69,70]

Chronic lymphocytic leukemia is the most common form of leukemia in the United States and Europe. Although prior practice favored splenectomy late in the course of the disease, recent studies have suggested earlier surgical intervention may yield more favorable results.[13]

Hairy cell leukemia is a rare chronic leukemia characterized by pancytopenia, circulating mononuclear cells with prominent cytoplasmic projections, and moderate to massive splenomegaly without significant lymphadenopathy.[71,72] The occurrence of neutropenia, thrombocytopenia and anemia has a negative impact on the prognosis for patients with hairy cell leukemia. Under such circumstances, splenectomy has been used in treatment with reported 5-year survival rates of between 60 and 70 per cent.[73-76]

The role of staging laparotomy in Hodgkin's disease has been accurate staging and delineation of subsequent treatment modalities.[77] Coker suggested three opportunities for restaging laparotomy in Hodgkin's disease: (1) at the completion of primary therapy to confirm remission of the disease; (2) at the time of suspected recurrence; and (3) at the time of a recurrence in a peripheral node to document coexistent abdominal disease.[77] Of note is the observation of Van Leeuwen et al.[78] who reported an increased risk of a second leukemia in patients with Hodgkin's disease who underwent splenectomy.

MISCELLANEOUS DISEASES

Felty's Syndrome

Felty's syndrome comprises chronic rheumatoid arthritis, splenomegaly, neutropenia, and occasionally anemia and thrombocytopenia. It usually affects middle-aged women who often show signs of arthritis prior to hematologic changes.[79]

Treatment modalities have included both corticosteroids and splenectomy. Whereas steroid therapy has failed to produce long lasting effects, splenectomy has been reported to produce good hematologic results.[80–82]

Gaucher's Disease

First described in 1882,[83] Gaucher's disease is an autosomal recessive disorder of sphingolipid metabolism. In 1965, Brady et al.[84] demonstrated that the disease was a result of a deficiency in the enzyme β-glucocerebrosidase. Patients with the disorder have massive splenomegaly and bone pain caused by deposition of glucocerebroside in the lysosomes of the reticuloendothelial cells of these organs.[85]

Splenectomy is the treatment of choice for the disease. Earlier teaching favored the use of total splenectomy.[86,87] However, because of the risk for lethal infection as well as the potential for acceleration of hepatic or bony involvement, partial splenectomy is a more reasonable option.[88,89] The results of the largest reported series of patients undergoing splenectomy for Gaucher's disease have indicated that total splenectomy is accompanied by more aggressive bone disease as well as a predisposition to malignancy.[90]

Sarcoidosis

Sarcoidosis is a chronic, granulomatous, multisystem disorder of unknown etiology. The disease is characterized by an accumulation of T lymphocytes and mononuclear phagocytes in the affected organs. The characteristic histologic appearance includes the presence of noncaseating epitheloid cell tubercles.

Approximately 25 per cent of patients with sarcoidosis develop some degree of hepatomegaly and splenomegaly. Although spontaneous recovery may occur in 50 per cent of the patients, splenectomy is considered for patients with splenomegaly who develop symptoms of hypersplenism, especially thrombocytopenic purpura.[52]

MISCELLANEOUS LESIONS

Ectopic Spleen

Although up to 30 per cent of the population may harbor an ectopic spleen, it is usually of no clinical consequence unless acute torsion of the pedicle occurs, in which circumstances surgical treatment is necessary.[52]

Splenic Artery Aneurysm

This is the second most common intra-abdominal aneurysm and is most commonly noted at autopsy. Women tend to be affected more than men, with the incidence of rupture increased during pregnancy.[2] As with other aneurysms, the optimal primary treatment is excision. The detection of a splenic artery aneurysm in a pregnant woman necessitates surgery.[91,92] Repair of the aneurysm usually necessitates splenectomy.

Splenic Cysts and Tumors

Splenic cysts are a rare entity and are often associated with parasitic infection.[13] In these instances, surgery is the preferred treatment. Nonparasitic cysts are less common and are classified as dermoid, epidermoid, epithelial, or pseudocysts.[2] Partial splenectomy has been determined to be the treatment of choice in these instances.[93]

Tumors of the spleen are quite uncommon with cavernous hemangioma being the most common benign neoplasm.[13] These hemangiomas usually are detected when they are either of sufficient size to cause pressure, spontaneously rupture, or result in splenomegaly. Treatment is splenectomy. Other benign tumors of the spleen include lipomas, hamartomas, and fibromas.[13,52]

Primary malignant tumors of the spleen are mainly hemangiosarcomas. Rarely tumors, including breast, lung, skin and colon, may metastasize to the spleen. As with most benign neoplasms, these tumors should be resected if the overall condition of the patient warrants intervention.[13]

Splenic Abscess

Although rare, the spleen occasionally is the site for an intra-abdominal abscess. Although the majority of abscesses are bacterial in origin, fungal abscesses are not uncommon.[94] It has been estimated that approximately 75 per cent of splenic abscesses are related to systemic bacteria, 15 per cent are secondary to trauma, and 10 per cent occur as a direct extension from an adjacent abscess, e.g., in the colon or stomach.[13]

In the past, treatment consisted of splenotomy and drainage of the abscess. Today, splenectomy and intravenous antibiotics are the primary forms of therapy.[13]

SPLENIC TRAUMA

Although the spleen is offered some protection in its position in the left upper quadrant, it is not immune from injury. Indeed, it is the most frequently injured abdominal organ in blunt trauma, and nearly 25 per cent of all blunt injuries of the abdomen involve the spleen.[52] Splenic injury may be classified into four categories: nonpenetrating (blunt) trauma, penetrating trauma, operative (iatrogenic) trauma, or spontaneous rupture.

Blunt trauma may result in a number of injuries including transverse fracture along an intersegmental plane, a stellate laceration, avulsion injuries from traction on either the upper or lower pole, or subcapsular hematomas.[13]

A five-tiered grading system has been developed in the evaluation of splenic injuries. Grade I injuries are those that involve capsular tears or ligament avulsion. Grade II involves a superficial laceration or fracture less than or equal to 2 cm deep. Deep lacerations or fractures greater than 2 cm are classified as Grade III. Grade IV describes splenic fragmentation into two segments or into an ischemic segment that requires resection. Grade V characterizes splenic fragmentation into multiple small pieces or the presence of a major hilar vascular injury.[4] Penetrating trauma to the spleen is usually a result of gunshot or stab wounds and exploratory laparotomy is indicated for such injuries.

Iatrogenic splenic injury is a relatively common problem during certain abdominal operations. Gastric, renal, esophageal, and aortic surgery are all procedures in which damage to the spleen is a potential occurrence. Olsen and Beaudoin[95] have described the common mechanism of splenic injury during gastric surgery especially in the area of the esophageal hiatus. They noted that traction on the stomach toward the right side of the abdomen is more likely to tear short gastric vessels or the splenic capsule. Similarly, downward traction on the splenic flexure of the colon may cause tension on the lienocolic ligament and produce a capsular tear. In certain instances, the spleen may be injured by a retractor. Although previous reports have noted a high percentage of splenectomies for iatrogenic trauma, a recent study by Coon[96] has demonstrated that the frequency of iatrogenic splenic trauma had decreased to 9 per cent.

Although spontaneous rupture is an uncommon event, it is frequently encountered in various hematologic disorders and often follows relatively trivial trauma. Malaria and infectious mononucleosis are diseases in which spontaneous rupture of the spleen occurs commonly.[1]

TECHNIQUE OF LAPAROSCOPIC SPLENECTOMY

Splenectomy

In patients who undergo laparoscopic splenectomy, it is crucial that necessary preoperative scans are performed to eliminate the possibility of accessory spleens since these may not be easily visible at laparotomy. In addition, to facilitate vascular control immediately prior to surgery, the splenic artery should be embolized with subsequent confirmation by angiography (Fig. 14-1).

The patient is placed in the supine position on the operating table. A small roll is placed under the left posterior costal margin to facilitate splenic exposure. Prior to surgery, a nasogastric tube is placed in the stomach.

In patients undergoing the procedure for hematologic disorders, a laparoscopic cholecystectomy may be indicated as a synchronous procedure. After this initial procedure (see Chapter 39), a fifth port located in the left lower quadrant is introduced to facilitate dissection in the parasplenic and gastric greater curve area (Fig. 14-2).

During the initial exploration, care should be taken to avoid iatrogenic trauma. This reflects the difficulty that surgeons face since many patients who undergo elective splenec-

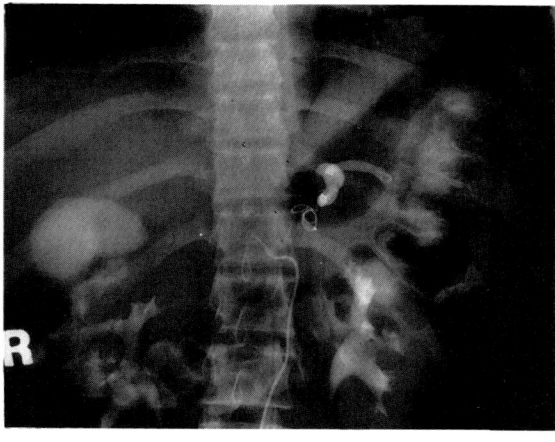

Figure 14-1. Preoperative postembolized celiac axis arteriogram of a patient with hereditary spherocystosis showing no flow in the splenic artery. (Photograph courtesy of M. M. Gazayerli, M.D., F.R.C.S.)

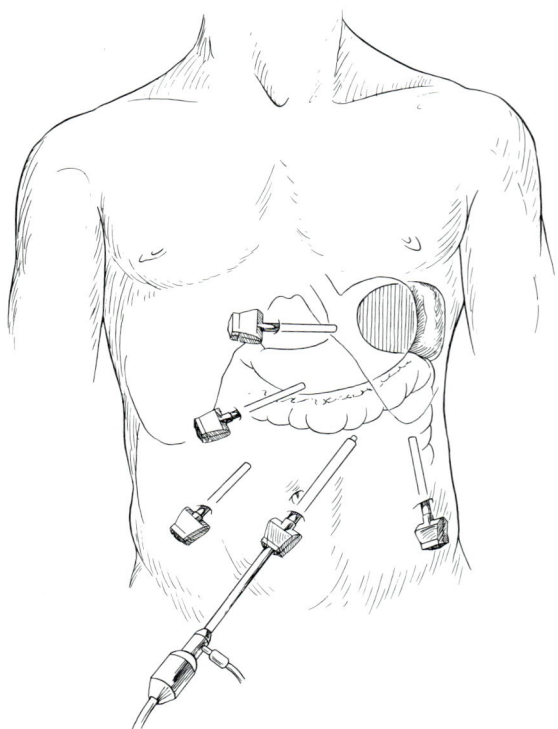

Figure 14-2. Positioning of the five ports used in a laparoscopic splenectomy.

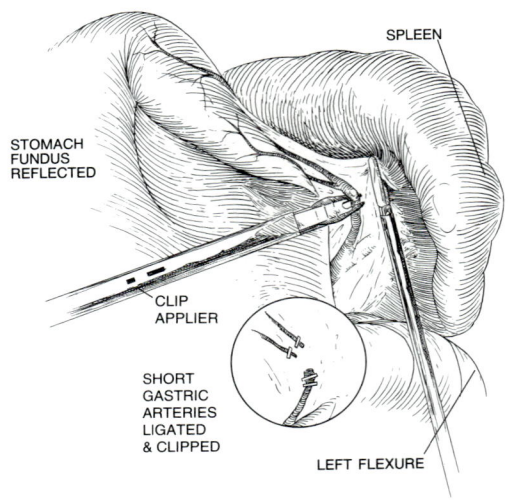

Figure 14-4. Short gastric vessels are clipped and cut.

tomy suffer from hematologic disorders or coagulation difficulties that may adversely influence surgery. In addition, the spleen may be particularly fragile (Fig. 14-3). After assessing size, consistency, and mobility of the organ, ligation of the short gastric arteries should be undertaken as the initial step (Fig. 14-4). Standard clips are adequate for this series of vessels. Once the short gastric arteries are ligated and dissected, the spleen is reflected laterally and superiorly to reveal the splenic artery and vein. An 0-ethibond suture can then be passed around the artery and vein, which are tied off with a suture ligature device (Fig. 14-5). An endoscopic gastrointestinal anastomosis stapling device is then introduced through the most appropriately sited port and positioned with a view for division of the main hilar arterial and venous vessels (Fig. 14-6). The instrument should be carefully positioned to ensure complete coverage

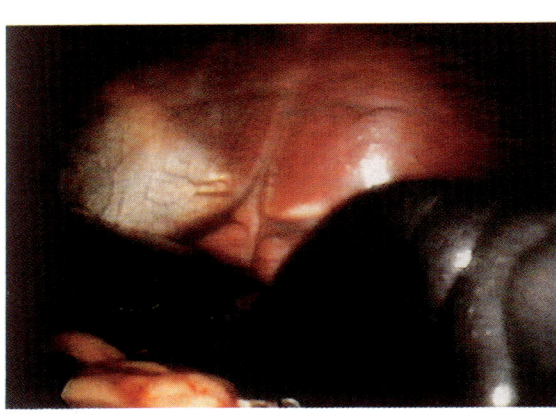

Figure 14-3. Intra-abdominal view revealing the enlarged spleen (right). (Photograph courtesy of M. M. Gazayerli, M.D., F.R.C.S.)

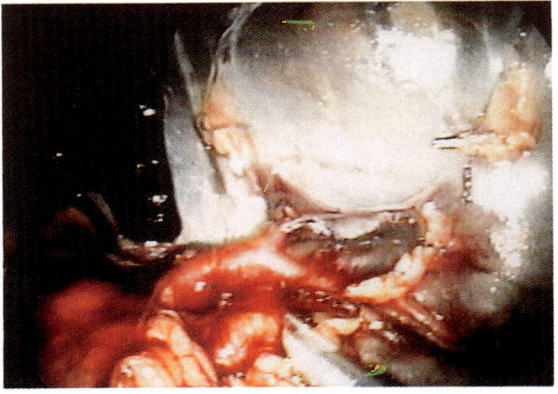

Figure 14-5. Splenic artery and vein are dissected. (Photograph courtesy of M. M. Gazayerli, M.D., F.R.C.S.)

Splenic Surgery

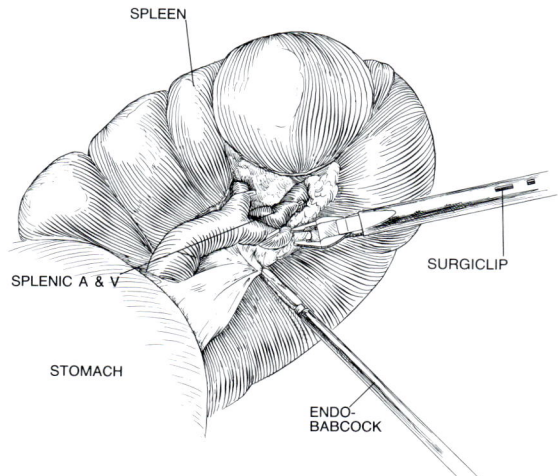

Figure 14-6. The splenic vessels are suture ligated.

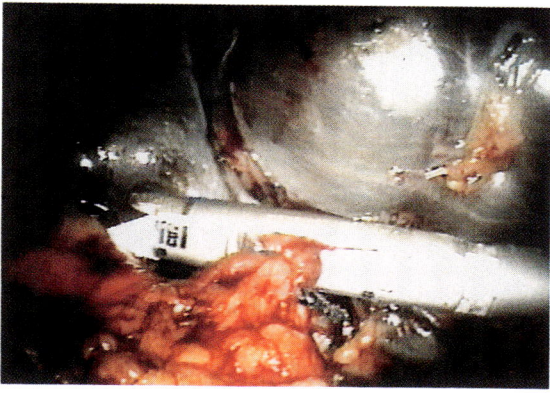

Figure 14-8. The ENDO GIA* 30 stapling device is fired across the vessels. (Photograph courtesy of M. M. Gazayerli, M.D., F.R.C.S.)

of all vascular structures prior to operation (Fig. 14-7). In the instance of a particularly wide or bulky splenic pedicle, two sequential firings of the stapler may be necessary (Fig. 14-8). Once the pedicle is severed, careful evaluation for bleeding should be undertaken and small individual branches may need to be clipped (Fig. 14-9). At this stage, one or two further short gastric arteries (Fig. 14-10) may need to be detached to completely free the spleen. Similarly, some peritoneal adhesions or ligaments may need to be coagulated, clipped, and divided to effect complete mobilization.

Once the spleen is free from all attachments and adhesions, it is placed into a bag and morsellated (Fig. 14-11). The bag and its contents can then be brought out through a widened trochar incision.

In instances in which total splenectomy is to be performed, the surgeon has several options available. Microwave coagulation and ultrasonic aspiration may prove to be more effective methods for removing the organ from the abdomen since their use avoids enlarging the trochar incision.

Splenic Salvage

In patients who have sustained splenic trauma, laparoscopic evaluation of the spleen

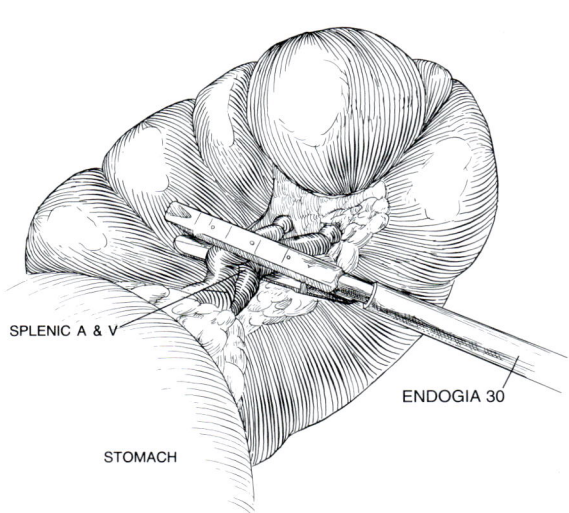

Figure 14-7. An ENDO GIA* 30 stapling device is placed across the vascular pedicle.

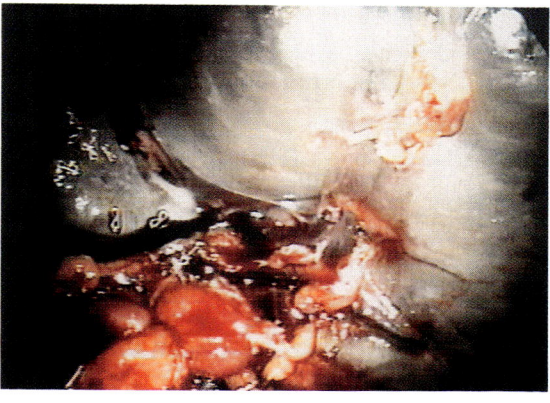

Figure 14-9. The splenic artery and vein are transected. (Photograph courtesy of M. M. Gazayerli, M.D., F.R.C.S.)

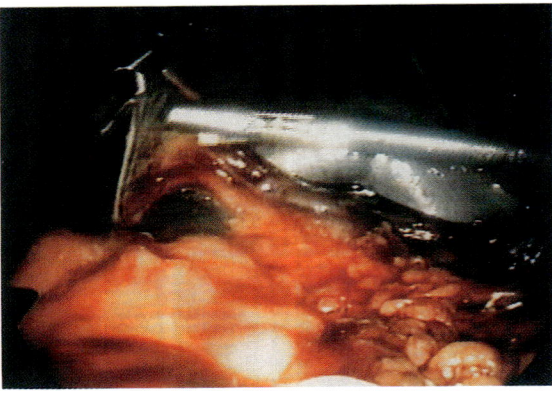

Figure 14-10. Additional short gastric vessels are ligated and cut. (Photograph courtesy of M. M. Gazayerli, M.D., F.R.C.S.)

is necessary prior to determination of treatment. If the splenic injury is low grade (Grade I, II, or III), splenic salvage may be an option. Patients with Grade IV or V splenic injury are primary candidates for splenectomy.

Trochar and laparoscope placement are identical to those described earlier. Once the laparoscope has been inserted, it is necessary for the surgeon to evaluate and quantitate the degree of splenic injury.

If the decision has been made to attempt splenic salvage, the surgeon should then decide upon the course of repair. The injured spleen should be initially mobilized by division of the various splenic ligaments. Capsular tears and ligament avulsions can be hemostatically sealed by spraying a thin layer of hemostatic agents such as fibrin glue, collagen, gelatin, or fibrin. Alternatively, the agent may be injected into the fractured splenic surface. With deep penetrating wounds of the spleen, deep injection of the hemostatic agent can be utilized. Injection of the agent is continued as the needle passes out of the spleen. Local pressure using cotton pads may be helpful in providing direct hemostasis.

After injection of the agent, it is recommended that the laparoscope remain in the abdomen for 30 to 60 additional minutes to visually confirm that appropriate hemostasis has occurred.

REFERENCES

1. Wolf BC, Neiman RS. Disorders of the Spleen, Vol 20, Major Problems in Pathology. Philadelphia, WB Saunders, 1989.
2. Schwartz SI, Adams JT, Bauman AW. Splenectomy for hematologic disorders. Curr Probl Surg, May 1971; pp 1–57.
3. Reigner O. Ueber einen Fall Von Exstirpation der Traumatisch Zerrissenen Milz. Berl Klin Wochenschr 1883; 30:177–181.
4. Kram HB, Del Junco T, Clark SR, et al. Techniques of splenic preservation using fibrin glue. J Trauma 1990; 30:97–101.
5. Franke EL, Neu HC. Postsplenectomy infection. Surg Clin North Am 1981; 61:135–155.
6. Traub AC, Perry JF. Splenic preservation following splenic trauma. J Trauma 1982; 22:496–501.
7. Sekikawa T, Shatney CH. Septic sequelae after splenectomy for trauma in adults. Am J Surg 1983; 145:667–673.
8. Morgenstern L, Shapiro SJ. Techniques of splenic conservation. Arch Surg 1979; 114:449–454.
9. Millikan JS, Moore EE, Moore GE, et al. Alternatives to splenectomy in adults after trauma. Am J Surg 1982; 144:711–716.
10. Toy FK, Reed WP, Taylor LS. Experimental splenic preservation employing microwave surgical techniques: A preliminary report. Surgery 1984; 96:117–120.
11. Delaney HM, Porreca F, Mitsudo S, et al. Splenic capping: An experimental study of a new technique for splenorrhaphy using woven polyglycolic acid mesh. Ann Surg 1982; 196:187–193.
12. Morgenstern L. Salvaging the spleen. Contemp Surg 1983; 23:27–34.
13. Bowdler AJ. The Spleen. Structure, Function and Clinical Significance. London, Chapman and Hall Medical, 1990.
14. Dresbach M. Elliptical human red corpuscles. Science 1904; 19:469.
15. Lipton EI. Elliptocytosis with hemolytic anemia: The effects of splenectomy. Pediatrics 1955; 15:67–83.
16. Blackburn EK, Jordan A, Lythe WJ, et al. Hereditary elliptocytotic haemolytic anemia. J Clin Pathol 1958; 11:316–320.
17. Cooley TB, Lee P. A series of cases of splenomegaly in children, with anemia and peculiar bone changes. Trans Am Pediatr Soc 1925; 37:29–30.

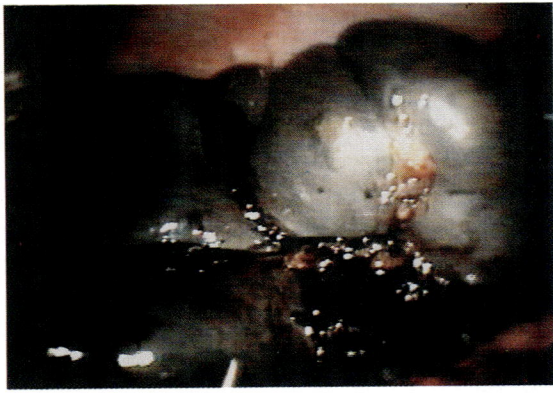

Figure 14-11. The spleen is shown completely detached from its vascular and fibrous attachments. (Photograph courtesy of M. M. Gazayerli, M.D., F.R.C.S.)

18. Brain MC, McCullouch PB. Current Therapy in Hematology-Oncology 1983-1984. New York, Brian C. Decker, 1983.
19. Reemtsma K, Elliot RHE Jr. Splenectomy in Mediterranean anemia; an evaluation of long-term results. Ann Surg 1956; 144:999-1007.
20. Politis C, et al. Partial splenic embolisation for hypersplenism of thalassemia major: Five year follow-up. Br Med J 1987; 294:665-667.
21. Herrick JB. Peculiar elongated and sickle-shaped red corpuscles in a case of severe anemia. Arch Intern Med 1910; 6:517.
22. Stewart WB. Sickle cell anemia. Report of a case with splenectomy. Am J Dis Child 1927; 34:72-80.
23. Shottom D, Crockett CL Jr, Leavell BS. Splenectomy in sickle cell anemia: Report of a case and review of the literature. Blood 1951; 6:365-371.
24. Sprague CC, Paterson JCS. Role of the spleen and effect of splenectomy in sickle cell disease. Blood 1958; 13:569.
25. Pinna AD, Argiolu FA, Marongiu L, Pinna DC. Indications and results for splenectomy for beta thalassemia in two hundred and twenty-one pediatric patients. Surg Gynecol Obstet 1988; 167:109-113.
26. Emond AM, Morais P, Venugopal S, et al. Role of splenectomy in homozygous sickle cell disease in childhood. Lancet 1984; I:88-90.
27. Chauffard MA, Troisier J. Anemie grave avec hemolysine dans le serum. Semain Med 1908; 28:904.
28. Doan CA, Bruce MD, Wiseman BK. Hypersplenic cytopenic syndromes: A 25 year experience with special reference to splenectomy. In Proceedings of the Sixth International Congress of the International Society of Hematology. New York, Grune & Stratton, 1958, p 429.
29. DeWeese MS, Coller FA. Splenectomy for hematologic disorders. West J Surg 1959; 67:129-138.
30. Schwartz SI, Bernard RP, Adams JT, Bauman AW. Splenectomy for hematologic disorders. Arch Surg 1970; 101:338-347.
31. Harrington WJ, Minnick M, Hollingsworth J, Moore CV. Demonstration of a thrombocytopenic factor in the blood of patients with thrombocytopenic purpura. J Lab Clin Med 1951; 38:1-10.
32. Doan CA, Bouroncle BA, Wiseman BK. Idiopathic and secondary thrombocytopenic purpura: Clinical study and evaluation of 381 cases over a period of 28 years. Ann Intern Med 1960; 53:861-876.
33. Coon WW. Splenectomy for idiopathic thrombocytopenic purpura. Surg Gynecol Obstet 1987; 164:225-229.
34. Ravikumar TS, Allen JD, Botha A Jr, Steele G Jr. Splenectomy. The treatment of choice for human immunodeficiency virus-related immune thrombocytopenia? Arch Surg 1989; 124:625-628.
35. Ratner L. HIV-1 associated thrombocytopenia. Presented at the AIDS Clinical Treatment Group Meeting, Washington, DC, July 1988.
36. Tyler DS, Shaunak S, Bartlett JA, Iglehart JD. HIV-1-Associated thrombocytopenia. Ann Surg 1990; 211:211-217.
37. Ferguson CM. Splenectomy for immune thrombocytopenia related to human immunodeficiency virus. Surg Gynecol Obstet 1988; 167:300-302.
38. Walsh C, Krigel R, Lennette E, Karpatkin S. Thrombocytopenia in homosexual patients. Ann Intern Med 1985; 103:542-545.
39. Walsh CM, Nardi MA, Karpatkin S. On the mechanism of thrombocytopenia purpura in sexually active homosexual men. N Engl J Med 1984; 311:635-639.
40. Moschcowitz E. An acute febrile pleiochromic anemia with hyaline thromboses of the terminal arterioles and capillaries: An undescribed disease. Arch Intern Med 1925; 36:89-93.
41. Amorosi EL, Ultmann JE. Thrombotic thrombocytopenic purpura: Report of 16 cases and review of the literature. Medicine (Baltimore) 1966; 45:139-159.
42. Schneider PA, Rayner AA, Linker CA, et al. The role of splenectomy in multimodality treatment of thrombotic thrombocytopenic purpura. Ann Surg 1985; 202:318-322.
43. Cuttner J. Thrombotic thrombocytopenic purpura: A ten year experience. Blood 1980; 56:302-306.
44. Dameshek W. Hypersplenism. Bull NY Acad Med 1955; 31:113
45. Jacob HS. Hypersplenism: Mechanisms and management. Br J Haematol 1974; 27:1-5.
46. Amorosi EL. Hypersplenism. Semin Hematol 1965; 2:249-285.
47. Doan CA. Hypersplenism. Bull NY Acad Med 1949; 25:625-650.
48. Child CG, Turcotte JG. Surgery and Portal Hypertension. In Child CG, ed. The Liver and Portal Hypertension. Philadelphia, WB Saunders Company, 1964, Chap 1.
49. Wantz GE, Payne MA. Experience with portacaval shunt for portal hypertension. N Engl J Med 1961; 265:721.
50. Rousselot LA, Panke WF, Bono RF, Moreno AH. Experiences with portacaval anastomosis. Analysis of 104 elective end-to-side shunts for the prevention of recurrent hemorrhage from esophago-gastric varices. Am J Med 1963; 34:297-307.
51. Tumen HJ. Hypersplenism and portal hypertension. Ann NY Acad Sci 1970; 170:332-344.
52. Schwartz SI. Principles of Surgery. New York, McGraw-Hill, 1989.
53. Silverstein MN. Agnogenic myeloid metaplasia. In Williams JW, Beutler E, Erslev AJ, et al., eds. Hematology, ed 3. New York, McGraw-Hill International Book Co, 1983, pp 214-218.
54. Ellis JT, Peterson P, Geller SA, et al. Studies of bone marrow in polycythemia vera and the evolution of myelofibrosis and second hematologic malignancies. Semin Hematol 1986; 23:144-155.
55. Silverstein MN. Agnogenic Myeloid Metaplasia. Acton, MA, Publishing Sciences Group, 1975, pp 109-114.
56. Silverstein MN. Postpolycythemia myeloid metaplasia. Arch Intern Med 1974; 134:113-116.
57. Mulder H, Steenbergen J, Haanen C. Clinical course and survival after elective splenectomy in 19 patients with primary myelofibrosis. Br J Haematol 1977; 35:419.
58. Silverstein MN, ReMine WH. Splenectomy in myeloid metaplasia. Blood 1979; 53:515-518.
59. Broe PJ, Comley CL, Cameron JL. Thrombosis of the portal vein following splenectomy for myeloid metaplasia. Surg Gynecol Obstet 1981; 152:488-492.
60. Brenner B, Nagler AM, Tatarski A, Hasmonai M. Splenectomy in agnogenic myeloid metaplasia and postpolycythemic myeloid metaplasia. A study of 34 cases. Arch Intern Med 1988; 148:250-255.
61. Ward HP, Block MH. The natural history of agnogenic myeloid metaplasia and a critical evaluation of its relationship with the myeloproliferative syndrome. Medicine (Baltimore) 1971; 50:357.
62. Coon WW, Liepman MK. Splenectomy for agnogenic myeloid metaplasia. Surg Gynecol Obstst 1982; 154:561-563.
63. Christiansen BE, Hansen LK, Kristensen JK, Vidabaek A. Splenectomy in hematology—Indications, results

and complications in 41 cases. Scand J Haematol 1970; 7:247–260.
64. Hyatt DF, Skarin AT, Moloney WC, Wilson RE. Splenectomy for lymphosarcoma. Surg Gynecol Obstet 1970; 131:928–932.
65. Mittelman A, Elias EG, Grace JT Jr. Further experience with splenectomy in Hodgkin's disease. J Surg Oncol 1969; 1:339–344.
66. Strumia M, Strumia PV, Bassert D. Splenectomy in leukemia—Hematologic and clinical effects on 34 patients and review of 229 published cases. Cancer Res 1966; 26:519–528.
67. Cooper TA, Ironside PN, Madigan JP, et al. The role of splenectomy in the management of advanced Hodgkin's disease. Cancer 1974; 34:408–417.
68. Adler S, Stutzman L, Sokal JE, Mittelman A. Splenectomy for hematologic depression in lymphocytic lymphoma and leukemia. Cancer 1975; 35:521–528.
69. Aisenberg AC. The staging and treatment of Hodgkin's disease. N Engl J Med 1978; 299:1228–1232.
70. Allison JG. The role of surgery in the management of lymphoma. JAMA 1981; 246:2843–2848.
71. Golomb HM, Vardiman JW. Response to splenectomy in 65 patients with hairy cell leukemia: An evaluation of spleen weight and bone marrow involvement. Blood 1983; 61:349–352.
72. Golomb HM, Catovsky D, Golde DW. Hairy cell leukemia: A clinical review based on 71 cases. Ann Intern Med 1978; 89:677–683.
73. Mintz U, Golomb HM. Splenectomy as initial therapy in twenty-six patients with leukemic reticuloendotheliosis (hairy cell leukemia). Cancer Res 1979; 39:2366–2370.
74. Jansen J, Herman J, Remme J, et al. Hairy cell leukemia, clinical features and effect of splenectomy. Scand J Haematol 1978; 21:60–71.
75. Van Norman AS, Nagorney DM, Martin JK, et al. Splenectomy for hairy cell leukemia. Cancer 1986; 57:644–648
76. Flandrin G, Sigaux F, Sebahoun G, Boufette P. Hairy cell leukemia: Clinical presentation and follow-up of 211 patients. Semin Oncol 1984; 11(Suppl 2):458–471.
77. Coker DD, Morris DM, Coleman JJ, et al. Restaging laparotomy for Hodgkin's disease. Ann Surg 1982; 197:79–83.
78. Van Leeuwen FE, Somers R, Hart AAM. Splenectomy in Hodgkin's disease and second leukemias. Lancet 1987; 2:210–211.
79. DeGruchy C. Diagnosis and treatment of Felty's syndrome. Geriatrics 1965; 20:219.
80. O'Neil JA Jr, Scott HW, Billings FT, Foster JH. The role of splenectomy in Felty's syndrome. Ann Surg 1968; 167:81–84.
81. Coon WW. Felty's syndrome: When is splenectomy indicated? Am J Surg 1985; 149:272–275.
82. Riley SM, Aldrete JS. The role of splenectomy in Felty's syndrome. Am J Surg 1975; 130:51–52.
83. Gaucher PCE. De l'epitheliome primitif de la rate. Theses de Paris, 1882.
84. Brady RO, Kanfer JN, Shapiro D. Metabolism of glucocerebrosides. II. Evidence of an enzymatic deficiency in Gaucher's disease. Biochem Biophys Res Commun 1965; 18:221–225.
85. Rodgers BM, Tribble C, Joob A. Partial splenectomy for Gaucher's disease. Ann Surg 1987; 205:693–699.
86. Salky B, Kreel I, Gelernt I, et al. Splenectomy for Gaucher's disease. Ann Surg 1979; 190:592–594.
87. Shiloni E, Bitran D, Rachmilewitz E, Durst AL. The role of splenectomy in Gaucher's disease. Arch Surg 1983; 118:929–932.
88. Bar-Maor JA, Govrin-Yehudian J. Partial splenectomy in children with Gaucher's disease. Pediatrics 1985; 76:398–401.
89. Rubin M, Yampolski I, Lambrozo R, et al. Partial splenectomy in Gaucher's disease. J Pediatr Surg 1986; 21:125–128.
90. Fleschner PR, Aufses AH Jr., Grabowski GA, Elias R. A 27-year experience with splenectomy for Gaucher's disease. Am J Surg 1991; 161:69–75.
91. Stanley JC. Pathogenesis and clinical significance of splenic artery aneurysms. Surgery 1974; 76:898–909.
92. Trastek VF. Splenic artery aneurysms. Surgery 1982; 91:694–699.
93. Morgenstern L. Partial splenectomy for nonparasitic cysts. Am J Surg 1980; 139:278–281.
94. Helton WS, et al. The diagnosis and treatment of splenic fungal abscesses in the immune-suppressed patient. Arch Surg 1986; 121:580–586.
95. Olsen WR, Beaudoin DE. Surgical injury to the spleen. Surg Gynecol Obstet 1970; 131:57–62.
96. Coon, WW. Iatrogenic splenic injury. Am J Surg 1990; 159:585–588.

Chapter 15
Approaches to Pancreatic Disease

Steven D. Leach
Irvin M. Modlin

The application of laparoscopic technology to the diagnosis and treatment of pancreatic disease remains in its infancy. A partial list of both current and theoretical applications is presented in Table 15-1. Although several of these procedures have become fairly commonplace in certain institutions, the majority of the procedures remain developmental and have been incompletely evaluated with regard to either feasibility or efficacy. At present, the development of laparoscopic approaches to pancreatic disease is hindered not only by a lack of appropriate instrumentation, but also by reluctance on the part of the surgeon. Intuitively, the experienced surgeon may exhibit caution in the application of laparoscopic techniques to pancreatic disease. Indeed, the pancreas remains relatively inaccessible from an anatomic point of view. Laparoscopic access to the pancreas is difficult for several reasons. These include the retroperitoneal position of this organ as well as the barrier of access to the lesser sac presented by the lesser omentum, stomach, greater omentum, and transverse mesocolon. The major vascular structures adjacent to the pancreas further complicate laparoscopic manipulation.

On the other hand, a number of theoretic arguments have been offered for developing minimally invasive approaches to neoplastic and inflammatory diseases of the pancreas. Primary among these is the relative ineffectiveness of currently available invasive therapies. In this context it should be noted that approximately 10,000 patients in this country each year are subjected to laparotomy for staging and possible resection of incurable pancreatic carcinoma. The positive contribution of this invasive approach to either quality of life or overall survival remains difficult to demonstrate. Thus, the development of less invasive methods for accurate diagnosis, staging, and appropriate palliation might be of benefit. In this chapter, we review the historical and technical aspects of laparoscopic pancreoscopy and discuss applications of this technique to the management of patients with both neoplastic and inflammatory diseases of the pancreas.

HISTORICAL ISSUES

Techniques for laparoscopic exposure and examination of the pancreas were initially described nearly two decades ago by a number of investigators.[1,2] Meyer-Burg[1] reported a technique for inspection, palpation, and biopsy of the pancreas during laparoscopy in 1972. His method, however, did not involve entry into the lesser sac and relied on visualization and needle biopsy of the pancreas through the lesser omentum. In 1973, Strauch, Lux, and Ottenjann[2] reported a more direct method of pancreatic inspection during laparoscopy which involved creation of a

Table 15-1. Partial List of Laparoscopic Applications in Pancreatic Surgery

Pancreatic Surgery	Laparoscopic Applications
Pancreatic carcinoma	Laparoscopic staging[a] Laparoscopic biopsy of the pancreas[a] Palliative laparoscopic gastrojejunostomy[b] Laparoscopic lymph node biopsy[c] Laparoscopic guided brachytherapy[c] Thoroscopic splanchnic nerve division for pain control
Islet cell neoplasms	Laparoscopic staging[c] Localization with laparoscopic ultrasound[c] Laparoscopic enucleation[c]
Acute pancreatitis	Diagnostic laparoscopy[a] Laparoscopic placement of lesser sac lavage catheters[c]
Chronic pancreatitis	Laparoscopic pseudocystgatrostomy[b]

[a] Procedures in which published experiences have been accrued.
[b] Procedures that have been performed but for which no published experience is available.
[c] Applications that still remain speculative.

window in the gastrocolic ligament through which the laparoscope could be advanced into the lesser sac. This method was referred to as an "infragastric pancreoscopy."[2]

These initial reports of supragastric and infragastric techniques for examination of the pancreas were subsequently refined by other investigators. In 1978, Cuschieri and co-workers[3] combined the technique of infragastric pancreoscopy with needle biopsy and laroscopic cholangiogram to study 23 patients with suspected pancreatic and periampullary neoplasms. Subsequent laparotomy confirmed the accuracy of laparoscopic findings in a majority of cases.

In 1983, Ishida[4] reported direct laparoscopic inspection of the lesser sac via creation of a window in the lesser omentum. This technique of "supragastric pancreoscopy" was applied to 124 patients with a variety of pancreatic diseases. Visualization of the pancreas combined with either needle or forceps biopsy was associated with a 3.3 per cent complication rate. The technique provided an accurate diagnosis in 50 per cent of patients with either acute or chronic pancreatitis and 60 per cent of patients with pancreatic carcinoma.

Initially, these techniques were primarily developed to enable biopsy of the pancreas without formal laparotomy. With the advent of computed tomography and percutaneous needle biopsy in the late 1970s, however, laparoscopic exposure of the pancreas became, until recently, a relatively uncommon event.

TECHNICAL ASPECTS

Following laparoscopic access to the peritoneal cavity, direct visualization of the pancreas may be attained through two different approaches: the supragastric and infragastric routes, which are equally successful in experienced hands. Animal studies have suggested that the supragastric approach may be optimal for examination of the pancreatic body and tail, while the infragastric approach facilitates examination of the pancreatic head. Experience with both techniques allows flexibility and adaptation to the anatomy of the individual patient.

Supragastric Approach

Initial inspection of the peritoneal cavity is carried out via an 10-mm trochar inserted at the umbilicus. The head of the table is then raised. An additional 10-mm trochar is introduced in a subxiphoid position, and two 5-mm trochars are inserted in the midclavicular line in each upper quadrant. The left lobe of the liver is elevated, and the stomach is retracted caudally and to the patient's left. The lesser omentum is thus placed on stretch, and an avascular area of the lesser omentum is identified. A window is created using a cautery forceps. The laparoscope is then withdrawn and reinserted through the subxiphoid port into the lesser sac, allowing for direct visualization of the pancreas. This technique is schematically displayed in Figure 15-1.

Infragastric Approach

Preliminary laparoscopy is performed via an 11-mm trochar placed 5 cm below the left costal margin in the midclavicular line. Additional 5-mm trochars are introduced through the umbilicus and in the upper midline. The gastrocolic ligament is retracted caudally. An avascular area in the gastrocolic ligament near the greater curvature is identified, and a window is created. The laparoscope is advanced directly into the lesser sac, and the pancreas is visualized. This technique is summarized in Figure 15-2.

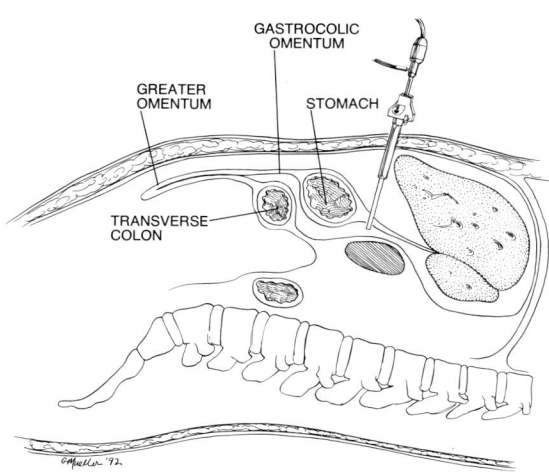

Figure 15-2. Schematic depiction of the infragastric technique for laparoscopic manipulation of the pancreas. Following the creation of a window in an avascular area of the gastrocolic omentum, the videolaparoscope is introduced into the lesser sac.

APPLICATIONS

Pancreatic Carcinoma

Pancreatic cancer remains a relatively common and highly lethal entity. Approximately 9 cases per 100,000 persons occur in the United States each year, accounting for 25,000 annual deaths.[5] The true prevalence of this disease may be much higher than generally appreciated, with some studies revealing either pancreatic carcinoma *in situ* or invasive carcinoma in as many as 10 per cent of all autopsies.[6] The prognosis for patients who develop pancreatic cancer remains abysmal, with a 5-year survival rate of 3.1 per cent.[2] Pancreatic cancer represents the second leading cause of death attributed to cancers of the gastrointestinal tract, and the fourth leading cause of death attributed to malignant disease of all types.

A significant component of this poor prognosis may be attributed to the inability to detect pancreatic carcinoma in its early stages. At the time of diagnosis, as many as 60 per cent of patients exhibit distant metastases, while in a further 14 per cent the disease has spread to regional lymph nodes.[7] Only 15 per cent of patients are seen with localized disease, and as few as 5 per cent may ultimately prove to have a resectable lesion. Resectable lesions tend to occur almost exclusively in the

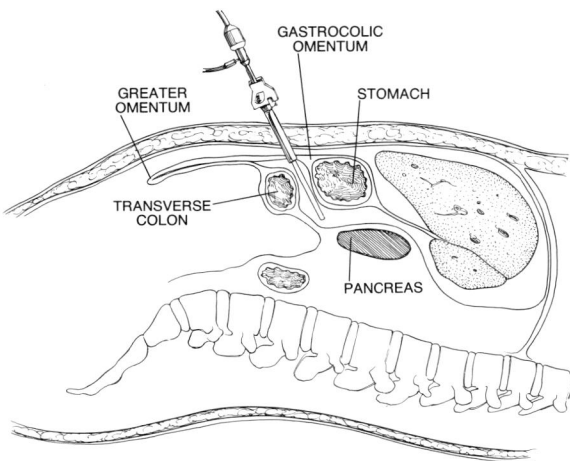

Figure 15-1. Schematic depiction of the supragastric technique for laparoscopic manipulation of the pancreas. Following creation of a window in the lesser omentum, the videolaparoscope is introduced through a subxiphoid port into the lesser sac.

head of the gland, whereas carcinomas arising in the body or tail of the pancreas typically are seen at an advanced stage.

Among patients who do undergo resection for cure, only a 15 to 20 per cent 5-year survival may be anticipated.[8,9] In an attempt to improve upon these results, some authors have advocated a wider area of resection than that defined by the traditional Whipple operation. In particular, total pancreatectomy has been advocated based upon pathologic data suggesting multicentricity of pancreatic carcinoma in up to 30 per cent of cases. It has become clear, however, that total pancreatectomy appears to provide no long term survival benefit over simple pancreaticoduodenectomy.[10,11] In addition, total pancreatectomy is associated with substantial additional morbidity in the form of surgically induced brittle diabetes. The introduction of an even more extended "regional pancreatectomy," involving *en bloc* resection and reconstruction of the intrapancreatic portal vein, has also failed to increase the likelihood of cure.[12,13] Thus, attempts to improve the outcome of patients with pancreatic cancer based upon increasingly aggressive resection have so far proven unsuccessful. Indeed, less extensive pylorus-preserving resections appear to have no adverse impact on long term survival.[14]

In patients with unresectable disease, various forms of palliation are available. Surgical decompression of the obstructed biliary tree with or without concomitant gastrojejunostomy remains the gold standard to which newer forms of therapy must be compared.[15] Nevertheless, dramatic improvements have been made in the ability to palliate biliary obstruction using nonsurgical techniques. The placement of transtumoral biliary stents may be accomplished either endoscopically or via a percutaneous, transhepatic approach. Initial success rates approach 90 per cent, although stent patency is typically limited to 3 to 6 months. While patients treated endoscopically have a decreased initial hospitalization time compared to surgically treated patients, they do require more frequent rehospitalization for stent occlusion and cholangitis.[16] The recent development of self-expanding stents as well as more less reactive biotechnology materials may further optimize these results. Thus, nonsurgical forms of palliation are currently an attractive option in those patients for whom a brief survival is anticipated.

With respect to other forms of therapy, combined radiation and chemotherapy may be of some benefit. In unresectable disease, the combination of external beam radiation with either 5-fluorouracil or Adriamycin appears to prolong survival.[17] A combination of radiation therapy and 5-fluorouracil is similarly effective in prolonging survival among patients who have undergone curative resection.[18] The addition of intraoperative radiation therapy to these regimens has been suggested to provide a modest incremental benefit.[19]

In spite of these discouraging results, it is clear that in selected patients with pancreatic carcinoma there is a reasonable chance of cure. In patients with tumors less than 2 cm in diameter, a 5-year survival rate of 30 per cent has been reported.[20] Similarly, a median survival period of 56 months has been reported for patients who are seen with resectable tumor and no lymph node metastases.[21] Thus, while the vast majority of patients with pancreatic carcinoma have unresectable, incurable disease, a small subset of patients clearly benefit from an aggressive surgical approach.

In order to distinguish between these different groups of patients, Warshaw et al.[22] have used staging laparoscopy combined with preoperative computed tomography (CT) and angiography to appropriately select patients for specific therapies. In a series of 55 consecutive patients with carcinoma in the head of the pancreas, 29 per cent had tumors that ultimately proved to be resectable. When laparoscopy, CT, and angiography results all were negative, a 78 per cent resectability rate was achieved. The finding of one or more positive studies resulted in a decrease in the rate of resectability to 5 per cent. In this series, laparoscopy proved to be a significant addition to CT and angiography alone, primarily by the identification of small peritoneal metastases undetected on CT scans, as well as by providing specimens for peritoneal cytology. Laparoscopy may thus already play an important potential role in the management of patients with pancreatic carcinoma. By increasing the accuracy with which patients may be identified as having unresectable disease, laparoscopy can be used to select patients with limited lifespans who may benefit from nonoperative therapy. Patients with unresectable tumors and distant metastases may best be served by endoscopic biliary stent placement. Patients with unresectable tumors but no distant metastases may benefit from a durable biliary-enteric bypass procedure in conjunction with gastrojejunostomy. On the other hand, patients who appear to have resectable disease following evaluation which includes staging laparoscopy should be offered the opportunity of surgical extirpation of the disease.

Further utilization of laparoscopic technology in the management of patients with pancreatic carcinoma currently remains speculative. It should be noted that the benefits of laparoscopy described earlier were attained without actual entrance into the lesser sac and visualization of the pancreas and peripancreatic tissues. Further refinements in laparoscopic technique may allow even more precise preoperative staging. In particular, laparoscopic biopsy of peripancreatic and periportal lymph nodes may allow predictions regarding resectability to be made with increasing accuracy. A similar benefit may be gained by assessing involvement of visceral vessels by way of laparoscopic duplex ultrasound. In addition, the development of radiolabeled monoclonal antibodies, which recognize pancreatic cancer-specific cell surface markers, may allow for the detection of micrometastases via a laparoscopic radioisotope detection device.

In patients with unresectable disease, the development of laparoscopic techniques for palliative therapy may eventually obviate the need for laparotomy. Utilizing laparoscopic suturing techniques, laparoscopic gastrojejunostomy has already been performed in the setting of unresectable pancreatic carcinoma. The availability of the ENDO GIA* stapling device and other similar devices may further simplify this procedure. Combined with the development of more durable endoscopic biliary prostheses, it is now feasible to provide both enteric and biliary bypass using minimally invasive techniques. Other palliative treatments may also be delivered in this manner. For example, it may become possible to directly apply palliative brachytherapy to pancreatic and peripancreatic tissues via the laparoscope. Thus, laparoscopy may effectively contribute to the diagnosis, staging, and palliation of pancreatic carcinoma. In this setting, open abdominal surgery would be reserved for those patients predicted to have curable disease.

Islet Cell Neoplasms

Neuroendocrine tumors of the pancreas continue to represent challenging entities for the pancreatic surgeon. An in-depth discussion of these neoplasms is beyond the scope of this chapter. The basic clinical features of the major islet cell neoplasms are summarized in Table 15-2.

For the majority of these tumors, biochemical diagnosis has become well established using plama hormone radioimmunoassays. Furthermore, the development of targeted pharmaceutical probes (e.g., somatostatin analog, omeprazole) has allowed for more effective palliation of symptoms. However, preoperative tumor localization remains a major impediment to effective surgical therapy. The development of highly discriminant imaging modalities, including CT, angiography, and selective venous sampling, has facilitated tumor localization,[23] but frequently small or aberrantly-located lesions are not identified. Thus, as many as 10 per cent of all insulinomas[24] and 30 per cent of gastrinomas[25] are not localized preoperatively.

In this setting, specialized ultrasound probes have become indispensable aids in the

Table 15-2. Clinical Features of the Major Pancreatic Endocrine Tumors

Tumor	Major Hormone	% Malignant	Symptoms	Eponym
Insulinoma	Insulin	10	Hypoglycemia	
Gastrinoma	Gastrin	90	Gastrointestinal ulceration Diarrhea	Zollinger-Ellison
Vipoma	Vasoactive intestinal polypeptide Pancreatic polypeptide	40	Watery diarrhea Hypokalemia Achlorhydria	Verner-Mornson
Glucagonoma	Glucagon	70	Diabetes, anemia Glossitis Migratory necrotizing erythema	

localization of small, nonpalpable tumors.[26] Endoscopic ultrasound allows for accurate visualization of pancreatic parenchyma when placed in either the stomach or duodenum. In a series of 12 patients with suspected pancreatic endocrine tumors at the Memorial Sloan-Kettering Cancer Center, endoscopic ultrasound provided accurate preoperative localization in 83 per cent.[26] In 5 patients with small tumors (0.5 to 2.0 cm) endoscopic ultrasound enabled preoperative visualization even when they were not seen with CT and angiography. In circumstances in which preoperative localization is unsuccessful, intraoperative ultrasound has proven invaluable in identifying nonpalpable tumors. In a series of 25 patients with insulinomas,[27] standard imaging modalities including CT, magnetic resonance imaging, and angiography provided preoperative tumor localization in only 48 per cent. Selective venous sampling provided additional localizing information in 77 per cent. Seven patients had nonpalpable tumors that were localized intraoperatively using intraoperative ultrasound. Using these combined modalities, the authors were able to perform curative resections in 24 of 25 patients.

A natural extension of these techniques is the use of laparoscopic sonography to provide further localization of pancreatic endocrine tumors prior to laparotomy. The development of such a technique may provide important information regarding the staging and resectability of islet cell neoplasms. Once localized, laparoscopic techniques may ultimately be applied to tumor excision. This may be especially valid for insulinomas, of which the majority are small benign adenomas and therefore curable by simple enucleation. Thus, the development of improved techniques and instrumentation may ultimately provide the means for insulinoma localization and excision using a purely laparoscopic approach. The higher malignant potential of other pancreatic endocrine tumors (see Table 15-2) typically mandates more traditional pancreatic resection and will probably remain in the realm of open abdominal surgery.

Acute Pancreatitis

Acute pancreatitis continues to represent an extremely vexing clinical entity. The pathobiology of the disease process is ill understood, and few effective therapies exist. A number of difficulties plague investigation of this disease. First, the clinical course of acute pancreatitis is extremely variable, and small numbers of patients with fulminant disease may be encountered in any single institution. Second, human pancreatic tissue remains essentially inaccessible for clinical investigation. Finally, there exists no ideal experimental model of the clinical disease process.

Nevertheless, in the last decade considerable evolution has occurred in the management of acute pancreatitis. These developments have recently been reviewed in detail.[28] They include the effective application of endoscopic papillotomy to fulminant gallstone pancreatitis,[29] the use of dynamic CT pancreatography[30] and percutaneous aspiration[31] to detect infected pancreatic necrosis, and the realization that not all cases of pancreatic necrosis require surgical debridement.[32] It should be noted, however, that these developments have largely been limited to addressing the complications of pancreatitis once they have already occurred; virtually no progress has been made in the primary treatment of acute pancreatitis.

In this context, the question of whether peritoneal lavage may provide effective therapy in acute pancreatitis has received considerable attention. Previous trials[33,34] produced conflicting results. While the prompt initiation of peritoneal lavage seems to lessen early cardiopulmonary morbidity, the demonstration of a decrease in late pancreatic sepsis or improved overall mortality has proven elusive. Recently, Ranson and Berman[35] have applied an extended (7-day) period of large volume lavage to selected patients with severe pancreatitis. In a randomized, prospective clinical trial involving a total of 29 patients with three or more signs of severity, 7-day lavage was found to be associated with a reduction in septic complications as well as overall mortality when compared to a 2-day period of lavage. While these data require further confirmation, the findings raise the possibility that peritoneal lavage may indeed favorably influence the outcome of acute pancreatitis. Whether there is any incremental benefit to lavage delivered directly into the lesser sac via surgically placed catheters (see Figure 15-2) remains a question for future investigation.[36]

The role of laparoscopy in the management of acute pancreatitis remains undefined. Technically, the application of laparoscopy in this setting may be problematic. Most patients with acute pancreatitis exhibit a significant ileus and often marked abdominal distention;

this fact alone may preclude the safe introduction of laparoscopic trochars. In addition, inflammatory adhesions may preclude adequate access to the lesser sac during acute pancreatitis.

In spite of these limitations, laparoscopy may ultimately prove to be useful in evaluating patients with acute pancreatitis. While the diagnosis of pancreatitis is usually straightforward, occasional uncertainty exists with respect to the possibility of confounding peptic ulcer disease or ischemic bowel. In this setting, diagnostic laparoscopy and examination of the pancreas may provide useful information. With respect to therapy, it is possible that laparoscopy may eventually allow for the placement of peritoneal lavage catheters directly into the lesser sac without the need for laparotomy. Given the high morbidity of traditional surgery in patients during the early stages of pancreatitis, this may confer a significant advantage. It should be stressed, however, that the feasibility and efficacy of such intervention currently remain speculative.

Chronic Pancreatitis

The primary sequelae of chronic pancreatitis include pain, malabsorption, and pancreatic pseudocyst. The application of CT scanning to patients with pancreatic pseudocysts has resulted in dramatic changes in management strategy. Previous recommendations regarding the need for surgical intervention were based on studies involving largely alcoholic populations seen with symptomatic pseudocysts; in such studies, the incidence of complications increased and the likelihood of spontaneous resolution decreased following 6 weeks of nonoperative observation.[37] Currently, pseudocysts are more likely to be seen in asymptomatic patients undergoing routine CT scanning. This expanded use of CT has made it clear that pseudocysts occur much more commonly than previously appreciated in patients with acute and chronic pancreatitis.[38] In addition, it appears that the natural history of asymptomatic pseudocysts demonstrated by CT may be much more benign than previously recognized. Two recent series[39,40] have reexamined the role of nonoperative pseudocyst management. In both reports, approximately 50 per cent of all pseudocysts were associated with significant symptoms requiring surgical intervention. The remaining 50 per cent comprised a combined total of 107 patients with asymptomatic, CT-documented pseudocysts who were managed nonoperatively. A combined pseudocyst-related complication rate of 6 per cent was reported in patients treated nonoperatively. Both series documented a 60 per cent rate of spontaneous pseudocyst resolution, with resolution often occurring long after 6 weeks of nonoperative intervention. These new insights into the natural history of pancreatic pseudocysts suggest that an initial nonoperative approach remains appropriate in selected asymptomatic patients.

Nevertheless, a subset of patients clearly require pseudocyst drainage, either because of pain, infection, or failure to resolve. While percutaneous pseudocyst drainage may be effective,[41] surgical therapy remains the standard approach. Recently, laparoscopic methods have been applied to the surgical treatment of pancreatic pseudocysts. Petelin (personal communication, 1992) has described a technique for laparoscopic pseudocyst-gastrostomy. Following the establishment of a pneumoperitoneum, a 10-mm trochar is introduced via the umbilicus. A second 10-mm port is placed in the left upper quadrant, along with a 5-mm port in the right upper quandrant, just lateral to the falciform ligament. An anterior gastrotomy is created using the neodymium-yttrium-garnet contact laser. A 1.5-cm diameter ellipse is excised from the posterior wall of the stomach, allowing for entrance into the cyst cavity and drainage of cyst contents. A series of hemostatic sutures are then placed circumferentially around the orifice of the cyst-gastrostomy. Intracorporeal knot-tying techniques are used to secure each suture. The anterior gastrotomy is then closed in layers.

Unlike purely endoscopic or percutaneous techniques for the management of pseudocysts, this laparoscopic method allows for aggressive irrigation and drainage of cyst contents, as well as the placement of hemostatic sutures around the edges of the cyst-gastrostomy. As such, it will probably provide an attractive alternative to traditional surgical methods in selected patients.

REFERENCES

1. Meyer-Burg J. The inspection, palpation, and biopsy of the pancreas by peritoneoscopy. Endoscopy 1972; 4:99–101.
2. Strauch M, Lux G, Ottenjann R. Infragastric pancreoscopy. Endoscopy 1973; 5:30–32.
3. Cuschieri A, Hall AW, Clark J. Value of laparoscopy

in the diagnosis and management of pancreatic carcinoma. Gut 1978; 19:672–677.
4. Ishida H. Peritoneoscopy and pancreas biopsy in the diagnosis of pancreatic diseases. Gastrointest Endosc 1983; 29:211–218.
5. National Cancer Institute. Annual Cancer Statistics Review 1973–1988. Bethesda, MD, Department of Health and Human Services, 1991.
6. Pour PM, Sayed S, Sayed G. Hyperplastic, preneoplastic, and neoplastic lesions found in 83 human pancreases. Am J Clin Pathol 1982; 77:137–152.
7. Baylor SM, Berg JW. Cross-classification and survival classification of 5000 cases of cancer of the pancreas. J Surg Oncol 1973; 5:335–358.
8. Cameron JL, Crist DW, Sitzmann JV, et al. Factors influencing survival after pancreaticoduodenectomy. Ann Surg 1991; 214:648–656.
9. Trede M, Schwall G, Saeger HD. Survival after pancreaticoduodenectomy. Ann Surg 1990; 211:447–458.
10. Brooks JR, Brooks DC, Levine JD. Total pancreatectomy for ductal cell carcinoma of the pancreas: An update. Ann Surg 1989; 209:405–410.
11. Van Heerden JA, McIlrath DC, Ilstrup MS, Weiland LH. Total pancreatectomy for ductal adenocarcinoma of the pancreas: An update. World J Surg 1988; 12:658–662.
12. Fortner JG. Regional pancreatectomy for cancer of the pancreas, ampulla, and other related sites. Ann Surg 1984; 199:418–425.
13. Sindelar WF. Clinical experience with regional pancreatectomy for adenocarcinoma of the pancreas. Arch Surg 1989; 124:127–132.
14. Grace PA, Pitt HA, Longmire WP. Pylorus preserving pancreatoduodenectomy: An overview. Br J Surg 1990; 77:968–974.
15. Sarr MG, Cameron JL. Surgical palliation of unresectable carcinoma of the pancreas. World J Surg 1984; 8:906–918.
16. Brandabur JJ, Kozarek RA, Ball TJ, et al. Nonoperative versus operative treatment of obstructive jaundice in pancreatic cancer: Cost and survival analysis. Am J Gastroenterol 1988; 83:1132–1139.
17. Gastrointestinal Tumor Study Group. Radiation therapy combined with Adriamycin or 5-fluorouracil for the treatment of locally unresectable pancreatic carcinoma. Cancer 1985; 56:2563–2568.
18. Gastrointestinal Tumor Study Group. Further evidence of effective adjuvant combined radiation and chemotherapy following curative resection of pancreatic cancer. Cancer 1987; 59:2006–2010.
19. Sindelar WF, Kinsella TJ. Randomized trial of intraoperative radiotherapy in unresectable carcinoma of the pancreas. Int J Radiat Oncol Biol Phys 1986; 12:148–149.
20. Tsuchiya R, Noda T, Harada M, et al. Collective review of small carcinomas of the pancreas. Ann Surg 1986; 203:77–81.
21. Cameron JL, Crist DW, Sitzmann JV, et al. Factors influencing survival after pancreaticoduodenectomy for pancreatic cancer. Am J Surg 1990; 161:120–124.
22. Warshaw AL, Gun ZY, Wittenberg J, Waltman C. Preoperative staging and assessment of resectability of pancreatic cancer. Arch Surg 1990; 125:230–233.
23. Fraker DL, Norton JA. Localization and resection of insulinomas and gastrinomas. J Am Med Assoc 1988; 259:3601–3605.
24. Katz BL, Aufses AH, Rayfield E, Mitty H. Preoperative localization and intraoperative glucose monitoring in the management of patients with pancreatic insulinoma. Surg Gynecol Obstet 1986; 163:509–512.
25. Norton JA, Doppmen JL, Collen MJ, et al. Prospective study of gastrinoma localization and resection in patients with Zollinger-Ellison syndrome. Ann Surg 1986; 204:468–479.
26. Lightdale CJ, Botet JF, Woodruff JM, et al. Localization of endocrine tumors of the pancreas with endoscopic ultrasonography. Cancer 1991; 68:1815–1820.
27. Doherty GM, Doppman JL, Shawker TH, et al. Results of a prospective study to diagnose, localize, and resect insulinomas. Surgery 1991; 110:989–996.
28. Leach SD, Gorelick FS, Modlin IM. New perspectives on acute pancreatitis. Scand J Gastroenterol 1992; 27(suppl. 192):29–38.
29. Neoptolemos JP, Carr-Lock DL, London NJ, et al. Controlled trial of urgent endoscopic retrograde cholangiopancreatography and endoscopic sphincterotomy versus conservative treatment for acute pancreatitis due to gallstones. Lancet 1988; 2:979–983.
30. Bradley EL, Murphy F, Ferguson C. Prediction of pancreatic necrosis by dynamic pancreatography. Ann Surg 1989; 210:495–504.
31. Gerzof SG, Banks PA, Robbins AH, et al. Early diagnosis of pancreatic infection by computed tomography-guided aspiration. Gastroenterology 1987; 93:1315–1320.
32. Bradley EL, Allen K. A prospective longitudinal study of observation versus surgical intervention in the management of necrotizing pancreatitis. Am J Surg 1991; 161:19–25.
33. Mayer DA, McMahon MJ, Corfield AP, et al. Controlled clinical trial of peritoneal lavage for the treatment of severe acute pancreatitis. N Engl J Med 1985; 312:399–404.
34. Stone HH, Fabian TC. Peritoneal dialysis in the treatment of acute alcoholic pancreatitis. Surg Gynecol Obstet 1980; 150:878–882.
35. Ranson JHC, Berman RS. Long peritoneal lavage decreases pancreatic sepsis in acute pancreatitis. Ann Surg 1990; 211:708–718.
36. Pederzoli P, Bassi C, Vesentini S, et al. Retroperitoneal and peritoneal drainage and lavage in the treatment of severe necrotizing pancreatitis. Surg Gynecol Obstet 1990; 170:197–203.
37. Bradley EL, Clements JL, Gonzales AC. The natural history of pancreatic pseudocysts: A unified concept of management. Am J Surg 1979; 137:135–141.
38. Walt AJ, Bouwman DL, Weaver DW, Sachs RJ. The impact of technology on the management of pancreatic pseudocyst. Arch Surg 1990; 125:759–763.
39. Yeo CJ, Bastidas JA, Lynch-Nyhan A, et al. The natural history of pancreatic pseudocysts documented by computed tomography. Surg Gynecol Obstet 1990; 170:411–417.
40. Vitas GJ, Sarr MG. Selected management of pancreatic pseudocysts: Operative vs. expectant management. Surgery 1992; 111:123–130.
41. VanSonnenberg E, Wittich GR, Casola G, et al. Percutaneous drainage of infected and noninfected pancreatic pseudocysts: Experience in 101 cases. Radiology 1989; 170:757–761.

Section IV
Surgery of the Biliary System

Chapter 16
Modern Treatment of Gallstones: Cholecystectomy

William C. Meyers
Gene D. Branum
Lawrence A. Saperstein

Laparoscopic cholecystectomy has rapidly become the popular method for treating gallstones in the United States and abroad. As surgeons learn the technique, safety improves and contraindications to the new procedure decrease. Through its evolution, however, complications inevitably occurred. In particular, the incidence of bile duct injury during the surgeon's learning phase with the procedure proved higher than with traditional cholecystectomy. Nevertheless, laparoscopic cholecystectomy offers a number of advantages over the open method of gallbladder extraction, and the overall safety of the procedure is comparable. As instrumentation, skill, and safety continue to improve, surgeons are finding easier methods to accomplish traditional procedures and are developing new ones.

A remarkable aspect of laparoscopic cholecystectomy is how quickly the radically new procedure gained acceptance. Credit goes to a number of surgeons, corporations, and the public, all of whom demanded the procedure. The initial skepticism of the academic community is being replaced with optimism.

DEVELOPMENT OF LAPAROSCOPIC CHOLECYSTECTOMY

The earliest treatments of gallstones were primarily medical. These probably began several thousand years ago in Japan where upper abdominal colic was treated with dried bear bile, the chemical equivalent of ursodeoxycholic acid. Hippocrates (circa 400 BC) attached great importance to diet and hygiene as the basis for medical therapy. His diet mandated avoidance of most fruits, vegetables, milk, and fish. Celsius (circa 50 AD) recommended surgical drainage of right upper quadrant abscesses, which probably represented gallstone fistulae. The illustrious 11th century Islamic scientist Avicenna (also known as Ibn Sima) provided the first definitive reports of drainage of biliary fistulae. Fabricius performed a cholecystolithotomy in 1618, but it is not clear whether this was on a living or dead person. Bobbs, an American, performed the first well documented cholecystolithotomy in Indiana in 1867. The procedure was indicated for hydrops of the gall-

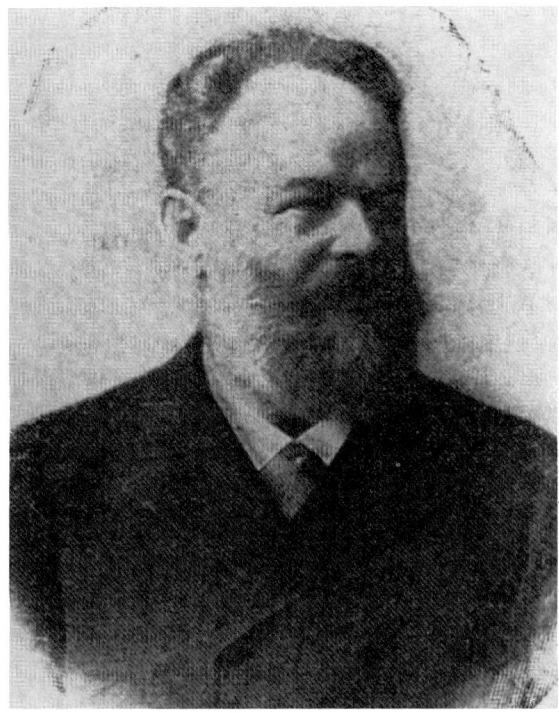

Figure 16-1. Carl Langenbuch, the German surgeon who performed the first cholecystectomy in 1882 at Lazarus Hospital in Berlin; he was 36 years old. (Reproduced with permission from Heimburger JL, King RD. Surgery and gallstones—From helplessness to triumph. Surgery 1965; 57:329.)

bladder and was performed in an apartment over a drugstore.

Langenbuch (to be distinguished from Langenbeck) performed the first successful cholecystectomy in 1882 (Fig. 16-1). Ohage performed the first cholecystectomy in the United States in 1886. Courvoisier is credited with the first choledochotomy in 1890, although the first choledochoduodenostomy was performed a year earlier. Halsted popularized gallbladder surgery before the turn of the century. One of his first operations was a cholecystolithotomy performed on his mother in the middle of the night in 1881. Ironically, Halsted died of complications of choledocholithiasis. Bakes first performed choledoscopy in 1923, and Mirizzi introduced intraoperative cholangiography in 1932. Glenn documented cholecystectomy as a safe surgical procedure in the 1940s and 1950s when cholecystectomy became the gold standard for the treatment of gallstones.[1]

Serious challenges to the established method of cholecystectomy came in the late 1970s and early 1980s with the reported success of dissolutional agents[2,3] and the shattering of gallstones with extracorporal lithotripsy.[4,5] Minor roles remain for these therapies today, however, because broad attempts to use them failed because of inconsistent effectiveness, cost, narrow indications, and the problem of recurrence.[6,7] Traditional treatment of gallstones, i.e., open cholecystectomy, had about a 0.5 per cent overall mortality and a 0.1 per cent mortality in low risk populations.[8]

The timing was right in the late 1980s for an effective, less invasive way of eliminating gallstones. Technological advancements in endoscopy alerted instrument companies to the possibilities of laparoscopy. Mouret from France performed the first laparoscopically assisted cholecystectomy in 1989. He ligated the cystic artery and duct laparoscopically and then made a small right upper quadrant incision to remove the gallbladder. Almost simultaneously Dubois in France and McKer-

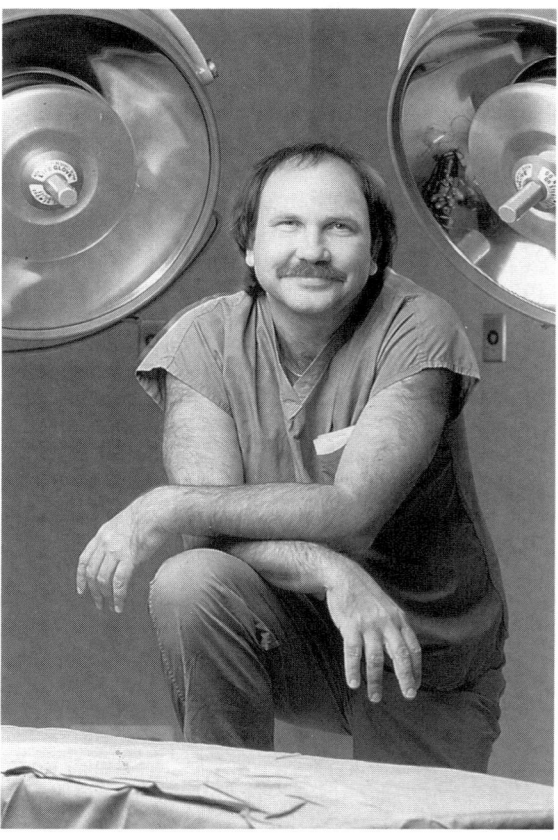

Figure 16-2. Eddie Joe Reddick, one of the originators of laparoscopic cholecystectomy. He helped popularize the technique in the late 1980s.

nan and Saye in Georgia (B. McKernan, personal communication) performed the first laparoscopic cholecystectomies as currently performed. Reddick and Olsen published a written account of the procedure the next year in the obscure journal *Laser Medical and Surgical News*[9] (Fig. 16-2). The authors followed that report with a comparison of laparoscopic cholecystectomy with conventional cholecystectomy performed through tiny incisions.[10] Thus, the first phase of popularization of laparoscopic cholecystectomy took place largely outside of academic settings (Table 16-1).

Data on large numbers of patients first came from the Southern Surgeons Club's prospective report of 1518 laparoscopic cholecystectomies performed by 59 surgeons in academic or private practice.[11] The short time (4 months) in which most of the cases were collected confirmed the new procedure's popularity and virtual replacement of conventional cholecystectomy at these hospitals. Most physicians began to accept laparoscopic cholecystectomy as the procedure of choice for the vast majority of patients with symptomatic gallstones. The procedure is still being refined, instrumentation continues to improve, and we are likely to see the development of reliable methods to manage common duct stones laparoscopically.

Indications for Laparoscopic Cholecystectomy

The primary indication for laparoscopic cholecystectomy is symptomatic gallbladder disease, i.e., abdominal pain, jaundice, or history of pancreatitis in conjunction with a consistent clinical history and documented gallstones. In their dramatic study of "silent" gallstones in 1980, Gracie and Ransohoff[12] shifted opinion in the United States away from prophylactic cholecystectomy toward nontreatment of asymptomatic stones. The same opinion, i.e., treatment of symptomatic stones only, also prevails for laparoscopic cholecystectomy. Ninety-nine per cent of patients in the Southern Surgeons Club's study had symptomatic gallstones. The other 1 per cent included patients with diabetes and several patients receiving immunosuppressive therapy after solid organ transplant. However, estimates reveal that the number of cholecystectomies in the United States increased last year, suggesting either a backlog of patients or a lowering of indications for surgery.

Laparoscopic cholecystectomy, like conventional cholecystectomy, is performed mainly for gallstones. Ninety-six per cent of patients in the Southern Surgeons Club's study had cholelithiasis and 4 per cent did not. Ninety per cent of patients had chronic cholecystitis and 10 per cent acute cholecystitis. The most popular method for documenting gallbladder abnormalities is clearly ultrasonography. Other methods include oral cholecystography, radionuclide scanning, cholecystokinin response tests, endoscopic retrograde cholangiopancreatography (ERCP), computed tomography, plain abdominal roentgenograms, and duodenal crystal examination.

Many of the once "absolute" contraindications to laparoscopic cholecystectomy are disappearing. Acute cholecystitis was infrequently tackled at the beginning of the Southern Surgeons Club's experience, yet ended up comprising 10 per cent of cases.

Table 16-1. History of the Surgical Treatment of Gallstones

Year	Surgeon	Treatment
1867	Bobbs	Cholecystolithotomy for hydrops of gallbladder
1882	Langenbuch	First successful cholecystectomy
1886	Ohage	First successful cholecystectomy in United States
1890	Courvoisier	First choledochotomy
1923	Bakes	First choledoscopy
1932	Mirizzi	Introduced intraoperative cholangiography
1940s/1950s	Glenn	Cholecystectomy established as gold standard
Late 1970s/early 1980s		Use of dissolutional agents and extracorporal shock wave lithotripsy
1988	Mouret	First laparoscopically assisted cholecystectomy
1988	McKernon and Saye	First total laparoscopic cholecystectomy
1989	Reddick and Olsen	Popularization of laparoscopic cholecystectomy

Experience plays a significant role in how a surgeon selects patients for laparoscopic cholecystectomy. In order to evaluate the question of patient suitability for laparoscopic cholecystectomy, a survey was conducted of Southern Surgeons Club members (unpublished data). The surgeons were asked to list specific contraindications to laparoscopic cholecystectomy (Table 16-2). When the survey was conducted, no laparoscopic suturing techniques were available. The presence of a preoperatively known gallstone fistula to the gastrointestinal tract (either duodenum or colon) was the only contraindication named by all 20 surgical groups. One group performed laparoscopic cholecystectomy on pregnant patients, and most surgeons felt the need for a concomitant open surgical procedure was a contraindication. However, two surgeons were performing incidental laparoscopic appendectomy as well as other intraabdominal procedures such as hysterectomy with laparoscopic cholecystectomy. For gynecologic procedures, open lower abdominal procedures were performed second in order to avoid leakage of the pneumoperitoneum.

The majority of surgeons initially viewed cirrhosis as another strong contraindication. However, a significant minority felt that patients with cirrhosis benefited substantially by avoidance of a large incision. A low threshold for conversion to open cholecystectomy was also stressed. Laparoscopic cholecystectomy is more difficult in a patient with cirrhosis because of the firmness of the liver with subsequent inability to suspend the gallbladder and liver normally and the presence of varices.

The presence of severe adhesions was addressed by this question: "Would you attempt laparoscopic cholecystectomy on a patient who had a previous right upper quadrant shotgun wound"? Several surgeons said it would still be worth a look, and two surgeons had already performed successful cholecystectomies in such patients. The majority of surgeons felt that laparoscopic cholecystectomy might be of special benefit in patients who were anticoagulated on coumadin or heparin and again noted the low threshold for conversion for these patients. Morbid obesity was considered an excellent indication for laparoscopic cholecystectomy because of greatly reduced morbidity relating to incision size. All surgeons agreed that patients in whom ERCP or other nonsurgical attempts to extract common duct stones failed would benefit most by open cholecystectomy and traditional common duct exploration.

It is reasonable to conclude from these data that seemingly logical barriers to laparoscopic cholecystectomy were already being crossed, and experience was undoubtedly an important factor in the selection of patients for the new procedure. There are clearly significant advantages of this technique in high risk patient groups. A low threshold for conversion reflects sound judgment.

INDICATIONS FOR CONVERSION

In experienced hands, the incidence of conversion from laparoscopic to conventional cholecystectomy is about 4 to 5 per cent.[11,13] The most common reason for conversion relates to inflammation in the region of the gallbladder. Inflammatory processes leading to conversion are either acute or chronic or a combination of the two. The primary reason that acute or chronic inflammation leads to conversion is inadequate visualization of anatomical landmarks, making dissection difficult. The second most common reason for conversion is the presence of adhesions from previous surgery. Conversion is now less common because of open methods for insufflation, such as use of the Hasson trocar as well as increased confidence in laparoscopic adhesiolysis.

The third most common reason for conversion is recognition of a complication during laparoscopy. Examples of these complications include bile duct and bowel injury, severe stone spillage, and bleeding. Other reasons for conversion are unexpected pathologic findings, such as carcinoma, the need for duct exploration, and mechanical problems

Table 16-2. Acute Cholecystitis

Situation	Contraindications	
	Yes	No
Gallstone fistula	20	0
Pregnancy	19	1
Need for other procedure	18	2
Hepatic cirrhosis	13	7
Prior right upper quadrant shotgun wound	13	7
Anticoagulation	9	11
Morbid obesity	3	17

such as a loss of video or a malfunctioning insufflator.

INJURY

The complications of any new surgical procedure, including laparoscopic cholecystectomy, must undergo critical assessment before the procedure is generally accepted. In all published accounts of laparoscopic cholecystectomy, death appears extremely unlikely, as with traditional cholecystectomy. Unpublished anecdotal accounts of deaths are more common. Inexperience with the technique seems to be a common denominator in most of these deaths. Causes of death resulting from inexperience include trocar injury to major blood vessels, carbon dioxide insufflation into major blood vessels, and sudden tension pneumothorax from laser perforation of the diaphragm. The one death in the Southern Surgeons Club series resulted from a mistake in diagnosis. This patient died of a ruptured 3-cm posterior abdominal aortic aneurysm inappropriately treated as subacute cholecystitis. The diagnosis may not have been apparent at open laparotomy. Overall, laparoscopic cholecystectomy clearly has a low incidence of death, hemorrhage, or cardiopulmonary problems compared with conventional cholecystectomy. In addition, the complication rate of about 5 per cent, including very minor problems, is favorable compared to minilaparotomy for cholecystectomy.

The most common complication of laparoscopic cholecystectomy is wound infection. This is typically superficial and involves the site of insertion of the umbilical trocar, the usual site of gallbladder removal. An important difference between laparoscopic cholecystectomy and conventional cholecystectomy is the lower incidence (about 2 per cent) of previously undetected common duct stones in the new procedure. Reviews of large numbers of conventional cholecystectomies indicate an incidence of 8 to 16 per cent.[14,15] Preoperative selection of patients undoubtedly contributes to the low incidence in laparoscopic procedures; however, an increasing number of patients with retained stones already are being seen (Southern Surgeons Club report). However, most retained stones can now be extracted by ERCP. Perhaps, the most compelling evidence for the safety of laparoscopic cholecystectomy is the readmission rate of less than 1 per cent. This compares favorably with conventional cholecystectomy, which has a 3 to 5 per cent readmission rate.[16,17]

Enthusiasm for laparoscopic cholecystectomy grew rapidly as reports detailed the ease, efficacy, and safety of the procedure. Introducing surgeons to the new technique, however, results in a learning period in which there is a higher complication rate than expected with more experience. The most common devastating complication within the learning curve is major biliary injury. In the Southern Surgeons Club experience the incidence of bile duct injury was 2.2 per cent within the first 13 procedures of any participant's experience compared to 0.1 per cent after the 13th procedure. The overall incidence of undetected common or hepatic duct injury was only 0.2 per cent; however, these complications caused significant morbidity.

The classic laparoscopic biliary injury results from inappropriately identifying the common duct as the cystic duct[18] (Fig. 16-3). A small vessel to the common duct is interpreted as the cystic artery and is ligated and divided. The proximal bile duct together with a portion of the common hepatic duct is then severed with the gallbladder. Thus, a segment of the patient's major biliary tree is missing, and this results in biliary ascites, obstruction, or, commonly, both. The injury is also associated with injury to the right hepatic artery because it usually crosses immediately beneath the common duct in what is thought to be the gallbladder bed. Review of videotapes of 15 such injuries demonstrates the occurrence of the arterial injury that often results in profuse hemorrhage. In the classic injury, separation of the proximal biliary system occurs above or below the bifurcation. We have seen it as high as the tertiary biliary radical arteries. Fortunately reconstruction was still possible in that patient. However, a similar patient at another hospital has been placed on a liver transplant waiting list.

A variant of the classic injury occurs when clips are placed on the common duct instead of the distal cystic duct. The proximal clips are correctly placed, and the cystic duct is divided close to its junction with the common duct. As expected, the complication causes a total biliary leakage from the divided, unligated stump of the cystic duct while the common duct is completely obstructed.

The second most common, initially unrecognized, major biliary injury in laparoscopic cholecystectomy is a burn resulting in biliary stricture (Fig. 16-4). The burn is a result of excessive use of cautery or laser during dis-

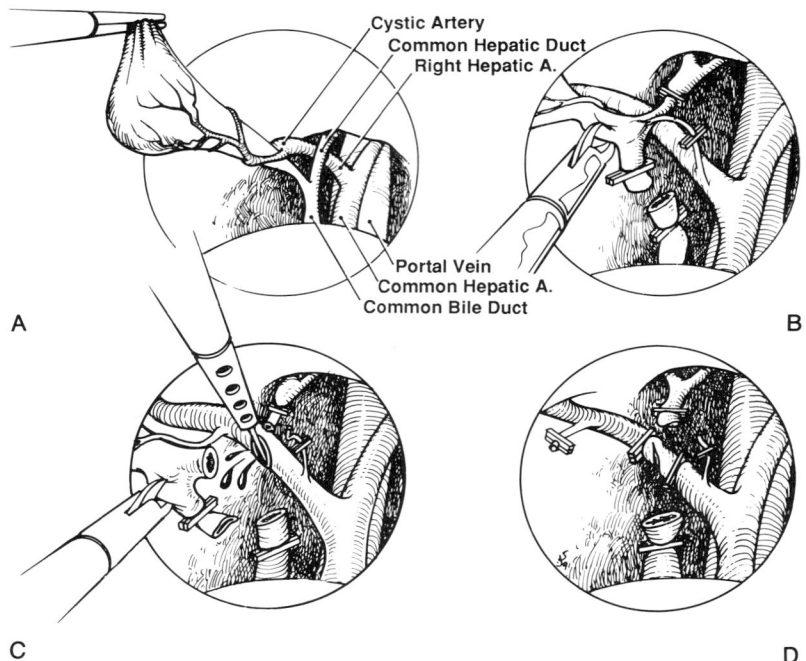

Figure 16-3. The classic laparoscopic biliary injury. A, Normal portal anatomy. B, Incorrect identification of the common bile duct as the cystic duct, with subsequent ligation and division. C, Incorrect identification of the small arterial supply to the common duct as the cystic artery, with subsequent ligation and division. Note also injury of the right hepatic artery, which occurred during proximal division of the common hepatic duct. D, Ligation of the right hepatic artery and complete obstruction of the biliary system. (Reproduced with permission from Davidoff AM, Pappas TN, Murray EA, et al. Mechanisms of major biliary injury during laparoscopic cholecystectomy. Ann Surg 1992;215(3):195–200.)

section of the gallbladder bed or cautery division of the cystic duct. Some of the first teaching tapes of laparoscopic cholecystectomy show division of the cystic duct with laser or cautery. Because of the potential for injury, this practice should be avoided.

Twenty-five major biliary injuries were managed at Duke University Medical Center over a 2-year period. All patients received definitive treatment after recognition of problems incurred during initial procedures. These patients were referred to the hospital and thus, their injuries occurred outside the Southern Surgeons Club experience. The videotapes of the original operations were available in all but 5 of these patients, facilitating the correlation of intraoperative events with subsequent pathologic conditions. The ability to visualize the injuries as they were occurring provided a unique opportunity to make strong recommendations for avoiding such complications.

Inadequate visualization of the operative field was an obvious common denominator in many of the films. Poor visualization was usually caused by both acute or chronic inflammation and the surgeon's inexperience with laparoscopy. Other factors contributing to injury included inadequate dissection of the gallbladder-cystic duct junction, grasping the common duct for traction rather than the ampulla of the gallbladder, excessive use of prograde (away from the common duct) rather than retrograde (toward the common duct) dissection, and excessive use of cautery or laser in the hilar region.

Major biliary system injury recognized during the procedure requires immediate conversion to open cholecystectomy. Most major biliary injuries go unrecognized at the initial operation. Clues to the existence of an injury during dissection include: (1) unexplained bile leakage, (2) peculiar anatomical structures, (3) a large unexplained ductal or vascular

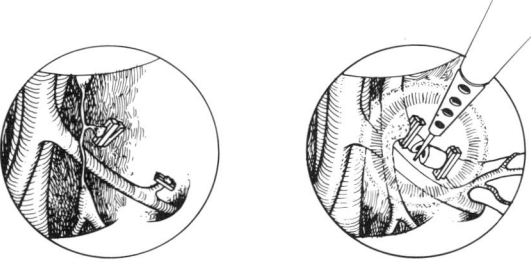

Figure 16-4. Thermal injury to the portal triad resulting in biliary stricture. (Reproduced with permission from Davidoff AM, Pappas TN, Murray EA, et al. Mechanisms of major biliary injury during laparoscopic cholecystectomy. Ann Surg 1992;215(3):195–200.)

structure encountered during "routine" dissection, and (4) hemorrhage. There are two principal clinical manifestations of bile duct injury: (1) bile leakage after the initial operation with pain and (2) biliary obstruction. Unexplained persistent pain was twice as common on clinical presentation of patients as biliary obstruction in the Duke series. The primary clue to early diagnosis of the problem after completion of the laparoscopic cholecystectomy is severe persistent abdominal pain out of proportion to what is expected. The pain is not necessarily associated with jaundice.

The following recommendations for avoidance of injury during laparoscopic cholecystectomy are noteworthy. Adequate visualization of the portal structures is essential. The cystic duct and cystic artery should be identified with certainty before ligation and division of any structures in the porta hepatis. It is more important to visualize the gallbladder-cystic duct junction than the cystic duct-common duct junction. The surgeon should not hesitate to use cholangiography to help define portal anatomy, particularly early in his or her experience. When acute inflammation and chronic scarring of the gallbladder bed restrict adequate identification of the anatomical features, early conversion to open cholecystectomy should be considered. Dissection should proceed away from the gallbladder *toward* the common duct, rather than in the other direction.

Common hepatic duct stricture usually results from thermal injury or excessive manipulation of the common duct during the laparoscopic procedure. Small caliber biliary systems are particularly susceptible to stricture formation by these mechanisms. Therefore, laser or cautery should be used judiciously during dissection in the portal region and manipulation of the common duct should be minimized.

The principles of management of injuries sustained during laparoscopic cholecystectomy are essentially the same as for those sustained during open procedures. These include early recognition of the injury, primary repair at the time of the initial laparoscopic procedure if possible, identification of the biliary anatomy prior to a secondary operative repair, and Roux-en-Y hepaticojejunostomy unless there is a compelling reason to do otherwise. Preoperatively placed percutaneous catheters into the biliary system are important in order to identify the injured ducts at surgery. They may also be useful if prolonged stenting is indicated. Preoperative computed tomographic drainage of intraperitoneal bile may convert the patient's condition to stability before operative intervention. At the time of corrective surgery, a coronary O ring may be placed on the Roux-en-Y segment and attached to the anterior abdominal wall. This is helpful if future access to the biliary system is necessary. In most patients hepaticojejunostomy is successful if there is no technical difficulty, cholangitis, or undiagnosed burn injury at the time of repair. An additional consideration at reconstruction is the possibility of an isolated draining major biliary radical artery that might not be incorporated into the hepaticojejunostomy.

CONTROVERSIES

Like any new procedure, laparoscopic cholecystectomy created a number of controversies. These were magnified because of the tremendous impact of the technique. Most controversies are resolving as individuals find that there are multiple ways to perform the procedure.

There are two principle positions for performing laparoscopic cholecystectomy. The surgeon may stand to the patient's left or between the patient's legs with the patient in the lithotomy position. Arguments persist concerning the use of disposable versus nondisposable instruments. Cautery has essentially replaced laser for dissection of the gallbladder bed. Cautery is cheaper, easier to use, and more familiar to most surgeons. Additional concerns pertain to the training of surgeons, the importance of trained assistants, and the implications for future training of residents in traditional procedures.

The indications and utility of cholangiography raise similar arguments, which have been longstanding for conventional cholecystectomy. The main argument concerns routine versus selective cholangiography. Most laparoscopic surgeons agree that routine cholangiography is beneficial early in one's experience. A minority of surgeons perform routine intravenous cholangiography prior to laparoscopic cholecystectomy. Routine preoperative ERCP is not indicated.[19]

Another important controversy pertains to the procedure indicated when a coincidental stone is found in the duct at laparoscopic cholecystectomy. Most surgeons presently do not perform laparoscopic common duct exploration. When laparoscopic common duct exploration is not possible, the choices are conversion to conventional cholecystectomy, postoperative ERCP, or simply expectant therapy (expecting the stone to pass spontaneously). Two important factors that influence the decision are the expertise of the individual performing ERCP and the size of the stone. The availability of individuals proficient in ERCP makes the surgeon more likely to end the laparoscopic procedure. The presence of large stones, which may be difficult to remove endoscopically, make the surgeon more likely to convert.

Conclusions

The main advantages of laparoscopic cholecystectomy are that it is less painful, it shortens hospital stay, it returns patients to active life sooner, and it causes minimal scarring. Nonetheless, laparoscopic cholecystectomy must be considered a major surgical procedure, carrying with it risks similar to those of conventional cholecystectomy. Moreover, with this type of surgery, as with conventional cholecystectomy, inexperience can lead to complications. Increasing experience leads to a lowering of contraindications. The experienced laparoscopic surgeon also has a low threshold for conversion to conventional cholecystectomy when the anatomical landmarks are obscure.

REFERENCES

1. Meyers WC, Jones RS. Disorders of the biliary system. *In* Meyers WC, Jones RS. Textbook of Liver and Biliary Surgery. Philadelphia, JB Lippincott, 1990, p 226.
2. Schoenfield LJ, Lachin JM, Baum RA, et al. Chenodiol (chenodeoxycholic acid) for dissolution of gallstones. The National Cooperative Gallstone Study. Ann Intern Med 1981; 95:257–282.
3. Thistle JL. Ursodeoxycholic acid treatment of gallstones. Semin Liver Dis 1983; 3:146–156.
4. Sackmann M, Delius M, Sauerbruch T, et al. Shock wave lithotripsy of gallbladder stones: The first 175 patients. N Engl J Med 1988; 318:393–397.
5. Paumgartner G, Delius M, Sauerbruch T, et al. Fragmentation of gallbladder stones by ESWL in humans. *In* Proceedings of the First International Symposium on Anesthesia and ESWL, Munich, 1986. New York, Springer-Verlag, 1987.
6. Erlinger S, Go AL, Husson JM, et al. Franco-Belgium cooperative study of ursodeoxycholic acid in the medical dissolution of gallstones: A double-blind, randomized, dose-response study, comparison with chenodeoxycholic acid. Hepatology 1984; 4:308–314.
7. Ferrucci JT. Biliary lithotripsy: What will the issues be? AJR 1987; 149:227–231.
8. Glenn F. Trends in surgical treatment of calculous disease of the biliary tract. Surg Gynecol Obstet 1975; 140:877–884.
9. Reddick EJ, Olsen DO, Daniel JF, et al. Laparoscopic laser cholecystectomy. Laser Med Surg News 1984; 7:38–40.
10. Reddick EJ, Olsen DO. Laparoscopic laser cholecystectomy: A comparison with mini-lap cholecystectomy. Surg Endosc 1989; 3:131–133.
11. Meyers WC. A prospective analysis of 1518 laparoscopic cholecystectomies. N Engl J Med 1991; 324:1073–1078.
12. Gracie WA, Ransohoff DF. The natural history of silent gallstones: The innocent gallstone is not a myth. N Engl J Med 1982; 307:798–800.
13. Cuschieri A, Dubois F, Moviel J, et al. The European experience with laparoscopic cholecystectomy. Am J Surg 1991; 161:385–387.
14. MacLean LD, Goldstein M, MacDonald JE, et al. Results of cholecystectomy in 1000 consecutive patients. Can J Surg 1975; 18:459–465.
15. Way LW. Retained common duct stones. Surg Clin North Am 1973; 53:1139–1147.
16. Roos LL Jr, Cayeorge SM, Roos NP. Centralization, certification, and monitoring: Readmissions and complications after surgery. Med Care 1986; 24:1044–1066.
17. Cohen MM, Young TK, Hammorstrand KM. Ethnic variation in cholecystectomy rates and outcomes. Manitoba, Canada, 1972–1984. Am J Public Health 1989; 79:751–755.
18. Davidoff AM, Pappas TN, Murray EA, et al. Mechanisms of major biliary injury during laparoscopic cholecystectomy. Ann Surg 1992; 215:196–202.
19. Cotton PB, Baillie J, Pappas T, Meyers WC. Laparoscopic cholecystectomy and the biliary endoscopist. Gastrointest Endosc 1991; 37:94–97.

Chapter 17
Management of Acute Cholecystitis

Karl A. Zucker
Robert W. Bailey
John L. Flowers

Laparoscopic cholecystectomy is now widely accepted as the procedure of choice for most patients with symptomatic gallbladder disease. The role of laparoscopic surgery in the management of acute cholecystitis, however, remains controversial. Many surgeons feel that the inflammation and edema present in such patients will distort the biliary ductal and vascular anatomical structures and result in a significantly higher complication rate. Some authors have even expressed concerns that laparoscopic intervention may be an absolute contraindication in the setting of acute inflammation.[1] Although most surgeons would agree that acute cholecystitis remains a relative contraindication for laparoscopic intervention, a number of recently published series have suggested that the most important factor in determining whether such patients should be offered this alternative is the experience of the surgical team.[2–4] These reports have all come from centers with extensive experience with both open and laparoscopic biliary tract surgery. The excellent results obtained by these surgeons indicate that with appropriate experience laparoscopic surgery may be safely performed in the setting of acute cholecystitis. In addition, these patients appear to benefit from many of the same advantages in terms of diminished hospitalization and rapid return to normal activities as those undergoing elective surgery.

At our institution the diagnosis of acute cholecystitis is reserved for those patients whose hospital admissions are unplanned and who have the following symptoms: acute abdominal pain, fever, leukocytosis, and abnormal biliary ultrasound or scintillation studies. Since 1990 all such patients seen at the University of Maryland Medical Center and its affiliated hospitals have routinely undergone laparoscopic surgery.[2] In nearly all patients surgery was performed within 48 hours of presentation—in the "acute" setting.

DEFINITION OF ACUTE CHOLECYSTITIS AND PREOPERATIVE PREPARATION

Intravenous fluids for rehydration and correction of electrolyte imbalances and broad spectrum antibiotics (usually a first or second generation cephalosporin) are administered and patients are given nothing by mouth. A nasogastric tube is used if there are indications of an accompanying ileus. A thorough explanation of the diagnosis and the various therapeutic alternatives is conducted with the patient; options discussed include continued medical management, traditional open laparotomy with cholecystectomy, and laparoscopic surgery. The explanation of the latter includes a detailed description of the procedure, its potential risks, and the possibility of converting the laparoscopic procedure to an open laparotomy. It is important that the patient understands that the decision to abort the laparoscopic approach does not necessarily indicate that a complication has occurred. Instead the patient must realize that the need for conversion to open laparotomy represents sound surgical judgment and will minimize the occurrence of operative complications.

The finding of common bile duct stones in patients seen with acute cholecystitis is extremely uncommon and, in most individuals, readily diagnosed prior to operative intervention. If choledocholithiasis is suspected, a decision must be made whether to attempt preoperative endoscopic retrograde cholangiopancreatography or proceed directly to cholecystectomy and possible common bile duct exploration. If the episode of acute inflammation is mild and rapidly responds to medical management, we will perform preoperative endoscopic retrograde cholangiopancreatography. Often the stone(s) will have already passed through the ampulla. Therefore, only individuals with strong indications of persistent choledocholithiasis such as common bile duct dilation (i.e., based on ultrasonography), continued abnormalities of liver function tests (alkaline phosphatase, hepatic transaminases, or bilirubin), or elevated pancreatic enzymes (i.e., amylase or lipase) will undergo preoperative biliary endoscopy. If the clinical signs of acute inflammation continue or even progress, a laparoscopic cholecystectomy and intraoperative cholangiogram are performed. If common bile duct stones are visualized with the radiographic study an open laparotomy and common bile duct exploration are performed.

OPERATIVE TECHNIQUE

Patients should be administered a general anesthetic with endotracheal intubation. Although regional epidural anesthesia has been successfully used for elective laparoscopic cholecystectomy, it has not proven feasible for patients undergoing emergency surgery.[5] Patients are prepared and draped for both a laparoscopic and open cholecystectomy. A major laparotomy instrument set is kept in the room. Nasogastric and urinary catheters are inserted to decompress the stomach and bladder. Although some surgeons have avoided using such catheters during elective surgery, we continue to advocate their use, especially in patients with acute cholecystitis.

The pneumoperitoneum is established using either the percutaneous approach or an open (i.e., Hasson) technique (see Chapter 9). In patients who have had prior upper abdominal surgery we prefer the open technique for insufflation and use one of the cannulas specially designed for this approach. Otherwise an insufflation needle (SURGINEEDLE*, United States Surgical Corporation, Norwalk, CT) is inserted through a small incision made in the upper folds of the umbilicus. Proper placement of the needle within the peritoneal cavity is confirmed (see Chapter 9), and insufflation with carbon dioxide is begun. After the abdomen is fully distended a 10.0- or 11.0-mm trocar and cannula are inserted through the upper folds of the umbilicus. We prefer using radiolucent sheathes because we routinely perform intraoperative cholangiography. The use of metal, radiopaque cannulas complicates this procedure (although it is possible to perform if one positions the cannulas away from the underlying bile ducts). After insertion of the umbilical sheath the

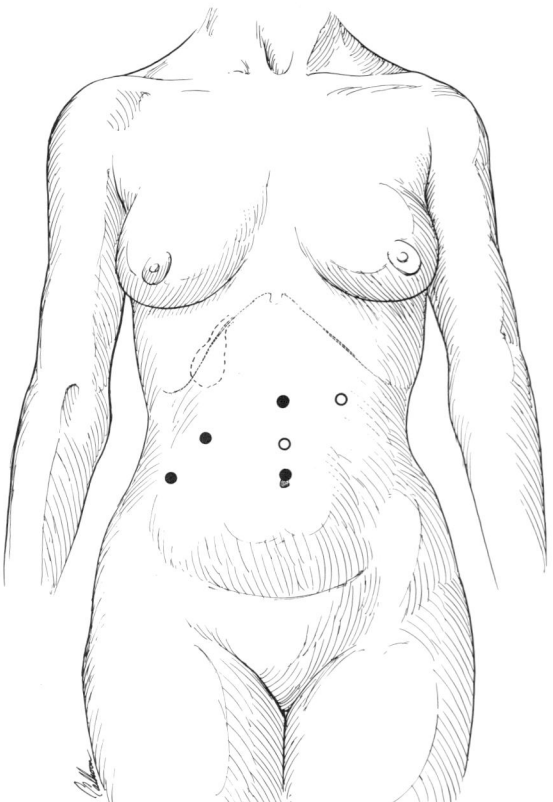

Figure 17-1. Insertion of additional cannulas is often necessary in patients seen with acute cholecystitis.

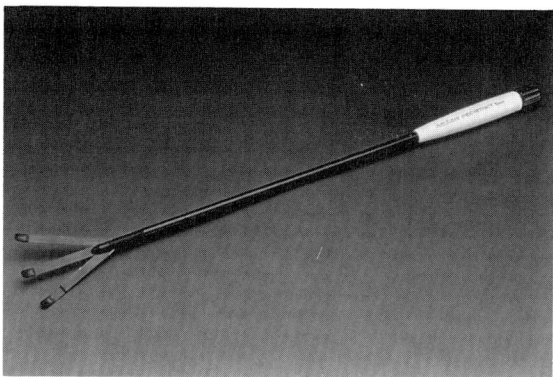

Figure 17-2. A recently designed fan-like retractor (ENDO RETRACT*, United States Surgical Corporation), which facilitates retraction of inflamed tissues in and around the porta hepatis.

laparoscope with attached video camera is introduced, and the peritoneal cavity is examined. The three accessary trocars and cannulas are then inserted through the abdominal wall under laparoscopic guidance. In patients with acute cholecystitis it is often necessary to insert a fifth cannula to obtain adequate exposure. The location of these additional punctures will vary depending upon the operative findings. The most common sites are in the midline halfway between the umbilical and subxiphoid sheaths or in the left subcostal space (Fig. 17-1). Additional instruments such as fan-like retractors or grasping forceps introduced through an extra portal will often improve the exposure and allow a procedure to be completed which otherwise may have been necessary to convert to an open laparotomy (Fig. 17-2). In our experience the placement of a fifth or even sixth cannula results in little or no additional postoperative discomfort or cosmetic deformity.

In addition to placing additional cannulas and instruments to facilitate the operative dissection, we also recommend using a side-viewing laparoscope. These are available with the viewing lens angled from 30 to 50 degrees and allow for greater versatility in visualizing the operative field. By rotating the laparoscope 360 degrees one can look up, down, left, or right and observe regions of the abdomen that are impossible with a forward-viewing telescope. A recently introduced semiflexible laparoscope (Fujinon Inc.) has been designed to improve on this concept (Fig. 17-3). These instruments allow the surgeon to deflect the tip of the telescope up to 70 degrees, and it can even be used to see around various structures or within spaces of the abdomen that are not accessible with traditional rigid laparoscopes.

In patients operated upon for acute cholecystitis the gallbladder is grasped and retracted cephalad toward the right shoulder in a manner similar to that used for elective procedures.[6] This maneuver, combined with elevating the head of the operating room table 20 to 30 degrees, facilitates exposure of the cystic duct and artery. Unfortunately, the inflamed gallbladder often proves difficult to grasp and hold. This may be because the tissues are too edematous and necrotic or the gallbladder may simply be too distended to allow the forceps to obtain an adequate bite. A tense, distended gallbladder or hydrops should be partially decompressed before at-

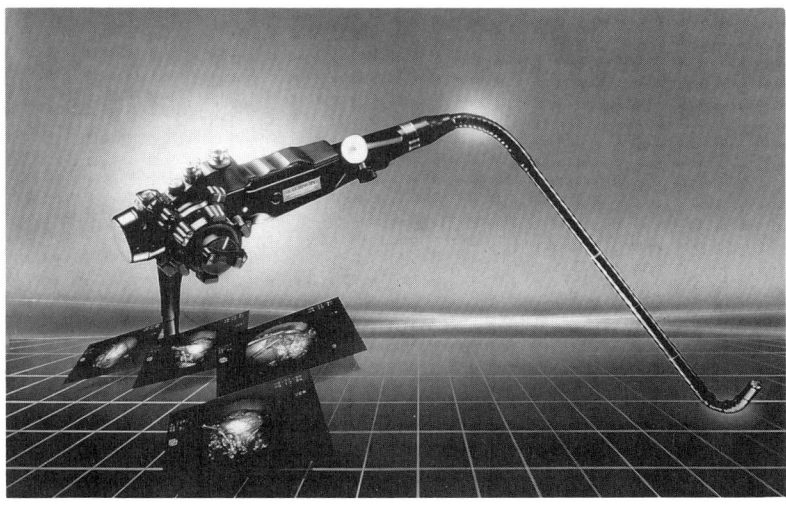

Figure 17-3. A flexible laparoscope produced by Fujinon allows viewing at angles up to 70°.

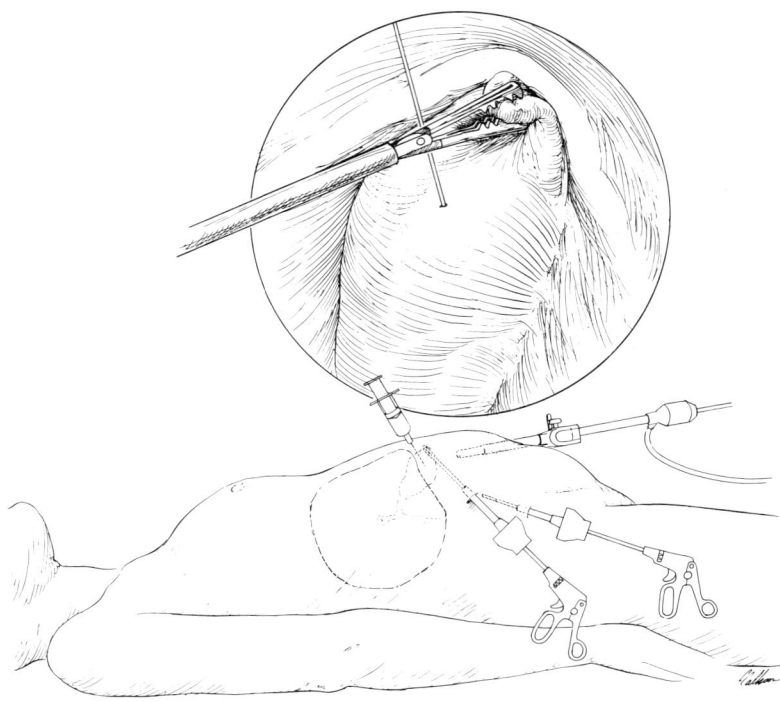

Figure 17-4. Percutaneous decompression of a distended gallbladder will often facilitate exposure of the cystic duct and artery.

tempting to retract it with either sharp or atraumatic forceps. This can be accomplished with a cyst aspiration needle (with a 5.0-mm upper shaft) inserted through one of the laparoscopic cannulas or with an 18-gauge (or larger) long needle guided percutaneously into the dome of the gallbladder (Fig. 17-4). The gallbladder should be decompressed enough to allow the forceps to grasp and retract it cephalad. Partial decompression of a distended gallbladder will also aid in the exposure of the cystic and common bile ducts. It should not be completely drained because an empty, flaccid gallbladder is more difficult to dissect away from the underlying liver bed. The puncture site is then occluded by applying the grasping forceps over the opening or with a pre-tied laparoscopic suture (Fig. 17-5).

A large selection of laparoscopic forceps have been designed specifically for retraction of an inflamed or necrotic gallbladder. The choice of which instrument to use will, of course, depend upon the intra-abdominal findings, but, for an edematous and inflamed gallbladder a sharp, penetrating forceps is often the best instrument to grasp and retract such tissues. These sharp forceps are readily available in both 5.0- and 10.0-mm diameter sizes; however, we prefer using the larger versions. To introduce these larger forceps the most lateral 5.0-mm cannula is replaced with a larger sheath (Fig. 17-6). Another method of providing adequate retraction is for the surgeon to place one or more large suture ligatures through the fundus of the gallbladder and lift upward. Although a pre-tied lapa-

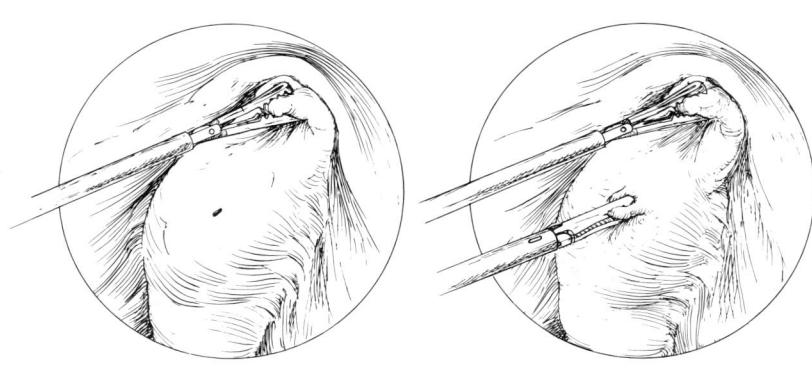

Figure 17-5. The puncture site should be occluded with a grasping forceps or a pre-tied laparoscopic suture (SURGITIE* disposable ligating, United States Surgical Corporation).

Management of Acute Cholecystitis 187

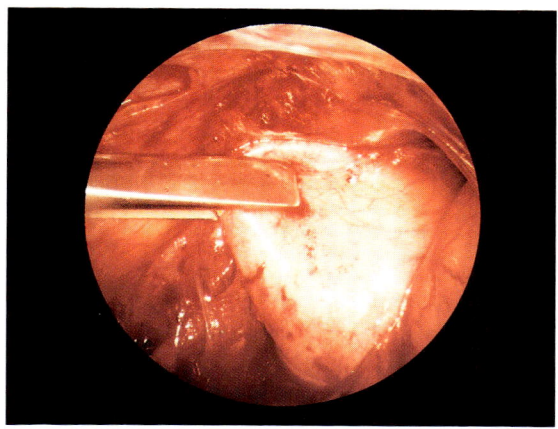

Figure 17-6. A large 10/11-mm sharp, penetrating forceps is used to retract the inflamed or necrotic gallbladder.

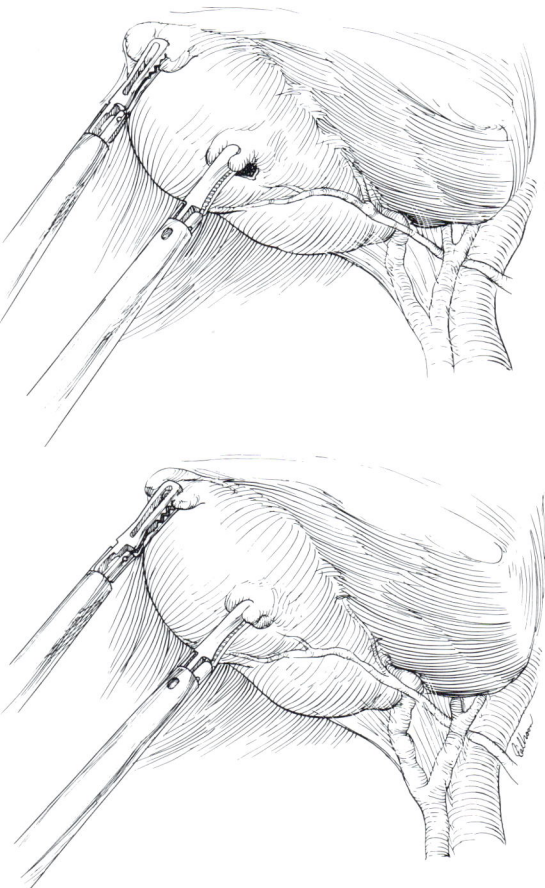

Figure 17-8. A small tear in the gallbladder may be occluded by reapplying the forceps.

roscopic suture may occasionally be used for this purpose, we prefer a deep, penetrating suture using a curved or straight needle. The suture may be pulled out through the abdominal wall or held with a grasping forceps (Fig. 17-7).

In addition to being difficult to grasp and retract, the acutely inflamed gallbladder is also more easily torn, resulting in bile or stone spillage. These injuries usually occur at the site where the grasping forceps has been applied for retraction. A tear into the gallbladder should be controlled as rapidly as possible. If the opening is small, it may be controlled by simply reapplying the same or larger forceps over the puncture site (Fig. 17-8). Larger tears generally require closure with either a suture ligature or a pre-tied laparoscopic suture (Fig. 17-9). Once again the gallbladder should not be allowed to drain completely empty. If bile or purulent fluid

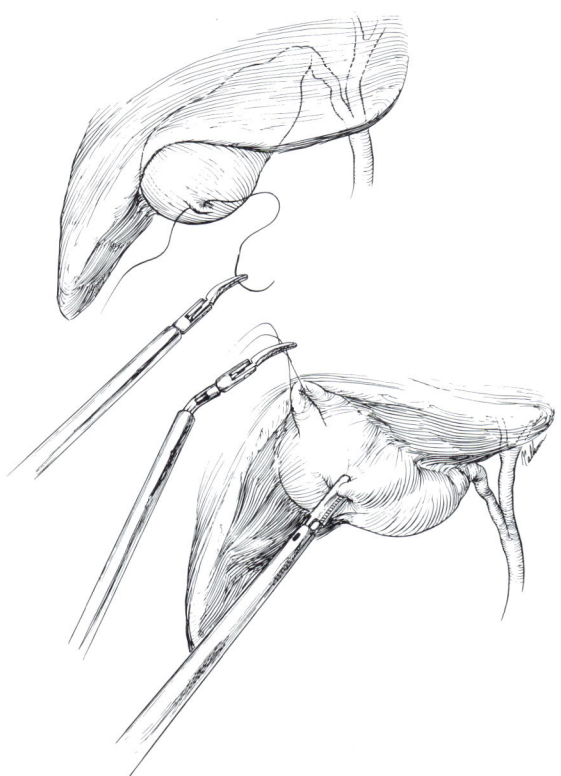

Figure 17-7. An alternative technique uses a deep, penetrating suture placed in the fundus of the gallbladder.

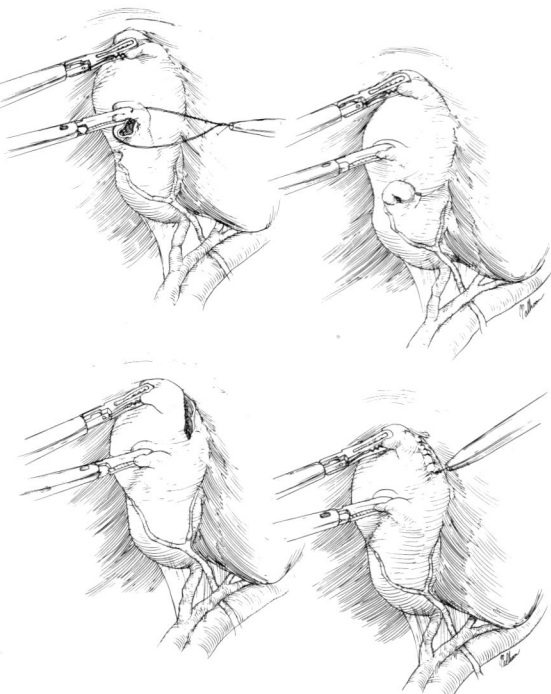

Figure 17-9. Larger openings will require a suture ligature or pre-tied suture to control the spillage.

nately, stones are often left behind despite vigorous attempts to remove them. In a recent report by Soper and Dunnegan[7] from St. Louis patients with documented bile or stone spillage which occurred during laparoscopic surgery were carefully followed and their postoperative course compared to individuals for whom no such incidents were apparent. Although the length of follow-up was limited, no significant sequelae were noted. Isolated cases of intra-abdominal abscess formation following gallbladder perforation have been reported, but such complications would appear to be uncommon considering the total number of laparoscopic procedures performed

has escaped, the peritoneal cavity should be copiously irrigated. Both 5.0- and 10.0-mm suction/irrigation devices are now available. Many incorporate a pool-tip configuration, which facilitates complete removal of the fluid. Stones that may have dropped into the peritoneal cavity should also be retrieved if possible. Small stones may be aspirated with irrigation/suction cannulas, but most will require extraction using forceps or balloon baskets (Fig. 17-10). If there are multiple or very large stones, it may be easier and faster to insert a sterile "bag" into the abdomen and place the calculi within it (Fig. 17-11). Use of this pouch minimizes the need to repeatedly remove the grasping forceps and reorient the video camera and laparoscope. Initially surgeons used gas-sterilized condoms or operating room gloves (one finger of a large-sized glove) to contain spilled stones but now commercially manufactured bags are available (Endo Catch, United States Surgical Corporation), which are easier to use. The bag and calculi may be removed through the larger, upper midline cannula or, if too distended, extracted at the end of the procedure through an enlarged umbilical fascial defect. Unfortu-

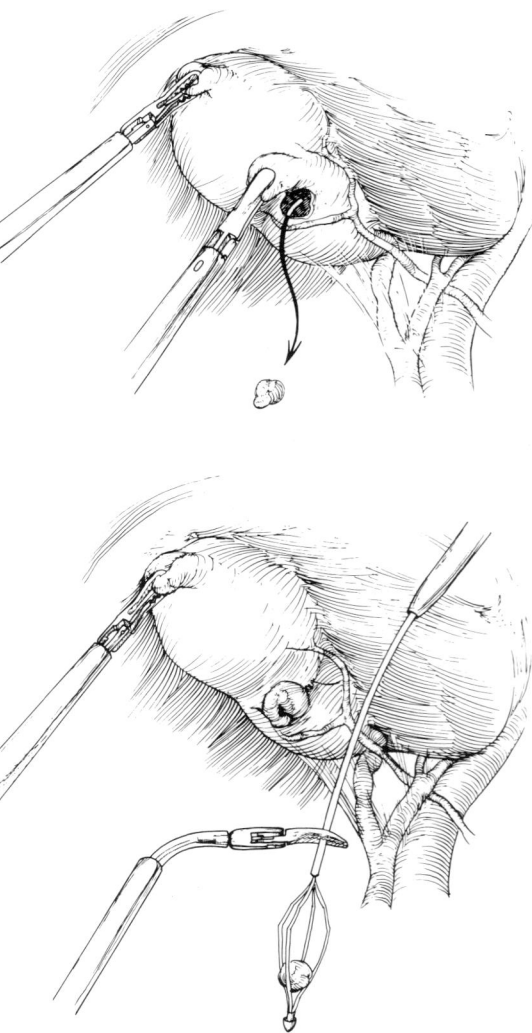

Figure 17-10. Extraction of gallstones that have escaped from the gallbladder.

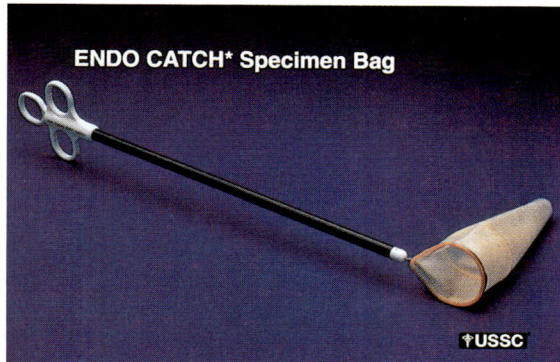

Figure 17-11. A sterile reservoir with a laparoscopic applicator sheath, which may be used within the abdomen to retrieve escaped gallstones.

over the past 5 years. In more than 600 laparoscopic procedures performed at the University of Maryland and Baltimore Veterans' Hospitals there has been only one clinically apparent problem resulting from gallstone spillage. This was a persistent draining sinus tract through the lateral puncture site, later found to communicate with a small gallstone that had adhered to the anterior abdominal wall.[8] In most instances bile and/or stone spillage alone should not be the sole reason for converting the procedure to an open laparotomy.

Meticulous dissection of the gallbladder and surrounding tissues is important in both emergency and elective laparoscopic biliary tract surgery. The inflammation and edema of the porta hepatis accompanying acute cholecystitis will often severely distort the ductal and vascular anatomical structures. As in the elective procedure the operative dissection begins high, near the fundus of the gallbladder, and proceeds distally toward the cystic and common bile ducts (Fig. 17-12). The dissection is continued close to the wall of the gallbladder with careful attention given at all times to hemostasis. Adhesive attachments to the gallbladder from the surrounding omentum, transverse colon, or duodenum are carefully exposed and divided. Often these inflammatory attachments can be removed with blunt dissection. Dense adhesions require sharp dissection using scissors or electrocautery. Many dissecting instruments are now designed to be used with monopolar electrocautery, and this has facilitated maintaining a bloodless operative field. In our experience 5.0- and 10.0-mm curved dissecting forceps (Maryland Dissector, American Surgical Instruments, Pompano Beach, FL) with insulated shafts and a monopolar cautery connectors have been useful instruments for freeing the gallbladder from these inflammatory adhesions. Other surgeons have reported the advantages of contact tip or free beam lasers for this portion of the operation. With either electrocautery or laser dissection care must be taken not to injure adjacent viscera, which may be hidden in the surrounding inflammatory tissues.

In addition to the acute inflammation and edema, the cephalad retraction of the gallbladder and right lobe of the liver will also distort the normal anatomy of the cystic and common bile duct junction (Fig. 17-13). It should be recognized that the common bile duct may be tented upward several centimeters from its normal position within the porta hepatis. The cystic and common bile duct juncture may therefore prove especially difficult to recognize when surrounded by dense and highly vascularized inflammatory adhesions. Occasionally the edematous reaction may mimic an enlarged cystic duct while in fact the ducts are of normal caliber. The operative dissection should continue distally until the complete course of the cystic duct along with its juncture to the common bile duct is readily apparent. Small cotton sponges or Kittners (endoscopic Kittner, OR Concepts, Roanoke, TX) may prove especially useful in dissecting edematous structures within the

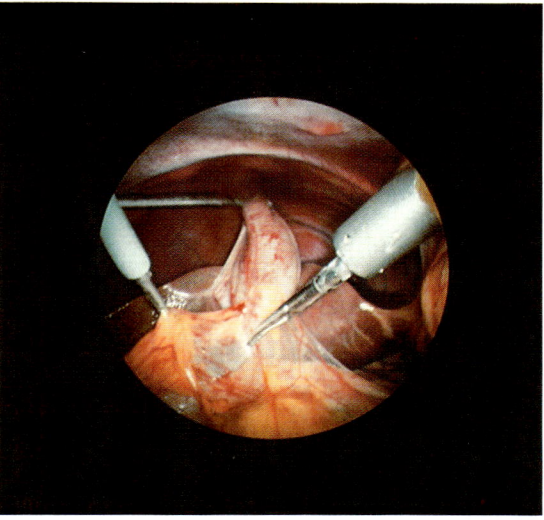

Figure 17-12. The operative dissection begins near the fundus of the gallbladder and continues distally toward the cystic and common bile ducts.

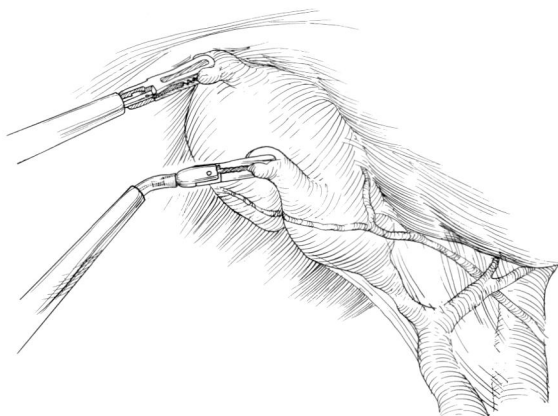

Figure 17-13. Cephalad and lateral retraction of the gallbladder and right lobe of the liver can severely distort the normal anatomy of the cystic-common bile duct juncture.

triangle of Calot (Fig. 17-14). A stroking or twisting motion with this cotton-tipped device will help separate and expose the tissue planes surrounding the cystic duct and artery. On more than one occasion a completely mobilized cystic duct has been shown, upon further dissection, to be the common bile duct. No presumed ductal or vascular structure should be divided until its anatomical features have been completely demonstrated. If the cystic duct and artery are not easily dissected free from the surrounding tissues, some authors have advocated attempting a retrograde dissection beginning at the fundus of the gallbladder.[9] This is not practiced by our group, and it is our impression that if the ductal and vascular structures are so obscured by dense inflammation as to preclude a safe antegrade dissection, then the procedure should be converted to an open laparotomy.

It is our policy to perform intraoperative cholangiography on all patients undergoing laparoscopic cholecystectomy. This is done not only to determine the presence of common bile duct stones but also to provide a road map of the ductal anatomy. Unusual or aberrant ductal anatomical features are often difficult to demonstrate in the setting of acute inflammation and edema. Intraoperative cholangiography will supply the surgeon with accurate details concerning the juncture of the cystic and common bile ducts as well as the presence of any accessary ducts that may be injured during the operative dissection (Fig. 17-15). Although there is a risk of common bile duct injury associated with cholangiogram catheter insertion, these injuries are usually easy to manage compared to complete division or even excision of the hepatic or common bile duct.

Occasionally one or more stones may be

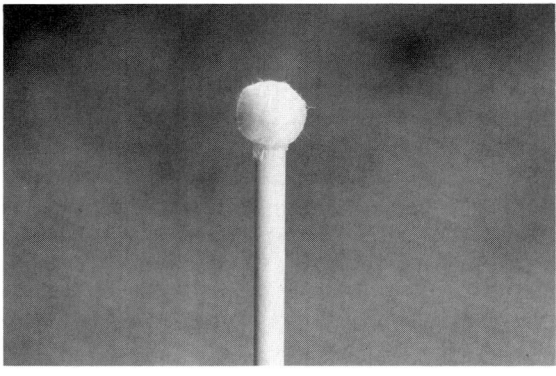

Figure 17-14. An endoscopic cotton-tipped dissector may prove useful in bluntly dissecting the cystic duct and artery. (Reproduced with permission from Zucker KA, Bailey RW. Laparoscopic cholangiography and management of choledocholithiasis. In Zucker KA, ed. Surgical Laparoscopy. St. Louis, Quality Medical Publishing, 1993, p 168.)

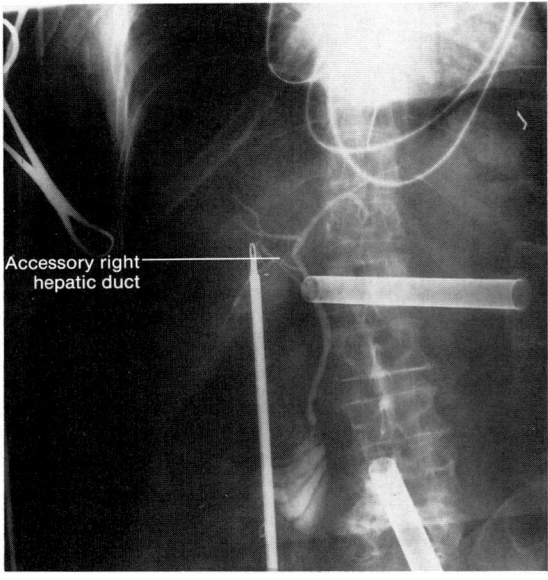

Figure 17-15. Intraoperative cholangiography demonstrating an accessary right bile duct. (Reproduced with permission from Bailey RW, Zucker KA. Laparoscopic cholangiography and management of choledocholithiasis. In Zucker KA, Bailey RW, Reddick EJ. Surgical Laparoscopy. St. Louis, Quality Medical Publishing, 1991, p 203.)

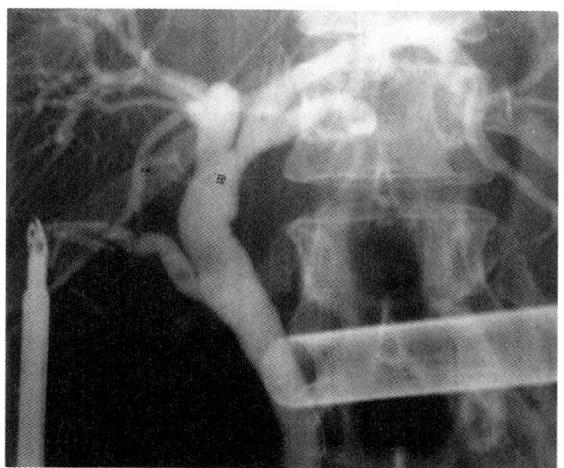

Figure 17-16. Intraoperative cholangiogram demonstrating a small stone impacted at the cystic and common bile duct juncture. (Reproduced with permission from Zucker KA. Laparoscopic cholangiography and management of choledocholithiasis. In Zucker KA, ed. Surgical Laparoscopy. St. Louis, Quality Medical Publishing, 1991, pp 201–226.)

identified within the distal cystic duct (Fig. 17-16). These stones should be removed because they may later pass into the common bile duct and cause symptoms. An atraumatic forceps can be used to "milk" them back into the gallbladder or out through the cystic duct opening. Rarely, a stone impacted at the common bile duct juncture will require the cystic duct to be opened down to this point to allow for direct removal.

After confirming the status of the ductal anatomy with the intraoperative cholangiogram the cystic duct may be ligated. During elective cholecystectomy the cystic duct is usually secured with multiple titanium staples and divided with laparoscopic scissors. If the tissues are severely edematous, the standard clips may not be large enough to completely occlude the cystic duct. Also, if the inflammation resolves rapidly following gallbladder removal, the clips might loosen and become dislodged. This may, in fact, be a factor in some cases of postoperative bile leaks. Therefore, if the cystic duct appears edematous or inflamed we prefer to use both surgical clips and pre-tied laparoscopic sutures (Fig. 17-17). A laparoscopic clip applier is introduced through the upper midline cannula and used to ligate the cystic duct. The duct is divided between the clips, and a pre-tied laparoscopic suture is introduced through the upper midline cannula and placed around the cystic duct stump. The clips and sutures must be carefully positioned on the cystic duct to avoid occluding the juncture with the common bile duct (Fig. 17-18).

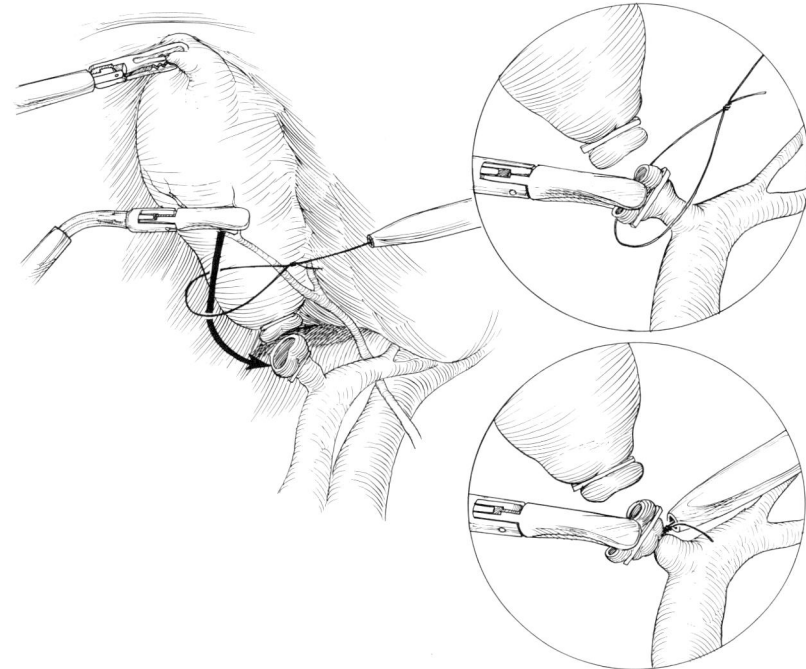

Figure 17-17. If the cystic duct appears edematous or inflamed, surgical clips are used to initially occlude it, followed by the application of a pre-tied laparoscopic suture.

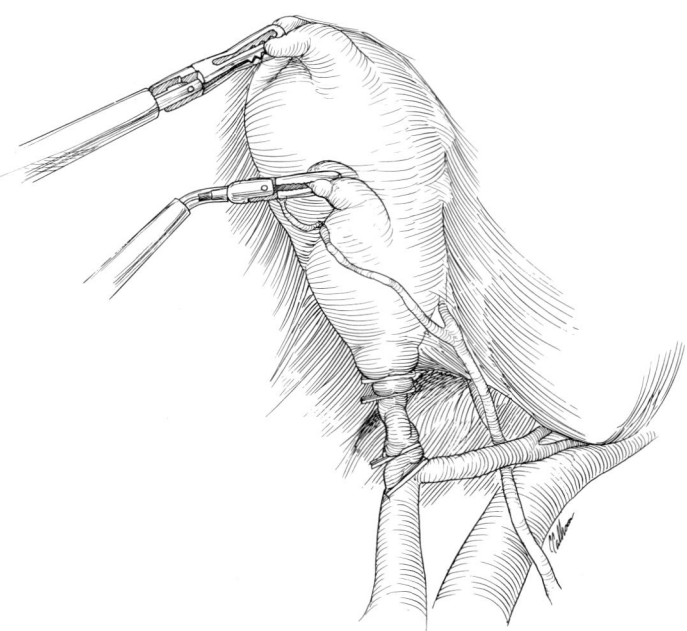

Figure 17-18. "Tenting" of the cystic and common bile duct junction may lead to inadvertent placement of clips or sutures across the common bile duct.

Prior to dividing the cystic duct the blood supply to the gallbladder should be identified and controlled. Consequently, if the cystic artery is torn during the course of its dissection, the intact ductal structures may keep the vessel from retracting back into the porta hepatis. The cystic artery is usually found medial and slightly posterior to the cystic duct. It should be carefully dissected free from the surrounding tissues with the same care in demonstrating the anatomical features as with the ductal structures. Acute and chronic inflammation occurring within the angle of Calot may render identification of the blood supply difficult. One of the most common causes of significant intraoperative bleeding during elective or emergency cholecystectomy is failure to identify the posterior branch of the cystic artery. Often the anterior branch is readily visualized coursing along the exposed surface of the gallbladder. The magnification of the video system as well as the direction of the image (from the umbilicus) can lead the surgeon to wrongly assume that this represents the main cystic artery trunk. If only the anterior branch is ligated and divided, the posterior branch may later be torn or avulsed as the gallbladder is being dissected from the underlying liver bed (Fig. 17-19). The cephalad retraction of the gallbladder combined with acute or chronic inflammation in the porta hepatis may also lead to inadvertent injury of the right hepatic artery. To avoid such injuries it is important to carefully dis-

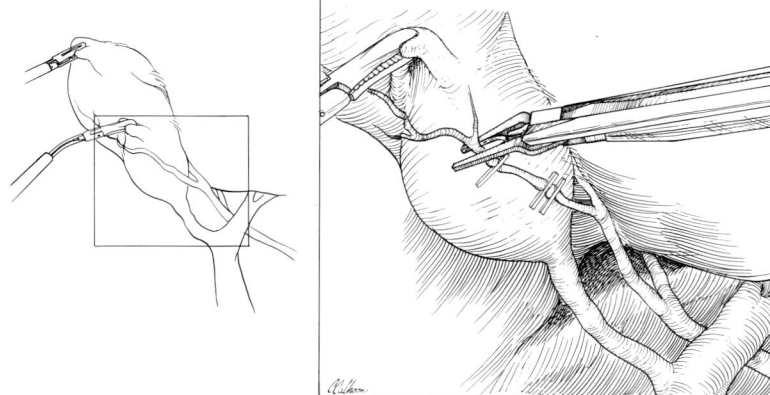

Figure 17-19. Acute and/or chronic inflammation may obscure an early takeoff of the posterior branch of the cystic artery. This vessel will then be later torn as the gallbladder is being dissected off the underlying liver bed.

sect and identify both branches of the cystic duct as well as the main trunk before any suspected vascular structures are divided.

After the cystic duct and artery are transected, the next step is to dissect the gallbladder from the underlying liver bed. This has also been described in the setting of acute inflammation using either electrocautery or laser energy.[10,11] The consensus of most surgeons is that both modalities have potential risks and benefits.[12,13] Each surgeon should use the device he or she feels most comfortable with and thoroughly study its advantages and disadvantages. At our institution electrocautery has been safely used in over 600 laparoscopic procedures, including those performed for acute cholecystitis. A variety of different monopolar cautery instruments have been used for dissecting the gallbladder from the liver, including hook-shaped devices, different configurations of blunt spatulas, and combinations of both designs. Some surgeons have reported that scissor dissection alone has proven successful in removing the gallbladder from the liver bed.[12] This technique has recently become more popular with the introduction of curved scissors with electrocautery capability (Endo-Shears, United States Surgical Corporation). These scissors are also disposable so that previous difficulties in keeping such instruments sharp are eliminated.

To minimize the risk of gallbladder perforation or liver injury it is important to maintain adequate exposure of the operative field. The most useful maneuver in our experience has been the "right-left twist" (Fig. 17-20). This is performed by the first assistant manipulating the two grasping forceps holding the gallbladder. The right twist exposes the medial aspect of the gallbladder and is accomplished by pushing the fundus toward the patient's left side and at the same time retracting the gallbladder neck to the patient's left. The left twist exposes the lateral attachments of the gallbladder to the liver and is performed by reversing the direction of each forceps. Successive right-left retraction of the gallbladder affords maximum exposure of the plane of dissection and thus avoids inadvertent gallbladder or liver injury.

In addition to cystic artery injuries, other possible sources of intraoperative blood loss include torn omental or mesenteric vessels, liver capsular tears, or bleeding from the liver bed. Torn mesenteric or omental vessels may occur during dissection of inflammatory adhesions away from the gallbladder and ductal structures (Fig. 17-21). These adhesive bands should be carefully removed using a combination of blunt and sharp dissection. Generally we use blunt dissection to separate these tissues from the anterior wall of the gallblad-

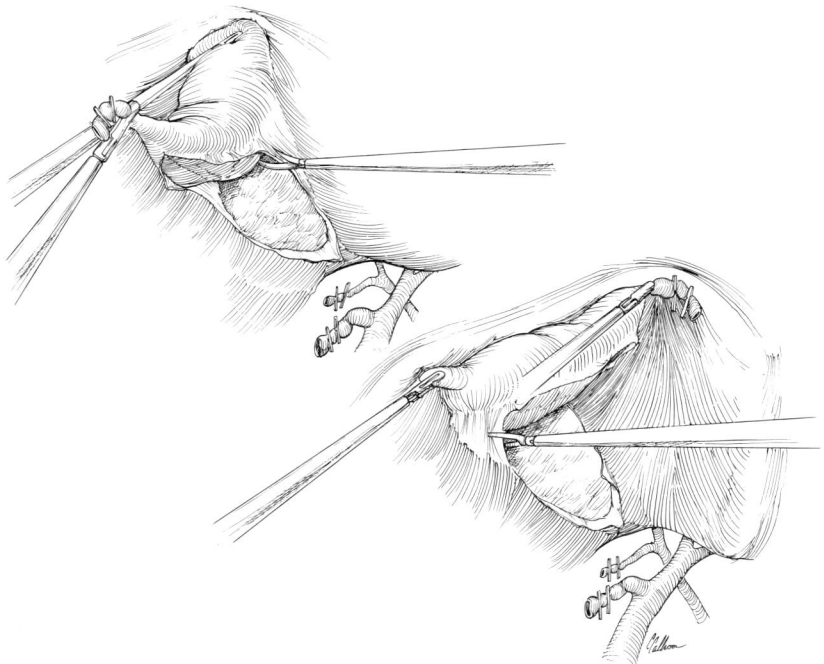

Figure 17-20. The right-left twist is used to alternatively expose the medial and lateral attachments of the gallbladder to the liver.

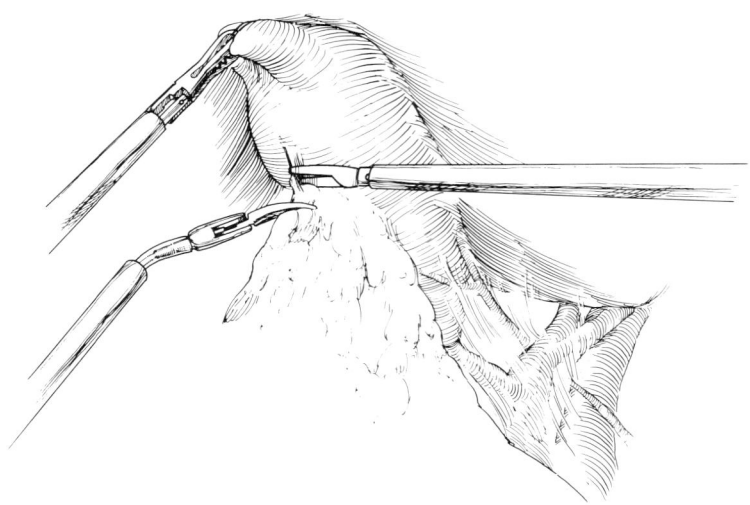

Figure 17-21. Inflammatory adhesions to the gallbladder should be removed with a combination of blunt and sharp dissection.

der. Dense or vascular adhesions are controlled with short bursts of monopolar cautery energy and then sharply divided. One must always assume that a loop of bowel or large blood vessel may be hidden within these inflammatory adhesions. Therefore, the extent of the sharp dissection or cauterization must be limited to those tissues that are under direct visualization.

Often the most difficult sources of bleeding to avoid in patients with acute cholecystitis is bleeding from the gallbladder fossa. These injuries occur because it is difficult to dissect between the posterior wall of the inflamed gallbladder and the small blood vessels within the liver bleed. If bleeding occurs it should be controlled immediately rather then waiting until the entire operative field is obscured. Often bleeding from within the liver bed can be controlled by judicious use of an electrocautery or laser energy device. The former modality appears to be more effective in controlling this type of bleeding, but once again, care must be taken to avoid injuring adjacent structures. Multiple, small superficial bleeding vessels may also be controlled by applying a collagen-like material to the liver bed. Avatine (MedChem Products Inc., Woburn, MA) is now available in a special applicator designed to simplify its application through a laparoscopic cannula. This material is placed in direct contact with the bleeding surface and held in place for several minutes. Bleeding vessels deep within the liver bed, however, may not be easily controlled with either electrocautery, laser coagulation, or collagen application. Although rarely necessary, the laparoscopic surgeon should develop the skills required to place occluding ligatures into the liver which can control such bleeding. If the injured vessel(s) cannot be controlled with such maneuvers, the procedure should be converted to an open laparotomy before other structures are injured or the patient's condition becomes unstable.

Prior to complete dissection of the gallbladder from the liver the peritoneal cavity should be copiously irrigated with saline and the operative field examined for any signs of persistent bleeding or bile leaks. With the gallbladder still attached to the liver the surgeon can easily maintain the proper exposure to inspect the gallbladder fossa and to ensure that the clips or sutures securing the duct and artery remain in place. If the gallbladder has already been freed from the liver, a fan-like retractor should be used to expose the opera-

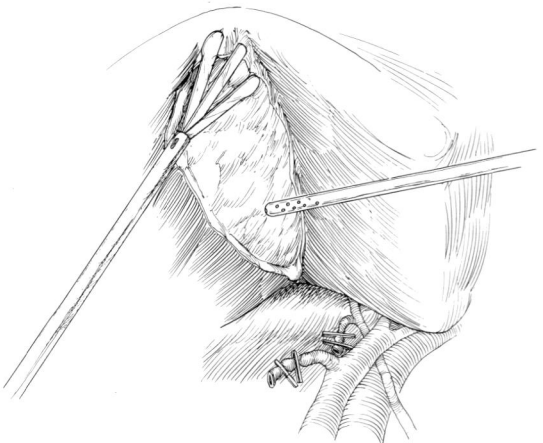

Figure 17-22. A fan-like retractor may be used to expose the liver bed if the gallbladder has been completely detached.

tive field (Fig. 17-22). A careful examination of the abdomen should be conducted to exclude other possible sources of bleeding or previously unrecognized bowel injuries.

We have rarely placed closed suction drains following elective laparoscopic cholecystectomy but have used them more often when operating on patients with acute cholecystitis. Indications for placing drainage catheters include bile spillage, persistent bile leakage, or bleeding from the liver bed. Although even moderate amounts of bleeding or bile loss from the liver bed should be controlled intraoperatively, occasionally persistent drainage of small quantities may be successfully managed with placement of closed suction catheters. This is especially true when a patient with an acutely inflamed gallbladder undergoes an operation. Smaller, closed suction drainage catheters may be introduced through the lateral 5.0-mm cannula (Fig. 17-23). The tip of the catheter is then held in place along the liver bed while the cannula is removed. Larger drains may be introduced through the upper midline 10/11-mm cannula, and after the pneumoperitoneum is reestablished, the distal portion of the catheter is appropriately positioned. The opposite end is then brought out through the lateral 5.0-mm sheaths and secured to the skin. With either technique the catheter should be trimmed to the desired length before inserting it into the abdomen.

Closed suction drains should be removed when they are no longer functioning. If the patient's postoperative course is uncomplicated, the catheters are usually removed within 24 to 48 hours.

After complete detachment of the gallbladder from the liver the video laparoscope is removed and replaced through the upper 10/11-mm cannula. This allows the surgeon to remove the gallbladder through the umbilical fascial defect (Fig. 17-24). The neck of the gallbladder is grasped with a larger (10/11 mm), penetrating forceps introduced through the umbilical cannula. As the gallbladder is pulled through the umbilical fascial defect, the entire sheath and forceps are removed from the abdomen. The neck of the gallbladder is then secured with a Kelly or Kocher clamp and pulled from the abdomen. In many patients operated upon for acute cholecystitis the gallbladder may not be easily removed through the standard umbilical fascial defect. This is especially true if the tissues are edematous and inflamed or, if the gallbladder contains very large stones. In such circumstances the periumbilical skin incision should be extended and the fascial opening dilated (Fig. 17-25). If the adjacent recti muscles are not incised, such a maneuver will result in minimal additional postoperative pain or cosmetic disfigurement. Recently, instruments designed to mechanically fragment

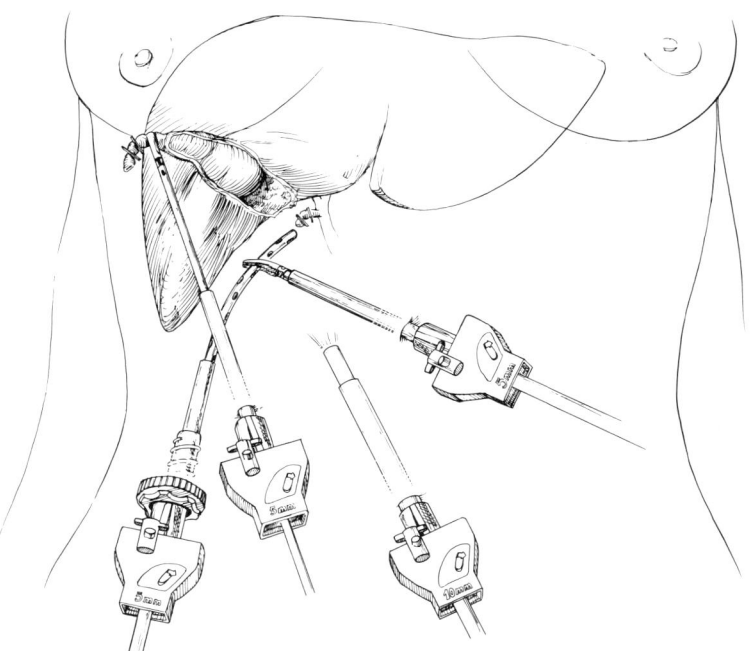

Figure 17-23. A small (5.5 mm or smaller diameter) closed suction drainage catheter may be inserted through the lateral cannula and positioned within the abdomen.

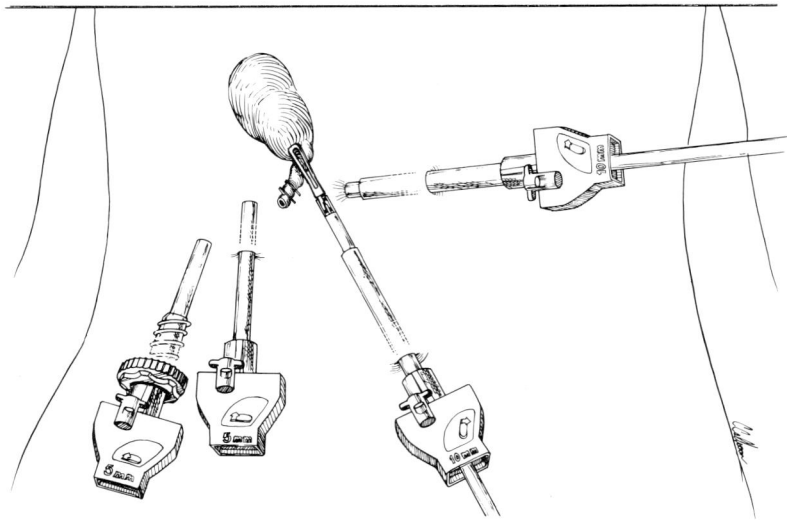

Figure 17-24. The laparoscope and attached video camera are moved to the upper midline cannula, and the gallbladder is extracted through the umbilical fascial defect.

large calculi while still within the gallbladder to facilitate their removal have become available (LaparoLith, Baxter Healthcare Corporation, Irvine, CA). Although the experience with such devices is still limited, their use is not recommended in the setting of acute cholecystitis because of the risk of peritoneal contamination. If the gallbladder has been torn and there is the possibility of further spillage during extraction, the gallbladder should be placed first within a sterile bag or glove. This will allow the gallbladder to be removed without additional stones, bile, or purulent fluid escaping into the peritoneal cavity.

Following gallbladder removal the remaining carbon dioxide is expelled from the abdomen and the umbilical fascial opening is closed with one or more large, absorbable sutures. This fascial defect is often distended beyond the initial 10 or 11 mm during gallbladder removal and failure to close this opening may lead to future hernia formation. The other 10/11-mm fascial openings are not routinely sutured unless the fascial defects are easily visualized. We do not advocate further extension of the skin incisions to close these accessary punctures because the likelihood of any subsequent problems is extremely low.

The urinary catheter is generally removed in the recovery room if the patient's condition appears to be stable. The nasogastric tube is not routinely removed at this time because many patients operated upon for acute cholecystitis will manifest signs of postoperative ileus. Usually this resolves within 24 to 48 hours. Intravenous antibiotics are continued postoperatively until the patient is afebrile and the white blood cell count returns to normal. Oral antibiotic therapy is then continued for 7 to 10 days.

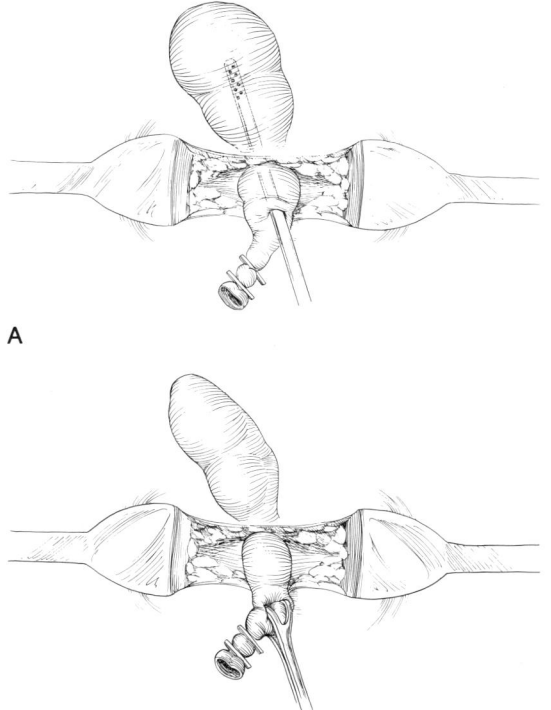

Figure 17-25. Enlarging the fascial defect will allow for the extraction of a thickened gallbladder (*top*) or one containing very large stones (*bottom*).

Table 17-1. Published Series Dealing with Laparoscopic Management of Acute Pancreatitis

Author (Ref.)	Number of Patients	Conversion to Laparotomy (%)	Length of Hospitalization (days)	Morbidity[a] (%)	Mortality (%)
Flowers et al.[2]	15	33	2.2	13	0
Unger[3][b]	55	7	2.6	11	0
Jacobs et al.[4][c]	79	15	4.0	1	0

[a] No major bile duct injuries were reported in three series.

[b] Approximately 25 per cent of patients underwent elective surgery and were then found to have evidence of acute cholecystitis at the time of laparoscopy.

[c] Authors did not indicate number of unplanned admissions.

Discussion

Although laparoscopic surgery has rapidly replaced traditional open laparotomy for the management of symptomatic gallbladder disease, there have been very few published reports dealing with its role in the management of acute cholecystitis. In a recent review of over 11,000 published laparoscopic cholecystectomies only 3 per cent were performed as emergencies. Findings from three articles that have specifically addressed this issue are summarized in Table 17-1.

In each of these series the conversion rate to open laparotomy was much higher than that reported for elective laparoscopic cholecystectomy (usually 5 per cent or less). Therefore, surgeons attempting to perform laparoscopic intervention in such patients should maintain a low threshold for aborting the procedure in favor of an open laparotomy. At our institution the general policy is that if the surgical team has not made significant progress in identifying the biliary anatomy within 1 hour, the procedure is converted to an open laparotomy. If the ductal and vascular structures are being demonstrated without undue difficulty, however, the procedure is continued well beyond this time frame. The average length of the operative procedure in the setting of acute inflammation in our experience has been approximately 2 hours (which includes intraoperative cholangiography).

Patients undergoing laparoscopic management of acute cholecystitis appear to enjoy many of the same benefits realized by those operated upon electively. The hospital stay is reduced with most patients returning home within 72 hours of surgery as compared to 7 days or more following open cholecystectomy. Patients also experience far less postoperative discomfort and are able to return to normal activities within 7 to 10 days of discharge. The most important issue, however, is that patients undergoing laparoscopic surgery for acute cholecystitis do not appear to be at a greater risk for major ductal or vascular injuries compared to those operated upon electively.

REFERENCES

1. Cameron JC, Gadacz TR. Laparoscopic cholecystectomy. Ann Surg 1991; 213:1–2.
2. Flowers JA, Bailey RW, Zucker KA. Laparoscopic management of acute cholecystitis: The Baltimore experience. Am J Surg 1991; 161:388–392.
3. Unger SW, Edelman DS, Scott JS, Unger HM. Laparoscopic treatment of acute cholecystitis. Surg Laparosc Endosc 1991; 1:14–16.
4. Jacobs M, Verdeja JC, Goldstein HS. Laparoscopic cholecystectomy in acute cholecystitis. Laparoendoscopy 1991; 1:174–175.
5. Hasnain JU, Matjesko J. Practical anesthesia for laparoscopic procedures. In Zucker KA, ed. Surgical Laparoscopy. St. Louis, Quality Medical Publishing, 1991, pp 77–86.
6. Zucker KA. Laparoscopic cholecystectomy using electrocautery dissection. In Zucker KA, ed. Surgical Laparoscopy. St. Louis, Quality Medical Publishing, 1991, pp 144–171.
7. Soper NJ, Dunnegan DL. Does intraoperative gallbladder perforation influence the early outcome of laparoscopic cholecystectomy? Surg Laparosc Endosc 1991; 1:156–161.
8. Cedric S, Rosengard B, Zucker KA. Persistent draining sinus tract following laparoscopic cholecystectomy. Surg Laparosc Endosc In press.
9. Cooperman AV. Laparoscopic cholecystectomy for severe acute, embedded and gangrenous cholecystitis. Laparoendoscopy 1990; 1:37–40.
10. Reddick E, Olsen D. Laparoscopic laser cholecystectomy: A comparison with mini-cholecystectomy. Surg Endosc 1989; 3:34–39.
11. Zucker KA, Bailey RW, Gadacz TR, Imbembo AL. Laparoscopic cholecystectomy: A plea for cautious enthusiasm. Am J Surg 1991; 161:36–44.
12. Corbitt JA. Laparoscopic cholecystectomy: Laser versus electrosurgery. Surg Laparosc Endosc 1991; 1:85–88.
13. Hertzmann P. Thermal instrumentation for laparoscopic general surgical procedures. In Zucker KA, ed. Surgical Laparoscopy. St. Louis, Quality Medical Publishing 1991, pp 57–75.

Chapter 18
Laparoendoscopic Management of Common Bile Duct Stones

Scott M. Graham
Thomas R. Scott

Over the past two decades, surgery has had a less prominent role in the management of common bile duct stones. Although good results for surgical treatment of choledocholithiasis have been reported,[1-15] the high complication rate among elderly and medically compromised patients[7,16] has been the motivation for less invasive approaches to the biliary tract. Endoscopic sphincterotomy has become established as the primary therapy for retained or recurrent choledocholithiasis. When this is unsuccessful, a variety of percutaneous or endoscopically guided devices can improve the chances of stone extraction. Ultrathin fiberscopes can now direct procedures within the biliary tract. In addition, with the use of extracorporeal shock wave lithotripsy, contact dissolution, or a permanent biliary endoprosthesis surgical common bile duct exploration may be avoided. The advent of minimally invasive surgery, however, has introduced laparoscopic approaches to the common bile duct. Surgeons, once again, find themselves at the cutting edge of therapy for common bile duct stones.

This chapter will detail endoscopic and laparoscopic approaches to the common bile stone. Particular attention will be given to efficacy and safety. It is important to recognize, however, that strict recommendations are problematic as patients referred for surgical and nonsurgical treatment have not had the same spectrum of problems.[17,18] Nevertheless, it is hoped that this examination will provide the clinician with information to select a technique or combination of techniques that is most suitable for the individual with common bile duct stones.

NONSURGICAL TREATMENT OF COMMON BILE DUCT STONES

Percutaneous Endoscopic Techniques

A variety of techniques can be applied in the nonsurgical management of retained common bile duct stones. In patients in whom a T-tube is present, calculi can be retrieved through the T-tube tract. Preparation for stone retrieval through the T-tube tract begins at the time of surgery. The tube should be at least 14 French in diameter, and the route to the skin should be as short and straight as possible.

Although common duct stones have been extracted through the T-tube tract since 1962,[19] a percutaneous endoscopic approach was first reported in 1976.[20] The main advantage of the endoscopic approach is that it permits a direct and, therefore, more accurate assessment of suspected radiologic defects. By providing direct visualization, it also enables the safer use of a variety of lithotripsy devices. Numerous series attest to its safety and efficacy.[21-27]

One disadvantage of relying on the T-tube tract is the 4- to 6-week delay required to allow tract manipulation. Because of this, early endoscopic sphincterotomy is being used in patients with T-tubes and retained stones.[21,28-34] Both percutaneous and peroral endoscopic methods effectively clear the common bile duct in the patient with a T-tube. Sphincterotomy, however, may carry a slightly higher risk[32] than the percutaneous approach and therefore might be reserved for patients in whom the percutaneous method has failed or is contraindicated.[35]

Endoscopic Sphincterotomy

In 1972, an impacted bile duct stone was crudely delivered from the ampulla of Vater endoscopically with a biopsy forceps.[36] During the next 2 years a variety of electrocautery devices[37-41] designed to gain more reliable access to pathologic conditions involving the common bile duct were successfully applied. These innovations opened the way for interventional endoscopy to replace surgery as the standard therapy for retained common bile duct stones.

Although improvements and refinements have been made in equipment, the basic technique of endoscopic retrograde cholangiopancreatography (ERCP) and endoscopic sphincterotomy has changed very little. Essentially, a side-viewing duodenoscope is introduced into the upper gastrointestinal tract and positioned in front of the papilla. Under visual and radiologic guidance a sphincterotome is inserted into the common bile duct (Fig. 18-1). The most widely used sphincterotome is one in which an electrosurgical wire bows from the end of a flexible catheter. Other sphincterotomes, however, have been designed to accommodate circumstances such as the difficult papilla (precut or knife) or unusual anatomic structures (Billroth II reverse papillotome). A prerequisite for safe papillotomy is the radiographic demonstration of the instrument in the common bile duct. Once confirmed, tension is applied to the wire, causing it to elevate the roof of the papilla (Fig. 18-2). Blended or cutting current is applied in short bursts to produce a well controlled incision (Fig. 18-3). The length of the incision should rarely exceed 1.0 to 1.5 cm; however, this will be modified by local anatomic constraints. It is important to note that the larger the opening the greater

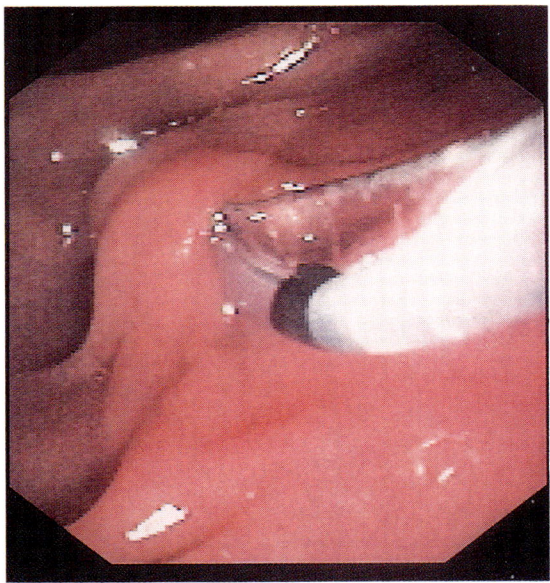

Figure 18-2. Once placement of the sphincterotome is confirmed, tension is applied to the cautery wire with elevation of the roof of the papilla.

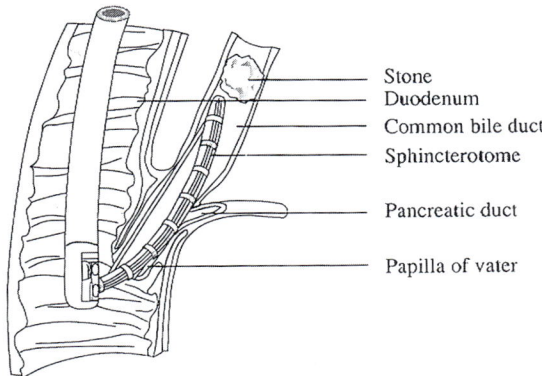

Figure 18-1. Diagram showing proper placement of a biliary sphincterotome into the common bile duct.

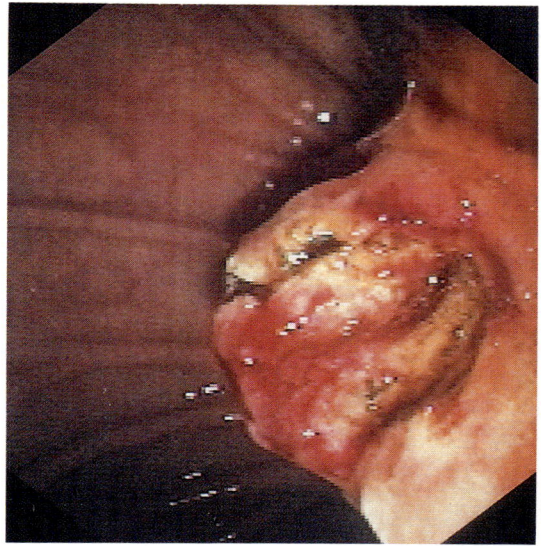

Figure 18-3. Completed sphincterotomy.

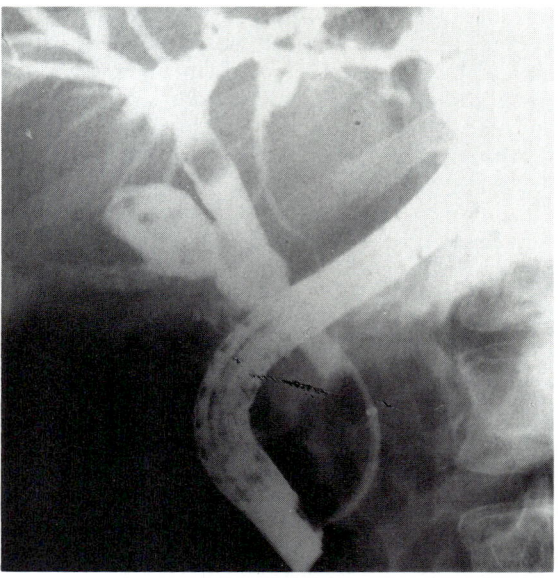

Figure 18-5. Balloon catheter approach for choledocholithiasis.

the risk of bleeding and retroduodenal perforation.

Once the sphincterotomy is completed, stones may be removed with the use of wire baskets and balloon catheters (Figs. 18-4 and 18-5). Most procedures are promptly completed by experienced surgeons; however, in up to 20 per cent of patients two or more procedures are required to extract stones.

The bile duct is cleared of stones in approximately 90 per cent of patients.[42] Anatomic restrictions such as prior gastric duodenal or biliary surgery and abnormalities of the papilla (Fig. 18-6) or duodenum account for the technical inability to achieve endoscopic sphincterotomy. Mechanical constraints such as a stone above a stricture, a large stone (greater than 1.5 cm), a common duct packed with stones, or inaccessible hepatic duct stones are common reasons why duct clearance fails (Fig. 18-7).

The immediate complications of endoscopic

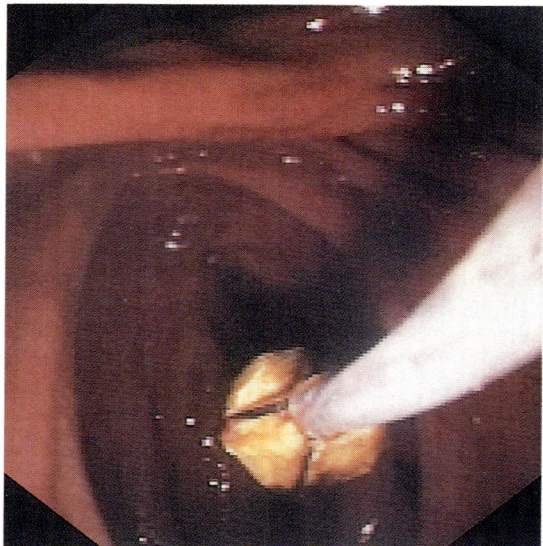

Figure 18-4. Common duct stone extracted with a wire basket.

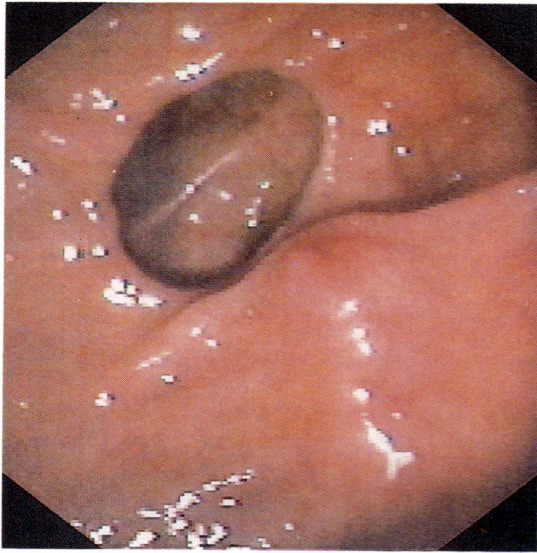

Figure 18-6. Juxtapapillary duodenal diverticulum may limit the safety of a sphincterotomy.

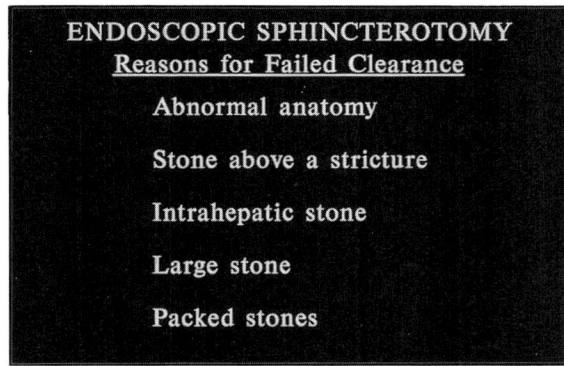

Figure 18-7. A list of the major obstacles to successful sphincterotomy and common duct stone clearance.

sphincterotomy include hemorrhage, cholangitis, pancreatitis, and perforation (Fig. 18-8). Such events can be anticipated in approximately 6 to 10 per cent of patients. The vast majority of these complications can be managed conservatively. Mortality is generally less than 2 per cent.[42,43]

The long term sequelae of sphincterotomy are related to cholangitis or jaundice from stricture formation or stone recurrence. Two studies[17,44] with the longest mean follow-up (49 and 96 months) show complication rates of 7 and 13 per cent, respectively. This suggests that, given sufficient time, the long term sequelae of sphincterotomy for common duct stones may be comparable to those of bile duct surgery.

Preoperative Endoscopic Sphincterotomy for Duct Clearance

There is little argument that endoscopic sphincterotomy is the procedure of choice for patients with acute cholangitis (Fig. 18-9, A and B) and retained common bile duct stones after cholecystectomy. Much debate, however, surrounds the idea of planned preoperative endoscopic sphincterotomy and duct clearance in the patient with suspected common bile duct stones and an intact gallbladder. Although the logic of this notion is compelling, its proven benefit remains unclear. Several retrospective studies favor preoperative endoscopic sphincterotomy.[45–47] Other studies,[5,48,52] three of which were prospective and randomized, have demonstrated either no advantage or some disadvantage with the use of preoperative biliary endoscopy.

Unfortunately, one cannot easily transfer these scholarly observations rooted in the prelaparoscopic era to guide current decision making. In the context of a patient's expectation of minimally invasive surgery, one can argue that the information gained by preoperative ERCP serves the desirable goal of diminishing the probability of open common duct exploration. Experience with this approach has been accumulating and indicates that stones are identified in one-third of patients in whom choledocholithiasis was clinically suspected (Fig. 18-10). Endoscopic sphincterotomy and duct clearance have been highly successful in reported cases with no significant morbidity and no mortality.[53–64] This information would appear to establish preoperative ERCP and sphincterotomy as a valid approach in patients with suspected common bile duct stones.

THE DIFFICULT COMMON BILE DUCT STONE REMOVAL

A number of endoscopically directed maneuvers can be used for common duct stones that cannot be removed with routine endoscopic sphincterotomy.[65] These include mechanical, electrohydraulic, and laser lithotripsy. In patients in whom sphincterotomy cannot be attained, a combined radiologic approach with a percutaneous transhepatic guide wire passed through the ampulla can

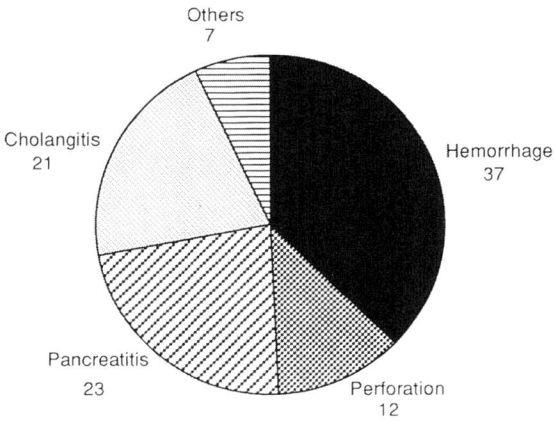

Figure 18-8. A graph illustrating the relative frequency of the major complications of endoscopic sphincterotomy.

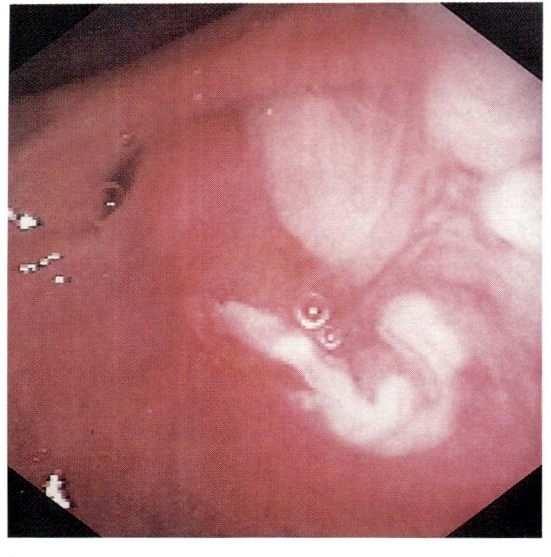 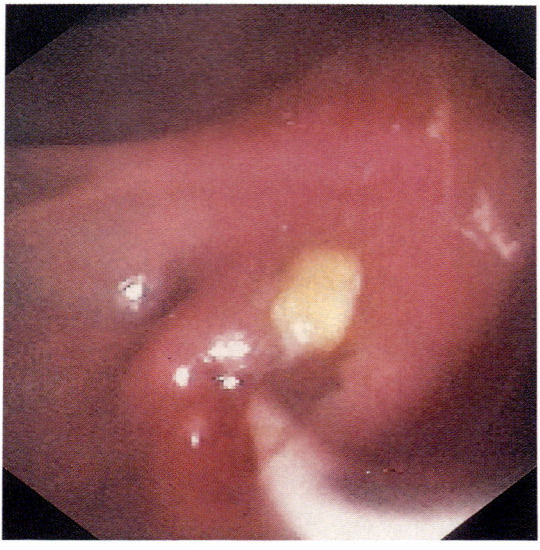

A B

Figure 18-9. A, Frank pus exiting the papilla of a patient with acute cholangitis due to choledocholithiasis. B, Postsphincterotomy removal of stones for acute cholangitis.

allow safe sphincterotomy (Fig. 18-11). Direct peroral endoscopic visualization of the pancreaticobiliary tree using ultrathin endoscopes passed through a duodenoscope can further facilitate bile duct manipulation[66] (Fig. 18-12, A and B). The integrated use of these modalities in conjunction with endoscopic sphincterotomy significantly improves ultimate duct clearance. It has been observed that with one or more of these methods nearly all patients can be treated successfully and probably

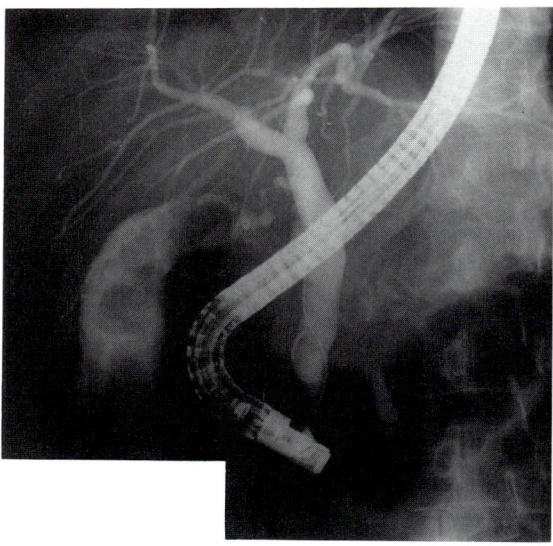

Figure 18-10. ERCP prior to laparoscopic cholecystectomy demonstrating choledocholithiasis. A guide wire has been placed to assist positioning of a sphincterotome.

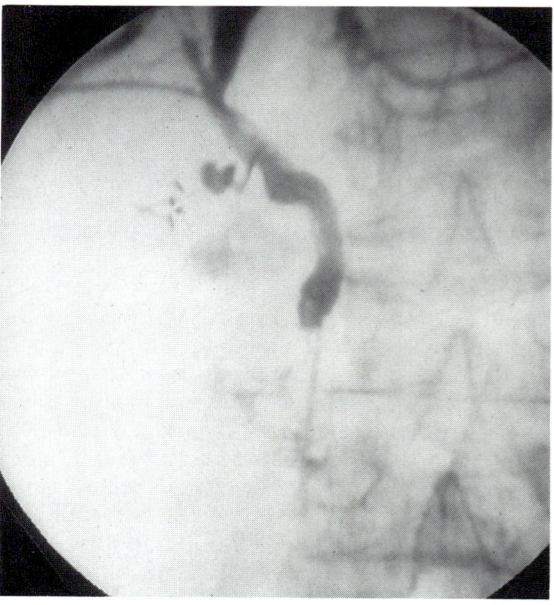

Figure 18-11. Percutaneous transhepatic placement of a catheter into the duodenum to assist endoscopic sphincterotomy and stone extraction in a patient with an abnormal periampullary anatomy.

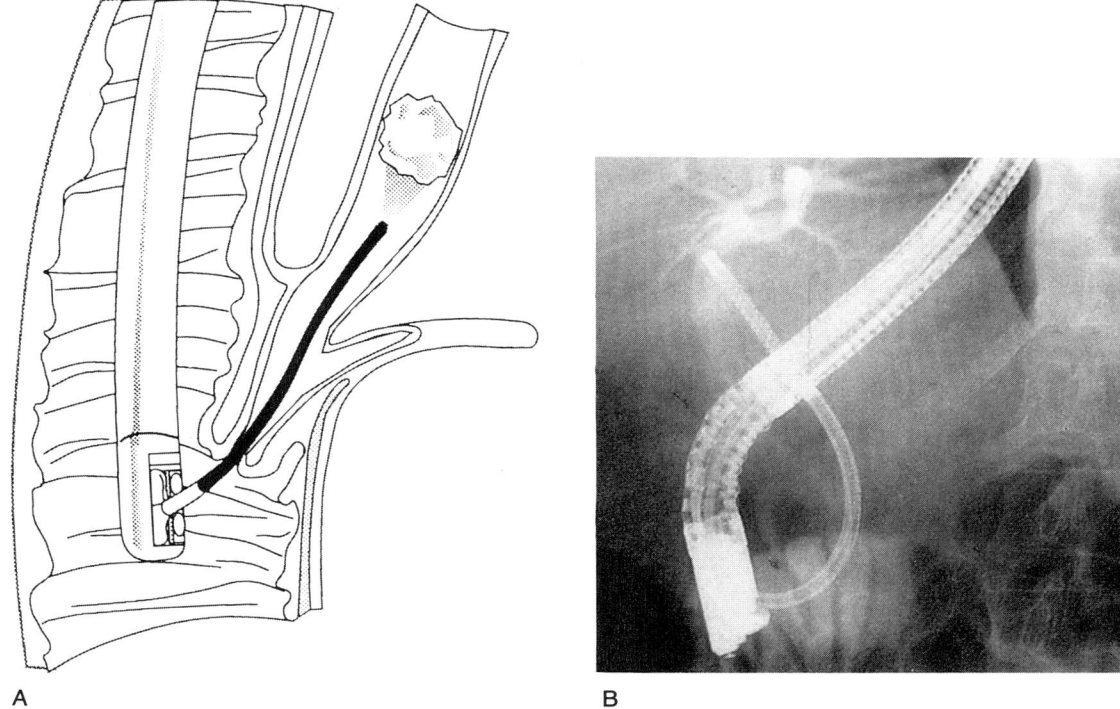

Figure 18-12. Diagram A, and radiographic B, demonstration of an ultrathin endoscope passed into the bile duct via the working channel of a duodenoscope.

fewer than 1 per cent of patients will require surgical exploration.[67] Duct clearance rates with these sophisticated methods vary between 70 and 90 per cent (Fig. 18-13). If surgery is contraindicated, the intransigent stone can be managed with a permanent endoscopically placed biliary stent.

Mechanical Lithotripsy

The first mechanical lithotriptor for common bile stones was introduced for clinical use[68,69] in 1982. This device is a heavy duty basket that is endoscopically guided into the common bile duct where it entraps a stone. The stone is then crushed by retracting the basket against the outer sheath of the apparatus. Following disintegration, the basket is removed and the rubble is evacuated (Fig. 18-14). With one exception,[70] ducts have been cleared in more than 80 per cent of attempts.[71-76] No center has reported significant morbidity, and no deaths have been attributed to this technique.

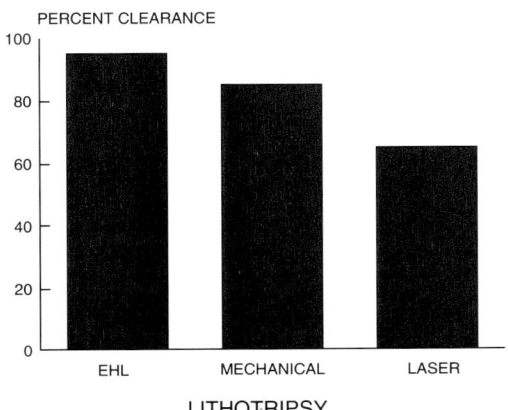

Figure 18-13. Graph summarizing the efficiency of three techniques of lithotripsy for difficult removal of common bile duct (CBD) stones.

Intracorporeal Electrohydraulic Lithotripsy

Intracorporeal electrohydraulic lithotripsy (EHL) has been used for urinary tract calculi for several decades. In 1975, Burhenne[77] suc-

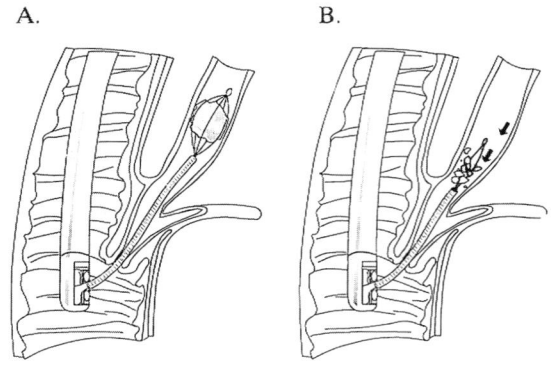

Figure 18-14. The technique of mechanical lithotripsy with which a stone within a sturdy basket A is crushed against a rigid coil spring sheath B.

cessfully used EHL to fragment a common bile duct stone through a T-tube tract under fluoroscopic guidance. This device creates a mechanical shock wave from an electrical discharge conducted in a fluid medium. This energy is absorbed by a stone within which pressure gradients and forces build with resultant fragmentation.

New basket and balloon EHL probes have been designed so that the electrode can be brought into direct contact with the target.[78,79] Saline must be infused into the bile duct to provide an ionic conducting medium for the electrical discharge. After confirming proper position fluoroscopically, the lithotriptor can be triggered (Fig. 18-15).

Despite precautions, a disadvantage of the fluoroscopic method is that it is relatively blind and absolute safety cannot be assured. Endoscopically guided EHL has been tried

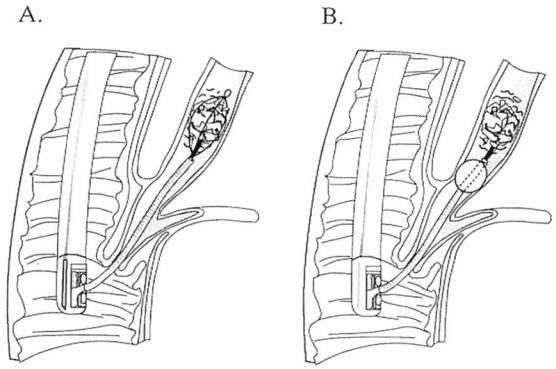

Figure 18-15. The technique of electrohydraulic lithotripsy with which the probe is centered against the stone with a basket A or balloon device B.

both percutaneously (T-tube or transhepatic) and perorally.[66] By either method, direct vision minimizes inadvertent injury by proper alignment of the probe. The results of cholangioscopic EHL indicate overall duct clearance of 90 per cent with no major morbidity or mortality.[70,80-89]

Endoscopic Laser Lithotripsy

A laser can be modified to deliver varying optical energies by manipulating its wavelength, pulse duration, pulse frequency, and pulse energy. The first laser used for common bile duct stones was a continuous wave neodymium-yttrium-aluminum-garnet (Nd:YAG) laser.[90] Its lack of efficacy, as well as a high potential for thermal injury, led to the development of pulsed laser systems that generate the power needed to fracture stones with less thermal dispersion.

Pulsed Nd:YAG and pulsed dye lasers are now in clinical use. As with EHL, the safest approach for directing laser energy is by cholangioscopy. Accumulated experience with endoscopic laser lithotripsy shows the rate of ductal clearance to be approximately 70 per cent.[91-95] The most recent experiences have improved the favorable outcome to 86 per cent.[93-95] Thus far there are no significant procedure-related complications or deaths. New devices in the early phases of development such as quality-switched Nd:YAG, alexandrite, erbium YAG, frequency doubled Nd:YAG and titan-sapphire lasers[96] may offer advantages over present technology.

THE INTRANSIGENT COMMON BILE STONE

A common bile duct stone will occasionally defy the surgeon's exhaustive attempts at retrieval. At this time, nonendoscopic methods such as extracorporeal shock wave lithotripsy[97] or contact solvents[98] may alleviate the problem. Other options for the intransigent common bile duct stone include surgery for the patient considered a good anesthetic risk and permanent biliary endoprosthesis for the patient considered a poor operative risk or the one with a short life expectancy.

Hollow stents of varying diameters and designs are placed through the papilla into the common bile duct over a guide wire with a positioning tube. The intracholedochal end is seated proximal to the obstruction and the distal end exits through the papilla into the duodenum (Fig. 18-16). Long term assessment of this therapy indicates that this conservative approach can be regarded as a definitive option in elderly high risk patients with unextractable stones.[99-104] An algorithm for the endoscopically directed management of retained common duct stones is suggested in Figure 18-17.

LAPAROSCOPIC MANAGEMENT OF COMMON BILE DUCT STONES

Laparoscopic Cholangiography

Cystic duct cholangiography can be performed during the course of laparoscopic cholecystectomy. Details of this method are presented later. Currently, opinions regarding its use are divided. Those who advocate its routine use[105] insist that it is a priority to identify both abnormal ductal anatomic features to avoid a surgical misadventure and to detect unsuspected common bile duct stones. As confidence with the safety of laparoscopic cholecystectomy grew, the routine use of

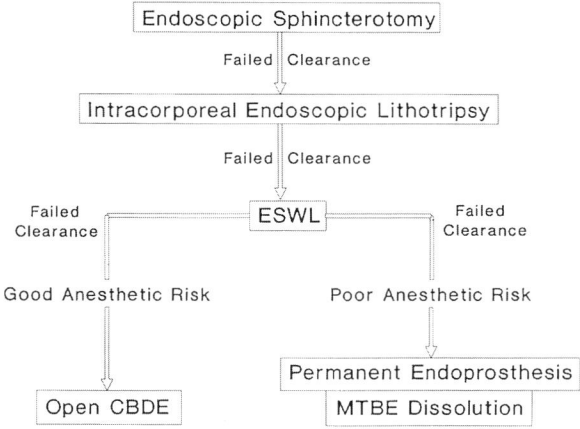

Figure 18-17. An algorithm for the management of retained common bile duct stones. ESWL, extracorporeal shock wave lithotripsy; CBDE, common bile duct exploration; MTBE, Methyl tertiary butyl ether.

cholangiography seemed less compelling and calls for selective use were heard.[62,106] Although debate will continue, a consensus statement of the National Institutes of Health requires surgeons to be familiar with the use of intraoperative cholangiography.[107] Intraoperative cholangiography during laparoscopic cholecystectomy has detected occult common duct stones in approximately 5 per cent of patients.[53-56,108-111]

Laparoscopic Common Bile Duct Exploration

When a common bile stone is encountered at cholangiography (Fig. 18-18), two options are available to the surgeon: delayed or immediate management. Delayed treatment includes observation or postoperative endoscopic retrieval. Immediate management includes common bile duct exploration (open or laparoscopic).

There are few data to support observation of common bile duct stones, although some have suggested that very small stones (less than 3.0 mm) might pass spontaneously or remain innocuous.[112] In the past, if a common bile duct stone was identified during open cholecystectomy, the common duct was explored. There is no reason why this time-honored approach should be relaxed during the laparoscopic era.

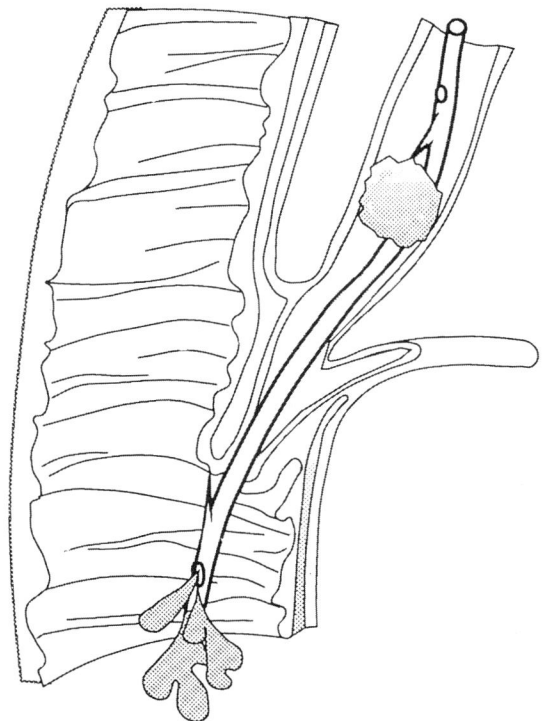

Figure 18-16. Diagram of the endoscopic placement of a biliary stent to drain a common duct obstructed by a stone.

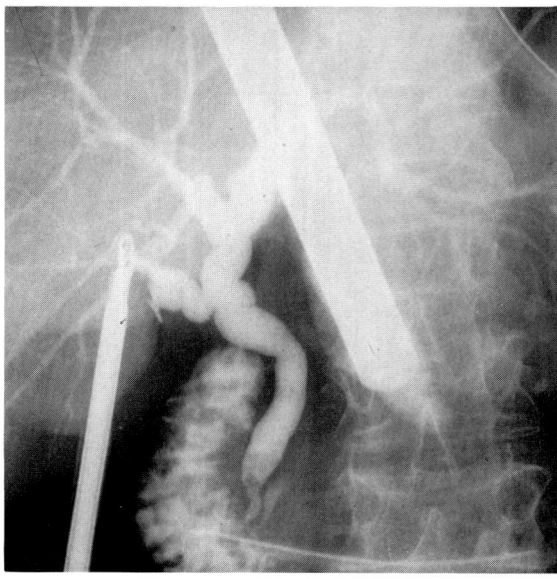

Figure 18-18. Laparoscopic intraoperative cholangiogram demonstrating unsuspected common duct stones.

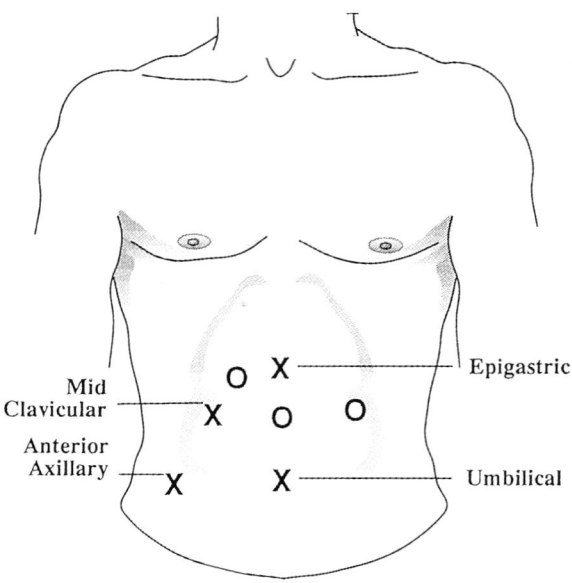

Figure 18-19. Diagram indicating the possible sites (O) for additional ports for transcystic or direct common duct exploration.

Two techniques for the laparoscopic clearance of common bile duct stones are in common use: indirect and direct. The indirect approach uses the cystic duct as a conduit to the common bile duct. Through the cystic duct catheters, balloons and baskets can be inserted, preferably with fluoroscopic assistance or under direct vision with a choledochoscope. In either case, an additional working port is often required to direct these maneuvers (Fig. 18-19). The cystic duct may need to be enlarged with rigid or balloon dilators to accommodate instruments (Figs. 18-20 and 18-21). Once visualized, stones can be extracted or advanced into the duodenum. The use of the flexible ultrathin choledochoscope allows greater security and safety in approaching common duct stones (Figs. 18-22 and 18-23, A and B). At the conclusion of the duct exploration the cystic duct can simply be ligated.

Direct laparoscopic choledochotomy requires additional dissection to define the anterior common duct wall and cystic duct-common duct junction (Fig. 18-24). Then, a longitudinal incision is made in the common duct for a distance of 1.0 to 2.0 cm, and exploration can proceed. At the conclusion of the exploration, a T-tube is placed, and the duct is securely closed with intracorporeal su-

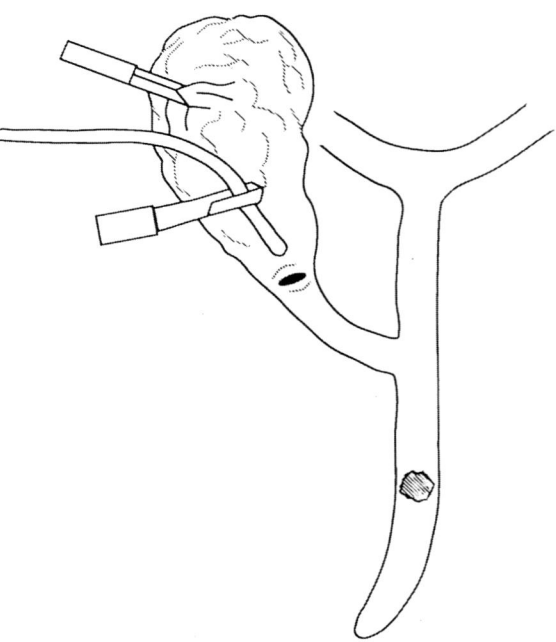

Figure 18-20. The cystic duct can be enlarged with rigid dilators to accommodate instruments for common duct manipulation.

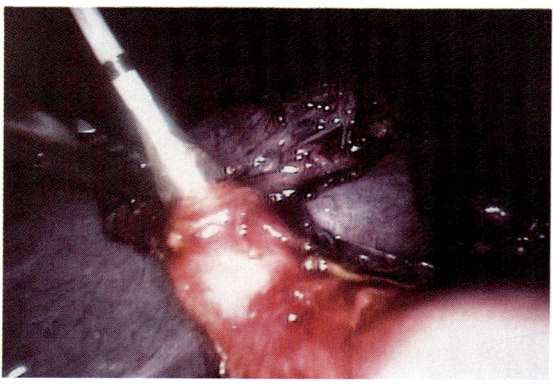

Figure 18-21. Photograph of a balloon dilation of the cystic duct in preparation for transcystic common duct exploration.

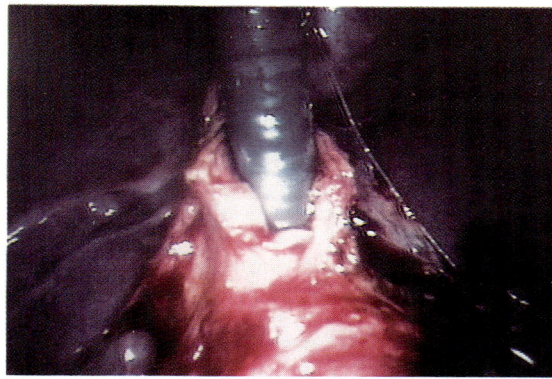

Figure 18-22. Photograph of a choledochoscope entering the cystic duct.

turing techniques (Fig. 18-25). Instruments for the efficient placement of T-tubes have been devised[113] (Fig. 18-26). It is recommended that a small drain be placed in the region of Morrison's pouch to control any drainage. It is evident that formal laparoscopic choledochotomy requires significant technical expertise and dexterity to be safely performed. Therefore, the surgeon who embarks on this approach must have considerable laparoscopic skill and confidence.

Published data on the laparoscopic management of common bile duct stones are still limited.[55,109,114–120] Excellent results, however, have been reported from centers with a special interest in advanced laparoscopic techniques. The majority of stones are being removed by the transcystic approach.

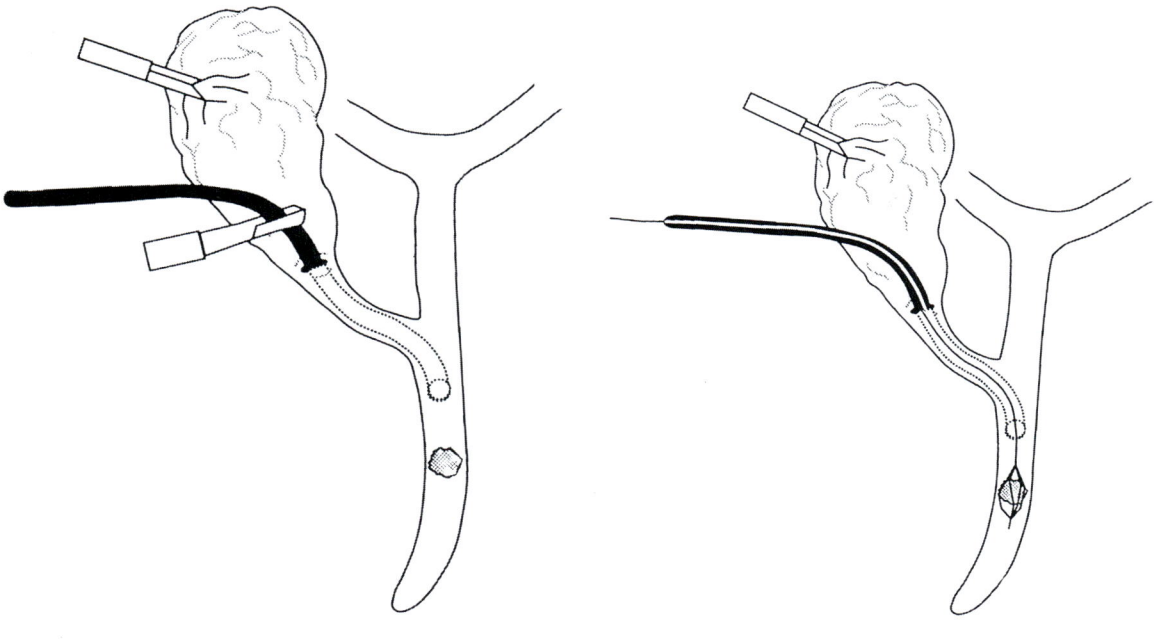

Figure 18-23. Representation of transcystic duct choledochoscopy A, and common duct stone extraction B.

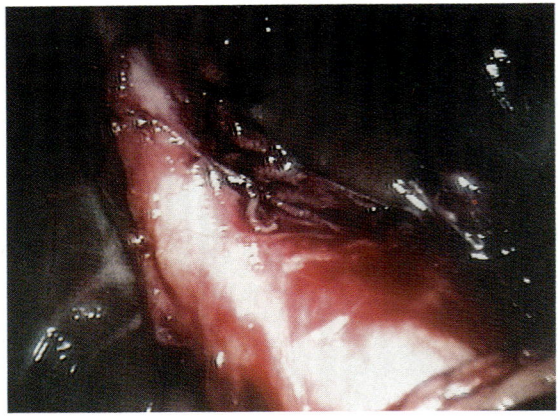

Figure 18-24. Photograph showing the common duct-cystic duct junction.

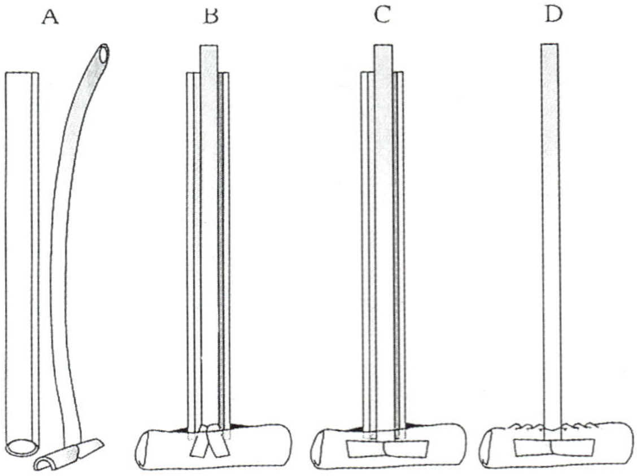

Figure 18-26. A method facilitating the laparoscopic placement of a T-tube.

If neither of these techniques is feasible, the surgeon may convert to an open common duct exploration. Patients selected for laparoscopic surgery are, by definition, considered good anesthetic risks and should tolerate an open procedure. An alternative, however, is to conclude the laparoscopic cholecystectomy and plan for a postoperative endoscopic extraction of retained stones. Intraoperative ERCP and sphincterotomy have been reported but with significant complications and inconsistent results.[110,117]

Experience with planned postlaparoscopic endoscopic sphincterotomy is limited,[53,55,58,61,114,115,121–123] yet in the vast majority of patients ductal clearance was successful and an open choledochotomy was avoided (Fig. 18-27). There has been no major morbidity or mortality associated with this approach. In addition, in several patients retained stones after unsuccessful laparoscopic common duct exploration have been successfully retrieved endoscopically.[116] Figure 18-28

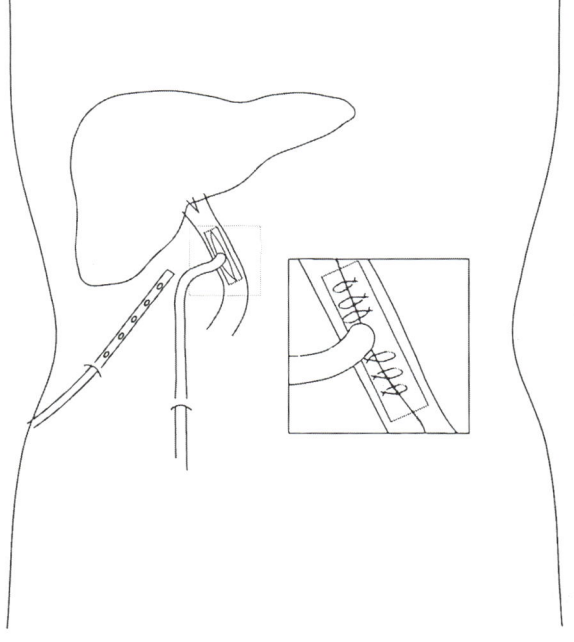

Figure 18-25. At the conclusion of common duct exploration, the choledochotomy is closed around a T-tube and a separate drain is placed in Morrison's pouch.

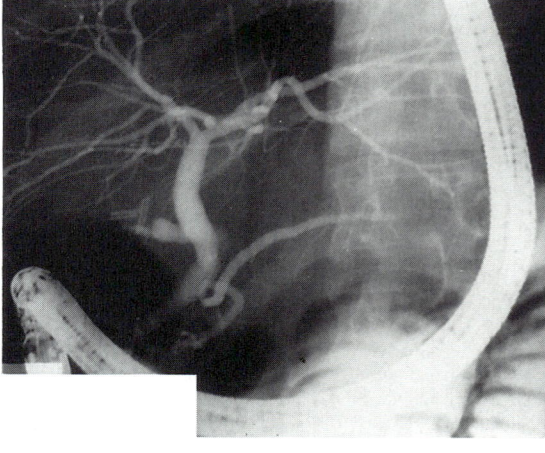

Figure 18-27. ERCP after laparoscopic cholecystectomy showing a retained common duct stone.

THE UNSUSPECTED COMMON BILE DUCT STONE

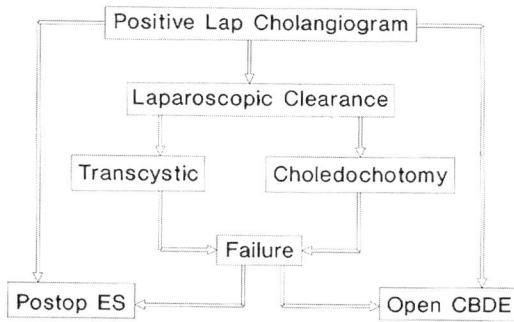

Figure 18-28. An algorithm for the management of common duct stones discovered by laparoscopic cholangiography. ES, endoscopic sphincterotomy; CBDE, common bile duct exploration.

suggests an algorithm for management of the common duct stone discovered during laparoscopic surgery.

REFERENCES

1. Pappas TN, Slimane TB, Brooks DC. 100 consecutive common duct explorations without mortality. Ann Surg 1990; 211:260–262.
2. Miller JS, Ferguson CM. Current management of choledocholithiasis. Ann Surg 1990; 56:66–70.
3. Thompson JE, Bennion RS. The surgical management of impacted common bile duct stones without sphincter ablation. Arch Surg 1989; 124:1216–1220.
4. Braghetto I, Csendes A, de la Cuadra R, et al. Treatment of residual common bile duct stones after cholecystectomy. Hepatogastroentology 1989; 36:123–127.
5. Miller BM, Kozarek RA, Ryan JA, et al. Surgical versus endoscopic management of common bile duct stones. Ann Surg 1988; 207:135–141.
6. Ganey JB, Johnson PA, Prillaman PE, McSwain GR. Cholecystectomy: Clinical experience with a large series. Am J Surg 1986; 151:352–357.
7. Roukema JA, Carol EJ, Liem F, Jakimowicz JJ. A retrospective study of surgical common bile duct exploration: Ten years experience. Neth J Surg 1986; 38:11–14.
8. Broughan TA, Sivak MV, Hermann RE. The management of retained and recurrent bile duct stones. Surgery 1985; 98:746–751.
9. Rogers AI, Farha GJ, Beamer RL, Chang FC. Incidence and associated mortality of retained common bile duct stones. Am J Surg 1985; 150:690–693.
10. Ratych RE, Sitzmann JV, Lillemoe KD, et al. Transduodenal exploration of the common bile duct in patients with nondilated ducts. Surg Gynecol Obstet 1991; 173:49–53.
11. Escudero-Fabre A, Escallon A, Sack J, et al. Choledochoduodenostomy: Analysis of 71 cases followed for 5 to 15 years. Ann Surg 1991; 213:635–644.
12. Gonma DJ, Konsten J, Soeters PB, et al. Long-term follow-up after choledochojejunostomy for bile duct stones with complex clearance of the bile duct. Br J Surg 1989; 76:451–453.
13. Baker AR, Neoptolemos JP, Leese T, Fossard DP. Choledochoduodenostomy, transduodenal sphincteroplasty and sphincterotomy for calculi of the common bile duct. Surg Gynecol Obstet 1987; 164:245–251.
14. Finan PJ, Hegarty JH, Donaldson DR, et al. Transduodenal exploration of the common bile duct. J R Coll Surg Edinb 1985; 30:34–38.
15. Ramsay G, Hehir M, McNeill AD. Routine transduodenal sphincterotomy for common bile duct exploration. J R Coll Surg Edinb 1985; 30:348–352.
16. Burdiles P, Csendes A, Diaz JC, et al. Factors affecting mortality in patients over 70 years of age submitted to surgery for gallbladder or common bile duct stones. Hepatogastroenterology 1989; 36:136–139.
17. Hawes RH, Cotton PB, Vallon AA. Follow-up 6 to 11 years after duodenoscopic sphincterotomy for stones in patients with prior cholecystectomy. Gastroenterology 1990; 98:1008–1012.
18. Cotton PB. Endoscopic management of bile duct stones (apples and oranges). Gut 1984; 25:587–597.
19. Mondet A. Tecnica de la extraccion incruenta de los calculos en la litiasis residual del coledoco. Bol Soc Cir 1962; 46:278–290.
20. Yamakawa T. Improved choledochofiberoscopic and nonsurgical removal of retained biliary calculi under direct visual control. Gastrointest Endosc 1976; 22:160.
21. Nussinson E, Cairns SR, Dowsett J. A 10-year single center experience of percutaneous and endoscopic extraction of stones with T-tube in situ. Gut 1991; 32:1040–1043.
22. Moss JP, Whelan JG, Dedman TC, Voyles RC. Postoperative choledochoscopy through the T-tube tract. Surg Gynecol Obstet 1980; 151:807–809.
23. Birkett DH, Williams LF. Postoperative fiber optic choledochoscopy. A useful surgical adjunct. Ann Surg 1981; 194:630–634.
24. Chen MF, Chou FF, Wang CS, Jan YY. Experience with and complications of postoperative choledochofiberoscopy for retained biliary stones. Acta Chir Scand 1982;148:503–509.
25. Chen MF, Jan YY. Percutaneous transhepatic removal of common bile duct and intrahepatic duct stones with a fiberoptic choledoscope. Gastrointest Endosc 1986; 32:347–349.
26. Yamakawa T. Percutaneous cholangioscopy for management of retained biliary tract stones and intrahepatic stones. Endoscopy 1989; 21:333–337.
27. Berci G, Hamlin JA. Intraoperative and postoperative biliary endoscopy (choledochoscopy). Endoscopy 1989; 21:279–284.
28. Soehendra N, Cempeneers I, Eichfuss HP. Early postoperative endoscopy after biliary tract surgery. Endoscopy 1981; 13:113–117.
29. Simpson CJ, Gray GR, Gillespie G. Early endoscopic sphincterotomy for retained common bile duct stones. J R Coll Surg Edinb 1985; 30:288–289.
30. O'Doherty DP, Neoptolemos JP, Carr-Locke DL. Endoscopic sphincterotomy for retained common bile duct stones in patients with T-tube in situ in the early postoperative period. Br J Surg 1986; 73:454–456.
31. Bickerstaff KI, Berry AR, Chapman RW. Early postoperative endoscopic sphincterotomy for retained

biliary stones. Ann R Coll Surg Engl 1988; 70:350–351.
32. Lambert ME, Martin DF, Tweedle DEF. Endoscopic removal of retained stones after biliary surgery. Br J Surg 1988; 75:896–898.
33. Danilowitz MD. Early postoperative endoscopic sphincterotomy for retained common bile duct stones. Gastrointest Endosc 1989; 35:298–299.
34. Tandon RK, Nijhawan S, Aurora A. Management of retained common bile duct stones in patients with T-tube in situ: Role of endoscopic sphincterotomy. Am J Gastroenterol 1990; 85:1126–1131.
35. Cotton PB. Retained bile duct stones: T-tube in place: Percutaneous or endoscopic management? Am J Gastroenterol 1990; 85:1075–1078.
36. Anazawa W, Takagi K, Kuno S. Endoscopic removal of gallstone impacted in the major papilla: A case report. Stomach Intest 1972; 7:641.
37. Demling L. Operative endoscopy. Med Welt 1973; 24:1253.
38. Classen M, Demling L. Endoskopische sphincterotomie der papilla Vateri und stein extraction aus dem choledochos. Dtsch Med Wochenschr 1974; 99:496–497.
39. Sohma S. Endoscopic papillotomy: A new approach for extraction of residual stones. Gastrointest Endosc 1974; 16:446.
40. Kawai K. Preliminary report of endoscopic papillotomy. J Kyoto Pref Univ Med 1973; 82:353–355.
41. Kawai K, Akasaka Y, Murakamy K, et al. Endoscopic sphincterotomy of the ampulla of Vater. Gastrointest Endosc 1974; 20:148–151.
42. Sivak MV. Endoscopic management of bile duct stones. Am J Surg 1989; 158:228–240.
43. Cotton PB, Lehman G, Vennes J, et al. Endoscopic sphincterotomy complications and their management: An attempt at consensus. Gastrointest Endosc 1991; 37:383–393.
44. Jacobsen O, Matzen P. Long-term follow-up study of patients after endoscopic sphincterotomy for choledocholithiasis. Scand J Gastroenterol 1987; 22:903–906.
45. Heinerman PM, Boeckl O, Pimpl W. Selective ERCP and preoperative stone removal in bile duct surgery. Ann Surg 1989; 209:267–272.
46. Ponchon T, Bory R, Chavaillon A, Fouillet P. Biliary lithiasis: Combined endoscopic and surgical treatment. Endoscopy 1989; 21:15–18.
47. Stiegmann GV, Pearlman NW, Goff JS, et al. Endoscopic cholangiography and stone removal prior to cholecystectomy. A more cost effective approach than other operative duct exploration? Arch Surg 1989; 124:787–790.
48. Neoptolemos JP, Davidson BR, Shaw DE, et al. Study of common bile duct exploration and endoscopic sphincterotomy in a consecutive series of 438 patients. Br J Surg 1987; 74:916–921.
49. Neoptolemos JP, Carr-Locke DL, Fossard DP. Prospective randomized study of preoperative endoscopic sphincterotomy versus surgery alone for common bile duct stones. Br Med J 1987; 294:470–474.
50. Neoptolemos JP, Shaw DE, Carr-Locke DL. A multivariate analysis of preoperative risk factors in patients with common bile duct stones: Implications for treatment. Am Surg 1989; 209:157–161.
51. Stain SC, Cohen H, Tsuishoysha M, Donovan AJ. Choledocholithiasis endoscopic sphincterotomy or common bile duct exploration. Am Surg 1991; 213:627–634.
52. Stiegmann GV, Gough JS, Mansour A, et al. Precholecystectomy endoscopic cholangiography and stone removal is not superior to cholecystectomy, cholangiography and common duct exploration. Am J Surg 1992; 163:227–230.
53. Graves HA, Ballinger JF, Anderson WJ. Appraisal of laparoscopic cholecystectomy. Ann Surg 1991; 213:644–664.
54. Stockmann PT, Soper NJ. Early results of laparoscopic cholecystectomy at a teaching institution. Persp Gen Surg 1991; 2:1–19.
55. Larson GM, Vitale FC, Casey J, et al. Multipractice analysis of laparoscopic cholecystectomy in 1983 patients. Am J Surg 1992; 163:221–226.
56. The Southern Surgeons Club. A prospective analysis of 1518 laparoscopic cholecystectomies. N Engl J Med 1991; 324:1073–1078.
57. Arregui ME, Davis CJ, Arkush AM, Nagan RF. Laparoscopic cholecystectomy combined with endoscopic sphincterotomy and stone extraction or laparoscopic choledochoscopy and electrohydraulic lithotripsy for management of cholelithiasis and choledocholithiasis. Surg Endosc 1992; 6:10–15.
58. Baird DR, Wilson JP, Mason EM, et al. An early review of 800 laparoscopic cholecystectomies at university affiliated community teaching hospital. Am J Surg 1992; 58:206–210.
59. Ellul JPM, Wilkinson ML, McColl I, Dowling RH. A predictive ERCP study of patients with gallbladder stones (GBS) and probable choledocholithiasis—Predictive factors. Gastrointest Endosc 1992; 38:266.
60. Vanneman W, Kingsbury R, Duberman E, Lee M. When is ERCP indicated before laparoscopic cholecystectomy? Gastrointest Endosc 1992; 38:265.
61. Graham SM, Flowers JL, Scott TR, et al. Laparoscopic cholecystectomy and common bile duct stones: The utility of planned perioperative ERCP and sphincterotomy. Experience with 63 patients. Ann Surg In press.
62. Barkun JS, Barkun AN, Fried GM, et al. Cholecystectomy without operative cholangiography: Implications for common bile duct injury and retained common duct stones. In Proceedings of the American Surgical Association, pp 51–53, A-15.
63. Brodish RJ, Fink AS. ERCP, cholangiography and laparoscopic cholecystectomy: SAGES opinion survey. Surg Endosc 1993; 7:3–8.
64. Vitale GC, Larson GM, Wieman TJ, et al. The use of ERCP in the management of common bile duct stones in patients undergoing laparoscopic cholecystectomy. Surg Endosc 7:9–11.
65. Graham SM, Flowers JL, Zucker KA. Endoscopic management of the difficult common bile duct stone. Surg Laparoendosc 1993; 3:54–59.
66. Ponsky JL, Scheeres DE, Simar I. Endoscopic retrograde cholangioscopy: An adjunct to endoscopic exploration of the common bile duct. Am Surg 1990; 56:235–237.
67. Gadacz TR. Reoperation versus alternatives in retained biliary calculi. Surg Clin North Am 1991; 71:93–108.
68. Demling L, Seuberth K, Riemann JF. A new mechanical lithotriptor. Endoscopy 1982; 14:100–112.
69. Riemann JF, Seuberth K, Demling L. Clinical application of a new mechanical lithotriptor for smashing common bile duct stones. Endoscopy 1982; 14:226–230.
70. Liguory C, Lefebvre JF, Bonnel D, Vitale GC. Crushing stones; mechanical, intracorporeal and extracorporeal lithotripsy in the clearance of common bile duct lithiasis. Can J Gastroenterol 1990; 4:628–631.

71. Higuchi T, Kon Y. Endoscopic mechanical lithotripsy for the treatment of common bile duct stone: Experience with the improved double sheath basket. Endoscopy 1987; 19:216–217.
72. Schneider MU, Matek W, Bower R, Domschke W. Mechanical lithotripsy of bile duct stones in 209 patients: Effective technical advances. Endoscopy 1988; 20:244–253.
73. Siegel JH, Ben-Zvi JS, Pullano WE. Mechanical lithotripsy of common duct stones. Gastrointest Endosc 1990; 36:351–356.
74. Shaw MJ, Dorsher PJ, Vennes JA. A new mechanical lithotriptor for the treatment of large common bile duct stones. Am J Gastroenterol 1990; 85:796–798.
75. Chung SCS, Leung JWC, Leong HT, et al. Endoscopic extraction of large common duct stones using a mechanical lithotripsy basket. Gastrointest Endosc 1991; 37:252.
76. Van Dam J, Sivak MV. Endoscopic mechanical lithotripsy of common bile duct stones. Gastrointest Endosc 1991; 37:258.
77. Burhenne HJ. Electrohydraulic fragmentation of retained common duct stone. Radiology 1975; 117:721–722.
78. Koch H, Stolze N, Walze V. Endoscopic lithotripsy in the common duct. Endoscopy 1977; 9:95–98.
79. Manegold BC, Mennicken G, Jung M. Endoscopic electrohydraulic disintegration of common bile duct concrements. Presented at the World Congress of Gastroenterology, Stockholm, Abstract 573, 1982.
80. Koch H, Rosch W, Walz V. Endoscopic lithotripsy in the common bile duct. Gastrointest Endosc 1980; 26:16–18.
81. Riemann JF, Demling L. Lithotripsy of bile duct stones. Endoscopy 1983; 15:191–196.
82. Mo LR, Wang MH, Yueh SK, et al. Percutaneous transhepatic choledochoscopic electrohydraulic lithotripsy (PTCS-EHL) of common bile duct stones. Gastrointest Endosc 1988; 34:122–125.
83. Leung JWC, Chung SSC. Electrohydraulic lithotripsy with peroral choledochoscopy. Br Med J 1989; 299:595–598.
84. Yoshimoto H, Ikeda S, Tenaka M, et al. Choledochoscopic electrohydraulic lithotripsy and lithotomy for stones in the common bile duct, intrahepatic ducts and gallbladder. Ann Surg 1989; 210:576–582.
85. Fan ST, Choi TK, Wong J. Electrohydraulic lithotripsy for biliary stones. Aust N Z J Surg 1989; 59:217–221.
86. Picus D, Weyman PJ, Marx MV. Role of percutaneous intracorporeal electrohydraulic lithotripsy in the treatment of biliary tract calculi. Radiology 1989; 170:989–993.
87. Josephs LG, Birkett DH. Electrohydraulic lithotripsy (EHL) for the treatment of large retained common duct stones. Am Surg 1990; 56:232–234.
88. Siegel JH, Ben-Zvi JS, Pullano WE. Endoscopic electrohydraulic lithotripsy. Gastrointest Endosc 1990; 36:134–136.
89. Chen MF, Jan YY. Percutaneous transhepatic cholangioscopic lithotripsy. Br J Surg 1990; 77:530–532.
90. Orii K, Nakahara A, Takase Y, et al. Choledocholithotomy by YAG laser with a choledochofiberoscope: Case reports of two patients. Surgery 1981; 90:120–122.
91. Ell C, Lux G, Hochberger J, et al. Laser lithotripsy of common bile duct stones. Gut 1988; 29:746–751.
92. Cotton PB, Putnam WS, Weinerth J, et al. Endoscopic laser lithotripsy of large bile duct stones. Gastrointest Endosc 1989; 35:163.
93. Hawes RH, Kopeci KK, Lieman GL, Sherman S. Prospective evaluation of the utility and safety of the pulsed dye laser in the management of difficult bile duct stones. Gastrointest Endosc 1991; 37:257.
94. Neuhaus H, Hoffmann W, Hogrefe A, Classen M. Cholangioscopic dye laser lithotripsy in the nonsurgical treatment of difficult bile duct stones. Gastrointest Endosc 1991; 37:254.
95. Ponchon T, Gagnon P, Valette PJ, et al. Pulsed dye laser lithotripsy of bile duct stones. Gastrointest Endosc 1991; 37:250.
96. Hockberger J. Laser lithotripsy—The new wave. Can J Gastroenterol 1990; 4:632–636.
97. Sauerbruch T, Stern M. Fragmentation of bile duct stones by extracorporeal shock waves. A new approach to biliary calculi after failure of routine endoscopic measures. Gastroenterology 1989; 96:146–152.
98. Neoptolemos JP, Hofmann AF, Moosa AR. Chemical treatment of stones in the biliary tree. Br J Surg 1986; 73:515–524.
99. Siegel JH, Yatto RP. Biliary endoprosthesis for the management of retained common bile duct stones. Am J Gastroenterol 1984; 79:50–54.
100. Cotton PB, Forbes A, Leung JWC, Dineen L. Endoscopic stenting for long-term treatment of large bile duct stones: Two to five year follow-up. Gastrointest Endosc 1987; 33:411–412.
101. Van Steenbergen W, Pelemans W, Ponette E, Feveri J. Endoscopic biliary endoprosthesis as definitive treatment of elderly patients with large bile duct stones. Neth J Med 1987; 30:107–116.
102. Kiil J, Cruse A, Rokkjaer M. Large bile duct stones treated by endoscopic biliary drainage. Surgery 1989; 105:51–56.
103. Foutch PG, Harland J, Sanowsky RA. Endoscopic placement of biliary stents for treatment of high risk geriatric patients with common duct stones. Am J Gastroenterol 1989; 84:527–529.
104. Soomers AJ, Nagengast FM, Yap SH. Endoscopic placement of biliary endoprosthesis in patients with endoscopically unextractable common bile duct stones: A long-term follow-up study of 26 patients. Endoscopy 1990; 22:24–26.
105. Flowers JL, Zucker KA, Graham SM, et al. Laparoscopic cholangiography: Results and indications. Ann Surg 215:209–216.
106. Soper NJ. Selective cholangiography during laparoscopic cholecystectomy. Presented at the Society of American Gastrointestinal Endoscopic Surgeons Postgraduate Course: Advances in Laparoscopic Surgery, 1991, Monterey, CA.
107. National Institutes of Health Consensus Development Conference Statement: Gallstones and laparoscopic cholecystectomy. J Laparoendosc Surg 1993; 3:77–90.
108. Bailey RW, Zucker KA, Flowers JL, et al. Laparoscopic cholecystectomy: Experience with 375 consecutive patients. Ann Surg 1991; 214:531–541.
109. Spaw AT, Reddick EJ, Olsen DO. Laparoscopic laser cholecystectomy: Analysis of 500 procedures. Surg Laparosc Endosc 1991; 1:2–7.
110. Berci G, Sackier JM. The Los Angeles experience with laparoscopic cholecystectomy. Am J Surg 1991; 161:382–384.
111. Nathanson LK, Shimi S, Cuschieri A. Laparoscopic cholecystectomy. The Dundee technique. Br J Surg 1991; 78:155–159.

112. Bergdahl C, Holmund DEW. Retained bile duct stones. Acta Chir Scand 1976;142:145.
113. Kitano S, Iso Y, Moriyama M, Sugimachi K. A rapid and simple technique for insertion of a T-tube into the minimally incised common bile duct at laparoscopic surgery. Surg Endosc 1993; 7:104–105.
114. Petelin JB. Laparoscopic approach to common duct pathology. Surg Laparosc Endosc 1991; 1:33–41.
115. Quattlebaum JK, Flanders HD. Laparoscopic treatment of common bile duct stones. Surg Laparosc Endosc 1991; 1:26–32.
116. Jacobs M, Verdeja JC, Goldstein HS. Laparoscopic choledocholithotomy. J Laparoendosc Surg 1991; 1:79–82.
117. Phillips E, Carroll B, Daykovsky L, et al. Management of common bile duct stones (CBD) encountered during laparoscopic cholecystectomy (LC). Gastrointest Endosc 1991; 37:245.
118. Stoker ME, Leveillee RJ, McCann JC, Maini BS. Laparoscopic common bile duct exploration. J Laparoendosc Surg 1991; 5:287–293.
119. Shapiro SJ, Gordon LA, Daykhovsky L, Grundfest W. Laparoscopic exploration of the common bile duct: Experience in 16 selected patients. J Laparoendosc Surg 1991; 1:333–341.
120. Hunter JG. Laparoscopic transcystic common bile duct exploration. Am J Surg 1992; 163:53–58.
121. Pruitt RE, Bailey AH, Faust TW, et al. Endoscopic retrograde cholangiography with sphincterotomy and common bile duct stone extraction combined with laparoscopic laser cholecystectomy: Our initial experience. Gastrointest Endosc 1991; 37:286.
122. Aliperti G, Edmundowicz SA, Soper NJ, Ashley SW. Combined endoscopic sphincterotomy and laparoscopic cholecystectomy in patients with cholepocholithiasis and cholecystolithiasis. Ann Intern Med 1991; 115:783–785.
123. Manoukian AV, Schmalz MJ, Geenen JE, et al. Endoscopic treatment of problems encountered after cholecystectomy. Gastrointest Endosc 1993; 39:9–14.

Section V
Surgery of the Lower Gastrointestinal Tract

Chapter 19
Appendectomy for Acute Appendicitis

Gerald M. Larson
William G. Cheadle
Hiram C. Polk, Jr.

The principal determinants of morbidity and mortality for appendectomy are the status of the appendix (perforated or not) and the age of the patient. Complications are always more frequent and the mortality rate higher following appendectomy if the acute appendicitis has proceeded to perforation. The mortality rate for appendicitis with a nonperforated appendix is about 0.1 per cent, whereas the mortality with a ruptured appendix increases to 3 to 5 per cent, and rates as high as 15 per cent have been reported for patients greater than 70 years of age.[1]

Reginald Fitz receives the credit for being the first to clearly define the clinical aspects of appendicitis in 1886 and emphasizing that early appendectomy is important for cure. Today, complications occur in 10 per cent of patients after appendectomy, with wound infection being the most common. The overall mortality rate for appendicitis is less than 1 per cent.[2] Death in those patients with a perforated appendix is usually related directly to appendicitis, while death in patients with an unperforated appendix is most commonly related to coexisting disease.[1]

For most of this century, the standard treatment for acute appendicitis has been appendectomy performed through a right lower quadrant incision. During the past decade laparoscopic removal of the appendix has been described and performed with increasing frequency. The purpose of this chapter is to review the results of laparoscopic appendectomy, to discuss the technique of laparoscopic appendectomy, and to compare those results to the record for the traditional appendectomy.

The first cases of laparoscopic appendectomy apparently were performed by surgeons in Germany in 1982 and 1983.[3,4] Since 1987 several reports have been published on experience with laparoscopic appendectomy for acute appendicitis and these results form the basis of this chapter.

TRADITIONAL OPEN APPENDECTOMY FOR ACUTE APPENDICITIS

Table 19-1 summarizes the results from three large surgical series of appendectomy. The series reported by Lewis et al.[1] is an analysis of 1000 consecutive appendectomy patients at the San Francisco General Hospital during January 1963 to June 1973. All age groups were included: 9 per cent of patients were less than 10 years of age and 10 per cent were greater than 50 years of age. The mortality rate in this study was 0.8 per cent, and all deaths occurred in patients over age 50. Five deaths occurred in patients with dif-

Table 19-1. Results for the Standard Open Surgical Appendectomy

Series	No. Cases	Perforated (%)	Nonperforated Appendix			Perforated Appendix		
			Mort	Compl	Wd Infx	Mort	Compl	Wd Infx
Lewis et al., 1975[1]	1000	21	0.4	10	6.6	2.5	0	17.5
Law et al., 1976[5]	216	29	0	10	8	0	33	15
Scher and Coil, 1980[6]	335	32	0	3	0.8	0.9	47	35

Mort, mortality; Compl, complications; Wd Infx, wound infection.

fuse peritonitis after perforation of the appendix.

Law et al.[5] evaluated appendectomy for acute appendicitis during 1972 and 1973 at the Denver General Hospital. All age groups were included. There was a 10 per cent complication rate in patients without perforation and 33 per cent in those with perforation. The study of Scher and Coil[6] is based on the experience at two community hospitals in Huntington, West Virginia. In each series there is a much higher complication rate and greater incidence of wound infection when a ruptured appendix was found at operation.

LAPAROSCOPIC APPENDECTOMY FOR ACUTE APPENDICITIS

In Table 19-2, we summarize the results from four reports on laparoscopic appendectomy. In three of the four series the preoperative diagnosis was acute appendicitis. We have excluded other studies for which the procedure started as a diagnostic laparoscopy for pelvic and/or abdominal pain. We have also indicated the percentage of patients with a gangrenous or perforated appendix and that percentage was lower than for the open surgical series.

Two German surgeons, Pier and Gotz, working at St. Joseph Hospital in Linnich, Germany, deserve much of the credit for demonstrating the feasibility and safety of laparoscopic removal of an acutely inflamed appendix in a large number of patients.[7,8] They describe a three-puncture technique using the standard laparoscopic approach. The appendix is skeletonized by coagulation of the mesoappendix and the vessels, and then, divided between loop ligatures. They have performed this procedure in more than 700 patients in all stages of appendicitis and have had to convert to an open laparotomy in only 14 patients (2 per cent).

The series reported by Saye et al.[9] consisted of 109 laparoscopic appendectomies performed primarily as incidental appendectomies secondary to other indications such as adhesions and endometriosis. The authors state that 10 per cent of these procedures were performed for acute appendicitis, one appendix was perforated, and no complications were observed. The study by Valla et al.[10] is unique and special because it is a children's series. Laparoscopic appendectomy was performed in 465 children at four medical centers in France. The ages of the patients ranged from 3 to 16 years with a mean of 10 years. Ninety per cent of the appendices were

Table 19-2. Results for Laparoscopic Appendectomy

Series	No. Cases	Gangrenous or Perforated (%)	Outcome (%)			Conversion Rate (%)
			Mort	Compl	Wd Infx	
Pier and Gotz, 1991[7]	625	3	0	1	2	2
Saye et al., 1991[9]	109	1	0	0	0	0
O'Regan, 1991[11]	40	15	0	5	0	17
Valla et al., 1991[10]	465 (children)	16	0	3	0	1

Mort, mortality; Compl, complications; Wd Infx, wound infection.

inflamed, and 16 per cent were gangrenous or perforated. The postoperative complications (rate 3 per cent) included wound drainage or hernia, obstructive symptoms, pain, ileus, and pelvic abscess. Their technique included ligating the base of the appendix with a surgical clip or a loop ligature and then dividing the appendix with scissors.

In the children, Valla et al.[10] used the same 5- and 10-mm instruments as for adults. As advantages for laparoscopic appendectomy, the authors list easy and rapid identification of the appendix regardless of its position, the chance for more complete exploration of the abdomen, and a reduction in the incidence of wound infection.

O'Regan[11] practices at University Hospital in Vancouver, British Columbia, and his personal experience (personal communication) with laparoscopic appendectomy for acute appendicitis comprises 40 patients. In 7 patients he converted to an open procedure because of advanced disease and a dissection that he considered too difficult or too dangerous. In each case he was able to see the appendix and confirm the diagnosis.

LAPAROSCOPIC APPENDECTOMY VERSUS OPEN APPENDECTOMY

To our knowledge only one prospective study comparing these two procedures has been performed. In 1991 McAnena et al.[12] studied appendectomy results in 65 consecutive patients who were assigned to either open (36 patients) or laparoscopic appendectomy (29 patients). Their comparative results for open versus laparoscopic appendectomy, respectively, were a postoperative stay of 4.8 versus 2.2 days, a mean anesthesia time of 52 versus 48 minutes, and a wound infection rate of 11 versus 4 per cent; they had to convert two laparoscopic procedures to open procedures. They maintain that the risk of wound infection for laparoscopic appendectomy is reduced because the appendix is removed through the cannula without touching the wound. The data on wound infection in Tables 19-1 and 19-2 also suggest that the incidence of wound complications is less following laparoscopic appendectomy. One must keep in mind, however, that these groups are not directly comparable. The open surgical series included all patients without selection, and many more of the patients in the open series had advanced disease with perforation, which adversely influences the complication rate. Obviously more controlled studies are needed.

TECHNIQUE

Most surgeons will have had experience with laparoscopic cholecystectomy at the time they start to perform laparoscopic appendectomy. While the procedures are similar, there are two differences in room setup and trochar position worth noting. First, it is most helpful to place the television monitor at the foot of the table or to the right side of the patient's knee rather than at the head of the table. With this arrangement the surgeon, standing on the patient's left side, has a straightforward view of the surgical dissection that is parallel to the orientation of his instruments. The assistant surgeon/camera operator stands on the patient's right as does the operating room nurse. The second difference is the location of the trochar cannulas. We prefer to place one working port in the suprapubic midline and a second port in the right upper quadrant. An extra cannula can be placed in the left lower or right upper quadrant if necessary for dissection of the appendix. A nasogastric tube and bladder catheter are inserted when the patient is asleep and before trochars are inserted (Fig. 19-1).

The pneumoperitoneum is established and a 10- or 11-mm trochar cannula is inserted through the umbilicus. A 10-mm forward-viewing laparoscope is then placed through this cannula, and a visual abdominal exploration is performed. Next, a 10-mm trochar cannula is inserted into the suprapubic midline and a 5-mm trochar cannula is inserted under direct vision in the right upper quadrant. Laparoscopic examination of the abdomen and particularly of the right lower quadrant is performed to locate the appendix and to look for other coexisting disorders. Exposing the appendix and the adnexa is facilitated by putting the patient in the Trendelenburg position and rotating the table slightly to the left. Generally the cecum is seen first and can be gently moved to show the appendix. Adhesions to the appendix and the cecum are common, and it may be necessary to free these as well as adjacent loops of ileum from the appendix before skeletonization of the appendix begins. In most cases it is possible to grasp the tip of the appendix with the right upper quadrant forceps, elevate it, and display the mesoappendix. Through the suprapubic port, the dissecting forceps is in-

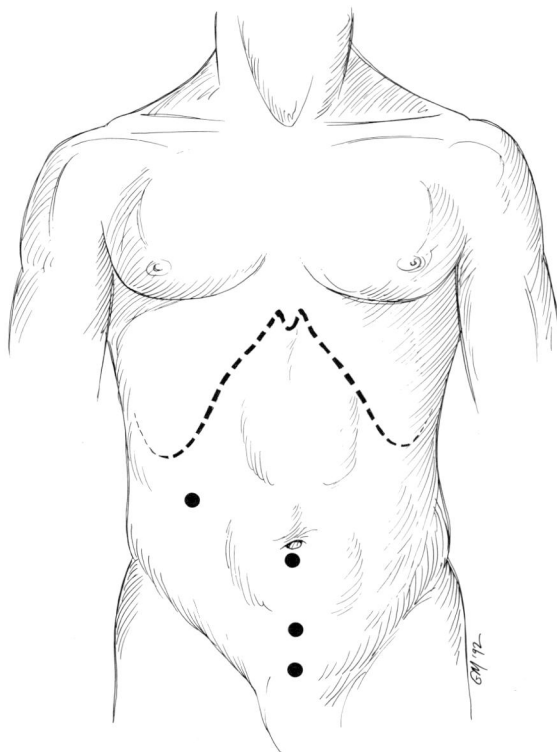

Figure 19-1. Recommended sites for trocar placement for a laparoscopic appendectomy.

serted to make openings in the mesoappendix and expose the vessels. Once the appendiceal artery and its branches have been identified, we use standard endoscopic clips to clip and divide the vessels. Others have described using laser energy to divide the mesentery and also to divide the base of the appendix.[9]

Once the appendix is isolated, two loop ligatures are inserted over the appendix to ligate the base, and a third loop is placed more distally on the appendix. With coagulation current delivered through a scissors, the appendix is divided between the ligatures. It is important that the coagulation cut be at least 5 mm from the ligature to avoid heat damage to it, which could be a potential cause of stump leakage (Fig. 19-2).

Occasionally the appendix is very thick and edematous and not easily grasped by a forceps. In that instance application of a pre-tied endoscopic loop ligature around the tip of the appendix will facilitate manipulation of the appendix. Appendices that are not greater than 10 mm are removed through the 10-mm port. For the appendix that is too large or tenuous to extract through a 10-mm port, alternative approaches include the use of a latex bag inserted into the abdomen into which the appendix is placed and then the bag is removed through a cannula or through enlargement of the puncture site in the abdominal wall.[9] For the large appendix,

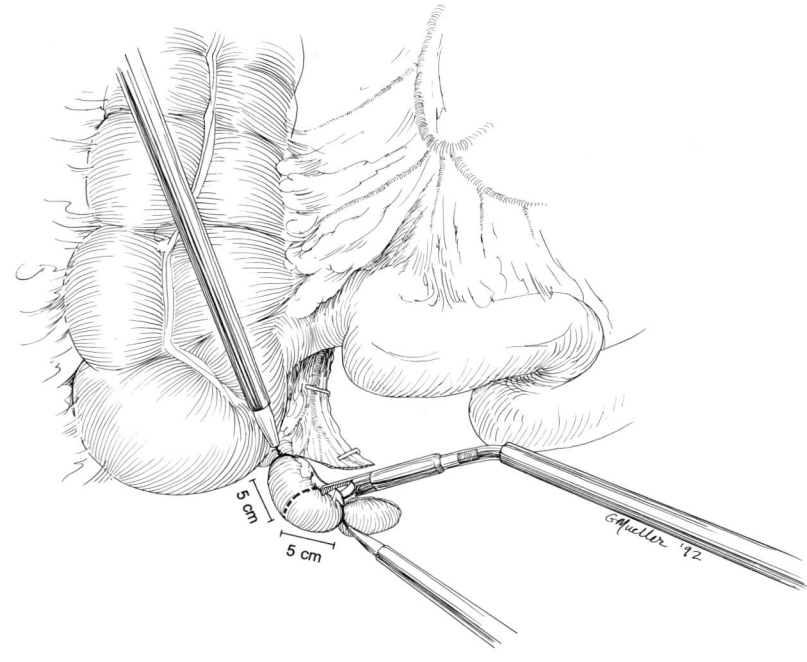

Figure 19-2. The appendix is divided between the ligatures with the electrocautery scissors.

O'Regan replaces the 10-mm cannula with a 15-mm cannula and then removes the appendix.[11] He has not encountered an appendix that would not pass through a 15-mm cannula. Endoscopic clips have not been designed for cross-clipping the appendix, and, in our opinion, currently available clips should not be used for that purpose. In most cases the clips are not large enough to securely cross the appendix.

Growing in popularity is the use of endoscopic gastrointestinal anastomosis stapling instruments to staple and divide the mesoappendix and the appendix.[13] There are no published results for this technique at the time of this writing but, based on a generally positive experience with the use of gastrointestinal anastomosis instruments for other intestinal procedures, this technique would seem to be satisfactory. The expense of the device is, however, a factor.

The appendiceal stump is either simply ligated or ligated and invaginated. Semm[3] recommended inverting the appendiceal stump with a pursestring suture. In the reports that followed, surgeons generally have just ligated the stump without adverse effects. In fact, two studies of this matter show no advantage to stump inversion compared to simple ligation of the appendix, and most surgeons find intracorporeal suturing to be somewhat time-consuming.[14,15]

SPECIAL CONSIDERATIONS

Stump Leakage and Fecal Fistula

Two cases of leakage from the appendiceal stump after laparoscopic appendectomy have been reported. Pier and Gotz[7] report a single case that occurred because the coagulation division of the appendix was too close to the loop ligature and caused thermal damage to the ligature. As a result, they recommend that the coagulation area must be 6- to 7-mm from the loop ligature. In the other instance, a fistula from the cecum was caused by heat damage to the cecum during endocoagulation of the mesoappendix.[4] Therefore, the incidence of this complication appears to be low.

Hospital Stay

All authors state that postoperative recovery is faster following laparoscopic appendectomy and that hospital stays are shorter. Comparative data are sparse. Saye et al.[9] report that most patients having an incidental appendectomy were discharged 23 hours following surgery compared to 36 hours for patients with acute appendicitis. In O'Regan's series[11] all patients returned to work in 1 week.

Conversion Rate

The rate of conversion from laparoscopic appendectomy to an open procedure ranges from 1 to 17 per cent.[7,10,11] As for laparoscopic cholecystectomy, this change in the operative plan is not to be considered a failure of the surgeon's laparoscopic technique, but rather an exercise of good judgment when the dissection is difficult, exposure is not adequate, or the laparoscopic appendectomy is taking too long. The reasons generally given for converting to an open procedure include adhesions, bleeding, an abnormal position of the appendix, abscess formation, and perforation.

Pregnancy

Although laparoscopic appendectomy has been performed in pregnant patients, this condition is considered by some to be a relative contraindication to the laparoscopic approach.[11,13] The issue of concern is what the effect of raised intra-abdominal pressure and the high concentration of intra-abdominal carbon dioxide will have on the fetus. Schrieber[16] has performed laparoscopic appendectomy with good results in six patients who were in the first and second trimesters of pregnancy.

Children

Laparoscopic appendectomy has been performed in children as young as 2 years of age.[7,10] Standard 5- and 10-mm trochar cannulas and instruments are used. Extra caution when placing trochars is in order, however, because of the generally thin abdominal wall in pediatric patients and the superficial and close proximity of the major abdominal vessels to the abdominal wall especially during trochar insertion. Because of the thin abdominal wall, there is a tendency for the cannulas to slip out of position and the use of screw-type anchors only partially solves this problem.[10]

Contraindications

As with laparoscopic cholecystectomy, the number of contraindications has decreased, and they are definitely related to the experience of the operating surgeon. The relative contraindications include pregnancy, a scarred-in right lower quadrant from previous surgery or trauma, and the rare patient who cannot tolerate general anesthesia.

Claimed Advantages

Since prospective controlled studies of laparoscopic appendectomy have not been performed, many of the claimed advantages will require documentation. Advantages frequently mentioned for laparoscopic appendectomy include: (1) a better view of the abdomen compared to the more limited examination through a small right lower quadrant incision; (2) identification and treatment of nonappendiceal lesions; (3) reduced tissue trauma and more rapid return of bowel function; (4) decreased postoperative pain, shorter hospital stays, and more rapid return to normal activity; (5) good exposure even in the obese patient; and (6) a lower incidence of postoperative wound infection because of the small puncture wounds.

Summary

It is a matter of record that the standard open appendectomy for acute appendicitis has been a very effective operation. Recognition of the natural course of acute appendicitis and the practice of early appendectomy for suspected appendicitis has lowered the mortality rate from a high of 50 per cent for perforated appendicitis at the turn of the century to a current overall mortality risk of less than 1 per cent and a complication rate of 10 per cent.[2] It is now also apparent that laparoscopic appendectomy can be safely performed in the majority of patients with acute appendicitis. Since more and more surgeons now perform operative laparoscopy, the merits of laparoscopic appendectomy for acute appendicitis are being considered. Surgeons who defend the open appendectomy maintain that it is a good operation that can be easily performed through a small incision with rapid recovery of the patient and a short hospital stay. Most surgeons who perform laparoscopic appendectomy accept those arguments but still maintain that the laparoscopic approach indeed decreases postoperative discomfort and allows patients to return to normal activity more rapidly. From a technical perspective, laparoscopic appendectomy is simpler to perform than cholecystectomy and does not have the potential risks of retained stones or injury to the common bile duct.

One of the most persuasive arguments for laparoscopic appendectomy is the low rate of wound infection, which is a consistent finding in all of the studies we have reviewed. There are no hard data to date on the cost-benefit analysis. Intraoperative costs may be greater for laparoscopic appendectomy because of the use of disposable instruments and because of the growing popularity of the endoscopic gastrointestinal anastomosis devices for appendectomy. Until more data from prospective controlled studies are available, the decision for a laparoscopic appendectomy will probably remain the surgeon's preference.

REFERENCES

1. Lewis FR, Holcroft JW, Boey J, Dunphy JE. Appendicitis: A critical review of diagnosis and treatment in 1,000 cases. Arch Surg 1975; 110:677–679.
2. Condon RE. Acute appendicitis. In Moody FG, Carey LC, et al., eds. Surgical Treatment of Digestive Disease. Chicago, Year Book Medical Publishers, Inc, 1986.
3. Semm K. Endoscopic appendectomy. Endoscopy 1983; 15:59–64.
4. Schreiber JH. Early experience with laparoscopic appendectomy in women: Surgical Endoscopy. 1987; 1:211–216.
5. Law D, Law R, Eiseman B. The continuing challenge of acute and perforated appendicitis. Am J Surg 1976; 131:533–535.
6. Scher KS, Coil JA. The continuing challenge of perforating appendicitis. Surg Gynecol Obstet 1980; 150:535–538.
7. Pier A, Gotz F. Laparoscopic appendectomy in 625 cases: From innovation to routine. Surg Laparosc Endosc 1991; 1:8–13.
8. Pier A, Gotz F. Laparoscopic appendectomy. Probl Gen Surg 1991; 8:416–425.
9. Saye WB, Rives DA, Cochran EB. Laparoscopic appendectomy: Three years' experience. Surg Laparosc Endosc 1991; 1:109–115.
10. Valla JS, Limonne B, Valla V, et al. Laparoscopic appendectomy in children: Report of 465 cases. Surg Laparosc Endosc 1991; 1:166–172.

11. O'Regan PJ. Laparoscopic appendectomy. Can J Surg 1991; 34:256–258.
12. McAnena OJ, Austin O, Hederman WP, et al. Laparoscopic versus open appendicectomy. Lancet 1991; 338:693.
13. Olsen DO. Laparoscopic appendectomy using a linear stapling device. Surg Rounds 1991; 14:873–883.
14. Engström L, Fenyö G. Appendicectomy: An assessment of stump invagination versus simple ligation: A prospective, randomized trial. Br J Surg 1985; 72:971–972.
15. Sinha AP. Appendicectomy: An assessment of the advisability of stump invagination. Br J Surg 1977; 64:499–500.
16. Schreiber JH. Laparoscopic appendectomy in pregnancy. Surg Endosc 1990; 4:100–102.

Chapter 20
Treatment of Lower Gastrointestinal Diverticular Disease

Walter E. Longo
Anthony M. Vernava, III

The use of laparoscopy in the surgical treatment of diseases of the abdomen and pelvis continues to escalate. Although use of the laparoscope as an operative tool has been traditionally limited to gynecologic procedures, it is now used in urologic, orthopedic, thoracic, and colon and rectal surgery. The benefit appears to be reduced length of hospitalization and recovery as well as the potential for a decreased financial burden to the patient.

Diverticular disease of the lower gastrointestinal tract has become increasingly common in western civilization. Whereas the risk of developing diverticulosis in the colon is 50 per cent by age 60, symptoms will develop in only 10 per cent of those with diverticulosis. Less common types of diverticula are also found in other sites within the gastrointestinal tract. Congenital and acquired diverticula of the jejunum and ileum in the adult occur in approximately 1 to 2 per cent of the population. The percentage of patients with small bowel diverticular disease that will become symptomatic is unclear. The major complications of jejunal-ileal and colonic diverticular disease requiring surgery are bleeding and infection. There is a group of patients with chronic symptoms unresponsive to medical therapy who will have persistent abdominal pain and require operative intervention.

Diverticulitis, a well-known complication of diverticulosis, both of the small bowel and colon, may be either a self-limited phenomenon or may progress to life-threatening sepsis. The diagnosis is not always straightforward both on clinical grounds as well as radiographically, and diverticulitis may occasionally be misinterpreted as appendicitis, a perforated peptic ulcer, or even cholecystitis. In the small bowel, it is rarely suspected preoperatively and at laparotomy is dealt with by resection and primary anastomosis. In the colon, especially in the sigmoid, controversy persists as to method of drainage of an established abscess, timing of resection, and need for stoma.

The potential roles for laparoscopy in the treatment of diverticular disease include diagnosis, control of sepsis, diversion, removal of the involved segment, and reconstruction, either primary or via a staged procedure. Furthermore, since this disease often affects the elderly, the potential for minimal access surgery without general anesthesia may be of further benefit.

COLONIC DIVERTICULAR DISEASE

It was Sir Erasmus Wilson who was the first to note the presence of a colonic diverticula in a specimen he examined in 1840.[1] Cruveilhier[2] is credited with the first detailed description of diverticula of the colon as a distinct pathologic entity in 1849. Diverticulitis was first described by Fraser[3] in 1899, but it was not until 1904 that Beer[4] described the pathologic and clinical features of colonic diverticulitis such as perforation and fistulization. Mayo[5] was an early proponent of a staged procedure with initial drainage of diverticular abscesses and colostomy followed by resection. Lockhart-Mummery[6] in 1938 and Smithwick[7] in 1942 established the safety of the three-stage procedure. Henri Hartmann[8] in 1921 advocated a sigmoid colectomy with sigmoid colostomy and closure of the rectosigmoid for tumors of the proximal rectum or distal sigmoid. Subsequently, this two stage operation has been used as the management of acute complicated diverticular disease. In the 1960s, Madden and Tan[9] suggested primary resection with end-to-end anastomosis for the treatment of acutely perforated diverticulitis. In 1964, Reilly[10] introduced longitudinal myotomy of the colon in hopes of interfering with the primary mechanism of the motor disorder.

Anatomy

The colonic mucosa is surrounded by an inner circular layer of smooth muscle and an outer longitudinal smooth muscle layer concentrated into three narrow bands known as teniae. These three teniae commence at the base of the appendix and run along the entire length of the colon until they coalesce to provide a complete longitudinal muscle coat for the rectum. The vasa recta, the nutrient blood supply to the bowel, are of two types: long and short. The long branches divide and encircle the colon with their terminal branches running in the bowel wall deep to the teniae and anastomose on the antimesenteric border. The short branches supply the mesocolic two thirds of the bowel circumference. These vessels, the nutrient supply to the colon, pierce the bowel adjacent to the teniae. Diverticulosis results from herniation of the mucosa through defects in the muscle coats located at sites where these blood vessels pierce the muscular wall to enter the submucous plane. These vessels enter just on the mesenteric side of the two lateral teniae, so diverticula commonly occur in two parallel rows along the bowel. Colonic diverticula are pseudodiverticula in that all layers of the intestinal wall are not present. As their wall lacks a muscle layer, the diverticula are unable to readily expel any fecal material.

Etiology and Pathogenesis

The pathogenesis of diverticulosis is thought to be multifactorial. Increased intraluminal pressure, segmentation, a low fiber diet, and defects in colonic wall strength have all been implicated in its development. Persistent or intermittent elevations of colonic pressure secondary to a motility disorder were thought to put stress on the colonic wall and eventually cause the colonic mucosa to herniate through its weakest points. Arfwidssen and Dock[11] found that patients with diverticular disease had significantly higher intraluminal pressure when compared with normal control subjects in the resting state and after meals. Painter and Truelove[12] did not find pressure differences in the resting state between normal persons and patients with diverticular disease, but did confirm abnormalities that occurred postprandially and after stimulation with prostigmine. Unfortunately, a motility disorder has not been identified in all patients with diverticurosis. Indeed, a normal pattern of motility has been documented in some patients with diverticular disease, while others with abnormal patterns of motility fail to develop diverticula.

Recently, studies of resected specimens have implicated abnormalities of elastin in the pathogenesis of diverticulosis. Whiteway and Morson[15] studied 25 specimens of sigmoid colon obtained from patients with symptomatic diverticulosis. The circular muscle layer and the teniae coli were thickened, but the muscle layer of the teniae were normal. This thickening of the circular muscle layer was due to an increase in elastin fibers. It was hypothesized that the stiffened muscle is first unable to relax and the inelastic bundles tend to produce intraluminal obstructive segments and thus raise intraluminal pressure. These pressure changes in response to eating or pharmacologic manipulation are responsible for the bulging of mucosa through breaks in the muscular wall normally perforated by the vasa recta with the formation of typical diverticular sacs.[16,17]

Location

Diverticulosis is most frequently seen in the sigmoid colon. Approximately 65 per cent of patients with diverticulosis have isolated involvement of the sigmoid colon while 30 per cent have involvement of the sigmoid colon and another segment of colon. Only 5 to 10 per cent of patients with diverticulosis do not have sigmoid colon involvement. The number of diverticula in the colon is highly variable. In the sigmoid colon, multiple diverticula are found. In contrast, isolated right-sided diverticulosis usually consists of a solitary diverticulum or at most a few diverticula. Pancolonic diverticulosis occurs in less than 10 per cent of patients. Only a few patients with rectal diverticula have been reported.[18]

Right-sided diverticulosis is encountered most commonly in the Orient. In the United States, it represents 1 to 2 per cent of cases of diverticulosis. In many instances the cecal diverticulum is a true diverticulum that contains all layers of the bowel wall. To date approximately 400 cases of cecal diverticulitis have been reported in patients with a solitary cecal diverticulum. Cecal diverticulitis is clinically indistinguishable from acute appendicitis although patients tend to be older, have a longer duration of symptoms, and present less often with nausea and vomiting.[19] Charges of diagnosis may be enhanced by barium enema. When the diagnosis of cecal diverticulitis is made, nonoperative supportive care as in sigmoid diverticulitis is undertaken. At surgery, the etiology of the right lower quadrant inflammatory mass is often unclear. It may be difficult to exclude the possibility of a performed cecal carcinoma. Thus, in these patients, a right hemicolectomy is usually performed. Some authors have advocated limited local diverticulectomy when there is no doubt about the diagnosis.

Complications of Colonic Diverticular Disease

The complications of diverticulosis are pain, felt to be secondary to spasm, bleeding, intestinal obstruction, hemorrhage, and inflammation. Diverticulitis, one of the most lethal complications, may be complicated by perforation, fistulization to adjacent viscera, and intra-abdominal abscesses. Some degree of chronic obstruction is common with advanced forms of diverticulitis. The criteria for the diagnosis of diverticulitis are left lower quadrant pain and local tenderness, acute constipation or diarrhea, fever, and leukocytosis. The annual risk for developing diverticulitis in the population with diverticulosis is 1 to 3 per cent. The differential diagnosis of acute diverticulitis includes carcinoma of the colon with localized perforation, ischemic colitis, appendicitis, or either ulcerative and granulomatous colitis. A chest roentgenogram and flat and upright roentgenograms of the abdomen are used to search for free intraperitoneal air. A small risk of perforation exists with contrast studies of the large bowel. There is little indication for flexible endoscopy. Computed tomographic (CT) scan is now the optimal diagnostic procedure, for it may reveal inflammation of the soft tissue suggesting an abscess or phlegmon. It also permits transcutaneous drainage of any localized septic process in the pericolic fat or pelvis.

An acknowledged use of laparoscopy is for the diagnosis of acute lower abdominal pain. Direct inspection of both the mesenteric and antimesenteric surfaces of the bowel for occult diverticula may be performed. In the case of diverticulitis of either the colon or small bowel, perforation may leave a yellowish-brown fluid seen in the gutters or in between loops of adjacent bowel. This can be aspirated and sent for Gram stain. If these findings are noted, one may proceed to either laparotomy or laparoscopic resection.[20]

EXTENT OF RESECTION AND RECURRENT DIVERTICULITIS

Diverticulitis generally involves a short segment of the colon. Resection of the involved segment of intestine provides symptomatic relief in the overwhelming majority of patients. Although diverticula may be seen above and below the inflamed area, only the thickened area where muscle hypertrophy has occurred is removed. Diverticulitis rarely occurs after resection. Of 136 patients followed for a mean of 9 years after resection for diverticular disease Wychulis et al.[21] reported 7 per cent suffered recurrent pain while 5 per cent had documented recurrent diverticulitis. Although these numbers are small, this problem can be frustrating for the surgeon. Proximal and distal lines of resection need to be established.

Proximally the diverticulosis may extend into the descending, transverse, or right colon. Do all diverticula-bearing segments of the colon need to be removed? In a study from the Mayo Clinic by Wolff and co-workers,[22] 61 patients who underwent elective resection for diverticular disease underwent barium enema in the perioperative period and within 5 years after resection. The average length of colon removed was 22 cm. Recurrent diverticulitis occurred in 11.4 per cent. Progression of diverticulosis into the proximal colon occurred in 14.7 per cent. Three of 61 patients (4.9 per cent) had both recurrent diverticulitis and progression of disease seen on barium enema. There was no association between the number of diverticula in the residual colon and the development of recurrent diverticulitis.

Does the distal anastomosis need to be to the rectum? Is an anastomosis to the distal sigmoid colon related to recurrent diverticulitis? A study of 501 patients who had a resection for colonic diverticular disease at the Mayo Clinic with an intestinal anastomosis (321 descending colosigmoidostomies and 180 descending colorectostomies) was performed.[23] The duration of follow-up was at least 5 years for 77 per cent of the group. Recurrent diverticulitis occurred in 30 of 132 patients (22.7 per cent) with descending colosigmoidostomies and in 5 of 81 patients (6.2 per cent) with descending colorectostomies. Another operation for diverticular disease was required in 15 patients: 11 in the sigmoidal group and 4 in the rectal group.

The requirements for decreasing the risk of recurrent diverticulitis are to perform an adequate sigmoid resection and to fashion a descending colorectal anastomosis. Complete removal of the thickened bowel and an anastomosis to soft pliable colon is necessary.[24] Due to the large, bulky nature of the sigmoid colon in diverticular disease, extracorporeal resection and anastomosis would be virtually impossible. Laparoscopic intracorporeal intestinal resection in diverticular disease may be feasible. The procedure could be initially begun laparoscopically, and if a redundant sigmoid is found, splenic flexure mobilization may not need to be performed. Because of foreshortening by scarring, the specimen will be small. The anus would be a potential port for the delivery of the specimen as well as introduction of the circular stapling device.

Hartmann's Procedure

Options for surgical treatment of colonic diverticulitis with abscesses include drainage alone, proximal diverting colostomy with drainage, or resection of the involved segment of colon with anastomosis or with an end colostomy. In the past, surgeons often treated complications of diverticulitis with a three stage procedure; drainage and construction of a colostomy, resection and finally closure of the colostomy. Unfortunately, this procedure did not remove the source of sepsis at the first operation and consequently was complicated by a 71 percent rate of morbidity and 11 percent rate of mortality.[25] More recently surgeons have preferred to treat patients with a two stage approach called a Hartmann procedure. In this technique the sigmoid colon, the source of sepsis, is resected and an end descending colostomy is constructed at the first procedure. The rectum is sutured or stapled closed. At the second operation the colostomy is taken down and a colorectostomy is constructed. This approach has diminished the rate of septic complications. Nonetheless, some surgeons remain reluctant to utilize this strategy because of the difficulties encountered with resection of the inflamed sigmoid colon and the subsequent closure of the colostomy. Similarly, primary resection with primary anastomosis has failed to gain widespread acceptance because of its high mortality rate and a morbidity rate which approaches 50 per cent.[26]

Despite the continued use of this procedure, especially in the acute setting, mortalities ranging from 1 to 10 per cent and a high morbidity is still encountered. Many of these complications relate to superficial wound infections. Kerner et al.[27] emphasized that limited excision of the acute disease process at the first operation is of paramount importance. The operation does not entail splenic flexure mobilization or opening the retrorectal space. In Kerner's study, 66 patients underwent Hartmann's procedure for acute complicated diverticulitis. The average age of patients was 65 years. Thirty-eight patients (58 per cent) had one or more complications during either the first or second stage of the procedure. One perioperative death occurred. The overall morbidity was 39 per cent for both operations, which is similar to previous reports.[28,29] The mortality rate is an improvement over the three-stage procedure[25] and resection with primary anastomosis.[9]

In the treatment of acute complicated sigmoid diverticulitis, Hartmann's procedure removes the sepsis and diverts the fecal stream. In the event that the procedure is definitive, an end-sigmoid colostomy is easy to care for. The second procedure, colostomy closure, has been simplified with the circular stapler and may be performed laparoscopically.

CT-Guided Percutaneous Drainage

Since percutaneous drainage of intra-abdominal abscesses was first reported in 1976, the interventional radiologist has played an important role in the management of diverticular abscesses. Percutaneous drainage of a pericolic or pelvic abscess caused by diverticulitis may prevent the need for emergency resection and end colostomy, which would require a second or even a third subsequent operation. Percutaneous drainage can control sepsis and may allow a subsequent one-stage resection and primary anastomosis. In certain instances, the abscess may not be able to be drained under radiographic guidance (e.g., deep interloop abscesses that are inaccessible because of surrounding bowel or incomplete liquefaction of a phlegmon). The generally accepted criteria for percutaneous drainage of an abscess include a well defined unilocular abscess with a safe route of drainage. Mueller et al.[30] reported 24 patients who had percutaneous drainage of a diverticular abscess, of which 14 (58 per cent) underwent single-stage resection within 10 days of drainage. Five patients required two-stage procedures because of residual inflammation. Neff et al.[31] reported among 16 patients that 11 (68 per cent) underwent single-stage resection. Stabile et al.[32] followed 19 patients for an average of 17.4 months after drainage. There were no complications related to catheter placement. Fourteen patients (74 per cent) underwent single-stage colectomy and primary anastomosis. These studies concluded that percutaneous drainage of diverticular abscesses is safe and effective and obviates the need for colostomy in the majority of patients.

The complications of percutaneous drainage are perforation of a hollow viscus and subsequent fistula or perforation of the ureter or major vessel. Laparoscopic visualization of the diverticular phlegmon with drainage under direct vision can potentially allow for complete eradication of the abscess without complication or recurrence. A larger bore catheter can be left in place for irrigation and drainage.

Colomyotomy

Reilly[10] proposed a sigmoid myotomy for the treatment of sigmoid diverticulosis based on the hypertrophy and thickening of the muscle found in specimens of sigmoid colon containing diverticular disease. The procedure consisted of incising the circular muscle coat down to the mucosa through a longitudinal incision in the line of one of the antimesenteric teniae. The incision is carried along to normal bowel above and below for a distance of about 10 to 20 mm. Perforation is a feared complication of this procedure and may go unrecognized until sepsis supervenes. Daniel[33] distended the colon by rectal air insufflation to reveal any microperforations and, if recognized, closed them with sutures or wrapped them with omentum. The clinical results showed that 95 per cent of patients were free of symptoms over a 1- to 5-year follow-up.

Hodgson[34] suggested that a transverse tenomyotomy was better therapy for diverticular disease than a longitudinal division of circular fibers. This type of myotomy would, in theory, allow for the sigmoid colon to lengthen itself. The operation consists of making a transverse cut in the two antimesenteric teniae at intervals of 2 cm starting on the anterior rectal wall at the peritoneal reflection and extending to just above the upper limit of the disease proximally. The cuts do not divide any circular muscle. This procedure does not sufficiently change the intraluminal pressure of the colon. Hodgson[34] reported at 2 to 3 years after transverse tenomyotomy only a 5 per cent recurrence of symptoms.

Kettlewell and Moloney[35] proposed combining a longitudinal and horizontal myotomy of the colon. This was felt to be a complete myotomy of the colon and is associated with satisfactory short term results, but carries the risk of mucosal perforation as does the sigmoid myotomy described by Reilly.

Castrini and Pappalardo[36] reported a new procedure, the L or horizontal T colomyotomy. The operation consists of transverse tenomyotomies performed alternatively every 3 cm on the medial and lateral antimesenteric tenia combined with a simultaneous vertical myotomy. They reported on seven patients with a history of advanced, symptomatic, and uncomplicated diverticulosis of the colon. There was no postoperative mortality or morbidity and patients had an average hospitalization of less than 8 days. In six patients, complete remission of preoperative symptoms was noted. Although the number of diverticula remained unchanged, follow-up motility studies showed that the mean motility index had significantly decreased after myotomy in both basal conditions and after pharmacologic stimulation.

One-Stage Resection

Belding in 1957[37] reported on four patients with perforated diverticulitis who underwent primary resection and anastomosis without a mortality. After a 0 per cent mortality was further reported by Madden and Tan[38] in six patients with perforating diverticulitis as contrasted to a 33 per cent mortality of those undergoing staged procedures, others reported increased morbidity and mortality among those undergoing staged procedures. This was felt to be a result of the fact that many elderly patients have numerous medical risk factors that may make staged procedures not appropriate.

The advent of percutaneous CT-guided drainage has allowed control of diverticular sepsis, and bowel rest, along with intravenous fluids and parenteral antibiotics, is the primary treatment before definitive surgical therapy. Following the resolution of sepsis, the patient may undergo mechanical bowel preparation and a one-stage colonic resection during the same hospital admission. Primary resection and anastomosis without a protecting colostomy has become the treatment of choice for diverticulitis complicated by a contained abscess.[39] Patient selection is of paramount importance in determining those who will fare well after a one-stage procedure.

JEJUNAL-ILEAL DIVERTICULAR DISEASE

The surgeon will encounter jejunal-ileal diverticular disease in a variety of clinical settings. It may be an incidental finding noted in the workup of the patient with already documented gastrointestinal disease or may be found radiographically as the cause of abdominal symptoms initially felt to be caused by another intra-abdominal pathologic condition. It may be an unsuspected finding as the cause of peritonitis when laparoscopy is performed in the patient with an acute abdomen. Diverticula of the jejunum and ileum are uncommon, and the majority are asymptomatic. These diverticula should not always be dismissed as incidental, for they may be the underlying cause of vague symptomatology. Complications arising directly from these lesions are rare, but their occurrence may produce uncertainty as to diagnosis and management.

Etiology

Small bowel diverticula were first described by Sommerring and Baillie in 1794.[40] In 1807, Sir Astley Cooper reported the first instance of jejunal diverticulosis in a monograph on hernias.[41] The first account of an operation for small bowel diverticula was published by Gordinier and Sampson in 1906.[42] Excluding the stomach, jejunal-ileal diverticula (non-Meckelian), represent the rarest form of gastrointestinal diverticular disease. The reported incidence is 0.5 to 2.3 per cent of small bowel contrast studies and 0.3 to 4.5 per cent of autopsy studies.[43,44] These diverticula are multiple, but the number decreases distally with a solitary diverticulum commonly found in the ileum. Nearly 80 per cent occur in the jejunum, approximately 15 per cent in the ileum, and 5 per cent in both. They are most frequently seen in the sixth and seventh decades of life and are more common in men.[45,46] Jejuno-ileal diverticula, except Meckel's diverticulum, are acquired false diverticula in that they lack a true muscular wall and are thin walled and fragile.

The pathogenesis of these lesions, as in colonic diverticular disease, is that an acquired pulsion diverticulum develops. The site of herniation appears to be where paired blood vessels penetrate the mesentery into the bowel wall.[47] An alternative theory has centered upon jejuno-ileal diverticula being a manifestation of abnormal contractions of the intestinal wall leading to ineffective, uncoordinated motor activity from an underlying dysmotility disorder.[46-48] Nearly 50 per cent of cases of jejuno-ileal diverticulosis are associated with colonic diverticula.[49]

Presentation and Diagnosis

The majority of patients with jejuno-ileal diverticular disease have no symptoms. When symptoms do occur, jejunal-ileal diverticular disease will present either as malabsorption, hemorrhage, inflammation, or obstruction. Chronic symptoms of intermittent abdominal pain, flatulence with episodes of diarrhea, and anemia are reported to occur in up to 30 per cent of patients.[50] Plain upright films of the abdomen will suggest the diagnosis from the presence of air-fluid levels in multiple diverticula throughout the small intestine. Contrast studies, including enteroclysis of the jejunum and ileum will demonstrate a large outpouching with retained contrast medium after the main lumen has become empty. The lumen of the intestine will be dilated in the area of the diverticula and the mucosal folds will be thickened and prominent.[51,52] The triad of obscure pain, anemia, and dilated loops of bowel on barium x-ray film suggest jejuno-ileal diverticulosis.[53]

Complications of Jejunal Diverticular Disease

The symptoms of jejunal diverticulosis are largely caused by an interference with normal peristalsis and propulsion of intestinal content along the bowel. Unexplained abdominal pain, steatorrhea, and megaloblastic anemia may suggest disease. Stasis resulting in an overgrowth of coliform organisms occurs, leading to the deconjugation of bile acids and the intraluminal metabolism of vitamin B_{12}.[54,55] The diagnosis is established by measurements of serum folate, vitamin B_{12}, and the use of the Schilling test. The identification of coliform organisms in the proximal intestinal aspirate is also useful.[56] A high protein, low residue diet with vitamin supplements is recommended. A trial of broad spectrum antibiotics, either tetracycline or metronidazole should be prescribed. If improvement is noted, a relapse after discontinuation of drug treatment may require long-term antibiotic prophylaxis. Chronic symptoms that are unresponsive to nonoperative therapy require surgical intervention.[57,58]

The first case of bleeding from jejunal diverticulosis was reported by Braithwaite[59] in 1923. Less than 60 cases of bleeding from jejunal diverticula have been reported.[47,56,60–63] These patients most commonly exhibit hematochezia but can also have melena and hematemesis. Preoperative localization may be difficult. Furthermore, coexisting colonic diverticula (50 per cent) will further confuse the picture. After initial colonoscopy and esophagogastroduodenoscopy fail to reveal an obvious source, selective mesenteric arteriography is undertaken. If arteriography does not reveal the source, a radionuclide scan and repeat upper and lower endoscopy are performed. If the patient's condition is stable and recurrent blood loss occurs, the patient should undergo a contrast study of the jejunum and ileum, i.e., enteroclysis. If jejunal diverticulosis is found, one resection should be scheduled. In patients who had jejunal diverticulosis that was ignored as the source of bleeding, recurrence has been high.[64] The exact definition of the bleeding point may be difficult. If the patient has an angiographic catheter in place, instillation of methylene blue through the catheter will aid in localization.[65] The treatment of choice in such cases is complete resection of the involved segment of small intestine with an end-to-end anastomosis.

Intestinal obstruction secondary to jejunal diverticula may be caused by volvulus, adhesions, enterolith formation, intussusception, or compression by a large diverticulum.[66–69] Adhesions from previous diverticular inflammation may lead to mechanical obstruction extraluminally or an intraluminal stricture. Volvulus and adhesions require resection of the involved intestinal segment.

Obstruction may also be a nonmechanical problem from dyskinesia.[70] Peristaltic activity of the jejunum can become uncoordinated and inefficient, producing the bloating sensation. In severe cases of jejunal dyskinesia, the clinical picture is identical to that of mechanical obstruction with a thickened jejunum and dilated proximal bowel. Symptoms in patients with jejunal dyskinesia have been effectively relieved after resection of the abnormally hypertrophied intestine including the diverticula.[58]

Perforation of an acquired jejunal diverticula may give rise to symptoms indistinguishable from those of a perforated peptic ulcer, pancreatitis, or cholecystitis. Localized peritonitis usually results because the diverticulum is walled off by adjacent small bowel mesentery. Generalized peritonitis may occur. The mortality from perforated small bowel diverticula has been reported to be between 21 and 40 per cent.[71] Acute inflammation in the absence of perforation is an uncommon finding.[72] It is extremely rare that the diagnosis of a perforated diverticulum is made prior to operation. In the patient with jejunal diverticulitis, a CT scan may reveal an inflammatory mass containing air with edema of the mesentery and intraluminal contrast material outlining an adjacent diverticulum.[73]

The occurrence of pneumoperitoneum without peritonitis is a well described complication of jejunal diverticula.[74,75] This is often due to rupture of a diverticulum or by transmural passage of air through the semipermeable membrane of a thin-walled diverticulum. In patients with peritonitis or pneumoperitoneum of obscure origin, laparoscopy may be used to examine the small bowel for jejunal diverticulosis. This may manifest as chronic nonlocalizing abdominal pain in a patient with a diagnosis of irritable bowel syndrome; the symptoms may be indirectly related to jejunal diverticulosis. In these patients, intestinal resection is indicated and may alleviate symptoms.

Complications of Ileal Diverticular Disease

Acquired ileal diverticulosis is an uncommon entity. Bristowe[76] in 1854 is credited with the first description of an acquired ileal diverticulum. The reported incidence of ileal diverticula ranges from 0.001 to 2 per cent.[77] In contrast to jejunal diverticulosis, these lesions appear to be solitary. Complications of ileal diverticula appear to be more catastrophic than those of jejunal disease with perforation, hemorrhage and diverticulitis most common.

Inflammation seen as acute diverticulitis or perforation is the most common presentation of symptomatic ileal diverticulosis. Most patients exhibit signs and symptoms indistinguishable from appendicitis.[78-82] Obviously, these patients should be operated upon promptly and a limited small bowel resection should be performed. A small group of patients will have recurrent bouts of abdominal pain, fevers, and failure to thrive.[83] Rarely ileal diverticulitis will be seen as a fistula either to the bladder or the jejunum.[84] Perforation of ileal as well as jejunal diverticula by foreign bodies has been reported.[85] Radiographically, a small bowel follow-through will reveal thickening of mucosa folds, a perforation with extravasation, or findings suggestive of an inflammatory mass.[86] The CT findings of thickening of the ileal mesentery or a mass in ileal diverticulitis can probably not be differentiated from those of other inflammatory processes in the right lower quadrant.[87]

At surgery, most of these patients have an inflammatory mass in the right lower quadrant.[88-92] In the absence of appendicitis or obvious Crohn's disease, one should consider a perforated ileal diverticulum and proceed with ileocolectomy. Since these lesions originate on the mesenteric side of the bowel, simple closure, excision, or invagination may be impossible in the presence of inflammation, and segmental resection is preferred.

As in the jejunum, ileal diverticula may present as a small bowel obstruction. This may be caused by stenosis and scarring caused by chronic diverticulitis of the distal ileum.[93] Volvulus, intussusception, and enteroliths also may occur.[94,95] A rare cause of obstruction has been the migration of bezoars that were found to be impacted in an ileal diverticulum.[96] In all cases, a resection of the small bowel bearing the diverticular segment is recommended.

Bleeding from ileal diverticula has been documented only three times and has always been associated with inflammation.[97,98] Two patients experienced hypotension due to erosion into major vessels, while the third had recurrent hematochezia. A diverticular source of blood loss was confirmed at laparotomy. As in jejunal diverticular disease the diagnosis may be elusive; however, when ileal diverticular disease is found intestinal resection and anastomosis should be performed.

MECKEL'S DIVERTICULUM

Johann Meckel first published the description of the congenital anomaly that bears his name in 1809.[99] Meckel's diverticulum is the most common congenital anomaly of the gastrointestinal tract. It is a remnant of the duct between the intestinal tract and the yolk stalk. Its incidence has been reported in various autopsy series to vary from 0.3 to 2.5 per cent.[100] In most reported series there is a male/female preponderance of approximately 2:1. The diverticulum is located on the antimesenteric border of the ileum, varies in shape, and is between 1 and 25 cm in length. It is situated 10 to 150 cm from the ileocecal valve and possesses a mesentery and an independent arterial supply from an arcade of the ileal vasculature. The lining of the diverticulum is the same as that of the ileum in most cases. However, heterotopic mucosa of either gastric, duodenal, colonic, or pancreatic tissue may occur either singly or in combination.[101]

Most Meckel's diverticula are asymptomatic, and of those patients who develop symptoms, 60 per cent will be seen at or below 10 years of age.[102] The common complications of Meckel's diverticulum are either hemorrhage from ulceration of adjacent ileum by ectopic gastric mucosa, inflammation from diverticulitis, or obstruction by intussusception, volvulus, or a fibrous band.[103-106] Rarely it will present as an umbilical fistula[107] or be found to contain a neoplasm.[108] The presence of a Meckel's diverticulum in a hernia sac is extremely rare and known as a Littre's hernia. Both the coexistence of Crohn's disease with extension of the ileal disease into a Meckel's diverticulum and primary Crohn's disease of a Meckel's diverticulum with microscopic normal ileum have been reported.[109] A Meckel's diverticulum may be found in the asymptomatic patient, either on a contrast study or as an incidental finding at surgery. Resection of a Meckel's diverticulum should be performed when it is the site of bleeding, obstruction, or diverticulitis.[110–112] In infants and children, it should be removed when found incidentally at laparotomy.[113] In the adult, a wide mouthed, thin walled, unattached diverticulum can be safely left alone. However, if it is attached to a mesodiverticular band, contains palpable thickening suggestive of ectopic tissue, or has a narrow base felt to be prone to lateral inflammation, it should be removed.[114,115]

Summary

The role of laparoscopy in the treatment of diverticular disease of the small bowel and colon will have many facets. In the immediate future it will aid in the diagnosis in the patient with persistent abdominal pain of unknown etiology or unexplained abdominal sepsis. Diverticular abscesses of the colon for which CT-guided drainage is not possible may potentially be drained laparoscopically. In colonic diverticular inflammation, whether it be perforation or abscess, the diverticular segment may be removed by a limited resection and Hartmann's procedure. Intestinal continuity may be restored laparoscopically by the use of the intraluminal circular stapler. Colomyotomy may be performed in the patient with refractory pain secondary to diverticular spasm, thereby avoiding a resection and anastomosis. Diverticulectomy through the laparoscope of the ileum, cecum, or a Meckel's diverticulum may avoid a laparotomy. In small bowel diverticular disease, an extracorporeal resection and primary anastomosis can potentially be performed. Since most patients afflicted with diverticular disease fall within the more advanced age groups. Minimally invasive surgical techniques for the treatment of diverticulitis will become increasingly more attractive as a means to diminish the high rates of morbidity and mortality associated with intervention in these patients.

REFERENCES

1. Nathan BN. Who first described colonic diverticula? Can J Surg 1991; 3:203.
2. Goligher JC. Surgery of the Anus, Rectum and Colon, 4th ed. London, Bailliére-Tindall, 1980, pp 200–214.
3. Fraser E. Über multiple falsche Darmdivertikel in der Flexura sigmoidea. Muench Med Wochenschr 1899; 46:74.
4. Beer E. Some pathological and clinical aspects of acquired (false) diverticula of the intestine. Am J Med Sci 1904; 128:135–145.
5. Mayo WJ. Acquired diverticulitis of the large intestine. Surg Gynecol Obstet 1907; 5:8–15.
6. Lockhart-Mummery JP. Late results in diverticulitis. Lancet 1938; 2:1401–1404.
7. Smithwick RH. Experiences with surgical management of diverticulitis of sigmoid. Ann Surg 1942; 115:969–985.
8. Hartmann H. Classic articles in colonic and rectal surgery. Henri Hartmann 1860–1952. New procedure for removal of cancers of the distal part of the pelvic colon. Dis Colon Rectum 1984; 27:273.
9. Madden JL, Tan PY. Primary resection and anastomosis in the treatment of perforated lesions of the colon, with abscess or diffusing peritonitis. Surg Gynecol Obstet 1961; 113:646.
10. Reilly M. Sigmoid myotomy. Proc R Soc Med 1964; 57:566.
11. Arfwidssen S, Dock NG. Pathogenesis of multiple diverticula of the sigmoid colon in diverticular disease. Acta Chir Scand 1964; 342(Suppl):5–68.
12. Painter NS, Truelove SC. The intraluminal patterns in diverticulosis of the colon. Gut 1964; 5:201–213.
13. Srivasta GS, Smith AN, Painter NS. Sterculia bulk-forming agent with smooth muscle relaxant use bran in diverticular disease. Br Med J 1976; 1:315–318.
14. Weinreich J, Anderson D. Intraluminal pressure in the sigmoid colon. II. Patients with sigmoid diverticula and related conditions. Scand J Gastroenterol 1976; 2:581–586.
15. Whiteway J, Morson BC. Elastosis in diverticular disease of the sigmoid colon. Gut 1985; 26:258–266.
16. Williams J. Changing emphasis in diverticular disease of the colon. Br J Radiol 1963; 36:393–406.
17. Schwartz JT, Graham DY. Diverticular disease of the large intestine. In Kirshner JB, ed. Diseases of the Colon, Rectum, and Anal Canal. Baltimore, Williams & Wilkins, 1988, pp 519–537.
18. Rege RV, Nahrwold DC. Diverticular disease. Curr Probl Surg 1989; 26:139–189.
19. Graham SM, Ballantyne GH. Cecal diverticulitis. A review of the American experience. Dis Colon Rectum 1987; 30:821–826.
20. Berci G. Emergency laparoscopy. In Salky BA, ed. Laparoscopy for General Surgeons. New York, Igaku-Shoin, 1990, pp 145–152.
21. Wychulis AR, Beahrs OH, Judd ES. Surgical management of diverticulitis of the colon. Surg Clin North Am 1967; 47:961–969.
22. Wolff BG, Ready RL, MacCarty RL, et al. Influence of sigmoid resection on progression of diverticular

disease of the colon. Dis Colon Rectum 1984; 27:645–647.
23. Benn PL, Wolff BG, Ilstrup DM. Level of anastomosis and recurrent colonic diverticulosis. Am J Surg 1986; 151:269–271.
24. Bell AM, Wolff BG. Progression and recurrence after resection for diverticulitis. In Veidenheimer MC, ed. Seminars in Colon and Rectal Surgery 1990; 1:99–102.
25. Classen JN, Bonardi R, O'Mara CS, et al. Surgical treatment of acute diverticulitis by staged procedures. Ann Surg 1976; 184:582–586.
26. Botsford TW, Zollinger RM Jr, Hicks R. Mortality of the surgical treatment of diverticulitis. Am J Surg 1973; 127:513–518.
27. Kerner BA, Oliver GC, Einsenstat TE, et al. Use of the Hartmann procedure in the treatment of complicated acute diverticulitis. In Veidenheimer MC, ed. Seminars in Colon and Rectal Surgery 1990; 1:87–92.
28. Howe EHJ, Casali RE, Westbrook KL, et al. Acute perforations of the sigmoid colon secondary to diverticulitis. Am J Surg 1979; 137:184–187.
29. Mallogna ET, Brummelkamp WH, Van Gulik TM, et al. The Hartmann procedure: Its role in acute complicated diverticulitis. Neth J Surg 1985; 38:171–174.
30. Mueller PR, Asini S, Wittenberg J, et al. Sigmoid diverticular abscess: Percutaneous drainage as an adjunct to surgical resection in 24 cases. Radiology 1987; 164:321–325.
31. Neff CC, van Sonnenburg E, Casola G, et al. Diverticular abscesses: Percutaneous drainage. Radiology 1987; 163:15–18.
32. Stabile BE, Poccio E, van Sonnenberg E, Neff CC. Preoperative percutaneous drainage of diverticular abscess. Am J Surg 1990; 159:99–105.
33. Daniel O. Sigmoid myotomy with peritoneal graft. Proc R Soc Med 1969; 62:39.
34. Hodgson J. Transverse tenomyotomy: A new surgical approach for diverticular disease. Ann R Coll Surg Eng 1974; 55:80.
35. Kettlewell MGW, Moloney GE. Combined horizontal and longitudinal colomyotomy for diverticular disease. Dis Colon Rectum 1977; 20:24.
36. Castrini G, Pappalardo G. A new technique of combined colomyotomy for diverticular disease. Int Surg 1981; 66:71–72.
37. Belding HH. Acute perforated diverticulitis of the sigmoid colon with generalized peritonitis. Arch Surg 1957; 74:511.
38. Madden JL, Tan PY. Primary resection and anastomosis in the treatment of perforated lesions of the colon, with abscess or diffusing peritonitis. Surg Gynecol Obstet 1961; 113:646.
39. Bonello J, Howerton RA. Single stage resection without colostomy in acute diverticulitis. In Veidenheimer MC, ed. Seminars in Colon and Rectal Surgery, 1990:1, pp 81–86.
40. Soemmering ST, Baillie M. Anatomie des krankhaften Baues von einigen der wichtigsten Theile im menschlischen Korper. Berlin, Vossiche Buchhandlung, 1794.
41. Cooper A. Anatomy and Surgical Treatment of Crural Umbilical Hernia. London, 1807.
42. Gordinier HC, Sampson JA. Diverticulitis (not Meckel's) causing intestinal obstruction. JAMA 1906; 46:1585.
43. Wilcox RD, Shatney CH. Surgical implications of jejunal diverticula. South Med J 1988; 81:1386.
44. Fisher JK, Fortin D. Partial small bowel obstruction secondary to ileal diverticulitis. Radiology 1971; 122:321.
45. Baskin RH, Mayo CW. Jejunal diverticulosis. Surg Clin North Am 1952; 32:1185.
46. Benson RE, Dixon CF, Waugh JM. Non-Meckelian diverticula of the jejunum and ileum. Ann Surg 1943; 118:377–393.
47. Mendonca HL, Vieta JO, Ling WSM. Jejunal diverticulosis with massive hemorrhage. Am J Gastroenterol 1978; 70:657–659.
48. Maull KI, Nicholson BW, Mendez-Picon G. Jejunoileal diverticulosis. South Med J 1981; 74:792–795.
49. Lee RE, Finby N. Jejunal and ileal diverticulosis. Arch Intern Med 1958; 102:97–102.
50. Nobles ER. Jejunal diverticula. Arch Surg 1971; 102:172–174.
51. Philips JHC. Jejunal diverticulosis. Some clinical aspects. Br J Surg 1953; 40:350.
52. Salomonowitz G, Wittich G, Hajek P, et al. Detection of intestinal diverticula by double contrast small bowel enema: Differentiation from other intestinal diverticula. Gastrointest Radiol 1983; 8:271–278.
53. Englund R, Jensen M. Acquired diverticulosis of the small intestine: Case reports and literature review. Aust N Z J Surg 1986; 56:51–54.
54. Donald JW. Major complications of small bowel diverticula. Ann Surg 1979; 190:183.
55. Knauer CM, Svoboda AL. Malabsorption and jejunal diverticulosis. Am J Med 1988; 44:610.
56. Khubchandani M, Berman L, Radolinski A. Non-Meckelian diverticulosis of the jejunum and ileum: A report of four cases, one with an arteriovenous malformation. NY State J Med 1986; 86:202–203.
57. Altmeier WA, Bryant LR, Wulsin JH. The surgical significance of jejunal diverticulosis. Arch Surg 1963; 86:732–744.
58. Williams RA, Davidson DD, Serota AI, Wilson SE. Surgical problems of diverticula of the small intestine. Surg Gynecol Obstet 1981; 152:621–626.
59. Braithwaite LR. A case of jejunal diverticula. Br J Surg 1923–24; 9:184.
60. Wilcox RD, Shatney CH. Massive rectal bleeding from jejunal diverticula. Surg Gynecol Obstet 1987; 165:425–428.
61. Spiegel RM, Schultz RW, Casarella WJ, Wolff M. Massive hemorrhage from jejunal diverticula. Radiology 1982; 143:367–371.
62. Shackelford, Marcus WY. Jejunal diverticula—A cause of gastrointestinal hemorrhage: A report of three cases and review of the literature. Ann Surg 1960; 151:930–938.
63. Baskin RH, Mayo CW. Jejunal diverticulosis. Surg Clin North Am 1952; 32:1185–1196.
64. Thomas CS, Tinsley EA, Brockman SK. Jejunal diverticula as a source of massive upper gastrointestinal bleeding. Arch Surg 1967; 95:89–92.
65. Rubio PA, Farrell EM. A new technique for identifying bleeding of the small bowel utilizing methylene blue infusion. Surgery 1979; 86:764.
66. Walker RM. The complications of acquired diverticulosis of the jejunum and ileum. Br J Surg 1944–45; 32:457.
67. Slater NS. Perforation and obstruction by enterolith complicating jejunal diverticulosis. Br J Surg 1954; 41:60.
68. Dunlop EE. Perforation of jejunal diverticulum associated with acute recurrent jejunogastric intussusception. Aust N Z J Surg 1952–54; 77:22.

69. Watson CM. Diverticula of the jejunum: A case with enterolith causing intestinal obstruction. Surg Gynecol Obstet 1924; 38:67.
70. McGrew W, Patel J, Miller P. Jejunal diverticulosis: Medical and surgical management. South Med J 1985; 78:533–535.
71. Roses DF, Gouge THE, Scher KS, Ranson JCH. Perforated diverticula of the jejunum and ileum. Am J Surg 1976; 132:649–652.
72. Herrington JL. Perforation of acquired diverticula of the jejunum and ileum. Surgery 1962; 51:426–433.
73. Greenstein S, Jones B, Fishman SK, et al. Small bowel diverticulitis: CT findings. AJR 1986; 147:271–274.
74. Dunn V, Nelson JA. Jejunal diverticulosis and chronic pneumoperitoneum. Gastrointest Radiol 1979; 4:165–168.
75. Herrington JL. Spontaneous asymptomatic pneumoperitoneum: A complication of jejunal diverticulosis. Am J Surg 1967; 113:567–570.
76. Bristowe JS. Trans Path. Soc Lond 1854; 6:191.
77. Parulekhar SG. Diverticulosis of the terminal ileum and its complications. Radiology 1972; 103:282–287.
78. Ackerman NB. Perforated diverticulitis of the terminal ileum. Am J Surg 1974; 128:426–428.
79. Sloan GM, Vineyard GC. Perforated diverticulum of the ileum. Am J Gastroenterol 1980; 74:447–450.
80. Cocks JR, Zino FJ. Acute diverticulitis of the terminal ileum. Br J Surg 1968; 55:45–49.
81. Kraus M, Sampson D, Wilson SD. Perforation of diverticulum of terminal ileum presenting as acute appendicitis. Surgery 1976; 79:724–725.
82. Jones D, McMillin R, Greene F. Complications of acquired diverticula of the ileum. Am Surg 1983; 43:218–220.
83. Bokhari SR, Resnick AM, Nemir P. Diverticulitis of the terminal ileum. Report of a case and review of the literature. Dis Colon Rectum 1982; 25:660–663.
84. Meng RL, Gardiner R, Banich T, Banich F. Ileovesical fistula: A rare complication of ileal diverticulitis. Can J Surg 1981; 24:74–76.
85. Lumdsen AB, Dixon JM. Tomato skins penetrating the small bowel. Br J Surg 1984; 71:648.
86. Miller WB, Felson B. Diverticula of the terminal ileum. AJR 1966; 96:361–365.
87. Gale ME, Birnbaum S, Gerzof, et al. CT appearance of appendicitis and its local complications. J Comput Assist Tomogr 1985; 9:34–37.
88. Clements JL, Berman M. Acute diverticulitis of the terminal ileum. Am J Gastroenterol 1970; 53:169–172.
89. Ikenaga T, Takeuchi Y. Acute diverticulitis of the terminal ileum. Am J Gastroenterol 1972; 57:68–73.
90. Bartone NF, Grieco RV. Acute diverticulitis of the terminal ileum. JAMA 1967; 202:1103–1105.
91. Crowley JG. Perforation in acquired diverticular disease of the terminal ileum. Am Surg 1973; 33:514–517.
92. Hoover EL, Natesha R, Soltani R, et al. Diverticulosis of the ileum with perforation. J Tenn Med Assoc 1988; 81:620–621.
93. Fisher JK, Fortin D. Partial small bowel obstruction secondary to ileal diverticulitis. Radiology 1977; 122:321–322.
94. Eckhauser FE, Zelenock GB, Freier DT. Acute complications of jejuno-ileal pseudodiverticulosis: Surgical implications and management. Am J Surg 1979; 138:320–323.
95. Resnick DJ, Raytich RE. Small intestinal diverticula. In Nyhus LM, ed. Shackleford's Surgery of the Alimentary Tract, 3rd ed. Philadelphia, WB Saunders, 1991, Vol 5, p 424.
96. Billings PJ, Farrington GH. Small bowel obstruction caused by bezoar from intestinal diverticula. Br J Surg 1987; 74:1186.
97. Delaney WE, Hedges RC. Acquired ileal diverticulosis and hemorrhagic diverticulitis. Gastroenterology 1962; 42:56–59.
98. Wilcox RD, Shatney CH. Surgical significance of acquired ileal diverticulosis. Am Surg 1990; 56:222–225.
99. Meckel JF. Ueber die divertikel am darmkanal. Arch Physiol 1809; 9:421–453.
100. Harkins HN. Intussusception due to invaginated Meckel's diverticulum. Ann Surg 1933; 98:1070–1095.
101. Taneja OP, Taneja S. Diseases of Meckel's diverticulum. Arch Surg 1965; 90:349–357.
102. Brian JE, Stair JM. Non-colonic diverticular disease. Surg Gynecol Obstet 1985; 161:189–195.
103. Ludtke FE, Mende V, Kohler H. Incidence and frequency of complications and management of Meckel's diverticulum. Surg Gynecol Obstet 1989; 169:537–542.
104. Moore T, Johnson B. Complications of Meckel's diverticulum. Br J Surg 1976; 63:453–454.
105. Weinstein EC, Cain JC, Remine WH. Meckel's diverticulum: 55 years of clinical and surgical experience. JAMA 1962; 182:251–253.
106. Ilbawi MN, Mishalany HG, Slim MS. Meckel's diverticulum review of a 30-year experience. Am J Proctol 1973; 24:237–244.
107. Yamaaguchi M, Takeuchi S, Awazu S. Meckel's diverticulum. Investigation of 600 patients in Japanese literature. Am J Surg 1978; 136:247–249.
108. Johnson HR. Carcinoma of Meckel's diverticulum. Cancer 1973; 31:742.
109. Solomons D, Halford MEH. Crohn's disease of a Meckel's diverticulum occurring in a case of jejunal diverticulitis. Br J Surg 1964; 51:910–913.
110. Leijonmarck C-E, Bonman-Sandelin K, Frisell J, et al. Meckel's diverticulum in the adult. Br J Surg 1986; 73:146–149.
111. Diamond T, Russell CFJ. Meckel's diverticulum in the adult. Br J Surg 1985; 72:480–482.
112. Passaro E, Richmond D, Gordon E. Surgery for Meckel's diverticulum in the adult. Arch Surg 1966; 93:315–318.
113. Schwartz H. Meckel's diverticulum; diverticulosis of the small intestine; umbilical fistulae and tumors. In Maingot's Abdominal Operations, 8th ed. Norwalk, CT, Appleton-Century-Crofts, 1985, p 1097.
114. Williams RS. Management of Meckel's diverticulum. Br J Surg 1981; 68:477–480.
115. Lang-Stevenson A. Meckel's diverticulum: To look or not to look; to resect or not to resect. Ann R Coll Surg Engl 1983; 65:218–220.

Chapter 21
Colorectal Cancer

Michele D. Davis
Garth H. Ballantyne

Cancer of the colon and rectum is the most common carcinoma of the gastrointestinal tract.[1] Colorectal cancer is second only to lung cancer as a leading cause of cancer deaths in the United States.[2] In 1989, approximately 150,000 new cases of colorectal cancer were diagnosed in the United States. At least 60,000 persons die of this disease yearly.[3] Indeed, in the United States, the incidence appears to be increasing.[4]

Unfortunately, the number of patients who develop colorectal cancers each year has been constantly increasing over the last half century.[5] The number of cases of colorectal cancer in the state of Connecticut, for example, has steadily increased (Fig. 21-1). During the period 1973 through 1985, 28,082 cases of colorectal cancer were reported to the Connecticut Tumor Registry. Between 1973 and 1985 the number of cases per year nearly doubled. Furthermore, the number of cases per year has linearly increased. As a result, it seems likely that this trend will continue for the foreseeable future.

The number of cases of colorectal cancer observed each year has increased faster than the growth of the population. The advancing age of the population accounts for part of this increased number of cases because the incidence of colorectal cancer increases with age.[6] Nonetheless, the age-adjusted incidence of colorectal cancer, which compensates for the changing age distribution of the population, has also increased (Fig. 21-2). Since the inception of the Connecticut Tumor Registry in 1935, the age-adjusted incidence of colorectal cancer has increased from 35.2 to 70.2 cases/100,000/year for men and from 32.1 to 49.2 cases/100,000/year for women. Unfortunately, this trend has continued both for men and for women. This trend has not been unique to Connecticut.

The incidence of colorectal cancer has also increased in other regions of the United States. The Surveillance, Epidemiology, and End Results (SEER) Program of the National Cancer Institute has calculated the age-adjusted incidence of colorectal cancer in five states and four metropolitan areas, which represent about 10 per cent of the population.[7] The SEER Program identified a 9.4 per cent increase in the age-adjusted incidence of colorectal cancer from 1973 to 1986. Age-adjusted incidence of colon and rectal cancer in 1986 for all groups was 50.5 cases/100,000/year, for men was 61.1 cases/100,000/year, and for women was 42.2 cases/100,000/year. Significant increases of incidence were noted since 1973 among all races as well as for both men and for women. The age-adjusted incidence for people over the age of 65 was 302.4 cases/100,000/year in 1973 and 333.5 cases/100,000/year in 1986. These results indicate that colorectal cancer is becoming an increasing danger for all segments of the United States population.

Unfortunately, end results for the treatment of colorectal cancer have changed very little

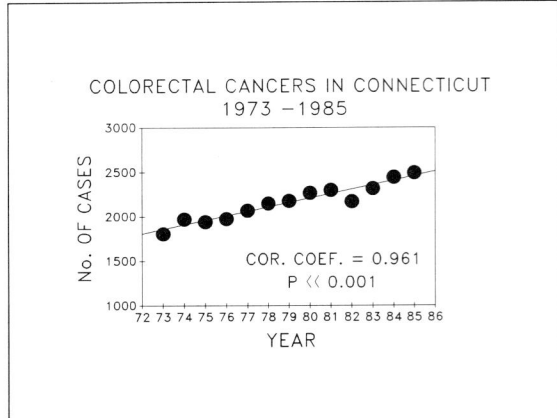

Figure 21-1. Number of new cases of colorectal cancer in Connecticut from 1973 through 1985. The number of cases has been linearly increasing. (Modified with permission from Vukasin AP, Ballantyne GH, Flannery JH, et al. Increasing incidence of cecal and sigmoid carcinoma: Data from the Connecticut tumor registry. Cancer 1990; 66:2442–2449.)

over the last 50 years. Despite countless numbers of publications, the relative benefits of various techniques of surgical resection for colorectal cancer remain undetermined. Indeed, discussion of the merits of these various approaches to colorectal resections among any group of surgeons often leads to lively debate. The recent advent of laparoscopic techniques for colorectal resections has rekindled these arguments.

The purpose of this chapter is to review current concepts of the surgical treatment of colorectal cancer. Specifically, areas of controversy will be highlighted so that the reader will be reminded that even in the era of "open surgical technique," there was no uniformity of approach to the treatment of colorectal cancer, and many critical issues remained unresolved. As a result, as we enter an era of "closed surgical technique," there should be no anticipation by anyone that surgeons will reach a consensus of opinion of what constitutes "good laparoscopic cancer surgery."

SURGICAL ANATOMY OF THE COLON AND RECTUM

The surgical treatment of colorectal cancer is based on anatomic resections of the involved portions of the large bowel. The extent of the resection is largely based on the normal blood supply and lymphatic drainage of the involved segment. Consequently, we will commence our discussion with a review of the normal blood supply and lymphatic drainage of the various segments of the colon and rectum.

Blood Supply and Lymphatic Drainage

RIGHT COLON

Blood supply to the right colon is delivered via the ileocolic and right colic arteries (Fig. 21-3). Venous drainage follows the arterial supply and eventually empties into the superior mesenteric vein, which leads to the portal vein (Fig. 21-4). Lymphatic drainage of the colon follows a course from intramural lymphatic vessels, to epicolic and paracolic lymph nodes, to regional lymph nodes, to nodes along the ileocolic and right colic vessels eventually terminating in nodes near the origin of the superior mesenteric artery (Fig. 21-5).[8-10] The ileocolic lymphatic drainage is segregated from the superior mesenteric drainage of the remainder of the small bowel by the avascular space of Treves, which runs on the medial side of the ileocolic vessels.[11] This zone provides a division in the direction of lymph flow since the distal portion of the ileal mesentery is devoid of both lymphatic and major vascular channels.

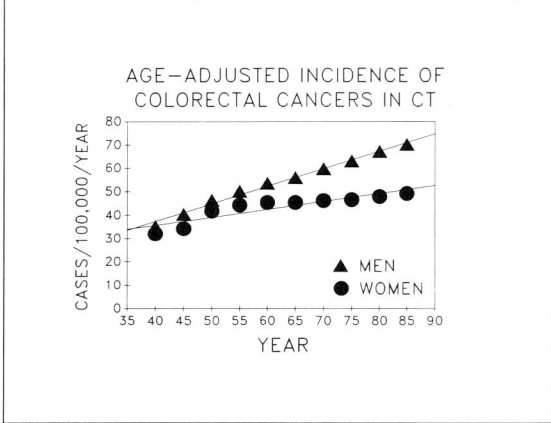

Figure 21-2. The age-adjusted incidence of colorectal cancers in Connecticut. Since 1935, the incidence of colorectal cancers for both men and women have been linearly increasing. (Modified with permission from Vukasin AP, Ballantyne GH, Flannery JH, et al. Increasing incidence of cecal and sigmoid carcinoma: Data from the Connecticut tumor registry. Cancer 1990; 66:2442–2449.)

shift by comparing distribution of large bowel cancer sites from resections that took place from 1928 through 1967. They showed a change in incidence of right colon cancers from 7 to 22 per cent and from 80 to 62 per cent for tumors of the sigmoid, rectosigmoid, and rectum. A trend toward lower stage tumors was also evident, possibly reflecting better methods of earlier detection or improved patient education. Similar reports of a left to right shift have been published by a number of institutions.[24-29]

This redistribution of colorectal cancers by percentage reflects the increasing incidence of colon cancers. Earlier in this century, colon cancers were uncommon. Since that time the incidence of rectum cancer has remained the same, while the incidence of colon cancers, particularly cecal and sigmoid cancers, has dramatically increased.[5] When distribution of lesions is calculated as a percentage, this appears to show a "shift to the right." In fact, the number of rectal cancers per population has remained unchanged, and the number of colon cancers, both right-sided and left-sided lesions, has substantially increased.

Patterns of Spread

Colorectal cancer can spread by direct extension through the bowel wall to invade surrounding tissues and organs, by lymphatic spread to local and regional nodes, and by way of hematogenous routes to local or distant metastatic sites. Spread through the peritoneal cavity, allowing adherence to the peritoneum, omentum, and serosa of organs, and specific metastases to the ovary have also been described.[3]

EXTENSION WITHIN THE BOWEL WALL

Invasion of a malignancy within the bowel wall may occur longitudinally, radially, or circumferentially. Intramural lymphatics form circumferential bands and then drain in a radial direction to the lymphatics of the mesentery. Consequently, invasive carcinomas tend to spread annularly and radially.[30] Indeed, the most direct route for spread of the carcinoma is by way of radial growth with contiguous extension into the deeper layers of the bowel wall and then extension to the pericolic or perirectal tissues and eventually invasive involvement of adjacent organs and tissues.

The extension of a colonic tumor may result not only in adherence to and invasion of surrounding structures, but alternatively in free perforation into the peritoneal cavity.[31] In contrast, rectal cancers do not usually gain access to the peritoneal cavity because of their retroperitoneal position in the pelvis.

Longitudinal growth of tumors has been intensively studied in lower colonic and rectal tumors because, in these sites, the risk of residual tumor at the distal site of resection is a critical issue. Scrutiny of longitudinal spread of colorectal cancer commenced in 1904 with a study by Clogg.[32] Since that time many authors have joined the debate.[4,33-36] In patients who have undergone curative resections, distal intramural spread of colorectal cancer is rare.[34,36,37] When it occurs, it is usually limited to within 2 cm of the primary lesion. Consequently, when a curative resection for sigmoid and rectal lesions is performed, a distal margin of 2 cm is satisfactory in more than 99 per cent of patients.

In patients with advanced colorectal cancers, the lesion may spread longitudinally for long distances. In these patients, obstruction of the usual patterns of lymphatic drainage causes retrograde flow of tumor-bearing lymph distally along the bowel wall in the submucosa. These patients exhibit an increased likelihood of extensive lymph node involvement. Often the tumor is poorly differentiated.[33,37] As a result, when a large bulky malignancy is encountered, 2 cm may not be adequate to ensure a tumor-free margin of distal resection.

LYMPHATIC EXTENSION

Patterns of lymphatic extension of colorectal carcinoma follow the anatomic route of lymphatic drainage of the large bowel. This proceeds from paracolic or pararectal lymph nodes to regional nodes to nodes of the origin of the mesenteric vessels. Skip lesions, which result from bypass of local or regional nodes to more proximal central nodes, are uncommon (less than 10 per cent of cases).[18,38]

The direction of lymphatic drainage of the large bowel cancers depends on the proximity of the major blood supply. Tumors lying near a major pedicle have a more predictable pattern of lymphatic spread while those lying between major pedicles may drain in a variety of different patterns and combinations.[18,30]

Miles[39] meticulously studied the lymphatic drainage of the rectum. He determined that the extramural lymphatic drainage of the rectum could be divided into three zones (Fig. 21-8).

1. The zone of downward spread includes the perianal skin, the ischiorectal fat, and the external sphincter muscle. The downward efferent lymphatics traverse the fatty tissue of the ischiorectal fossa following the path of the inferior hemorrhoidal vessels. The lymphatics enter Alcock's canal and then pass to the internal iliac nodes.

2. The zone of lateral spread encompasses the levator ani muscles, the coccyx muscles, the pelvic peritoneum, the prostate gland, the base of the bladder, the cervix uteri, and the base of the left broad ligament and the internal iliac glands. The lateral efferents enter a plexus situated between the levator ani muscles and the pelvic fascia. From this plexus, they pass through the obturator node situated at the obturator formen and hence to the internal iliac nodes.

3. The zone of upward spread includes the retrorectal nodes, the pelvic mesocolon, the paracolic nodes, the nodes at the bifurcation of the left common iliac artery, and the median lumbar node. The upward main efferent lymphatics accompany the superior hemorrhoidal veins. They pass through the lowermost mesocolic nodes and then follow the inferior mesenteric vein. As emphasized by Miles:

> Since the majority of the efferent lymphatics, which form the intramural lymphatic system, either pass through or terminate in the structures contained in this zone, it follows that these structures constitute the principal paths by which cancer cells spread from primary growths in the rectum. In fact this is the most constant and, therefore, the most important of all routes of spread.

VASCULAR SPREAD

Distant metastases in colorectal cancer patients develop by way of hematogenous spread. The sites most commonly involved are the liver, lung, bone, and ovary. A study undertaken by Russell et al.[40] examining sites of dissemination of carcinomas of the large bowel located above the peritoneal reflection showed that 80 per cent of patients with disseminated disease at the time of diagnosis had evidence of liver metastases. In 32 per cent of these patients, the liver was the only site of spread. Seventeen per cent had other sites of extra-abdominal metastases, the lung being the most common.

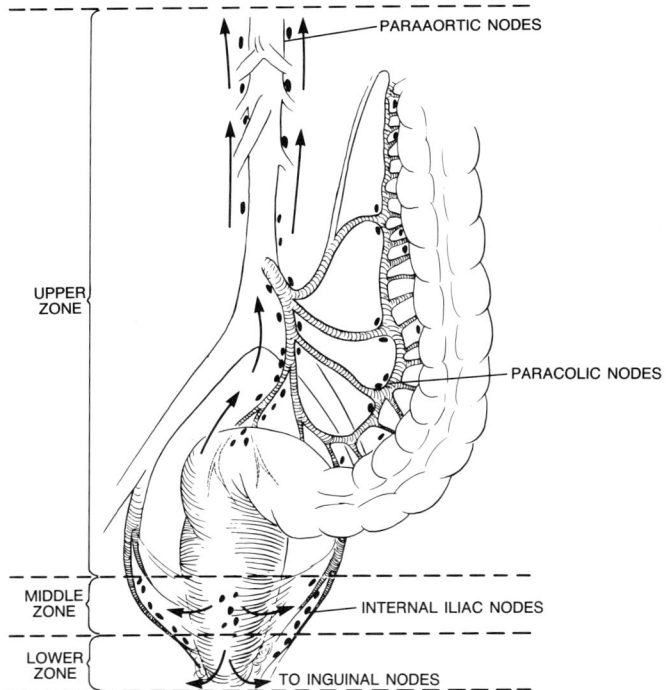

Figure 21-8. The zones of lymphatic drainage of the rectum as divided by Miles.

In a study of patients with disseminated rectal carcinoma, Dionne[41] found that 83 per cent of patients had liver metastases and in 73 per cent the liver was the sole focus of distant spread. He also found that 15 per cent of these patients had lung metastases with 8.7 per cent having the lung as the only distant metastatic site. Lower rectal cancers may have a greater propensity toward sole pulmonary metastases than tumors in the colon because there is access to the systemic circulation (bypassing the portal system) via the middle and inferior rectal veins.[42]

OVARIAN METASTASES

The mechanism by which colorectal cancer metastasizes to the ovary is poorly understood.[3] These fairly common metastases are often subcapsular and bilateral, suggesting they originated via hematogenous spread.[3,43] In an effort to explain this frequency of ovarian metastases, Alford et. al.[44] examined hormone receptors (estrogen and other steroids) in colon carcinomas. They found that 70 per cent of 33 colon carcinomas displayed these receptors, suggesting that some tumor cells spreading hematogenously may favor the "hormonal environment" of the ovary.

SURGICAL MANAGEMENT

The goals of surgical management of cancer of the colon and rectum include removal of all cancerous tissue while assuring minimal perioperative morbidity and mortality and leaving the patient with a reasonably good quality of life. The primary tumor and an adequate margin should be excised along with any possible regional lymphatic spread or direct invasion of adjacent tissues. This approach may be influenced by a variety of factors including (1) the general condition of the patient, (2) the age of the patient, (3) the acuteness of the presentation, (4) the adequacy of the bowel preparation, (5) the involvement of adjacent organs or metastatic sites, and (6) the experience of the surgeon.

Preoperative assessment of the patient with a large bowel tumor using computed tomography, endoluminal ultrasonography, and colonoscopy as well as a general medical assessment and carcinoembryonic antigen level determination may be helpful to the surgeon in making operative plans. Principles in the management of perioperative issues such as infection control, nutritional supplementation, preoperative bowel preparation, choices in adjuvant therapy, and timing of surgery must also be carefully considered by the surgeon. These issues, however, will not be discussed further in this chapter. Factors influencing decisions concerning choice of operation, margins of resection, and high ligation of vascular trunks will be discussed. Topics directly concerning patient survival such as rates of recurrence, morbidity and mortality, complications, and survival status will also be reviewed.

History

Although surgery of the colon dates back to 1776 when the first successful cecostomy was constructed,[45] the first successful resection and anastomosis was not performed until 1823 by Reybard.[46] Prior to this, exteriorization was the mainstay for the treatment of large intestine disease or injury until colostomy was instituted as a palliative procedure around 1839. Mortality rates for colonic resections were as high as 60 per cent during these times; therefore, intra-abdominal resection and anastomosis were abandoned for the staged, extraperitoneal procedure.[47-49] By 1900, the mortality rate for colon surgery had dropped to 37 per cent.[50] New operative procedures developed toward the end of the nineteenth century as a result of advances in anesthesia and aseptic technique.

In 1908, Miles[51] developed a new procedure for the treatment of cancer of the rectum: the combined abdominoperineal proctectomy became the standard of therapy for this disease. In 1922 a two-stage procedure was developed by Hartmann to avoid some of the problems of complications, morbidity, and mortality caused by the Miles procedure. Hartmann's method of resecting the sigmoid and intraperitoneal rectum did not include an extensive nodal dissection as the abdominoperineal resection described by Miles; however, many patients were cured and seemed to tolerate this procedure better.[52,53] Dixon[54] introduced the low anterior resection and sutured anastomosis for colorectal cancer in 1930. Prior to 1940, most surgeons did not advocate the use of intraperitoneal primary anastomosis for colon cancer operations. Instead, resection was usually preceded by colostomy or performed using a two-stage procedure.

By the 1950s, Allen[55] and others had demonstrated significant improvement in operative mortality. Attention to factors in perioperative care such as replacement of fluids, electrolytes, and blood, the use of antibiotics, nasogastric suction, and respiratory care, and improved anesthetic management aided in the reduction of operative mortality.

Since the 1950s, quality of life has become an important concern in the treatment of patients with colorectal cancer. The accomplishment of a procedure that allows retention of anal sphincter function and ensures an adequate curative resection has been the primary goal of surgeons in the treatment of large bowel tumors. Methods such as pull through procedures and abdominosacral resections have generally been replaced by the use of the low anterior resection either with a handsewn or stapled anastomosis.[56-60] Procedures such as local excision, electrodesiccation, trans-sphincteric resection, posterior proctectomy, and intracavitary radiation therapy were also developed for the purpose of sphincter preservation. However, they should be reserved for the treatment of small cancers, polypoid lesions, or villous adenomas, rather than as standard cancer operations.[61-65] Mucosal proctectomy has proven useful in the treatment of patients with premalignant conditions, such as inflammatory bowel disease and multiple polyposis syndromes, and certain small rectal cancers.[66-68]

Although the goals in the treatment of colorectal cancer have not changed, more emphasis is being placed on early detection, removal of premalignant lesions, and improvement in quality of life. As was done in the past, surgeons should continue to seek better methods for treating their patients with colorectal cancer not only to decrease morbidity, mortality, and complications perioperatively, but also to strive to improve survival by improving detection and removal of early lesions. From a historical point of view, great advances have been made since the late nineteenth century and with the more recent development of stapling devices and state-of-the-art equipment for use in laparoscopic surgery of the large bowel, surgeons can look forward to improved techniques in treating their patients with large bowel cancer.

Carcinoma of the Colon

CHOICE OF OPERATION

The main considerations in resecting colon tumors include (1) determination of sufficient margins to prevent recurrence, (2) ligation of vascular and lymphatic pedicles to ensure adequate clearance of lymphatic drainage routes, and (3) assurance that remaining tissue maintains an adequate blood supply to allow viability. As stated previously, the site or location of the tumor along the course of the large intestine determines not only its vascular supply, but also its lymphatic drainage. Whether the tumor is located adjacent to or between major pedicles determines with some probability what course of lymphatic drainage it will utilize. Tumors that are located directly adjacent to the major vascular pedicle are more likely to have a very direct route of drainage. Tumors located between major pedicles may drain in a variety of patterns; thus, wider mesenteric clearance may be necessary for these cancers. For this reason attention must be paid to the location of the tumor and operative plans be made accordingly.

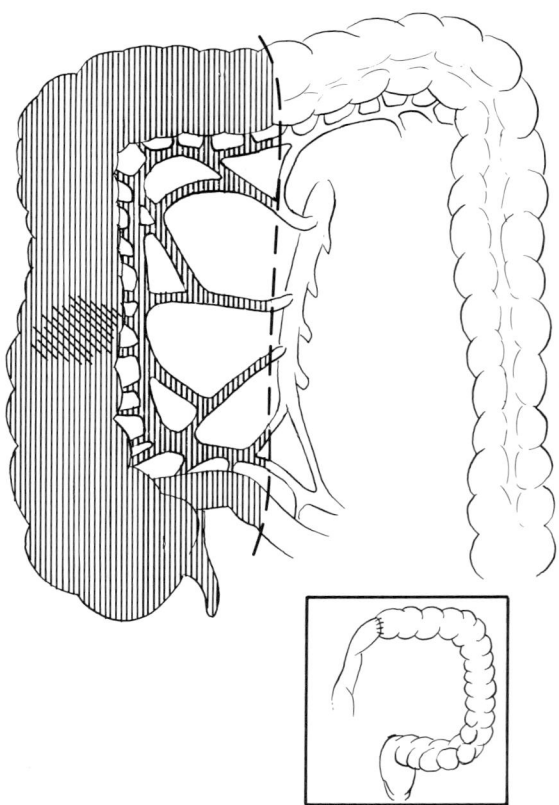

Figure 21-9. Right hemicolectomy for cecal, ascending colon, and hepatic flexure carcinomas with ligation of the ileocolic artery, the right colic artery, and the right branch of the middle colic artery.

CANCER OF THE RIGHT COLON

Adenocarcinomas of the cecum, ascending colon, and hepatic flexure are generally treated by right hemicolectomy (Fig. 21-9).[69–72] Tumors of the cecum generally drain along the ileocolic group of lymph nodes while tumors in the ascending colon and hepatic flexure generally drain along the right colic and middle colic groups of nodes, respectively. Depending on the location of the tumor in relation to the major lymphovascular pedicle, the tumor may share adjacent routes of drainage. Ligation and division of the lymphovascular pedicles of the ileocolic, right, and middle colic vessels are generally performed without difficulty, except occasionally in the obese patient. The extent of the resection generally runs from a point 10 cm proximal to the ileocecal valve to approximately the middle of the transverse colon. Primary anastomosis following right hemicolectomy is generally safe as long as no damage to the remaining vascular trunks has occurred.

CANCER OF THE TRANSVERSE COLON

Adenocarcinomas that arise in the region of the transverse colon to the splenic flexure generally drain and metastasize to lymph nodes that lie along the arterial arcade between the middle and left colic arteries. Depending on the location of the tumor along this length of colon, the pattern of drainage and metastases may occur along a variety of routes terminating in nodes at the origin of the superior mesenteric artery, inferior mesenteric artery, or periaortic region.

If the cancer appears to be metastasizing by way of the middle colic artery system, the transverse colon can be resected from the hepatic flexure to the splenic flexure (Fig. 21-10). The middle colic lymphovascular pedicle is ligated at its origin. In some situations, this would cause a colocolonic anastomosis that may not be tension-free. For this reason in this setting the entire right colon should also be resected to avoid the morbidity associated with an ischemic colocolonic anastomosis. Although there are no data that support either approach over the other, most authors prefer the security of a well perfused ileocolostomy even if it means a wider resection of colonic tissue.[69,71,72]

If the tumor is in an area of the distal transverse colon or splenic flexure that would permit drainage along the left colic artery or

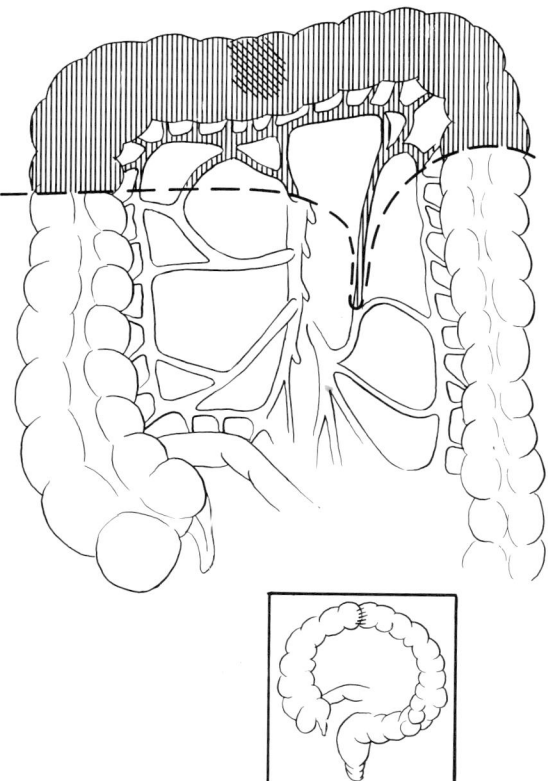

Figure 21-10. Segmental resection of the transverse colon with ligation of the middle colic artery at its origin for a transverse colon carcinoma.

if lymphatic metastases in this area are evident, more extensive resection is warranted. Ligation of the ileocolic and right and left colic lymphovascular trunks is performed and resection of the ascending, transverse, and descending colon is followed by ileosigmoid anastomosis.[70]

CANCER OF THE DESCENDING COLON

Tumors of the left colon drain and metastasize to nodes along the left colic artery and eventually to nodes around the origin of the inferior mesenteric artery and aorta. Most authors agree that left hemicolectomy is the procedure of choice for a carcinoma in this region of the bowel (Fig. 21-11). This procedure involves ligation of the inferior mesenteric lymphovascular pedicle and resection of the left transverse colon, splenic flexure, descending colon, and sigmoid colon.[69,70,72] Clearly, a large portion of normal colon is removed with this procedure, although it offers the widest clearance of the lymphatic-bearing mesentery. Even though no specific

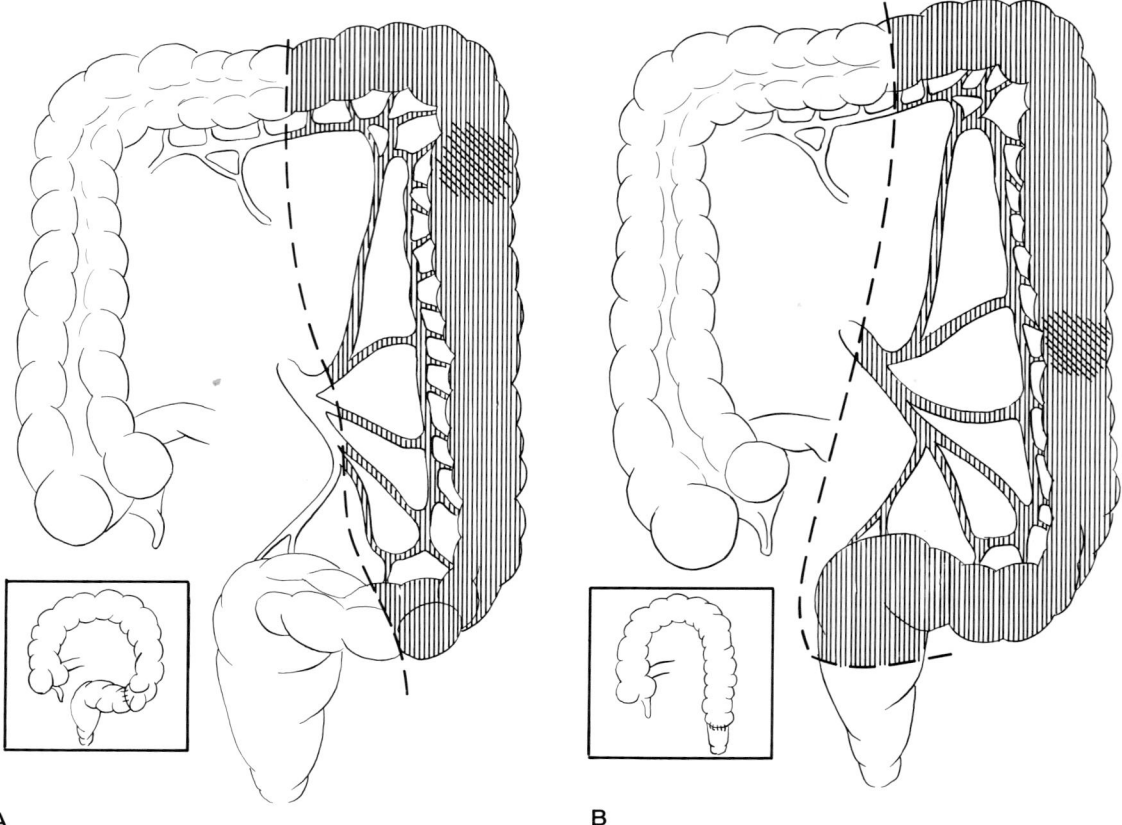

Figure 21-11. Left hemicolectomy with high ligation of the inferior mesenteric artery for a descending colon carcinoma. With: A, preservation of the inferior mesenteric artery and B, high ligation of the inferior mesenteric artery.

morbidity is associated with the dissection of the origin of the inferior mesenteric artery, the risk of surgical trauma associated with dissection of the splenic flexure and mobilization of the hepatic flexure to allow colorectal anastomosis must be considered. With this circumstance in mind, one may elect to perform a segmental resection of the involved segment of bowel and mesentery while still achieving adequate margins.

Rosi et al.[73] compared the results of left hemicolectomy and segmental resection for patients with tumors in the region of the descending colon and sigmoid colon (143 of 545 patients or 26.2 per cent). They found an increase in the 5-year survival rate by using left hemicolectomy (76.8 per cent) rather than segmental resection (63.0 per cent). One must keep in mind that this was not a randomized study and that the two groups were operated on during different time periods (segmental resection—1945 to 1950; left hemicolectomy —1950 to 1955). Also, other methods were initiated during the latter time period that may account for improvement in survival.

CANCER OF THE SIGMOID COLON

The sigmoid colon receives its blood supply by way of the sigmoidal arteries, which are low branches of the IMA. Lymphatic drainage of this portion of bowel parallels this course. The standard operation for cancers in this portion of the bowel is sigmoid resection or high anterior resection with primary anastomosis of the colon. This operation preserves the left colic artery, sacrificing only the sigmoidal branches of the inferior mesenteric artery (Fig. 21-12). Some authors advocate the use of left hemicolectomy, especially for proximal sigmoid lesions, which involves high ligation of the inferior mesenteric lymphovascular trunk and the construction of a sometimes technically difficult transverse colorectal anastomosis.[70,73] Depending on the location of

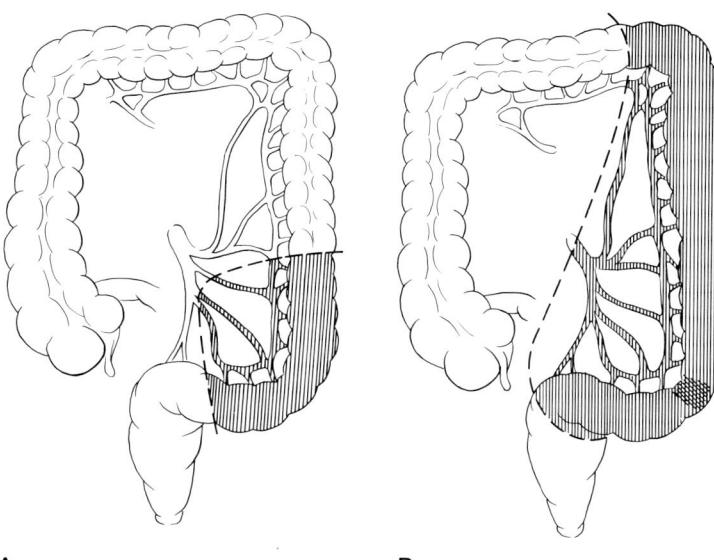

Figure 21-12. A, Sigmoid colectomy with preservation of the left colic and inferior mesenteric artery for a sigmoid carcinoma. B, Left hemicolectomy with high ligation of the inferior mesenteric artery for a sigmoid carcinoma.

the tumor, one may also choose a segmental resection that does not sacrifice the upper branches of the left colic artery. This preserves the blood supply to the splenic flexure and descending colon, but still allows adequate clearance of tumor with wide margins and substantial mesentery.[69,71,72] This procedure also avoids the possible hazards associated with additional dissection of the splenic flexure. Regardless of which of these procedures the surgeon elects to use, it is essential that the anastomosis is under no tension and has an adequate blood supply from proximal and distal sources. Surgical treatment for tumors of the rectosigmoid will be discussed in the section with surgical treatment for tumors of the rectum.

SURGICAL TECHNIQUE

Determination of Resectability

The determination of whether or not a patient has curable or resectable disease usually rests on the presence of tumor beyond the boundaries of resectability. These tumor deposits may be found on preoperative evaluation or at the time of laparotomy. They may be present in the liver, greater omentum, ovaries, contiguous structures, or other parts of the colon. Isolated metastases in the liver or lung do not necessarily indicate incurability, just as contiguous involvement of adjacent structures does not mean a tumor is unresectable. It is generally accepted that en bloc resections may be performed as a potentially curative procedure.

Extent of Resection

The extent of resection for cancers of the colon has been the topic of debate for some time. This issue does not carry with it certain ramifications that affect the patient's quality of life as resection of carcinoma of the rectum does. The prospect of possessing a permanent colostomy is not welcomed by most patients if it can be avoided and if the prognosis for the patient is not affected. In most circumstances involving nonemergency surgery for cancer of the colon, resection with colostomy formation is not necessary since primary resection may be performed followed by immediate reconstitution of bowel integrity through anastomosis.

The determination of whether extended resection is necessary for tumors of the colon may be made by examining not only the anatomy of the bowel itself, but also the biology of the tumor. The rationale for extensive lymphatic resection developed as more detailed information about the anatomy of the bowel wall and lymphatic system was uncovered. Gilchrist and David[122] found lymphatic metastases in postmortem specimens from patients who had undergone large bowel resection for cancer. Most of these lymphatic metastatic sites were located 1.5 cm or less from the bounds of the standard resection. They offered the idea that perhaps potential cure could be achieved by a wider lymphatic resection. This led other investigators to examine the progression of spread of tumor through the lymphatics. Gabriel, Dukes, and Bussey found that cancer did not spread erratically along the lymphatics, but that lymphatic metastases occurred in an orderly fashion along the lymph node chain toward the major vascular pedicle.[141] As mentioned previously "skip metastases" may occur, but only in approximately 5 per cent of the population. Concern about other patterns of metastatic spread led Grinnell[74] to study "retrograde lymphatic metastases" caused by blockage of normal drainage routes of colorectal tumors by infiltration with cancer cells. He found examples of this type of spread in 4.2 per cent of the 913 specimens that were examined.

High Ligation of the Inferior Mesenteric Artery

The identification of lymph node metastases by Grinnell near the origin of the inferior mesenteric artery gave rise to enthusiasm for performing radical lymphadenectomy in an attempt to perform a potential curative resection by removing as many cancerous nodes as possible. Studies by Rosi et al.[73] and McElwain et al.[75] demonstrated an increase in the incidence of positive nodes within specimens from patients who had undergone this extended lymphadenectomy. Bacon et al.[76] suggested by clinicopathologic correlation that some patients could benefit from this approach in terms of 5-year survival. Other authors have also demonstrated improvements in survival by using extended lymph node dissection for patients with left colonic and rectal cancer.[73,77,78]

Not all surgeons have agreed with the use of radical hemicolectomy for treating colon cancer. Ferguson et al.[79] suggested that survival of patients having undergone radical procedures was comparable with those having conservative operations. Harvey and Auchincloss[80] believed that extensive resections should be performed only when there was little additional risk added to the procedure since radical procedures offered little in prolonging patient survival. Even Grinnell[74] found that his patients with retrograde lymphatic metastases would not benefit in terms of survival from the use of a radical procedure. Thus, although the rationale for the use of this extensive lymphatic dissection is well based, clinical support for this radical technique has not been clear-cut. Unfortunately, a randomized control study that would clarify this issue has not been accomplished.[81]

Evaluation of the "No-Touch" Technique

The "no-touch" technique involves ligation of the lymphovascular pedicle prior to any manipulation of the tumor theoretically to prevent tumor emboli from being disloged during operation. Advocates of this technique believed that these tumor emboli to the liver were important causes of treatment failure in colorectal cancer.[82-84] This procedure had already been described by Barnes in 1952[85]; nevertheless, in 1967 Turnbull et al.[84] published survival statistics using this approach in patients who had colon cancer. In this study comparisons were made between the "no-touch" technique, as practiced by Turnbull, and the conventional methods used by his colleagues. The crude survival rates for all classes of tumor were 51 and 35 per cent at 5 years and 40 and 29 per cent at 10 years with the patients undergoing resection using the "no-touch" technique doing better. Turnbull also included in this publication a new staging designation for patients with residual tumor following resection—class D tumors. Stage-specific actuarial survival for patients with A tumors was 98.9 per cent, for patients with B tumors was 85 per cent, and for patients with C tumors was 67.3 per cent.

Criticism of Turnbull's technique and results have been widespread. The results of the study are often challenged because this was not a randomized trial; only the results of a controlled trial can resolve this issue. Clearly it has been shown that the same results are obtainable by other surgeons who do not use this technique.[86] Other areas of debate concerning the "no-touch" technique have been undertaken, including examination of peripheral or portal venous blood for cancer cells during operation[87-89]; however, none of these data either support or negate the use of the no-touch technique in the surgical treatment of large bowel cancer. Until data from controlled clinical trials are available, techniques such as these should only be used if no harm will be caused to the patient. In the next section, margins of resection and high ligation of the lymphovascular pedicle will be discussed.

Prophylactic Oophorectomy

Ovarian metastases often develop in female patients with colorectal cancers. Indeed, macroscopic evidence of ovarian metastases is found in 3 to 8 per cent of women during operations for large bowel cancers.[90] Prospective studies in which all women patients underwent prophylactic oophorectomy determined that the incidence of macroscopic or microscopic ovarian metastases ranged from 7 to 11 per cent.[91] Because of the high mortality associated with ovarian metastases, a number of groups have advocated routine prophylactic oophorectomy in all women treated for colorectal malignancy.[92,93] A study from the Mayo Clinic supported the concept that a 3 to 8 per cent improvement in survival might be achieved with prophylactic oophorectomy.[94] Unfortunately, the size of the study limited the significance of the findings. Thus, at present, the benefit of prophylactic oophorectomy in women with colorectal cancer remains unconfirmed.

Local Excision

Some colon cancers that are found in a polyp are adequately treated by colonoscopic polypectomy.[95] In general, these lesions should be pedunculated, less than 2 cm in diameter, and be able to be excised in one piece with snare cautery. Histologic review should demonstrate that the lesion is well differentiated, the tumor is not near the margin of resection, and no vascular invasion is present. Under these circumstances long term survival can be anticipated in more than 95 per cent of patients.[96–99]

The introduction of laparoscopic techniques for colonic resections makes the possibility of local excisions of colonic cancers a potential future option. The success of endoscopic polypectomy in the treatment of malignant polyps and the success of local excision of early rectal cancers (see next section) suggest that local excision of early colon cancers may prove an appropriate treatment strategy. This issue will require careful evaluation in the future.

SURGICAL MANAGEMENT FOR CARCINOMA OF THE RECTUM

Determination of Resectability

The principles for determining resectability for cancers of the rectum are similar to those for colon cancers. The determination of whether a cancer is curable lies in the observation that tumor spread does not extend beyond the limits of resection. Often this cannot be accurately assessed until the time of laparotomy when the liver, omentum, pelvic structures, ovaries, and the remainder of the colon are examined. Although a preoperative computed tomographic scan of the pelvis may add much information to the initial clinical assessment, the final decision as to the resectability of a cancer is made at the time of laparotomy.

The determination of resectability is generally made on observations obtained at the initial operation. These include the presence of metastases in the liver, peritoneum, or other sites and the fixity of tumor to surrounding structures. While metastases to the liver, lung, or ovary do not imply incurability,[4,100,101] an assessment of the number and extent of metastatic disease should be made intraoperatively by the surgeon to determine if curative resection is technically possible. A study by Durdey et al.[102] demonstrated that fixation of the tumor in the pelvis or to an adjacent organ does not necessarily mean that there is contiguous spread of cancer. They showed that 27 per cent of the 625 patients in the study had fixation with 20 per cent attributed to malignant invasion. In the remaining 7 per cent of patients inflammatory tissue was the cause for attachment, which did not seem to decrease survival or increase the likelihood of recurrent disease.

Choice of Operation

The selection of the appropriate operative procedure for patients with rectal cancer depends on a variety of issues. Factors that have proven helpful in determining this choice include the level of the lesion, the macroscopic appearance, the fixity, the degree of circumferential involvement, the degree of differentiation, the status of lymph nodes, body habitus, sex, age, and the presence of metastatic or systemic disease.

The major controversy surrounding the surgical treatment of rectal cancer is the debate concerning treatment of tumors of the middle and lower portions of the rectum. The objective of any cancer operation is to provide the patient with the best chance of cure or optimal long term survival and minimal complications without interfering with the patient's overall quality of life. Certainly sacrifice of the anal sphincter falls into this category. Thus, in the following discussion each of the previous factors will be examined to determine whether low anterior resection (as a sphincter-preserving operation) should be used instead of abdominoperineal resection in patients with low rectal cancers. Local treatment for these lesions will also be discussed.

Surgical Technique

LEVEL OF THE LESION

The location of the cancer in the rectum is probably the most important factor in determining whether a sphincter-preserving operation is technically feasible. The distance of the tumor from the anal verge has a direct bearing on the amount of tissue available for construction of the anastomosis. It has been customary and practical when discussing location of tumors in the rectum to refer to cancers as lying in the lower, middle, or upper third of the rectum. Generally, distance from the anal verge defines boundaries for the upper third (from 11 to 15 cm from the anal verge), the middle third (from 7 to 11 cm from the anal verge), and the lower third of the rectum (less than 7 cm from the anal verge). These distances are measured using the sigmoidoscope with great care being taken to measure the distance from the anal verge not from where it emerges from the buttock. In general, tumors of the upper third of the rectum are treated by low anterior resection. Tumors of the lower third of the rectum are often treated using abdominoperineal resection. Treatment of lesions of the middle third of the rectum provides the greatest area of debate. In this segment, the clinician must take into consideration all factors that may affect outcome when deciding between abdominoperineal resection and low anterior resection for patients with these tumors.

MARGINS OF RESECTION

What constitutes a reliably safe distal margin has been under much debate. The "5-cm rule" of distal margin was the standard of practice for many years. This was based on the interpretation of studies that addressed the risk of distal (retrograde) intramural spread of the tumor (Table 21-1).[103,104] With the advent of stapling devices that made low rectal anastomoses more easily and safely ac-

Table 21-1. Degree of Distal Intramural Spread in Curative versus Palliative Resections for Tumors 5 to 18 cm from the Dentate Line

	Curative Resections	Palliative Resections
Number of cases	76/93 (82%)	17/96 (18%)
Cases with distal intramural spread >5 mm	9/76 (12%)	9/17 (53%)
Maximum extent of spread (cm)	4.0	7.0
Average extent of spread (cm)	2.0	3.0

Data from Grinnell RS. Distal intramural spread of carcinoma of the rectum and rectosigmoid. Surg Gynecol Obstet 1954; 99:421–428.

complished, this issue was reexamined. Indeed, pathologic and anatomic studies have supported the concept that this type of tumor spread is rarely a problem and that for low grade (Broder's 1 and 2) tumors, a margin of 2 to 2.5 cm beyond the macroscopic margin of tumor would be sufficient to include that microscopic spread within the bowel wall.[105-107]

Survival data support the use of a 2-cm rule for distal margins. Pollett and Nicholls[108] demonstrated that a distal margin of less than 2 cm for rectal cancers does not adversely affect local recurrence or survival. Similarly, Wilson and Beahrs[109] found similar rates of survival and local or pelvic recurrence in groups of patients with distal margins greater than 5 cm or less than 2 cm. In some patients, anastomosis as low as the levator ani muscles has been performed.[110] However, lesions of high grade malignancy (poorly differentiated) have a greater chance of distal intramural spread and a greater margin (perhaps up to 6 cm) should be allowed.[103,106]

DETERMINATION OF PROXIMAL MARGINS

The site of the proximal transection of the colon during resections for rectal cancers is mandated by the level of vascular ligation. An adequate blood supply for the proximal side of the anastomosis must be guaranteed. If the inferior mesenteric vessels and at least some of the sigmoid branches are preserved, an anastomosis between the proximal sigmoid and distal rectum can be constructed (Fig. 21-13). If the ascending branch is preserved,

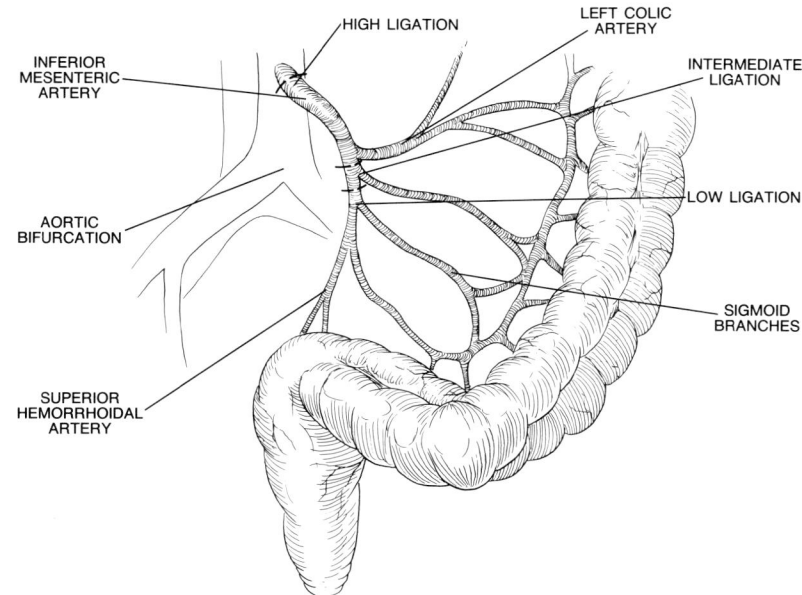

Figure 21-13. During low anterior resection or abdominoperineal resection for rectal carcinoma the inferior mesenteric artery can be ligated at three levels: 1, high ligation; 2, intermediate ligation; and 3, low ligation.

the descending colon can be utilized. If a high ligation of the inferior mesenteric vessels is accomplished, the distal transverse colon will be used for the anastomosis.

THE LEVEL OF VASCULAR AND LYMPHATIC LIGATION

Several groups have insisted that ligation of the inferior mesenteric artery flush with the aorta improves survival of patients afflicted with cancers of the rectum.[80,111,112] Many of these reports advocate use of high ligation without any support from survival analysis. Some recent investigations, however, suggest that there is no advantage in terms of 5-year survival in performing a high ligation of the inferior mesenteric artery in treating patients with rectal cancer.[75,113,114] Certainly no difference in survival with high ligation should be expected for patients with Dukes A and B tumors since there is no lymph node involvement.

The effect of high ligation on survival of patients with lymph node involvement remains hotly debated. To evaluate the effect of high ligation on patients with Dukes C tumors, Surtees et al.[115] used a highly selected group of patients. Following analysis using a variety of pathologic variables, no survival benefit was demonstrated for patients with Dukes C rectal cancer who underwent high vascular ligation of the inferior mesenteric artery. It has been suggested that by the time the tumor has spread to lymph nodes at the origin of the inferior mesenteric artery, further spread to other nodes and sites "beyond the reach of cure by surgery" has also occurred.[113]

LATERAL MARGINS

The need for dissection of the lateral pelvic wall for extended lymph node resections remains controversial. This radical dissection was encouraged originally because of the identification of positive iliac nodes in some patients who had undergone abdominopelvic lymphadenectomy.[116–118] Indeed, Waugh and Kirklin[119] suggested that the poor survival rate seen for patients with low rectal cancer was a result of the lateral spread of tumor. Also, others showed that there was in fact lateral lymphatic spread of some tumors probably caused by blockage of the usual routes of lymphatic drainage by extensive metastatic disease.[41,120–122]

Long term follow-up of patients does not seem to support the use of radical pelvic dissections. Stearns and Deddish[77] showed, for example, that not only did this extended lymphatic dissection show no benefit for patients in terms of survival, but actually increased the morbidity associated with rectal excision by increasing the rate of urologic complications, the length of hospital stay, and the transfusion rate per patient. Similar findings by other groups have led some surgeons to abandon this procedure.[123] Nonetheless, others continue to advocate radical lateral dissections.[124]

RESECTION OF THE DISTAL MESORECTUM

The fascia propria, which enveils the mesorectum, may act as a barrier to the spread of rectal cancer. In addition, rectal cancers may metastasize to lymph nodes in the rectal mesentery, which are more than 2 cm distal to the gross margin of the tumor. Based on these two concepts, Heald and colleagues[125] have argued that in the performance of a low anterior resection, the entire mesorectum should be excised along with the specimen.

Heald's group implemented complete mesorectal excision as part of their standard technique for low anterior resection. Since the entire blood supply of the rectum is excised, the anastomosis is constructed within 3 to 4 cm of the anal canal. Heald and colleagues[126] reported 5-year results on 115 patients. Only 3.7 per cent of patients had developed local pelvic recurrences; this is the lowest rate of pelvic recurrence ever reported. Unfortunately, the morbidity of this procedure is high. The devascularization of the rectum leads to a high leak rate from the colorectal anastomosis. In addition, functional results after this procedure are poor in many patients. Overall Heald's results are promising but require further substantiation from other investigators.

OTHER DETERMINING FACTORS

There are other factors that may help the surgeon in determining which procedure to use when treating patients with rectal cancer. The macroscopic appearance of the tumor during endoscopy may indicate the aggressiveness or the invasiveness of the tumor. If a lesion is polypoid, small, and exophytic, it may be adequately excised by less radical means than a large infiltrative or ulcerated tumor. Similarly, more aggressive tumors are more likely to exhibit more extensive growth patterns, causing the tumor to occupy a greater circumference of the bowel. The degree of fixation of the tumor in the pelvis may also encourage the surgeon to use a more aggressive approach to eliminate the chance of local recurrence. This may include en bloc resection of surrounding structures with low anterior resection (LAR) or abdominoperineal resection (APR) or the option of preoperative radiation therapy may be considered. A biopsy prior to operative intervention will also give the surgeon information needed to choose an appropriate procedure. As mentioned previously, tumors that are low grade (well or moderately well differentiated) tend to be less aggressive and require minimal margins for cure. However, if a cancer is more anaplastic or poorly differentiated, more generous distal margins are probably necessary. Preoperative evaluation using digital examination or intrarectal ultrasound may also give information as to the extent of spread of the lesion.

ABDOMINOPERINEAL RESECTION VERSUS LOW ANTERIOR RESECTION

There are numerous reports showing that APR and sphincter-preservation surgery for cancer of the middle third of the rectum have comparable 5-year survival rates as well as morbidity and mortality figures.[127-135] One of these studies by Slanetz et al.[130] showed that patients undergoing LAR were less likely to suffer postopertive morbidity than those undergoing APR (56 per cent versus 68 per cent) especially in terms of cardiovascular complications (4.8 per cent versus 12 per cent) and genitourinary complications (14 per cent versus 35 per cent).[130] Mortality figures demonstrated that 50 per cent of the deaths of patients who underwent APR were caused by cardiopulmonary disasters, whereas sepsis was the leading cause of death in those undergoing LAR. The authors also noted that mortality figures from LAR have significantly decreased in the more recent portion of the study. Comparison of local recurrence rates between the two groups showed that rates for LAR were slightly lower than for APR. Although most reports comparing the two procedures are not controlled trials, they do support the concept that sphincter-saving operations are a good alternative for properly selected patients with carcinoma of the middle third and perhaps some with carcinoma of the distal third of the rectum.

FAILURE OF RADICAL SURGICAL TECHNIQUES

During the last 50 years, surgeons have been frustrated by their failure to improve the survival of patients with rectal cancer. Consequently, a variety of radical techniques that strived to eliminate all regional disease by more and more extensive resections have been implemented by some surgeons. Unfortunately, no clear advantage in survival outcome has been consistently confirmed for any of these techniques.

Sugarbaker and Corlew[136] from the National Institutes of Health compiled a review to examine the evidence that certain surgical techniques may influence survival rates for patients with colorectal cancer. They examined data concerning the following factors of surgical treatment: (1) distal margins, (2) the presence of adhesions in adjacent structures, (3) the difference between segmental resection and radical hemicolectomy, (4) the no-touch technique, and (5) techniques to control intraluminal tumor cells. No consistent evidence could be found to suggest that distal margins less than 5 cm in patients undergoing LAR decreased survival. Likewise, no statistically significant differences could be found in survival rates between patients undergoing segmental resection or radical hemicolectomy for similar colon or rectal disease. It was apparent, however, that significantly increased rates of morbidity were associated with the use of radical surgical treatment of rectal carcinoma. No evidence to support the use of the no-touch technique or techniques to control the spread of intraluminal cancer cells could be found. The en bloc excision of adjacent adhesed structures was deemed important in improving survival in a small distinct group of patients. This review evaluated important aspects of techniques used for colorectal cancer surgery; however, it is clear that more controlled trials are needed to examine special techniques in cancer surgery to determine their impact on patient survival.

LOCAL EXCISION

The lack of improved survival associated with radical resections has led some surgeons to attempt more limited resections. These surgeons hoped to improve the results of treatment of rectal cancer by decreasing the morbidity and mortality produced by the operation and also to improve the quality of life of rectal cancer patients.

Local excision for the treatment of rectal cancer is limited to lesions that meet strict criteria.[137-142] There may even be a specific patient population with rectal cancer for whom local excision is the treatment of choice.[143,144] The lesions most amenable to treatment by local excision are small, exophytic, movable, low grade tumors. They should ideally lie in the distal third of the rectum, with no evidence of deep infiltration or regional lymph node involvement either clinically or radiographically.

Following local excision, pathologic examination of the tumor may reveal that it was not completely excised or that it is a poorly differentiated tumor. In this case, it is wise to consider additional modalities of treatment, either surgery or radiation therapy.[144] The combination of local excision and adjuvant therapy may also be useful in patients who require palliative therapy or are too debilitated to undergo a major operation.[133]

Results of local excision have been reviewed by several groups. Unfortunately, it is often difficult to compare results of these different series owing to the variance in criteria for patient selection.[131,137,140,141,143-147] Survival in these studies ranged from 47 to 100 per cent at 5 years (mixed crude and corrected rates) with the rate of local recurrence ranging from 6 to 36 per cent. A review by Graham et al.[148] of invasive cancers of the rectum located within 6 cm of the anal verge showed a cancer-specific survival rate of 82 to 100 per cent and a local recurrence rate from 0 to 27 per cent. Of the patients who had local recurrence, 22 to 100 per cent were cured with further surgical treatment. The overall results of local excision for rectal cancer have been encouraging. The identification of the ideal strategy for the use of adjuvant therapy in combination with local excision, however, will require further investigation in the future.

COMPLICATIONS OF SURGERY OF THE COLON AND RECTUM

Colorectal resections are fraught with complications. In the remainder of this chapter we will review the full spectrum of complications associated with colorectal resections. As we enter the era of laparoscopic colon surgery, it will be particularly important to scrutinize the rates of complications generated by these new procedures and to compare them to those encountered during the performance of these operations using open techniques.

Intraoperative Complications

Complications resulting from iatrogenic injury of surrounding organs and tissues are a major concern in colorectal cancer surgery. Considering the locations of the colon and rectum within the abdominal cavity, just about any organ or tissue may be subjected to iatrogenic injury. The organs or tissues that appear to be most often at risk include the urinary tract, vascular structures, or adjacent small bowel. Small bowel injuries that are recognized at the time of operation are usually dealt with easily by using standard techniques of repair. The realm of possibilities for iatrogenic injury is wide; however, only those structures listed previously will be included here.

INJURY TO THE URINARY TRACT

Ureteral Injury. One of the greatest concerns that many surgeons face when performing abdominal and pelvic surgery is avoiding injury to the ureter. Such an injury usually takes place at one of three points during the procedure.[149-152] The first is during the ligation of the inferior mesenteric vessels. The left ureter should be identified and moved laterally so that it is not included in the ligature or damaged during division of the pedicle. This is particularly important during laparoscopic procedures since the loss of depth perception in the two dimensional video image compounds this risk. The second point of risk is deep in the pelvis during the division of the lateral stalks. One must be particularly concerned with this type of injury when a synchronous two-team approach is used during abdominoperineal resection. Graham and Goligher[153] have reported that this approach may increase the chance of injuring the ureter during perineal dissection. Some surgeons prefer preoperative assessment using an intravenous pyelogram or placement of ureteral catheters to prevent injury, while others prefer to identify the ureters throughout their course and retract them laterally when they are at risk because of difficult dissection.[154] The third danger point puts both ureters at risk. In abdominoperineal resection the ureters may be injured during mobilization or closure of the peritoneum at the pelvic floor. Care must be taken to visualize both ureters and displace them laterally so that they are not included in or kinked by the suture.

Ureteral injury is most often detected in the postoperative period.[155] If ureteral injury is suspected intraoperatively, however, injection of indigo carmine dye (5 ml of an 0.8 per cent solution intravenously) may reveal the site of insult.[149,154] If ligation without disruption of the ureter is questioned, antegrade insertion of a ureteral catheter may be used to ensure patency.[156] Injury to or ligation of the ureter may be recognized postoperatively because of copious serous or serosanguinous drainage through the wound or drains or flank pain, leukocytosis, and fever, respectively. Devascularization secondary to inadvertent dissection too close to the ureter may cause necrosis and formation of a urinary fistula.[149] Regardless of the type of injury to the ureter, the colorectal surgeon or any surgeon working in the pelvis should be fully prepared and trained to deal with these situations.

Injury to the Mid and Upper Ureter, Bladder, and Urethra. Injuries to the mid and upper ureter as well as to the bladder and urethra do occur, however, on a much smaller scale. Direct extension of tumor, anatomic variation, or overzealous dissection may account for these injuries, and the surgeon should take care to avoid them. If they do occur, however, the surgeon should make every effort to construct the best repair possible. Often consultation with a urologist either intraoperatively or postoperatively may be invaluable.

VASCULAR COMPLICATIONS

The most common type of vascular complication is hemorrhage. Meticulous attention to hemostasis and careful dissection should minimize blood loss. Nevertheless, there are a number of sites from which bleeding may arise. The astute surgeon identifies and corrects these sites of hemorrhage prior to the patient's leaving the operating room. Depending on the area of dissection, specific areas should be inspected. If the splenic flexure has been dissected, one must observe that the spleen is not torn nor its pedicle injured by dissection or retraction. Dissection in the pelvis for lower sigmoid or rectal cancers may also cause bleeding at specific sites. Damage to both the prostatic venous plexus and the middle sacral vein may cause troublesome bleeding. Generally this type of venous bleeding is more difficult to control and more dangerous than arterial bleeding. Attempts to clamp or suture the vessel should be avoided; direct pressure with heated abdominal packs and thrombin-soaked Gelfoam as well as patience usually controls excessive bleeding.

Presacral hemorrhage may also cause problems for the surgeon working in the pelvis. Bleeding in the pelvis during mobilization of the rectum may occur if the presacral vein is torn. This may be controlled by using packing, electrocautery, or a stick tie.[157,158] Blunt dissection of the posterior rectum may give rise to severe hemorrhage from the basivertebral vein. This site of bleeding is usually located between S3 and S5 where it connects to the internal vertebral vein in approximately 15 per cent of patients.[159] Unlike bleeding from the presacral vein, this is not easily controlled by the techniques mentioned previously. The use of titanium thumbtacks placed at the bleeding site, which may be identified by a small dimple in the sacrum, may permanently halt this life-threatening hemorrhage.[159,160] Damage to both the presacral and basivertebral vein may be avoided by the use of sharp rather than blunt dissection of the posterior rectum to eliminate disruption of the presacral fascia.

Postoperative Complications

Postoperative complications from surgery of the colon and rectum are varied. Because of the nature and location of the organ, the surgeon must be concerned with problems of infection, ischemia, and those caused by dissection of surrounding tissues including neuronal dysfunction. Prevention of potential complications may begin with knowledge of anatomy and physiology of the large bowel. Understanding of the causes and management of the complications associated with each procedure, however, is essential. This portion of the chapter will outline the most commonly seen complications in the postoperative period.

ANASTOMOTIC COMPLICATIONS

Anastomotic Bleeding. Hemorrhage from the anastomotic site occurs in approximately 1 per cent of patients.[161] If bleeding from the anastomotic site is caused by inadequate hemostasis, one may expect to see signs of hemorrhage within the first 48 hours. Bleeding may not become evident for 10 days to 2 weeks, however, if it is a result of rupture of a pelvic hematoma through the posterior wall of the anastomosis.[149] In both of these cases the surgeon must be concerned about the integrity of the anastomosis and consider exploration if warranted by the clinical picture.

Anastomotic Leak. Anastomotic leaks that are associated with sepsis and fecal fistula are major concerns in the postoperative period. Earlier reports suggested a complication rate of between 15 and 77 per cent.[161–170]; however, more recent reports suggest an incidence of less than 10 per cent.[171,172] Healing of the anastomosis is dependent not only on the patient's condition but also on several technical factors involved in the construction of the anastomosis. The risk involved is generally worsened in patients who (1) are malnourished, (2) are diabetic, (3) have undergone previous irradiation, (4) have suffered severe blood loss or are exhibiting signs of shock, or (5) have not had adequate bowel preparation.[173] Technical factors that contribute to anastomotic dehiscence include (1) inadequate blood supply, (2) tension on the suture line, (3) stool in the lumen of the bowel, (4) diseased ends of bowel (inflammation, ischemia, or thickening), and (5) technique to prevent trauma, inaccurate suture placement, or obtaining an impregnable seal.[163,166,169,173,174] The use of drains in the region of the anastomosis has also been associated with an increased risk of breakdown.[175,176]

Most anastomotic breakdowns are evident within 5 to 7 days postoperatively. Generally signs associated with sepsis (fever, leukocytosis, and tachycardia) and/or generalized peritonitis (abdominal distention, tenderness, and ileus) are seen. If anastomotic dehiscence occurs early and is obvious by these signs, immediate laparotomy is necessary. If this complication occurs late and the patient's condition allows further study, Gastrografin enema usually is the most accurate means of identifying a leak. Investigation using a plain radiograph, computed tomographic scan, or endoscopy may or may not be helpful in identifying a leak.[173]

Anastomotic Stricture. Anastomotic stricture from benign disease is usually a result of fibrosis following anastomotic dehiscence.[149] Recurrence of malignancy may also be the cause of stricture; therefore, this possibility must be ruled out by the use of a biopsy and computed tomographic scan. In this case surgical resection should be considered; however, with benign stricture only patients in whom conservative therapy has failed need to undergo further resection. The use of stool softeners or suppositories may initially help these patients; however, dilatation either manually or with dilators should be undertaken to eliminate symptoms. Transanal lysis in the posterior midline may also be attempted before another operation is considered.[149]

COMPLICATIONS OF THE URINARY TRACT AND SEXUAL DYSFUNCTION

Urinary Retention. Although permanent bladder dysfunction following colorectal surgery is rare, urinary retention and urinary tract infection are the most common complications associated with these procedures. An incidence of 20 to 34 per cent has been reported in patients following rectal procedures.[177,178] Disruption of the micturition reflex through damage to the parasympathetic nerves (detrusor muscle) or sympathetic nerves (bladder neck, trigone, or urethra) in the pelvis is the most likely reason for urinary retention. Also, autonomic nerve injury may cause bladder dysfunction. Other factors that may contribute to this problem include loss of support followed by prolapse of the bladder into the pelvis and preexisting prostatic hypertrophy.

A study of patients undergoing rectal procedures by Kinn and Ohman[179] has shown that the complication of bladder dysfunction is fairly short-lived postoperatively. After 6 months, no parasympathetic denervation or detrusor paralysis could be demonstrated, which probably indicates that there is a time-related nerve regeneration in the postoperative period. Improvement of bladder dysfunction probably occurs gradually; nevertheless, in patients with pelvic dissection, use of a Foley catheter for 5 to 7 days postoperatively is important. If urinary function is not normal following this interval, heralded by high postvoiding residuals, the Foley catheter should be reinserted. If after 5 to 7 more days the patient is still unable to void, medical therapy with bethanechol chloride (Urecholine) to improve detrusor muscle tone should be instituted. Urologic evaluation with urodynamic studies is also prudent.[149]

Sexual Dysfunction. Injuries to nerves and vasculature may also give rise to impotence and infertility. Impotence is defined by Masters and Johnson as the inability to obtain or maintain an erection of sufficient firmness to permit coitus to be maintained or completed.[180] In a review of the literature, Walsh and Schlegel[181] demonstrated the incidence of erectile dysfunction to be 46 per cent for men undergoing abdominoperineal resection and 15 per cent for those undergoing low anterior resection and a lesser difference in terms of ejaculatory dysfunction (35 per cent and 44 per cent, respectively). They also found the rate of sexual dysfunction in men undergoing rectal resection to be lower (approximately 5 to 6 per cent). Perhaps this is due to the fact that these patients are younger and tend to have fewer preexisting disease states that may contribute to impotence.

The complicated processes involved in normal sexual function are mediated by a coordinated series of vascular and neurologic events. Parasympathetic nerves (nervi erigentes) generally play a role in initiating the vascular events required to achieve erection; however, the somatic nerves (pudendal nerves) are also involved. Sympathetic nerves originating in the thoracolumbar region, which travel from the spinal cord to the sympathetic ganglia, hypogastric nerves, and pelvic plexus, mediate ejaculation.[181] Injury to any one of these groups of nerves from excessive dissection, traction, or cautery may occur and result in dysfunction in erection and ejaculation. Impotence can also be caused by vascular damage if there is ligation of the anterior or distal branches of the internal iliac artery or the internal pudendal vessels.[181]

Regardless of the mechanism of injury, it is important to note that for most patients experiencing sexual dysfunction after pelvic surgery, function gradually returns during the first year.[181] It is appropriate to discuss the risk of impotence with the patient preoperatively because patients who have borderline sexual function before surgery may be more apt to suffer from impotence postoperatively even if there is minimal trauma.[149]

COMPLICATIONS IN WOUND HEALING AND INFECTION

Abdominal Wound Infection. The development of an abdominal wound infection requires the interaction of a variety of factors including the contamination of the wound with pathogenic organisms, the susceptibility of the host, the presence or absence of antibiotics in the wound tissue, and the condition of the wound tissue. The role of mechanical bowel preparation and broad-spectrum prophylactic antibiotics in reducing the incidence of wound infection has been shown by many authors.[182-189] The incidence of wound infection is directly related to the level of contamination of the wound. The incidence of infection in a clean (Type I) wound is about 1 to 3 per cent while with Type II (clean contaminated), Type III (contaminated), and Type IV (dirty) wounds, the risk increases to between 3 and 16 per cent.[185]

Since nosocomial infection is a major concern in wound infection, the Centers for Disease Control have outlined a few preventative guidelines for preparing patients for surgery.[190] These include (1) treatment of all identified sources of infection preoperatively, (2) limitation of the preoperative hospital stay, (3) preoperative nutritional support when warranted, and (4) preoperative preparation with an appropriate antiseptic solution. Other measures may be taken to reduce the risk of infection. However, the surgeon must keep in mind the need for adequate hemostasis, debridement of devitalized tissue, careful tissue handling, irrigation, and the limitation of operative time to limit the rate of infection in the patient.[149]

Perineal Wound Problems. The major complications associated with the perineal wound include infection and dehiscence. The infected perineal wound may be the result of contamination owing to fecal spillage, perforation, or previous perineal disease. It may also be caused by an infected hematoma.[149] The patient generally develops signs of sepsis postoperatively and once the source is found, the wound should be explored, thoroughly drained, and allowed to heal by secondary intention.

A controlled trial by Irvin and Goligher[191] found that primary closure with closed suction drainage yields the best results. In 45 to 95 per cent of patients, primary healing is successful[192–195]; however, 4 to 20 per cent of perineal wounds that open because of infection or that are left open to close secondarily are still unhealed at 1 year postoperatively.[196] Patients with unhealed perineal wounds should certainly undergo further evaluation to determine the cause of the healing problem, whether it be from recurrence of carcinoma or the presence of a foreign body. In certain patients reconstructive surgery using a muscle flap procedure may be possible.[173]

Other local complications including perineal hemorrhage, necrotic colostomy, perineal hernia, stomal problems, pelvic abscess, fecal fistula, incontinence, and irregular bowel habits may also be problematic; however, they will not be further discussed here.

OTHER COMPLICATIONS

Postoperative Intestinal Obstruction. Mechanical small bowel obstruction is a common clinical problem not only in the overall patient population, but especially in patients who have undergone certain abdominal procedures. The development of early small bowel obstruction in patients who have had operations on organs cephalad to the transverse colon is uncommon. In the series of Stewart et al.,[197] 1.5 per cent of patients who underwent right colectomy and 3 per cent of patients who underwent left colectomy and resection of the rectum suffered postoperative small bowel obstruction. Similarly, Goligher et al.[198] found the incidence of obstruction to be 3 per cent of 1302 patients who had undergone abdominoperineal resection.

One of the more common mechanisms of small bowel obstruction following abdominoperineal resection is herniation of the small bowel below the pelvic floor. This may occur when a suture breaks or pulls through the peritoneum, leaving a defect in the pelvic floor. A loop of small bowel may then slip through this hole and become entrapped. Strangulation, gangrene, or herniation through the perineal wound may also take place; however, instances of these are rare.[149] Some authors advocate leaving this space open to avoid possible herniation[199]; however, one must keep in mind the possibility of postoperative radiation therapy of the pelvis and the benefit of keeping the small bowel out of the field of treatment. Another mechanism of herniation within the peritoneal cavity is herniation through the lateral colostomy space (through a defect in the lateral gutter). Certainly one must remember that adhesive bands are a common cause of postoperative small bowel obstruction in the patient undergoing laparotomy for any cause. In a series of 101 patients with small bowel obstruction, Pickleman and Lee[200] found that 61 per cent of 23 patients undergoing exploratory laparotomy for unresolved obstruction had obstructive bands.

The diagnosis of postoperative obstruction may be difficult. Typically, the patient cannot tolerate removal of the nasogastric tube after 7 days or has been started on a diet and develops abdominal distention, nausea, and vomiting. The patient may also complain of colicky abdominal pain. Abdominal films may show dilated loops of small bowel with or without air-fluid levels. Management of this problem should consist of conservative measures initially with nasogastric suction and replacement of fluid and electrolytes. Pickleman and Lee[200] reported that small bowel obstruction resolved with conservative treatment in 78 of 101 patients (70 per cent within the first week).[200]

The decision to operate on this group of patients for unresolved obstruction of or circulatory damage to the bowel is based solely on the clinical judgment of the surgeon. In many patients the diagnosis of the latter may be inferred by the development of noncolicky abdominal pain, fever, leukocytosis, abdominal tenderness, and systemic signs such as tachycardia or metabolic acidosis.[201,202] Evaluation of other parameters such as the presence of bloody bowel movements, the duration of symptoms, the location of abdominal pain, and the patient's surgical history may aid in the decision of whether or not to take the patient to the operating room.[202]

Postoperative or adynamic ileus involves both the small and large bowel to some degree and occurs after every abdominal operation.[203] Temporary motor dysfunction generally resolves at different rates in the gastrointestinal tract with the small bowel recovering first (12 hours), followed by the stomach (12–24 hours), and the colon (3 to 5 days). The degree of postoperative ileus may be extended because of inhibition of the neuromuscular apparatus caused by a wide variety of local and systemic factors including intraperitoneal inflammation, retroperitoneal pathologic conditions, thoracic lesions, or systemic disorders in electrolyte or acid-base balance as well as certain medications.[203] Thus, prolonged postoperative ileus may be the first sign to the clinician that an abnormal condition may be developing. Whether it is a result of prolongation of intestinal ileus caused by one or many factors or a mechanical obstruction, the surgeon should continue to evaluate the patient for development of any life-threatening condition.

Anastomotic Obstruction. Obstruction at the site of anastomosis may occur in the early or late postoperative period. In the immediate postoperative period, edema at the suture line as well as intestinal ileus can contribute to the cause of the obstruction. Certainly technical factors involved in creating the anastomosis must be taken into consideration. Narrowing of the lumen owing to the "purse-string" effect of a running suture, puckering of the bowel wall to allow fit of two unequal ends, or use of a closed type of anastomosis by an inexperienced surgeon must be recognized and avoided.[201] Modern stapling devices, when used properly, have abolished these problems for the most part by allowing proper alignment and efficient creation of anastomosis in areas of the abdomen and pelvis that are not always easily accessible.

Late obstruction at the suture line may be caused by fibrosis and scar tissue; nevertheless, recurrence of malignancy must be excluded as a cause. Once this has been done, most patients benefit from gradual dilatation of the lumen at the suture line over a period of several months. This is a rare complication, which infrequently requires another operation.[201]

Complications of the Stapled Anastomosis. The three most common complications of the stapled anastomosis are hemorrhage, stricture, and breakdown.[204] The problem with hemorrhage, which appeared to be a function of the early single-row staplers, has been largely corrected by the introduction of the newer interlocking, double-row staplers.[205] This is even less of a problem with the endoscopic stapling devices that have three rows of staples.

Anastomotic stricture also poses a problem. This is probably a result of the same problem of breakdown and fibrosis as seen with a conventional sutured anastomosis and not an inherent problem with the staples.[149] The concern that the use of the circular stapler leads to narrowed anastomoses has prompted investigators to examine their results with this method. Depending on the definition of stricture (allowing passage of a 15- or 19-mm sigmoidoscope), narrowings from 1 to 30 per cent have been recorded.[206–221] Stenosis may be attributable to ischemia caused by overzealous clearing of surrounding tissues, including the blood supply to that portion of tissue which will be placed in the stapling device.[133] Alternatively, it may be caused by excessive tension on the anastomosis. Certain authors have noted that by limiting the amount of tissue that is cleared from the bowel, the incidence of recurrence of malignancy may be significantly reduced.[133]

The incidence of anastomotic breakdown after use of a stapling device may be defined according to breakdowns that are clinically or radiographically evident. Clinical leakage rates range from 0 to 16 per cent.[206–221] In contrast, the rate of leaks demonstrated radiographically by using Gastrografin enemas has been shown to be 2 to 3 times higher.[210,213,216,218,221,222]

Comparison of the stapling method with

hand-sewn anastomosis has yielded mixed results. In three studies, stapled anastomoses were less likely to break down than their hand-sewn counterparts.[222–224] On the other hand, incidences of equal rates of breakdown for both techniques have been reported by others.[173,225,226] Clearly the advantage of circular stapling, which diminishes the need for abdominoperineal resection,[222,227–229] has offset any of the other complications that may be attributible to this device specifically. Other complications include rectovaginal fistula, serosal tears, incomplete donuts, instrument failure, and difficulty extracting the instrument.

Pulmonary Complications. Pulmonary complications may follow any procedure requiring general anesthesia or laparotomy. They may be manifested in the form of respiratory failure, atelectasis, or pulmonary edema. Because the pathophysiologic features of respiratory failure are complex, a full discussion will not be undertaken here. The pathogenetic mechanisms of respiratory difficulties following laparotomy are numerous and varied. Hypoventilation from muscle weakness or changes in respiratory mechanics from abdominal distention or pain may last for many days following a procedure. Aspiration of gastric contents may occur despite attempts by the anesthesiologist to maintain airway control. Fluid overload with pulmonary edema, microemboli, fat emboli, and pulmonary infection also interferes with gas exchange. Increases in bronchial secretion as well as the presence of vomitus, blood, or other material may lead to obstruction of the tracheobronchial tree. The development of atelectasis in the distal lung segment may follow, which may increase the risk of bronchopneumonia. Preexisting lung disease from smoking, asthma, emphysema, or other chronic lung disease may contribute to the development of postoperative atelectasis. The patients inability to cough effectively also may aid in the onset of atelectasis. General anesthesia, narcotics, immobilization, and splinting owing to pain interfere with the patient's ability to cough and breathe deeply.

Adult respiratory distress syndrome is a serious form of respiratory insufficiency that may occur in the patient postoperatively. Sepsis appears to be one of several etiologic factors in the development of this life-threatening complication. Aggressive respiratory support must be undertaken to ensure the best possible outcome for the patient.[230]

The incidence of postoperative pulmonary complications may be reduced by attention to factors influencing respiratory function in the perioperative period. Preoperatively the patient should be instructed to stop smoking 2 weeks prior to the procedure and should be given instruction in deep breathing and coughing exercises. Postoperative pain should be controlled to allow comfortable deep breathing. Respiratory therapy with the use of deep breathing and coughing exercises, continuous positive airway pressure, and the administration of inhalation medications, such as bronchodilators, mucolytics, and expectorants, may be particularly helpful in preventing and treating atelectasis. Changes in body positioning and early ambulation may also aid in the mobilization of secretions and prevention of atelectasis. For those patients with more severe respiratory dysfunction, more aggressive therapy is appropriate. This might include nasotracheal suctioning, postural drainage, bronchoscopy, and administration of supplemental oxygen. Patients with respiratory failure who require ventilatory support should be monitored closely with particular attention to oxygen delivery and the pathophysiologic condition causing the state of respiratory insufficiency.[230]

Recurrence

RECURRENCE OF COLON CARCINOMA

There are a number of factors that may contribute to recurrence of carcinoma of the colon. Possibilities include the presence of residual lymphatic metastases or the mobilization of tumor emboli into venous channels at the time of operation, which may lead to dissemination or contamination of margins by exfoliated tumor cells.[231] Early recurrences at the anastomotic site are probably a result of implantation rather than the development of a metachronous lesion.[232] To examine patterns of recurrence and recurrence rates more closely, a differentiation between local and distant recurrence must be made. The local pattern of recurrence generally refers to cancer growth in an area directly adjacent to or contiguous with the previously excised tumor bed or at the site of bowel anastomosis. Distant metastases occur at sites remote from the primary site and are probably a result of unrecognized dissemination of disease at the time of initial primary resection. It is also possible for any patient to exhibit both of these patterns of recurrence simultaneously.

The incidence of local and distant recurrence appears to depend upon certain pathologic features of the original surgical specimen. Increased depth of invasion of the bowel wall and lymph node positivity indicate a higher probability of recurrence. Three studies comparing crude recurrence rates for local disease and local plus distant disease (overall recurrence) demonstrate this point.[233–235] Patients with disease confined to the bowel wall with no demonstrated lymph node metastases had a local recurrence rate of 2.5 to 5.2 per cent and a overall recurrence rate of 6.1 to 9.4 per cent at 5-year follow-up. However, patients with disease extending beyond the bowel wall (still with negative lymph nodes) showed recurrence rates of 17.5 to 17.7 per cent (local) and 28.4 to 34.5 per cent (overall) at 5 years. The addition of positive lymph nodes increased the rate of local recurrence to 22 to 33 per cent and the rate of overall recurrence to 42.3 to 60.7 per cent at 5 years. In a review by Devesa et al.,[236] 30 to 50 per cent of patients in whom recurrence was seen showed local recurrence while 80 per cent manifested distant recurrence. The most frequent site of distal involvement was the liver.

Time to recurrence has been reported as ranging from 1 to 102 months,[233,235,237] with 60 to 84 per cent of recurrences becoming apparent within the first 2 years after initial operation and 90 per cent being detected within 4 years.[233,236] Presentation of patients who have recurrence is varied. One would hope that aggressive follow-up programs using colonoscopy, barium enema, and/or carcinoembryonic antigen level determination would detect most of these recurrences so that treatment for recurrent disease may occur earlier in its course. However, this is not always the case.

Many patients are seen with vague symptoms of malaise, anorexia, weight loss, abdominal discomfort, or changes in bowel habits. Physical examination often does not reveal the presence of recurrence and in some instances, further examination using barium enema or colonoscopy fails to do so as well. Hope for improving survival in these patients may depend on detecting recurrent disease not only in the symptomatic but also in the asymptomatic population.

RECURRENCE OF RECTAL CARCINOMA

There are a number of factors that may contribute to the development of recurrent disease in the pelvis following rectal resection. These include incomplete excision of the primary lesion, implantation at or near the anastomotic site, or development of a metachronous lesion at the anastomotic site.[133] Variables that have been found to be associated with an increase risk of recurrence are advanced Dukes stage, higher grade of tumor, ulceration, location below the peritoneal reflection, limited margin of clearance, and venous and perineural invasion.[161,238] The recurrence rate for carcinoma of the rectum upon the area of the rectum that is involved, with patients with proximal lesions faring better than those with lesions of the lower rectum.[243] Similarly, McDermott et al.[239] showed that the incidence of recurrence was less with lesions in the upper third of the rectum (14 per cent) than in the middle (21 per cent) and lower thirds (26 per cent).

The rate of recurrence of rectal carcinoma also depends on tumor stage, similar to colon carcinoma. Studies have shown that in patients with local recurrence from tumor that was confined to the bowel wall the crude recurrence rate was between 6.1 and 11.1 per cent at 5-year follow-up and the recurrence rate at all sites was between 16.7 and 18.4 per cent.[235,240,241] Certain studies have shown, however, that local recurrence rates of 4 per cent for this stage of lesion may be found.[58,242] Recurrence rates at 5-year follow-up for patients with tumors that extended through the bowel wall with no nodal metastases are somewhat worse. Local recurrence ranged from 24 to 30.8 per cent and overall recurrence (including all sites) varied from 41.1 to 47.5 per cent. The addition of positive lymph nodes increased recurrence rates to 26.3 to 50 per cent in the local recurrence only group and to 52.6 to 70.5 per cent in the local plus distant recurrence group.

As one might expect, a wide range of recurrence rates for rectal carcinoma has been reported, depending on the procedure performed. A review by Philipsen[243] found that the incidence of recurrence ranged from 12 to 32 per cent following abdominoperineal resection. Published series do not support the assumption that low anterior resection is followed by a higher pelvic recurrence rate. Indeed, several studies compared recurrence following these two procedures using matched controls and found no significant difference between the two rates of recurrence.[141,244,245] Schiessel et al.[246] also showed comparative rates between low anterior resection and abdominoperineal resection (14.4 and 16.7 per cent, respectively); however, the recurrence rate for these rectal carcinomas was significantly higher than after resection for colon cancer (4.4 per cent). Despite these reports, others have published reports of even lower recurrence rates of approximately 3 per cent following resection of cancer of the rectum, which the authors attribute to increased clearance of the mesorectum.[247,248] Thus, available information suggests that there is no intrinsic advantage of abdominal perineal resection over low anterior resection for the treatment of rectal carcinoma.

Regardless of whether abdominoperineal resection or low anterior resection was performed for treatment of a rectal cancer, the patient may be seen with symptomatic or asymptomatic recurrence. Symptoms suspicious for a recurrence in the pelvis following low anterior resection include bleeding, pain, or a change in bowel habits. In patients having undergone abdominoperineal resection, symptoms are likely to be pain or pressure in the pelvis, abdomen, or back or a disturbance of the urinary tract. Follow-up examination of the asymptomatic patient may reveal a mass, a perineal recurrence, or another irregularity; however, regular investigations using sigmoidoscopy, carcinoembryonic antigen level determination, and especially computed tomographic scanning should be planned.[133]

THE ROLE OF LAPAROSCOPIC TECHNIQUE IN THE TREATMENT OF COLORECTAL CANCER

Many techniques of the treatment of colorectal cancer have remained of unproven benefit for the last fifty years. Consequently, the principles of proper oncologic surgical technique for the treatment of colorectal cancer remain undetermined. Unfortunately, it is unlikely that these issues will be resolved in the forseeable future. Obviously, the introduction of laparoscopic techniques of colorectal resections will not alter this fact.

The role of laparoscopic techniques in the treatment of colorectal cancers has not been defined. In the application of this new technology to large bowel malignancies surgeons should follow the same principles of cancer surgery to which they have adhered in the past. In the performance of laparoscopic resections for malignancy, the surgeon should accomplish exactly the same type of resection that he or she would have performed through a large abdominal incision. If it has been the habit of the surgeon to perform a high ligation of the inferior mesenteric artery, he or she should continue to use this technique during laparoscopic procedures. If at any time the surgeon is uncertain that the accustomed standard of technique can be achieved, the laparoscopic procedure should be converted to an open operation.

In the next decade, the results of laparoscopic procedures for colorectal cancers must be meticulously assessed. Surgeons should enroll their patients into prospective registries so that end-result data will become available for these procedures as soon as possible. In the discussion of these results, however, the focus of the debate should be the impact of laparoscopic technique on outcome, not the relative importance of various radical techniques of resection, which has remained undetermined for decades.

REFERENCES

1. Schwartz SI, Shires GT, Spencer FC. Principles of Surgery. New York, McGraw-Hill Book Co, 1989, pp 1270–1314.
2. Luk GD. Colorectal cancer. Gastroenterol Clin North Am 1988; 17:655–967.
3. Fry DR, Fleshman JW, Kodner IJ. Colorectal cancer. Clin Symp 1989; 41:1–32.
4. Soybel DI, Bliss DP, Wells SA. Colon and rectal carcinoma. Curr Probl Cancer 1987; 11:259–356.
5. Vukasin AP, Ballantyne GH, Flannery JH, et al. Increasing incidence of cecal and sigmoid carcinoma: Data from the Connecticut tumor registry. Cancer 1990; 66:2442–2449.
6. De Leon MP, Antoniolli A, Ascari A, et al. Incidence and familial occurrence of colorectal cancer and polyps in a health-care district in Northern Italy. Cancer 1987; 60:2848–2859.
7. Centers for Disease Control. Trends in colorectal cancer incidence—United States, 1973–1986. MMWR 1989; 38:728–731.
8. Goligher JC, Duthie HL. Surgical anatomy and physiology of the colon, rectum and anus. In Goligher JC, ed. Surgery of the Anus, Rectum and Colon, 4th ed. London, Baillière Tindall, 1980, pp 1–47.
9. Nivatvongs S, Gordon PH. Surgical anatomy. In Gordon PH, Nivatvongs S, eds. Principles and Practice of Surgery for the Colon, Rectum and Anus. St. Louis, Quality Medical Publishing, Inc, 1992, pp 3–38.
10. Goss CM, ed. Gray's Anatomy of the Human Body, 29th ed. Philadelphia, Lea & Febiger, 1973, pp 759–766.
11. Slanetz CA Jr, Herter FP. The large intestine. In Haagensen CD, Feind CR, Herter FP, et al. The Lymphatics in Cancer. Philadelphia, WB Saunders Co, 1972, pp 489–559.
12. Goligher JC. The blood supply to the sigmoid colon and rectum. Br J Surg 1949; 37:157–162.
13. Enquist IF, Block IR. Rectal cancer in the female: Selection of proper operation based upon anatomic studies of rectal lymphatics. Prog Clin Cancer 1966; 2:73–85.

14. Ballantyne GH. The rectosigmoid sphincter of O'Beirne. Dis Colon Rectum 1986; 29:525–531.
15. Fenoglio CM, Kaye GI, Lane N. Distribution of human colonic lymphatics in normal, hyperplastic and adenomatous tissue. Gastroenterology 1972; 64:51–66.
16. Kaye GI, Fenoglio CM, Pascal RR. Comparative electron microscopic features of normal, hyperplastic and adenomatous human colonic epithelium. Variations in cellular structure relative to the process of epithelial differentiation. Gastroenterology 1973; 64:926–945.
17. Deschner EG. Adenomas: Preneoplastic events, growth characteristics and development. Pathol Annu 1983; 13:205–219.
18. Herter FP, Slanetz CA. Patterns and significance of lymphatic spread from cancer of the colon and rectum. In Weiss L, Gilbert HA, Ballon SC, eds. Lymphatic System Metastases. Boston, GK Hall Medical Publishers, 1980, pp 275–307.
19. Cole PP. The intramural spread of rectal carcinoma. Br Med J 1913; 1:431–433.
20. Black WA, Waugh JM. The intramural extension of carcinoma of the descending colon, sigmoid and rectosigmoid. Surg Gynecol Obstet 1948; 87:457–464.
21. Goligher J. Surgery of the Anus, Rectum and Colon, 5th ed. London, Ballière Tindall, 1984, pp 465–779.
22. Griffiths JD. Extramural and intramural blood supply of the colon. Br Med J 1961; 1:323–326.
23. Cady B, Perrson AV, Monson DO, et al. Changing patterns of colorectal carcinoma. Cancer 1974; 33:422–426.
24. Rhodes JB, Holmes FF, Clark GM. Changing distribution of primary cancers in the large bowel. JAMA 1977; 238:1641–1643.
25. Abrams JS, Reines HD. Increasing incidence of right-sided lesions in colorectal cancer. Am J Surg 1979; 137:522–526.
26. Rosato FE, Marks G. Changing site distribution patterns of colorectal cancer at Thomas Jefferson University Hospital. Dis Colon Rectum 1981; 24:93–95.
27. Beart RW, Melton LJ, Maruta M, et al. Trends in right and left sided colon cancer. Dis Colon Rectum 1983; 26:393–398.
28. Greene FL. Distribution of colorectal neoplasms. Am Surg 1983; 49:62–65.
29. Slater GI, Haber RH, Aufses AH. Changing distribution of carcinoma of the colon and rectum. Surg Gynecol Obstet 1984; 158:216–218.
30. Grinnell RS. The spread of carcinoma of the colon and rectum. Cancer 1950; 3:641–652.
31. Hamilton SR. Pathologic diagnosis of colorectal and anal malignancies: Classification and prognostic features of pathologic findings. In Beahrs OH, et al., eds. Colorectal Tumors. Philadelphia, JB Lippincott Co, 1986, pp 107–112.
32. Clogg HS. Some observations on carcinoma of the colon. Practitioner 1904; 72:525–544.
33. Grinnell RS. Distal intramural spread of carcinoma of the rectum and rectosigmoid. Surg Gynecol Obstet 1954; 99:421–430.
34. Quer EA, Dahlin DC, Mayo CW. Retrograde intramural spread of carcinoma of the rectum and rectosigmoid. Surg Gynecol Obstet 1953; 96:24–30.
35. Hughes TG, Jenevein EP, Poulos E. Intramural spread of colon carcinoma. Am J Surg 1983; 146:697–699.
36. Williams NS, Dixon MF, Johnston D. Reappraisal of the 5 centimetre rule of distal excision for carcinoma of the rectum: A study of distal intramural spread and patients' survival. Br J Surg 1983; 70:150–154.
37. Lazorthes F, Voigt JJ, Roques J, et al. Distal intramural spread of carcinoma of the rectum correlated with lymph nodal involvement. Surg Gynecol Obstet 1990; 170:45–48.
38. Grinnell RS. The lymphatic and venous spread of carcinoma of the rectum. Ann Surg 1942; 116:200–216.
39. Miles WE. Cancer of the Rectum. Being the Lettsomian Lectures. London, Harrison and Sons, Ltd, 1926, pp 1–72.
40. Russell A, Tong D, Dawson LE, et al. Adenocarcinoma of the proximal colon: Sites of initial dissemination and patterns of recurrence following surgery alone. Cancer 1984; 53:360–367.
41. Dionne L. The pattern of blood-borne metastasis from carcinoma of the rectum. Cancer 1965; 18:775–781.
42. Batson OV. The function of the vertebral veins and their role in the spread of metastasis. Ann Surg 1940; 112:138–149.
43. Birnkrant A, Sampson J, Sugarbaker PH. Ovarian metastasis from colorectal cancer. Dis Colon Rectum 1986; 29:767–771.
44. Alford TC, Do HM, Geelhoed GW, et al. Steroid hormone receptors in human colon cancers. Cancer 1979; 43:980–984.
45. Pillore de Rouen. Quoted in Wangensteen OH, Wangensteen SD. The Rise of Surgery. Minneapolis, University of Minnesota Press, 1978, pp 85–88.
46. Reybard JF. Memoire sur une tumeur cancereuse affectant l'iliaque du colon: Ablation de la tumeur et de l'intestin. Bull Acad Natl Med (Paris) 1844; 9:1031.
47. Bloch OT. Om extra-abdominal behandlung af cancer intestinates (rectum derfra und taget) med en frem stillung afde for denne sygdom foretagne operationaer og deres resultater. Nord Med Ark 1892; 24:1–10.
48. Paul FT. Colectomy. Br Med J 1895; 1:1136–1139.
49. von Mikulicz J. Chirurgische erjahrun uber das darmcarcinom. Arch Klin Chir Berl 1903; 69:28–47.
50. Morgan CN. The management of carcinoma of the colon. Ann R Coll Surg Engl 1952; 10:305–323.
51. Miles WE. A method of performing abdominoperineal excision for carcinoma of the rectum and terminal portion of the pelvic colon. Lancet 1908; 2:1812.
52. Hartmann H. Chirurgie du Rectum. Paris, Masson et Cie, 1931.
53. McKittrick LS. Touching all bases. Am J Surg 1965; 109:57–62.
54. Dixon CF. Surgical removal of lesions occurring in the sigmoid and rectosigmoid. Am J Surg 1939; 46:12.
55. Allen AW. The development of surgery for cancer of the colon. Ann Surg 1951; 134:786–796.
56. Bacon HE. Anus-Rectum-Sigmoid Colon. Diagnosis and Treatment, 3rd ed. Philadelphia, JB Lippincott Co, 1949, Vol 1.
57. Cutait DE, Figlioni FJ. A new method of colorectal anastomosis in abdominoperineal resection. Dis Colon Rectum 1961; 4:335–342.
58. Localio SA, Eng K, Coppa GF. Abdomino-sacral resection for midrectal cancer. A 15 year experience. Ann Surg 1983; 198:320.
59. Ravitch MM, Steichen FM. Staplers in gastrointestinal surgery. In Schwartz SI, Ellis H, eds. Maingot's

Abdominal Operations, 8th ed. Norwalk, CT, Appleton-Century-Crofts, 1985, p 1537.
60. Waugh JM, Miller EM, Kurzweg FT. Abdominoperineal resection with sphincter preservation for carcinoma of the midrectum. Arch Surg 1954; 68:469.
61. Lock MR, Cairns DW, Ritchie JK, Lockhart-Mummery HE. The treatment of early colorectal cancer by local excision. Br J Surg 1978; 65:346.
62. Madden JL, Kandalaft S. Clinical evaluation of electrocoagulation in the treatment of cancer of the rectum: A continuing study. Am J Surg 1971; 122:347–352.
63. Mason AY. Transphincteric surgery for lower rectal cancer. In Malt RA, ed. Surgical Techniques Illustrated, Boston, Little, Brown and Co, 1977, Vol 2, No 2, p 71.
64. Papillon J. Rectal and Anal Cancers: Conservative Treatment by Radiation—An Alternative to Radical Surgery. New York, Springer-Verlag, 1982.
65. Sischy B. The place of radiotherapy in the management of rectal adenocarcinoma. Cancer 1982; 50(suppl):2631–2637.
66. Beart RW Jr, Dozois RR, Kelly KA. Ileoanal anastomosis in the adult. Surg Gynecol Obstet 1982; 154:826–828.
67. Peck DA. Rectal mucosal replacement. Ann Surg 1980; 191:294–303.
68. Parks AG, Percy JP. Resection and sutured coloanal anastomosis for rectal carcinoma. Br J Surg 1982; 69:301–304.
69. Bouwman DL, Weaver DW. Colon cancer: Surgical therapy. Gastroenterol Clin North Am 1988; 17:859–871.
70. Rosi PA. Selection of Operations for Carcinomas of the Colon. pp 221–230.
71. Steele G Jr, Osteen RT. Surgical treatment of colon cancer. In Colorectal Cancer. New York, Marcel Dekker, 1986, pp 127–162.
72. Fazio VW, Pilipshen SJ. Techniques for the resection of colon cancer: An appraisal of the no-touch isolation technique. In Beahrs OH, Higgins GA, Weinstein JJ, eds. Colorectal Tumors. Philadelphia, JB Lippincott Co, 1986, pp 159–169.
73. Rosi PA, Cahill WJ, Carey J. A ten-year study of hemicolectomy in the treatment of carcinoma of the left half of the colon. Surg Gynecol Obstet 1962; 114:15–24.
74. Grinnell RS. Lymphatic block with atypical and retrograde lymphatic metastasis and spread in carcinoma of the colon and rectum. Ann Surg 1966; 163:272–280.
75. McElwain JW, Bacon HE, Trimpi HD. Lymph node metastases: Experience with aortic ligation of inferior mesenteric artery in cancer of the rectum. Surgery 1954; 35:513–531.
76. Bacon HE, Dirbas F, Myers TB, Ponce de Leon F. Extensive lymphadenectomy and high ligation of the inferior mesenteric artery for carcinoma of the left colon and rectum. Dis Colon Rectum 1958; 1:457–465.
77. Stearns MW Jr, Deddish MR. Five-year results of abdominopelvic lymph node dissection for carcinoma of the rectum. Dis Colon Rectum 1959; 2:169–172.
78. Grinnell RS, Hiatt RB. Ligation of the inferior mesenteric artery at the aorta in resections for carcinoma of the sigmoid and rectum. Surg Gynecol Obstet 1952; 94:526–534.
79. Ferguson LK, Boland JP, Thomen FJ. Anterior segmental resection for carcinoma of the upper rectum, rectosigmoid, and sigmoid. Surgery 1962; 52:741–746.
80. Harvey HD, Auchincloss H. Metastases to lymph nodes from carcinomas that were arrested. Cancer 1968; 21:684–691.
81. Sugarbaker PH, Corlew S. Influence of surgical techniques on survival in patients with colorectal cancer. A review. Dis Colon Rectum 1982; 25:545–557.
82. Ault GW. Technique for cancer isolation and extended dissection for cancer of the distal colon and rectum. Surg Gynecol Obstet 1958; 106:467–477.
83. Cole WH, Roberts SS, Strehl FW. Modern concepts in cancer of the colon and rectum. Cancer 1966; 19:1347–1358.
84. Turnbull RB Jr, Kyle K, Watson FR, Spratt J. Cancer of the colon: The influence of the no-touch isolation technique on survival rates. Ann Surg 1967; 166:420–427.
85. Barnes JP. Physiologic resection of the right colon. Surg Gynecol Obstet 1952; 94:722–726.
86. Stearns MW, Schottefeld D. Techniques for the surgical management of colon cancer. Cancer 1971; 28:165–169.
87. Griffiths JD, McKinna JA, Rowbotham HD, et al. Carcinoma of the colon and rectum: Circulating malignant cells and five-year survival. Cancer 1973; 31:226–236.
88. Engell HC. Cancer cells in the blood. A five- to nine-year follow-up study. Ann Surg 1959; 149:457–461.
89. Moore GE, Sako K. The spread of carcinoma of the colon and rectum: A study of invasion of blood vessels, lymph nodes and peritoneum by tumor cells. Dis Colon Rectum 1959; 2:92–97.
90. Graffner HOL, Alm POA, Oscarson JEA. Prophylactic oophorectomy in colorectal carcinoma. Am J Surg 1983; 146:233–235.
91. MacKeigan JM, Ferguson JA. Prophylactic oophorectomy and colorectal cancer in premenopausal patients. Dis Colon Rectum 1979; 22:401–405.
92. Barr SS, Valiente MA, Bacon HE. Rationale for bilateral oophorectomy concomitant with resection for carcinoma of the rectum and colon. Dis Colon Rectum 1962; 5:450–452.
93. Antoniades K, Spector HB, Hecksher RH Jr. Prophylactic oophorectomy in conjunction with large-bowel resection for cancer: Report of two cases. Dis Colon Rectum 1977; 20:506–510.
94. Ballantyne GH, Reigel M, Wolff B, Ilstrup DM. Oophorectomy and colon cancer: Impact on survival. Ann Surg 1985; 202:209–214.
95. Bilchik AJ, Ballantyne GH. Should malignant polyps of the colon and rectum be treated conservatively? In Gitnick G, ed. Debates in Medicine. Chicago, Year Book Medical Publishers, Inc, 1990, Vol 3, pp 254–287.
96. Haggitt RC, Glotzbach RE, Soffer EE, et al. Prognostic factors in colorectal carcinomas arising in adenomas: Implications for lesions removed by endoscopic polypectomy. Gastroenterology 1985; 89:328–336.
97. Cranley JP, Petras RE, Carey WD, et al. When is endoscopic polypectomy adequate therapy for colonic polyps containing invasive carcinoma? Gastroenterology 1986; 91:419–427.
98. Contee CC. Management of endoscopically removed malignant colon polyps. J Surg Oncol 1987; 36:116–121.
99. Nivatvongs S, Rojanasakul A, Reiman HM, et al.

The risk of lymph node metastasis in colorectal polyps with invasive adenocarcinoma. Dis Colon Rectum 1991; 34:323–328.
100. Cutait R, Lesser ML, Enker WE. Prophylactic oophorectomy for large bowel cancer. Dis Colon Rectum 1983; 26:6–11.
101. Birnkrant A, Sampson J, Sugarbaker PH. Ovarian metastases from colorectal cancer. Dis Colon Rectum 1986; 29:767–771.
102. Durdey P, Williams NS. The effect of malignant and inflammatory fixation of rectal carcinoma on prognosis after rectal excision. Br J Surg 1984; 71:787–790.
103. Grinnell RS. Distal intramural spread of carcinoma of the rectum and rectosigmoid. Surg Gynecol Obstet 1954; 99:421–430.
104. Goligher JC. Surgery of the Anus, Rectum and Colon, 3rd ed. London, Ballière Tindall, 1975.
105. Williams NS, Dixon MF, Johnston D. Reappraisal of the 5 centimetre rule of distal excision for carcinoma of the rectum: A study of distal intramural spread and patient survival. Br J Surg 1983; 70:150–154.
106. Quer EA, Dahlin DC, Mayo CW. Retrograde intramural spread of carcinoma of the rectum and rectosigmoid. Surg Gynecol Obstet 1953; 96:24–30.
107. Kirwan WO, Drumm J, Hogan JM. Determining safe margin of resection in low anterior resection for rectal cancer. Br J Surg 1988; 75:720.
108. Pollett WG, Nicholls RJ. The relationship between the extent of distal clearance and survival and local recurrence rates after curative anterior resection for carcinoma of the rectum. Ann Surg 1983; 198:159–163.
109. Wilson SM, Beahrs OH. The curative treatment of carcinoma of the sigmoid, rectosigmoid and rectum. Ann Surg 1976; 183:556–565.
110. Localio SA, Eng K, Coopa GF. Abdominosacral resection for midrectal cancer: A fifteen-year experience. Ann Surg 1983; 198:320–324.
111. McElwain JW, Bacon HE, Trimpi HD. Lymph node metastases: Experience with aortic ligation of inferior mesenteric artery in cancer of the rectum. Surgery 1954; 35:513–531.
112. Whittaker M, Goligher JC. The prognosis after surgical treatment for carcinoma of the rectum. Br J Surg 1976; 63:384–388.
113. Grinnell RS. Results of ligation of inferior mesenteric artery at the aorta in resection of carcinoma of the descending and sigmoid colon and rectum. Surg Gynecol Obstet 1965; 120:1031–1036.
114. Pezim ME, Nicholls RJ. Survival after high or low ligation of the inferior mesenteric artery during curative surgery for rectal cancer. Ann Surg 1984; 200:729–733.
115. Surtees P, Ritchie JK, Phillips RKS. High versus low ligation of the inferior mesenteric artery in rectal cancer. Br J Surg 1990; 77:618–621.
116. Deddish MR. Therapeutic trends and management in advanced carcinoma of the colon and rectum. NY State J Med 1950; 50:2047–2049.
117. Sauer I, Bacon HE. A new approach for the excision of the lower portion of the rectum and anal canal. Surg Gynecol Obstet 1952; 95:229–242.
118. Enker WE, Laffer UT, Block GE. Enhanced survival of patients with colon and rectal cancer is based upon wide anatomic resection. Ann Surg 1979; 190:350–360
119. Waugh JM, Kirklin JW. The importance of the level of the lesion in the prognosis and treatment of carcinoma of the rectum and low sigmoid colon. Ann Surg 1949; 129:22–33.
120. Coller FA, Kay EB, MacIntyre RS. Regional lymphatic metastasis of carcinoma of the rectum. Surgery 1940; 8:294–311.
121. Grinnell RS. The lymphatic and venous spread of carcinoma of the rectum. Ann Surg 1942; 116:200–216.
122. Gilchrist RK, David VC. A consideration of pathological factors influencing 5-year survival in radical resection of the large bowel and rectum for carcinoma. Ann Surg 1947; 126:421–438.
123. Glass RE, Ritchie JK, Thompson HR, et al. The results of surgical treatment of cancer of the rectum by radical resection and extended abdominosacral lymphadenectomy. Br J Surg 1985; 72:599–601.
124. Enker WE, Pilipshen SG, Heilweil ML, et al. En bloc pelvic lymphadenectomy and sphincter-preservation in the surgical management of rectal cancer. Ann Surg 1986; 203:426–433.
125. Heald RJ, Husband EM, Ryall RDH. The mesorectum in rectal cancer surgery: The clue to pelvic recurrence? Br J Surg 1982; 69:613–616.
126. Heald RJ, Ryall RDH. Recurrence and survival after total mesorectal excision for rectal cancer. Lancet 1986; 1:1479–1480.
127. Jarvinen HJ, Ovaska J, Mecklin JP. Improvements in the treatment and prognosis of colorectal carcinoma. Br J Surg 1988; 75:25–27.
128. McDermott F, Hughes ESR, Pihl E, et al. Long term results in restorative resection and total excision for carcinoma of the middle third of the rectum. Surg Gynecol Obstet 1982; 154:833–837.
129. Nicholls RJ, Ritchie JK, Wadsworth J, Parks AG. Total excision or restorative resection for carcinoma of the middle third of the rectum. Br J Surg 1979; 66:625–627.
130. Slanetz CA, Herter FP, Grinnell RS. Anterior resection versus abdominoperineal resection for cancer of the rectum and rectosigmoid. Am J Surg 1972; 123:110–117.
131. Stearns MW Jr. The choice among anterior resection, the pull through and the abdominoperineal resection of the rectum. Cancer 1974; 34:969–971.
132. Williams NS, Durdey P, Johnston D. The outcome following sphincter-saving resection and abdominoperineal resection for low rectal cancer. Br J Surg 1985; 72:595–598.
133. Gordon PH. Malignant neoplasms of the rectum. In Gordon PH, Nivatvongs S, eds. Principles and Practice of Surgery for the Colon, Rectum and Anus. St. Louis, Quality Medical Publishing Inc., 1992, pp 591–654.
134. Williams NS, Johnston D. Survival and recurrence after sphincter-saving resection and abdominoperineal resection for carcinoma of the middle third of the rectum. Br J Surg 1984; 71:278–282.
135. Wolmark N, Fisher B. An analysis of survival and treatment failure following abdominoperineal resection and sphincter-saving resection of Dukes' B and C rectal carcinoma. Ann Surg 1986; 204:480–487.
136. Sugarbaker PH, Corlew S. Influence of surgical techniques on survival in patients with colorectal cancer. Dis Colon Rectum 1982; 25:545–547.
137. Cuthbertson AM, Kaye AH. Local excision of the rectum, anus and anal canal. Aust N Z J Surg 1978; 48:412–415.
138. Deddish MR. Local excision. Surg Clin North Am 1974; 54:877–880.
139. Morson BC, Bussey HJ, Samoorian S. Policy of local excision for early cancer of the colorectum. Gut 1977; 18:1045–1050.
140. Hager TH, Gall FP, Hermanek P. Local excision of

cancer of the rectum. Dis Colon Rectum 1983; 26:149–151.
141. Grigg M, McDermott FT, Pihl EA. Curative local excision in the management of carcinoma of the rectum. Dis Colon Rectum 1984; 27:81–83.
142. Jackman RJ. Conservative management of selective patients with carcinoma of the rectum. Dis Colon Rectum 1961; 4:429–434.
143. Killingback MJ. Indications for local excision of rectal cancer. Br J Surg 1985; 72S:S54–S56.
144. Whiteway J, Nicholls RJ, Morson BC. The role of local excision in the treatment of rectal cancer. Br J Surg 1985; 72:694–697.
145. Heberer C, Denecke H, Demmel N, et al. Local procedures in the management of rectal cancer. World J Surg 1987; 11:499–503.
146. Biggers OR, Beart RW Jr, Ilstrup DM. Local excision of rectal cancer. Dis Colon Rectum 1986; 29:374–377.
147. Gerard A, Pector JC, Ferreira J. Local excision as conservative treatment for small rectal cancer. Eur J Surg Oncol 1989; 15:544–546.
148. Graham RA, Garsney L, Jessup JM. Local excision of rectal carcinoma. Am J Surg 1990; 160:306–312.
149. Corman ML. Colon and Rectal Surgery. Philadelphia, JB Lippincott Co, 1984, Chap 11, pp 329–411.
150. Bandler CG, Roen PR. Urologic complications of left colon surgery. Ann Surg 1948; 128:80–88.
151. Baumrucker GO, Shaw JW. Urologic complications following abdominoperineal resection of the rectum. Arch Surg 1953; 67:502–513.
152. Cass AS, Bubrick MP. Ureteral injuries in colonic surgery. Urology 1981; 18:359–364.
153. Graham JW, Goligher JC. The management of accidental injuries and deliberate resections of the ureter during excision of the rectum. Br J Surg 1954; 42:151–160.
154. Beahrs JR. Urologic complications of colorectal and anal malignant tumors. In Beahrs OH, Higgins GA, Weinstein JJ, eds. Colorectal Tumors. Philadelphia, JB Lippincott Co, 1986, pp 271–279.
155. Zinman LM, Libertino JA, Roth RA. Management of operative ureteral injury. Urology 1978; 12:290–303.
156. Zollinger RM, Sheppard MH. Carcinoma of the rectum and rectosigmoid: A review of 729 cases. Arch Surg 1971; 102:335–338.
157. Metzger PP. Modified packing technique for control of presacral pelvic bleeding. Dis Colon Rectum 1988; 31:981–982.
158. Zama N, Fazio VW, Jagelman DG, et al. Efficacy of pelvic packing in maintaining hemostasis after rectal excision for cancer. Dis Colon Rectum 1988; 31:923–928.
159. Wang O, Shi W, Zhaw Y, et al. New concepts in severe presacral hemorrhage during proctectomy. Arch Surg 1985; 120:1013–1020.
160. Nivatvongs S, Fang DT. The use of thumbtacks to stop massive presacral hemorrhage. Dis Colon Rectum 1986; 29:589–590.
161. Manson PN, Corman ML, Coller JA, et al. Anterior resection for adenocarcinoma: Lahey clinic experience from 1963 through 1969. Am J Surg 1976; 131:434–441.
162. Clark CG, Harris J, Elmasri S, et. al. Polyglycolic acid sutures and catgut in colonic anastomosis. Lancet 1972; 2:1006–1007.
163. Debas HT, Thomson FB. A critical review of colectomy with anastomosis. Surg Gynecol Obstet 1972; 135:747–752.
164. Dunphy JE. The cut gut. Am J Surg 1970; 119:1–8.
165. Goligher JC, Graham NG, DeBombal FT. Anastomotic dehiscence after anterior resection of the rectum and sigmoid. Br J Surg 1970; 57:109–118.
166. Hawley PR. Infection—The course of anastomotic breakdown: An experimental study. Proc R Soc Med 1970; 63:752.
167. Irvin TT, Goligher JC. Aetiology of disruption of intestinal anastomosis. Br J Surg 1973; 60:461–464.
168. Morgenstern L, Yamakawa T. Anastomotic leakage after low colonic anastomosis: Clinical and experimental aspects. Am J Surg 1972; 123:104–109.
169. Schrock TR, Deveney CW, Dunphy JE. Factors contributing to leakage of colonic anastomosis. Ann Surg 1973; 177:513–518.
170. Sehapayak S, McNatt M, Carter HG, et al. Continuous sump-suction drainage of the pelvis after low anterior resection: A reappraisal. Dis Colon Rectum 1973; 16:485–489.
171. Heberer G, Denecke H, Pratschke E, et al. Anterior and low anterior resection. World J Surg 1982; 6:517–524.
172. Hunt TK. Anastomotic failure. In Simmons RL, ed. Topics in Intra-abdominal Surgical Infection. Norwalk, CT, Appleton-Century-Crofts, 1982, p 101.
173. Nivatvongs S. Complications of anorectal and colorectal operations. In Gordon PH, Nivatvongs S, eds. Principles and Practice of Surgery for the Colon, Rectum and Anus. St. Louis, Quality Medical Publishing, Inc, 1992, Chap 36.
174. Ballantyne GH. Intestinal suturing: Review of the experimental foundations for traditional doctrines. Dis Colon Rectum 1983; 26:836–843.
175. Goldstein M, Duff JH. Reconsideration of colostomy in elective left colon resection. Surg Gynecol Obstet 1972; 134:593–594.
176. Manz CW, LaTendresse C, Sako Y. The detrimental effects of drains on colonic anastomosis: An experimental study. Dis Colon Rectum 1970; 13:17–25.
177. Marks CG, Ritchie JK. The complications of synchronous combined excision for adenocarcinoma of the rectum at St. Mark's Hospital. Br J Surg 1975; 62:901–905.
178. Guice SL, Brannan W. Urologic complications of colon and rectal surgery. In Ferrari BT, Ray JE, Gathright JB, eds. Complications of Colon and Rectal Surgery: Prevention and Management. Philadelphia, WB Saunders Co., 1985, pp 15–24.
179. Kinn AC, Ohman U. Bladder and sexual dysfunction after surgery for rectal cancer. Dis Colon Rectum 1986; 29:43–48.
180. Masters WH, Johnson VE. Human Sexual Inadequacy. Boston, Little, Brown and Co, 1970.
181. Walsh PC, Schlegel PN. Radical pelvic surgery with preservation of sexual dysfunction. Ann Surg 1988; 208:391–400.
182. Clarke JS, Condon RE, Bartlett JG, et al. Preoperative oral antibiotics reduce septic complications of colon operations; Results of prospective, randomized, double-blind clinical study. Ann Surg 1977; 185:251–259.
183. Herter FP, Colacchio TA. The influence of antibiotics on infection and anastomotic recurrence after colon resection for cancer. World J Surg 1982; 6:188–194.
184. Keighly MRB, Crapp AR, Burdon DW, et al. Prophylaxis against anaerobic sepsis in bowel surgery. Br J Surg 1976; 63:538–541.
185. Nichols RL. Postoperative wound infection. N Engl J Med 1982; 307:1701–1702.
186. Palumbo LT, Sharpe WS. Anterior versus abdominoperineal resection: Resection for rectal and rectosigmoid carcinoma. Am J Surg 1968; 115:657–660.

187. Sandusky WR. Use of prophylactic antibiotics in surgical patients. Surg Clin North Am 1980; 60:83–92.
188. Washington JA, Dearing WH, Judd ES, et al. Effect of preoperative antibiotic regimen on development of infection after intestinal surgery: Prospective, randomized, double-blind study. Ann Surg 1974; 180:567–572.
189. Nichols RL, Holmes JWC. Prophylactic and therapeutic antibiotics in colon and rectal surgery. Perspect Colon Rectal Surg 1990; 3:183–195.
190. Polk HC Jr, Simpson CJ, Simmons BP, et al. Guidelines for prevention of surgical wound infection. Arch Surg 1983; 118:1213–1217.
191. Irvin TT, Goligher JC. A controlled clinical trial of three different methods of perineal wound management following excision of the rectum. Br J Surg 1975; 62:287–291.
192. Baudot P, Keighley MRB, Alexander-Williams J. Perineal wound healing after proctectomy for carcinoma and inflammatory disease. Br J Surg 1980; 67:275–276.
193. Elliot M, Todd IP. Primary suture of the perineal wound using constant suction and irrigation following rectal excision for inflammatory bowel disease. Ann R Coll Surg Engl 1985; 67:6–7.
194. Oakley JR, Fazio VW, Jagelman DG, et al. Management of the perineal wound after rectal excision for ulcerative colitis. Dis Colon Rectum 1985; 28:885–888.
195. Tompkins RG, Warshaw AL. Improved management of the perineal wound after proctectomy. Ann Surg 1985; 202:760–765.
196. Anthony JP, Mathes SJ. The recalcitrant perineal wound after extirpation. Arch Surg 1990; 125:1371–1377.
197. Stewart RM, Page CP, Brender J, et al. The incidence and risk of early postoperative small bowel obstruction. Am J Surg 1987; 154:643–647.
198. Goligher JC, Lloyd-Davies OV, Robertson CT. Small gut obstructions following combined excision of the rectum, with special reference to strangulation around the colostomy. Br J Surg 1952; 38:467–473.
199. Harshaw DH, Gardner B, Vives A, et al. The effect of technical factors upon complications from abdominal perineal resections. Surg Gynecol Obstet 1974; 139:756–758.
200. Pickleman J, Lee RM. The management of patients with suspected early postoperative small bowel obstruction. Ann Surg 1989; 210:216–219.
201. Chassin JL, Mulholland JH. Complications of surgery of the colon. Surg Clin North Am 1954: 1337–1345.
202. Sarr MG, Buckley GB, Zuidema GD. Preoperative recognition of intestinal strangulation obstruction: Prospective evaluation of diagnostic capability. Am J Surg 1983; 145:176–182.
203. Schwartz SI. Manifestations of gastrointestinal disease. In Schwartz SI, Shires GT, Spencer FC, eds. Principles of Surgery, 5th ed. New York, McGraw-Hill Book Co, 1989, Chap 24, p 1084.
204. Ballantyne GH, Beart RW Jr. Maschinelle anastomosen in der colorectalen Chirurgie: Indikationen und ergebnisse. Chirurg 1985; 56:223–226.
205. Heald RJ, Leicester RJ. The low stapled anastomosis. Dis Colon Rectum 1981; 24:437–444.
206. Belli L, Beati CA, Frangi M, et al. Outcome of patients with rectal cancer treated by stapled resection. Br J Surg 1988; 75:422–424.
207. Zannini G, Renda A, Lepore R, et al. Mechanical anterior resection for carcinoma of the mid rectum: Long term results. Int Surg 1987; 72:18–19.
208. Antonsen HK, Kronberg O. Early complications after low anterior resection for rectal cancer using the EEA stapling device. Dis Colon Rectum 1987; 30:579–583.
209. Hedberg SE, Helmy AH. Experience with gastrointestinal stapling at the Massachusetts General Hospital. Surg Clin North Am 1984; 64:511–528.
210. Fazio VW. Advances in the surgery of rectal carcinoma utilizing the circular stapler. In Spratt JS, ed. Neoplasms of the Colon, Rectum and Anus. Philadelphia, WB Saunders, 1984, pp 268–288.
211. Isbister WH, Beasley SW, Dowle CS. The EEA stapler—A Wellington experience. Coloproctology 1983; 6:323–326.
212. Vezeridis M, Evans TJ, Mittelman A, et al. EEA stapler in low anterior anastomosis. Dis Colon Rectum 1982; 35:364–367.
213. Polglase AL, Cunningham GE, Hughes ESR, et al. Initial clinical experience with the EEA stapler. Aust N Z J Surg 1982; 52:71–75.
214. Leff EI, Hoexter B, Labow SB, et al. The EEA stapler in low colorectal anastomoses: Initial experience. Dis Colon Rectum 1982; 25:704–707.
215. Helm W, Rowe PH. Rectal anastomosis with the EEA stapling instrument. Ann R Coll Surg Engl 1982; 64:356–357.
216. Hamelmann H, Thiede A, Jostarndt L, et al. Stapler anastomosis in low rectal third. In Heberer G, Denecke H, eds. Colorectal Surgery. Berlin, Springer-Verlag, 1982, pp 115–119.
217. Goligher JC. The use of circular staples for the construction of colorectal anastomoses after anterior resection. In Herberer G, Denecke H, eds. Colorectal Surgery. Berlin, Springer-Verlag, 1982, pp 107–113.
218. Heald RJ, Leicester RJ. The low stapled anastomosis. Br J Surg 1981; 68:333–337.
219. Cutait DE, Cutait R, DaSilva JH, et al. Stapled anastomosis in colorectal surgery. Dis Colon Rectum 1981; 24:155–160.
220. Cade D, Gallagher P, Schofield PE, et al. Complications of anterior resection of the rectum using the EEA stapling device. Br J Surg 1981; 68:339–340.
221. Kirkegaard P, Christiansen J, Hjortrup A. Anterior resection for midrectal cancer with the EEA stapling instrument. Am J Surg 1980; 140:312–314.
222. Goligher JC, Lee PWR, Lintott DJ. Experience with the Russian model 249 suture gun for anastomosis of the rectum. Surg Gynecol Obstet 1979; 148:517–524.
223. Aldoff M, Arnaud JP, Beehary S. Stapled versus sutured colorectal anastomosis. Arch Surg 1980; 115:1436–1438.
224. Scher KR, Scott-Conner C, Jones CW, et al. A comparison of stapled and sutured anastomosis in colonic anastomoses. Surg Gynecol Obstet 1982; 155:489–493.
225. Beart RW Jr, Kelly KA. Randomized prospective evaluation of the EEA stapler for colorectal anastomosis. Am J Surg 1981; 141:143–147.
226. McGinn FP, Gartell PC, Clifford PC, et al. Staples or sutures for low colorectal anastomoses. Br J Surg 1985; 73:603–605.
227. Jarvinen HJ, Ovaska J, Mecklin JP. Improvements in the treatment and prognosis of colorectal carcinoma. Br J Surg 1988; 75:25–27.
228. Heald RJ. Towards fewer colostomies—The impact of the circular stapling devices on the surgery of

rectal cancer in the district hospital. Br J Surg 1980; 67:198–200.
229. Odou MW, O'Connell TX. Changes in the treatment of rectal carcinoma and effects on local recurrence. Arch Surg 1986; 121:1114–1116.
230. Schwartz SI. Complications. *In* Schwartz SI, et al., eds. Principles of Surgery, 5th ed. New York, McGraw-Hill Book Co, 1989, pp 473–481.
231. Sugarbaker PH, Gunderson LL, Wittes RE. Colorectal cancer. *In* DeVita VT Jr, Hellman S, Rosenberg SA, eds. Cancer Principles and Practice of Oncology, 2nd ed. Philadelphia, JB Lippincott Co, 1985, pp 795–884.
232. Umpleby HC, Williamson RCN. Anastomotic recurrence in large bowel cancer. Br J Surg 1987; 74:873–878.
233. Russell A, Tong D, Dawson LE, et al. Adenocarcinoma of the proximal colon: Sites of initial dissemination and patterns of recurrence following surgery alone. Cancer 1984; 53:360–367.
234. Willett CG, Tepper JE, Cohen AM, et al. Failure patterns following curative resection for colonic carcinoma. Ann Surg 1984; 200:685–690.
235. Malcolm AW, Perencerich NP, Olson RM, et al. Analysis of recurrence patterns following curative resection for carcinoma of the colon and rectum. Surg Gynecol Obstet 1981; 152:131–136.
236. Devesa JM, Morales V, Enriquez JM. Colorectal cancer: The basis for a comprehensive follow-up. Dis Colon Rectum 1988; 31:636–652.
237. Boey J, Cheung HC, Lai CK, et al. A prospective evaluation of serum carcinoembryonic antigen (CEA) levels in the management of colorectal cancer. World J Surg 1984; 8:279–286.
238. Feil W, Wunderlich M, Kovatz E, et al. Rectal cancer: Factors influencing the development of local recurrence after radical anterior resection. Int J Colorectal Dis 1988; 3:195–200.
239. McDermott FT, Hughes ESR, Pihl E, et al. Local recurrence after potentially curative resection for rectal cancer in a series of 1008 patients. Br J Surg 1985; 72:34–37.
240. Stearns MW, Binkley GE. The influence of location on prognosis in operable rectal cancer. Surg Gynecol Obstet 1957; 96:368–370.
241. Rich T, Gunderson LL, Lew R, et al. Patterns of recurrence of rectal cancer after potentially curative surgery. Cancer 1983; 52:1317–1329.
242. Follett WG, Nicholls RJ. The relationship between extent of distal clearance and survival and local recurrence rates after curative anterior resection for carcinoma of the rectum. Ann Surg 1983; 198:159–163.
243. Philipsen S. Cancer of the rectum: Local recurrence. *In* Fazio VW, ed. Current Therapy in Colon and Rectal Surgery. Toronto, Brian C Decker, 1990, pp 137–149.
244. Fick ThE, Baeten CGMI, von Meyenfeldt MF, et al. Recurrence and survival after abdominoperineal and low anterior resection for rectal cancer without adjuvant therapy. Eur J Surg Oncol 1990; 16:105–108.
245. Williams NS, Durdey P, Johnston D. The outcome following sphincter-saving resection and abdominoperineal resection for low rectal cancers. Br J Surg 1985; 72:595–598.
246. Schiessel R, Wunderlich M, Herbst F. Local recurrence of colorectal cancer: Effect of early detection and aggressive surgery. Br J Surg 1986; 73:342–344.
247. Pihl E, Hughes ESR, McDermott FT, et al. Recurrence of carcinoma of the colon and rectum at the anastomotic suture line. Surg Gynecol Obstet 1981; 153:495–496.
248. Heald RJ. Rectal cancer: Anterior resection and local recurrence—A personal review. Perspect Colon Rectal Surg 1988; 1:1–26.

Chapter 22
Preoperative and Intraoperative Staging of Colorectal Cancer

Michele D. Davis
Garth H. Ballantyne

Staging systems for colorectal cancer were originally introduced to demonstrate that surgical resections of colorectal cancers cured certain subgroups of patients. In the last several decades, staging systems have been used to stratify groups of patients into different treatment protocols. Whereas most staging systems provide reliable prognostic information when applied to large populations of patients, they have proven unreliable in the prediction of individual patient outcome. More recently, multivariate analysis of large data banks of patient information have identified a series of independent clinical and pathologic variables that when used together generate accurate outcome predictions for individual patients. The rapid insertion of new technology into the practice of surgery, which has been catalyzed by videolaparoscopy, has remarkably improved our ability to preoperatively and intraoperatively stage colorectal cancers. As a result, in the immediate future surgeons will be able to select appropriate surgical techniques for the resection of colorectal cancers based on accurate outcome predictions for the individual patient. The purpose of this chapter is to review the historical development of staging systems of colorectal cancer and then to describe the capabilities of the methods by which the information needed for these staging systems is acquired. The introduction of minimally invasive techniques for the resection of colorectal cancers and recent advances in our capabilities in pre- and intraoperatively staging these lesions demand a reevaluation of current strategies for the surgical treatment of colorectal cancer.

HISTORY OF STAGING

The first attempts to classify patients with rectal cancer came in the early 1900s. Because of the excessive mortality associated with surgical resection of rectal cancers, surgeons hoped that they could identify the small group of patients who might best benefit from these operations.[1] In 1904, Clogg[2] was among the first to notice that certain pathologic features of disease correlated with outcome. He traced 41 patients to the autopsy room and tried to develop an understanding of the natural history of this disease. In addition, Cloggs reported 6 patients (of 14) who were alive 10 months to 6 years after resections of rectal cancers. Clogg became convinced that many rectal cancers could be successfully treated by operative resection and that visceral involvement occurred late in the course of the disease.

The Spread of Rectal Cancer

Miles[3] carefully characterized the spread of rectal cancer early in the twentieth century. Based on extensive autopsy studies Miles concluded that:

> . . . a cancerous growth in the rectum spreads in three directions, and invades the tissues either in the nature of direct permeation, or as a separate metastases; at any rate so far as naked-eye appearance shows. The directions of spread are downward, lateral, and upward, and take place in zones traversed by the lymphatic vessels.

Miles postulated that extirpation of rectal cancers could be accomplished by an operation that removed the rectum and all the tissues in these three zones of spread. He substantiated this new concept by reporting his early results with this operation. Among 24 patients treated with abdominoperineal resection, 10 died during the perioperative period. Of the remaining 14, however, 12 were alive and free of disease: 8 for more than 18 months and 3 for more than 3 years.

Broders' Classification

The success of Miles in the treatment of rectal cancer prompted surgeons at the Mayo Clinic to attempt surgical treatment of colon cancer. By 1926, Rankin[4] reported 509 operations for colon cancers. The operative mortality for the 333 patients who underwent "curative" resections (i.e., no residual macroscopic tumor) was 19.6 per cent. Overall survival, however, was a startling 49.5 per cent at 5 years.

The surgeons at the Mayo Clinic attempted to identify a method by which they could preoperatively stage colon cancer. They hoped to identify the group of patients who might be cured by an operative resection and spare patients with incurable disease the high perioperative mortality. They divided factors that influenced the outcome of surgical treatment into "extrinsic" and "intrinsic" influences. The extrinsic factors included age, general condition of the patient, duration of symptoms, and, in addition, gross characteristics of the lesion such as the size, mobility, lymphatic involvement, distal metastases, fibrosis, lymphocytic infiltration, and hyalinization. The intrinsic influences were represented by the activity of the tumor cells themselves. It was suggested that degree of differentiation reflected the rate at which tumor cells multiplied: cells that multiplied slowly would have enough time to achieve a mature appearance whereas rapidly dividing cells would retain an immature histologic appearance.[5] Broders,[6] a pathologist at the Mayo Clinic, believed that the rapidly proliferating cells with the immature appearance were unable to control their own growth whereas the more slowly dividing cells demonstrated a greater level of control.

In 1928, Rankin and Broders[7] applied the idea of histologic grading to rectal carcinoma, defining tumors on the basis of differentiation. In this system in Grade 1, the cancer cells were almost completely differentiated; in Grade 2, the cells were less well differentiated; in Grade 3, the cells were less mature in appearance, and acinar formation was irregular, and in Grade 4, the cells were undifferentiated and acini were ill defined. The major advantage of this system of classification, which remains true today, is that it can be used to stratify patients into different groups prior to operation and consequently can be used in the selection of the optimum surgical technique for the treatment of the tumors in individual patients.

The Epithelial Origin of Carcinomas

The systems of classification of colorectal cancer that dominated the second and third quarters of the twentieth century derive from the postulate that all colorectal cancers originate from the epithelial cells of the intestinal mucosa. Two seminal theories contributed to the acceptance of this concept: the unicellular origin of cancers, as proposed by Bauer,[8] and the progression of benign polyps into cancers, as advocated by Dukes.[9] Together these theories lead to the general belief that colorectal cancers spread in an orderly and predictable fashion: lesions that had originated in the mucosa penetrated first into the submucosa and subsequently into the muscularis propria and pericolic or perirectal soft tissues. Once free of the constraints of the bowel wall, the cancer spread first to the local lymph nodes and then to regional lymph nodes. Finally, the cancer escaped the confines of the lymphatic barriers and dispersed to the liver and other distant sites. This view of the orderly spread of colorectal cancer continues to form the basis of present day staging systems.

Staging Systems

LOCKHART-MUMMERY (1927)

J. P. Lockhart-Mummery, a surgeon at St. Mark's Hospital in London, treated rectal cancer by perineal excision (Fig. 22-1). In 1926, he reported his results with this approach in the treatment of 200 patients.[10] He was anxious to identify a system for the prediction of prognosis for his patients. Consequently, he proposed a classification system for rectal tumors based on the depth of tumor invasion into the rectal wall. Lesions were classified as follows:

Class A: Tumors are small, freely movable with no invasion of muscular coat or glands, very favorable prognosis with 5-year survival of 73.7 per cent.
Class B: Tumors involve muscular coat with no fixity of rectal wall and no extensive glandular involvement, moderate prognosis with 5-year survival of 44.1 per cent.
Class C: Tumors are fixed to surrounding structures with extensive glandular involvement; very poor prognosis with 5-year survival of 44.4 per cent.

This system was based exclusively on the histologic features of the lesion as characterized by the surgical pathologist after the operation. It ignored all clinical features such as the condition of the patient or the presence of any distant metastases. Consequently, this classification system could only be used to advise the patient about prognosis after the operation was accomplished and could not be utilized in the preoperative selection of different treatment alternatives. Nevertheless, this system set the pattern of classification for the next 50 years.

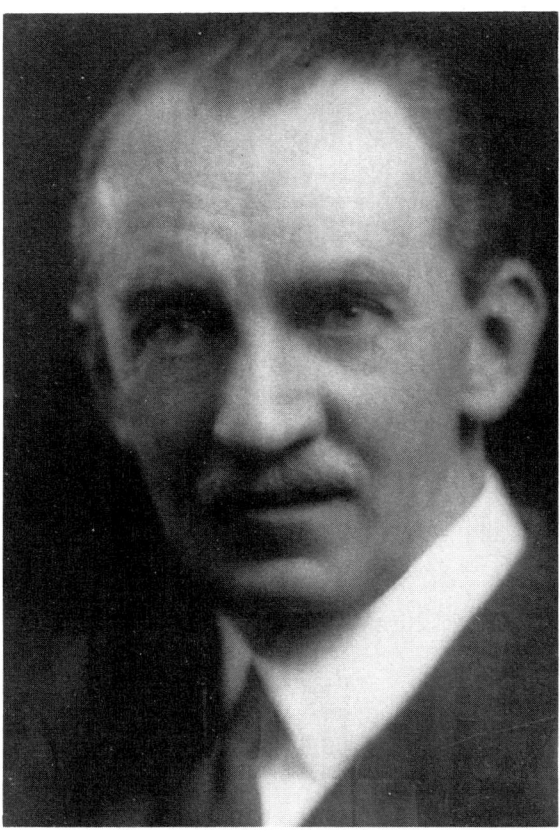

Figure 22-1. J. P. Lockhart-Mummery who practiced surgery at St. Mark's Hospital in London first proposed a staging system for rectal cancer based on the depth of penetration of the cancer into the rectal wall and the status of lymph node involvement.[10]

DUKES (1930)

Cuthbert E. Dukes, the surgical pathologist at St. Mark's Hospital, picked up the gauntlet from Lockhart-Mummery and became the primary spokesman for staging of colorectal cancer throughout the remainder of his career. The staging system suggested by Lockhart-Mummery was altered by Dukes in 1930.[11] He believed that it was important to distinguish the group of patients in whom "the stage in the slow erosion of neighboring tissues that the more rapid spread into lymphatics (had) commenced." In this publication, Dukes reported the results of careful dissection of 100 surgical specimens of rectal cancers and divided the lesions into the following categories:

A: Malignant tumors in which the growth extends into the submucosa, but not into the muscle coat.
B: Malignant tumors in which the growth extends into the muscular coat, but has not spread by direct continuity into the perirectal tissue. B tumors can be further subdivided into:
  B1: Circular muscle limits growth.
  B2: Longitudinal muscle has been reached.
C: Malignant tumors that have spread by direct continuity into perirectal tissues. C tumors may also be subdivided into:
  C1: Without glandular involvement.
  C2: With metastases to lymph nodes.

Among the 100 patients, none of the A ($n = 1$) or B ($n = 24$) lesions had lymphatic metastases, while lymph node involvement was found in association with 40 of the 75 C lesions. Consequently, Dukes concluded that lymphatic metastases rarely occurred until the cancer had spread by direct continuity beyond the intestinal wall into the perirectal tissues.

DUKES (1932)

In 1932, Dukes published his classic article defining what is generally referred to now as the Dukes classification system.[12] This modification stressed Dukes' belief that lymph node involvement was rare until the full thickness of the rectal wall had been penetrated by tumor. In this article, Dukes classified 215 rectal cancers into three categories as follows (Fig. 22-2):

A: Carcinoma limited to the wall of the rectum, there being no extension into the extrarectal tissues and no metastases to the lymph nodes.
B: Carcinoma spread by direct continuity to the extrarectal tissues, but no regional lymph node involvement.
C: Carcinoma that has metastasized to regional lymph nodes.

Dukes' main concern was to formulate a staging system that allowed the best prognostication of outcome for patients afflicted with rectal cancer. He reported the 3-year survival for 52 of these 215 patients divided into his three categories: A, 80 per cent; B, 73 per cent; and C, 7 per cent.[12] He also compared this classification system to that defined by Broders, which used grade of differentiation as the major criteria. Dukes found no consistent relationship between these two systems and was unable to find a reliable prediction of survival for patient groups divided on the basis of histologic grading.

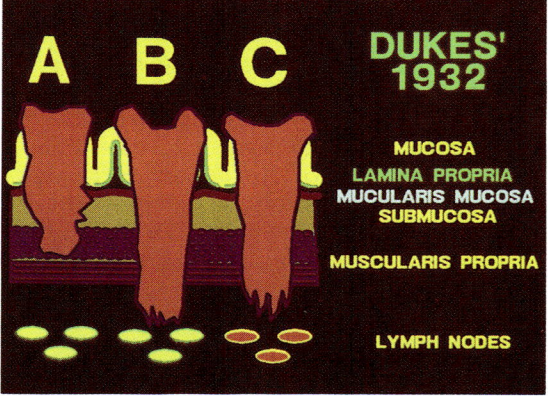

Figure 22-2. The classification system proposed by Dukes in 1932 stressed the orderly and predictable progression of rectal cancer. Dukes was convinced that rectal cancers rarely spread to the lymph nodes until they had penetrated through the rectal wall into the perirectal fat.[12]

GABRIEL, DUKES, AND BUSSEY (1936)

A further modification of Dukes' system was published in 1936 by Gabriel, Dukes, and Bussey.[13] In this system, the three categories of A, B, and C were unchanged as described in the 1932 article. The C category, however, was divided into two groups:

C1: Tumors in which regional lymph nodes are involved, or those in which the upward spread has not yet reached the glands at the point of ligature of the blood vessels.
C2: Tumors in which the glandular spread has reached up to the level of the point of ligature of the blood vessels.

The purpose of this classification system was to more carefully define the usual sequence of lymphatic spread of rectal cancer. This paper proposed that in the same way that rectal cancer spreads in an orderly manner through the layers of the rectal wall, it spreads in an orderly and predictable manner along the lymphatic vessels of the rectal mesentery. This implied that rectal cancer could be cured by rectal resection as long as the malignancy had not as yet reached the apex of the dissection.

SIMPSON AND MAYO (1939)

In 1939, Simpson and Mayo[14] applied Dukes' principles of depth of penetration of the tumor in the classification of patients with colonic cancers. They wished to determine if the same methods that had been successfully applied to rectal cancers would prove useful in the classification and prediction of prognosis for colon cancers. Their classification included three categories:

A: No penetration through the submucosa; 5-year survival 100 per cent ($n = 10$).
B: No penetration beyond the muscularis; 5-year survival 61.9 per cent ($n = 21$).
C: Penetration through the muscularis; 5-year survival 49.4 per cent ($n = 89$).

They also found that besides depth of penetration or degree of differentiation, extent of lymph node involvement by tumor also helped to predict survival.[14]

KIRKLIN, DOCKERTY, AND WAUGH (1949)

During the 1940s, surgeons at the Mayo Clinic began to advocate anterior resection for rectosigmoid carcinomas and coloanal pull-through procedures for midrectal cancers. Many other surgeons insisted that these lesions should be treated with an abdominoperineal resection because they held a clinical impression that lesions below the peritoneal reflection carried a worse prognosis. In 1949, Kirklin et al.[15] deemed the muscularis propria as an important anatomic landmark by which tumors should be differentiated. They designed a study to specifically assess the role of the location of the tumor in relation to the peritoneal reflection in the prognosis for patients with rectal carcinoma. In doing so, the cases were limited to include those that were Broder's Class 2 and did not have metastases. Lesions were divided into four categories:

A: Lesions limited to the mucosa.
B1: Lesions that extended into the muscularis propria but did not penetrate through it.
B2: Lesions that penetrated through the muscularis propria.
C: Lesions of either type B1 or B2 that also had involvement of the lymph nodes.

They found no significant difference between the 5-year survival for patients with cancer located above (54.4 per cent) and below (59.4 per cent) the peritoneal reflection. The results, which compared the stage-specific classification of these two groups, were also similar. This study not only was the first to name the muscularis propria as an important anatomic landmark in classifying tumors on the basis of invasion, but also showed that the location of the tumor in relation to the peritoneal reflection was not important in determining survival. This supported the use of sphincter-saving resections for treatment of cancers of the rectosigmoid and rectum.[16]

ASTLER AND COLLER (1954)

The conclusions reached by Kirklin, Dockerty, and Waugh were not accepted by many surgeons. Astler and Coller[17] reexamined this issue several years later because they remained convinced that lesions below the peritoneal reflection carried a worse prognosis than those above it. Their foray into this controversy produced the modification of Dukes original classification system that is most widely used today. In support of their contention, Astler and Coller quoted the results of Gilchrist and David (1943)[18] on the lymphatic spread of rectal cancer. In their own analysis of these data, Astler and Coller calculated that overall 5-year survival for patients with tumors above the peritoneal reflection was 65 per cent and for those below was 51 per cent. They concluded from this that the serosa found above the peritoneal reflection was an important barrier to the spread of disease. The Astler-Coller modification was devised to support this hypothesis by subdividing the C category of tumors on the basis of penetration through the bowel wall. They retained the A, B1, and B2 classifications as proposed by Kirklin and colleagues.[15] In addition, they divided lesions with positive lymph nodes into two categories:

C1: Lesions limited to the bowel wall with positive lymph nodes.
C2: Lesions that extended through all layers of the bowel wall with positive lymph nodes.[17]

Patients with widely metastatic disease were excluded. Astler and Coller reported the 5-year survival of 352 patients as follows: A 100 per cent ($n = 1$); B1 66.6 per cent ($n = 48$); B2 53.9 per cent ($n = 104$); C1 22.4 per cent ($n = 14$); and C2 22.4 per cent ($n =$

125) with an overall 5-year survival for all patients of approximately 44 per cent. Just as Kirklin and colleagues[15] had used their system to justify the use of sphincter preservation surgery for patients with rectal carcinoma below the peritoneal reflection, so did Astler and Coller use their data to advocate the opposite belief. Astler and Coller believed that they had substantiated "the need for radical extirpation of perirectal tissues if delayed local recurrence is to be conquered."

TURNBULL, KYLE, WATSON, AND SPRATT (1967)

Studies by surgeons at the Cleveland Clinic disclosed the presence of malignant cells in the bloodstream during resections of colorectal cancers.[19] In hopes of obviating dissemination of colorectal metastases at the time of operation, Rupert Turnbull designed a "no touch technique" for the removal of colorectal cancers. Turnbull insisted that the lymphovascular pedicles should be divided and the colon divided at the chosen sites of resection before the cancer-bearing section was handled or mobilized. In order to support the use of his no touch technique, Turnbull and colleagues reported the long term follow-up of 896 patients with colonic cancers that had been treated at the Cleveland Clinic. The patients were divided into four categories (Fig. 22-3):

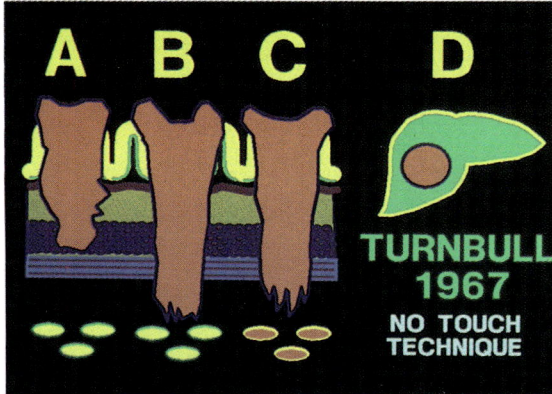

Figure 22-3. Rupert Turnbull and colleagues modified the Dukes classification of 1932[12] to include a D category for lesions with distant metastases and advanced local disease.[19] This added clinical data to what was previously an entirely pathologic staging system.

A: Tumor confined to the colon and its coats.
B: Tumor extension into pericolic fat.
C: Tumor metastases to regional mesenteric lymph nodes, but no evidence of distant metastases.
D: Lesions with tumor metastases to liver, lung, or bone; lesions with seeding of tumor into the abdominal cavity; lesions that were irremoveable because of parital invasion; lesions that invaded directly into contiguous organs.

The patients were divided into those who had undergone traditional surgical resections and those treated by Turnbull with his no touch technique. Turnbull's patients achieved a 50.9 per cent overall 5-year survival while only 34.8 per cent treated by conventional techniques survived for 5 years. The system utilized in this paper retained the A, B, and C classifications from Dukes 1932 system. In contrast, this system added a designation to the classification system for distant tumor metastases or more advanced local disease. Thus, this study was the first to add information based on clinicosurgical observations to that obtained by histopathologic observations.[20]

GUNDERSON AND SOSIN (1974)

In 1974, Gunderson and Sosin developed a modification of the Astler-Coller system based on the need to identify patients that might benefit from adjuvant radiation therapy following surgical resection.[21] They retained the A, B1, B2, C1, and C2 classifications of the Astler-Coller system but also added subgroups to designate microscopic or gross extension through the bowel wall. In addition, two new designations, B3 and C3, were added to classify tumors that were locally invasive into adjacent structures.

A: Lesions limited to the mucosa, lymph nodes negative.
B1: Lesions that extend through mucosa but are confined within the bowel wall, lymph nodes negative.
B2: Lesions that extend through the entire bowel wall without invasion of surrounding tissues or organs, lymph nodes negative.
  B2m: Microscopic extension through the bowel wall only.
  B2m&g: Extension through the bowel wall both microscopically and grossly.
B3: Lesions that were adherent to or in-

vaded adjacent organs or structures submitted with the surgical specimen, lymph nodes negative.

C1: Lesions with positive lymph nodes but limited to the bowel wall.

C2: Lesions with positive lymph nodes that extend through the entire bowel wall.

   C2m: Lesions that extend microscopically through the bowel wall only.

   C2m&g: Lesions that extend through the bowel wall both microscopically and grossly.

C3: Lesions with positive lymph nodes that were adherent to or invaded into adjacent organs or structures submitted with the pathologic specimen.

The purpose of this complex system was to identify patients who might benefit from adjuvant radiotherapy. The creation of the B3 and C3 categories served to retrieve these patients from the D category proposed by Turnbull. This system also challenged the underlying concept that underpinned the earlier Dukes systems: namely the concept that rectal cancer advanced in an orderly and predictable manner through the layers of the bowel wall and up the rectal lymphatic vessels.

AUSTRALIAN CLINICO-PATHOLOGY SYSTEM

The Australian system[22] attempted to include clinical, operative, and pathologic observations in a single staging system:

ACPS A: Lesions that have spread into the bowel wall but not beyond the muscularis propria, lymph nodes negative.

ACPS B: Lesions that have spread beyond the muscularis propria into adjacent tissues in continuity or into adjacent organs, lymph nodes negative.

ACPS C: Lesions that may have varying spread into or through the bowel wall, but one or more lymph nodes contain cancer. There are no distant metastases.

ACPS D: Evidence (clinical or microscopic) of residual tumor after the resection either locally or distantly.

ACPS O: Lesions confined to the mucosa in a patient who has undergone a bowel resection.

ACPS X: Lesions treated by local excision or other local procedures accomplished without a lymphadenectomy.

ACPS Y: Lesions for which pathologic details are unknown.

On comparison of this system with that of Dukes,[23] Astler and Coller,[23] or TMN,[24] the Australian system was found to have a better predictive and discriminant power than the others.

TNM SYSTEM

Denoix proposed the TNM (tumor-node-metastasis) system in 1954.[25] The TNM system is more complicated than earlier systems. It categorizes tumors on the basis of depth of invasion (T), nodal metastases (N), and metastases (M) (Table 22-1). Then it groups these categories together to form specific stages that have predictive value. This system, adapted by the American Joint Committee for Cancer Staging and End Results, is complex, but has advantages over the Dukes' systems.[16] By using new nomenclature (TNM), it avoids confusion caused by continual changes of the ABCD designation and it

Table 22-1. TNM Classification Union Internationale Contre le Cancer

Stage	Characteristics
TX	Minimum requirements to assess the primary tumor cannot be met
T0	No evidence of primary tumor
Tis	In situ carcinoma
T1	Tumor extends into submucosa
T2	Tumor extends into muscularis propria
T3	Tumor extends through muscularis propria into subserosa or nonperitonealized pericolic or perirectal tissues
T4	Tumor perforating visceral peritoneum or direct extension in adjacent organs or tissues
NX	Minimum requirements to assess regional lymph nodes cannot be met
N0	No lymph node metastases
N1	Metastases from 1 to 3 pericolic or perirectal lymph nodes
N2	Metastases in one to three pericolic, may or may not be relevant
N3	Metastases to any other sites (organs, tissues) along
MX	Minimum requirements to assess distant metastatic sites
M0	No distant metastasis
M1	Distant metastasic disease

also includes clinical information about metastases.[25] There has also been a designation based on clinical-surgical data (csTNM) and staging based on pathologic data obtained from the surgical specimen (pTNM). Because preoperative assessment using the csTNM system is often inaccurate and incorrect, it has not been highly recommended.[26,27]

METHODS USING MULTIVARIATE STATISTICAL ANALYSIS

The classification systems derived from Dukes classification essentially rely upon pathologic data obtained from the surgical specimen. Some include evidence of distant metastases. As a group, however, they ignore the importance of other clinical information. Two groups have approached this problem by using sophisticated methods of statistical analysis in hopes of identifying the clinical and pathologic factors that independently influence the prognosis for the patient. Chapuis and colleagues[28] subjected data from 709 patients to multivariate analysis. They identified seven factors: clinical pathologic stage, patient age, tumor grade, venous invasion, patient sex, direct spread into adjacent structures, and intestinal obstruction.

The Large Bowel Cancer Project used similar techniques in their analysis of data from 2524 patients.[29] They found that the factors of greatest statistical importance influencing long term prognosis after curative resection and excluding postoperative deaths were lymph node status, depth of primary tumor penetration, intestinal obstruction, and tumor fixation. The computer analysis of these data has produced formulas that allow accurate predictions of individual patient outcomes. Indeed, in the immediate future, computer software based on these findings will be available for use by surgeons in their offices (L. P. Fielding, personal communications). This will allow the calculation of extremely accurate predictions of prognosis for individual patients. The role of such computer-based systems in the selection of different modalities of therapy in the future remains to be explored.

FUTURE DIRECTIONS

The future aim is to establish a reliable staging system for colorectal cancer at the international level. A subcommittee of the American Society of Colon and Rectal Surgeons (in the United States) and the Cancer Coordinating Committee (in the United Kingdom) are working to develop a data-gathering system and to produce a clinicopathologic staging system that is comprehensive, statistically sound, and internationally acceptable.[16]

STAGING COLORECTAL CANCER

Conventional staging of colorectal cancer occurs during and after operative intervention. During the operative procedure the surgeon has the opportunity to examine the contents of the abdominal cavity carefully, making note of metastases, perforation of the bowel, or any other features that may affect the outcome for the patient. Following removal of the tumor, the pathologist examines, dissects, and samples particular areas of the tumor, lymph nodes, and surrounding tissue. Depending on the institution or individual pathologist, special clearance techniques for lymph nodes or special staining or sectioning techniques may or may not be used in processing the tissues. Following microscopic examination and evaluation of the tumor, lymph nodes, and other tissues, the pathologist decides with relative certainty the stage, grade, and other relevant pathologic characteristics of the tumor. The surgeon and/or oncologist may then decide whether any adjuvant therapy is warranted.

Technologic advances offer new possibilities in the staging of colorectal cancer, not only intraoperatively but also preoperatively, allowing novel treatment alternatives. Accurate preoperative determination of the depth of penetration of rectal cancers, for example, allows the selection of appropriate groups of patients for the use of preoperative radiation therapy. The remainder of this chapter will examine methods of evaluating tumor stage, some of which are time-honored and others of which are on the brink of insertion into clinical practice.

METHODS OF EVALUATION

Digital Rectal Examination

The digital rectal examination has been the mainstay in the identification and evaluation of rectal tumors for centuries. This evaluation of the lower rectum is easily performed and is often the initial assessment providing invaluable information to the astute clinician. As many as 20 per cent of colorectal tumors may be identified using this method,[30] and it also may provide the experienced examiner with information about the regional extent of disease.

The reliability and reproducibility of assessments from one examiner to another using this technique have not been objectively evaluated. Nonetheless, it is possible to use this method as a means for clinical staging. Nicholls et al.[31] and Beynon et al.[32] showed that experienced examiners correctly assessed tumors in the lower two-thirds of the rectum 70 to 80 per cent of the time when judging regional spread, annularity, ulceration, and invasion beyond the bowel wall. Despite the valuable clinical information that examiners may gain in performing the routine digital rectal examination, many still rely upon other methods of evaluation of tumor growth and pathologic features to facilitate preoperative decision-making.

Computed Tomography

Computed tomographic (CT) scanning has been used as a method for not only the preoperative staging of rectal tumors, but also as a means of evaluating patients with rectal carcinoma postoperatively. Although conventional means of evaluating the rectum and rectosigmoid colon, such as physical examination, barium enema, and rectosigmoidoscopy, are easily used, these techniques provide very little insight into the stage of the disease. Consequently, the use of CT scanning in the estimation of the extent of disease has been investigated in hopes of more accurately staging tumors preoperatively.

Initial reports indicated that CT scanning was an accurate means for the staging of colon and rectal cancers.[33-35] Many of these reports, however, used a staging method that had been developed specifically for use with CT scanning.[36,37] Based on this classification system, accuracy has been reported to be as high as 82.5 to 92 per cent.[36,37] Nevertheless, the accuracy in the assessment of the depth of intramural invasion or detection of lymph node metastases as demanded by more conventional staging methods (e.g., the Astler-Coller modification of the Dukes system) has been shown to be less than adequate.[34,36,38-40] Furthermore, whereas the use of CT scanning allows detection of enlarged (greater than 1.5 cm) lymph nodes, its reliability in revealing smaller lymph nodes that may contain metastases is questionable.[40,41] Indeed, lymph nodes containing metastases are often less than 5 mm in size.[42] Freeny et al.[40] found that when using the Dukes' classification, CT scanning correctly staged colorectal cancer in patients only 47.5 per cent of the time and most tumors (83.3 per cent) were down-staged. Thus, the CT scanner cannot be used reliably to detect or exclude the possibility of lymph node metastases in patients with colorectal cancer. Although many believe that CT scanning for preoperative assessment in colorectal cancer patients provides useful clinical information, the dependability of staging information obtained by this imaging method should not be overestimated because of its poor reliability in the evaluation of the local extent of disease.

Preoperative CT scanning may be of some benefit in the detection of liver metastases. This is an important issue because liver metastases are the primary reason for treatment failure in patients with colorectal cancer. As new treatments for liver metastases become available, it may prove important to identify and characterize the extent of hepatic disease involvement preoperatively. Not only is it important to identify metastases, but the number, size, and location of these lesions should also be accurately described. CT scanning has been somewhat useful in this regard, with accuracy reports varying between 73 and 94 per cent in the detection of hepatic metastases.[40,43-45] Most of the metastases that were missed by CT scanning were small, usually noted to measure less than 1.5 cm at the time of surgery. Some success in improving the sensitivity of liver CT scanning for metastases in the 1 to 2 cm range has been noted by the use of an oil emulsion liver contrast medium.[46] Despite these advances, however, the CT scanner remains an unreliable method for the detection of small colorectal metastases in the liver.

The most reliable use for CT scanning is the detection of recurrences in patients after resection for colorectal cancer.[40,41,47-51] Some difficulties have been identified, however, when an attempt is made to distinguish local recurrence from postoperative changes (e.g., fibrosis or hematoma).[48,52-54] Nevertheless, postoperative evaluation of patients with colorectal cancer by CT scans at regularly scheduled intervals is accepted as being clinically useful and accurate in detecting or confirming tumor recurrence.[40,41] It is important to bear in mind that the use of magnetic resonance imaging in evaluating patients with colorectal cancer has not been shown to be superior to evaluation using CT scans.[55]

Ultrasonography

ULTRASONOGRAPHY FOR RECTAL CANCER

The use of endoluminal ultrasonography, especially intrarectal ultrasound (IRUS), has gained much popularity in the preoperative assessment of patients with rectal cancer. This method allows more accurate determination of the depth of tumor invasion in the rectal wall by radially scanning the rectum and surrounding tissue. Normally, the rectal wall appears as five distinct rings (two hypoechoic and three hyperechoic), which represent interfaces between tissues of different densities (Fig. 22-4). The interfaces between the instrument and the mucosa, the mucosa and the muscularis, and the muscularis and the perirectal fat are hyperechoic with two intervening hypoechoic areas representing the anatomic layers of the mucosa (inner line) and muscularis (outer line). During assessment of a tumor, interruption of any of these interfaces corresponds to extension of the tumor through the corresponding layer.

Based on the TNM system proposed by the Union Internationale Contre le Cancer, local invasion of tumors as defined by ultrasound assessment may be classified as follows:

uT1: Tumor confined to the mucosa and submucosa.
uT2: Tumor confined to the rectal wall.
uT3: Tumor penetrating into the perirectal fat.
uT4: Tumor penetrating the surrounding organs.[56]

By using this system, direct comparison may be made to the pathologic stage defined by histopathologic examination of the excised specimen. Perirectal blood vessels and lymph nodes may be differentiated from one another and evaluated using dynamic scanning techniques.[57]

Despite the learning curve associated with gaining familiarity in using this method, many investigators have found intrarectal ultrasonography to be a reliable method in the preoperative assessment of patients with rectal cancers.[57-66] Accuracy rates between 76 and 94 per cent have been reported when comparing depth of penetration determined by ultrasound to histopathologic staging of the resected specimen.[57-64,66] Hildebrandt and colleagues[57] compared preoperative staging with endorectal ultrasonography to postoperative histopathologic staging of the excised specimen in 89 patients. They found that sonographic assessment of tumor invasiveness was correct in 90 per cent (80 of 89) patients with rectal tumors. In 8 of the cases that were incorrectly assessed, the tumor was overstaged rather than understaged. Other reports have also shown that when ultrasound evaluation of depth of tumor penetration is incorrect, the result is more likely to be an overstaged rather than understaged tumor.[58-61,64] Comparison of this technique with digital rectal examination has shown that even when the tumor is within reach of the examiner's finger, subjective assessment is correct less than 50 per cent of the time.[58,62] Assessment using CT scanning does not appear to add any useful information over digital examination in the evaluation of tumor invasion.[31,58,61] While there have been some pitfalls in the evaluation of certain tumors, continued upgrading of transducers and equipment to improve resolution along with broadened experience of examiners should provide a more valuable tool for the assessment of rectal tumors.

The assessment of lymph node involvement with tumor using IRUS has not been as promising. Accuracy reports have ranged from 38.1 to 70 per cent when an attempt is made to identify lymph nodes that contain metastases.[60,62-64,66] Milsom and Graffner[62] examined specificity and sensitivity rates for the evaluation of lymph nodes adjacent to rectal cancer using IRUS. By combining their data with those from five other studies, they showed a sensitivity and specificity of 81 and 80 per cent, respectively.[67-71] Perirectal lymph nodes as small as 0.3 cm may be detected; however, the ability of this method to distinguish metastatic lymph nodes from inflam-

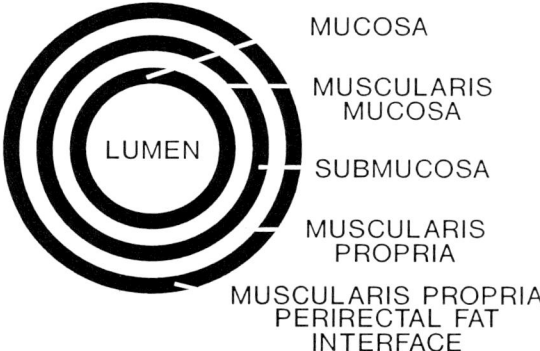

Figure 22-4. The layers of the rectal wall appear as five distinct concentric layers during endoluminal ultrasonography (IRUS).

matory or enlarged nodes is not dependable.[60,61,63] Despite the uncertainty associated with lymph node appraisal using IRUS, it certainly surpasses the accuracy reported by using digital examination, CT scanning, or magnetic resonance imaging.[62,64]

ULTRASONOGRAPHY FOR COLONIC CANCERS

More recently, instrumentation allowing endoluminal ultrasonic evaluation of colonic tumors has become available. The ultrasound colonoscope is a flexible forward-viewing instrument with a radial scanning ultrasound transducer (Fig. 22-5). Once colonoscopy is performed with visualization of a specific lesion, endosonography may be performed by establishing an interface between the transducer and the colon wall by either filling the lumen with water or instilling water into a latex balloon which covers the transducer. Similar to the ultrasound image of the rectum, there are five distinct layers visualized in the colonic wall. In addition, portions of adjacent structures, such as liver, kidneys, pancreas, and bladder, may also be seen.[72,73]

Early experience with colonoscopic ultrasonography suggests that this technique will offer the same level of accuracy for the staging of colonic cancers as observed with ultrasonography for rectal lesions (Fig. 22-6). In an early report Cho et al.[74] correctly assessed the depth of tumor penetration in only 75 per cent of 62 patients with colonic tumors. In contrast, Shimuzu et al.[63] correctly assessed depth of invasion of colonic tumors in 85 per cent of 53 patients. In this study, however, only 38 per cent of paraintestinal lymph node metastases were detected. More impressively, a more recent study reports an accuracy of 93 per cent for colonic tumors (30 cases). As in the study of Shimuzu and colleagues, the assessment of lymph node involvement with tumor was accurate only 67 per cent of the time. Once again, it was demonstrated that the size of the lymph nodes detected did not correlate with the prevalence of metastastic involvement.[66] Other authors have found endosonography useful for the evaluation of large adenomatous polyps that had no evidence of invasive carcinoma on biopsy.[73] This modality has also been shown to be useful in the detection of anastomotic recurrences of colon cancers when compared to CT scanning and endoscopy.[73]

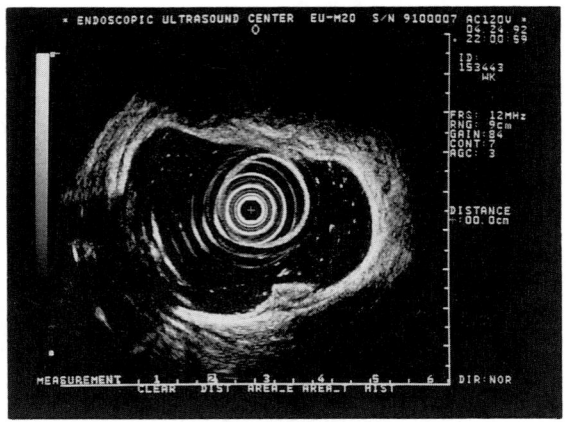

Figure 22-6. Endoscopic image of a malignant colonic polyp. The pathologic examination demonstrated a T1 lesion. The five layers of the colonic wall remain intact in the areas adjacent to the polyp. (Courtesy of Gregory A. Boyce, M.D., M.D.C., Division of Gastroenterology, Cleveland Clinic, Cleveland, Ohio.)

ULTRASOUND PROBES

Endoscopic ultrasound probes are being developed for use as alternatives to dedicated ultrasound endoscopic instruments. The probes pass through the instrument channel of standard fiberoptic or video endoscopes. They allow high resolution of focal lesions by direct application of the probe to the surface. As a result these probes are not useful for examining large areas of tissue. A further limitation of these devices is their poor penetration of surrounding tissues. This limits

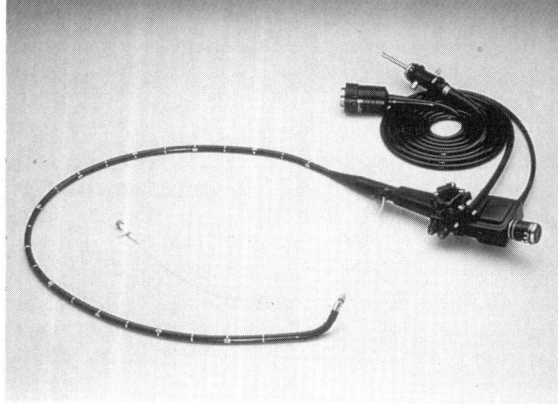

Figure 22-5. The Olympus Corporation has developed an instrument that serves as both a colonoscope and endoluminal ultrasound device.

their ability to identify lymph nodes. This technology has entered a period of rapid development and as it evolves, its future role in clinical practice will be defined.[75]

THREE-DIMENSIONAL ULTRASOUND

Another new technique in hollow organ imaging is computerized three-dimensional (3-D) ultrasound. This technique involves reconstruction of two-dimensional (2-D) images generated by intraluminal ultrasound into a 3-D image by computer. The 3-D image is generated by collecting a series of consecutive, longitudinally aligned 2-D images of a hollow organ, which are then processed by a personal computer-based image analysis system to produce a reproduction of luminal and transmural morphology in a 3-D image. This new technology lends itself to many exciting diagnostic applications and possibilities. Future studies will refine this system and will determine the indications and applications for its clinical use.[76]

INTRAOPERATIVE ULTRASOUND DETECTION OF HEPATIC METASTASES

The use of conventional ultrasound to screen for hepatic metastases has produced mixed results. Preoperative ultrasound may be hindered by a number of factors including the presence of gas in hollow organs, the patient's condition (e.g., obesity), or lack of cooperation from the patient. Other shortcomings of the procedure result from its inability to detect small (less than 2 cm) lesions, lesions that are smooth and thin, or lesions that have an echogenic nature similar to surrounding tissue.

The direct application of the ultrasound probe onto the liver bypasses many of the problems of transabdominal ultrasonography. Intraoperative surveillance of the liver using an ultrasound probe has proven very sensitive. Since no energy is lost traversing the abdominal wall, resolution is enhanced, allowing detection of smaller intrahepatic tumors. Needle biopsy of intrahepatic lesions may also be performed under ultrasound guidance. Intraoperative ultrasonography has clearly been shown to be more accurate as well as to have a better specificity, sensitivity, and predictive value in detecting hepatic metastases than preoperative ultrasound, preoperative CT scanning, and surgical exploration.[77]

LAPAROSCOPIC ULTRASONOGRAPHY

With the resent upsurge in laparoscopic procedures, it was only natural that laparoscopic ultrasound probes would be soon developed. To further enhance the utility of these instruments, ultrasonography has been linked with other imaging modalities. Echolaparoscopic prototypes are presently available. Under the direct guidance of a small laparoscope, the echographic probe is placed directly on the surface of the organ to be examined (Fig. 22-7). This direct application of the probe eliminates any interference from other structures. Preliminary results using this technique to detect small hepatic metastases have been promising. The instrument obtains a high resolution image with fine detail without being hindered by the need for deep penetration.[78,79] Low frequency probes are also being developed for better examination of deeper layers. These instruments may prove useful for ultrasound-guided biopsy to obtain tissue diagnoses. The technique of echolaparoscopy is still in the experimental stage; nevertheless, the prospects for practical application of this technology are exciting and may be soon forthcoming.[80]

Radioimmune Detection of Cancer

SCANNING TECHNIQUES

Monoclonal antibodies directed against tumor-associated antigens, which have been radiolabeled with gamma-emitting isotopes, have been used in the presurgical staging of patients with colorectal cancer. This procedure generally entails intravenous injection of the radiolabeled antibody, for example anticarcinoembryonic antigen (CEA), 791T/36, or B72.3, followed by external scanning a few days later to detect tumor deposits localized by the tumor-specific antibody.

The use of this technology as a diagnostic tool in the colorectal cancer patient population has been investigated by a number of groups.[81-85] Doerr et al.[81] showed that colorectal cancer in 70 per cent of patients was detected correctly using this technique and, in addition, showed that detection of occult disease changed the surgical intervention in 12 per cent of patients. Similarly, Duda et al.[82]

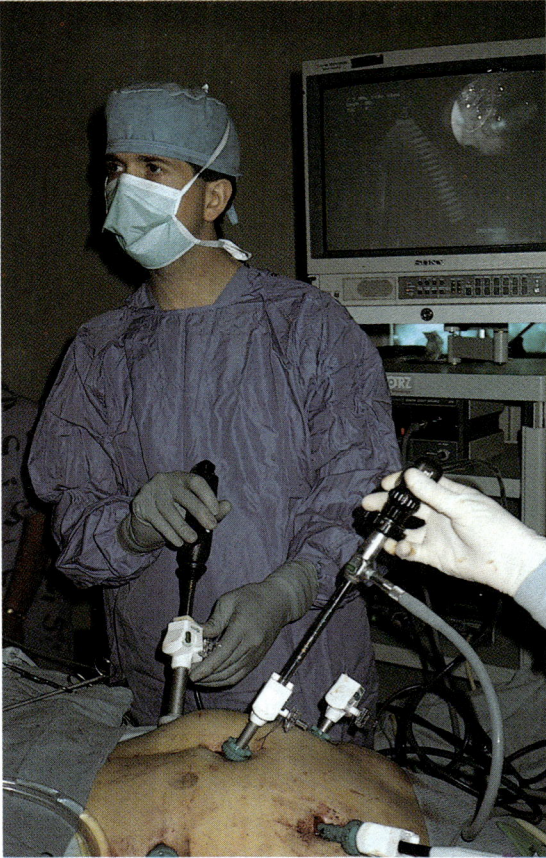

Figure 22-7. A. Laparoscopic ultrasound probes are inserted into the abdomen through 10 mg trocars and can be used to find occult metastases in the liver. B. In the Endomedix System the ultrasound image and the laparoscopic image are both projected on the video monitor. (Courtesy of Allan Siperstein, MD, San Francisco, CA.)

showed that detection of occult metastases using this method may assist the surgeon in facilitating operative exploration.

LIMITATIONS OF SCANS

While initial results were promising,[86,87] the technique itself presented many specific and difficult problems.[88] Some patients experience adverse effects after injection of the radiolabeled antibody, such as specific sensitivity reactions or damage to the thyroid gland.[88] Interpretation of scans was often difficult because of background radioactivity, which required the development of subtraction techniques to circumvent the problem.[89] Radiolocalization was also affected by the characteristics of the antibody such as antibody-tumor binding specificity or features of tumor morphology such as size, density, or vascularity.[88] Further difficulty in the use of this scan arose because of its inability to detect small lesions less than 2 cm in diameter. This was probably a result of insufficient concentration of antibody within the tumor to allow detection.[87–89] One of the major limitations is defined by the inverse square law $(S = So/D^2)$.[90] This law states that the sensitivity (S) of the device is inversely proportional to the square of the distance (D) from the device to the source (So); in this case the source would be the tumor, which is emitting energy from the radiolabel. In the case of deeply seated tumors, it may be impossible to get the scanner close enough to detect these sites accurately. With the introduction of more advanced scanning devices that can be used intraoperatively and placed directly over the radioactive site as well as the development of more specific monoclonal antibodies, sensitivity and specificity of this localization technique may be enhanced.[91]

HAND-HELD GAMMA SCANNING DEVICES

The problems associated with the use of external scanning gave rise to the development of hand-held gamma scanning devices, which can be used intraoperatively to detect occult tumor metastases.[90,91] Experimental work in nude mice showed that tumors that were too small to be detected by external scanning could be detected with a portable device of this type.[92] The probe most commonly used today is produced by the Neoprobe Corporation (Columbus, OH). It is a hand-held gamma detection probe (GDP) that may be used intraoperatively to detect tumor loci of any size since it can be placed in close proximity to a suspicious area. An incorporated microprocessor eliminates background interference from circulating levels of antibody. The antibody most commonly used with this system is ^{125}I-labeled B72.3, which recognizes the mucin glycoprotein TAG-72. One milligram of this antibody (2 mCi of ^{125}I) has been shown to be relatively nontoxic. The Neoprobe system has been evaluated in Phase I/II studies.

The radioimmunoguided surgery (RIGS) system with the Neoprobe GDP developed by Martin et al. has been used to study patients with not only primary colorectal tumors, but also those with recurrent disease.[93–99] Preliminary results from this group were encouraging. In 37 patients (6 with primary and 31 with recurrent colorectal cancer) the use of ^{125}I-labeled B72.3 antibody allowed localization of 89 per cent of the primary tumors and 82 per cent of recurrent tumors using the GDP intraoperatively. Occult tumor deposits were localized in 26 per cent of patients.[95] These results were supported by Nieroda et al.[98] in a study of 10 patients with rectal or low sigmoid cancers. In an extended study designed to assess tumor localization, detection of occult sites and toxicity, only 1 of 105 patients displayed a hypersensitivity reaction to the antibody during a skin test.[98] In this study of 104 patients with primary or recurrent colorectal cancer, sensitivity and positive predictive value of the RIGS system were 77 and 78 per cent, respectively. In 26 patients, 30 occult tumor sites were localized by the RIGS system in the pelvis (8), the retroperitoneum infrapancreatic region (6), the periportal region (6), the liver (5), the retroperitoneal retro- or suprapancreatic region (3), the cecum (1), and the supraclavicular nodes (1). These were not apparent on routine physical examination, x-ray films, or surgical exploration. The impact of this technique on surgical decision-making was also of interest. Of patients who appeared to have unresectable disease, the decision for the 27 per cent of the patients who did not undergo curative resection was based on information gained by use of the GDP. Similarly, of the patients who were deemed to have resectable disease, 23 per cent underwent extended resection based on data gathered by use of the GDP.

The majority of published studies with the Neoprobe GDP used the monoclonal antibody B72.3. Much work has been performed in developing more specific monoclonal antibodies and fragments in conjunction with the use of this intraoperative probe in patients with colorectal cancer.[99–101] In one study, anti-CEA monoclonal antibody (A5B7) localized 97.8 per cent of primary tumors and 88.8 per cent of the principal tumor in second look procedures.[99] Dukes stage was correctly predicted by RIGS in 77 per cent of the first look procedures. The use of this technique appears to be more dependable in localizing clinically occult tumor deposits than other methods especially when used during second look procedures. The role this method will play in the future depends not only on further refinement of the system (and development of a more specific antibody label), but also on information gained from expanded studies and follow-up series.

The detection of lymph node metastases using the RIGS system has been questionable. Apparently, there have been occasions when positive reactivity of lymph nodes by the GDP was not confirmed by histologic examination. Whether this reactivity is caused by occult metastases that were not detected by routine sectioning and histologic examination or by sequestration of antigen is not clear.[100] The determination of lymph node positivity clearly affects treatment options for the patient with colorectal cancer. Another imaging technique that uses monoclonal antibodies to define and examine lymphatic drainage of tumors is immunolymphoscintigraphy. This technique has been used along with the RIGS system to evaluate lymphatic invasion of tumor in patients with breast cancer.[102–104] The principle of the technique is to administer a radiolabeled antibody into the lymphatic drainage field, which then sequesters in the metastastic sites within the lymph nodes.[105] This technique shows promise, but has not yet been refined.

LAPAROSCOPIC HAND-HELD GDP

While significant progress has been made in the preparation and development of antibodies, no tumor-specific antibody has been discovered. The hand-held GDP produced by Neoprobe has been further modified so that it can be used through a trocar during laparoscopic procedures (Fig. 22-8). It may allow better decision-making at the time of both first and second look operations, which may not only extend the originally planned operation, but may also limit other procedures if

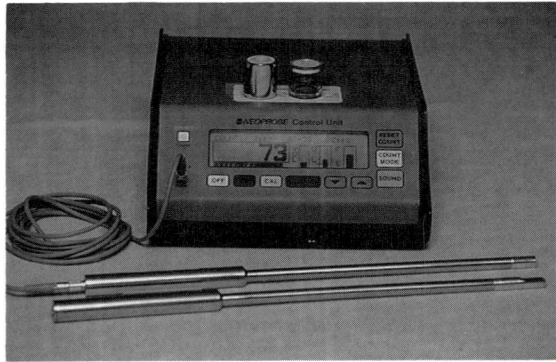

Figure 22-8. The Neoprobe Corporation has developed a hand-held gamma detection device, which may be useful for the detection of primary colorectal cancers, lymph nodes bearing metastatic carcinoma, and other metastatic lesions during laparoscopic procedures.

the new information demonstrates a bleaker picture. With further refinements of this system and combination of this technology with others (e.g., echolaparoscopic GDP), more accurate intra- and preoperative staging of colorectal cancer will be possible, which can only enhance our ability to treat and cure patients with this disease.

THE FUTURE

In the past, staging systems for colorectal cancers were used to prove retrospectively that various surgical techniques could cure large numbers of patients with early lesions. More recently, staging systems have been used to stratify patients in different treatment arms of prospective randomized trials that have tested the efficacy of adjuvant radiotherapy and chemotherapy. These staging systems are based on pathologic observations obtained by the surgical pathologist from the resected surgical specimen after the operation. These conventional systems, which are largely derived from those proposed by Lockhart-Mummery and Dukes more than 60 years ago, are limited by two overwhelming flaws: (1) these pathologic staging systems cannot be used to select different forms of surgical therapy since the stage of the lesion is determined after the operation; and (2) these staging systems cannot reliably predict outcome for an individual patient. These shortcomings are not surprising since these conventional staging systems were never designed or intended to achieve these goals.

Recent advances in several areas suggest that we may soon enter a new era in the treatment of colorectal cancers. The utilization of multivariate statistical techniques in the analysis of data from large numbers of colorectal cancers has identified a number of individual clinical and pathologic factors, which individually influence outcome of patients afflicted with this cancer. Improvements in imaging with CT scanners and ultrasonography now allow accurate preoperative determination of the depth of bowel wall penetration by colorectal cancers. The Neoprobe hand-held gamma detector probe may prove able to detect lymph node and hepatic metastases during operations. The combination of these technologies will allow accurate intraoperative staging of colorectal cancers before the operative technique has been selected. Furthermore, computer-generated multivariate formulas utilizing both clinical and morphological information will generate reliable predictions of prognosis for individual patients. Based on the prognosis associated with specific lesions, the surgeon will then be in a position to decide what surgical technique will best treat the individual patient.

In the past, tumors in various locations of the colon and rectum were generally treated by standard operations. Right colon cancers were treated by right hemicolectomies. Left colon cancers were treated with left hemicolectomies. Rectal cancers were treated with abdominoperineal resections. These standard operations were used regardless of the stage or condition of the patient.

Recently, alternative operations have been offered to patients with early rectal cancers. Intrarectal ultrasonography has promoted the application of these limited resections by the accurate illumination of the depth of rectal wall invasion by the rectal lesion. Excellent survival rates have been achieved in patients with lesions limited to the submucosa or muscularis propria.

The advent of laparoscopic techniques for colon resections portends an era of new alternatives in the surgical treatment of colorectal cancers. In the past, once a large abdominal incision was made, the surgeon felt compelled to accomplish an extensive "cancer" resection. This was reasonable since prognostic data were not available until after the completion of the operation. The new modalities discussed previously have changed this situation. The combination of intraluminal or laparoscopic ultrasonography and the hand-held laparoscopic Neoprobe gamma detector (or other novel technologies) may make available to the surgeon complete data on prognosis for the patient while only several laparoscopic trocars have been inserted. It may prove appropriate to treat early colon cancers that are limited to the submucosa or muscularis propria and have not spread to regional lymph nodes by local or limited resections. Similarly, patients with advanced lesions may be best served by limited laparoscopic procedures. In addition, the patients who will most benefit from extensive resections will also be identified. This approach will require very careful evaluation before it can be widely advocated or implemented.

REFERENCES

1. Ballantyne GH. Theories of carcinogenesis and their impact on surgical treatment of colorectal cancer: An historical review. Dis Colon Rectum 1988; 31:513–517.
2. Clogg HS. Some observations on carcinoma of the colon. Practitioner 1904; 72:525–544.
3. Miles WE. The radical abdomino-perineal operation for cancer of the rectum and of the pelvic colon. Br Med J 1910; 2:941–943.
4. Rankin FW. Surgery of the Colon. New York, Appleton, 1926, pp 263–351.
5. Ochsenhirt NC. The significance of mucus-forming cells in carcinoma of the rectum. Surg Gynecol Obstet 1928; 47:32–35.
6. Broders AC. Cancer's self control. Med J Rec 1925; 121:133–135.
7. Rankin FW, Broders AC. Factors influencing prognosis in carcinoma of the rectum. Surg Gynecol Obstet 1928; 46:660–667.
8. Bauer KH. Mutationstheorie der Geschwulstentstehung. Ubergang von Korperzellen in Geschwulstzellen durch Gen-Anderung. Berlin, Springer, 1928.
9. Dukes C. Simple tumours of the large intestine and their relation to cancer. Br J Surg 1924–1925; 13:720–733.
10. Lockhart-Mummery JP. Two hundred cases of cancer of the rectum treated by perineal excision. Br J Surg 1926–1927; 14:110–124.
11. Dukes CE. On the spread of cancer in the rectum. Br J Surg 1929–1930; 17:110–124
12. Dukes CE. The classification of cancer of the rectum. J Pathol Bacteriol 1932; 35:323–332.
13. Gabriel WB, Dukes CE, Bussey HJR. Lymphatic spread in cancer of the rectum. Br J Surg 1936; 23:395–413.
14. Simpson WC, Mayo CW. The mural penetration of the carcinoma cell in the colon: Anatomic and clinical study. Surg Gynecol Obstet 1939; 68:872–877.
15. Kirklin JW, Dockerty MB, Waugh JM. The role of the peritoneal reflection in the prognosis of carcinoma of the rectum and sigmoid colon. Surg Gynecol Obstet 1949; 88:326–331.
16. Fielding LP, Ballantyne GH. Classification systems for staging colorectal cancer. Past, present and future. Probl Gen Surg 1987; 4:39–53.
17. Astler VB, Coller FA. The prognostic significance of direct extension of carcinoma of the colon and rectum. Ann Surg 1954; 139:846–851.
18. Gilchrist RK, David VC. A consideration of pathological factors influencing five year survival in radical resection of the large bowel and rectum for carcinoma. Ann Surg 1943; 126:421–438.
19. Turnbull RB, Kyle K, Watson FR, Spratt J. Cancer of the colon: The influence of the no-touch isolation technique on survival rates. Ann Surg 1967; 166:420–427.
20. Rubio CA, Emas S, Nylander G. A critical reappraisal of Dukes' classification. Surg Gynecol Obstet 1977; 145:682–684.
21. Gunderson LL, Sosin H. Areas of failure found at operation (second or symptomatic look) following "curative surgery" for adenocarcinoma of the rectum. Cancer 1974; 34:1278–1292.
22. Davis NC, Newland RS. The reporting of colorectal cancer: The Australian clinico-pathological staging system. Aust N Z J Surg 1982; 52:395–397.
23. Chapuis PH, Fisher R, Dent OF, et al. The relationship between staging methods and survival in colorectal carcinoma. Dis Colon Rectum 1985; 28:158–161.
24. Chapuis PH, Dent OF, Newland RC, et al. An evaluation of the American Joint Committee (pTNM) staging method for cancer of the colon and rectum. Dis Colon Rectum 1986; 29:6–10.
25. Zinkin LD. A critical review of the classification and staging of colorectal cancer. Dis Colon Rectum 1983; 26:37–43.
26. Sugarbaker PH, Gunderson LL, Wittes RE. Colorectal cancer. In DeVita VT Jr, Hellmann S, Rosenberg SA, eds. Cancer: Principles and Practice of Oncology, 2nd ed. Philadelphia, JB Lippincott Co, 1985, pp 795–884.
27. American Joint Committee on Cancer. Beahrs OH, Myers MH, eds. Manual for Staging of Cancer, 2nd ed. Philadelphia, JB Lippincott Co, 1983, pp 73–80.
28. Chapuis PH, Dent OF, Fisher R, et al. A multivariate analysis of clinical and pathological variables in prognosis of resection of large bowel cancer. Br J Surg 1985; 72:698–702.
29. Fielding LP, Phillips RKS, Frye JS, Hittinger R. The prediction of outcome after curative resection for large bowel cancer. Lancet 1986; 2:904–907.
30. Horm JW, Asire AJ, Young JL Jr, et al. SEER Program: Cancer Incidence and Mortality in the United States 1973–1981. NIH Publication No. 85–1837. Bethesda, MD, U.S. Department of Health and Human Services, Public Health Service, National Institutes of Health, National Cancer Institute, 1984.
31. Nicholls RJ, Mason AY, Morson BC, et al. The clinical staging of rectal cancer. Br J Surg 1982; 69:404–409.
32. Beynon J, Mortensen NJM, Foy DMA, et al. Preoperative assessment of local invasion in rectal cancer: Digital examination, endoluminal sonography or computed tomography? Br J Surg 1985; 73:1015–1017.
33. Mayes GB, Zornoza J. Computed tomography of colon carcinoma. AJR 1980; 135:43–46.
34. Dixon AK, Fry IK, Morson BC, et al. Preoperative computed tomography of carcinoma of the rectum. Br J Radiol 1981; 54:655–659.
35. Zaunbauer W, Haertel M, Fuchs WA. Computed tomography in carcinoma of the rectum. Gastrointest Radiol 1981; 6:79–84.
36. Thoeni RF, Moss AA, Schnyder P, Margulis AR. Detection and staging of primary rectal and rectosigmoid cancer by computed tomography. Radiology 1981; 141:135–138.

37. van Waes PFGM, Koehler PR, Feldberg MAM. Management of rectal carcinoma: Impact of computed tomography. AJR 1983; 149:241–246.
38. Grabbe E, Lierse W, Winkler R. The perirectal fascia: Morphology and use in staging rectal carcinoma. Radiology 1983; 149:241–246.
39. Adalsteinsson B, Glimelius B, Graffman S, et al. Computed tomography in staging rectal carcinoma. Acta Radiol 1985; 26:45–50.
40. Freeny PC, Marks WM, Ryan JA, Bolen JW. Colorectal carcinoma evaluation with CT: Preoperative staging and detection of postoperative recurrence. Radiology 1986; 158:347–353.
41. Thompson WM, Halvorsen RA, Foster WL Jr, et al. Preoperative and postoperative CT staging of rectosigmoid carcinoma. AJR 1986; 146:703–710.
42. Herrera-Ornelas L, Justiniano J, Castillo N, et al. Metastases in small lymph nodes from colon cancer. Arch Surg 1987; 122:1253–1274.
43. Alderson PO, Adams DF, McNeil BJ, et al. Computed tomography, ultrasound, and scintigraphy of the liver in patients with colon or breast carcinoma: A prospective comparison. Radiology 1983; 149:225–230.
44. Smith TJ, Kemeny MM, Sugarbaker PH, et al. A prospective study of hepatic imaging in the detection of metastatic disease. Ann Surg 1982; 195:486–491.
45. Knopf DR, Torres WE, Fajman WJ, et al. Liver lesions: Comparative accuracy of scintigraphy and computed tomography. AJR 1982; 138:623–627.
46. Sugarbaker PH, Vermess M, Doppman JL, et al. Improved detection of focal lesions with computerized tomographic examination of the liver using ethiodized oil emulsion (EOE-13) liver contrast. Cancer 1984; 54:1489–1495.
47. Leer JWH, Scholten ET, Tjho-Heslinga RE, et al. Role of computed tomography in the diagnosis and radiotherapy planning of recurrent rectal carcinoma. Diagn Imaging Clin Med 1980; 49:208–213.
48. Husband JE, Hodson NJ, Parsons CA. The use of computed tomography in recurrent rectal tumors. Radiology 1980; 134:677–682.
49. Moss AA, Thoeni RF, Schynder P, et al. Value of computed tomography in the detection and staging of recurrent rectal carcinomas. J Comput Assist Tomogr 1981; 5:870–874.
50. Beart RW Jr, O'Connell MJ. Postoperative follow-up of patients with carcinoma of the colon. Mayo Clin Proc 1983; 58:361–363.
51. Moss AA. Computed tomography in the staging of gastrointestinal carcinoma. Radiol Clin North Am 1982; 20:761–780.
52. Kelvin FM, Korobkin M, Heaston DK, et al. The pelvis after surgery for rectal carcinoma: Serial CT observations with emphasis on nonneoplastic features. AJR 1983; 141:959–964.
53. Lee JKT, Stanley RJ, Sagel SS, et al. CT appearance of the pelvis after abdomino-perineal resection for rectal carcinoma. Radiology 1981; 141:737–741.
54. Reznek RH, White FE, Young JWR, et al. The appearances on computed tomography after abdomino-perineal resection for carcinoma of the rectum: A comparison between the normal appearances and those of recurrence. Br J Radiol 1983; 56:237–240.
55. Hodgman CG, MacCarty RL, Wolff BG, et al. Preoperative staging of rectal carcinoma by computed tomography and 0.15T magnetic resonance imaging. Dis Colon Rectum 1986; 29:446–450.
56. Spiessel B, Hermanek P, Scheibe O, Wagner G. UICC-TNM Atlas. New York, Springer-Verlag, 1985, pp 110–111.
57. Hildebrandt U, Feifel G. Intrarectal ultrasound in the evaluation of cancer of the rectum. In Nelson RL, ed. Problems in General Surgery: Controversies in Colon Cancer, 1987, Vol 4, No 1, pp 71–75.
58. Hildebrandt U, Feifel G. Preoperative staging of rectal cancer by intrarectal ultrasound. Dis Colon Rectum 1985; 28:42–46.
59. Beynon J, Foy DMA, Roe AM, et al. Endoluminal ultrasound in the assessment of local invasion in rectal cancer. Br J Surg 1986; 73:474–477.
60. Jochem RJ, Reading CC, Dozois RR, et al. Endorectal ultrasonographic staging of rectal cancer. Mayo Clin Proc 1990; 65:1571–1577.
61. Roubein LD, David C, DuBrow, et al. Endoscopic ultrasonography in staging rectal cancer. Am J Gastroenterol 1990; 85:1391–1394.
62. Milsom JW, Graffner H. Intrarectal ultrasonography in rectal cancer staging and in the evaluation of pelvic disease. Ann Surg 1990; 212:602–606.
63. Shimizu S, Tada M, Kawaii K. Use of endoscopic ultrasonography for the diagnosis of colorectal tumors. Endoscopy 1990; 22:31–34.
64. Cohen JL, Grotz RL, Welch JP, Deckers PJ. Intrarectal sonography: A new technique for the assessment of rectal tumors. Am Surg 1991; 57:459–462.
65. Napoleon B, Pujol B, Berger F, et al. Accuracy of endosonography in the staging of rectal cancer treated by radiotherapy. Br J Surg 1991; 78:785–788.
66. Tio TL, Coene PPLO, van Delden OM, Tytgat GNJ. Colorectal carcinoma: Preoperative TNM classification with endosonography. Radiology 1991; 179:165–170.
67. Saitoh N, Okui K, Sarashina H, et al. Evaluation of echographic diagnosis of rectal cancer using intrarectal ultrasonic examination. Dis Colon Rectum 1986; 29:234–242.
68. Candio GD, Mosca F, Campatelli A, et al. Endosonographic staging of rectal carcinoma. Gastrointest Radiol 1987; 12:289–295.
69. Beynon J, Mortensen NJ, Foy DMA, et al. Preoperative assessment of mesorectal lymph node involvement in rectal cancer. Br J Surg 1989; 76:276–279.
70. Rifkin MD, Ehrlich SM, Marks G. Staging of rectal carcinoma: Prospective comparison of endorectal US and CT. Radiology 1989; 170:319–322.
71. Hildebrandt U, Feifel G, Schwartz HP, et al. Endorectal ultrasound: Instrumentation and clinical aspects. Int J Colorectal Dis 1986; 1:203–207.
72. Boyce GA, Sivak MV Jr. New approaches to the diagnosis of malignant and premalignant lesions: Colonoscopic endosonography and laser-induced fluorescence spectroscopy. Semin Colon Rectal Surg 1991; 2:17–21.
73. Rosch T, Lorenz R, Classen M. Endoscopic ultrasonography in the evaluation of colon and rectal disease. Gastrointest Endosc 1990; 36:S33–S39.
74. Cho E, Yasuda K, Kioyta K, et al. Endoscopic ultrasonography in the diagnosis of colorectal cancer invasion. Gastrointest Endosc 1988; 24:203–208.
75. Kimmey MB, Martin RW, Silverstein FE. Endoscopic ultrasound probes. Gastrointest Endosc 1990; 36(2S):S40-S46.
76. Cavaye DM, Tabbara MR, Kopchok GE, et al. A new technique for intraluminal hollow organ imaging: Three-dimensional ultrasound. J Laparoendosc Surg 1991; 1:259–268.

77. Machi J, Isomoto H, Yamashita Y, et al. Intraoperative ultrasonography in screening for liver metastases from colorectal cancer: Comparative accuracy with traditional procedures. Surgery 1987; 101:678–684.
78. Ohta Y, Fujiwara K, Sato Y, et al. New ultrasonic laparoscope for diagnosis of intra-abdominal diseases. Gastrointest Endosc 1983; 4:289–294.
79. Fukuda M, Mima S, Tanabe T, et al. Endoscopic sonography of the liver—Diagnostic application of the echolaparoscope to localize intrahepatic lesions. Scand J Gastroenterol 1984; 19(S102):24–38.
80. Dagnini G. Laparoscopy and Imaging Techniques. Pearcey S, trans. Berlin, Springer-Verlag 1990, pp 19–32.
81. Doerr RJ, Abdel-Nabi H, Krag D, Mitchell E. Radiolabeled antibody imaging in the management of colorectal cancer: Results of a multicenter study. Ann Surg 1991; 214:118–124.
82. Duda RB, Zimmer AM, Rosen ST, et al. Radioimmune localization of occult carcinoma. Arch Surg 1990; 125:866–870.
83. Mach J-P, Chatal J-F, Lumbroso J-D, et al. Tumor localization in patients by radiolabeled monoclonal antibodies against colon carcinoma. Cancer Res 1983; 43:5593–5600.
84. Sullivan DC, Silva JS, Cox CE, et al. Localization of I-131-labeled goat and primate anti-carcinoembryonic antigen (CEA) antibodies in patients with cancer. Invest Radiol 1982; 17:350–355.
85. Epenetos AA, Mather S, Granowska M, et al. Targeting of I-123-labeled tumour-associated monoclonal antibodies to ovarian, breast, and gastrointestinal tumours. Lancet 1982; 2:999–1005.
86. Goldenberg DM, DeLand F, Kimm E, et al. Use of radiolabeled monoclonal antibodies to carcinoembryonic antigen for the detection and localization of diverse cancers by external photoscanning. N Engl J Med 1978; 298:1384–1388.
87. Goldenberg DM, Kim EE, DeLand FH, et al. Radioimmune detection of cancer with radioactive antibodies to carcinoembryonic antigen. Cancer Res 1980; 40:2984–2992.
88. Rankin EM, McVie JG. Radioimmunedetection of cancer: Problems and potential. Br Med J 1983; 287:1402–1404.
89. Begent RHJ, Keep PA, Green AJ, et al. Liposomally entrapped antibody improves tumour imaging with radiolabeled (first) antitumour antibody. Lancet 1982; 2:1347–1348.
90. Aitken DR, Hinkle GH, Thurston MO, et al. A gamma-detecting probe for radioimmune detection of CEA-producing tumors: Successful experimental use and clinical case report. Dis Colon Rectum 1984; 27:279–282.
91. Martin DT, Hinkle GH, Tuttle S, et al. Intraoperative radioimmune detection of colorectal tumor with a hand-held radiation detector. Am J Surg 1985; 150:672–675.
92. DeLand FH, Kim EE, Simmons G, Goldenberg DM. Imaging approach in radioimmune detection. Cancer Res 1980; 40:3046–3048.
93. Sickle-Snatanello BJ, O'Dwyer PJ, Mojzisik C, et al. Radioimmunoguided surgery using the monoclonal antibody B72.3 in colorectal tumors. Dis Colon Rectum 1987; 30:761–764.
94. Martin EW Jr, Mojzisik CM, Hinkle GH, et al. Radioimmunoguided surgery using monoclonal antibody. Am J Surg 1988; 156:386–392.
95. Nieroda CA, Mojzisik CM, Sardi A, et al. The impact of radioimmunoguided surgery (RIGS) on surgical decision-making in colorectal cancer. Dis Colon Rectum 1989; 32:927–932.
96. Cohen AM, Martin EW Jr, Lavery I, et al. Radioimmunoguided surgery using iodine 125 B72.3 in patients with colorectal cancer. Arch Surg 1991; 126:349–352.
97. Dawson PM, Blair SD, Begent RHJ, et al. The value of radioimmunoguided surgery in first and second look laparotomy for colorectal cancer. Dis Colon Rectum 1991; 34:217–222.
98. Sardi A, Agnone CM, Nieroda CA, et al. Radioimmunoguided surgery in recurrent colorectal cancer: The role of carcinoembryonic antigen, computerized tomography and physical examination. South Med J 1989; 82:1235–1239.
99. Sardi A, Workman M, Mojzisik C, et al. Intraabdominal recurrence of colorectal cancer detected by radioimmunoguided surgery (RIGS system). Arch Surg 1989; 124:55–59.
100. Lavery IC. Radioimmunoguided surgery for colon cancer. Semin Colon Rectal Surg 1991; 2:54–57.
101. O'Dwyer PJ, Mojzisik CM, Hinkle GH, et al. Intraoperative probe-directed immunodetection using a monoclonal antibody. Arch Surg 1986; 121:1391–1394.
102. Thompson CH, Stackler SA, Salehi N, et al. Immunoscinigraphy for detection of lymph node metastases from breast cancer. Lancet 1984; 2:1245–1247.
103. DeLand FH, Kim EE, Corgan RL, et al. Axillary lymphoscintigraphy by radioimmunodetection of carcinoembryonic antigen in the breast. J Nucl Med 1979; 20:1243–1250.
104. Nieroda CA, Mojzisik CM, Sardi A, et al. Staging of carcinoma of the breast using a hand-held gamma-detecting probe and monoclonal antibody B72.3. Surg Gynecol Obstet 1989; 169:35–40.
105. Weinstein JN, Stellar MA, Keenan AM, et al. Monoclonal antibodies in the lymphatics. Selective delivery to lymph node metastases of solid tumors. Science 1983; 223:423–426.

Chapter 23
Intestinal Obstruction

L. Peter Fielding
Ozuru O. Ukoha

"Intestinal obstruction" is the term used to describe a decrease or cessation in the migration of intestinal contents along the gut. It has been recognized as a clinical entity since the days of Hippocrates who considered it "a physician's repository" and recommended treatment with a combination of "enemas and inflation of the rectum."[1]

Over the last 70 years much has been written on this subject because of the grave consequences of delayed or inadequate treatment.[2-6]

CLINICAL FEATURES

Acute abdominal conditions that require a review by a surgeon are common, and intestinal obstruction accounts for about 20 per cent of such surgical admissions[7] and for 5 per cent of all general surgical admissions.

The classification of this group of conditions can be achieved in a number of ways based on etiology (Table 23-1). However, additional adjectives are often applied for descriptive purposes (i.e., degree of obstruction: partial or complete; duration of symptoms: acute or chronic; anatomical site of lesion: high or low small bowel and large bowel).

In countries where elective surgical procedures are carried out frequently, bowel "adhesions" are the most common cause of small bowel obstruction for all age groups; hernia and neoplasia are the second and third, respectively. These three causes combined account for more than 80 per cent of all cases of intestinal obstruction.[1,7,8]

Mechanical small bowel obstruction caused by adhesions can occur after any abdominal operation but are found most frequently after gynecologic procedures[9] and operations on the colon and small bowel. Obstruction is relatively rare after operations on the stomach or the biliary system.

The time between the abdominal operation and the subsequent intestinal obstruction varies widely from years to decades with an average of 6 to 10 years and a median of 1 to 2 years.[1]

At the turn of this century, the mortality rate for intestinal obstruction was about 60 per cent. Improvements in patient resuscitation with fluid and electrolyte therapy, tube decompression of the stomach, antibiotic therapy, and changes in surgical technique have been associated with a reduction in mortality rate to about 5 per cent for patients with a nonstrangulating obstruction who are operated on within 24 hours of presentation.[7,10]

However, a delay in treatment resulting in complications of the obstruction greatly increases mortality rate; strangulation alone raises the rate from 5 to 37 per cent.[1,7] It must be emphasized that at present there are no reliable methods to identify the onset or

Table 23-1. Classification of Bowel Obstruction Based on Etiology

1. Simple mechanical obstruction
   a. Intrinsic lesions
   b. Extrinsic lesions
   c. Intraluminal bodies

2. Complex mechanical obstruction
   a. Obstruction associated with ischemia
   b. Closed-loop obstruction

3. Neuromuscular defects
   a. Paralytic ileus
      i. Inhibition of motility
      ii. Humoral factors (inflammation)
      iii. Metabolic derangements
      iv. Ischemia
   b. Spastic ileus
   c. Aganglionic bowel segments
   d. "Idiopathic" pseudomechanical obstruction

4. Vascular occlusion
   a. Arterial
   b. Venous
   c. Both arterial and venous

the presence of bowel ischemia or even bowel necrosis, although acid-base balance disturbances are more common in the presence of these complications.

One reason for following a nonoperative approach to treat adhesion obstruction is that a significant number of patients will not require surgery, at least during the current episode of obstruction. Furthermore, if the problem resolves, then the patient avoids the pain and suffering and potential complications of a major abdominal incision. The dilemma, of course, is that a nonoperative approach may risk progression to bowel ischemia and even infarction with its greatly increased risk of mortality and morbidity.

Thus, a method of investigation that might have therapeutic value and could be done at an early phase in the development of intestinal obstruction (namely, laparoscopy) is conceptually very attractive if it could be shown to achieve a number of goals: (a) be therapeutic in some or many patients; (b) avoid a major abdominal incision; and (c) diminish the incidence of bowel strangulation by early intervention. If successful, laparoscopic-assisted treatment of adhesive small bowel obstruction would have the added benefit of a reduced postoperative hospital stay, which currently averages 10 to 15 days.

Large bowel obstruction occurs most commonly on the left side of the colon (70 per cent) and is caused by carcinoma in half to three quarters of the patients, volvulus (15 to 25 per cent), and diverticular disease (5 to 10 per cent). In most series, acute intestinal obstuction is the presenting symptom of colon carcinoma in 20 per cent of cases.[1,11]

Although there may be a history of bowel resection for cancer, a presentation of bowel obstruction should not be attributed to inoperable tumor. Many of these patients have nonmalignant adhesive obstruction and in others, the tumor recurrence causing the obstruction (which may be single or multiple) can usually be treated by palliative bypass or resection, returning a good quality of life to the patient, at least for a period of time.

Sigmoid volvulus, which accounts for 70 to 80 per cent of all cases of volvulus, is usually caused by redundancy of the sigmoid colon and can be treated by endoscopic or hydrostatic decompression, with a 43 per cent recurrence rate. By contrast, cecal volvulus is caused by a congenital anomaly of poor or absent fixation of the cecum to the posterior abdominal wall, resulting in torsion around the pedicle of the ileocolic vessels. Nonoperative decompression is less feasible for cecal volvulus.

PATHOPHYSIOLOGY OF MECHANICAL BOWEL OBSTRUCTION

The constant clinical finding of bowel obstruction is the accumulation of gas and fluid proximal to the site of obstruction. Vomiting, which causes additional fluid and electrolyte problems, occurs more rapidly in more proximal bowel obstruction, while abdominal distention is more marked in distal lesions.

The reason for the presence of gas and fluid in the obstructed proximal bowel has been investigated, but the precise mechanisms for these accumulations are not fully understood.

The upper gastrointestinal tract secretes 5 to 6 liters of fluid per day. Eighty per cent of this fluid is absorbed in the small gut before reaching the colon, leaving only 100 to 200 ml in the feces.[5] In the interdigestive period, the small gut is essentially empty. However, under conditions of bowel obstruction there is a change in the balance of secretion to absorption, leading to a net accumulation of fluid within the lumen of the bowel. The precise reasons for this change in balance are unclear. However, some substances have been implemented in this net hypersecretory state: vasoactive intestinal peptide,[12] prostaglandin,[7] and bile salts. A working hypothesis to explain these findings is that bacterial overgrowth occurs proximal to the site of obstruction, which induces a secretory state with the local fermentation products loosening the tight junctions between the enterocytes, thus allowing the basement membrane of the enterocytes to be influenced by luminal contents. The net secretory stimulatory outcome results in the clinical feature of intraluminal fluid accumulation. It is not known whether the normal absorptive capacity of the small bowel is blocked during this process, and further investigations are needed to elucidate these mechanisms.

The origin of most intestinal gas is from swallowed air.[7] Thus, 70 per cent is nitrogen, of which a negligible amount is absorbed from the normal gut. The bacterial fermentation proximal to the site of obstruction leads to the accumulation of some methane and hydrogen gases.[7]

Thus, in theory, a better understanding of the mechanisms associated with the cycle of bowel distention and secretion, which result in gas and fluid accumulation, might lead to development of therapeutic agents that could retard fluid secretion, increase fluid absorption, and therefore help reverse the "cycle" of deterioration. There is some preliminary experimental data suggesting that increasing fractional inspired oxygen might retard or even reverse the accumulation of gas and fluid found in the obstructed segment.[13] Furthermore, on theoretical grounds, new compounds that could increase the integrity of intercellular tight junctions and that could inhibit gut secretion under these conditions might be helpful during the resuscitation phase of patient management. We can hypothesize that such new agents could prevent deterioration of the patient's condition and possibly facilitate laparoscopically assisted surgery by reducing the volume of both gas and fluid within the bowel lumen at the time of surgery.

The additional effects of strangulation and ischemia, which can result in bowel perforation, and local or systemic sepsis (particularly in those with the closed-loop variety of obstruction) are beyond the scope of this chapter. However, in the context of laparoscopic-assisted abdominal surgery, early inspection of the abdominal contents may reduce the definitive treatment time delay, which has such a devastating effect on mortality and morbidity.

Although laparoscopy may help early diagnosis, it is likely that complex bowel obstruction, potentially associated with local sepsis and/or perforation, will need to be treated by open techniques. It would be helpful if we could establish methods to identify such patients before surgery so that we might deploy laparoscopic-assisted techniques in the appropriate patient population. Unfortunately, no such clinical or biochemical markers exist. On clinical grounds we can assume that laparoscopic methods of treatment will not be suitable for patients who have had multiple operations on the abdomen and those who have been treated with irradiation (particularly a combination of endocavity and external beam irradiation). The picture of sepsis, both clinically and using the objective data derived from Swan-Ganz catheterization, is also not a reliable way to identify ischemia or perforation, despite the knowledge that derangements of acid-base balance and central and peripheral vascular disturbance are more common in the presence of ischemia and perforation.

Perhaps one of the most useful aspects of the laparoscopic technique is the opportunity to visualize the gut early in the pathogenesis of ischemia and thus reduce the mortality and morbidity associated with delay in its treatment.

OPERATIVE FINDINGS

Until recently there seemed to be little reason to classify the most common operative findings found in patients with bowel obstruction caused by adhesions who required emergency or urgent surgery. Indeed, no formerly accepted method of classification has been published because the central clinical decision has rested on indications for or against surgery without regard to the probable findings at laparotomy. However, in the emerging era of laparoscopic-assisted gut surgery there will be those patients who can be readily treated by this new method and those in whom it would be unwise (at least with our current state of knowledge and experience) to attempt using the new technology. Ten clinical scenarios of bowel obstruction can be recognized:

1. Simple band adhesion (one or a few) without local ischemia.

This form of obstruction would appear to be the type most suitable for laparoscopically assisted treatment. Once the band can be identified with proximally dilated and distally collapsed bowel, it would be a simple matter to relieve the obstruction by band division (Fig. 23-1).

Proximal decompression of the bowel might be possible by a number of methods: nasogastric suction; direct bowel puncture obliquely through the bowel wall to aspirate intraluminal gas (the puncture site could then be closed if necessary with a single suture repair); or transoral passage of a long endoscope to travel into the upper small bowel to decompress the gut but under direct vision from the laparoscope.

It is clear that if methods can be developed to remove the intraluminal gas and fluid, then the mechanical difficulty of exploring the abdominal cavity by laparoscopy in patients who have an obstructed bowel would be largely ameliorated. Furthermore, the theoretical possibility of development of drugs that might reduce the volume of the gas and fluid accumulation in the bowel will be an interesting subject for future research.

2. Simple band adhesion (one or a few) with the addition of an ischemic segment of bowel.

If the vascular supply to the bowel immediately beneath the obstructed band (or at the site of the hernial orifice) has been compromised, then it would be wise to oversew this "band" of ischemia. This maneuver can be achieved by current technology using laparoscopic instrumentation by either the interrupted or perferably the continuous suture technique. Alternatively if a short segment of bowel is ischemic, extracorporeal local resection and anastomosis can be performed.

3. Simple band adhesion with local bowel perforation.

The likelihood of large volumes of obstructed succus entericus entering the peritoneal cavity in this circumstance strongly suggests that these patients should be operated upon immediately by "open" technique to contain the leakage and then proceed with bowel resection.

4. Multiple "light" adhesions.

These lesions are common and often occur in combination with band adhesion although sometimes they are the only cause of intestinal obstruction. Here the process of "taking down" these diffuse adhesions would be difficult laparoscopically. However, with increased expertise and the development of bowel-moving and bowel-holding instrumentation, this form of bowel obstruction might be able to be treated laparoscopically.

5. Dense adhesions.

It seems likely that multiple sites of densely adherent bowel, one to another or to the abdominal wall, would be very difficult to treat without open laparotomy. In these patients much of the procedure depends upon direct contact and feel of the anatomical structures by the surgeon's hand; therefore, a laparoscopic approach would be rather difficult.

6. Dense small bowel adhesions associated with irradiated tissue.

The pathobiologic cause of adhesions associated with irradiated tissue is local ischemia generated by endarteritis obliterans. Thus, the chances of major bowel content spillage under these conditions is high, and laparoscopic treatment would seem contraindicated in patients with bowel obstruction following irradiation therapy unless simple bypass is contemplated.

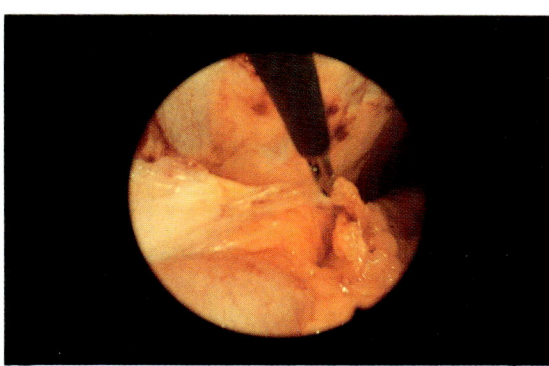

A

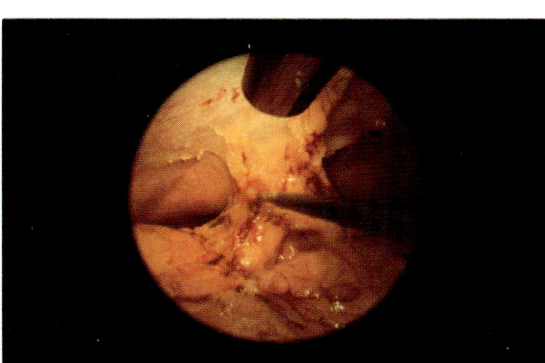

B

Figure 23-1. Laparoscopic lysis of simple adhesions, which had produced partial and uncomplicated intestinal obstruction

7. Large bowel obstruction caused by a primary cancer.

The use of the colonoscope for stricture management by tumor dilatation or laser debulking will become commonplace for the initial treatment and biopsy of patients with large bowel obstruction caused by cancer. Once decompression of the more proximal bowel can be achieved by these methods, the patient can be resuscitated and then prepared for elective surgery in the usual fashion, making it possible, once the surgeon has gained appropriate experience, to carry out an elective laparoscopically assisted colorectal resection.

8. Bowel obstruction caused by or associated with recurrent intra-abdominal cancer.

Although recurrent tumor may be present in the abdomen (e.g., liver metastases), it is not possible to determine preoperatively if the obstruction is being caused by a benign adhesive process, recurrent tumor, or a combination of these processes. A preliminary exploration by laparoscope might identify a few patients who could be managed by this method although the majority will probably require open surgery.

9. Large bowel obstruction caused by diverticulitis.

A diverticular disease phlegmon, often associated with local bowel perforation and local sepsis, could be difficult to treat without open laparotomy. However, percutaneous abscess drainage, trephine, or laparoscopically assisted loop stoma to decompress and defunction the acute diverticular disease phlegmon might represent a useful alternative to full open laparotomy. However, many of these patients have complex intra-abdominal septic foci and may have a combination of large and small bowel obstruction that will continue to require open surgery for the forseeable future.

10. Volvulus.

The ability to intubate a volvulus so that the bowel may be decompressed depends on the gentleness and persistence of the surgeon to pass the tube through the twisted gut. It may be that with a laparoscope in situ, the frequency of volvulus decompression (of either the sigmoid colon or the cecum) will increase. Once achieved, this will allow for patient resuscitation and bowel preparation so that a semielective laparoscopically assisted colon resection will become feasible. If the volvulus cannot be intubated, bowel decompression without untwisting the gut might be possible under direct vision of the distended loop by needle puncture. Once the bowel is partially decompressed, the likelihood of endoluminal endoscopic intubation will increase.

Summary

The era of laparoscopic enterolysis has started.[14] Some patients with bowel obstruction will, of course, be more easily treated by laparoscopically assisted techniques than others with simple single-band adhesion at one end of the spectrum and ischemic post-irradiation obstruction at the other. A combination of both intraluminal and laparoscopic endoscopic techniques will, no doubt, be developed to make bowel decompression possible and thus increase the likelihood of treating the primary cause by intra-abdominal laparoscopic methods.

The possibility of the development of new pharmaceutical agents to ameliorate the accumulation of proximal gas and fluid is a subject worthy of pursuing in the laboratory.

Equipment to hold, to move, and to stabilize the bowel during surgery suitable for use through 12- to 15-mm ports will gradually be developed. This will increase our ability to treat the more complex cases of bowel obstruction.

With the assumption that improvements in the equipment and the development of techniques will continue at the present pace, it is clear that many patients with bowel obstruction will undergo early intervention. The absence of an abdominal wound will allow for social and financial advantages associated with rapid rehabilitation.

Because there are inherent problems and dangers of both morbidity and mortality associated with the development and deployment of such new techniques, it seems essential to establish and maintain a registry of patients treated by these new methods. Such a registry, the purpose of which is to identify problems and allow others to benefit from the "learning curve", represents an important professional responsibility. Those interested in developing the subject need to take the time and the trouble to devise, refine, and publish their experience based on documentation of all cases so treated in this rapidly developing area of general surgery.

REFERENCES

1. Holder WD Jr. Intestinal obstruction. Gastroenterol Clin North Am 1988; 17:317–340.
2. Moynihan B. Abdominal operations. Philadelphia, WB Saunders, Vol. 2, Chap 31, 1926.

3. Wangensteen OH. Intestinal Obstruction, 3rd ed. Springfield, IL, Charles C Thomas, 1955.
4. Ellis H. Intestinal obstruction. New York, Appleton-Century-Croft, 1982.
5. Fielding LP, Welch J. Intestinal Obstruction. Edinburgh, Churchill Livingstone, 1987.
6. Welch J. Bowel obstruction. Philadelphia, WB Saunders, 1990.
7. Schwartz SI. Manifestations of gastrointestinal disease. *In* Principles of Surgery, 5th ed. New York, McGraw-Hill, 1989 p. 1061–1101.
8. Mucha P Jr. Small bowel obstruction. *In* Cameron JL, ed. Current Surgical Therapy, 3rd ed. Philadelphia, BC Decker, 1989.
9. Krebs HB, Goplerud DR. Mechanical intestinal obstruction in patients with gynecologic disease: A review of 368 patients. Am J Obstet Gynecol 1987; 157:577–583.
10. Pickleman J, Lee RM. The management of patients with suspected postoperative small bowel obstruction. Ann Surg 1989; 210:216–219.
11. Phillips RKS, Hittinger R, Fielding LP. Malignant large bowel obstruction. Br J Surg 1985; 72:296–302.
12. Basson MD, Fielding LP, Bilchik AJ, et al. Does vasoactive intestinal polypeptide mediate the pathophysiology of bowel obstruction? Am J Surg 1989; 157:109–115.
13. Crandall CW, Fielding LP. Effects of oxygen on the accumulation of gas and fluid in small bowel obstruction. Surg Res Commun 1989; 5:133–140.
14. Silva PD, Cogbill TH. Laparoscopic treatment of recurrent small bowel obstruction. Wis Med J 1991; 90:169–170.

Chapter 24
Functional Disorders of the Colon

John H. Pemberton
Andrea Ferrara

The clinical spectrum of functional disorders of the colon and rectum is ill defined. As our knowledge of the related physiopathology evolves, however, so will the understanding of the clinical entities that have a functional etiology. At the same time, the development of minimally invasive surgery will surely redefine the indications and choice of operation for these problems; our operative approach to full thickness rectal prolapse, solitary rectal ulcer, colitis cystica profunda, internal intussusception of the rectum, colonic pseudo-obstruction, and intractable constipation may be altered by minimally invasive techniques. Of no small importance is the fact that patients with functional bowel disorders have benign diseases and not life-threatening malignancies; utilization of laparoscopic surgical techniques may offer advantages in these patients without fear of incomplete or unsafe dissections.

RECTAL PROLAPSE

Definitions

Distinguishing between mucosal prolapse, internal intussusception (occult internal prolapse) and complete rectal prolapse (procidentia) is important before embarking on discussions of etiology and management.

MUCOSAL PROLAPSE

Mucosal prolapse is caused by looseness of the connective tissue between the submucosa of the rectum and anal canal and underlying muscle. With progression more anal canal mucosa and distal rectal epithelium protrude, leading to the characteristic picture of linear mucosal furrows and absence of a perianal sulcus. Mucosal prolapse is considered part of the spectrum of hemorrhoidal disease and does not progress to complete rectal prolapse. Nonsurgical treatment consists of avoiding straining and using stool-bulking agents. Surgical treatment is hemorrhoidectomy with removal of the excess prolapsed mucosa.

INTERNAL INTUSSUSCEPTION

Internal intussusception (occult rectal prolapse) is a distinct clinical entity and may represent the precursor of complete rectal prolapse. Occult rectal prolapse in which the rectum prolapses to but not through the anal canal (rectal-anal occult prolapse) is probably a precursor of complete rectal prolapse. Occult rectal prolapse that does not prolapse to the anal canal (rectorectal occult prolapse) probably does not lead to complete rectal prolapse later.

Occult rectal prolapse is only diagnosed reliably by a defecating proctogram. However, completely asymptomatic rectal intussusception on a defecating proctogram has been observed in 50 per cent of a group of healthy volunteers. It is centrally important to understand that patients having symptoms from internal intussusception (tenesmus, incomplete emptying, or rectal pain) respond poorly indeed to surgical treatment. Measures to treat symptoms including avoidance of straining, use of stool-bulking agents, and biofeedback are indicated in these patients.

COMPLETE RECTAL PROLAPSE

Complete rectal prolapse (procidentia) is caused by intussusception of the full thickness of the rectum through the anal canal.

Etiology and Diagnosis of Complete Rectal Prolapse

The etiology of complete rectal prolapse is unknown, but motor dysfunction of the pelvic floor may play an important role. Intense straining against a nonrelaxed pelvic floor may facilitate intussusception of the rectal wall. Prolonged straining could lead to stretching of the pelvic floor muscles, perineal descent, and stretching of the pudendal nerve, which over time may result in denervation of the external anal sphincter and puborectalis muscle. Then the interesting clinical picture of fecal incontinence occurring after years of constipation and straining at stool may be present. Incontinence is also aggravated by the presence of the prolapsed rectum which dilates the anal canal and causes mucus leakage.

Diagnosis of complete rectal prolapse is obvious; the rectum is prolapsed or protrudes upon straining to defecate. Characteristically concentric rings of mucosa are present, the tip of the protrusion is displaced posteriorly, a double thickness of the rectal wall is palpated, and a sulcus is present (Fig. 24-1). Colonoscopy or barium enema is indicated to rule out concomitant abnormalities. Anorectal

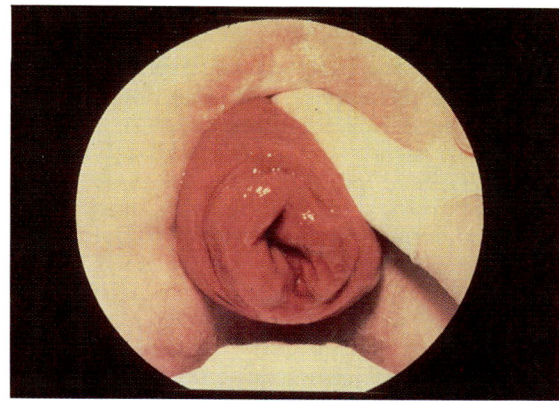

Figure 24-1. Complete rectal prolapse. Note the characteristic "concentric ring" appearance of the folds of the rectal wall. The examining index finger is placed near the junction of the skin and mucosa appreciating the sulcus between the prolapse and the perineal skin.

manometry is a useful examination; if patients cannot augment their resting anal canal pressures during a squeeze effort, incontinence may occur after repair of the prolapse, necessitating further management with biofeedback and/or sphincteroplasty.

Several anatomical features are associated with complete rectal prolapse (but are not the cause of prolapse) and are listed in Table 24-1.

Clinical Features

The true incidence of rectal prolapse in the general population is unknown. In adults, the condition occurs much more frequently in women, with incidence varying from 3 to 10 times that in men. In women, the incidence increases with age, peaking in the sixth and

Table 24-1. Anatomic Abnormalities Associated with Complete Rectal Prolapse

Abnormally deep rectosigmoid or rectovesical pouch
Lax and atonic pelvic floor musculature
Lack of normal sacral fixation of the rectum
Redundant rectosigmoid colon
Lax and atonic anal sphincter

Reproduced with permission from Levin KE, Pemberton JH. Rectal prolapse: Pathogenesis and management. In Benson JT, ed. Investigation and Management of Female Pelvic Floor Disorders. New York, Norton Medical Books, WW Norton & Company, 1993 (in press).

seventh decades, but in men the incidence does not increase after age 40.[1] In the past, multiparity was proposed as a possible etiologic factor. However, a higher incidence is actually seen in nulliparous women.[2] Several additional factors predispose to the development of rectal prolapse such as poor bowel habits, chronic constipation with long-standing laxative abuse, and prolonged straining at stool. Such straining may be the consequence of an underlying disorder of the pelvic floor which may lead to the prolapse in the first place or may be caused by the prolapse itself. Ihre and Seligson[3] reviewed 90 patients with rectal intussusception and found that 61 per cent had obstructed defecation, 33 per cent had pain on defecation, 34 per cent had bleeding, and diarrhea was present in 18 per cent.

Diseases of the nervous system, such as multiple sclerosis, tabes dorsalis, and lesions of the cauda equina may also contribute.[4] Patients in psychiatric hospitals and nursing homes are commonly afflicted. Rectal prolapse may also be a consequence of a number of anorectal surgical procedures: injury to the puborectalis muscle during anal fistulotomy or pull-through operations may predispose to either mucosal or true prolapse. Uterine prolapse is commonly found coincident with rectal prolapse.[1]

Symptoms

The most frequent primary complaint of patients with rectal prolapse is referable to the prolapse itself and 75 per cent of the patients complain of protrusion. In addition, feelings of incomplete evacuation after bowel movement and fecal incontinence are nearly always present. Constipation with straining is associated with prolapse in 50 per cent of patients.[5]

Incontinence becomes increasingly likely the longer the protrusion is present and the larger it becomes. Early on the patient may have internal intussusception and the sensation of incomplete evacuation, fullness, or obstruction in the rectum. Most patients suffer long-standing constipation and spend up to several hours per day straining to have a bowel movement. Difficulty in defecation often leads the patient to apply manual perineal pressure or to digitally remove stool to achieve evacuation.[5] Later in its course, protrusion may be present only with straining at stool or when lifting heavy objects. In time, the rectum may prolapse when the patient simply assumes an upright position or walks. Attempts by the patient to reduce the prolapse manually become increasingly difficult until finally the rectum protrudes continuously. At this time, a constant mucoid discharge, fecal incontinence, and frequent bleeding from irritation of the exposed mucosa are present.

Differential Diagnosis

A protruding complete rectal prolapse is easy to diagnose. At times, however, it may be difficult to distinguish it from mucosal prolapse or prolapsed third-degree internal hemorrhoids. Although it may appear that the entire rectal wall is protruding, the mucosal folds are arranged in a radial fashion to the level of the anal skin in patients with mucosal prolapse. With prolapsed hemorrhoids, edema and thrombosis may give the impression of complete rectal prolapse; however, radial grooves are usually present between the masses of hemorrhoidal tissue, down to the anal skin. In true rectal prolapse, concentric rings of intact mucosa are evident throughout the circumference of the protruding mass. A complete rectal prolapse protrudes for varying distances but usually 4 to 5 cm. It is rare for mucosal prolapse to protrude more than 1 to 2 cm. The protruding mass in mucosal prolapse is very thin, consisting only of a double layer of mucosa.

Rarely, a villous polyp or carcinoma of the rectum may intussuscept and protrude through the anus. Differentiation is usually easy after reduction of the prolapse and endoscopic visualization of the lesion.

Syndromes Related to Rectal Prolapse

Solitary rectal ulcer and colitis cystica profunda may be considered disorders caused by some chronic traumatic insult to the rectal mucosa.[6] These conditions are usually associated with occult or complete rectal prolapse. Intense and prolonged straining expose the rectal wall to intraluminal pressures exceeding 300 mm Hg with resulting decreased local mucosal blood flow, congestion, fibrosis, and ulceration. Currently, only if these abnormalities are associated with complete rectal prolapse is surgical treatment indicated (repair of the prolapse).

Surgical Therapy

An impressive number of surgical procedures have been designed to treat complete rectal prolapse (Table 24-2). Generally, however, there are three approaches: perineal, transabdominal and transsacral repair. The most popular abdominal operations are anterior resection and proctopexy (Ripstein). The perianal operation of choice is perineal rectosigmoidectomy (Altemeier). Anal encirclement (Thiersch) is rarely performed except in bedridden patients. The introduction of laparoscopic surgery may have a significant impact upon these several approaches for complete rectal prolapse since all of the anatomical characteristics associated with rectal prolapse (see Table 24-1) can potentially be dealt with by laparoscopic dissection and resection.

PERINEAL RECTOSIGMOIDECTOMY

Patients who are at high risk for complications from abdominal surgery are usually the best candidates for perineal rectosigmoidectomy. Few surgeons consider this procedure of choice for all patients. With the patient in the lithotomy position, the rectum is grasped and fully prolapsed. A full thickness circumferential incision is made starting 2 cm proximal to the dentate line, the cut edge of the proximal bowel is then unfolded, the mesentery is divided, and the rectum and sigmoid colon pulled to the anus. The perineum is entered, repaired, and attached to the pulled-through sigmoid anteriorly. The redundant rectum and sigmoid are resected and the cut edges anastomosed outside of the anus. The anastomosis then retracts back into the pelvis.

Although the operation is very well tolerated, there are several problems. First, it is not always easy to achieve satisfactory prolapse of the bowel with perineal traction alone. Second, the recurrence rate has been reported to be as high as 60 per cent. These problems could be addressed by utilizing the laparoscope to assist in mobilizing the rectum and sigmoid colon. When a satisfactory segment of bowel has been prolapsed, the sigmoid could be stapled to the sacrum through the laparoscope using the powered fascial stapler.[5] This combined perineal/laparoscopic approach should facilitate prolapsing the bowel completely. Moreover, recurrence might be decreased by addition of the sigmoidopexy.

Table 24-2. Operative Procedures for Complete Rectal Prolapse

1. Perineal procedures
   Anal encirclement (Thiersch)[a]
   Perineal rectopexy (Wyatt)[a]
   Mucosal sleeve resection (Delorme)
   Perineal rectosigmoidectomy (Altemeier)[a]
   Gracioplasty (Atri)

2. Transabdominal procedures
   A. Repair of pelvic floor defects
      Obliteration of the pouch of Douglas (Moschcowitz)
      Restoration of the pelvic floor (Graham)
      Abdominoperineal levator repair (Hughes)
   B. Suspension or fixation of the rectum
      Sigmoidopexy (Pemberton-Stalker)
      Presacral suture proctopexy (Cutait)[a]
      Presacral fascia lata proctopexy (Orr)[a]
      Ivalon sponge implant (Wells)[a]
      Anterior Teflon sling rectopexy (Ripstein)[a]
      Puborectalis sling rectopexy (Nigro)[a]
   C. Rectal wall stenting
      Rectal plication (Devadhar)
      Ivalon stint (Wedell)
   D. Rectosigmoid resection
      Low anterior resection (Muir)[a]
      Anterior resection with proctopexy (Frykman-Goldberg)[a]

3. Transsacral procedures
   Transsacral resection and fixation (Thomas)

Reproduced with permission from Levin KE, Pemberton JH. Rectal prolapse: Pathogenesis and management. *In* Benson JT, ed. Investigation and Management of Female Pelvic Floor Disorders. New York, Norton Medical Books, WW Norton & Company, 1993 (in press).
[a] Could be laparoscopically performed or assisted.

ANAL ENCIRCLEMENT

In selected patients anal encirclement could be performed using the usual technique,[7] but a rectopexy could be performed with the laparoscope concomitantly. Again, recurrence should be decreased.

ANTERIOR RESECTION

Anterior resection can be performed laparoscopically and details of the technique are reported in Chapter 43. The anatomical derangements associated with rectal prolapse (see Table 24-1) should make the pelvic dissection and resection of the rectosigmoid actually easier. In addition, since prolapse is a benign disease, the dissection need not be wide. Once the anterior resection has been completed, rectopexy could be added with the fascial stapler.

SLING RECTOPEXY

Similarly, sling rectopexy (Ripstein) could be performed laparoscopically. The midportion of the Marlex sling would be stapled to the presacral fascia. The limbs of the sling could then be passed around the sides of the rectum, the rectum elevated out of the pelvis, and the mesh stapled or clipped to the rectum. The major complication of this operation has always been fecal impaction and worsening of the constipation; consequently the sling should be left open anteriorly.

Current Approach

At the Mayo Clinic, the abdominal operation of choice in patients with complete rectal prolapse is anterior resection. For patients who are in poor general health and therefore have a high risk for complications during abdominal surgery, a perineal approach is advocated. In this circumstance we favor performing a perineal rectosigmoidectomy (Altemeier procedure). High anterior resection for rectal prolapse has been performed at the Mayo Clinic since 1952. After anterior and posterior rectal dissection and mobilization of the lateral ligaments, the anastomosis is performed at the level of the abdominal wall. This is accomplished by tenting the rectum firmly out of the pelvis and transecting it flush with the abdominal wall. The point of transection of the sigmoid/descending colon is likewise determined by stretching the colon out of the abdomen firmly and transecting it flush with the abdominal wall. In this way, the redundant sigmoid colon is resected. The anastomosis is then performed and at completion of the operation, the rectum will lie in the natural curve of the pelvis without tension. This type of anastomosis is a high anterior anastomosis. Postoperative fibrosis in the pelvis and at the site of the anastomosis will fix the rectum to the sacrum. In a group of 52 patients with complete rectal prolapse treated by high anterior resection, the recurrence rate was 3 per cent at 2 years, 6 per cent at 5 years, and 14 per cent at 10 years.[8] The morbidity was 19 per cent. In order to be widely accepted, laparoscopically assisted high anterior resection for rectal prolapse should improve these results significantly.

Perineal rectosigmoidectomy for rectal prolapse is particularly useful in high risk patients or in patients exhibiting strangulation. This procedure may be performed in the lithotomy or prone position. The lithotomy position is associated with fewer ventilatory problems and is generally favored. The choice of anesthesia for perineal proctosigmoidectomy is either local, spinal or general, depending on the particular clinical situation. A mechanical and antibiotic bowel preparation should always be performed except in patients requiring urgent surgery for incarceration or strangulation of the prolapsed segment.

Complications with the perineal approach are infrequent. The excellent results reported by Altemeier et al. in 1971[9] stimulated enthusiasm for this procedure. He reported a 19-year experience in a series of 106 consecutive cases with no mortality and only 3 recurrences. Although more recent series confirm the low morbidity and mortality rates, long term follow-up is either not reported at all,[10,11] or if it is, documents recurrence rates as high as 60 per cent.[5] The addition of a laparoscopic rectopexy or rectal suspension should at least match the low morbidity and significantly reduce the long term recurrence rate in order to be justifiable.

Comment

Rectal prolapse is an uncommon problem the etiology of which still remains incompletely understood. Although a number of abdominal and perineal approaches are presently used to treat rectal prolapse and several laparoscopic procedures are, in principle, appropriate, the goal common to all techniques is to achieve fixation of the rectum to the sacrum by means of postoperative fibrosis or rectopexy.

INTRACTABLE CONSTIPATION

Constipation is a complex condition with multiple causes. The manifestations vary from mild to truly incapacitating. The term "constipation" encompasses both infrequent defecation as well as difficulty with defecation. Ob-

Functional Disorders of the Colon **295**

jectively, constipation should be defined as two or fewer stools per week and/or repeated straining at stool.

In the United States, it is estimated that over 4 million people complain of frequent constipation. This corresponds to a prevalence of about 2 per cent. Constipation is by far the most common digestive complaint; it is three times more common in women than in men and markedly increases in incidence with age.[12]

While the majority of patients are treated medically with success, in some the condition is refractory to therapy. When repeated attempts to treat constipation medically fail, the surgeon should utilize advances in evaluation to define indications for successful surgery.

Patient Assessment

When a patient with incapacitating constipation is evaluated, it is critically important to identify the underlying pathophysiologic cause. We have developed an algorithm as a guide in the evaluation and treatment of constipated patients (Fig. 24-2). The goal of such testing is to classify patients into diagnostic categories. The first step is to determine if there is an extracolonic (Table 24-3) or colonic (Table 24-4) cause of constipation. The colonic causes of chronic severe constipation are further divided into colonic dysmotility and disordered defecation.

Extracolonic causes of constipation are numerous. Faulty diet and habits can cause mild or moderate constipation. Metabolic, endocrine, and pharmacologic causes are uncommon but easy to correct. Anxiety and depression may be etiologic factors and also affect the result of therapy.

Colonic Dysmotility

Slow transit constipation affects young women primarily and is an idiopathic disorder characterized by a radiographically *normal* colon with greatly prolonged transit time. The interval between bowel movements in-

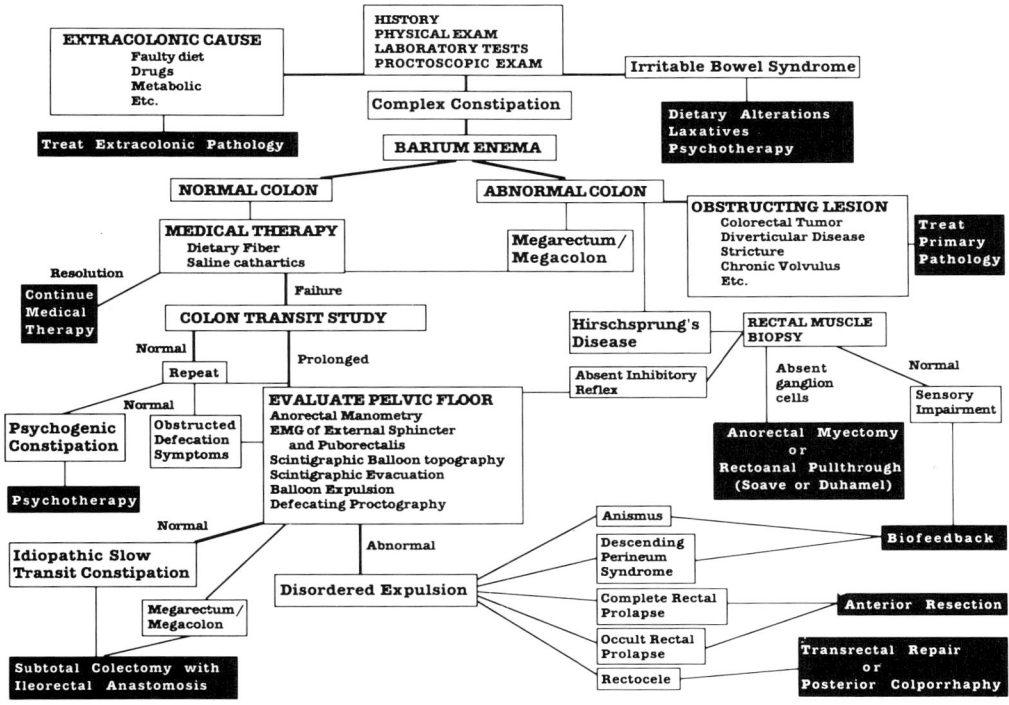

Figure 24-2. Algorithm of diagnosis and management of constipation in the adult. (Reproduced with permission from Pemberton JH, Levin KE. The surgery of intractable constipation. In Ogilvie E, ed. Current Practice in Surgery, Edinburgh, Churchill Livingstone, 1990, Vol 2, pp 117–124.)

Table 24-3. Extracolonic Causes of Chronic Constipation

Faulty diet and habits
  Inadequate bulk (fiber)
  Excessive ingestion of foods which harden stools (e.g., cheese)
  Lack of exercise
  Ignoring the call to stool

Pharmacologic
  Analgesics
  Antacids
  Anticholinergics
  Anticonvulsants
  Antidepressants
  Antiparkinsonian drugs
  Diuretics
  Ganglionic blockers
  Hypotensive agents (monoamine oxidase inhibitors)
  Iron
  Laxative abuse
  Metallic intoxication (arsenic, lead, mercury, phosphorus)
  Opiates (especially codeine)
  Psychotropic drugs (especially phenothiazines)

Metabolic and Endocrine
  Diabetes mellitus, uremia, hypothyroidism, hypercalcemia, hypokalemia, hyperparathyroidism, amyloidosis, hypopituitarism, pheochromocytoma, pregnancy, porphyria

Psychiatric
  Depression, psychoses, anorexia nervosa

Neurologic
  Iatrogenic: resection of nervi erigentes, immobilization
  Spinal: neoplasm, lumbosacral cord trauma, paraplegia, multiple sclerosis, tabes dorsalis, Shy-Drager syndrome, meningocele
  Cerebral: neoplasm, stroke, Parkinson's disease
  Peripheral: autonomic neuropathy, ganglioneuromatosis (von Recklinghausen's disease)

Reproduced with permission from Pemberton JH, Levin KE. The surgery of intractable constipation. *In* Ogilvie E, ed. Current Practice in Surgery. Edinburgh, Churchill Livingstone 1990, Vol 2, pp 117–124.

Table 24-4. Functional Causes of Chronic Severe Constipation in Adults

Colonic Dysmotility	Disordered Defecation
Slow transit	Anismus
Constipation-predominant irritable bowel syndrome	Descending perineum syndrome
	Hirschsprung's disease
	Disturbed rectal sensation
	Occult rectal prolapse
	Procidentia (complete prolapse)
	Rectocele
	Posterior rectal hernia

Reproduced with permission from Pemberton JH, Levin KE. The surgery of intractable constipation. *In* Ogilvie E, ed. Current Practice in Surgery. Edinburgh, Churchill Livingstone, 1990, Vol 2, pp 117–124.

myenteric plexus, deficient rectal sensation, and laxative abuse.

Normal transit constipation (irritable bowel syndrome) is characterized by abdominal pain, distention, and alternating periods of constipation and diarrhea. The probable etiology is enhanced colonic response to meals, stress, and luminal distention. Gut transit time tends to be normal. Treatment usually consists of a high fiber diet, stool-bulking agents, and antispasmodic agents. Psychotropic drugs are sometimes of benefit.

Disordered Defecation

ANISMUS

The major physiologic abnormality in this condition is failure of the pelvic floor muscles to relax upon straining to defecate. The clinical findings include inability to initiate defecation, incomplete evacuation, need for manual disimpaction, and laxative and enema abuse. On examination, the patient often cannot push the perineum downward and relax the puborectalis muscle. These patients may even contract the external anal sphincter and puborectalis against the examining finger while straining to defecate.

DESCENDING PERINEUM SYNDROME

Patients with this disorder strain at stool but still complain of incomplete evacuation.

creases steadily over years until it is a week or more. Most patients take laxatives in increasing amounts until they are completely unable to defecate spontaneously. Etiologic factors may include an abnormality of the

The perineum bulges upon straining, reflecting a lack of pelvic floor support. The cause of abnormal perineal descent may be related to injury to the sacral nerves innervating the levator ani muscles or to direct damage to those muscles during childbirth or chronic straining. Inability to empty leads to a constant feeling of fullness and more straining, which leads to progressive denervation of the external anal sphincter, the puborectalis muscle and, in turn, incontinence.

ADULT HIRSCHSPRUNG'S DISEASE

Aganglionosis in the adult is a rare condition, but it must be considered in any patient with intractable constipation. This is a congenital disease and almost all patients have had symptoms since birth.

OCCULT AND COMPLETE RECTAL PROLAPSE

These entities have been discussed in detail earlier in this chapter. Severe constipation may cause rectal prolapse with chronic forceful straining. However, once full prolapse has developed, patients are often incontinent.

DISTURBED RECTAL SENSATION

Sometimes patients will ignore the sensation that stool is in the rectum. If this becomes a habit, large volumes of stool accumulate that are difficult or painful to pass. This may be secondary to behavioral problems or may occur in older patients. Read et al.[13] found that 30 per cent of young women who were constipated did not have a desire to defecate and very large volumes of rectal distention were required to induce sensation.

RECTOCELE

Rectocele is a ballooning or herniation of the anterior rectal and posterior vaginal walls caused by weakness in the rectovaginal septum. When the rectocele is functionally significant, stool will preferentially fill it instead of being evacuated. Some patients need to place a finger in the vagina and push backward while straining in order to defecate, while others digitally extract stool from the rectocele. While it is clear that rectocele can cause difficult defecation, many women with rectocele have no difficulties with defecation.

Evaluation and Management

Physical examination and barium enema are the starting points of the diagnostic process (see Fig. 24-1). Colonoscopy is also satisfactory in identifying obstructing lesions of the colon (e.g., neoplasms, diverticular disease, or stricture); however it is not as helpful as is the barium enema in identifying Hirschsprung's disease or megarectum/megacolon.

Colon transit studies quantify the colon transit time of small radiopaque ingested markers.[14] If the colon transit time is prolonged (greater than 72 hours), then a diagnosis of quantifiably significant constipation has been established. The next step in the evaluation scheme is to determine whether the patient has a coexistent disorder of pelvic floor function. A series of different anorectal function tests is performed because the result of no single study is, as yet, pathognomic of pelvic floor dysfunction. Pelvic floor evaluation is also indicated when the colon transit time is within normal range, and there is a suggestion that the rectosigmoid segment is slow while the other segments are normal, or if symptoms of disordered expulsion, such as tenesmus, incomplete evacuation, fullness, and finger disimpaction are present.

PELVIC FLOOR EVALUATION

These tests have been recently developed and are evolving (see Fig. 24-1). New tests or modifications of already existing tests are continuously added to improve the understanding of the pelvic floor function. Currently we utilize: (1) anorectal manometry with three-dimensional analysis of the anal sphincters, (2) ambulatory, long term recording of anorectal motility,[15] (3) electromyography, (4) scintigraphic balloon topography,[16] (5) scintigraphic evacuation,[17] (6) balloon expulsion, and (7) defecating proctography (Fig. 24-3).

On the basis of these tests, we classify patients in the following way:

1. Abnormal colonic transit and normal pelvic floor function (slow transit constipation).

DEFECATING PROCTOGRAPHY

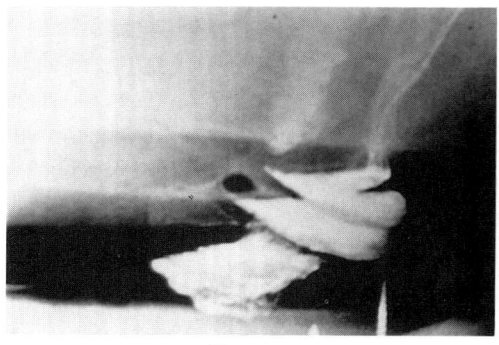
Rest

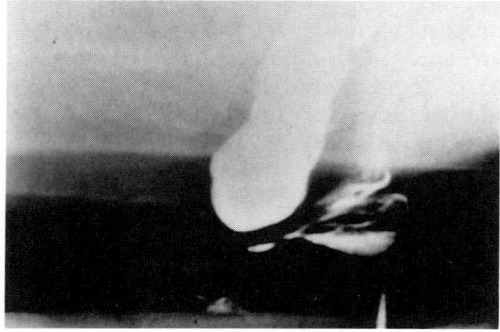
Strain

Figure 24-3. Defecating proctography. Liquid or semisolid barium is infused into the rectum and the subject defecates on a radiolucent commode during fluoroscopic monitoring and recording on videotape. This test defines the physiologic anatomy of the rectum and anal canal during defecation straining. The test is helpful in elucidating the cause of symptoms in disordered defecation, especially in determining the presence of occult rectal prolapse rectocele. Puborectalis accentuation on defecating proctography provides evidence for anismus as a contributing factor in a constipated patient. In the patient shown here, during straining there is significant posterior bulging of the rectum and ineffective expulsion.

2. Normal colonic transit, abnormal pelvic floor function (disordered defecation).
3. Abnormal colonic transit and abnormal pelvic floor dysfunction (combined disorder).
4. Normal transit constipation (irritable bowel syndrome).

ABNORMAL COLONIC TRANSIT AND NORMAL PELVIC FLOOR FUNCTION

Patients with prolonged transit time and normal pelvic floor function have a primary disorder of colonic motility termed idiopathic slow transit constipation. If symptoms are disabling and all medical treatment modalities have been exhausted, then abdominal colectomy with ileorectal anastomosis (IRA) is indicated.[18] In doing this procedure, the anastomosis is made at the level of the sacral promontory, where the rectum has good blood supply and an adequate rectal reservoir is preserved. Because the pelvic floor functions well in such patients, the operation has an excellent chance of success. Most failures in the past have probably resulted from undiagnosed pelvic floor abnormalities.

Patients requiring ileoreal anastomosis for slow transit constipation may be ideal candidates for laparoscopic colectomies. They are usually young women of normal or below average weight and may welcome the advantage of avoiding an abdominal scar. Moreover, the dissection is basically limited to the abdominal colon, and there is no need for rectal dissection or mobilization. The resected colon could be extracted transrectally, through a large percutaneous port or through a small incision. A transanally stapled ileorectal anastomosis would complete the operation. Acceptance of surgical therapy in this group of patients might be enhanced by proposing laparoscopic colectomy versus the traditional open resection.

Failure to relieve constipation following ileorectal anastomosis is usually caused by unrecognized pelvic floor dysfunction or by whole gut dysmotility (pseudo-obstruction of the small bowel). Whether or not small bowel manometry and gastric emptying studies should be administered routinely preoperatively in patients considered for colectomy is controversial. Subtotal colectomy and ileorectal anastomosis, however, are not contraindicated in some patients with whole gut pseudo-obstruction.[18]

In the few patients who develop a megarectum and impaired rectal sensation after ileorectal anastomosis, completion proctectomy with ileal pouch anal anastomosis and permanent ileostomy are surgical alternatives. Total proctocolectomy is a major abdominal procedure but laparoscopic surgery could be proposed to selected patients as experience is gathered in this technique. The transperineal access to the abdominal cavity during proctectomy would facilitate the dissection. If an ileostomy is performed, this could be done through one of the trocar ports. If an ileoanal anastomosis is indicated, an ileal pouch could be constructed, exteriorizing the terminal ileum through a small incision or through a large port and the ileoanal anastomosis could then be performed using the transanal circular stapler.

Patients with idiopathic megacolon with prolonged colon transit time and normal pelvic floor function are candidates for surgical treatment if medical modalities do not relieve the severe constipation. Since the results of localized resection have been disappointing, subtotal colectomy with ileorectal anastomosis is presently the recommended procedure also for this group of patients.

ABNORMAL COLONIC TRANSIT AND PELVIC FLOOR DYSFUNCTION

This is a combined disturbance of delayed transit and disordered expulsion. The transit delay may be secondary to the inability to empty the rectum. If no anatomical abnormalities such as rectal prolapse, rectocele, or descending perineum syndrome have been discovered, the patient probably has anismus. This usually can be confirmed by electromyography, scintigraphic balloon topography, and defecating proctography. Operations designed to treat anismus by anorectal myectomy or puborectalis division have met with mixed results.[19,20] Instead, a new approach aimed at retraining the muscles of the pelvic floor by biofeedback is becoming increasingly popular.[21] If retraining is successful, and the patient can be taught to evacuate efficiently, the colon transit study is repeated. In a few patients the transit will return to normal. In others, the colon transit will remain prolonged; in such patients colectomy and ileorectal anastomosis are indicated if symptoms are severe.

ANATOMICAL ABNORMALITIES

Rectal prolapse should be repaired (see earlier). Patients with descending perineum syndrome should be referred for pelvic floor retraining. If these patients become incontinent, operations such as sphincteroplasty and anterior and/or posterior anal repair may be indicated. Physiologically significant rectoceles should be repaired. Patients with Hirschsprung's disease should undergo a Duhamal procedure.

Current Approach

We have recently reported on 277 patients referred to the Mayo Clinic for severe symptoms of chronic intractable constipation.[18] The algorithm previously described was used to identify patients suitable for surgery. Patients underwent colon transit studies, anorectal manometry, measurement of anorectal angle movements, efficiency of evacuation, balloon expulsion studies, electromyography of the pelvic floor, and defecating proctograms. Based on these studies, patients were categorized into four different groups: slow transit constipation (STC), 29 patients; pelvic floor dysfunction (PFD), 37 patients; combined SCT and PFD, 14 patients; and normal transit constipation, 197 patients (71 per cent). Patients with STC underwent abdominal colectomy and ileorectal anastomosis. Patients with PFD underwent pelvic floor retraining (biofeedback) only, while patients with PFD and STC underwent pelvic floor retraining followed by abdominal colectomy. Patients with normal transit constipation were treated medically. Thirty-eight patients (STC and STC and PDF) were operated on without mortality. Prolonged ileus developed in 13 per cent and small bowel obstruction in 11 per cent of the patients. With a mean follow-up of 20 months after ileorectostomy, no patient was constipated, none required laxatives, and none was incontinent.

To achieve predictable success in managing constipated patients then, it is important that underlying pathophysiologic processes are identified objectively; in this way patients for whom aggressive surgical or medical intervention is suitable can be identified. Tests of colonic and pelvic floor function distinguished severely constipated patients with slow transit who are candidates for operation from those with pelvic floor dysfunction and normal transit constipation who are not. Patients with slow transit constipation may represent the ideal candidates for laparoscopic colectomy.

REFERENCES

1. Kupfer CA, Goligher CA. One hundred consecutive cases of complete rectal prolapse of the rectum treated by operation. Br J Surg 1970; 57:481–487.

2. Goligher J. Surgery of the anus, rectum and colon. London, Baillière-Tindall, 1984, pp 246–284.
3. Ihre T, Seligson U. Intussusception of the rectum-internal procidentia: Treatment and results in 90 patients. Dis Colon Rectum 1975; 18:391–396.
4. Schoetz DJ, Veidenheimer MC. Rectal prolapse: Pathogenesis and clinical features. In Henry MM, Swash M, eds. Coloproctology and the Pelvic Floor: Pathophysiology and Management. London, Butterworths, 1985, pp 303–339.
5. Corman ML. Rectal prolapse. In Corman ML, ed. Colon and Rectal Surgery. Philadelphia, JB Lippincott Co, 1989, pp 209–247.
6. Nelson H, Pemberton JH. Solitary rectal ulcer. In Fazio VW, ed. Current Therapy in Colon and Rectal Surgery. Toronto, BC Decker, Inc, 1990, pp 98–102.
7. Dietzen CD, Pemberton JH. Perineal approaches for the treatment of complete rectal prolapse. Neth J Surg 1989; 41:140–144.
8. Schlinkert RT, Beart RW Jr, Wolff BG, Pemberton JH. Anterior resection for complete rectal prolapse. Dis Colon Rectum 1985; 28:409–412.
9. Altemeier WA, Culbertson WR, Schwengerdt C, Hunt J. Nineteen years experience with the one-stage repair of rectal prolapse. Ann Surg 1971; 173:993–1006.
10. Wassef R, Rothenberg DA, Goldberg SM. Rectal prolapse. Curr Probl Surg 1986; 23:402–451.
11. Prasad ML, Pearl RK, Abcarian H, et al. Perineal proctectomy, posterior rectopexy and postanal levator repair for the treatment of rectal prolapse. Dis Colon Rectum 1986; 29:547–552.
12. Sonnenberg A, Koch TR. Epidemiology of constipation in the United States. Dis Colon Rectum 1989; 32:1–8.
13. Read NW, Timms JM, Barfield LJ, et al. Impairment of defecation in young women with severe constipation. Gastroenterology 1986; 90:53–60.
14. Metcalf AM, Phillips SF, Zinsmeister AR, et al. Simplified assessment of segmental colon transit. Gastroenterology 1987; 92:40–47.
15. Ferrara A, Pemberton JH, Hanson RB. Coordination between ileal pouch and anal canal motor activity preserves continence after ileoanal anastomosis. Am J Surg. In press.
16. Barkel DC, Pemberton JH, Pezim ME, et al. Scintigraphic assessment of the anorectal angle in health and after ileal pouch-anal anastomosis. Ann Surg 1988; 208:42–49.
17. Pemberton JH, Phillips SF. Constipation and diarrhea. In Moody FG, ed. Surgical Treatment of Digestive Disease. Chicago, Year Book Medical Publishers, 1990, pp 39–52.
18. Pemberton JH, Rath DM, Ilstrup DM. Evaluation and surgical treatment of severe chronic constipation. Ann Surg 1991; 214:403–413.
19. Barnes PRH, Hawley PR, Lennard-Jones JE. Experience of posterior division of the puborectalis muscle in the management of severe constipation. Br J Surg 1985; 72:475–477.
20. Kamm MA, Hawley PR, Lennard-Jones JE. Lateral division of the puborectalis muscle in the management of severe constipation. Br J Surg 1988; 75:661–663.
21. Bleijenberg G, Kuijpers HC. Treatment of the spastic pelvic floor syndrome with biofeedback. Dis Colon Rectum 1987; 30:108–111.

Chapter 25
Volvulus of the Colon

David N. Armstrong
Garth H. Ballantyne

Volvulus is defined as an abnormal twisting of a segment of bowel on itself, along its longitudinal axis. This results in occlusion of the proximal bowel and a closed loop obstruction within the segment. Compromised blood supply to the involved segment, together with the increase in intraluminal pressure, leads to gangrene and perforation if unrelieved.

Worldwide, the incidence of volvulus of the large bowel varies widely, according to the population studied. In an advanced Western population, large bowel volvulus accounts for 1 to 5 per cent of all large bowel obstructions. In these populations, the most common site of large bowel torsion is the sigmoid colon (80 per cent), followed by cecum (15 per cent), transverse colon (3 per cent), and splenic flexure (2 per cent). The condition is common in regions of Africa, Southern Asia, and South America. In the "volvulus belt" of Africa and the Middle East, 50 per cent of large bowel obstructions result from volvulus, almost exclusively of the sigmoid colon. In Northern Iran sigmoid volvulus accounts for 85 per cent of large bowel obstructions.

In the vast majority of patients, sigmoid volvulus is an acquired condition, resulting from elongation of the sigmoid loop and stretching of the sigmoid mesocolon. This is in contrast to cecal volvulus, which results most commonly from failure of retroperitoneal fixation of the cecum.

SIGMOID VOLVULUS

Etiology

In the West, sigmoid volvulus occurs from sigmoid elongation, resulting in a redundant loop. Most commonly it results from long term neurologic or psychiatric disease. Associations with Parkinson's disease, multiple sclerosis, and spinal cord injuries are well known. Psychotropic drugs or sedatives interfere with colonic motility and are etiologically implicated in the high incidence of volvulus seen in psychiatric institutes. The high incidence in nursing homes and mental institutions led Ronka et al. to describe the condition as the "Bedford syndrome," after the Veterans Administration institute that had a high proportion of psychiatric patients who developed sigmoid volvulus.

A second major etiologic factor is the excessive use of laxatives, cathartic agents, and enemas. This may merely represent another manifestation of the chronic constipation and prolonged recumbency seen in long term care facilities. In developing countries, a high fiber diet results in overloading of the sigmoid colon, which twists around its mesentery, resulting in volvulus.

Rarer conditions predisposing to volvulus include Chagas' disease and Hirschsprung's disease, both of which result in destruction of the myenteric plexus and culminate in megacolon. A pelvic mass may displace the sigmoid colon sufficiently to cause it to twist. This explains the association of sigmoid volvulus with pregnancy and massive ovarian tumors.

Rarely, an elongated mesocolon may provide excess mobility to the sigmoid colon. This may be a result of abnormal congenital fixation. An interesting association between volvulus of the stomach, splenic flexure of colon, and sigmoid colon has been described. The latter association is referred to as a "traveling volvulus." This association probably reflects an uncommon elongation of the mesenteric fixation of intraperitoneal organs.

Classically, sigmoid volvulus occurs in a clockwise direction, although the authors are not aware of any reported experience describing the ratio of clockwise to a counterclockwise volvulus. In contrast, and with the same provisos, cecal volvulus occurs in anticlockwise direction.

Volvulus of the sigmoid colon occurs in the face of three conditions: (1) elongation of the sigmoid colon; (2) narrowing of the base of the sigmoid mesocolon; and (3) a torque force to the sigmoid colon, which initiates the torsion process.

The base of the sigmoid mesocolon becomes foreshortened as a result of repeated episodes of torsion. Many of these episodes are subacute and self-limiting, and the patients never seek medical attention. More than 50 per cent of patients seen with volvulus give a history of previous episodes. As a result of foreshortening of the mesocolon, the narrow base acts as a fulcrum, about which the sigmoid colon may twist. In addition, adhesive bands develop between the two limbs of the sigmoid, creating a paddle-like configuration. This chronic "mesosigmoiditis" is visible in the root of the sigmoid mesentery in most patients in whom a sigmoid volvulus occurs (Fig. 25-1).

Chronic constipation in Western cultures results in an overloaded sigmoid loop, whose weight provides the momentum to initiate volvulus. In African and Middle Eastern societies, a high fiber diet results in a bulky sigmoid colon, which provides the necessary impetus. A shift in the relative positions of the intra-abdominal organs, as seen in pregnancy or in the presence of large pelvic tumors, may precipitate an episode of sigmoid volvulus.

Sigmoid volvulus has a definite age and sex predilection. In a review by Ballantyne, sigmoid volvulus was more common in men (63.7 per cent of 571 patients), the lower incidence in women being attributed to a wider pelvis. In Western cultures, volvulus is a disease of the sixth decade, but it occurs 15 to

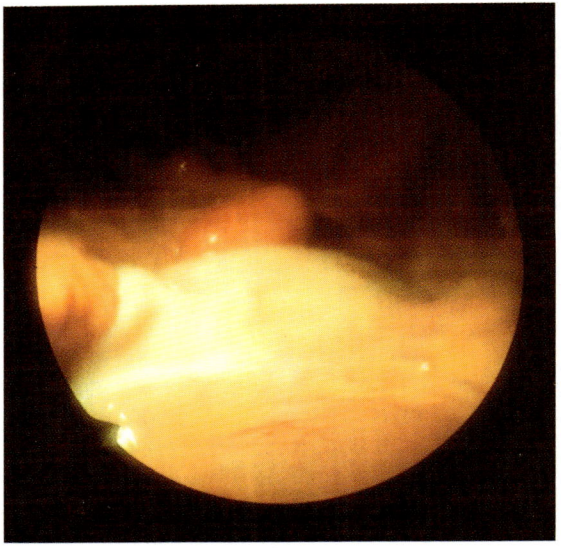
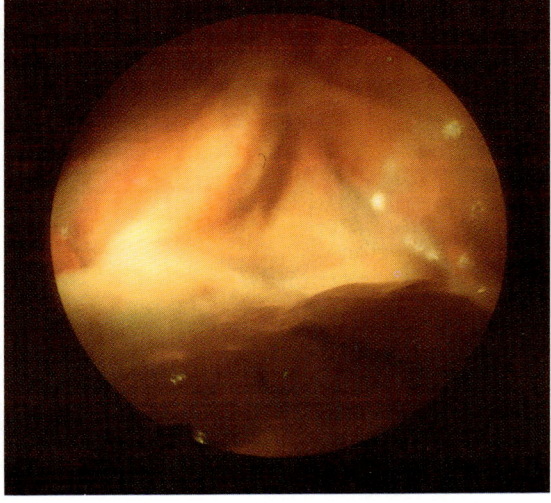

A
B

Figure 25-1. A, Dense scarring of the root of the sigmoid mesentery caused by chronic mesosigmoiditis. The fibrosis extends down toward the common iliac vessels. B, A closer view of the confluent scarring at the base of the sigmoid mesentery.

20 years earlier in developing nations. A racial trend was also noted, with 67 per cent of patients being black and 33 per cent white.

Diagnosis

The patient with volvulus is often debilitated and bedridden. Because of the frequent association with neurologic or psychiatric impairment, a reliable history is often not available. The patient or his or her attendant may give a history of previous episodes of abdominal pain and distention, with the inability to pass flatus. An unknown proportion of these episodes of volvulus are self-limiting. With each episode of volvulus, the base of the mesocolon becomes increasingly narrow and therefore predisposed to recurrent bouts. Abdominal distention is frequently massive and characteristically tympanitic over the gas-filled, thin-walled sigmoid loop. Overlying tenderness or peritonism raises the concern of ischemic or perforated bowel. Depending on the extent of ischemia or leakage, systemic toxicity may be apparent.

Diagnosis of sigmoid volvulus is usually obvious from a plain abdominal radiograph, which shows the characteristic "omega" or "inverted loop" sign. In doubtful cases a limited Gastrografin enema will reveal the characteristic "beaked" appearance of the apex of the volvulus in the distal sigmoid.

Treatment—Resuscitation

The first priority is resuscitation of the patient. This should be performed in a well staffed facility, which is equipped for radiography, invasive monitoring, and rigid sigmoidoscopy. Vomiting and third space fluid loss into the sigmoid colon results in hypovolemic shock, which must be corrected with intravenous balanced salt solutions such as Ringer's lactate solution. Fluid resuscitation should be initiated before any attempts are made to reduce the volvulus. In the event of inadvertent perforation, the patient will be more adequately perfused, and any further delay to optimize the patient's general condition before surgery will be minimized.

Hypovolemic shock may be compounded by sepsis in the presence of ischemic bowel. For the same reasons given previously, broad spectrum antibiotics (aerobic and anaerobic) should be given to preempt a sigmoidoscopic perforation. The patient is laid in the left lateral position to improve venous return, which may be compromised as a result of massive abdominal distention. Oxygen is given, since splinting of the diaphragm impedes respiratory efforts and results in "shunting" of blood through the pulmonary circulation. A Foley catheter is inserted to assess fluid balance and a nasogastric tube should be placed if vomiting is a prominent symptom or the radiograph reveals significant small bowel obstruction.

Rationale for Definitive Treatment

The treatment of sigmoid volvulus has evolved over the past decades from immediate surgical correction, which carries a high mortality, to immediate sigmoidoscopic reduction and elective surgery with its attendant lower mortality. Even from the time of Hippocrates, reduction of the volvulus was attempted using a long suppository—"10 digits long"—inserted into the rectum. This mode of deflating the volvulus was suggested again in 1859 by Gay in England, but did not gain widespread acceptance until the middle of the next century. In the latter part of the twentieth century, percutaneous deflation of the loop using trochars was described by Crisp, who performed his studies on cadavers. Open reduction of the volvulus at laparotomy was first described by Atherton in 1883, although recurrence rates were high (Table 25-1), and fixation or resection of the sigmoid was attempted. Emergency resection carried a mortality rate of well over 50 per cent (Table 25-2), and a high rate of recurrence was found with sigmoidopexy (Table 25-3). The failure of sigmoidopexy was illustrated during reexploration of the abdomen for recurrent volvulus, which often revealed little evidence of the attempted fixation. In 1947 Bruusgaard revived the technique of transanal deflation using sigmoidoscopy. By providing the means of averting the high mortality incurred by urgent laparotomy, it was with relief that sigmoidoscopic decompression gained widespread acceptance (Table 25-4). More recently the use of the flexible sigmoidoscope or colonoscope provides a further weapon in the armamentarium of the surgeon attempting nonoperative reduction of the sigmoid loop.

After successful endoscopic deflation, the question of whether or not subsequent surgery is required arises. Simple deflation, without operative fixation or resection, is followed by subsequent episodes of volvulus in

Table 25-1. Operative Derotation of Sigmoid Volvulus

Authors	Year	Recurrence (%)	Mortality (%)
Shepherd	1968	40	16
Taha	1980	13	
Ballantyne	1982	18	16
Pahlman	1986	44	
Mangiante	1988		10
Peoples	1990		17

Table 25-2. Emergency Resection of Sigmoid Colon for Volvulus

Authors	Year	Type of Resection	Mortality (%)
Gabriel	1953		86
Farringer	1955		67
Wuepper	1966		58
Shepherd	1968	Primary anastomosis	50
		Hartmann's	12
		Paul Mikulicz	45
Ball	1981		100
Ballantyne	1982	Primary anastomosis	25
		Hartmann's	50
		Paul Mikulicz	36
Pasch	1985		57

Table 25-3. Decompression and Sigmoidopexy of the Sigmoid Colon for Volvulus

Author	Year	Recurrence (%)	Mortality (%)
Shepherd	1968	38	8

Table 25-4. Sigmoidoscopic Decompression of Sigmoid Volvulus

Authors	Year	Recurrence (%)	Mortality (%)
Drapanas	1961	60	
Hines	1967	90	
Shepherd	1968	40	0
Knight	1980	43	21
Bak	1986	70	22
Pahlman	1989	70	21

over half of the patients, with attendant complications and mortality. Elective resection, during the same hospital stay is advocated by Bak, who cites a 6 per cent operative mortality, compared to a mortality of 30 per cent from recurrent episodes of volvulus (Table 25-5).

These statistics are disputed by Arnold et al., who cite an operative mortality of 15 per cent from resection after the first episode, yet a lower mortality (9 per cent) from recurrent episodes of volvulus requiring surgery. The authors further stratified their patients according to age (younger than 70 and older than 70 years of age) and found, not surprisingly, that two-thirds of the deaths occurred in the older population. They concluded that resection should be performed after the first episode only in patients younger than 70 years of age, and in patients older than 70, resection should be deferred until the second or subsequent episode. The lower operative mortality for recurrent episodes was attributed to an increase in the blood supply as a result of recurrent episodes of volvulus.

The experience of Arnold et al. can be interpreted another way. The elderly (older than 70 years), debilitated patient may not live long enough for another episode of volvulus to develop, and this subgroup thus is removed from the equation. Yet the less debilitated septuagenarians may survive long enough to experience one or many further episodes. If resection is performed only in this healthier subgroup, the operative mortality will naturally be lower. Candidates for elective resection should therefore be selected not only on basis of age greater or less than 70 years, but on the usual cardiorespiratory and metabolic criteria that determine fitness for surgery. It is unlikely that patients older than age 70 who are in reasonable health will benefit from recurrent episodes of volvulus, not to mention the humanitarian and financial burden placed on them from repeated admissions to the hospital. In addition, it is difficult to define a "first" episode of volvulus, since many patients (approximately 50 per cent) give a history of similar, self-resolving episodes in the past. Finally, as demonstrated by the Mayo Clinic, an operative mortality at or near 0 per cent can be achieved with even elderly patients when they undergo elective sigmoid resection after nonoperative decompression. Thus, most patients regardless of age should undergo elective sigmoid resection during the same hospitalization after nonoperative resection of the volvulus.

In the past 2 years, another historic treatment for sigmoid volvulus has gained popularity, with the renewed use of percutaneous deflation of the sigmoid loop described by Salim. He reported a 100 per cent success rate using percutaneous deflation of the sigmoid loop, followed by perianal intubation and elective band sigmoidopexy. This regimen had 0 per cent mortality and 5 per cent morbidity, compared with 13 per cent morbidity and 13 per cent mortality with conventional sigmoidoscopic reduction and elective sigmoid resection.

The recent explosion of laparoscopic surgery provides another dimension to the evolving treatment of sigmoid volvulus. Although laparoscopic intervention in its current mode will not play a role in reduction of the acute volvulus, its use in elective resection of the redundant sigmoid loop may be facilitated by anatomic considerations. The base of the mesocolon is foreshortened and contracted, facilitating its mobilization and division. The mobile nature of the sigmoid loop itself may also facilitate its mobilization and reduce the risk of damage to adjacent structures. Lastly, the close apposition of the proximal rectum and distal left colon (as a result of the short-

Table 25-5. Reduction and Elective Resection of the Sigmoid Colon for Volvulus

Authors	Year	Recurrence (%)	Mortality (%)
Arnold	1972	0	15
Ball	1981	0	25
Pasch	1985	0	20
Mangiante	1988	0	5
Peoples	1990	0	13
Salim	1991	0	13

ened mesosigmoid) may facilitate the performance of a stapled end-to-end anastomosis.

Sigmoidoscopic Reduction

With the patient in the left lateral position, a rigid sigmoidoscope is advanced into the rectum under direct vision, with adequate illumination. Air is insufflated into the rectum at frequent intervals. This assists in identifying the apex of the volvulus and, by expanding the rectal ampulla, helps prevent inadvertent perforation. Occasionally the air pressure itself may reduce the twist. The apex of the volvulus is identified by a spiraling of the rectal mucosa, which is often edematous. The tip of a well-lubricated no. 32 rubber rectal tube is pushed *gently* into the apex of the spiral and advanced into the obstructed segment. If initial attempts are unsuccessful, use a larger, not smaller, diameter tube and apply constant pressure at the apex. Try moving the patient into alternate positions, such as the knee-elbow position, if the patient's condition permits. This allows the colon to fall away and opens up the angle of the volvulus. Do not be tempted to push a narrow, rigid probe into the apex, as this will perforate the already compromised bowel wall. If visibility is poor, place the end of the sigmoidoscope directly on the apex and, without moving the sigmoidoscope, slide the tube up the scope and the tip will then lie at the apex. Never use undue force and never probe blindly. There will be no doubt when decompression has been achieved. A polythene-lined bucket should be on hand to avoid unnecessary spillage from the sudden, forceful rush of gas and liquid stool.

Surgery for Sigmoid Volvulus

The timing and nature of surgery for sigmoid volvulus are determined by two main factors: first, the suspected presence of ischemic or necrotic bowel; and second, the success or failure of sigmoidoscopic reduction.

SUSPECTED ISCHEMIC OR NECROTIC BOWEL

The suspicion of ischemic or necrotic bowel mandates laparotomy and resection of the compromised segment. This will usually take the form of a Hartmann's resection, since the distal margin at the rectosigmoid junction is often too short to permit its mobilization onto the anterior abdominal wall as a mucous fistula.

SUCCESSFUL SIGMOIDOSCOPIC REDUCTION

Sigmoidoscopic decompression is successful in more than 90 per cent of patients. Decompression should be confirmed radiologically and the rectal tube taped securely to the buttocks. Retorsion occurs in up to 50 per cent of patients who do not undergo surgery, and elective surgery should be performed during the same admission. In the interim, the patient's condition can be further stabilized and assessed for surgery. A mechanical bowel preparation is given and broad spectrum antibiotics are administered, irrespective of the planned procedure. This allows for a change in tactics (sigmoid resection, instead of planned sigmoidopexy) if the need arises.

LAPAROTOMY FOR SIGMOID VOLVULUS

The patient is placed in Lloyd-Davis stirrups. The marginal loss of elbow room for the surgeon and his or her assistants is more than made up for by the ability to pass an end-to-end anastomosis stapling device per anum, if an unexpectedly low anastomosis is necessary. Both abdomen and perineum are prepared separately in the standard fashion. The perineum remains draped until it becomes necessary to pass the stapling device. A low midline incision is mandatory to provide necessary exposure and reduction of an often enormously dilated sigmoid loop. The first priority is to reduce the volvulus. The sigmoid colon generally twists in a counterclockwise direction.

If the colon is clearly viable, the surgical options are sigmoidopexy or resection. If the colon appears ischemic, apply warm packs and wait for a timed 5 minutes. In the presence of frank gangrene or nonviable bowel, resection is mandatory. Several options are available: (1) Paul-Mikulicz exteriorization and resection, (2) Hartmann's procedure, or (3) resection and primary anastomosis.

COLOPEXY

Several techniques of colopexy have been described. The simplest involves suturing the sigmoid colon to the lateral abdominal wall using interrupted sutures. More elaborate methods include enclosing the sigmoid in a lateral retroperitoneal "pouch," plicating the mesentery (mesenteropexy), Gortex banding of the sigmoid colon to the abdominal wall, and sigmoid colostomy. All these techniques have recurrence rates similar to those in patients who do not undergo surgery and are often more time consuming than a simple resection.

RESECTION: SIGMOID COLECTOMY

This is the simplest approach and has the lowest rates of recurrence of volvulus.

HOW MUCH TO RESECT?

As a result of foreshortening of the mesentery, the peritoneal reflection of the rectum and the descending colon are brought into close proximity. Recurrence rates are lowest after simple resection of the omega loop of the sigmoid, and more extensive resections are unnecessary. The inferior mesenteric artery is divided at its most accessible location, since this is a benign disease process. The remaining blood supply is divided up to the edge of the colon, so as not to compromise viability of the suture line. The sites of transection are chosen to allow a well perfused, tension-free anastomosis.

FAILED SIGMOIDOSCOPIC REDUCTION OR SUSPECTED ISCHEMIC BOWEL: PAUL-MIKULICZ RESECTION

This involves exteriorization of the nonviable segment through a lateral oblique incision. The sigmoid loop is amputated distal to crushing clamps. A double-barreled colostomy is fashioned using interrupted sutures which encompass all layers of the bowel wall and subdermal layer of the skin. A few interrupted sutures are placed between the two adjacent limbs of the colostomy. This is largely of historic interest, as the distal stoma is usually too short to allow exteriorization.

HARTMANN'S PROCEDURE

Exteriorization of the proximal colon and closure of the rectal pouch may be necessary if the viability of the bowel beyond the limits of resection is in doubt. Prior perforation of the sigmoid and significant peritoneal soiling would also make this the procedure of choice. A primary anastomosis in this setting carries a high incidence of anastomotic leak.

RESECTION AND PRIMARY ANASTOMOSIS

In selected patients this has resulted in a satisfactory outcome with low leak rates. Absence of peritoneal soiling and viable bowel ends are prerequisites.

LAPAROSCOPIC SURGERY FOR SIGMOID VOLVULUS

The role of laparoscopic surgery for sigmoid volvulus is not yet defined. Since the abdomen is often already massively distended during the acute stages of the volvulus, laparoscopic procedures are impractical. After successful sigmoidoscopic decompression, stabilization of the patient, and an adequate bowel preparation, laparoscopy may have a role in elective resection of the sigmoid colon. Two factors make this procedure an attractive adjunct to the surgical armamentarium. First, the patients are generally elderly and debilitated and would potentially benefit to a large degree from minimally invasive surgery. Second, the long sigmoid mesocolon seen in sigmoid volvulus lends itself to easy laparoscopic mobilization of the redundant omega loop. Furthermore, the base of the mesocolon is foreshortened, so the proximal and distal ends of the colon are easily brought together, facilitating a stapled primary anastomosis. Two techniques can be used for elective laparoscopically assisted sigmoid resection in patients in whom the volvulus has been nonoperatively reduced.

LAPAROSCOPICALLY ASSISTED SIGMOID RESECTION WITH A SIDE-TO-SIDE FUNCTIONAL END-TO-END ANASTOMOSIS

In patients that have severe scarring of the root of the sigmoid mesentery from chronic mesosigmoiditis, intracorporeal division of the

308　Surgery of the Lower Gastrointestinal Tract

sigmoid vessels is difficult. In addition, the long redundant sigmoid colon makes exposure of these vessels problematic. In these patients, a modification of the Paul Mikulicz resection is easily accomplished.

The patient undergoes a standard mechanical and antibiotic bowel preparation. In the operating room, the patient is placed in a supine position with legs supported by Lloyd-Davies stirrups. The lower legs are wrapped with pneumatic compression boots. After induction of general endotracheal anesthesia, a nasogastric tube and urinary catheter are inserted. The abdomen is prepared and draped in a sterile fashion. The patient is dropped into a deep Trendelenburg position. A carbon dioxide pneumoperitoneum is established with a Veress needle inserted in a supraumbilical position. The Veress needle is replaced with a 10-mm trocar. The abdomen is inspected with the 10-mm 0-degree laparoscope. Four additional 10-mm trocars are inserted: two in the right lower quadrant and two in the left lower quadrant (Fig. 25-2).

The small bowel is pulled out of the pelvis with grasping instruments. The deep Trendelenburg position causes the small bowel to roll up toward the diaphragm. From the right side of the patient, the assistant surgeon in-

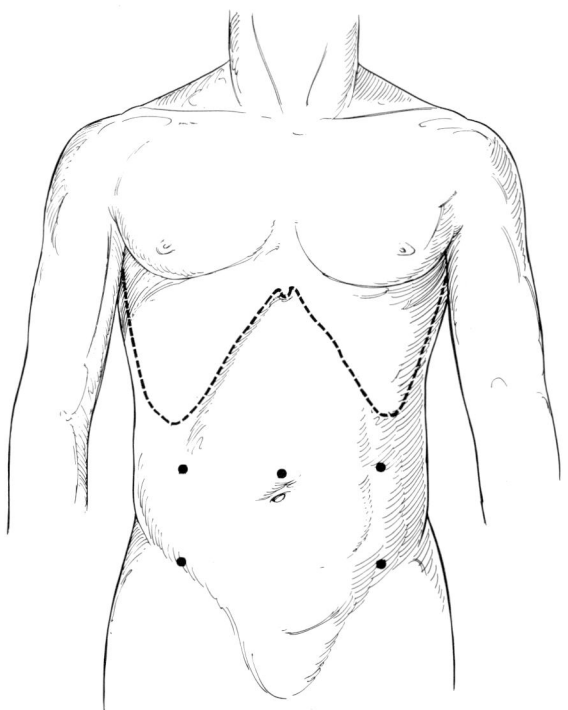

Figure 25-2. Sites of trocar placement for a laparoscopically assisted sigmoid resection.

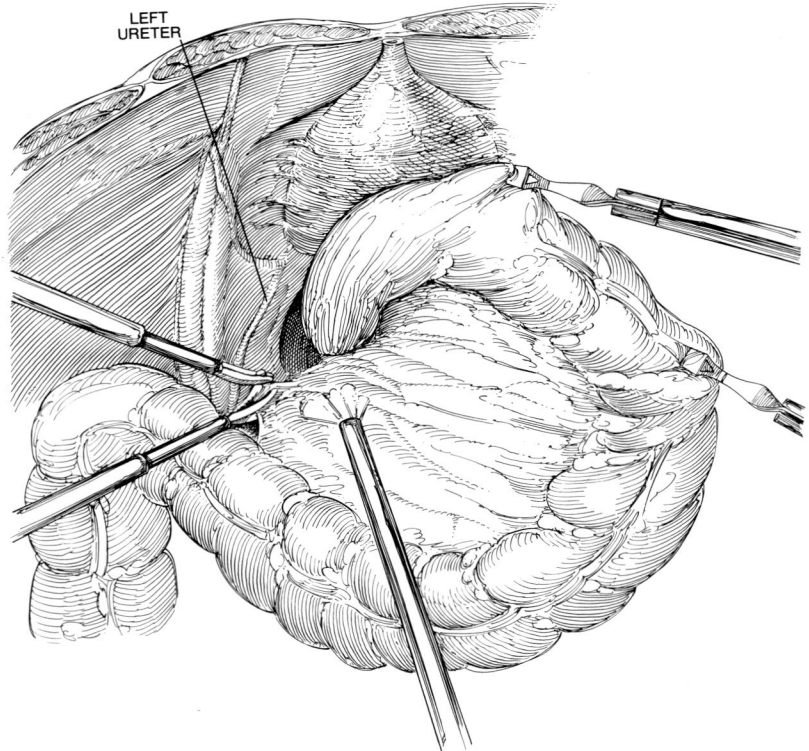

Figure 25-3. Exposure of the retroperitoneum lateral to the sigmoid. Two Endo Babcock clamps retract the rectosigmoid and distal sigmoid colon medially and anteriorly.

serts two ENDO BABCOCK* clamps (United States Surgical Corporation, Norwalk, CT) and grasps the distal sigmoid colon and proximal rectum, retracting them medially and anteriorly. This exposes the left iliac vessels and the root of the sigmoid mesentery (Fig. 25-3). If the adhesions are scant or moderate in density, the rectum and distal sigmoid mesentery are divided intracorporeally and an end-to-end anastomosis is constructed (in the following discussion). If the mesosigmoiditis is severe, the resection is accomplished extracorporeally.

In patients with dense adhesions, the rectosigmoid and descending colon are mobilized. The surgeon, on the left side of the patient, uses ENDO SHEARS* (United States Surgical Corporation) and a grasping instrument to incise the retroperitoneum (Fig. 25-4). The left ureter is exposed. The retroperitoneal incision is extended down the left side of the pelvis and then up the left gutter. The rectum, sigmoid, and descending colon are bluntly swept medially using the shafts of the ENDO SHEARS*. The rectum and descending colon are mobilized enough that they can be pulled up to the abdominal wall for construction of an extracorporeal anastomosis.

The surgeon and assistant surgeon trade sides. The retroperitoneum of the sacral promontory is incised with electrocautery scissors, giving the rectosigmoid additional mobility. Dissection is continued until the

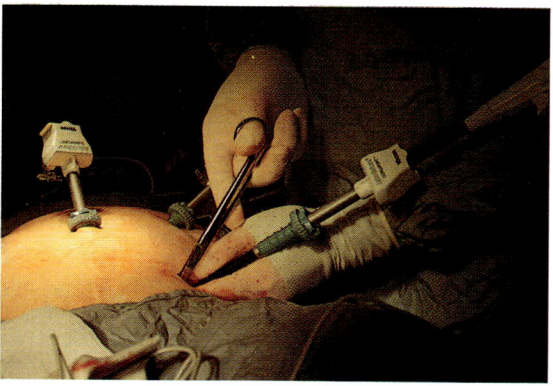

Figure 25-5. Withdrawal of the sigmoid colon through a left lower quadrant trocar site using an Endo Babcock clamp. The trocar is pulled out of the abdominal wall over the shaft of the Endo Babcock clamp.

rectosigmoid can be elevated easily up to the planned site of incision in the left lower quadrant.

An ENDO BABCOCK* clamp is inserted through the caudad trocar in the left lower quadrant and used to grasp the apex of the sigmoid loop. The trocar is pulled out of the abdominal wall over the shaft of the ENDO BABCOCK* clamp (Fig. 25-5). A transverse incision about 1.5 inches in length is made through the trocar site. The apex of the sigmoid colon and then the entire sigmoid loop are pulled through the incision (Fig. 25-6).

Two enterotomies are made in the antimesenteric sides of the proximal rectum and distal descending colon. A GIA* 60 stapling device (United States Surgical Corporation) is inserted through the enterotomies and used to construct a side-to-side, functional end-to-end anastomosis (Fig. 25-7). The staple line is inspected for hemorrhage. The edges of the enterotomy are apposed with Allis clamps and closed with a TA* 90 stapling device (United States Surgical Corporation) (Fig. 25-8). The sigmoid mesentery is included within the staple line. Thus, firing the stapling device both closes the enterotomy and ligates the sigmoid mesentery. Care is taken not to injure the inferior mesenteric vessels. This will ensure an excellent blood supply for the colorectal anastomosis. The sigmoid colon and sigmoid mesentery are resected and handed off the field. The specimen is opened within the operating room by a surgical pathologist.

The anastomosis is dropped back into the abdomen. The abdomen is liberally irrigated

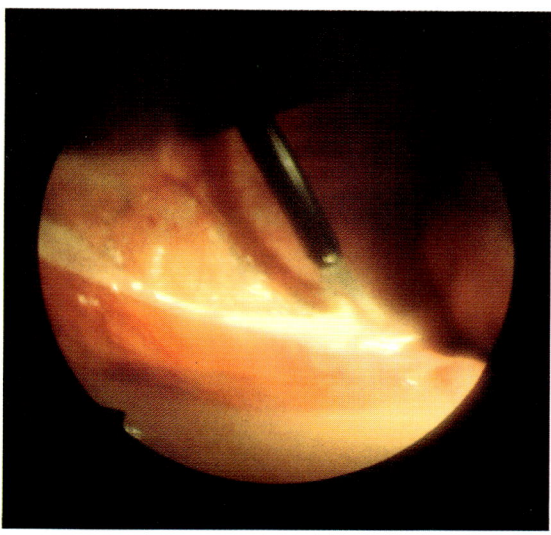

Figure 25-4. Incision of the retroperitoneum over the common iliac vessels in preparation for the identification of the left ureter.

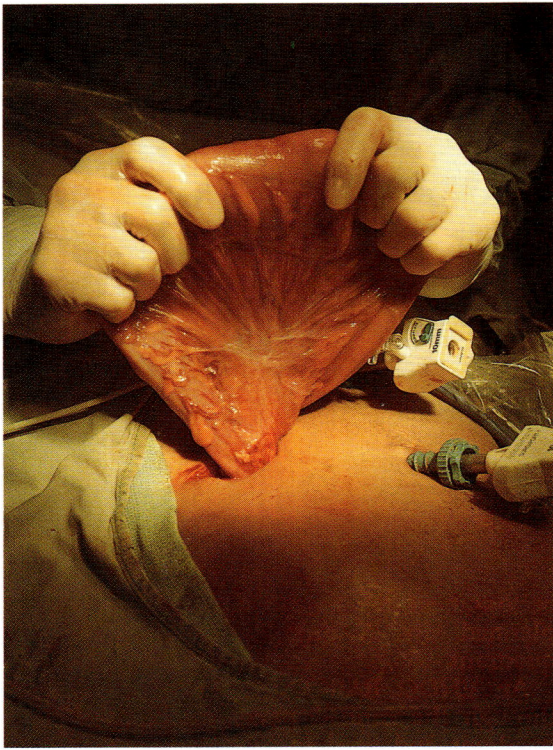

Figure 25-6. The exteriorized sigmoid colon. Chronic mesosigmoiditis caused scarring of the sigmoid mesentery in this patient who developed a sigmoid volvulus.

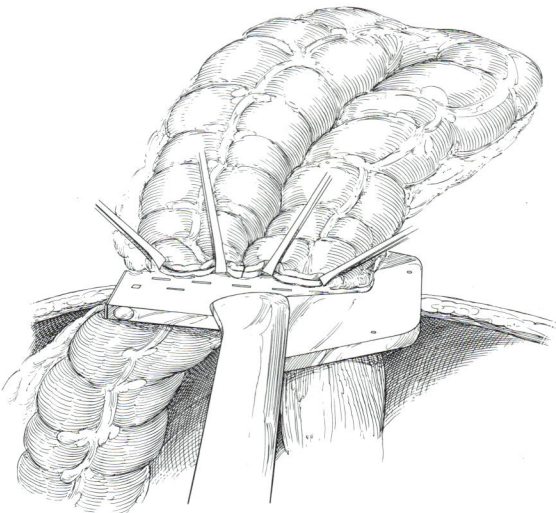

Figure 25-8. Closure of the remaining enterotomy with a TA* 90 stapling device. The sigmoid mesentery is ligated at the same time.

through the incision with warmed saline. This facilitates removal of any clots that have accumulated within the operative field. The incision is closed with interrupted sutures. The pneumoperitneum is reinflated. The anastomosis is scrutinized. The colon is traced proximally to make sure that a volvulus was not generated during construction of the anastomosis. A colonoscope is passed transanally to examine the anastomosis (Fig. 25-9). The colon is insufflated and checked for evidence of leaks.

The trocars are removed one at a time. The fascial defects are closed with interrupted sutures. The skin edges are apposed with skin

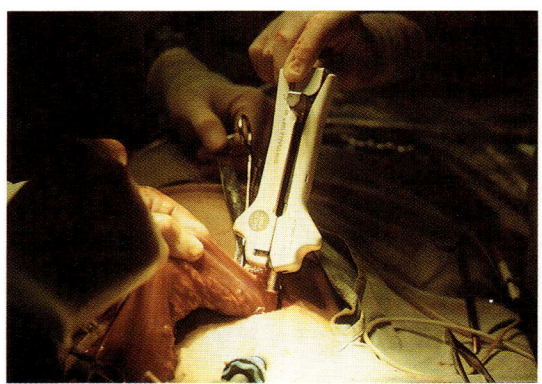

Figure 25-7. Construction of the side-to-side, functional end-to-end anastomosis with the GIA* 60 stapling device.

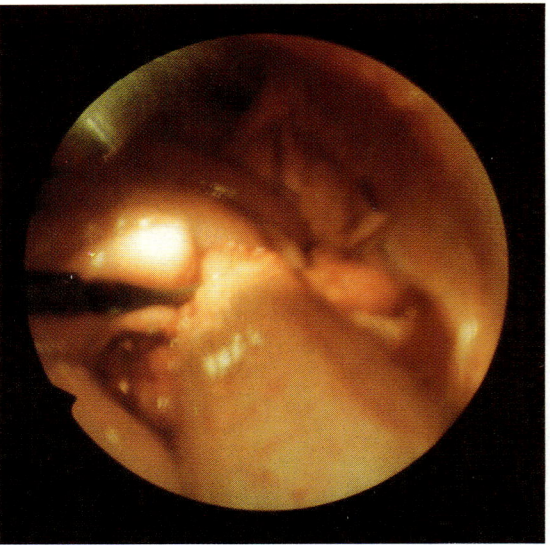

Figure 25-9. Inspection of the anastomosis with a colonoscope. The light of the colonoscope is visible through the wall of the colon.

staples. Band-Aids (Johnson & Johnson, Inc.) are applied over the wounds.

LAPAROSCOPIC SIGMOID RESECTION WITH END-TO-END ANASTOMOSIS

In patients with little scarring of the sigmoid mesentery, a more standard type of sigmoid resection can be accomplished. The patient is prepared and positioned as described previously. The pneumoperitoneum is insufflated. Five 10-mm trocars are inserted as shown in Figure 25-2. The retroperitoneum is incised, and the left ureter is identified. The proximal rectum, sigmoid, and descending colon are mobilized medially. The retroperitoneum on the right is incised over the sacral promontory. The presacral space is entered between the fascia propria and the retrorectal (Waldeyer's) fascia. The inferior mesenteric and superior hemorrhoidal vessels are identified.

The feasibility of exposing the distal sigmoid branches is assessed. The redundancy of the sigmoid colon and limited space for retraction within the abdominal cavity make this difficult. If space proves inadequate, an extracorporeal resection is performed (see preceding discussion). If visualization is satisfactory, intracorporeal transection of the proximal rectum and division of the distal sigmoid branches are performed.

The assistant surgeon grasps the proximal rectum on either side of the planned point of transection with two ENDO BABCOCK* clamps. The caudad 10-mm trocar in the right lower quadrant is replaced with a 12- or 15-mm trocar. The rectum is transected and closed with multiple applications of the ENDO GIA* 30 stapling device (United States Surgical Corporation) or a single firing of the ENDO GIA* 60 stapling device (United States Surgical Corporation) (Fig. 25-10). The staple lines are inspected for hemorrhage.

Traction on the two rectal staple lines exposes the proximal rectal and distal sigmoid mesentery. The mesenteric vessels are divided between clips or with serial applications of the ENDO GIA* 30 stapling device using white vascular cartridges. The inferior mesenteric and superior hemorrhoidal vessels are carefully preserved since the blood supply of the anastomosis will be based on these vessels. Division of the sigmoid branches continues while exposure is satisfactory.

An ENDO BABCOCK* clamp is inserted through the caudad trocar in the left lower

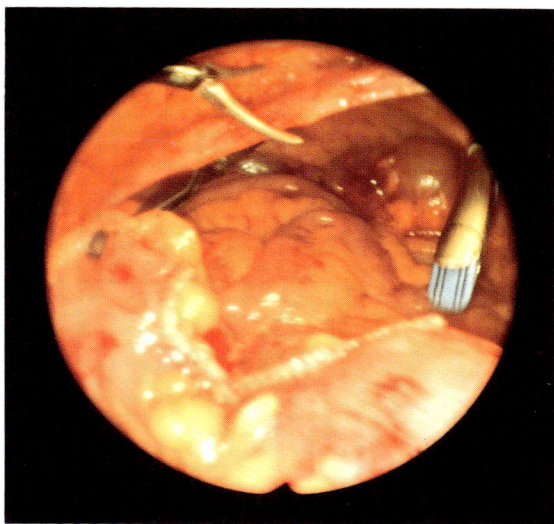

Figure 25-10. The proximal rectum is divided with multiple applications of the ENDO GIA* 30 stapling device.

quadrant. The trocar is pulled out of the abdominal wall over the shaft of this instrument. A 1-inch transverse incision is made through this trocar site. The end of the specimen and then the entire sigmoid colon is pulled through the incision. Any remaining proximal sigmoid vessels are divided between clamps and ligated (Fig. 25-11).

The point of proximal resection is selected. The mesenteric fat is cleared for a distance of 1 inch around the circumference of the colon at this point. The Automatic PURSESTRING* device (United States Surgical Corporation) is fired (Fig. 25-12). The colon is transected. The specimen is opened within the operating room. The diameter of the colon is sized. The anvil-shaft assembly of the Premium CEEA* stapling device is inserted into the lumen of the colon (Fig. 25-13). The low profile anvil and modified shaft are used. The modified shaft has an additional groove which facilitates grasping of the shaft with an Endo Babcock clamp. The purse-string suture is tied, and the bowel is placed back into the abdomen. The tip of the anvil-shaft assembly is positioned in the pelvis so that it points directly at the rectal stump.

The abdomen is liberally irrigated through the incision. The incision is closed with interrupted sutures. The pneumoperitoneum is reinflated. The anus is dilated to admit four fingers. The head of the CEEA* stapling device is introduced through the anus and advanced up through the rectum. The white

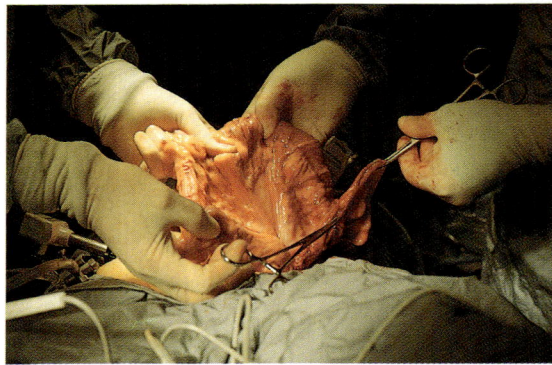 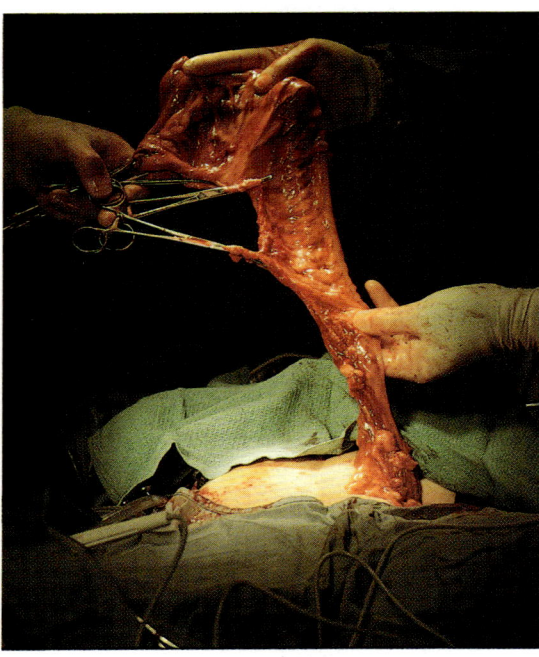

Figure 25-11. A. Delivery of the sigmoid colon through an incision in a left lower quadrant trocar site. The proximal rectum was divided intracorporeally with an ENDO GIA* stapling device. B. The proximal sigmoid mesentery is divided more easily outside of the abdominal cavity because of space limitations within the abdomen.

trocar tip is screwed out through the previous stapled closure of the rectum. It is lassoed with a pre-tied laparoscopic ligature and withdrawn out through the 12- or 15-mm trocar. The anvil-shaft assembly is grasped with an ENDO BABCOCK* clamp and docked into the orange collar of the cartridge of the Premium CEEA* stapling device (Fig. 25-14). The CEEA* stapling device is screwed closed, fired, and then removed. The donut-like rings of the anastomosis contained within the stapling device are checked. A colonoscope is inserted through the anus and advanced up to the anastomosis. The colon is insufflated and checked for evidence of air leakage under water.

The trocars are removed, and the fascial defects are closed. The skin edges are apposed with skin staples. Band-Aids cover the wounds.

CECAL VOLVULUS

Cecal volvulus may be organoaxial (true volvulus) or mesentericoaxial (cecal bascule). The former involves the distal ileum and ascending colon twisting around each other, in much the same way as a sigmoid volvulus. Mesentericoaxial volvulus (cecal bascule) involves the cecum "folding" in an axis at right angles to the mesentery. Cecal volvulus is less

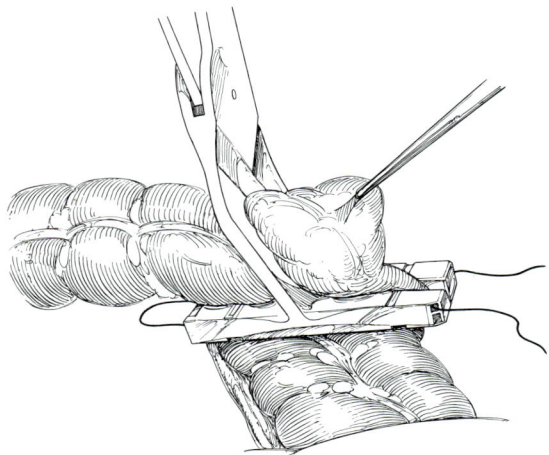

Figure 25-12. An Automatic PURSESTRING* device staples a purse-string suture onto the distal descending colon.

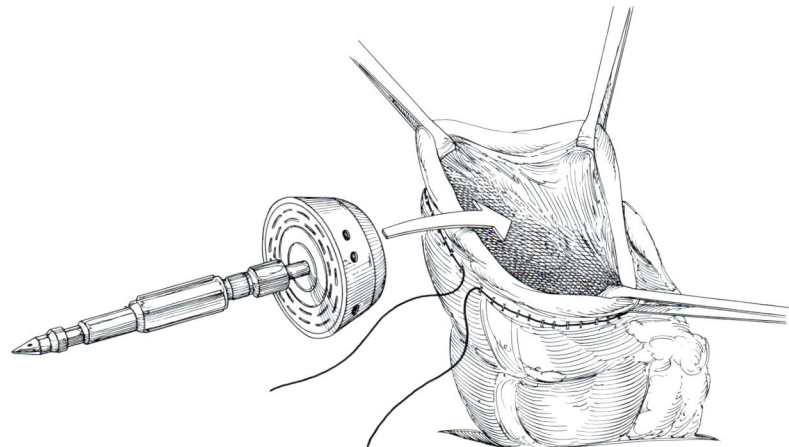

Figure 25-13. The anvil-shaft assembly of the Premium CEEA* stapling device is secured in the distal descending colon with a purse-string suture.

common than its sigmoid equivalent (one-seventh to one-tenth as common), and its demographic features appear to have changed over the last half-century from a condition of both sexes in the second or third decade, to one affecting predominately women in the sixth decade.

In contrast to sigmoid volvulus, which is usually an acquired condition, cecal volvulus is caused by congenital incomplete retroperitoneal fixation of the cecum or ascending colon. In an autopsy study by Anson, more than 10 per cent of ascending colons had a mobile mesentery, permitting volvulus to occur. In a further 25 per cent of cadavers, the cecum alone was sufficiently mobile to permit cecal bascule to occur. Further anomalies included undescended right colon and previous surgical mobilization of the cecum, both permitting sufficient mobility for volvulus.

In contrast to sigmoid volvulus, cecal volvulus occurs in a counterclockwise direction, although no data exist to support this anecdotal observation.

As in sigmoid volvulus, a space-occupying lesion in the pelvis, such as a gravid uterus or an ovarian tumor may precipitate an episode of cecal volvulus by altering the relative positions of the intra-abdominal organs.

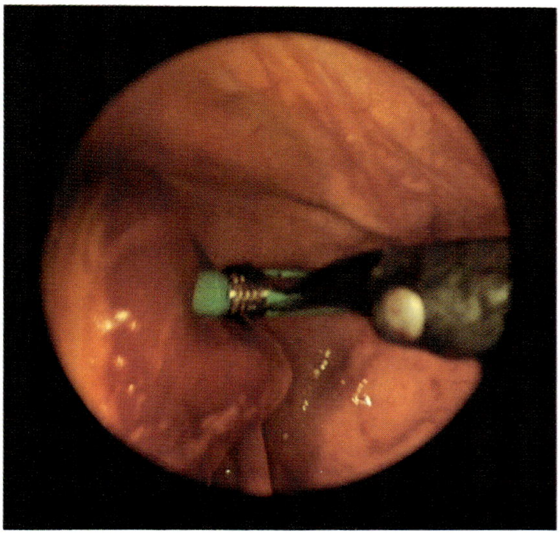

Diagnosis

Low intestinal obstruction and a distended, tympanitic abdomen are the hallmarks of cecal volvulus. The diagnosis is rarely made clinically, and only 50 per cent of radiographs show the characteristic "coffee-bean" (cecal volvulus) or "tear-drop" (bascule) appearances. Contrast studies with barium or water-soluble contrast media have a risk of bowel perforation, owing to the extensive insufflation required to get the contrast medium to the right colon. Water-soluble contrast medium can be delivered via the colonoscope, in the event of diagnostic uncertainty. However, by this stage in the diagnostic workup, laparotomy will nearly always be required, irrespective of the nature of the obstruction. Diagnostic colonoscopy reveals a cul-de-sac at the hepatic flexure in cases of volvulus, and in cecal bascule, a broad-based obstructing fold is seen in the ascending colon. The role of colonoscopy is debatable, since perforation

Figure 25-14. The anvil-shaft assembly is laparoscopically docked into the orange collar of the Premium CEEA* stapling device.

is a hazard, and surgery will usually be required, whatever the findings.

Treatment

REDUCTION OF THE VOLVULUS

Detorsion of the cecum and operative fixation or resection are the goals of treatment. Colonoscopic decompression of the cecum is more frequently unsuccessful in patients with cecal volvulus compared to sigmoid volvulus. Because of the poor rate of success and of the inherent risks colonoscopic decompression is not recommended as a routine.

Percutaneous deflation of the cecum was described in 1987 by Patel et al. The authors used a simple intravenous cannula inserted via an anterior approach. The cecum deflated, and the cannula was removed after a few minutes. Spontaneous detorsion occurred, and no further surgery was performed. The patient died 3 months later from unrelated causes. Percutaneous deflation of the colon has been successful used in colonic pseudo-obstruction (Ogilvie's syndrome) via a retroperitoneal approach; however, decompression of a free intraperitoneal cecum has attendant risks of leakage. Although more experience is required, the procedure may prove to be a useful alternative in poor risk patients who may not tolerate surgery.

FIXATION OR RESECTION?

Surgical options for cecal volvulus in the absence of gangrene include cecopexy, cecostomy, and right colectomy. Simple operative detorsion alone is generally considered prone to recurrence, although Anderson found only a 4 per cent recurrence rate after simple operative detorsion (Table 25-6). Other authors report similar results, but the follow-up period is short and the true incidence of life time recurrence of volvulus is probably higher. Furthermore, because of edema in the bowel wall, simple detorsion often does not completely relieve the obstruction, making resection necessary.

Cecopexy can be achieved by simple suturing of the cecum to the lateral paracolic gutter or fixation using a peritoneal flap. Recurrence after cecopexy remains a problem: Anderson et al. reported a 20 per cent incidence of recurrence of volvulus after cecopexy (Table 25-7). Rabinovici et al. found similar recurrence rates (12 to 13 per cent) after cecopexy and operative detorsion alone. The authors concluded that fixation of the cecum is unnecessary; however, a more adequate technique of cecopexy, such as a peritoneal flap, is probably what is really required.

Cecostomy as a mode of cecal fixation has received mixed reviews (Table 25-8). Jacobs et al. describe cecostomy (combined with cecopexy) as "the procedure of choice." In contrast, Rabinovici et al. conclude that cecostomy "should be abandoned" because of its high rate of complications such as wound infection, abdominal wall necrosis, and leakage. In their series of 561 reported cases of cecal volvulus, recurrence rates, morbidity, and mortality were higher than those with any other procedure, including resection. Despite the controversy, cecostomy provides a viable option for decompressing the cecum and providing some degree of fixation in circumstances where resection is inappropriate.

Resection for nongangrenous bowel eliminates the possibility of recurrence. Reported mortality rates, however, vary widely (Table 25-9). Since the bowel is already completely mobilized, resection can usually be performed expeditiously. Resection also offers the distinct advantage that the obstructed segment of bowel is removed and consequently ongoing bacterial translocation is ablated. The authors consider resection as the therapy of choice in patients who can tolerate the procedure.

Resection is required in the presence of nonviable or excessively friable bowel. Resection of the right colon avoids the risks of recurrence and deals definitively with ischemic bowel as a potential source of sepsis. Primary anastomosis should be avoided in the

Table 25-6. Detorsion of the Cecum for Volvulus

Authors	Year	Recurrence (%)	Morbidity (%)	Mortality (%)
Anderson	1975	4		36
Ballantyne	1985	11		33
Rabinovici	1990	12	15	13

Table 25-7. Cecopexy for Cecal Volvulus

Authors	Year	Recurrence (%)	Morbidity (%)	Mortality (%)
Ballantyne	1985	0		9
Anderson	1986	20		10
Rabinovici	1990	3	15	10

Table 25-8. Cecostomy for Cecal Volvulus

Authors	Year	Recurrence (%)	Morbidity (%)	Mortality (%)
Ballantyne	1985	0		0
Anderson	1986	25		33
Rabinovici	1990	14	52	32

Table 25-9. Resection (Right Hemicolectomy) for Cecal Volvulus

Authors	Year	Recurrence (%)	Morbidity (%)	Mortality (%)
Ballantyne	1985	0		12
Anderson	1986	0		40
Rabinovici	1990	0	29	22

presence of peritoneal contamination from perforation by the use of a diverting ileostomy. The distal end can be brought out as a mucous fistula or stapled and returned to the peritoneal cavity. Mortality rates for cecal volvulus are primarily determined by the degree of bowel ischemia; they vary from 12 per cent for viable bowel and increase almost 3-fold to 32 per cent in the presence of gangrene.

Laparoscopic Surgery for Cecal Volvulus

As with sigmoid volvulus, there is little experience with laparoscopic surgery for cecal volvulus. As a result of the abdominal distention present in the acute stages, it is unlikely that laparoscopic resection will have a significant role in emergency resection because of the risks of perforation of the closed loop during introduction of the cannulas and the difficulties of maneuvering within the abdomen in the presence of a dilated thin-walled cecum.

After successful colonoscopic detorsion of the loop, however, elective laparoscopic right hemicolectomy has the same potential advantages as in sigmoid volvulus, including reduction in postoperative ileus and reduced analgesic requirements. The technique is facilitated by the presence of a mobile cecum and ascending colon, minimizing the amount of retroperitoneal dissection required, and close proximity of the proximal and distal sites of anastomosis.

Volvulus of Transverse Colon

This constitutes only 4 per cent of cases of volvulus of the large bowel and affects predominately young women. Predisposing conditions include a long mesocolon, close proximity of hepatic and splenic flexures or hepatodiaphragmatic interposition of the colon (Chilaiditi's syndrome). Distal colonic obstruction elongates and expands the transverse colon, with the potential for volvulus.

Treatment includes laparotomy and resection. Detorsion alone is followed by recurrence in 75 per cent of cases. Segmental resection of the transverse colon or extended right hemicolectomy are the preferred options. Elaborate techniques of colopexy are described, but the simplest and most reliable option remains resection.

VOLVULUS OF SPLENIC FLEXURE

The splenic flexure is the least common site for volvulus in the large bowel. The majority of reported cases are in women (2:1, women/men). As in volvulus elsewhere, predisposing conditions are previous abdominal surgery and distal colonic obstruction or megacolon. The options available are detorsion alone, cecopexy with or without colostomy, or resection. The rarity of the condition prevents a large surgical experience. On an empiric basis, however, resection has the advantage of eliminating recurrent volvulus and removes suspect bowel.

BIBLIOGRAPHY

Anderson JR, Lee D. The management of acute sigmoid volvulus. Br J Surg 1981; 68:117–120.

Anderson JR, Welch GH. Acute volvulus of the right colon: An analysis of 69 patients. World J Surg 1986; 10:336–342.

Arnold GJ, Nance FC. Volvulus of the sigmoid colon. Ann Surg 1972; 177:527–537.

Bak MP, Boley SJ. Sigmoid volvulus in elderly patients. Am J Surg 1986; 151:71–75.

Ballantyne GH. Review of sigmoid volvulus. Clinical patterns and pathogenesis. Dis Colon Rectum 1982; 25:823–830.

Ballantyne GH. Review of sigmoid volvulus: History and results of treatment. Dis Colon Rectum 1982; 25:494–501.

Ballantyne GH. Sigmoid volvulus: High mortality in county hospital patients. Dis Colon Rectum 1981; 24:515–520.

Ballantyne GH. Volvulus of the splenic flexure. Dis Colon Rectum 1981; 24:630–632.

Ballantyne GH, Brandner MD, Beart RW Jr, Ilstrup DM. Volvulus of the colon. Incidence and mortality. Ann Surg 1985; 202:83–92.

Drapanas T, Stewart JD. Acute sigmoid volvulus. Am J Surg 1961; 101:70–77.

Farringer JL, Wilson H. Volvulus of the sigmoid colon. Am J Surg 1955; 90:588–592.

Gabriel LT, Campbell DA, Musselman MM. Volvulus of the sigmoid colon. Gastroenterology 1953; 24:378–384.

Hines JR, Geurkink RE, Bass RT. Recurrence and mortality rates in sigmoid volvulus. Surg Gynecol Obstet 1967; 124:567–570.

Knight J, Bokey EL, Chapius PH, Pheils MT. Sigmoidoscopic reduction of sigmoid volvulus. Med J Aust 1980; 2:627–628.

Mangiante EC, Croce MA, Fabian TC, et al. Sigmoid volvulus. A four-decade experience. Am Surg 1989; 55:41–44.

Pahlman L, Enblad P, Rudberg C, Krog M. Volvulus of the colon. A review of 93 cases and current aspects of treatment. Acta Chir Scand 1989; 155:53–56.

Pasch AR, Adams JT. Acute volvulus of the sigmoid colon: Current management. Contemp Surg 1985; 26:65–68.

Peoples JB, McCafferty JC, Scher KS. Operative therapy for sigmoid volvulus. Identification of risk factors affecting outcome. Dis Colon Rectum 1990; 33:643–646.

Rabinovici R, Simansky DA, Kaplan O, et al. Cecal volvulus. Dis Colon Rectum 1990; 33:765–769.

Salim AS. Percutaneous deflation and colopexy for volvulus of the sigmoid colon: A new approach. J Royal Coll Surg Edinb 1990; 35:356–359.

Shepherd JJ. Treatment of volvulus of the sigmoid colon. Br Med J 1968; 1:280–283.

Smith WR, Goodwin JN. Cecal volvulus. Am J Surg 1973; 126:215–222.

Taha SE, Suleiman SI. Volvulus of the sigmoid colon in the Gezira. Br J Surg 1980; 67:433–435.

Wuepper KD, Otteman MG, Stahlgren LH. An appraisal of the operative and nonoperative treatment of sigmoid volvulus. Surg Gynecol Obstet 1966; 122:84–88.

Section VI
Surgery for Other Disorders

Chapter 26
Diagnostic Laparoscopy

Lawrence E. Harrison
Anne C. Mosenthal
Philip F. Caushaj

A resurgence of interest in minimally invasive surgery has focused attention once again on diagnostic laparoscopy as a potential tool of the general surgeon. Twenty years ago it was used primarily for diagnosis of liver disease when its accuracy and complication rate were superior to those for percutaneous biopsy.[1-3] However, the increased sophistication of radiologic diagnostic modalities such as computed tomography, ultrasound, and magnetic resonance imaging have caused a loss of favor of diagnostic laparoscopy for this indication. Subsequently, in the 1970s and 1980s laparoscopy has been advocated for diagnosis of chronic and acute abdominal pain,[4-6] staging of malignancies,[7,8] and more recently, the diagnosis of abdominal pathologic conditions in trauma[9-11] or critically ill patients.[12,13] Newer technology now allows for increased therapeutic interventions through the laparoscope. It is hoped that its diagnostic role can become broadened as well, resulting in fewer laparotomies with normal findings, shorter patient stays, and better control of costs. To accomplish these goals diagnostic laparoscopy must be used selectively and rationally (Table 26-1); its use is presently confined to those patients in whom a laparotomy can be avoided based on its findings. This chapter will review the current techniques and indications for diagnostic laparoscopy in general surgery.

TECHNIQUE

Patients are prepared and evaluated preoperatively as for other surgical procedures. Coagulation profile, hematocrit, platelet count, chest radiograph, and electrocardiogram are obtained, as well as any other preoperative studies the patient's condition dictates. Laparoscopy under local anesthesia with sedation has been well described particularly in the elective situation.[14,15] We prefer general anesthesia since the stretching of the peritoneum and diaphragm can cause a great deal of discomfort as well as vasovagal response during insufflation. There are a few absolute contraindications to laparoscopy: abdominal wall infection or large hernias, peritonitis, pregnancy, and severe comorbid disease are examples. Multiple previous operations can be a relative contraindication but often access to the abdomen can be obtained with the laparoscope in a lateral quadrant away from any incisions or adhesions; however, if visibility is limited within the peritoneum, the examination is obviously nondiagnostic. Similarly, morbid obesity provides a challenge to the laparoscopist because the trocars and instruments may not be long enough to provide adequate exposure. While many consider this to be a contraindication, we have found that careful planning of the placement of the camera and trocars can allow adequate exam-

Table 26-1. Indications for Diagnostic Laparoscopy

Abdominal pain
Acute abdomen
Cancer staging
Ischemic colitis
Acalculus cholecystitis
Acute cholecystitis
Trauma

ination of the peritoneal cavity, provided the often fatty omentum can be mobilized and retracted.

The abdomen is prepared and draped widely; should a laparotomy become necessary during the procedure the field need not be changed. All patients receive gastric and urinary bladder decompression by the appropriate catheters. The periumbilical area is selected for the site of insertion of the Veress needle in most instances. If the patient has had multiple lower abdominal or right upper quadrant procedures, we have found the left upper quadrant to be the area most consistantly free of adhesions and we then insert the Veress needle there. Confirmation of entry into the peritoneal cavity is made by the presence of a low pressure and the saline drop test. Carbon dioxide is insufflated to an intra-abdominal pressure of 14 to 15 mm Hg. A 10-mm trocar is then inserted in the same site following a 1.5-cm skin incision. The camera is passed through the trocar, and inspection of the peritoneal cavity is performed.

A systematic inspection of the peritoneal cavity should be performed during any laparoscopy just as it is during a laparotomy. The surgeon should utilize all patient positions to facilitate examination of organs. With the patient in the reverse Trendelenburg position the liver, falciform ligament, and gallbladder are inspected. By lateral rotation the stomach, spleen, duodenum, and head of pancreas can be visualized. Depending on which pathologic condition is suspected, it is useful to introduce a second trocar in the right upper quadrant so that a probe may be used to retract the liver up and examine its undersurface. This probe can be used to retract the omentum and colon so that the spleen, diaphragm, and its hiatus can be inspected. If a pancreatic pathologic condition is suspected, the probe can be replaced by a dissector and a small window made in the gastrocolic omentum to allow introduction of the laparoscope directly into the lesser sac; the entire pancreas can then be seen in this fashion.

To inspect the pelvis and lower abdomen the patient should be placed in the Trendelenburg position. This allows the small intestine and omentum to fall cephalad so that the uterus, ovaries, cecum, and appendix can be observed. Again the insertion of a second 5-mm trocar is helpful (we prefer the suprapubic area) to allow the use of a probe or dissector for retraction. The iliac fossa, ureter, rectum, and pouch of Douglas can then be seen with minimal dissection.

Biopsy is an important adjunct to diagnostic laparoscopy. Solid organs such as the liver are easily sampled using a Trucut needle placed directly through the abdominal wall. Larger surface lesions on the liver, omentum, or mesentery can be sampled for biopsy using laparoscopic forceps; some of these may require the introduction of an additional large (10 or 11 mm) trocar to retrieve the specimens. Caution should be exercised in the control of bleeding from biopsy sites as cautery can damage underlying tissues, particularly the intestine.

If cytologic examination is indicated, the abdomen can be lavaged with saline or peritoneal fluid can be aspirated. Saline (500 ml) should be injected via an irrigator; the patient should be rotated so all areas are lavaged and the fluid aspirated into a trap by the suction apparatus. Brush biopsies of solid organs or peritoneal deposits can also be done through a trocar.

Cultures should be obtained if indicated. Fluid can be aspirated directly through the abdominal wall using a syringe and needle; inoculation of the abdominal wall resulting in cellulitis or fasciitis is a theoretic possibility, but we have not yet seen it described. Cultures can also be aspirated via the suction apparatus as described for cytologic specimens.

The evaluation of ascites for malignancy or liver disease is occasionally necessary. Ascites is not a contraindication to laparoscopy. A 2- to 3-cm skin incision is made in the periumbilical region. The Veress needle is inserted with care since the small bowel may float on the surface of the fluid. Carbon dioxide is insufflated, but usually smaller quantities are needed since there is already increased intra-abdominal pressure caused by the ascites. Dissection down to the fascia is carried out. The open technique as described by Hasson[16] can be used. Sutures should always be placed around the site of trocar insertion to allow closure of the fascial defect to prevent ascitic leak. If visualization is poor because of fluid, 500 ml can be aspirated and replaced with carbon dioxide. The anesthesiologist should be alerted to intravascular fluid shifts if this is done.

INDICATIONS

Staging of Abdominal Malignancies

The selection of patients with gastrointestinal malignancies for curative and palliative surgery remains a challenge for the general surgeon. The benefit of a curative resection must be balanced by the risk of morbidity and mortality. The presence of metastatic disease may not justify the perioperative risk in some cases. Proper preoperative staging usually allows for adequate selection of patients for surgery; despite modern radiologic tests occasionally patients will undergo laparotomy only to reveal unsuspected incurable disease.

Laparoscopy is used for (1) diagnosis and biopsy of a primary tumor, (2) assessment of operability, (3) evaluation of metastatic disease, and (4) the search for an unknown primary tumor.[17] While computed tomography, ultrasound, and magnetic resonance imaging have improved preoperative evaluation, lesions less than 1 cm in the abdomen are typically undetected by these modalities. Laparoscopy permits easy identification and biopsy for tissue diagnosis. Laparoscopy has been used with varying success for the evaluation of malignancies of the pancreas, stomach, esophagus, colon, and liver as well as lymphoma.

ESOPHAGUS

Cancer of the esophagus portends a very poor outcome for the patient. More than half of patients with this disease have unresectable tumors. Unresectability is determined by either locally advanced disease or intra-abdominal metastases. In these patients the tumor is best treated by nonoperative palliation such as intra-esophageal stenting or radiation. Curative surgery is possible for limited cancers but carries a relatively high morbidity and mortality. Clearly accurate staging is critical to properly select patients.

The use of laparoscopy in staging esophageal cancer has been reported. Dagnini et al.[18] evaluated 369 patients with cancer of the esophagus and cardia with laparoscopy. Laparoscopy demonstrated intra-abdominal metastases in 52 patients (14 per cent) and regional disease in 36 patients (9.7 per cent). In addition, severe portal hypertension was noted in 25 patients (6.7 per cent) which precluded curative resection. However, laparoscopy failed to demonstrate intra-abdominal metastases in 11 patients (3.0 per cent). In another study, Watt et al.[19] compared the sensitivity, specificity, and accuracy of laparoscopy, ultrasound, and computed tomography in 90 patients with esophageal cancer. Although all techniques showed a high specificity for metastases, laparoscopy was more sensitive and accurate with regard to hepatic disease. Moreover, while ultrasound and computed tomography scan did not detect any peritoneal metastases, laparoscopy detected eight of nine.

Laparoscopy for staging esophageal cancer is performed via a periumbilical approach. Detailed inspection of the liver surfaces for metastatic deposits is performed as well as exploration of the anterior gastric wall, cardia, gastrohepatic ligament, and diaphragm for extension of disease.

While this technique is accurate, its clinical application is, in reality, limited. Only patients who are candidates for curative resection based on computed tomography scan can benefit; in 14 per cent of these additional pathologic lesions will be found. In summary, therapy will not be changed based on the findings at laparoscopy in the majority of patients.

STOMACH

Gastric carcinoma also portends a poor prognosis and has a low resectability rate (21 to 58 per cent).[20] Palliative surgery, however, is a more feasible option than esophageal resection. Many patients require surgery for symptoms of obstruction or bleeding regardless of the stage or curability of the tumor. For this reason, preoperative staging before laparotomy may be helpful only in those patients with asymptomatic lesions.

Laparoscopic evaluation begins with careful inspection of the peritoneal surfaces, diaphragm, and liver. Ascites is noted as well and sent for cytologic evaluation. The entire stomach surface and the omentum should be inspected. Specific attention should be directed toward demonstrating criteria for unresectability: serosal infiltration, tumor fixation, lymph node metastases, peritoneal dissemination, and hepatic metastases. By lifting the left lobe of the liver with a retractor, the lesser curve, the gastrohepatic omentum, cardia, and the duodenum can be examined. The posterior wall of the stomach can be evaluated by placing the laparoscope through an aperture made in an avascular area of the greater omentum into the lesser sac. It is difficult to evaluate the celiac axis and retroperitoneum for posterior fixation of the tumor. This is a critical area for the determination of resectability and does limit the value of laparoscopy in this setting.

The results of this technique have been described in the literature.[8,21,22] Kriplani and Kapur[8] performed laparoscopy in 40 patients with otherwise resectable gastric cancer. Laparoscopy disclosed unrecognized distant metastases in 5 patients (12.5 per cent) and locally advanced, unresectable disease in 11 patients (27.5 per cent). Overall, unnecessary laparotomy was avoided in 16 patients (40 per cent). The diagnostic accuracy of laparoscopy was 91.6 per cent. Possik et al.[22] studied the value of laparoscopy for staging of gastric cancer and the detection of hepatic metastases in 360 patients. Hepatic metastases were most accurately detected by laparoscopy as compared to liver scintigraphy and ultrasound; the latter had a higher false positive rate. No comparison to computed tomography was done. Whereas these studies have shown laparoscopy to be accurate in staging, it is still relatively poor for establishing resectability because posterior fixation is hard to evaluate. Since many patients with advanced stages of gastric cancer still undergo resection for palliation and some without disseminated disease do not undergo resection because of local extension, laparoscopy probably does not replace laparotomy at this time.

PANCREAS

Carcinoma of the pancreas is often diagnosed at an advanced stage. Ductal cancers can be resected 10 to 20 per cent of the time although ampullary tumors can be resected more often (60 to 80 per cent). Preoperatively computed tomography or angiography in combination with percutaneous biopsy for tissue diagnosis was considered the standard to evaluate metastatic disease and resectability of the primary lesion. Palliation for unresectable or metastatic disease can be accomplished either nonoperatively with internal biliary stents or percutaneous transhepatic drainage or operatively by biliary enteric bypass. Laparotomy may not always be necessary in some patients; it is this group of patients with incurable disease who can benefit most from laparoscopy.[7,23]

Warshaw et al.[24] reviewed 88 patients with pancreatic cancer for preoperative assessment of resectability. Patients underwent computed tomography, angiogram, magnetic resonance imaging, and laparoscopy. Laparoscopy was used only to detect liver or peritoneal metastases and not to evaluate the primary tumor itself. Laparoscopy detected metastases in 22 of 23 patients (96 per cent). This was more sensitive than computed tomography, which identified only 2 of 27 patients with liver or peritoneal metastases. The authors felt that the combined modalities of computed tomographic scan, angiogram, and laparoscopy were more accurate than any one alone in predicting resectability. Eighty-nine per cent of unresectable tumors and 90 per cent of resectable tumors were accurately identified.

The laparoscope has also been used to inspect the pancreas directly when cancer is suspected but not diagnosed. Meyer-Burg[25] and Ishida et al.[26] have described a supragastric approach. The patient is placed in the reverse Trendelenburg position, the left lobe of the liver is retracted, and an opening is established in the gastrohepatic ligament; the laparoscope is inserted into the lesser sac, the pancreas is inspected, and a biopsy specimen is taken directly if necessary. The clinical application of a laparoscopic biopsy, now that percutaneous biopsy of pancreatic cancer is well established, is of questionable value. However, the controversy of seeding the biopsy tract with tumor cells may be obviated by laparoscopy.

LIVER

Laparoscopy has been used extensively in the past for the evaluation of pathologic conditions of the liver, both benign and malignant.[1,27-30] In recent years, the sophistication of computed tomographic- and ultrasound-guided percutaneous biopsy has largely eliminated laparoscopy as a primary diagnostic tool for liver pathologic conditions. Computed tomography and ultrasound can image intraparenchymal lesions; ultrasound can determine portal vein thrombosis. However, laparoscopy is more sensitive for small capsular hepatic lesions of 1 cm or less that are beyond the resolution of radiologic studies. Brady et al.[28] studied 25 patients with known primary malignancies with elevated liver function tests and ascites but no evidence of metastases by computed tomographic scanning. Laparoscopy detected metastatic lesions in 12 of 25 patients (48 per cent). Laparoscopy may still have a role in the differentiation of cirrhosis and small benign lesions from malignant disease. In addition, it may facilitate directed biopsies.

In summary, although refinements of computed tomography and ultrasound have improved detection of hepatic lesions (metastatic or primary), there still are indications for laparoscopy in the evaluation and directed biopsy of liver tumors, especially when other imaging studies fail to detect any abnormalities in a suspicious clinical situation.

LYMPHOMA

The staging laparotomy was originally developed to determine the subdiaphragmatic presence of Hodgkin's disease. The rationale was to alter treatment, by appropriately staging disease in patients and altering their chemotherapy. Laparoscopy represents an alternative diagnostic procedure to laparotomy. DeVita et al.[31] and later Bagley et al.[32] were early champions of diagnostic laparoscopy in the evaluation of Hodgkin's lymphoma. Beretta et al.[33] studied 121 patients with Hodgkin's lymphoma with staging laparoscopy and needle bone marrow biopsy and found extranodal liver or marrow involvement in 9 per cent of patients. The use of laparoscopy in the staging of Hodgkin's lymphoma is warranted only if laparotomy is contemplated for direction of therapy. In patients with suspicious computed tomographic results directed liver biopsy and lymph node sampling can be performed, but biopsy of the spleen is generally considered unsafe. With the evolution and rapid advancement of laparoscopic technique, staging of Hodgkin's lymphoma may include laparoscopic splenectomy, as well as liver and node biopsy, thus eliminating the need for open laparotomy.

COLORECTAL CANCER

The use of laparoscopy in the evaluation of colorectal cancer is currently undergoing experimental investigation. Sotnikof and Agamov[34] in the Soviet Union have demonstrated its efficacy in staging rectal cancer. Its clinical value in directing specific therapy has not been conclusively demonstrated because the majority of patients with colorectal cancer require laparotomy regardless of the stage of their tumor. Nevertheless, it does have great potential value in subsets of patients with recurrent colorectal cancer, elevated carcinoembryonic antigen, and resectable metastases to the lung or liver, but no data are available at this time.

MISCELLANEOUS CANCERS

Laparoscopy may help in the evaluation of other malignancies as well. Laparoscopic features and staging of gallbladder cancer have been described. Gynecologic malignancies can be staged laparoscopically, e.g., ovarian carcinoma at the initial diagnosis, as well as being used for subsequent "second-look" operations.

LAPAROSCOPY IN THE DIAGNOSIS OF TRAUMA

The diagnosis of abdominal injury after blunt or penetrating trauma may be elusive. Peritoneal lavage, introduced by Root in 1965, is a very reliable predictor of intraabdominal injury. However, false positive results can lead to laparotomies with negative results. In addition, some intraperitoneal injuries do not necessarily require operative intervention, such as minor liver lacerations or minor mesenteric vascular injuries. Computed tomography has a high sensitivity and specificity, but false negative results occur; in particular, injuries to hollow organs can be missed.

Laparoscopy has been described in the diagnosis of abdominal trauma in the past.[9-11,35,36] Its use has been reported for both penetrating and blunt trauma. Laparoscopy offers the advantage of direct intra-abdominal visualization, as well as the possibility of therapeutic intervention.

The laparoscopic examination is performed in the emergency ward, intensive care unit, or the operating room. After adequate local anesthesia, the Veress needle is introduced in the infraumbilical position, and a pneumoperitoneum is created. The patient's vital signs and additional hemodynamic monitoring are obtained as dictated by the patient's clinical status throughout the procedure. After adequate insufflation, the Veress needle is removed and the trocar for the laparoscope is introduced through the same puncture site. A second trocar is placed in the right upper quadrant for retracting purposes. A systematic exploration of the abdomen is done, including inspection of the small and large bowel and the liver and spleen. Biliary or small bowel injury will show a characteristic bile staining. The source of hemorrhage can be evaluated and operative or nonoperative therapies planned.

A prospective trial comparing peritoneal lavage to laparoscopy in 55 patients was reported by Cuschieri et al.[35] Both procedures were highly sensitive for the detection of significant intra-abdominal injury (100 per cent). However, the specificity was 83 per cent for lavage and 94 per cent for laparoscopy. There were fewer false positive results in the laparoscopy group (8 per cent) than in the lavage group (27 per cent).

Although some data show that laparoscopy is more accurate in the diagnosis of intra-abdominal trauma, it is more cumbersome than peritoneal lavage. Up to now it has not gained wide acceptance, but ongoing protocols may demonstrate its potential.

LAPAROSCOPY FOR ABDOMINAL PAIN

The use of diagnostic laparoscopy in the evaluation of right lower quadrant pain has been well described, particularly in the young female patient.[5,6,37,38,39,40] History, physical examination, ultrasound, and laboratory tests are neither sensitive nor specific for the diagnosis of acute appendicitis. The differential diagnosis includes several entities that can be treated nonoperatively: pelvic inflammatory disease, tubo-ovarian abscess, mesenteric adenitis, ileitis, and ovarian cyst. While the surgeon hopes to minimize the rate of negative results on laparotomy, perforated appendicitis is to be avoided as well.

Laparoscopy is performed by a periumbilical approach. The patient is placed in left lateral decubitus and Trendelenburg position. A second trocar is placed in the suprapubic or right lower quadrant position for insertion of a probe for retraction. An inflamed appendix is erythematous and thickened and appears hypervascular with edema. Some may have a whitish exudate. It is important to visualize the entire appendix, which sometimes can be difficult. Clarke et al.[39] describe three additional signs that suggest appendicitis: adherent omentum to the right iliac fossa, cecal inflammation, or turbid fluid in the right pelvis. These all warrant appendectomy laparoscopically or via laparotomy if the appendix cannot be adequately visualized. Leape et al.[40] prospectively studied 234 patients admitted with a diagnosis of suspected appendicitis. Fifty per cent improved spontaneously without any invasive diagnostic modality; 87 of 234 (37 per cent) had clear clinical criteria for appendicitis and underwent laparotomy. Of these only one had a normal appendix. In 32 of 234 (13 per cent) the diagnosis was equivocal, and laparoscopy was performed. Seventeen patients had appendicitis; 12 patients who had a normal appendix were spared laparotomy. However, 2 patients had false negative results on laparoscopy and subsequently underwent appendectomy via laparotomy. The overall incidence of removing a normal appendix was 1 per cent, a significant reduction from the expected 5 to 10 per cent.

Other authors also found laparoscopy to be useful in this setting, but there was no reduction in the rate of negative results on appendectomy when patients were selected for laparoscopy based on clinical criteria.[5,41] This was primarily because laparoscopy was not 100 per cent accurate in visualizing the appendix.

Laparoscopy is indicated in the evaluation of right lower quadrant pain in selected patients. Those with confounding variables in the clinical picture such as steroid use, previous antibiotic treatment, or a lengthy history of symptoms may be ideal candidates. Patients also at the extremes of age or with other severe illness that preclude laparotomy may also benefit. Finally, women in whom infertility is a risk should undergo laparoscopy. The role of laparoscopy in men with right lower quadrant pain is less obvious. However, since laparoscopic appendectomy is now an option in many centers, the indication for diagnostic laparoscopy in this setting has broadened. More studies are needed to define the false negative and positive rate of laparoscopy in the diagnosis of appendicitis and its true impact on overall outcome.

Conclusions

Diagnostic laparoscopy historically has proved accurate in the staging of malignancy and diagnosis of trauma and right lower abdominal pain. Its true clinical applicability for these indications is controversial in some cases in view of ever increasing sophistication of less invasive diagnostic tests. Selected patients clearly can benefit. The recent explosion of therapeutic laparoscopy in general surgery will certainly broaden its utility in diagnosis, particularly in such areas as mesenteric ischemia[12] and acalculous cholecystitis in the critically ill patient and intra-abdominal hemorrhage in the trauma patient.

REFERENCES

1. Cushieri A. Value of laparoscopy in hepatobiliary disease. Ann R Coll Surg 1975; 57:33–38.
2. Friedman IH, Wolff WI. Laparoscopy—A safe method for liver biopsy in the high risk patient. Am J Gastroenterol 1977; 67:319–323.
3. McCallum RW, Berci G. Laparoscopy in hepatic disease. Gastrointest Endosc 1976; 23:20–24.
4. Wood RAB, Cuscheri A. Laparoscopy for chronic abdominal pain. Br J Surg 1979; 60:900.
5. Whitworth CM, Whitworth PW, Sanfillipo J, Polk HC Jr. Value of diagnostic laparoscopy in young women with possible appendicitis. Surg Gynecol Obstet 1988; 167:187–190.
6. Paterson-Brown S, Eckersley JRT, Sim AJW, Dudley HAF. Laparoscopy as an adjunct to decision making in the 'acute abdomen.' Br J Surg 1986; 73:1022–1024.
7. Warshaw AL, Tepper JE, Shipley WU. Laparoscopy in the staging and planning of therapy for pancreatic cancer. Am J Surg 1986; 151:776–780.
8. Kriplani AK, Kapur BML. Laparoscopy for pre-operative staging and assessment of operability in gastric carcinoma. Gastrointest Endosc 1991; 37:441–443.
9. Gazzaniga AB, Slanton WEW, Bartlett R. Laparoscopy in the diagnosis of blunt and penetrating injuries to the abdomen. Am J Surg 1976; 131:315–318.
10. Carnevale N, Baron N, Delaney HM. Peritoneoscopy as an aid in the diagnosis of abdominal trauma: A preliminary report. J Trauma 1977; 17:634–641.
11. Berci, Dunkelman D, Michel SL, et al. Emergency minilaparoscopy in abdominal trauma: An update. Am J Surg 1983; 146:261–265.
12. Iberti TJ, Salky BA, Onofrey D. Use of bedside laparoscopy to identify intestinal ischemia in postoperative cases of aortic reconstruction. Surgery 1989; 105:686–689.
13. Cortesi N, Zambarda E, Manenti A, et al. Laparoscopy in routine and emergency surgery. Am J Surg 1979; 137:647–649.
14. Berci G, Cuschieri A. *Practical Laparoscopy*. London: Bailliére-Tindall, 1986, pp 82–94.
15. Saleh JW. Laparoscopy. Philadelphia, WB Saunders, 1988.
16. Hasson HM. Modified instrument and method for laparoscopy. Am J Obstet Gynecol 1971; 110:856–887.
17. Coupland GAE, Towend DM, Martin CJ. Peritoneoscopy—Use in assessment of intra-abdominal malignancy. Surgery 1981; 89:645–649.
18. Dagnini G, Caldironi MW, Marin G. Laparoscopy in abdominal staging of esophageal carcinoma. Gastrointest Endosc 1986; 32:400–402.
19. Watt I, Stewart I, Anderson D, et al. Laparoscopy, ultrasound and computed tomography in cancer of the oesophagus and gastric cardia: A prospective comparison for detecting intra-abdominal metastases Br J Surg 1989; 76:1036–1039.
20. Craven JL. International variations in the results of treatment of gastric cancer. *In* Fielding JWL, Newman CE, Ford CHJ, Jones BG, eds. *Gastric Cancer.* Oxford, Pergamon Press, 1981, pp 219–229.
21. Gross E, Bancewicz J, Ingram G. Assessment of gastric cancer by laparoscopy. Br Med J 1984; 288:1577.
22. Possik RA, Franco EL, Pires DR, et al. Sensitivity, specificity, and predictive value of laparoscopy for the staging of gastric cancer and for the detection of liver metastases. Cancer 1986; 58:1–6.
23. Cuschieri A, Hall W, Clark J. Value of laparoscopy in the diagnosis and management of pancreatic cancer. Gut 1978; 19:672–677.
24. Warshaw AL, Gu Z, Wittenberg J, Waltman AC. Preoperative staging and assessment of resectability of pancreatic cancer. Arch Surg 1990; 125:230–233.
25. Meyer-Burg J. The inspection, palpation and biopsy of the pancreas by peritoneoscopy. Endoscopy 1972; 4:99.
26. Ishida H, Furukawa Y, Kuroda H, et al. Laparoscopic observation and biopsy of the pancreas. Endoscopy 1981; 13:68–73.
27. Ishida H, Dohzono T, Furukawa Y, et al. Laparoscopy and biopsy in the diagnosis of malignant intra-abdominal tumors. Endoscopy 1984; 16:140–142.
28. Brady PG, Peebles M, Goldschmid S. Role of laparoscopy in the evaluation of patients with suspected hepatic or peritoneal malignancy. Gastrointest Endosc 1991; 37:27–30.
29. Jori GP, Peschle C. Combined peritoneoscopy and liver biopsy in the diagnosis of hepatic neoplasm. Gastroenterology 1972; 63:1016–1019.
30. Mansi C, Savarino V, Piccotta A, et al. Comparison between laparoscopy, ultrasonography, and computed tomography in widespread and localized liver disease. Gastrointest Endosc 1982; 28:83–85.
31. DeVita VT, Bagley CM, Goodell B, et al. Peritoneoscopy in the staging of Hodgin's disease. Cancer Res 1971; 31:1746–1750.
32. Bagley CM, Thomas LB, Johnson RE, et al. Diagnosis of liver involvement by lymphoma: Results in 96 consecutive peritoneoscopies. Cancer 1973; 31:840–847.
33. Beretta G, Spinelli P, Rilke F, et al. Sequential laparoscopy and laparotomy combined with bone marrow biopsy in staging Hodgkin's disease. Cancer Treat Rep 1976; 60:1231–1237.
34. Sotnikov VN, Agamov AG. Laparoscopic diagnosis of metastases in cancer of the rectum. Sov Med 1974; 10:108–110.
35. Cuschieri A, Hennessy TPJ, Stephens RB, Berci G. Diagnosis of significant abdominal trauma after road traffic accidents: Preliminary results of a multicentre clinical trial comparing minilaparoscopy with peritoneal lavage. Ann R Coll Surg Eng 1988; 70:153–155.
36. Sherwood R, Berci G, Austin E, Morgenstern L. Minilaparoscopy for blunt abdominal trauma. Arch Surg 1980; 115:672–673.
37. Diehl JT, Eisenstat MS, Gillinov S, Rao D. The role of peritoneoscopy in the diagnosis of acute abdominal conditions. Clevel Clin Q 1981; 48:325–330.

38. Anteby SO, Schenker JG, Polishuk WZ. The value of laparoscopy in acute pelvic pain. Ann Surg 1975; 181:484–486.
39. Clarke PJ, Hands LJ, Gough MH, Kettlewell MGW. The use of laparoscopy in the management of right iliac fossa pain. Ann R Coll Surg Engl 1986; 68:68–69.
40. Leape LL, Ramenofsky ML. Laparoscopy of questionable appendicitis—Can it reduce the negative appendectomy rate? Ann Surg 1980; 191:410–413.
41. Gomel V. Laparoscopy in general surgery. Am J Surg 1976; 131:319–323.

Chapter 27
The Acute Abdomen

S. Paterson-Brown
H. A. F. Dudley

Performance in management of the acute abdomen has come under close scrutiny during the last two decades following evidence from computer-aided diagnosis (CAD) studies that have shown clinical diagnostic accuracy in terms of cause to be no more than 75 per cent[1] and often much lower.[2] The use of computers clearly improved these figures by up to 20 per cent. However, in surgical decision-making, it is ultimately the decision whether to operate or not made irrespective of the diagnostic probability that is most important.[3]

A recent prospective audit of acute abdominal pain has demonstrated that the overall in-hospital mortality is on the order of 4 per cent, rising to 8 per cent for perioperative deaths, and peaking for particular conditions at 23 per cent for perforated peptic ulcers and 71 per cent for leaking abdominal aneurysms.[4] Additional data from this study associated the mortality from perforated peptic ulcers with elderly patients and those in whom there had been a delay in presentation or treatment.[5] Similar results can be seen for the treatment of acute appendicitis, not only for mortality[6] but also for perforation[7] and its sequelae.[8] Attempts to reduce what some studies have termed "bad management errors"[2] have inevitably been associated with a certain number of unnecessary operations, which for appendicitis remains around 20 per cent[9] and rises to more than 40 per cent in young women.[10] It is difficult to evaluate the complications of a "negative" laparotomy, but the incidence of complications following an unnecessary appendectomy range between 13 and 17 per cent.[9,11]

ADJUNCTIVE TECHNIQUES TO IMPROVE DECISION-MAKING IN THE PATIENT WITH AN ACUTE ABDOMEN

Over the years a number of additional techniques have been added to clinical assessment of the patient with an acute abdomen and the traditional investigations associated with it. CAD, already mentioned briefly, improves diagnostic accuracy and consequently decision-making. For example, CAD has reduced the incidence of perforation in acute appendicitis, bad management errors (i.e., delay), and also the number of unnecessary laparotomies.[2] However, a large part of its success is the consequence of the use of structured patient data sheets,[12] and it would be fair to say that CAD has not proved popular among clinicians.[13] Ultrasonography is of proven value in the assessment of acute biliary tract disease and acute cholecystitis in particular.[14] The acutely inflamed appendix may be detected using ultrasonography in 86 per cent of patients,[15] but, because the diagnosis relies on visualizing a swollen and edematous appendix, the perforated appendix is less easily seen. Other investigations include peritoneal lavage[16] and fine catheter aspiration peritoneal cytology,[17] both of which provide reliable information on the presence of peritoneal inflammation but cannot predict whether an operation is required. It is only laparoscopy that is in a position to solve all these problems in the patient with an acute abdomen. Not only may the causative diagnosis be established, but in patients in whom the need for surgery is uncertain, laparoscopy will allow the surgeon to look without resorting to laparotomy.

DIAGNOSTIC LAPAROSCOPY

Although first suggested as far back as 1942 for the assessment of blunt abdominal trauma,[18] the use of laparoscopy in the management of the patient with an acute abdomen was not formally evaluated for a further 33 years. At that time, a group of surgeons in America demonstrated that preoperative laparoscopy (before laparotomy) could reduce the incidence of unnecessary laparotomies.[19] Since then other studies, which concentrated primarily on lower abdominal and pelvic pain, have confirmed these results.[20-24] However, until recently there have been few reports on the place of laparoscopy in the patient with an acute abdomen given that all would agree it should not be used on every patient with this problem.

Influence of Laparoscopy on Decision-Making in the Patient with an Acute Abdomen

To identify the role of laparoscopy in the patient with an acute abdomen we classified patients, after initial assessment by the admitting surgeon, according to their need for surgery: A—definitely requires operation; B—definitely does not require operation; and C—need for operation uncertain. This approach is operational rather than diagnostic, which conforms with what is usually in the surgeon's mind. A decision was made in group C whether the surgeon would normally "look and see" (exploratory laparotomy) or "wait and see" (observation/investigation) and then this group underwent laparoscopy under general anesthesia. Early results showed that the potential decision error rate in the uncertain group could be reduced from 19 to 0 per cent using laparoscopy.[25]

Further studies showed that the unnecessary appendectomy rate in the certain group reached 22 per cent compared to only 8 per cent in the uncertain group submitted to laparoscopy.[26] Further analysis revealed that without laparoscopy the combined rate of unnecessary appendectomies in all groups would have been 39 per cent in women compared to only 15 per cent in men. We concluded from these results that all women with suspected appendicitis should undergo laparoscopy before appendectomy irrespective of the certainty of the surgeon, and this view has been supported by studies from other centers.[27,28]

Indications for Diagnostic Laparoscopy in the Patient with an Acute Abdomen

The results from our studies indicate that laparoscopy should be used to assess patients with acute abdominal pain in whom the decision to operate remains uncertain after clinical assessment and in all women with suspected appendicitis. Further improvements to this protocol can be achieved using structured data sheets for initial patient assessment,[29] and these should become routine.[30] Other benefits from laparoscopy include the ability to make a diagnosis in many more patients. The overall incidence of nonspecific abdominal pain of 23 per cent in our studies[31] contrasts with incidences in excess of 40 per cent from others.[32] This ability to make a substantive diagnosis by laparoscopy (Table 27-1) also allows the surgeon to let symptomatic patients go home confident that an intra-abdominal condition requiring surgery is not undetected. Acute appendicitis can be reliably excluded by laparoscopy as the normal appendix can be visualised at laparoscopy in at least three-quarters of patients[33] and with experience this proportion rises to nearly 100 per cent.[27,34] Failure to visualize the appendix does not necessitate removal, as laparoscopic signs of right iliac fossa inflammation usually indicate the presence of acute appendicitis or an alternative cause for the patient's symptoms may be identified. Early recognition of gynecologic conditions such as pelvic inflammatory disease and the Fitz-Hugh and Curtis syndrome[35] (perihepatitis secondary to gynecologic infection) permits early treatment, which is important if the complications of these conditions (e.g., infertility) are to be reduced.[36]

Table 27-1. Diagnosis in 125 Patients with Acute Abdominal Pain Undergoing Laparoscopy in Whom the Clinical Decision to Operate was Uncertain

Diagnosis	No. of Patients
Acute appendicitis	48
Pelvic inflammatory disease	24
Nonspecific abdominal pain	23
Ovarian cysts	14
Peritoneal adhesions	4
Metastatic disease	3
Perforated diverticulitis	2
Ectopic gestation	2
Mesenteric infarction	1
Empyema of gallbladder	1
Torsion of appendix epiploica	1
Primary peritonitis	1
Retrograde menstruation	1

Table 27-2. Patients with Acute Abdominal Pain in Whom Laparoscopy Should Not Be Performed

Contraindications to laparoscopy
  Severe cardiorespiratory disease
  Morbid obesity[a]
  Intestinal obstruction
  Large hiatal and external hernias
  Multiple previous abdominal operations[a]
  Clotting abnormalities[a]
  Children (unless a pediatric laparoscope is available)[a]
Presumptive clinical diagnosis in which diagnostic laparoscopy is unlikely to be helpful
  Acute pancreatitis
  Renal tract disease
  Visceral perforation (proven by free intraperitoneal gas on plain x-ray films)[b]

[a] Relative contraindications.
[b] Perforated peptic ulcers can now be treated laparoscopically.

As long as gynecologists and abdominal surgeons share the predecision management of patients with acute lower abdominal pain, there will also be circumstances in which a condition, such as an ectopic pregnancy or a leaking pyosalpinx, is suspected in a female patient. On both sides the diagnosis and therefore the subsequent management may be wrong. In consequence, we believe that there is now adequate evidence from clinical experience that a female patient with acute lower abdominal pain, whatever the antecedent history and physical examination, should be seen in consultation by a gynecologist and abdominal surgeon with a view to a joint decision on laparoscopy.

As in other fields of laparoscopic surgery, there are patients with acute abdominal pain in whom diagnostic laparoscopy is either contraindicated or unlikely to be helpful. The criteria used in our studies are shown in Table 27-2, and patients falling into these categories represented one-third of all patients admitted with acute abdominal pain.

Acute Abdominal Conditions and Therapeutic Laparoscopic Surgery

The role of laparoscopic surgery for acute abdominal conditions remains to be formally established. Laparoscopic appendectomy is becoming increasingly popular,[37] and the procedure of diagnostic laparoscopy followed by laparoscopic appendectomy is likely to become commonplace. Whether a similar scenario could be envisaged for perforated peptic ulcers and acute diverticular disease remains to be seen. Reports on peptic ulcers have described the use of fibrin sealant and omental patches to seal small perforations, with gastrostomy being used for large ulcers in the stomach[38]; we have used intraperitoneal sutures to apply the omental patch. The advantage of laparoscopically performed peritoneal lavage in these patients is easily understood, and one option that should be explored is whether all patients with suspected perforated peptic ulcers should undergo upper gastrointestinal contrast studies before surgery to provide evidence of any persistent leak.[39] If a leak is not shown, then laparoscopy, lavage, and drainage only may suffice. By the same token, patients with acute diverticulitis in whom abscess or perforation is suspected should undergo a contrast enema to reveal any pericolic leak.[40] Laparoscopy could then be used to examine the diverticular segment wih the ability to proceed to drainage or resection. Severity of disease will decide how much can be done through the laparoscope.

Adhesions are often divided at laparoscopy, usually to improve access and exposure. However the value of adhesiolysis in patients with chronic abdominal pain remains controversial.[41] Laparoscopy is unlikely to become first line treatment for patients with established adhesive intestinal obstruction and this is, in fact, considered a contraindication in our own practice.

Endoscopic techniques and technology have improved, and most laparoscopic surgeons do not now consider acute cholecystitis a contraindication to laparoscopic cholecystectomy. Although the conversion rate to open operation is much higher than for patients with nonacute conditions, the morbidity and mortality do not differ.[42] When the gallbladder is frankly gangrenous, open operation is indicated to prevent the much higher risk of rupture during laparoscopic mobilization and dissection.

Conclusion

Emergency admissions constitute by far the largest proportion of the overall general surgical workload and use of available resources in the United Kingdom.[43] Incorporation of laparoscopy and laparoscopic surgery into patient management is likely to have important benefits on the costs of delivery of surgical care.

We suggest that laparoscopy should be routine in the management of patients with acute abdominal pain in whom the decision to operate is uncertain and in all women with suspected appendicitis, irrespective of the certainty with which the diagnosis is made, because of the high error rate in this group. The decision to proceed to laparoscopic therapy depends on many factors, of which surgical experience, severity of disease, and the logistics of performing emergency laparoscopic surgery "out of normal hours" currently are the most pertinent. Laparoscopy is safe, relatively simple to learn, and, following the enthusiastic acceptance of laparoscopic cholecystectomy, has already become much more familiar to surgeons than was the case even 5 years ago. The complication rate associated with gynecologic laparoscopy has been approximately 3 per cent with a mortality of 8 per 100,000 procedures.[44] These figures include both diagnostic and operative (mainly tubal surgery) laparoscopic procedures.

Conditions causing acute abdominal pain in which laparoscopy (with or witnout laparoscopic therapy) has a role include acute appendicitis, acute gynecological conditions, adhesions without overt intestinal obstruction, acute diverticulitis, perforated peptic ulcer, and acute cholecystitis. Laparoscopy may also be a benefit in the management of patients with other conditions such as mesenteric infarction and disseminated malignancy presenting as acute abdominal pain. As the use of diagnostic laparoscopy becomes more popular in patients with an acute abdomen, the opportunity to perform other emergency laparoscopic procedures will be presented.

REFERENCES

1. de Dombal FT, Leaper DJ, Staniland JR, McCann AP, Horrocks JC. Computer-aided diagnosis of acute abdominal pain. Br Med J 1972; 2:9–13.
2. Adams ID, Chan M, Clifford PC, et al. Computer aided diagnosis of acute abdominal pain: A multicentre study. Br Med J 1986; 293:800–804.
3. Dudley HAF, Paterson-Brown S, Thompson JN, Eckerssey JRT. Prospective scenarios: A method of evaluating new decision tools. World J Surg 1989; 13:277–280.
4. Irvin TT. Abdominal pain: A surgical audit of 1190 emergency admissions. Br J Surg 1989; 76:1121–1125.
5. Irvin TT. Mortality of perforated peptic ulcer: A case for risk stratification in elderly patients. Br J Surg 1989; 76:215–218.
6. Hunter IC, Paterson JG, Davidson AI. Deaths from acute appendicitis: A review of twenty-one cases in Scotland from 1974–1979. J R Coll Surg Edinb 1986; 31:161–163.
7. Moss JG, Barrie JL, Gunn AA. Delay in surgery for acute apppendicitis. J R Coll Surg Edinb 1985; 30:290–293.
8. Mueller BA, Daling JR, Moore DE, et al. Appendectomy and the risk of tubal infertility. N Engl J Med 1986; 315:1506–1508.
9. Deutsch AA, Shani N, Reiss R. Are some appendectomies unnecessary? J R Coll Surg Edinb 1983; 28:35–40.
10. Woodward A, Hemingway D, Greaney G, Murphy C. Which patients should undergo laparoscopy? (Letter). Br Med J 1988; 296:1740.
11. Chang PC, Hogle HH, Welling DR. The fate of the negative appendix. Am J Surg 1973; 126:752–754.
12. Lawrence PC, Clifford PC, Taylor IF. Acute abdominal pain: Computer aided diagnosis by non-medically qualified staff. Ann R Coll Surg Engl 1987; 69:233–234.
13. Sutton GC. Computer-aided diagnosis: A review. Br J Surg 1989; 76:82–85.
14. Ralls PW, Colletti PM, Lapin SA, et al. Real-time sonography in suspected acute cholecystitis. Radiology 1985; 5:767–771.
15. Ooms HWA, Koumans RKJ, Ho Kang You PJ, Puylaert JBCM. Ultrasonography in the diagnosis of acute appendicitis. Br J Surg 1991; 78:315–318.
16. Hoffmann J. Peritoneal lavage in the diagnosis of the acute abdomen of non-traumatic origin. Acta Chir Scand 1987; 153:561–565.
17. Stewart RJ, Gupta RK, Purdie GL, Isbister WH. Fine-catheter aspiration cytology of peritoneal cavity improves decision-making about difficult cases of acute abdominal pain. Lancet 1986; 2:1414–1415.
18. Estes WL. Nonpenetrating trauma of the abdomen. Surg Gynecol Obstet 1942; 70:419–424.
19. Sugarbaker PH, Bloom BS, Sanders JH, Wilson RE. Preoperative laparoscopy in diagnosis of acute abdominal pain. Lancet 1975; 1:442–445.
20. Anteby SO, Schenker JG, Polishuk WZ. The value of laparoscopy in acute pelvic pain. Ann Surg 1975; 181:484–486.

21. Leape LL, Ramenofsky ML. Laparoscopy for questionable appendicitis; can it reduce the negative appendectomy rate? Ann Surg 1980; 191:410–413.
22. Anderson JL, Bridgewater FHG. Laparoscopy in the diagnosis of acute lower abdominal pain. Austr N Z J Surg 1981; 51:462–464.
23. Deutsch AA, Zelikovsky A, Reiss R. Laparoscopy in the prevention of unnecessary appendectomies: A prospective study. Br J Surg 1982; 69:336–337.
24. Clarke PJ, Hands W, Gough MH, Kettlewell MG. The use of laparoscopy in the management of right iliac fossa pain. Ann R Coll Surg Engl 1986; 68:68–69.
25. Paterson-Brown S, Eckersley JRT, Sim AJWS, Dudley HAF. Laparoscopy as an adjunct to decision-making in the "acute abdomen." Br J Surg 1986; 73:1022–1024.
26. Paterson-Brown S, Thompson JN, Eckersley JRT, et al. Which patient with suspected appendicitis should undergo laparoscopy? Br Med J 1988; 296:1363–1364.
27. Spirtos NM, Eisenkop SM, Spirtos TW, et al. Laparoscopy as a diagnostic aid in cases of suspected appendicitis. Its use in women of reproductive age. Am J Obstet Gynecol 1987; 156:90–94.
28. Foster HMcA. Which patients should undergo laparoscopy? (Points) Br Med J 1988; 297:489.
29. Paterson-Brown S, Vipond MN, Simms K, et al. Clinical decision making and laparoscopy versus computer prediction in the management of the acute abdomen. Br J Surg 1989; 76:1011–1013.
30. Paterson-Brown S. Strategies for reducing inappropriate laparotomy rate in the acute abdomen. Br Med J 1991; 303:1115–1118.
31. Paterson-Brown S. The acute abdomen: The role of laparoscopy. In Williamson RCN, Thompson JN, eds. Gastrointestinal Emergencies, Part I. London, Ballière Tindall, 1991, pp 691–703.
32. Gray DWR, Collin J. Non-specific abdominal pain as a cause of acute admission to hospital. Br J Surg 1987; 74:239–242.
33. Paterson-Brown S, Olufunwa SA, Galazka N, Simmons SC. Visualisation of the normal appendix at laparoscopy. J R Coll Surg Edinb 1986; 31:106–107.
34. Crichton D. Ultrasonography for diagnosing acute appendicitis (Points). Br Med J 1988; 297:857.
35. Wood JJ, Bolton JP, Cannon SR. Biliary-type pain as a manifestation of genital tract infection: The Curtis-Fitz and Hugh syndrome. Br J Surg 1982; 69:251–253.
36. Pearce JM. Pelvic inflammatory disease. Br Med J 1990; 300:1090–1091.
37. Leahy PF. Technique of laparoscopic appendectomy. Br J Surg 1989; 76:616.
38. Mouret P, Francois Y, Vignal J, et al. Laparoscopic treatment of perforated peptic ulcer. Br J Surg 1991; 77:1006.
39. Crofts TJ, Park KGM, Steele RJC, Chung SSC, Li AKC. A randomized trial of non-operative treatment for perforated peptic ulcer. N Engl J Med 1989; 320:970–973.
40. Kourtesis GJ, Williams SE. Acute diverticulitis: Safety and value of contrast studies in predicting need for operation. Austr N Z J Surg. 1988; 58:801–804.
41. Alexander-Williams J. Do adhesions cause pain? Br Med J 1987; 294:659–660.
42. Domergue J, Fabre JM, Guillon F, et al. Laparoscopic cholecystectomy in acute and non-acute chlolecystolithiasis. Res Surg 1991; 3:147–149.
43. Ellis BW, Rivett RC, Dudley HAF. Extending the use of clinical audit data: A resource planning model. Br Med J 1990; 301:159–162.
44. Chamberlain GVP, Carron Brown JA. The Report of the Working Party of the Confidential Enquiry into Gynaecological Laparoscopy. London, Royal College of Obstetricians and Gynaecologists, 1978.

Chapter 28
Inguinofemoral Hernias

Titus D. Duncan
Edward M. Mason

More than 100 years have passed since the first true hernia repair was performed by the Italian surgeon Edourdo Bassini. Prior to the revolutionary work of Bassini, inguinal hernias were repaired by simply ligating or excising the hernial sac at the external inguinal ring, leaving the external oblique aponeurosis undisturbed.[1] In 1884 the field of hernia repair was inspired by introducing a revolutionary concept that has since been the basis of modern-day hernia repair. The technique reconstructs the "floor" of the inguinal canal by suturing the conjoined tendon to the inguinal ligament after high ligation of the hernial sac. A recurrence rate of less than 10 per cent was reportedly achieved with this procedure when surgeons of the time were accustomed to failure rates up to 50 per cent and an associated mortality rate of up to 7 per cent.[2] More importantly, however, for the first time in surgical history, the results could be reproduced by other well-trained surgeons.

Shortly thereafter numerous modifications of this technique were rapidly introduced, each using the inguinal ligament as a primary anchoring structure. Techniques described by Bull and Cooley[3], and later by Ferguson and Andrews[3,4], all relied on the strength of the inguinal (Poupart's) ligament for success, the sole difference among these repairs being the positioning of the spermatic cord. Consequently, this breakthrough focused surgical attention onto the posterior wall of the inguinal canal as a vital element in the successful repair of groin hernias. It is interesting that little has been added to this very basic concept of hernia repair since this innovation was introduced more than 100 years ago.

ETIOLOGY

The etiology of most inguinal hernias is a congenital persistence of the embryologic processus vaginalis. By definition, this congenital persistence constitutes an indirect inguinal hernia. Whether an indirect hernia is present at birth or develops later in life, the causative factor, a persistent processus vaginalis, is the same.

Direct inguinal hernias, which occur medial to the inferior epigastric vessels, are thought to be associated with both congenital and environmental factors.[5] For example, patients who have a relatively high arch of their transversus aponeurosis are at increased risk for direct herniation. Despite common beliefs held by the general public, there is little evidence to support the suggestion that trauma associated with heavy lifting or heavy straining is a causative factor in any type of hernia. However, increased intra-abdominal pressure combined with a weak posterior inguinal wall is important in the development of acquired hernias.

Age plays a major role in the occurrence of

inguinal hernia. The peak incidence of indirect hernia is during infancy when about 50 per cent of men have a patent vaginal process.[6] The direct inguinal hernia is seen almost entirely in the elderly as this group has a greater predisposition to attenuated fascial structures.

Sex is important as a predisposing factor to various hernias. The descent of the testis to the scrotum can account for the higher incidence of indirect hernias in the male population. Femoral hernias are three times more common in women than in men. And finally direct inguinal hernias are much more common in the elderly male than it is in the female population.

TREATMENT

Over one-half million Americans undergo inguinal herniorrhaphy each year in the United States.[2] Of that number 5,000 to 50,000 repairs are done for hernia recurrence. Unfortunately, this rate of recurrence contributes to increased health care costs as well as to increased patient morbidity. This cost is further amplified by physician fees and the employer-employee losses from work-related hernias and time out of work.

Fortunately, serious complications are uncommon in hernia surgery, but they do occur. Complications of hernia repair are primarily related to surgical manipulation and dissection in the inguinal area. These include inadvertent severance of contents within the inguinal canal, i.e., vas deferens, sensory nerves, testicular blood supply, and injury to adjacent structures such as bowel, urinary bladder, or femoral vessels.

Conventional herniorrhaphy, consisting of repair of the posterior inguinal wall, has been the mainstay of therapy since the landmark work of Edourdo Bassini in 1896. With improved surgical skills and technique overall results have improved and the complication rate has substantially decreased. However, conventional repair is still accompanied by a significant rate of recurrence, postoperative discomfort, and loss of economic gains. Recent studies show that recurrence after traditional hernia repair ranges from 7 to 21 per cent, with a rate as high as 20 per cent after first time repair of recurrent hernias.[6] These factors related to traditional hernia repair have led surgeons and patients to consider alternative approaches to the conventional methods of repair.

Laparoendoscopic Surgery

In an attempt to address some of the current drawbacks to conventional surgery, recent efforts have been made to find less invasive surgical techniques. The use of laparoendoscopic surgery is rapidly growing, and it is becoming a popular alternative to conventional surgery for a variety of surgically treated disorders. The most noted of late in this arena has been laparoscopic cholecystectomy for gallbladder disease. Other minimally invasive procedures such as laparoscopic appendectomy, laparoscopic endoscopic gynecologic procedures, and laparoscopic bowel surgery are being done and accepted with increasing frequency. With continuing improvement in technology we are finding that when done safely, laparoendoscopic surgery in certain settings can be associated with decreased postoperative pain, earlier return to normal levels of physical activity, and less cosmetic deformity.

Anatomy and Definitions

The conventional treatment for inguinal hernia has always been surgical repair. Whether repair involved high ligation of the hernial sac or detailed reconstruction of the inguinal floor, thorough and accurate "anatomical knowledge" of the inguinal region is mandatory for effective hernia repair.

Although herniorrhaphy is one of the most common surgical procedures performed in the United States today, the anatomy of the inguinal canal is still one of the most controversial and misunderstood areas in the field of general surgery. This is evidenced by the variety of procedures used today to essentially effect the same objective reconstruction of the defective inguinal floor.

It is astonishing that few surgeons are versed in the anatomy of the inguinal region. Training in hernia surgery has historically involved instruction on a "hand-me-down" basis. In most teaching institutions, the technique is typically taught by a senior surgical house officer who instructs a junior level resident in suturing two opposing fascial structures to reconstruct the anatomic defect. In addition, textbook illustrations, by necessity, portray the inguinal anatomy in a two-dimensional image, leading to distortion of anatomic relations. A three-dimensional mental conception of structural relations must be acquired if one is to understand groin anat-

334 Surgery for Other Disorders

omy and the fundamental features of a groin hernial repair[7] (Fig. 28-1).

Finally, there is the problem of nomenclature. Controversy over labels of anatomic structures within the literature continues to be a source of perpetual misunderstanding in hernial anatomy. Adherance to strict definition of these terms is of vital importance.

Definitions

The term *aponeurosis* in the context of inguinal anatomy implies a flat, dense, white tendon of insertion of one of the three flat muscles of the lateral abdominal wall: external oblique, internal oblique, and transverse abdominal. These aponeuroses join in the lower abdomen to form the anterior rectus muscle sheath.[7] An aponeurosis, being a tendon, is composed of strong collagenous tissue. The individual fiber bundles within the flat tendon can easily be seen.

A *fascia* is a condensation of connective tissue into a definable homogeneous layer. Fascia may vary from a thin transparent layer of no intrinsic strength to a more easily observed thicker layer of tissue. Such tissues invest the muscular and aponeurotic layers of the groin, but lack the organization and intrinsic tensile strength of the thicker aponeurosis.

The term *ligament* is applied to any definable tissue that bands two or more structures, whether bony or visceral, and may refer to structures of either areolar or aponeurotic consistency.

When pertaining to inguinal hernias one must take care not to confuse the similar terms transversus abdominis aponeurosis and transversalis fascia. Unfortunately, these terms are often erroneously used interchangeably. Transversalis fascia varies in density and possesses little intrinsic strength. It can be thin, is often transparent, and by itself has little capacity to secure an effective barrier from hernial protrusion. Transversus aponeu-

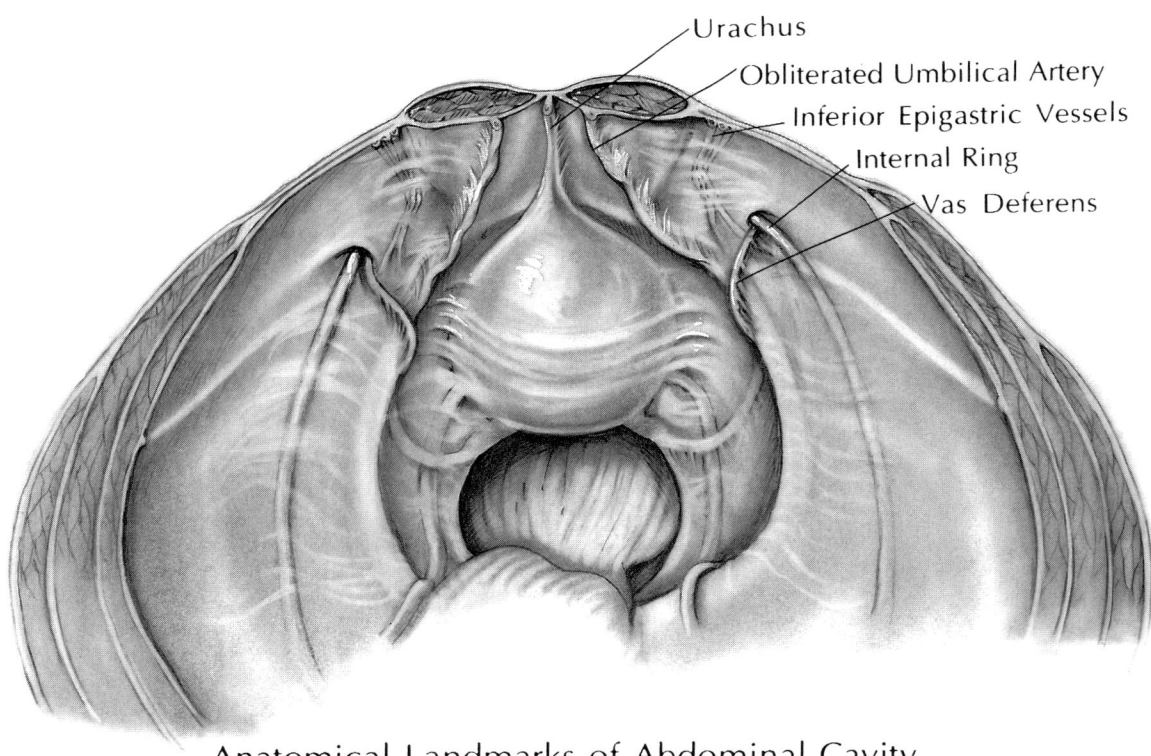

Figure 28-1. Surface anatomy of the anterior abdominal wall showing the cardinal landmarks utilized in laparoscopic hernia repairs.

rosis is a thicker, stronger fibrous band of tissue that when used in the proper setting can provide adequate foundation of a secure inguinal hernia repair.

LAPAROSCOPIC HERNIA REPAIR

Laparoscopic inguinal hernia repair was first felt to be a possibility following the merging of three separate historical events in the field of general surgery: (1) introduction of the preperitoneal approach to groin hernias, (2) introduction of synthetic mesh materials, and (3) utilization of the laparoscope.

Preperitoneal Approach

Thomas Annadale (1876) of Edinburgh pioneered the modern transabdominal preperitoneal approach. In 1891 Tait described the advantages of this posterior approach. These included ease of pulling out rather than pushing back herniated bowel, less hemorrhage, facilitated bowel resection, and no damage to the inguinal canal and its contents.[8] Bates further advanced the concept of this approach and used "transversalis fascia" in the repair.[9]

The definitive preperitoneal procedure for the repair of groin hernias was first described by Cheatle in 1921. Henry renewed interest in the approach and pursued study of the technique in 1936. A number of other surgeons during the 1940s and 1950s pursued the procedure with sporadic results. This method failed to flourish until Nyhus (1955) began to use the technique and reported favorable results in primary inguinal repair.

Prosthetic Repair

The use of prosthetic material has now become well established in the surgical armamentarium of hernia repair. Despite the application of appropriate surgical judgment and proper technique in primary herniorrhaphy, some hernias recur following primary repair. Recurrence after inguinal herniorrhaphy usually results from undue tension at the suture line or inadequate intrinsic strength of the tissues. In an effort to reduce this recurrence rate, the concept of a "tension-free" 24-hour hernia repair was introduced by Lichtenstein et al.[10] Prior to the work of Lichtenstein, mesh was used primarily in those patients with very large hernias or recurrent hernial defects. However, reports of excellent results from those using mesh repair techniques have recently inspired increased popularity of these materials in primary hernia repair. Encouraging results have been produced with this approach with recurrence rates of less than 2 per cent and minimal complications.

Laparoscopy

Endoscopic surgery has rapidly become a popular alternative to traditional operative procedures for a variety of diseases. Laparoscopic appendectomy, laparoscopic biliary procedures, and laparoscopic gynecologic procedures have all become accepted endoscopic procedures. When performed safely these minimally invasive techniques can offer substantial savings in total health care costs and decrease postoperative pain and morbidity over that provided with conventional open procedures.

Specifically for groin hernia repair, laparoscopy provides excellent visualization of the posterior inguinal wall without the morbidity and pain of extensive groin dissection. Combining this mode of visualization with accepted preperitoneal techniques of repair and prosthetic reinforcement has led to a new approach to groin hernia repair.

Several authors have recently reported their experience with laparoscopic inguinal hernia repair. Popp[11] reported the incidental repair of a direct inguinal hernia during a laparoscopic myomectomy using a dura mater patch graft over the defect. The graft was anchored into place using endoscopic suture to the peritoneum overlying the defect. Ger et al.[12] reported his study on laparoscopic repair of indirect inguinal hernias in beagle dogs using a special stapling device that approximates and closes the peritoneal opening of the hernial sac. Leonard Schultz has performed laparoscopic hernia repair by placing polypropylene mesh material into the inguinal canal after dissection of the peritoneal sac. The peritoneum is closed over this mesh with staples. The logic behind this approach is to obliterate the inguinal canal, thereby inhibiting visceral herniation. John Corbitt performs a repair by transecting the peritoneal sac and opening into the preperitoneal space. A piece of prosthetic mesh is rolled into a plug and inserted into the canal. Another piece of polypropylene mesh is then secured over the ring, and the peritoneum is reapproximated. Fitzgibbons places a generous piece of polypropylene mesh over the defect, but places it intraperitoneally.[13] The sac is left in situ and the mesh is secured to the peritoneum. To decrease adhesions he then sutures an absorbable adhesion barrier made of oxidized regenerated cellulose directly to the abdominal side of the prosthesis. It is too soon to extract meaningful data from any of these series.

Laparoscopic Preperitoneal Mesh Repair

To further reduce the incidence of recurrence after hernia repair, the use of synthetic mesh has become vital. The addition of mesh permits tension-free reconstruction of the posterior inguinal wall that when used in the proper setting produces permanent tightness of the posterior wall with minimal complications.[14]

The site of superficial emergence of inguinofemoral hernias depends directly on the type of hernia (e.g., an indirect hernia emerges lateral to the inferior epigastric vessels). However, without exception, each inguinofemoral hernia begins by passing through the posterior inguinal wall. For this reason, it has become apparent that the posterior inguinal wall represents the optimal depth to conduct repair of the inguinal defect. The procedure providing the most direct access to this posterior inguinal structure is the preperitoneal approach. Additionally, this procedure avoids complications secondary to trauma to the superficial inguinal nerves and testicular blood supply that both reside in the inguinal region.

Nonetheless, access to the groin using the preperitoneal approach still requires dissection through layers of subcutaneous tissue, fascia, and muscle. To avoid this soft tissue trauma, access to this area through the laparoscope seems to be the logical solution to this problem. Laparoscopy provides excellent exposure with ease in identification of anatomic structures and avoiding extensive soft tissue dissection. It provides a more direct approach, traversing only the peritoneal layer to access the posterior inguinal wall.

Laparoscopic Preperitoneal Hernia Repair

Repair of inguinal hernias using the preperitoneal approach can be accomplished through the laparoscope. Detailed understanding and working knowledge of anatomy is essential in using this approach.

INDIRECT HERNIA

Upon entering the abdominal cavity with the laparoscope, access to the preperitoneal space is accomplished. Once entry to this space has been gained, preperitoneal hernia repair can be done in one of two ways. In the first method, described by Nyhus,[15] the peritoneum is dissected as shown in (Fig. 28-2). Dissection is carried laterally and the indirect sac (peritoneum) is transected, leaving the inguinal portion of the sac in situ. Identification of anatomic landmarks and vital structures is essential using this technique to avoid costly injuries to major adjacent structures, i.e., iliac vessels or bladder. The peritoneum is incised medial and inferior to the internal ring (Fig. 28-2). Dissection is then carried out caudad to identify Cooper's ligament and the iliopubic tract (Fig. 28-3). We completely dissect the peritoneum and connective tissue from the iliac vein for complete exposure. Careful and accurate identification of these major structures is vital to avoid injury. After excising the proximal peritoneal sac, the dilated internal ring is tightened by sutures placed through the transversalis fascial ring (Fig. 28-4).

A second technique uses synthethic mesh as an inlay graft secured into place over the posterior inguinal wall after high ligation of the sac. After excision of the proximal peritoneal sac, a synthetic inlay mesh graft is secured to the iliopubic tract or Cooper's ligament inferiorly and the transversus aponeurosis superiorly. The mesh is then applied over the internal ring and secured laterally to the transversus superiorly and iliopubic tract inferiorly (Fig. 28-5). The peritoneum is then closed over the mesh effecting high ligation of the hernia sac. This obviates the need for tedious suturing and essentially creates a tension-free repair.

There are several benefits to using an "inlay" mesh repair (Fig. 28-5), where the prostheses is placed in the preperitoneal space as a buttress against positive intra-abdominal pressure. In contrast, with an "onlay" patch repair (Fig. 28-6) the mesh is secured in an anterior fashion to the posterior inguinal wall as classically described by Lichtenstein et al.[10] The inlay repair uses Pascal's principle (Fig. 28-6), which states that a gas or liquid at rest in a closed container transmits a pressure

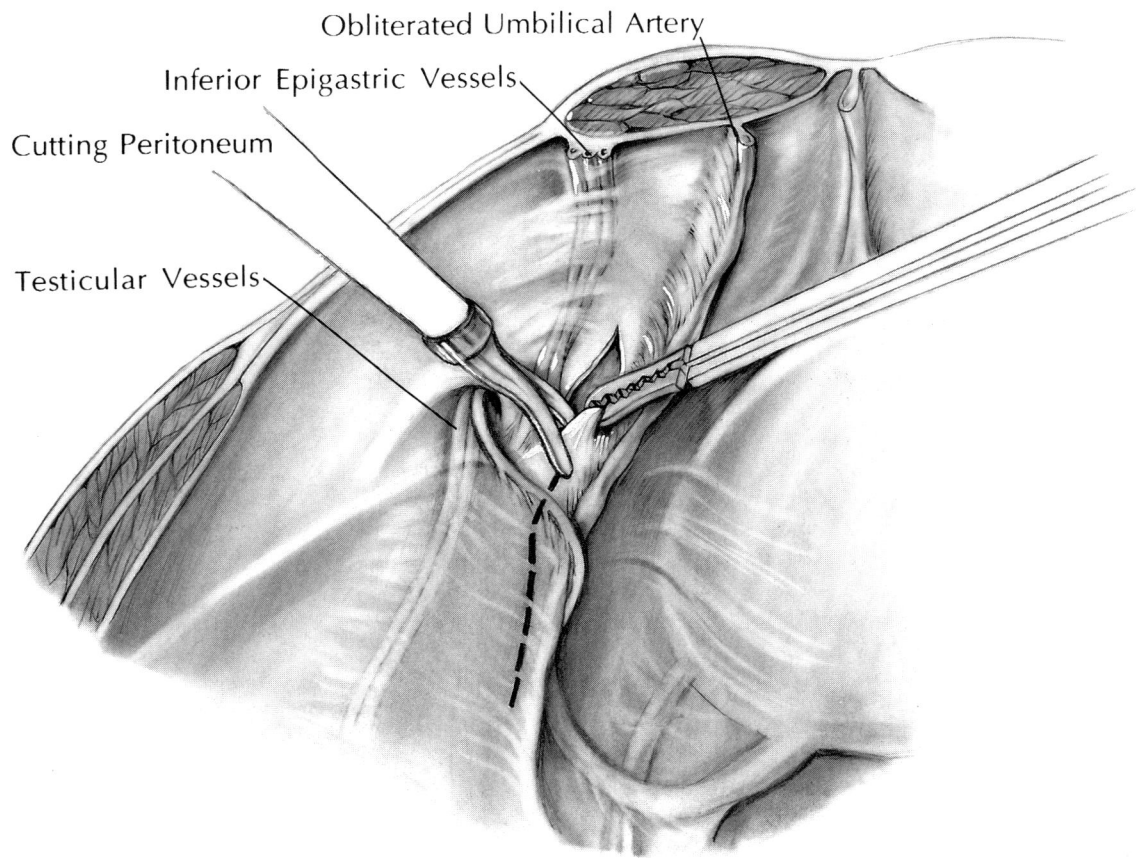

Figure 28-2. Dissection of the peritoneum for entry into the preperitoneal space.

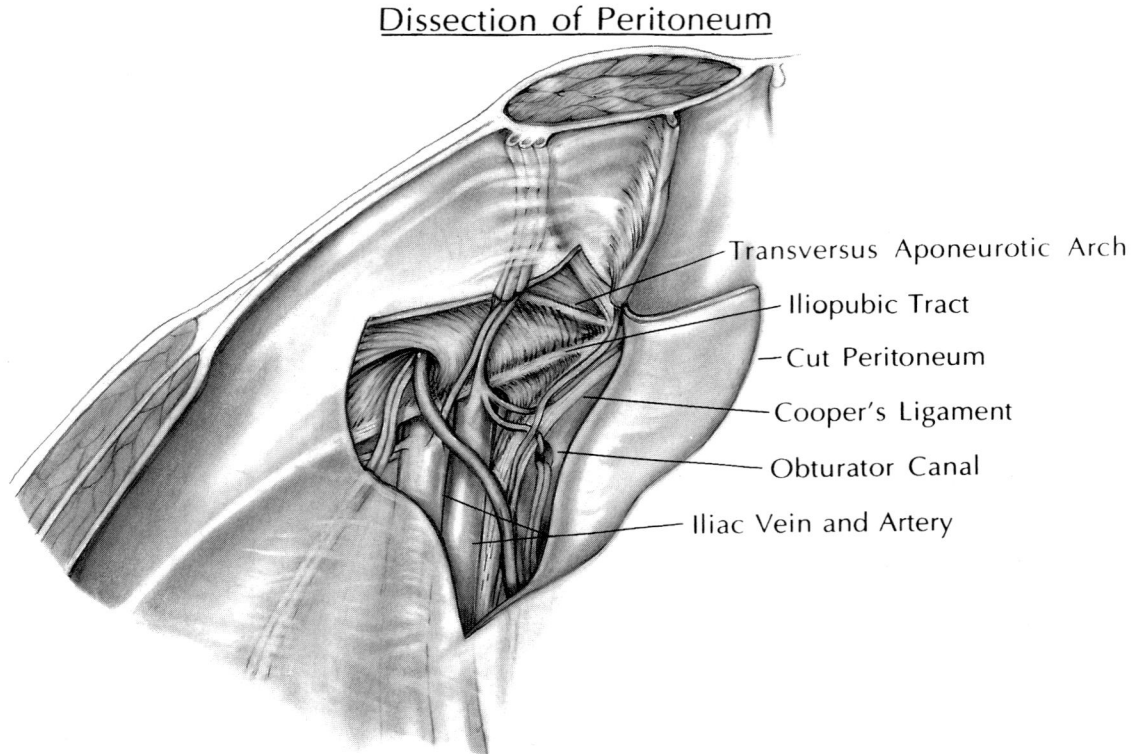

Figure 28-3. Identification of Cooper's ligament and the iliopubic tract.

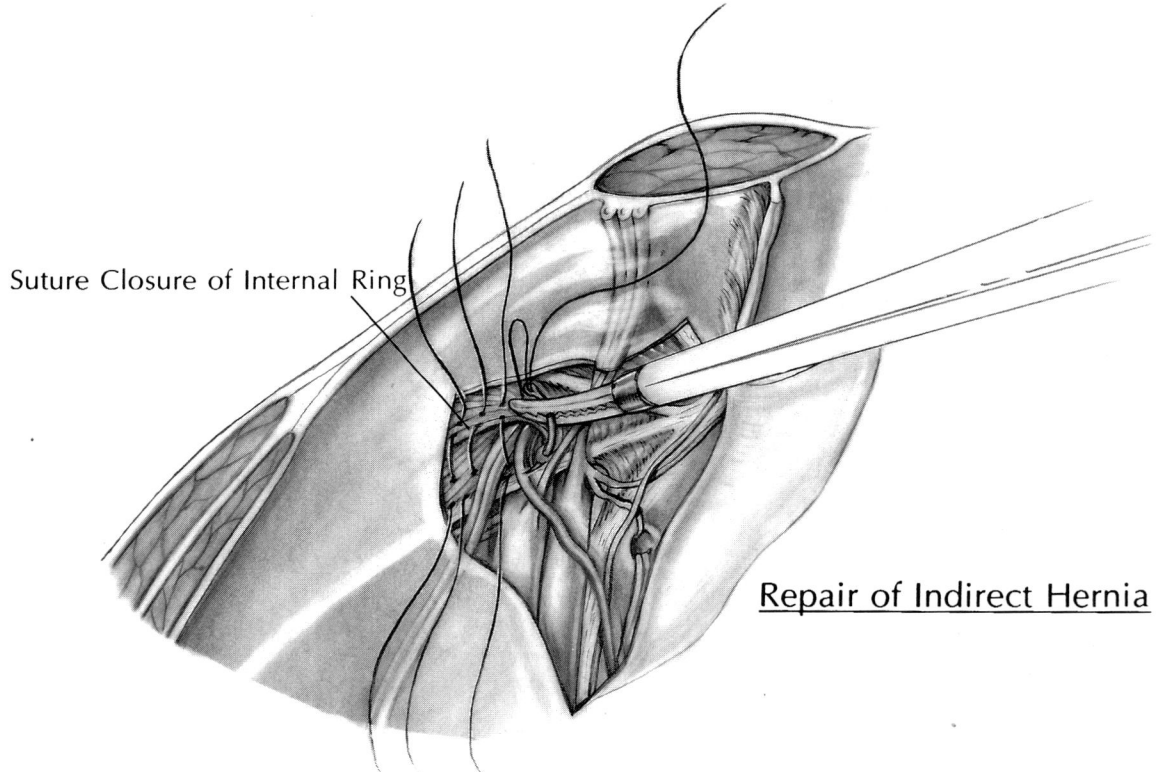

Figure 28-4. Tightening of the internal ring with interrupted sutures.

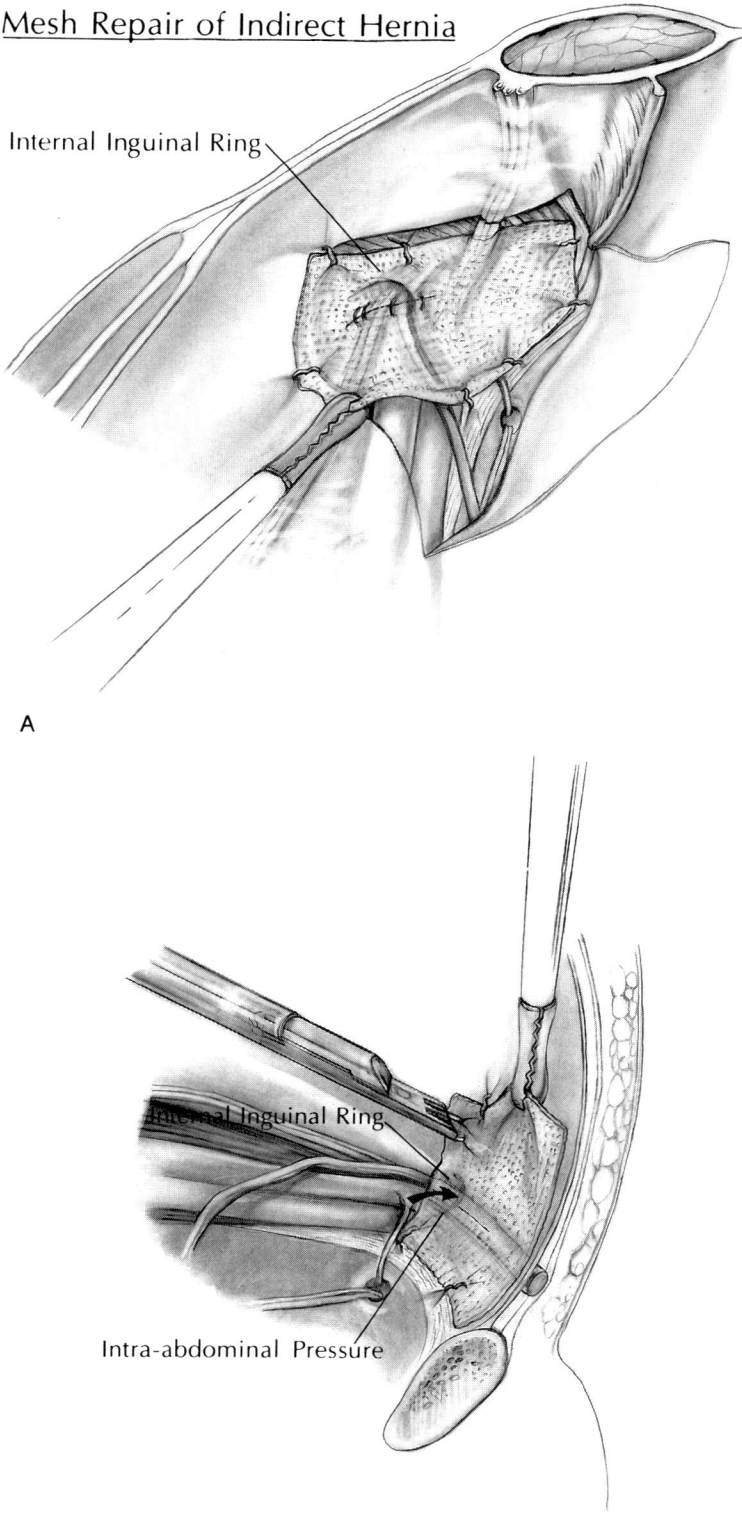

Figure 28-5. Preperitoneal repair using an "inlay" mesh repair. A. The mesh graft is secured to Cooper's ligament, the transversus aponeurosis, and the iliopubic tract. It covers the internal inguinal ring. B. Intra-abdominal pressure pushes the mesh against the internal ring.

change in one part without loss to the walls of the container. The principle further states that the pressure in a gas or fluid at rest is the same on all directions and that the pressure is the same on all planes passing through a specific point. These advantages can be seen graphically in Figure 28-6.

DIRECT HERNIA

Direct hernias occur medial to the inferior epigastric vessels and are lateral to the border of the rectus abdominis muscle. These defects usually have a relatively wide orifice and require a slightly different therapeutic approach. Again the peritoneum is incised and anatomic structures are carefully identified. We secure the mesh in a similar fashion to the transversus aponeurosis and to Cooper's ligament (Fig. 28-7). We feel that because of the size of the orifice of these hernias, there is a risk for the mesh to slide within the hernial cavity. We therefore reduce the pressure of pneumoperitoneum to 7 to 8 mm Hg before securing the mesh into place. This maneuver helps to avoid relaxation of the mesh into the cavity. Once the mesh is in place, the peritoneum is closed over the prosthesis.

Suture techniques for direct inguinal hernia repair are shown in Figure 28-8.

FEMORAL HERNIA

The femoral canal is located lateral and superior to Cooper's ligament and posterior to the iliopubic tract. The defect can be readily seen through the laparoscopic approach. Once the peritoneum is dissected an inlay patch is placed and secured to the iliopubic tract and interiorly to Cooper's ligament (Fig. 28-9). The suture technique would approximate Cooper's ligament and iliopubic tract as shown in Fig. 28-10.

Conclusion

Repair of inguinal hernias using the laparoscopic preperitoneal approach has several theoretical advantages over the traditional approach. The decrease in postoperative pain and shortened recovery are significant in comparison to the conventional anterior approach. With a significant decrease in time off from work one would theoretically expect a significant decrease in overall health care dollars spent in treatment of this entity. Only long term follow-up and study will allow us to evaluate these theoretical advantages and allow us to weigh the risk to benefit ratio.

We must clearly exercise extreme caution in our comparison of this technique to tradi-

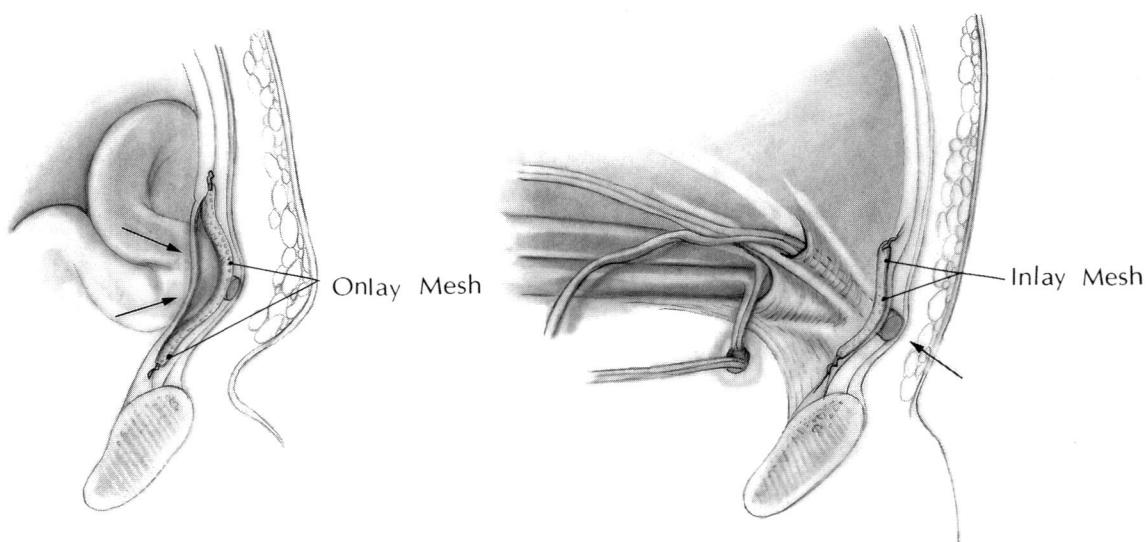

Figure 28-6. Differences between "onlay" and "inlay" mesh repairs of inguinal hernias. The "inlay" mesh takes advantage of Pascal's pressure principle.

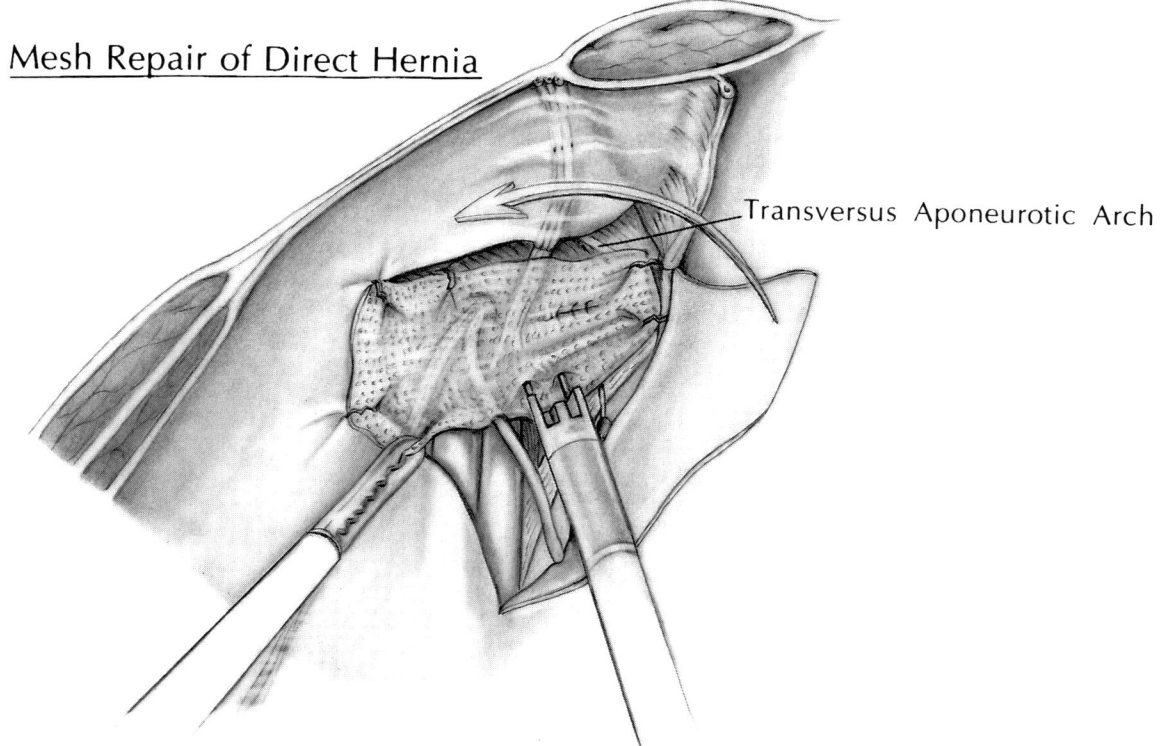

Figure 28-7. Preperitoneal mesh repair of a direct inguinal hernia. The mesh is secured to the transversus aponeurosis and to Cooper's ligament.

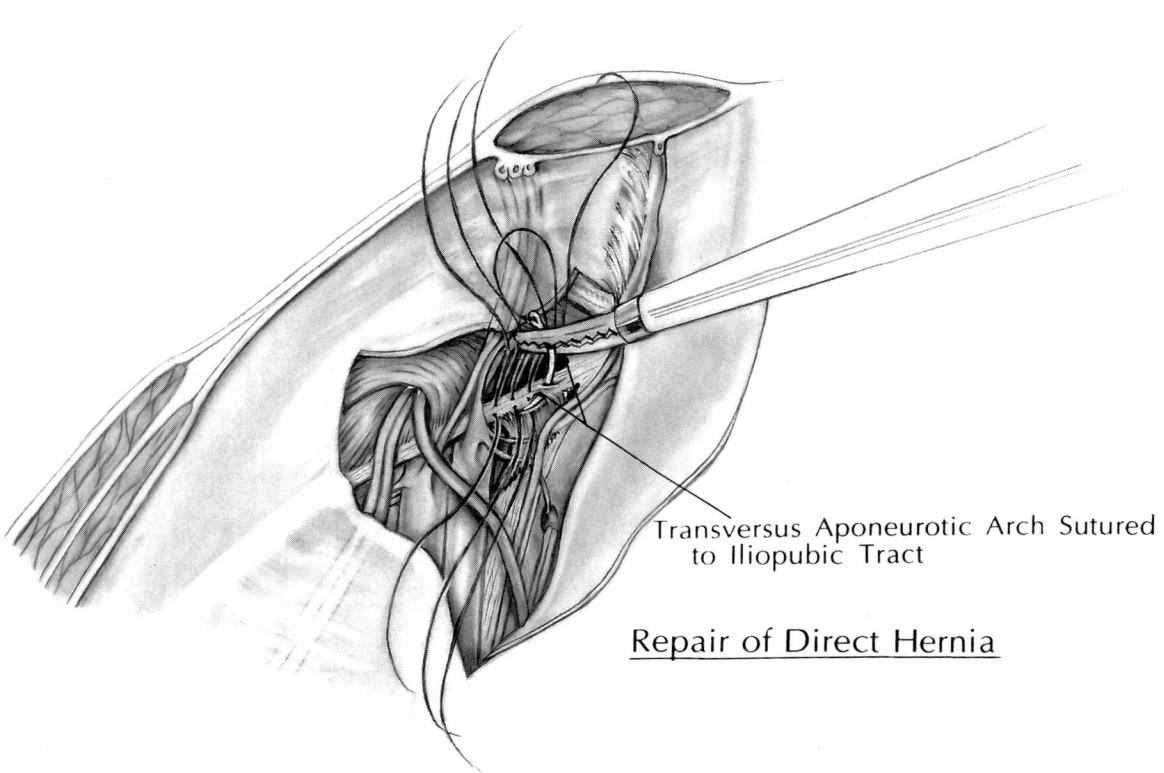

Figure 28-8. Sutured preperitoneal repair of a direct inguinal hernia.

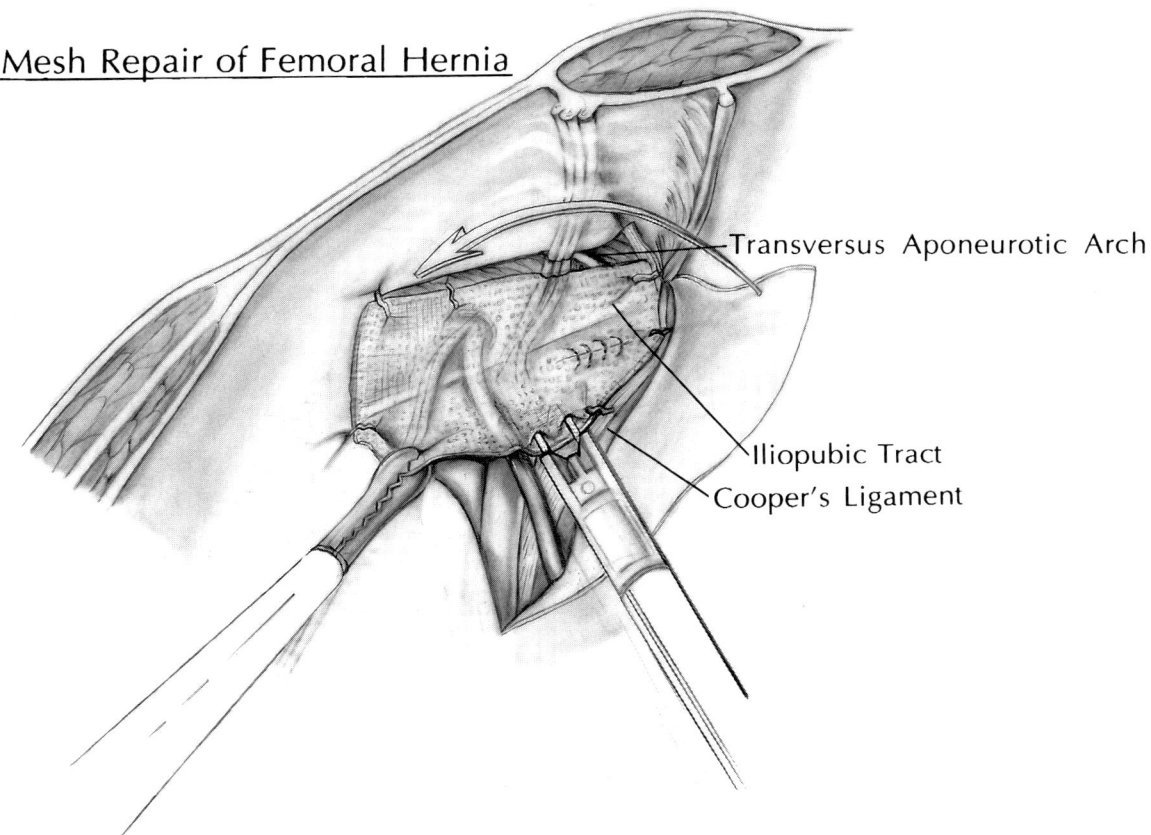

Figure 28-9. Preperitoneal mesh repair of a femoral hernia. The mesh is stapled to the iliopubic tract and Cooper's ligament.

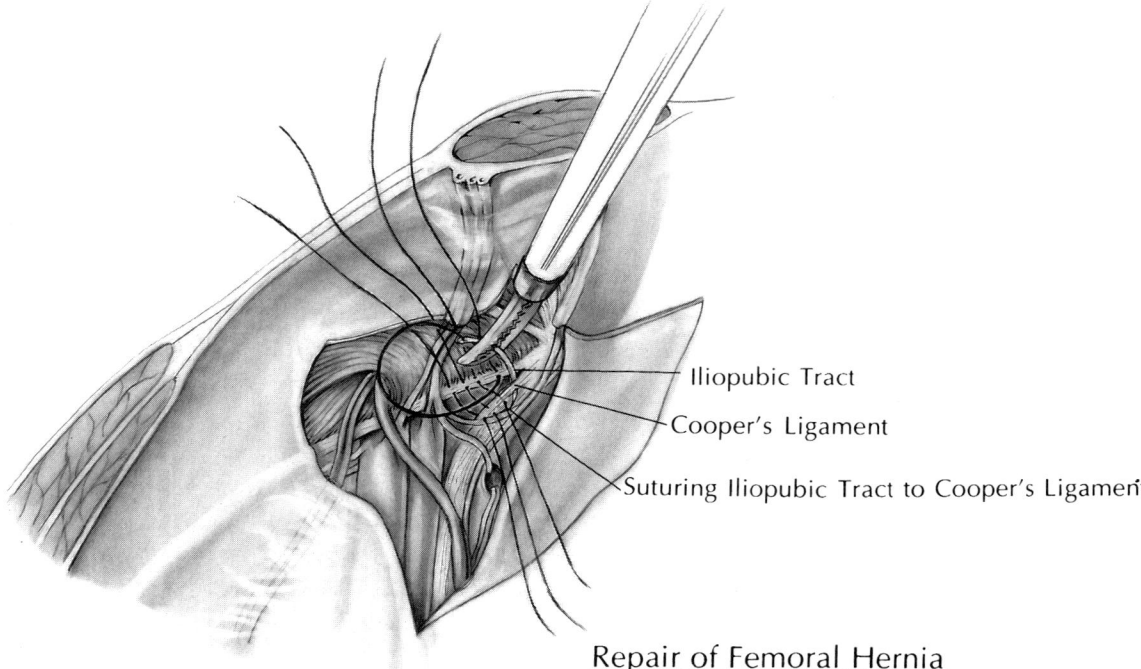

Figure 28-10. Preperitoneal mesh repair of femoral hernia with interrupted sutures. The sutures close the defect by apposing the iliopubic tract to Cooper's ligament.

tional methods now used as this method is still under investigation. It must again be stressed that one key factor significant to this type of hernia repair is the heavy reliance upon thorough understanding of the regional anatomy of the area.

REFERENCES

1. Read RC. Historical survey of the treatment of hernia. *In* Nyhus LM, Condon RE, eds. *Hernia*, 3rd ed. Philadelphia, JB Lippincott Co., 1989, pp 5–6.
2. Lichtenstein IL. Hernia repair with polypropylene mesh. AORN J 1990; 52:559–565.
3. Bull WT. Notes on cases of hernia which have relapsed after various operations for radical cure. N Y Med J 1981; 53:615.
4. Ferguson AH. Oblique inguinal hernia: Typical operation for its radical cure. JAMA 1899; 33:6.
5. Halverson K, McVay CB. Inguinal and femoral hernioplasty. Arch Surg 1970; 1901:127.
6. Spaw AT. Laparoscopic hernia repair: The anatomic basis. J Laparoendosc Surg 1991; 1:269.
7. Condon RE. The anatomy of the inguinal region and its relation to groin hernia. *In* Nyhus LM, Condon RE, eds. *Hernia*, 3rd ed. Philadelphia, JB Lippincott Co., 1989, pp 18–20.
8. Tait L. A discussion of treatment of hernia by median abdominal section. Br Med J 1891; 2:685–691.
9. Read RC. Groin hernias. *In* Cameron JL, ed. Current Surgical Therapy. Philadelphia, BC Decker, 1989, pp 408–411.
10. Lichtenstein IL, Shulman AG, Amid PK. The tension-free hernioplasty. Am J Surg 1989; 157:188–193.
11. Popp LW. Endoscopic patch repair of inguinal hernia in a female patient. Surg Endosc 1990; 4:10–12.
12. Ger R, Monroe K, Duvivier R, Mishrck A. Management of indirect inguinal hernias by laparoscopic closure of the neck of the sac. Am J Surg 1990; 159:371–373.
13. Salerno GM, Fitzgibbons RJ, Filipi CJ. Laparoscopic inguinal hernia repair. *In* Zucker K, ed. *Surgical Laparoscopy*. St. Louis, Quality Medical Publishing, Inc, 1991, pp 281–293.
14. Stoppa RE, Warlaumont CR. The preperitoneal approach and prosthetic repair of groin hernia. *In* Nyhus LM, Condon RE, eds. *Hernia*, 3rd ed. Philadelphia, JB Lippincott Co., 1989, pp 199–225.
15. Nyhus LM. The preperitoneal approach and iliopubic tract repair of inguinal hernia. *In* Nyhus LM, Condon RE, eds. *Hernia*, 3rd ed. Philadelphia, JB Lippincott Co., 1989, pp 154–188.

Chapter 29
Diagnostic and Therapeutic Thoracoscopy

Juan A. Sanchez
John C. Baldwin

Nearly a century following the introduction of the concept of thoracoscopy, the recent development of a sophisticated array of endoscopic instruments has made it possible to transform the technique from a state of relative obscurity as a diagnostic tool to a safe and effective therapeutic modality with expanding application. Current enthusiasm revolves around the vastly improved ability to examine the pleural cavity with video technology, as well as the capacity to carry out pulmonary resection and other invasive maneuvers safely.

Visualization of the pleural cavity by the introduction of cystoscopes through an open wound was carried out sporadically during the 1900s. Thoracoscopy was first consistently used in the division of adhesions to the chest wall in therapeutic pneumothorax for the treatment of pulmonary tuberculosis. This technique first appeared in the literature when described by Jacobleus in 1910.[1] With the decline in the incidence of tuberculosis following the introduction of antituberculous medication, the role of thoracoscopy was relegated chiefly to the diagnosis of pleural diseases. In the last two decades, directed poudrage with various sclerosing agents for recurrent pneumothorax was described but did not gain wide acceptance.[2-4]

There are many advantages to minimally invasive surgery in the chest. Thoracotomy incisions are well known to be among the most painful and to result in marked limitations in pulmonary function. By contrast, thoracoscopy is relatively painless and the large amount of tissue injury inherent in division of the thoracic musculature is avoided. Tissue trauma and pain are comparable to that experienced with multiple tube thoracostomies. These are especially important concerns in patients with poor pulmonary reserve, poor nutritional states, poor wound healing or any compromise of the immune system. In addition, recent clinical experience has shown that high resolution video technology thoracoscopy often provides better visualization of the entire pleural space than thoracotomy.

APPLICATIONS

Diagnostic

The excellent visualization of the pleural space afforded by thoracoscopy makes this an ideal method for diagnosis of diseases involving the pleura.[5-7] Biopsy of the parietal pleura or of pleural-based lung lesions is simple and reliable. Biopsy of lung parenchyma can be performed with endoscopic stapling instruments under direct visualization.[8] The diagnostic capacity of thoracoscopy in pulmonary diseases has been demonstrated in various infectious, and neoplastic processes, as well as in other conditions such as sarcoidosis occupational diseases, and idiopathic pulmonary fibrosis.[9,10] In addition to providing tissue diagnosis, thoracoscopy is an ideal adjunctive method for staging various neoplasms and, in particular, for establishing chest wall or pleural involvement in bronchogenic carcinoma or mesothelioma.[11]

The diagnosis of mediastinal disease outside the scope of mediastinoscopy may be facilitated with thoracoscopic techniques. With the ability to dissect the mediastinal pleura, biopsy of mediastinal masses can be obtained. This may be helpful for staging bronchogenic carcinoma, as well as for distinguishing lymphoma from other mediastinal tumors that would require excision. Evaluation of thoracic and mediastinal injury following both blunt and penetrating trauma, sulcus contusions, and lacerations of the pulmonary parenchyma as well as diaphragmatic rupture can readily be accomplished thoracoscopically.[12] In addition, identification of aortic pathologic conditions such as dissection may be possible. Transdiaphragmatic liver biopsy is feasible in selected patients.

Therapeutic

Thoracoscopy remains useful for etiologic diagnosis and treatment of recurrent pneumothorax. Resection of blebs and closure of peripheral parenchymal air leaks can often be accomplished using endoscopic graspers, stapling devices, and tissue scissors. Directed chemical pleurodesis and mechanical pleurodesis are well established thoracoscopic maneuvers, and definitive pleurectomy is now possible.

The recent advent of endoscopic stapling devices has greatly expanded the therapeutic potential of thoracoscopy. Wedge resection of peripheral masses within the outer third of the pulmonary parenchyma is relatively simple and can be accomplished with the stapler, the neodymium-yttrium-aluminum-garnet laser, or laser-assisted stapling.[12] The ability to perform more formal anatomic resections, such as lobectomies, is currently being explored. Development of instruments for endoscopic suture ligation with a needle as well as a wide complement of endoscopic staplers will result in more widespread use of this modality to perform major pulmonary resections (Table 29-1).

With the use of endoscopic tissue scissors, dissectors, and graspers, thoracoscopic pericardiectomy or creating a pericardial window has proven safe and effective.[13] Dorsal thoracic sympathectomy has also been performed successfully.[14] Injury to the thoracic duct with chylothorax has been repaired by thoracoscopic methods.[15,16] Empyema cavities have been drained, and debridement has been carried out under direct visualization.[17] Drainage of spinal and mediastinal abscesses has also been reported.[16] Some centers are reporting ligation of patent ductus arteriosus in infants and children using video thoracoscopy methods.[18] It is anticipated that endoscopic approaches to additional procedures, such as esophagomyotomy and other treatments for benign esophageal problems, will be common.

TECHNIQUE

In preparation of the patient for thoracoscopy the necessity for conversion to an open procedure should be anticipated. This should include frank discussions with the patient about this possibility. Although general anes-

Table 29-1. Recommended Instrumentation for Thoracoscopy

Telescope, 0 degrees
Video camera
Modular beam-splitter
35 mm camera adaptor (optional)
Video cassette recorder (optional)
Biopsy forceps, insulated
Coagulating electrode
Palpation probe
Grasping forceps
Dissecting scissors
Mixter dissecting forceps
Endoscopic staplers with reloadable cartridges, 2.5- and 3.5-mm staples
Babcock clamps (Endo Babcock; United States Surgical Corp.)
Tissue thickness gauge (Endogauge, United States Surgical Corp.)
Cannula/trocar assemblies; 5, 11, and 12 mm

thesia is necessary in most procedures, simple diagnostic thoracoscopy may be conducted in an awake adult with proper analgesia and sedation. In these patients, a stellate ganglion block may inhibit the cough reflex often produced with manipulation of the pleura. Use of a double-lumen endotracheal tube is important to achieve satisfactory visualization. Alternatively, silicone endobronchial tubes with "blocking" balloon catheters in the relevant bronchus (Univent; Vitaid, Lewiston, NY) may be used. Appropriate positioning of these tubes should always be verified bronchoscopically following patient repositioning.

Proper positioning of the patient is also essential for good results. In general, the lateral decubitus position with the involved side up is used. This allows access to the anterior and posterior thorax for placement of cannulas. In addition, it produces a shift of mediastinal and hilar structures away, permitting safer introduction of trocars and instruments. The chest is prepared with antiseptic solution and draped for thoracotomy in the eventuality of an open procedure. Sterile adhesive skin barriers do not present a problem and are encouraged.

Unless thoracoscopy is undertaken for visual inspection of the pleural space only, most patients will require a minimum of three trocar insertion sites (Fig. 29-1). One site accommodates the scope, and the others are used for instruments. Prior to inserting the first trocar, the involved lung is deflated with the double-lumen tube by balloon isolation of the appropriate bronchus and opening that lumen to air. The introduction of the first cannula is preceded by a stab wound made only slightly larger than the diameter of the intended cannula. The wound is then developed as for tube thoracostomy with entrance into the pleural space by "popping" through the parietal pleura. Alternatively, a needle can be carefully introduced into the pleural space allowing air to enter. This can be readily accomplished with a Veress needle which contains a spring-loaded blunt tip in order to reduce the incidence of laceration to the pulmonary parenchyma. The needle can be loaded with a drop of sterile saline solution or a small syringe containing air to alert the operator that entrance into the pleural cavity has been achieved. Passive collapse of the lung is accomplished slowly and one should avoid the temptation of forcing air through the needle via syringe for fear of producing mediastinal displacement under tension and attendant hemodynamic compromise.

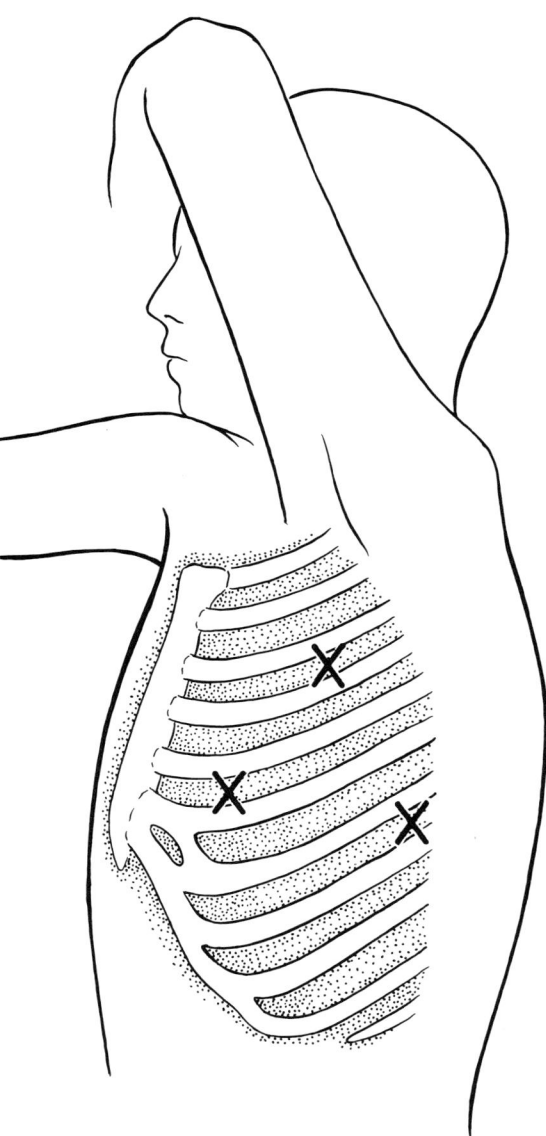

Figure 29-1. Suggested sites for trocar insertion in the chest. The actual arrangement will depend on the intended procedure.

A single trocar and cannula is introduced through the chest wall with care. In general, this should be through the fifth intercostal space at the anterior axillary line. Of course, some procedures may require creative positioning of the cannulas. The trocar is introduced over the superior border of the rib to avoid injury to the neurovascular bundle. Once the trocar is removed, the scope is inserted through the cannula for a general orientation and identification of topographic landmarks. The surgeon must maintain reference to these landmarks throughout the procedure.

Insufflation of the pleural space with carbon dioxide, while essential in the abdominal cavity, is not mandatory in the chest. However, carbon dioxide is generally recommended to achieve more complete and uniform collapse of all lung segments, a maneuver which brings out abnormalities on the lung parenchyma. Insufflation of air is not desirable, especially if use of cautery is anticipated. The gas is delivered via side ports on the cannulas. It is important to maintain gas pressures under eight mm Hg to prevent the possibility of hemodynamic embarrassment. This pressure is monitored through the insufflator.

A second trocar and cannula are inserted under endoscopic intrapleural visualization. For most procedures, this should be approximately 5 cm posteriorly, corresponding roughly with the posterior axillary line. A third cannula is required for most therapeutic manipulations. This cannula is inserted a few interspaces caudad, again under direct visualization, resulting in an inverted triangle pattern for the three sites. However, cannula positioning depends on many factors, including the patient's topography and the intended procedure.

If pleural fluid is encountered, it should be evacuated thoroughly by suction. The fluid can be collected in a Leukens-style trap for cultures or cytologic analysis. A single handheld instrument that can provide both suction and irrigation is ideal. Suction and irrigation should always be directly observed to avoid any injury to the surrounding pulmonary parenchyma. No instrument should be introduced or left unattended in a position where it cannot be observed with the camera.

The standard laparoscope usually affords satisfactory illumination and optics, both essential components for successful thoracoscopy. High resolution cameras and monitors are preferable, and the use of two video monitors on opposite sides of the operating table is ideal. This allows easy observation of a monitor by all members of the operating team. A beam-splitter adaptor allows visualization directly through the scope, as well as via video. Video recording capability is helpful for documentation and for educational purposes. Worn or frayed coaxial cable linkages are often the source of video malfunction and should be inspected periodically.

Fogging of the lens within the chest can be prevented by the application of antifogging fluid to all lens surfaces. Once in the chest, fogging of the distal lens can often be eliminated by lightly touching the visceral pleura with the end of the scope. It is also important to immerse the scope in warm saline solution prior to insertion to prevent condensation of water vapor.

Pleural adhesions can be divided sharply with scissors or, preferably, with cautery. It is desirable to achieve complete collapse of the lung for optimal exposure. Exposure of the inferior hilum and the inferior pulmonary vein may require division of the pulmonary ligament, which can also be accomplished with cautery.

The ability to apply the endoscopic stapler across lung tissue depends on tissue thickness. Once the segment of lung targeted for resection is tented by tissue graspers, a so-called "waist" becomes apparent. The tissue thickness at this level should be measured (ENDOGAUGE*, United States Surgical Corp., Norwalk, CT) to select the appropriate staple size, either 2.5 or 3.5 mm. In general, tissues that are more vascular require the use of smaller vascular staples. In the usual circumstance, more than one cartridge of staples is required to transect a given segment (Fig. 29-2). In cases of extreme thickness, the use of lasers such as neodymium-yttrium-aluminum-garnet or CO_2 can attenuate the amount of tissue at the waist in order to accommodate the stapler. This laser-assisted maneuver is depicted in Figure 29-3.

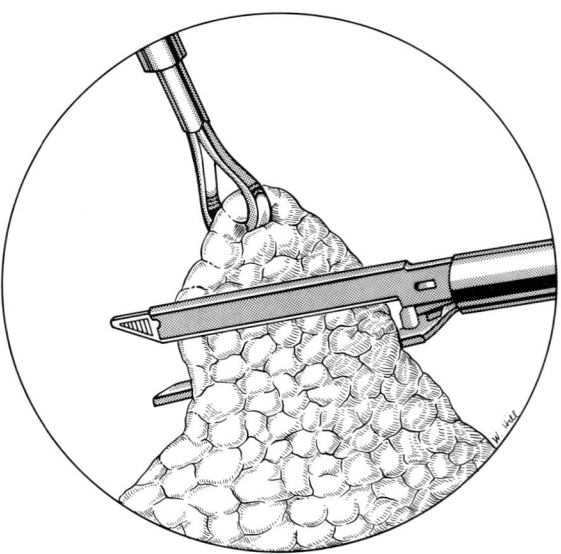

Figure 29-2. Application of the endoscopic stapler across pulmonary parenchyma.

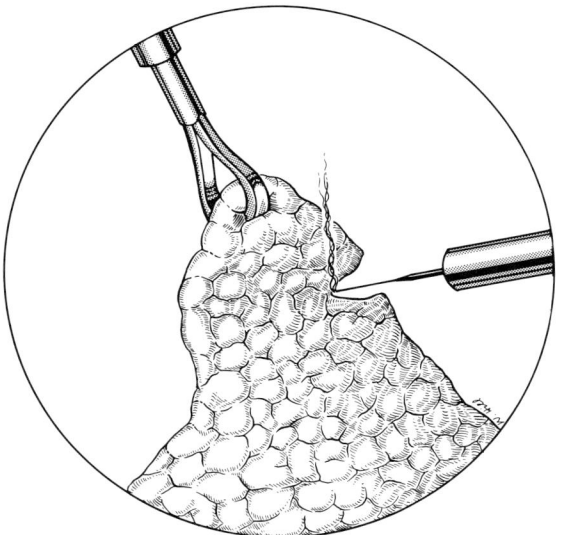

Figure 29-3. Laser-assisted techniques. The laser is used to attenuate lung tissue in order to accommodate the stapler.

Creation of fenestrations in the pericardium can be relatively simple in the absence of inflammation and adhesions between the pericardium and the epicardium. Forceps are used to separate the pericardium from the heart. Scissors are used to incise the pericardium with a lifting motion away from the heart (Fig. 29-4). Extreme care should be taken to visualize the phrenic nerve at all times. Bleeding from the free edge of pericardium can be cauterized provided it is not in close proximity to the heart.

Upon completion of the procedure, a chest tube is introduced via one of the cannula sites. Ideally, a large cannula should be placed in the intended chest tube site. This should accommodate a 28- to 32-French tube easily. The tube is grasped with an instrument and guided under direct visualization to its ultimate destination. Finally, the other wounds are closed using absorbable sutures for both the subcutaneous and subcuticular layers.

REFERENCES

1. Jacobeus VHC. Ueber die Moglichkeit die Zystoskopie bei Unteersuchung seroser Hohlungen anzuwenden. Muench Med Wochenschr 1910; 57:2090.
2. Keller R, Gutersohn J, Herzog H. The management of persistent pneumothorax by thoracoscopic procedures. Thoraxchirurgie 1974; 22:457–460.
3. Daniel TM, Tribble CG, Rodgers BM. Thoracoscopy and talc poudrage for pneumothoraces and effusions. Ann Thorac Surg 1990; 50:186–189.
4. Hansen MK, Kruse-Andersen S, Watt-Boolsen S, Andersen K. Spontaneous pneumothorax and fibrin glue sealant during thoracoscopy. Eur J Cardiothorac Surg 1989; 3:512–514.
5. Rodgers BM, Ryckman FC, Moazam F, Talbert JL. Thoracoscopy for intrathoracic tumors. Ann Thorac Surg 1981; 31:414–420.
6. Raffenberg M, Mai J, Loddenkemper R. Results of thoracoscopy in localized lung and chest wall diseases. Pneumologie 1990; 44(Suppl 1):182–183.
7. Boutin C, Astoul P, Seitz B. The role of thoracoscopy in the evaluation and management of pleural effusions. Lung 1990; 168(Suppl 1):113–121.
8. Miller DL, Allen MS, Trastek VF, et al. Video thoracoscopic wedge resections of the lung. Ann Thorac Surg 54(3):410–414.
9. Schaberg T, Suttmann-Bayer A, Loddenkemper R. Thoracoscopy in diffuse lung diseases. Pneumologie 1989; 43:112–115.
10. Trusov A, Rymko LP, Perelman MI. A method of thoracoscopic electrosurgical biopsy in the diagnosis of diffuse lung diseases. Klin Med (Mosc) 1990; 68:53–56.
11. Liewald F, Sunder-Plassmann L, Dienemann H, Mezger J: Pleural mesothelioma—Problems in diagnosis and clinical course in 25 patients. Langenbecks Arch Chir 1989; 374:105–110.
12. Kearney PA, Rouhana SW, Burney RE. Blunt rupture of the diaphragm: Mechanism, diagnosis, and treatment. Ann Emerg Med 1989; 18:132–136.
13. Vogel B, Mall W. Thoracoscopic pericardial fenestration—Diagnostic and therapeutic aspects. Pneumologie, 1990; 44(Suppl 1):184–185.
14. Guerin JC, Demolombe S, Brudon JR. Thoracic sympathectomy by thoracoscopy: Apropos of 15 cases. Ann Chir 1990; 44:236–238.
15. Morita R, Akaogi E, Suzuki Y, et al. A case of postoperative chylothorax successfully treated by thora-

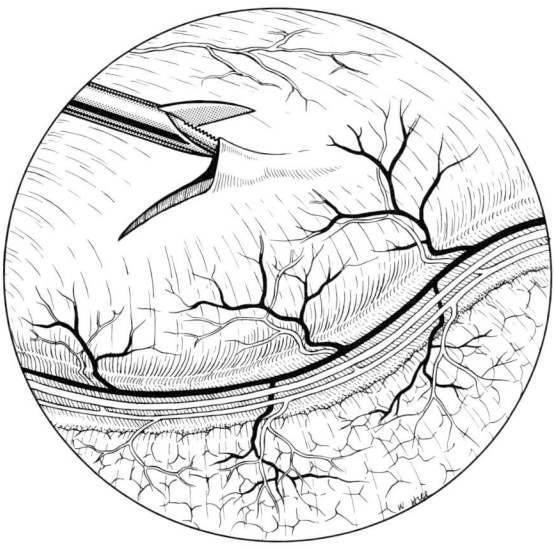

Figure 29-4. Creation of a pericardial window with dissecting scissors. The intrapericardial blade pulls the pericardium away from the heart.

coscopic fibrin gluing. Nihon Kyobu Geka Gakkai Zasshi (J Jpn Assoc Thorac Surg) 1990; 30:2465.
16. Mack M, Aronoff R, Acuff T, et al. The present role of thoracoscopy in the diagnosis and treatment of diseases of the chest. Presented at the Twenty-Eighth Annual Meeting of the Society of Thoracic Surgeons, February 3–6, 1992.
17. Hutter J, Hurari D, Bainbridge M. The management of empyema thoraces by thoracoscopy and irrigation. Ann Thorac Surg 1988; 39:517–520.
18. Laborde F, Noirhomme P, Karam J, et al. A new video thoracoscopy surgical technique for interruption of patent ductus arteriosus in infants and children. Presented at the Seventy-second Annual Meeting of the American Association for Thoracic Surgery, April 26–29, 1992.

Chapter 30
Urologic Disorders

Michael Pontari
William Morgan

LAPAROSCOPIC PELVIC LYMPH NODE DISSECTION

The value of pelvic lymphadenectomy for patients with genitourinary malignancies is well recognized. The nerve-sparing, potency-preserving radical prostatectomy described by Walsh and Donker[1] has popularized the retropubic approach to radical prostatectomy. Pelvic lymphadenectomy is routinely performed using the same incision. The role of pelvic lymphadenectomy in bladder cancer has recently changed. Patients with limited pelvic lymph node metastasis often undergo a cystectomy and pelvic lymph node dissection for cancer; they would probably not have had a cystectomy prior to the advent of effective platinum-based chemotherapy.[2] Pelvic lymphadenectomy is also an important staging tool in selected patients with advanced urethral or penile carcinoma. With the advent of laparoscopic techniques, the morbidity of pelvic lymph node dissection has been decreased. Consequently, clinicians have begun to modify further the indications for pelvic lymphadenectomy.

Role of Pelvic Lymphadenectomy in Staging and Prognosis of Prostate Cancer

The presence of metastatic deposits in the pelvic lymph nodes of patients who appear to have localized adenocarcinoma of the prostate is an important prognostic factor. The presence of positive lymph nodes has historically been a harbinger of further systemic spread, including bony metastases. Prout et al.[3] performed pelvic lymphadenectomies in 92 patients with clinically localized adenocarcinoma of the prostate who also underwent either radical prostatectomy or ^{125}I radioactive seed implantation. With a mean follow up of 43 months, progression (usually osseous disease) occurred in 18 of 32 patients with positive lymph nodes. In those with no spread of disease to the lymph nodes, only 6 of 60 showed progressive disease.

By 5 years, at least 75 per cent of patients with positive pelvic lymph nodes will have developed bony metastases.[4] Gervasi et al.[5] followed 511 patients after bilateral pelvic lymph node dissection and irradiation. The incidence of metastatic disease at 10 years was 31 per cent for patients with no lymph node metastases, and 83 per cent for those with disease in the nodes. The chance of dying from cancer was 17 per cent at 10 years in the node-negative group, and 57 per cent for those with nodes involved by prostate cancer.

Once nodal metastasis has occurred, the rate of tumor progression may be related to the volume of nodal disease. Smith and Middleton[6] showed that patients with gross evidence of disease at the time of pelvic lymphadenectomy for prostate cancer did poorly compared to patients with only microscopic disease. Whether patients with lesser amounts of microscopic disease, i.e., one positive lymph node, do better than patients with multiple positive nodes is still unresolved. In the report of Smith and Middleton,[6] patients with one positive lymph node had a more favorable outcome when compared with those with multiple positive nodes. At 5 years disease had progressed in 44 per cent of the multiple node group compared to 27 per cent of those with a single positive node. However, with longer follow-up, this difference becomes less apparent. Zincke and associates[7] reported a 92 per cent 5-year survival for patients with a single positive lymph node who underwent a radical prostatectomy and pelvic lymph node dissection. However, approximately half of these patients also received early hormonal therapy. In the Houston series,[5] patients with a single positive lymph node had a rate of progression and cancer-specific mortality similar to patients with more extensive nodal metastases. Disease in patients with more than one node positive progressed more rapidly than in those with multiple positive nodes (mean interval to progression 43 versus 30 months). However, at 10 years 84 per cent of those with multiple positive nodes and 80 per cent of those with one positive node had recurrent disease.

Influence of Tumor Grade and Clinical Stage on Incidence of Pelvic Lymph Node Metastases

The risk of lymph node involvement in patients with clinically localized prostate cancer is closely related to the histologic grade and clinical stage of the tumor (Table 30-1).

Tumor grade is a very important predictor of lymph node status. Smith and colleagues[10] from Utah explored this issue in 33 patients with clinical stage A2 disease. In this series, positive lymph nodes were found in none of the patients with well differentiated tumors. In contrast, positive lymph nodes were identified in 5 of 19 patients with moderately differentiated tumors and in 3 of 7 patients with poorly differentiated lesions. In clinical B1 disease, metastases to the lymph nodes were seen in only 2 of 53 patients with well differentiated tumors. For the clinical B2 lesions, 5 of 27 well differentiated, 29 of 106 moderately differentiated, and 9 of 21 poorly differentiated tumors were found to have spread to the pelvic lymph nodes. Several authors have reported the incidence of pelvic lymph node metastases in clinically localized prostate cancer based on grade alone. The results of several of these reports are summarized in Table 30-2.

Noninvasive Methods to Detect Lymph Node Status

The lymph nodes most commonly opacified by pedal lymphangiography are the external iliac, common iliac, and periaortic lymph nodes. Deposits in these groups can be identified with some accuracy. However, some authors contend that there is difficulty in visualizing nodes in the obturator lymphatics (medial chain of external iliac nodes), which are among the most commonly involved by

Table 30-1. Pelvic Lymph Node Dissection Stage (Clinical) and Positive Lymph Node Status

Author	A2	B1	B2	C
Gervasi et al.[5]	29/101	35/165	37/100	51/116
Elfving and Lundgren[8]	1/14	3/14	8/16	16/20
McDowell et al.[9]	4/8			82/147
Smith et al.[10]	8/33	18/156	43/154	36/68
Donohue et al.[11]	10/44	20/104	29/58	
Fowler and Whitmore[12]		5/75	56/129	58/96
Grossman, HB et al.[13]		0/18	6/25	28/33
Grossman, IC et al.[14]	25/47	3/18	4/14	5/19
Brendler et al.[15]	3/22	11/58	14/27	10/17
Bruce et al.[16]	0/3	0/6	5/13	6/8
Lieskovsky et al.[17]	1/8	3/16	12/39	11/17
McLaughlin et al.[18]		4/19	5/17	2/24
Totals	81/280	102/649	219/592	305/565
% lymph node positive	29	16	37	54

Table 30-2. Pelvic Lymph Node Dissection Grade versus Lymph Node Status: All Clinically Localized Disease

Author	% Positive Lymph Nodes with Each Grade		
	Well	Moderately	Poorly
Gervasi et al.[5]	29/196	55/177	52/84
Elfving and Lundgren[8]	4/9	11/25	13/20
McDowell et al.[9]	5/26	63/112	33/43
Paulson[19]	0/31	26/84	27/29
Grossman, IC et al.[14]	10/45	20/37	7/9
Totals	48/307	175/435	132/185
% lymph node positive	16	40	71

early disease extension from prostate cancer, thus leading to a high false negative rate for lymphangiography.[18,20] Others have disputed this finding.[21] The internal iliac lymph nodes, also commonly involved in early disease, are visualized about 50 per cent of the time.[22] On lymphangiograms, it is not possible to distinguish benign nodal abnormalities (such as replacement by connective, fatty, or inflammatory tissue) from those due to metastatic tumor.[23] Loening et al.[22] performed lymph node dissections in 40 patients after pedal lymphangiograms. They found a 59 per cent false positive rate and a 36 per cent false negative rate for lymphangiography. The sensitivity of lymphangiography has been shown to range from 33 to 75 per cent, with a specificity from 21 to 93 per cent.[24] Castellino[25] reported a positive predictive value of 81 per cent and a negative predictive value of 78 per cent.

The evaluation of lymph node status by computed tomographic (CT) scan is limited as well. Metastatic nodal disease is identified by an increase in size, rather than by changes in nodal architecture. Nodes larger than 1.5 cm are considered likely to be malignant, while nodes greater than 1 cm are suspect.[26] The sensitivity of CT scans compiled from several series by Hricak[27] was 50 to 75 per cent, the specificity was 86 to 100 per cent, and the overall accuracy was 83 to 93 per cent. Much lower estimates of the efficacy of CT scans can be found in the literature, with sensitivities of 0 to 14 per cent reported.[28,29] Magnetic resonance imaging has proved to be of no greater value than CT scanning and also is limited to evaluation of lymph node size.[26] The sensitivity, specificity, and overall accuracy of magnetic resonance imaging are comparable to those for CT.[30,31] Another modality that has been used for imaging lymph nodes in patients with prostate cancer is radiolabeled prostatic acid phosphatase. Results of early reports have been favorable and have found a sensitivity of 100 per cent and a specificity of 86 to 100 per cent.[32,33] In addition, radiolabeled monoclonal antibodies to prostatic antigens are being studied at our institution and others. However, early clinical trials suggest limited success using these modalities.

Lymphatic Anatomy

The anatomy of the pelvic lymphatics is clouded by a lack of uniformity in the terms used to describe pelvic lymphatic structures. The lymphatic drainage from the prostate courses through four major pathways to end in three nodal groups: the external iliac nodes, the hypogastric (or internal iliac) nodes, and the nodes of the sacral promentory.[34,35]

The external iliac lymphatics are made up of three chains: lateral, intermediate, and medial.[36] The lateral chain runs along the lateral surface of the external iliac artery and contains one to three lymph vessels. The intermediate chain is the least important of the three and runs between the external iliac artery and vein. The medial or internal lymph chain is the most important and contains the greatest number of lymph nodes and vessels. It is located medial and posterior to the external iliac vein and superior to the obturator nerve. The node most urologists refer to as the "obturator" node during lymphadenectomy is really the middle node of the medial iliac chain; there is no distinct obturator node chain which corresponds to any standard anatomic description.

The internal iliac or hypogastric lymph nodes usually number four to eight and are located along the internal iliac artery and its branches. These nodes are often involved in the early spread of prostate cancer.[9] Included in the internal group are the lateral sacral nodes (presciatic nodes), which are found along the lateral sacral arteries opposite the second and third sacral foramina. Reports have been published of these nodes containing solitary metastatic deposits of prostate cancer.[37]

The nodes of the sacral promentory are also known as the medial group of the common iliac nodes and consist of two to four nodes located near the L5-S1 intervertebral disc. Most surgeons do not routinely remove these nodes during lymphadenectomy, but some have advocated this.[37]

Resection Margins for Pelvic Lymph Nodes in Prostate Cancer

The location of lymph node metastases from prostate carcinoma can be obtained from series in which the external iliac and hypogastric lymph nodes were removed during pelvic lymphadenectomy at the time of radical prostatectomy. McLaughlin et al.[18] found that 87 per cent of lymph node metastases in patients with prostate cancer were in the obturator and hypogastric nodes alone or in combination with other groups of nodes, 9 per cent were in the external iliac nodes alone, and only 4 per cent were in the common iliac nodes alone. Metastatic disease was bilateral in 57 per cent of patients. Fowler and Whitmore[12] reported on 115 patients with prostate cancer metastatic to the lymph nodes. In their series, 77 per cent had disease in the hypogastric and obturator area alone or with external iliac involvement, and 23 per cent had external iliac nodes alone involved. Of 35 patients with a solitary focus of nodal metastases, 61 per cent were in the hypogastric and obturator area, and 39 per cent were in the external iliac area. Bruce et al.[16] reported that 91 per cent of patients with lymph nodes involved with prostate cancer had disease in the hypogastric and obturator area, and in 55 per cent the external iliac nodes were involved as well. Most authors agree that rarely has tumor spread to common iliac or para-aortic lymph nodes without also having involved the external or internal iliac lymph nodes. Prostate cancer rarely "skips" over the first echelon of nodes.[19,38] Saitoh et al.[39] has described two patterns of lymph node metastases from prostate cancer. In Type 1, pelvic and para-aortic nodes are involved. In Type 2, the para-aortic nodes only are involved. He postulated that the Type 2 pattern arises through spread via the vertebral vein bypass and is associated with hematogenous metastases as well. A closer look at this series of 753 autopsy specimens with metastatic prostate cancer is revealing.

In 476 cancer had spread to the lymph nodes. In 12 positive para-aortic nodes without pelvic node involvement were found, but in 6 of these involvement of other nodes including inguinal and clavicular areas, which were probably clinically apparent, was found. Thus, the incidence of truly isolated para-aortic nodal disease may be only 6 in 476, or 1.3 per cent.

Historically, a standard pelvic lymph node dissection involved removal of the three external iliac lymph node chains (the lateral, intermediate, and medial chains) as well as the internal iliac nodes lateral to and overlying the hypogastric artery.[3,12] This excludes the presciatic group of internal iliac lymph nodes and the sacral lymph nodes. With this dissection, the margins were: laterally, the genitofemoral nerve; medially, the bladder wall and ureter; posteriorly, the obturator nerve and vessels; and distally, the superficial circumflex iliac vessels and Cooper's ligament. Superiorly, the dissection was carried up to (and sometimes just beyond) the bifurcation of the common iliac artery. Whitmore began modifying the lymphadenectomy by omitting the dissection of the nodal tissue surrounding and lateral to the external iliac artery.[40] This made the lateral limit of the dissection the lateral margin of the external iliac vein rather than the genitofemoral nerve. This technique was termed the modified pelvic lymphadenectomy. Whitmore found no change in the incidence of positive lymph nodes when compared to the classical dissection. Others have reported similar rates of lymph node involvement using the two techniques.[15] Besides a smaller area of dissection, another benefit of the newer technique is the decreased incidence of postoperative lymphedema. Standard pelvic lymphadenectomy had been associated with prepelvic, groin, and genital lymphedema in approximately 50 per cent of patients, as well as occasional severe lower extremity edema.[40] The modified pelvic lymphadenectomy has by now become the accepted standard technique[10,17] and is the technique performed through the laparoscope.

Pelvic Lymphadenectomy in Other Genitourinary Malignancies

Other urologic malignancies for which pelvic lymphadenectomies are performed include bladder, urethral, and penile cancers. The role of pelvic lymph node dissection in bladder cancer has been markedly altered by the use of newer chemotherapeutic regimens. Lymphadenectomy was previously undertaken as a therapeutic effort in addition to cystectomy for muscle-invasive disease[41] or as a means of selecting candidates for radical cystectomy. Today, the status of the lymph nodes often does not change the initial surgical management of the disease. It does, however, identify patients who would benefit from postcystectomy systemic cytotoxic chemotherapy. Methotrexate, vinblastine, Adriamycin, and cisplatinum (MVAC) has been shown to produce a 69 per cent complete and partial response rate in patients with advanced transitional cell carcinoma.[42] Skinner et al.[2] performed a randomized trial in patients with stage P3 or greater disease and found a significant delay in the time to progression after cystectomy in patients treated with cisplatinum, doxorubicin, and cyclophosphamide, when compared to cystectomy alone.

Hence patients requiring a lymphadenectomy and cystoprostatectomy usually undergo the procedure regardless of the status of the nodes and then receive adjuvant chemotherapy if indicated. Thus, the role of laparoscopic pelvic lymphadenectomy would appear to be limited in these patients since they require an open operation regardless of the lymph node status.

Penile cancer spreads to the inguinal lymph nodes first and to the pelvic nodes only in advanced cases.[43] In patients with clinically positive inguinal nodes (still present after a 6-week course of oral antibiotic therapy), pelvic lymph node metastases have been reported in up to one-third of them.[44] Some surgeons believe that a pelvic lymphadenectomy should be performed prior to an inguinal lymph node dissection. The presence of positive pelvic nodes may obviate the need for the inguinal procedure, thereby sparing the patient the considerable morbidity associated with the inguinal dissection.[45,46] A laparoscopic pelvic lymphadenectomy may therefore be a good choice for the first procedure.

TECHNIQUE OF LAPAROSCOPIC PELVIC LYMPHADENECTOMY

Preoperative Preparation

Patients are admitted on the day of surgery after consuming a clear liquid diet and undergoing a mechanical bowel preparation at home the day before. Because the pelvic veins can produce a rapid, substantial blood loss if injured during the procedure, patient's blood is typed and cross-matched for two units of blood. Evidence suggests that preoperative and perioperative use of a minidose of subcutaneous heparin contributes to an increased rate of postoperative lymphocele formation in open lymphadenectomy,[47] so we use instead pneumatic compression stockings to decrease the risk of perioperative thromboembolic complications. One dose of a first-generation cephalosporin is given before the start of the procedure.

Operative Technique

The patient is placed in the supine position on the operating room table. A urethral catheter is placed. This allows for urine output monitoring, as well as decompression of the bladder, thus reducing the chance of bladder injury. A rolled towel is placed under the sacrum to achieve a 10 degree angle of flexion and the table is placed in mild Trendelenburg position (10 to 15 degrees). A nasogastric tube is placed by the anesthesiologist to decompress the stomach and avoid gastric injury. Most surgeons make an infraumbilical incision. However, in our experience the placement of the Veress needle via this approach sometimes results in a pneumoretroperitoneum because of the reflection of the peritoneal cavity around the urachus. For this reason, we advocate a supraumbilical incision 1 to 2 cm in length, approximately 4 mm cephalad to the umbilicus. Towel clips are placed on either side of this incision, and the abdominal wall is lifted away from the body to facilitate placement of the Veress needle. The needle is advanced at a 75-degree angle to the abdominal wall, angling slightly toward the pelvis. The needle is advanced until a palpable "pop" is felt, indicating that the needle has passed through the fascia. At this point resistance to the advancement of the needle will decrease. Carbon dioxide is then insufflated. If initial insufflation pressures are higher than 2 to 3 mm Hg, one should suspect that the needle has been improperly placed. It should be removed and reinserted. Following adequate insufflation a trochar is placed at the supraumbilical site after the needle is removed. This trocar should be 10 to 12 mm in size and should accommodate the camera. The remaining trocars are then placed under vision. In general, a 12-mm trocar is placed in the right lower quadrant just lateral to McBurney's point. This site is just lateral to the rectus muscle and therefore avoids traumatizing the inferior epigastric vessels. A 10-mm trochar is placed in a similar fashion on the opposite side. These large ports allow for the use of a stapling device from either side. A small 5-mm trocar is placed in the midline at a point one-third of the way cephalad between the pubis and the umbilicus. After exploration of the abdomen, the umbilical ligament is identified and an incision is made using electrocautery through the peritoneal reflection, just lateral to the umbilical ligament. The peritoneum is then bluntly dissected, identifying the vas deferens, which is doubly ligated with clips and then divided. At this point further dissection will identify the landmarks readily appreciated during open lymphadenectomy. The obturator nerve and external iliac vein are identified. Using blunt dissection, the nodal tissue package is dissected free from the inferior surface of the external iliac vein. It is similarly dissected away from the side wall and the surface of the obturator nerve. Visualization is enhanced by retracting the umbilical ligament and the ends of the vas deferens. As the dissection proceeds caudally one must search for the presence of an accessory obturator vein and avoid injuring this structure.

Similarly, the obturator artery and vein coursing just beneath the obturator nerve can be injured if not identified and preserved. Small bleeding vessels and lymphatic channels are controlled with cautery. Once the lymph node bearing tissue to be removed has been completely separated it can be extracted via one of the large ports using a grasping instrument. During the proximal portion of the dissection the proximity of the ureter must be appreciated, and this structure preserved. Electrocautery should be used sparingly in this vicinity. The contralateral side is dissected in a similar fashion. After the obturator fossa has been inspected for bleeding and hemostasis is deemed adequate, the trocars are removed under direct vision and the incisions are closed with a running subcuticular absorbable suture.

Postoperative Care

Patients are currently being kept overnight for observation. It is conceivable that this operation may soon be performed on an outpatient basis. Typically, oral liquids can be started in the evening. Patients are discharged the next morning and are given an oral cephalosporin for 5 to 7 days and pain medication. Activity is resumed in approximately 1 week.

LAPAROSCOPIC VARICOCELE LIGATION

A varicocele is an abnormal dilatation of the pampiniform plexus within the spermatic cord. The incidence of varicocele in men being evaluated for infertility is 19 to 41 per cent.[48] However, not all men with varicoceles are infertile. Varicoceles are present in 8 to 23 per cent of the general population.[49] Kursh[50] examined 100 men with proven fertility (one or more children) presenting for vasectomy and found a varicocele in 61 per cent.

Anatomy and Etiology of Varicocele

The majority of varicoceles are on the left side. In 870 varicocelectomy procedures, Dubin and Amelar[51] found 56 per cent bilaterally, 40 per cent only on the left, and 4 per cent solely on the right. The left internal spermatic vein enters the left renal vein at a right angle, while the right internal spermatic vein enters the vena cava obliquely. Hence, the left internal spermatic vein is 8 to 10 cm longer than the right. It is thought that its increased length and manner of insertion contribute to a higher hydrostatic pressure within the system.[52] Also, Ahlberg et al.[53] in a postmortem examination of 84 specimens found an absence of valves in 40 per cent of left internal spermatic veins and in 23 per cent of right internal spermatic veins.

Another proposed mechanism for the development of varicoceles is the "nutcracker phenomenon."[54] The left renal vein may become trapped between the abdominal aorta and superior mesenteric artery in the upright position. Varicoceles can also result from compression of the spermatic vein by retroperitoneal tumors. Patients presenting with an isolated right-sided varicocele should be evaluated for the presence of a retroperitoneal mass.

Pathophysiology of Varicoceles

Most men with varicoceles do not have abnormal semen parameters.[55] However, in some, abnormal spermatogenesis occurs, and defects in motility and morphology and low sperm counts can be observed. However, no one pattern appears to be diagnostic for the presence of varicoceles.[56] An explanation for the effect of varicoceles on sperm production and function is not known. Hypotheses include an elevation in testicular temperature, and reflux of toxic metabolites from the kidney and adrenal gland to the testes (including prostaglandin PE_2 and $PF_{2\alpha}$).[57] Other proposals include alterations in the hypothalamic-pituitary-gonadal axis.[58]

Diagnosis

Physical examination remains the best method of diagnosis. The patient is examined standing to accentuate the filling of the spermatic veins. The Valsalva maneuver will increase intra-abdominal pressure, therefore increasing filling as well. The patient is then examined supine to assess changes in the examination from the standing position. Bilateral thickening of the cord when standing, which resolves when supine, may represent bilateral varicoceles. Other methods used to detect varicoceles include Doppler ultrasound,[59] nuclear medicine scans,[60] and contact thermography.[61] Venography has been the gold standard. However, if the study is performed after the venous catheter is advanced into the gonadal vein, valves may be bypassed, leading to a false positive result.[62]

Treatment Options

Treatment options include surgical ligation and percutaneous embolization using various sclerosing agents, Gelfoams, coils, or balloons. Various surgical approaches have been described, including scrotal and retroperitoneal (high ligation of Palomo),[63] and inguinal (Ivanissevich approach).[64] The success rate of surgical treatment has been compiled from many series by Mordel et al.[65] A mean improvement in the semen analysis was seen in 57 per cent, with a mean pregnancy rate of 36 per cent. The recurrence rate after surgery ranges from 5 to 20 per cent[66] with a complication rate of 5 per cent.[67] Percutaneous spermatic vein occlusion is associated with a recurrence rate of 3 to 9 per cent[68,69] and a complication rate of 1 to 30 per cent.[70,71] A pregnancy rate of 39.7 per cent has been reported.[72] Both of these techniques can be performed under local anesthesia on an outpatient basis.[72,73]

Indications for Varicocele Repair

Varicocele ligation is appropriate as a treatment for infertility in patients with an abnormality in one or more semen parameters and no endocrine abnormalities. These couples should have been engaging in unprotected intercourse for at least 1 year, and female partners should have undergone a gynecologic workup for infertility. Marks et al.[74] suggested that preoperative parameters associated with a greater rate of postoperative pregnancy include: a lack of testicular atrophy, sperm density greater than 50 million, at least 60 per cent motile sperm, and a follicle-stimulating hormone level of less than 300 ng/ml. Men with symptomatic varicoceles are also included.

The treatment of bilateral varicoceles is controversial. In patients with left-sided varicocele, bilaterality of varicoceles has been found in up to 62 per cent[75] in surgical series and in up to 60 per cent of those evaluated by venography.[76] Amelar and Dubin[77] treated 41 men who had persistently poor semen quality after a left varicocelectomy. Following right varicocelectomy, semen parameters improved in 56 per cent, and 43 per cent achieved a pregnancy.

The entity of subclinical varicocele is also controversial. Yarborough et al.[78] performed gonadal venography in 40 infertile men without clinical varicocele, and diagnosed 22 "subclinical" varicoceles (19 left and 3 right). In the 13 patients followed for at least 6 months, a small but significant improvement in sperm count was observed. No pregnancy rate was available.

Technique of Laparoscopic Varicocele Ligation

Preparation and initial technique are similar to that described for lymphadenectomy.

OPERATIVE PROCEDURE

The 11-mm trochar is inserted supraumbilically. The camera is placed through this port, and the remaining ports are placed under direct vision. Generally, an additional 11-mm port is placed halfway between the umbilicus and the symphysis pubis, and a 5.5-mm port is placed between the umbilicus and the anterior superior iliac spine ipsilateral to the varicocele(s).

The landmarks are identical to those for pelvic lymph node dissection. The spermatic vessels are visualized beneath the peritoneum, and the peritoneum is opened transversely. The internal spermatic vein is sharply dissected free from the testicular artery. The artery must be identified. A few drops of papaverine on the vessels may be helpful in that the artery will spasm and the vein will not. Aaberg et al.[79] describe placing a Doppler flow probe over the ipsilateral hemiscrotum. Each vessel is gently occluded with an atraumatic grasper. The effect of this maneuver on the arterial pulse is monitored to determine the identity of each vessel. The veins are then doubly clipped and divided.

RESULTS

Early studies of the efficacy of this method are now being published. Long term follow-up is unavailable. Aaberg et al.[79] published a report of 4 patients who underwent bilateral outpatient laparoscopic varicocelectomies. All 4 resumed regular activity the day after surgery. In one patient the testicular artery could not be identified, and all the vascular structures in the spermatic cord were ligated. At 3 months, this patient had a normal testes volume, symmetric with the contralateral gonad. Hagood et al.[80] reported on 10 patients, 4 of whom had had a bilateral varicocele. Normal activity was resumed in 2 days, and in all patients varicoceles resolved clinically. The most complete follow-up comes from Donovan and Winfield[81] who performed laparoscopic varix ligation in 14 patients (5 bilaterally). In each patient the varicocele resolved postoperatively. Mean interval to resuming normal activity was 3.4 days. All procedures but one were performed on an outpatient basis. One patient required hospitalization from excessive anesthesia. In one patient the spermatic artery could not be identified and was presumably ligated. Four patients have achieved pregnancy postoperatively.

CRYPTORCHIDISM

Approximately 3.4 to 5.8 per cent of full term male newborns are born cryptorchid.[82] The incidence in premature male babies is higher, up to 9 to 30 per cent.[83] After 1 year, the incidence decreases to 0.8 per cent and remains the same through puberty. One-quarter of cryptorchid boys have bilaterally undescended testes. Cryptorchidism leads to several clinical problems: infertility (in both unilateral and bilaterally cryptorchid patients),[84] an approximately 20-fold increase in the risk of malignancy,[85] and an increased risk of developing testicular torsion.[86]

As early as the second year of life, 38 per cent of cryptorchid testes have completely lost their germ cells because of impaired transformation of the gonocyte.[82] Also, peritubular fibrosis can be seen in biopsies from cryptorchid testes in patients as young as 1 year of age.[87] Thus, most pediatric urologists believe treatment to restore the testes to an intrascrotal location should begin at 1 year of age.

Palpable undescended testes are easily treated by orchidopexy, and success with standard orchidopexy techniques approaches 95 per cent.[88] It is the impalpable gonad that presents the greatest diagnostic and therapeutic challenge and in these more difficult cases that laparoscopy plays a role. Prior to declaring a gonad impalpable, an examination must be done under optimal conditions. A warm examining room, warm hands, and a relaxed patient are mandatory. Placing the boy in a cross-legged position may increase the chances of successful palpation.[89] Also, we have found that some testes that were initially impalpable in the office become palpable under general anesthesia prior to a planned laparoscopy.

In those individuals with bilateral impalpable testes, a β-human chorionic gonadotropin (HCG) stimulation test has been used to signal the presence of testicular tissue. A negative test suggests the patient is truly anorchic. In boys with a normal karyotype, the presence of markedly elevated gonadotropins (luteinizing hormone and follicle-stimulating hormone) strongly suggests anorchism.[83] This method is not without its drawbacks, and false negative results have been reported.[90] These authors point out that a lack of response may be indicative of Leydig cell failure rather than complete absence of the testes. Thus, some feel that those with a negative β-HCG stimulation test should also undergo diagnostic laparoscopy.

Cryptorchidism can be treated either surgically or hormonally. Hormonal therapy has been used more widely in Europe. β-HCG was the first hormone used to induce testicular descent, followed by gonadotropin-releasing hormone. Hormone therapy is often ineffective in truly undescended testes; however, boys with retractile testes tend to respond.[91]

Laparoscopy in cryptorchidism is currently most useful as a diagnostic tool. The success of other diagnostic tests in localizing impalpable undescended testes has been limited. In one surgical series only 1 of 8 impalpable testes was identified by ultrasound, results which proved to be no better than those with a careful physical examination.[92] CT scanning has been used but is also of limited value in young children who lack the adequate amount of retroperitoneal fat required to delineate the testes.[93,94] CT scanning is also less attractive because of its associated radiation exposure and expense.

Venography may identify a blind-ending testicular vein, which is usually associated with an absent testes. However, this is an invasive technique, which can be technically demanding in pediatric patients, who often require general anesthesia.[95] The use of magnetic resonance imaging has met with some success in the localization of cryptorchid testes[96]; however, more data are needed to determine its efficacy. The long scanning time (often poorly tolerated by children) and need for sedation to prevent motion in children under the age of 5 make magnetic resonance imaging a less attractive option.

The use of laparoscopy for diagnosis and localization of impalpable testes was first reported in 1976.[97] Prior to its advent, the standard procedure for impalpable gonads was an inguinal exploration, which could be expanded to an intra-abdominal exploration if testes were not found in the inguinal area. Laparoscopy has several obvious advantages. The success rate for determining the presence or absence of a testis is 88 to 94 per cent.[98-101] In addition, with laparoscopy testes missed by a groin exploration can be identified, obviating the use of a large incision. In the series by Boddy et al.[98] laparoscopy was performed on 13 patients who had undergone a negative groin dissection for impalpable testes. An intra-abdominal testis was found in 5 of these patients. The use of laparoscopy can also prevent a needless exploration. Up to 64 per cent of impalpable testes are absent,[94] and thus almost two-thirds of patients who undergo evaluation for an impalpable gonad may be spared an unnecessary open procedure.

At the time of laparoscopy, the path of testicular descent can be carefully evaluated under direct vision. Absence of the testis has been called the "vanishing testis syndrome" and is thought to be secondary to a vascular catastrophe such as torsion or vascular occlusion during testicular descent.[102] The testes originate as retroperitoneal organs and descend along the gubernaculum. They remain at the abdominal end of the inguinal canal until the 7th month of gestation. They then pass through the inguinal canal and reach the scrotum by the 8th month.[103] Thus, the cryptorchid testis can be present at any point along the path of descent. However, the testis is most commonly located at the internal ring during the latent phase of descent[89] and finding it in a more cephalad position is uncommon. Ectopic testes are those that descend normally through the external inguinal ring, but are misdirected in their subsequent descent to a superficial inguinal, perineal, prepenile, or femoral location.[82]

The location of testes and findings at laparoscopy from several series are shown in Table 30-3.

The frequency of successful identification of testicular tissue in patients with impalpable testes varies considerably from series to series. With increasing experience, an examiner will miss fewer inguinal testes, thus increasing the percentage of absent testes in the impalpable group. Hence, these frequencies may vary with the skill of the examining physicians. Once a testis is identified laparoscopically,

Table 30-3. Location of Testes and Findings at Laparoscopy

Series	No. of Impalpable Testes	No. Absent	Location of Testes	
			Abdominal Inguinal	Ectopic
Castilho[105]	45	18 (40%)	5 (11.1%)	22 (49%)
Weiss and Seashore[95]	33	21 (64%)	5 (15%)	7 (21%)
Boddy et al.[99]	55	29 (53%)	19 (35%)	7 (13%)
Lowe et al.[102]	36	10 (28%)	14 (39%)	12 (33%)
Malone and Guiney[106]	45	5 (11%)	19 (42%)	21 (47%)
Manson et al.[102]	17	1 (6%)	5 (29%)	11 (65%)

appropriate treatment is dictated by its location. Testes found in the inguinal canal are best treated with a standard orchidopexy. The treatment options for an abdominal testis include standard orchidopexy if one finds a long testicular artery,[89] often facilitated by bringing the testis medial to the inguinal canal[106]; a Fowler-Stephens procedure, in which the testicular artery is divided relying on collateral blood low through the deferential artery[107]; a staged orchidopexy[108]; and testicular autotransplant with a microvascular anastomosis.[109] Of these treatment options for the high intra-abdominal testis, laparoscopy has its greatest application in the Fowler-Stephens orchidopexy. Bevan[110] first proposed the idea of orchidopexy by spermatic vessel transection in 1903. Because of poor results, the procedure lost popularity. In 1959, Fowler and Stephens[107] used intraoperative angiography to demonstrate vascular collateral vessels. Their findings, as well as those of others,[111] have shown that the testicular artery communicates with the vasal artery and the cremasteric artery. The vasal artery has a large caliber communication with the testicular artery in 87 per cent of patients.[111] This connection arises from the distal part of the vessel at the level of the cauda epididymidis. The cremasteric artery contribution to testicular blood flow most often arises as a solitary vessel located near the lower pole of the testis.

Fowler and Stephens[107] reported success in 8 of 12 patients treated by ligation of the spermatic vessels and primary orchidopexy. In a more recent series, Kogan et al.[112] reported an 89 per cent success rate in 38 similar cases. Necessary principles have been outlined by Gibbons et al.[113] for successful performance of this procedure: (1) one should leave a wide, medially based peritoneal strip attached to the vas deferens; (2) the surgeon should divide the testicular artery above the origin of the branch that will anastomose with the vasal artery; (3) the procedure is usually unsuccessful when performed as an afterthought following an extensive cord mobilization; and (4) direct injury to the vasal artery during cord dissection should be avoided.

Duckett first suggested that preliminary *in situ* ligation of the testicular vessels might improve the results of the Fowler-Stephens technique.[114] Pascual et al.[115] showed experimentally that spermatic vessel ligation *in situ* produces an initial decrease in blood flow of 80 per cent to the testes at 1 hour, but by 30 days normal flow is restored, and the integrity of the testis is usually preserved. On microscopic examination normal Leydig and Sertoli cell populations were seen with only mild tubular disturbances. Delaying testicular mobilization until a later date avoids traumatizing the testicle during the period of vascular compromise. Additionally, mobilization results in some element of tension on the vas deferens and remaining vessels, potentially further reducing the blood supply.

Bloom[114] reported on 7 patients in whom laparoscopy revealed an intra-abdominal testis. An endoscopic clip ligation of the spermatic vessels was performed through the laparoscope. Six months later a vas-based orchidopexy was done. An excellent result was obtained in six patients. In the seventh patient, who had undergone 2 previous inguinal explorations and ligation of the vas deferens, the procedure was unsuccessful. In their original paper, Fowler and Stephens felt a long loop-type vas deferens was necessary when a single-stage procedure was performed. Not all abdominal testes fit this criterion. Only 3 of 7 patients in the preceding series had a looping vas. This suggests that a two-step procedure with clip application is suitable for most abdominal gonads regardless of the vas length. Abdominal testes found at laparoscopy that appear to be nonviable and unlikely to produce sperm should be removed, because of an increased risk of malignancy in these testes. The orchidectomy can be performed laparoscopically.

Technique of Laparoscopy for Cryptorchidism

The patient is placed in the supine position. After the induction of general anesthesia, a small infraumbilical incision is made down to the level of the fascia. Using towel clips, upward traction is placed on either side of the umbilicus. The Veress needle is inserted through the incision, at a right angle to the abdomen, into the peritoneum. An audible "pop" is encountered in going through the fascia. The needle is connected to a carbon dioxide insufflator. Initial pressures of greater than 2 to 3 mm Hg indicate that the needle is not in the correct position, and it should be removed and reinserted.

We use the pressure of carbon dioxide insufflation as our guide to needle position and feel that this is reliable. Other authors advocate using the saline aspiration test.[89] A 10-ml syringe filled with 5 ml of saline is placed on the Luer lock of the Veress needle. Aspiration at this point should not produce gas bubbles or blood. The saline is then injected through the needle, and aspiration is repeated. If the needle is in the correct position, no saline will be aspirated. If the needle is extraperitoneal, some of the fluid will be aspirated back into the syringe. If the needle has been inserted into the bowel, then stool-stained saline will return. Once a pneumoperitoneum is established, the trochar is inserted along the same line and angle as the Veress needle.

The important anatomic landmarks in laparoscopy for impalpable testes are the medial and median umbilical ligaments, the internal rings, vasa, and spermatic vessels. In a patient with a unilateral impalpable testis, the normal side is inspected first. Traction on the testis may facilitate identification of the vessels. The goal is visualization of the spermatic vessels. Findings can be classified into three categories: (1) discovery of an intra-abdominal testis, (2) discovery of blind-ending testicular vessels, and (3) demonstration of a vas deferens and vessels entering the internal ring through a hernia or patent processus vaginalis. In our experience, which is supported by the literature, no testes have been found separate from blind-ending testicular vessels. Since the seminiferous tubules of the testis are of genital ridge origin and must fuse with the efferent ductules of the epididymis, nonfusion can occur and result in a testis separate from the epididymis.[116] Thus, a blind-ending vas deferens does not necessarily indicate absence of the testis. Nonfused testes, although unable to contribute to fertility, can produce hormones, and therefore this finding may warrant attempts to salvage them. In our experience, a hernia or patent processus vaginalis has not been observed in association with either an absent testis or a high abdominal testis. In every instance in which a hernia has been observed laparoscopically, a testis has been found at the level of the internal ring or more distally. Thus, an inguinal exploration is indicated in all patients in whom a hernia or patent processus vaginalis is visualized. Laparoscopic nonvisualization of the spermatic vessels is an indication for an intra-abdominal exploration.

Contraindications to laparoscopy for cryptorchidism include previous abdominal surgery, bleeding disorders, and prune belly syndrome, in which the testes are known to be in a high intra-abdominal position.

LAPAROSCOPIC NEPHRECTOMY

Clayman et al.[117] described the first laparoscopic nephrectomy in August 1991. This first procedure was performed for a tumor (proven to be an oncocytoma pathologically). Four trocars were placed with the patient in the supine position: an 11-mm trocar 2 inches above the umbilicus in the midline; an 11-mm trocar in the midclavicular line 4 inches above the umbilicus; a 5-mm trocar in the midclavicular line 1 inch below the umbilicus, and a 5-mm trocar 2 inches above the umbilicus. The fifth trocar was placed after the patient was repositioned in the lateral decubitus position (an 11-mm trocar in the anterior axillary line 2 inches above the umbilicus). After the right colon was reflected, the ureter was identified with the help of a ureteral catheter, which had been placed cystoscopically just prior to the procedure. The ureter was used for traction, and the renal vessels were dissected close to the medial border of the kidney. The segmental end vessels were clipped and divided. After the division of the ureter and dissection of the perirenal attachments, the kidney was free within the abdomen. It was then placed in an impermeable sterile sack inserted via an 11-mm trocar. The mouth of the sack was pulled up through the trocar, and the trocar was removed, leaving the neck of the sack protruding from the abdominal wall. The kidney was morcellated and aspirated from within the sack. Unfortunately, pathologic evaluation is limited with this technique, in that the margins are undetectable. Concerns over the potential for tumor spillage have also been raised. Many believe the laparoscopic approach seems best suited to patients who undergo nephrectomy for benign renal disease.

OTHER APPLICATIONS IN UROLOGY

Other uses for laparoscopy in urology have been proposed or described. Wickham[118] has described laparoscopic extraction of a ureteral calculus by ureterotomy which was left open, drained by a Penrose drain, and allowed to close by secondary intention. Another case of laparoscopic ureterolithotomy has since appeared in the literature.[119] Laparoscopy has been used to monitor and retract the bowel during the percutaneous removal of a staghorn calculus in a pelvic kidney.[120] Another described application is investigation of intersex disorders with gonadal biopsy.[121] There are many additional potential applications, including ureteral ligation for ureteral fistulas, retroperitoneal lymph node sampling for selected cases of testicular cancer, and bladder neck suspensions.

COMPLICATIONS

Complications during Laparoscopy for Urologic Disease

The possible complications during laparoscopy for urologic disease encompass those related to any laparoscopic procedure. These include intractable bleeding and injury to the bowel and intra-abdominal organs. One interesting complication of urologic interest is pneumoscrotum, occurring during varicocelectomy when carbon dioxide dissects through the internal ring and into the scrotum. This could also be expected to occur during hernia repairs. It causes no significant problems and can be reduced by squeezing the scrotum to compress the carbon dioxide back into the peritoneal cavity.

Complications Involving Urologic Organs

Urologic organs are at risk during laparoscopy. Grainger et al.[123] reviewed the 13 reported cases of ureteral injury during gynecologic laparoscopy. Four occurred during laparoscopic sterilization, 4 during treatment of endometriosis, 3 during lyses of adhesions, 1 during uterine sacral ligament transection, and 1 during trocar placement. Ureteral injury was clinically apparent soon after the procedure, within 48 to 72 hours. The most common clinical scenario included abdominal pain associated with peritoneal signs, an elevated white blood cell count, and fever. An intravenous pyelogram is a sensitive means for the identification of this complication.

Most of these injuries can be managed initially with endoscopic or percutaneous treatment, possibly obviating an open operation. Except for the trocar injury, each case of ureteral injury was associated with the use of electrocoagulation. This includes the use of bipolar coagulation, which was used during five of the procedures. The site of injury was most commonly in the area of the uterine sacral ligaments. Although the ureter may often be visualized through the peritoneum in the upper pelvis, it is less easily identified in its distal portion near these ligaments. The ureter is at increased risk during procedures for processes that distort the anatomy or thicken the peritoneum, such as endometriosis.

The bladder is also at risk during laparoscopy. Placement of a Foley catheter preoperatively reduces the likelihood of bladder injury. Bladder injury is usually related to trocar placement. Treatment of mild bladder injuries may be accomplished by Foley catheter placement alone. Severe injuries require open repair. Interestingly, one case of laparoscopic bladder repair following an iatrogenic injury has been reported.[124] As technical capabilities with endoscopic suturing mature, this may become a more common scenario. One case of peritonitis following injury to a vesicourachal diverticulum has been reported.[125]

REFERENCES

1. Walsh PC, Donker PJ. Impotence following radical prostatectomy: Insight into etiology and prevention. J Urol 1982; 128:492.
2. Skinner DG, Daniels J, Russell CA, et al. The role of adjuvant chemotherapy following cystectomy for invasive bladder cancer: A prospective comparative trial. J Urol 1991; 145:459.
3. Prout GR, Heaney JA, Griffen, PP, et al. Nodal involvement as a prognostic indicator in patients with prostatic carcinoma. J Urol 1980; 124:226.
4. Smith JA, Haynes TH, Middleton RG. Impact of external irradiation on local symptoms and survival free of disease in patients with pelvic lymph node metastasis from adenocarcinoma of the prostate. J Urol 1984; 131:705.
5. Gervasi LA, Mata J, Easley JD, et al. Prognostic significance of lymph nodal metastases in prostate cancer. J Urol 1989; 142:332.
6. Smith JA, Middleton RG. Implications of volume of nodal metastasis in patients with adenocarcinoma of the prostate. J Urol 1985; 133:617.
7. Zincke H, Fleming TR, Furlow WR, et al. Radical retropubic prostatectomy and pelvic lymphadenectomy for high-stage cancer of the prostate. Cancer 1981; 47:1901.
8. Elfving P, Lundgren R. Pelvic lymphadenectomy as staging before definitive treatment of prostatic carcinoma. Scand J Urol Nephrol 1988; 110(Suppl):155.
9. McDowell GC, Johnson JW, Tenney DM, Johnson DE. Pelvic lymphadenectomy for staging clinically localized prostate cancer: Indications, complications, and results in 217 cases. Urology 1990; 35:475.
10. Smith JA, Seaman JP, Gleidman JB, Middleton RG. Pelvic lymph node metastasis from prostatic cancer: Influence of tumor grade and stage in 452 consecutive patients. J Urol 1983; 130:290.

11. Donohue RE, Faurer HE, Whitesel JA, et al. Prostatic carcinoma: Influence of tumor grade on results of pelvic lymphadenectomy. Urology 1981; 28:435.
12. Fowler JE, Whitmore WF. The incidence and extent of pelvic lymph node metastases in apparently localized prostatic cancer. Cancer 1981; 47:2941.
13. Grossman HB, Batata M, Hilaris B, Whitmore WF. ^{125}I implantation for carcinoma of the prostate: Further follow-up of the first 100 cases. Urology 1982; 20:591.
14. Grossman IC, Carpiniello V, Greenberg SH, et al. Staging pelvic lymphadenectomy for carcinoma of the prostate: Review of 91 cases. J Urol 1980; 124:632.
15. Brendler CB, Cleeve LK, Anderson EE, Paulson DF. Staging pelvic lymphadenectomy for carcinoma of the prostate: Risk versus benefit. J Urol 1980; 124:849.
16. Bruce AW, O'Cleireachain F, Morales A, Awad SA. Carcinoma of the prostate: A critical look at staging. J Urol 1977; 117:319.
17. Lieskovsky G, Skinner DG, Weisenburger T. Pelvic lymphadenectomy in the management of carcinoma of the prostate. J Urol 1980; 124:635.
18. McLaughlin AP, Saltzstein SL, McCullough DL, Gittes RF. Prostatic carcinoma: Incidence and location of unsuspected lymphatic metastases. J Urol 1976; 115:89.
19. Paulson DF. The prognostic role of lymphadenectomy in adenocarcinoma of the prostate. Urol Clin North Am 1980; 7:615.
20. Flocks RH, Culp D, Porto R. Lymphatic spread from prostate cancer. J Urol 1959; 81:194.
21. Merrin C, Wajsman Z, Baumgartner G, Jennings E. The clinical value of lymphadenectomy: Are the nodes surrounding the obturator nerve visualized? J Urol 1977; 117:762.
22. Loening SA, Schmidt JD, Brown RC, et al. A comparison between lymphangiography and pelvic node dissection in the staging of prostatic cancer. J Urol 1977; 117:752.
23. Correa RJ, Kidd CR, Burnettt L, et al. Percutaneous pelvic lymph node aspiration in carcinoma of the prostate. J Urol 1981; 126:190.
24. Liebner EJ, Stefani S. Uro-Oncology Research Group. An evaluation of lymphangiography with nodal biopsy in localized carcinoma of the prostate. Cancer 1980; 45:728.
25. Castellino RA. Lymphography in clinically localized prostate cancer. NCI Monogr 1988; 7:37.
26. McCarthy P, Pollack HM. Imaging of patients with stage D prostatic carcinoma. Urol Clin North Am 1991; 18:35.
27. Hricak H. Noninvasive imaging for staging of prostate cancer: Magnetic resonance imaging, computed tomography and ultrasound. NCI Monogr 1988; 7:31.
28. Friedland GW, Chang P. The role of imaging in prostate cancer. Radiol Clin North Am 1991; 29:581.
29. Sawczuk IS, de Vere White R, Gold RP, Olsson CA. Sensitivity of computed tomography in evaluation of pelvic lymph node metastases from carcinoma of bladder and prostate. Urology 1983; 21:81.
30. Bezzi M, Kressel HY, Allen KS, et al. Prostatic carcinoma: Staging with MR imaging at 1.5 T. Radiology 1988; 169:339.
31. Singer JS, McClennan BL. The diagnosis, staging, and follow-up of carcinomas of the kidney, bladder, and prostate: The role of cross-sectional imaging. Semin Ultrasound CT MR 1989; 10:481.
32. Leroy M, Teillac P, Rain JJ, et al. The use of iodine 123 (^{123}I)-labeled monoclonal anti-prostatic acid phosphatase (PAP) 227A F (Ab) 2 antibody fragments in vivo. Cancer 1989; 64:1.
33. Kontturi M, Lukkarinen O, Vihko P, Vihko R. Radioimaging of lymph node involvement in prostatic carcinoma. Scand J Urol Nephrol 1988; 110(Suppl):113.
34. Rouviere H. Anatomy of the Human Lymphatic System. Ann Arbor, Edwards Brothers, Inc, 1938.
35. Clouse ME, Wallace J, eds. Lymphatic Imaging: Lymphography, Computer Tomography and Scintigraphy, 2nd ed. Baltimore, Williams & Wilkins, 1985.
36. Morgan WR, Lieber MM. Pelvic lymphadenectomy. In Crawford ED, Das S, eds. Current Genitourinary Cancer Surgery. Philadelphia, Lea & Febiger, 1990.
37. Golimbu M, Morales P, Al-Askari S, Brown J. Extended pelvic lymphadenectomy for prostatic cancer. J Urol 1979; 121:617.
38. Castellino RA, Ray G, Blank N, et al. Lymphangiography in prostatic carcinoma: Preliminary observations. JAMA 1973; 223:877.
39. Saitoh H, Yoshida K, Uchijima Y, et al. Two different lymph node metastatic patterns of a prostatic cancer. Cancer 1990; 65:1843.
40. Herr HW. Pelvic lymphadenectomy and iodine-125 implantation. In Jonson, DE, Boileau MA, eds. Genitourinary Tumors: Fundamental Principles and Surgical Techniques. New York, Grune and Stratton, 1982.
41. Lieskovsky G, Skinner DG. Role of lymphadenectomy in the treatment of bladder cancer. Urol Clin North Am 1984; 11:709.
42. Sternberg CN, Yagoda A, Scher H. et al. M-VAC (methotrexate, vinblastine, doxorobicin, and cisplatin) for advanced transitional cell carcinoma of the urothelium. J Urol 1988; 139:461.
43. Srinivas V, Morse MJ, Herr HW, et al. Penile cancer: Relation of extent of nodal metastasis to survival. J Urol 1987; 137:880.
44. Schellhammer PF, Grabstald H. Tumors of the penis. In Walsh PC, Gittes RF, Perlmutter AD, Stamey T, eds. Campbell's Urology. Philadelphia, WB Saunders Company, 1986.
45. Young MJ, Reda D, Waters WB. Penile carcinoma: A twenty five year experience. Urology 1991; 38:529.
46. Crawford ED, Das S. Carcinoma of the penis: Management of the regional lymphatic drainage. In Crawford ED, Das S. Current Genitourinary Cancer Surgery. Philadelphia, Lea & Febiger, 1990.
47. Catalona WJ, Kadmon D, Crane DB. Effect of minidose heparin on lymphocele formation following extraperitoneal pelvic lymphadenectomy. J Urol 1980; 123:890.
48. Dubin L, Amelar RD. Varicocele. Urol Clin North Am 1978; 5:563.
49. Greenberg SH. Varicocele and male fertility. Fertil Steril 1977; 28:699.
50. Kursh ED. What is the incidence of varicocele in a fertile population? Fertil Steril 1987; 48:510.
51. Amelar RD, Dubin L. Therapeutic implications of left, right, and bilateral varicocelectomy. Urology 1987; 30:53.
52. Pryor JL, Howards SS. Varicocele. Urol Clin North Am 1987; 14:499.
53. Ahlberg NE, Bartley O, Chidekel N. Right and left gonadal veins: An anatomical and statistical study. Acta Radiol 1966; 4:593.
54. Coolsaet, BLRA. The varicocele syndrome: Venogra-

phy determining the optimal level for surgical management J Urol 1980; 124:833.
55. Takihara H,. Sakatuku J, Cockett ATK. The pathophysiology of varicocele in male infertility. Fertil Steril 1991; 55:861.
56. Pryor JL, Howards SS. Varicocele. Urol Clin North Am 1987; 14:499.
57. Takihara H, Sakatuku J, Cockett ATK. The pathophysiology of varicocele in male infertility. Fertil Steril 1991; 55:861.
58. Greenberg JH. Varicocele and male fertility. Fertil Steril 1977; 28:699.
59. Greenberg JH, Lipshultz LI, Morganroth J, Wein AJ. The use of the Doppler stethoscope in the evaluation of varicoceles. J Urol 1977; 117:296.
60. Wheatley JK, Bergman WA, Green B, Walther MM. Transvenous occlusion of clinical and subclinical varicoceles. Urology 1991; 37:362.
61. Lewis RW, Harrison RM. Contact scrotal thermography. II: Use in the infertile male. Fertil Steril 1980; 34:259.
62. Pryor JL, Howards SS. Varicocele. Urol Clin North Am 1987; 14:499.
63. Palomo, A. Radical cure of varicocele by a new technique: Preliminary report. J Urol 1949; 61:604.
64. Ivanissevich O. Left varicocele due to reflux: Experience with 4,470 operative cases in forty-two years. J Int Coll Surg 1960; 34:742.
65. Mordel N, Mor-Yosef S, Margalioth BJ, et al. Spermatic vein ligation as treatment for male infertility: Justification by postoperative semen improvement and pregnancy rates. J Reprod Med 1990; 35:123.
66. Murray RN, Mitchell SE, Kadir J, et al. Comparison of recurrent varicocele anatomy following surgery and percutaneous balloon occlusion. J Urol 1986; 135:286.
67. Dubin L, Amelar RD. Varicocelectomy: 986 cases in a twelve-year study. Urology 1977; 10:446.
68. Reidl P, Lungimayr G, Stackl W. A new method of transfemoral testicular vein obliteration for varicocele using a balloon catheter. Radiology 1981; 139:323.
69. Marsman WP. Clinical versus subclinical varicocele: Venographic findings and improvement of fertility after embolization. Radiology 1985; 155:635.
70. Kaufman SL, Kadir J, Barth KH, et al. Mechanisms of recurrent varicocele after balloon occlusion or surgical ligation of the internal spermatic vein. Radiology 1983; 147:435.
71. Porst H, Bahren, W, Lenz, M, Altwin, JE. Percutaneous sclerotherapy of varicoceles—An alternative to conventional surgical methods. Br J Urol 1984; 56:73.
72. Kaye KW. Modified high varicocelectomy: Outpatient microsurgical procedure. Urology 1988; 32:13.
73. Braedel HU, Steffens J, Ziegler M, Polsky MS. Outpatient sclerotherapy of idiopathic left-sided varicocele in children and adults. Br J Urol 1990; 65:536.
74. Marks JL, McMahon R, Lipshultz LI. Predictive parameters of successful varicocele repair. J Urol 1986; 136:609.
75. Cockett ATK, Takihara H, Consentino MJ. The varicocele. Fertil Steril 1984; 41:5.
76. Naragan P, Amplatz K, Gonzales R. Varicocele and male subfertility. Fertil Steril 1981; 36:92.
77. Amelar RD, Dubin L. Right varicocelectomy in selected infertile patients who have failed to improve after previous left varicocelectomy. Fertil Steril 1987; 47:833.
78. Yarborough AA, Burns JR, Keller FS. Incidence and clinical significance of subclinical scrotal varicoceles. J Urol 1989; 141:1372.
79. Aaberg RA, VanCaille TG, Schuessler WW. Laparoscopic varicocele ligation: A new technique. Fertil Steril 1991; 56:776.
80. Hagood PG, Mehan DJ, Worischenk JH, et al. Laparoscopic varicocelectomy: Preliminary report of a new technique. J Urol 1992; 147:73.
81. Donovan JF, Winfield HN. Laparoscopic varix ligation. J Urol 1992; 147:77.
82. Hadziselimovic F. Testicular development. In Gillenwater JY, Grayhack JT, Howards SS, Duckett JW, eds. Adult and Pediatric Urology. St. Louis, CV Mosby, 1991.
83. Levitt SB, Kogan JJ, Schneider K, et al. Endocrine tests in phenotypic children with bilateral impalpable testes can reliably predict "congenital" anorchism. Urology 1978; 11:11.
84. Cortes D, Thorup J. Histology of testicular biopsies taken at operation for bilateral maldescended testes in relation to fertility in adulthood. Br J Urol 1991; 68:285.
85. Cromie WJ. Cryptorchidism and malignant testicular disease. In Hadziselimovic F, ed. Cryptorchidism: Management and Implications. New York, Springer-Verlag, 1983.
86. Anderson L, Willie-Jorgenson PA. Torsion of the testis: A 5-year material. Scand J Urol Nephrol 1990; 24:91.
87. Mininberg DT, Rodger JC, Bedford MJ. Ultrastructural evidence of the onset of testicular pathologic conditions in the cryptorchid testis within the first year of life. J Urol 1982; 128:782.
88. Youngson GG, Jones PF. Management of the impalpable testis: Long term results of the preperitoneal approach. J Pediatr Surg 1991; 26:618.
89. Elder JS. Laparoscopy and Fowler-Stephens orchiopexy in the management of the impalpable testis. Urol Clin North Am 1989; 16:399.
90. Bartone FF, Huseman CA, Maizels M, Firlit CF. Pitfalls in using human chorionic gonadotropin stimulation test to diagnose anorchia. J Urol 1984; 132:563.
91. Rajfer J, Handelsman DJ, Swerdloff RS, et al. Hormonal therapy of cryptorchidism: A randomized, double-blind study comparing human chorionic gonadotropin and gonadotropin-releasing hormone. N Engl J Med 1986; 314:466.
92. Weiss RM, Carter AR, Rosenfield AT. High resolution real-time ultrasonography in the localization of the undescended testis. J Urol 1986; 135:936.
93. Wolverson MK, Jagannadharao B, Sundaram M, et al. CT in localization of impalpable cryptorchid testes. AJR 1980; 134:725.
94. Weiss RM, Seashore JH. Laparoscopy in the management of the nonpalpable testis. J Urol 1987; 138:382.
95. Weiss RM, Glickman MG. Venography of the undescended testis. Urol Clin North Am 1982; 9:387.
96. Fritzsone PJ, Hricak H, Kogan BA, et al. Undescended testis: Valve of MR imaging. Radiology 1987; 164:169.
97. Cortesi N, Ferrari P, Zambarda E, et al. Diagnosis of bilateral abdominal cryptorchidism by laparoscopy. Endoscopy 1976; 8:33.
98. Boddy SM, Corkery JJ, Gornall P. The place of laparoscopy in the management of the impalpable testis. Br J Surg 1985; 72:918.
99. Hamidinia A, Nold S, Amankwah KS. Localization and treatment of nonpalpable testes. Surg Gynecol Obstet 1984; 159:439.
100. Lowe DH, Brock W, Kaplan GW. Laparoscopy for localization of nonpalpable testes. J Urol 1984; 131:728.

101. Manson AL, Terhune D, Jordan G, et al. Preoperative laparoscopic localization of the nonpalpable testis. J Urol 1985; 134:919.
102. Abeyaratne RR, Aherne WA, Scott JES. The vanishing testis. Lancet 1969; 2:822.
103. Tanagho W. Embryology of the genitourinary system. In Tanagho WA, McAninch JA, eds. *General Urology*. Norwalk, Appleton and Lange, 1988.
104. Castilho LN. Laparoscopy for the nonpalpable testis: How to interpret the endoscopic findings. J Urol 1990; 144:1215.
105. Malone PS, Guiney EJ. The value of laparoscopy in localising the impalpable undescended testis. Br J Urol 1984; 56:429.
106. Prentiss RJ, Weickgenant CJ, Moses JJ, Frazier DB. Undescended testis: Surgical anatomy of spermatic vessels, spermatic surgical triangles and lateral spermatic ligament. J Urol 1960; 83:686.
107. Fowler R, Stephens FD. The role of testicular vascular anatomy in the salvage of high undescended testes. Aust N Z J Surg 1959; 29:92.
108. Steinhardt GF, Kroovand RL, Perlmutter AD. Orchiopexy: Planned 2-stage technique. J Urol 1985; 133:434.
109. Silber SJ, Kelly J. Successful autotransplantation of an intra-abdominal testis to the scrotum by microvascular technique. J Urol 1976; 115:452.
110. Bevan AD. The surgical treatment of undescended testicle: A further contribution. JAMA 1903; 41:178.
111. Lee LM, Johnson HW, McLoughlin MG. Microdissection and radiographic studies of the arterial vasculature of the human testes. J Pediatr Surg 1984; 19:297.
112. Kogan SJ, Houman BZ, Reda EF, Levitt SB. Orchiopexy of the high undescended testis by division of the spermatic vessels: A critical review of 38 selected transections. J Urol 1989; 141:1416.
113. Gibbons MD, Cromie WJ, Duckett JW. Management of the abdominal undescended testicle. J Urol 1979; 122:76.
114. Bloom DA. Two-step orchiopexy with pelviscopic clip ligation of the spermatic vessels. J Urol 1991; 145:1030.
115. Pascual JA, Villanueva-Meyer J, Salido B, et al. Recovery of testicular blood flow following ligation of testicular vessels. J Urol 1989; 142:549.
116. Nowak K, Failure of fusion of epididymis and testicle with complete separation of the vas deferens. J Pediatr Surg 1972; 7:715.
117. Clayman RV, Kavoussi LR, Soper NJ, et al. Laparoscopic nephrectomy: Initial case report. J Urol 1991; 146:278.
118. Wickham JEA, ed. Urinary Calculous Disease. Edinburgh, Churchill Livingstone, 1979.
119. Adley R, Ferzli GS, Ioffreda R, Albert PS. Laparoscopic ureterolithotomy. Urology 1992; 39:223.
120. Eshghi AM, Roth JS, Smith AD. Percutaneous transperitoneal approach to a pelvic kidney for endourological removal of staghorn calculus. J Urol 1985; 134:525.
121. Scott JES. Laparoscopy as an aid in the diagnosis and management of the impalpable testis. J Pediatr Surg 1982; 17:14.
122. Grainger DA, Soderstrom RM. Schiff SF, et al. Ureteral injuries at laparoscopy: Insights into diagnosis, management, and prevention. Obstet Gynecol 1990; 75:839.
123. Neich H, McGlynn F. Laparoscopic repair of bladder injury. Obstet Gynecol 1990; 76:909.
124. Yong BL, Prabhakaren K, Lee YS, Ratham SS. Peritonitis following diagnostic laparoscopy due to injury to a vesicourachal diverticulum: Case report. Br J Obstet Gynaecol 1989; 96:365.

Chapter 31
Obstetric and Gynecologic Disorders

James Haebe
Dan C. Martin

In the last several years laparoscopic techniques have been introduced to general surgery. This minimally invasive surgery has added much to the surgeon's armamentarium. Indeed, a revolution of sorts is ongoing at the present. With the increased use of laparoscopy, surgeons will be encountering unexpected findings in the pelvis. It is important to the general surgeon to be able to recognize normal and pathologic conditions of the pelvis.

NORMAL ANATOMY

In order to recognize pathologic conditions of the pelvis, it is important to know the basic anatomy. On viewing the pelvis one can appreciate the close approximation of the uterus, the sigmoid colon, and the bladder (Figs. 31-1 and 31-2). The uterus is a muscular hollow organ measuring, in a nulliparous woman, 9.0 cm in length, 6.5 cm in width, and 3.5 cm in thickness. It is pyriform in shape and supported in an anteflexed and anteverted position.

The supporting ligaments of the uterus can be easily identified. The broad ligament is a filmy double layer of peritoneum through which important blood vessels, nerves, and lymphatics travel to the uterus. This ligament extends from the lateral margin of the uterus to the pelvic sidewall. At the base of the broad ligaments there is condensation of connective tissue running from the junction of the cervix and uterus to the lateral pelvic wall. These ligaments are known as the cardinal or Mackenrodt's ligaments. In the upper border of the broad ligament run three diverging structures, the most anterior being the round ligament. This muscular ligament runs from the uterine fundus just below and anterior to the insertion of the fallopian tube to the internal inguinal ring. The round ligament then runs through the inguinal canal to insert on the connective tissue of the labia majora. The ovarian ligament runs through the broad ligament posteriorly and connects the inner, lower pole of the ovary to the cornua of the uterus.

Other structures in the anterior peritoneal compartment are the vesicular ligament, the lateral umbilical ligaments, and the inferior epigastric vessels. The vesicular ligament is an inconstant horizontal peritoneal fold extending from side to side and crossing over the

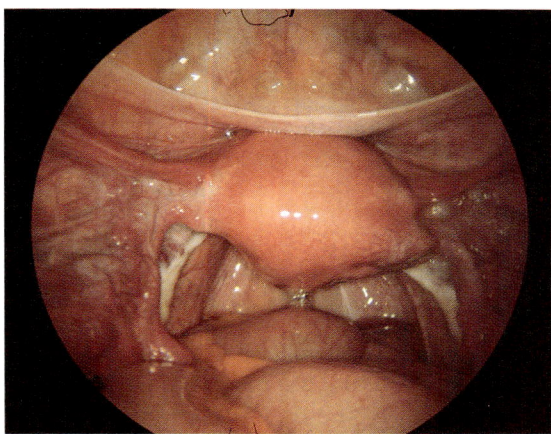

Figure 31-1. This is a normal pelvis with the uterus in mid position. The vesicular ligament is anterior to the uterus, and the bladder is beneath this. Below the uterus is the bowel and lateral are the tubes and ovaries.

round ligaments. The lateral umbilical ligaments are the remnant of the umbilical veins and extend from the umbilicus to the external iliac arteries near the inguinal rings. The inferior epigastric artery and vein are branches from and to the external iliac artery and vein and run between the peritoneum and rectus muscle near the lateral margin of the rectus muscle. When lower lateral punctures are placed, this artery and its associated veins are viewed directly in order to avoid damage to them.

Also running through the superior portion of the broad ligament is the fallopian tube. It is the most superior and central structure extending from the cornua out and back along the free upper margin of the broad ligament. The tube normally measures 10 to 12 cm in length and consists of four distinct portions. The interstitial portion is the shortest and narrowest segment, and it traverses the thickness of the myometrium. Next is the isthmus, which is 2 to 3 cm in length and 1 to 2 mm in luminal diameter. The walls of the isthmus are thick with muscle. The ampulla is the longest segment of tube, 6 to 7 cm, and is wider in diameter. The most distal portion of the infundibulum is trumpet shaped and has the fimbria, which sweep over the ovary to pick up the ovum. The ovaries are solid ovoid structures approximately 3 to 4 by 2.5 by 2 cm and weigh 4 to 8 g. The size of the ovary varies with time of the menstrual cycle. The ovaries appear pearly grey with a slightly corrugated surface. With aging come changes. A prepubertal ovary is small and elongated, while in the postmenopausal period, the ovary atrophies and its irregular contour is exaggerated. The ovaries are the only intraabdominal structures not covered by peritoneum. They are located below the tubes and attached to the posterior leaf of the broad ligament by the mesoovarium.

The uterosacral ligaments (Fig. 31-3) are condensations of endopelvic fascia, which connect the medial aspect of the cardinal ligaments and the uterus to the sacrum posteriorly. They can be seen as two folds of peritoneum running from the cervicouterine junction to the parietal peritoneum lateral to the rectum. This appearance is accentuated by using the uterine manipulator to push the uterus up and stretch the uterosacral ligaments. The uterosacral ligaments form the lateral boundaries of the pouch of Douglas or the posterior cul-de-sac. The anterior boundary of the cul-de-sac is the posterior vaginal wall and posteriorly lies the upper end of the rectum.

With laparoscopy, the course of the ureter can be traced in the pelvis (Fig. 31-4). This

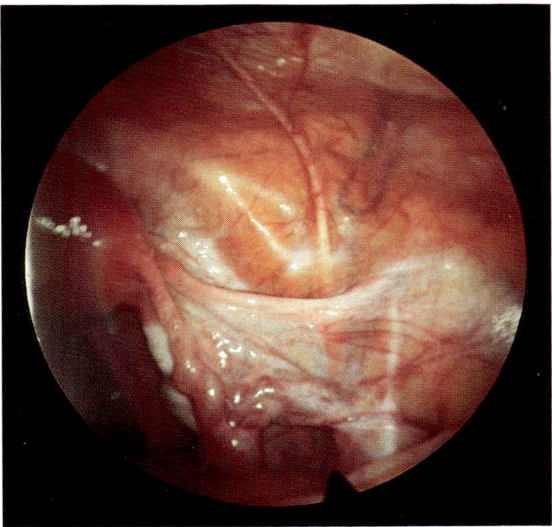

Figure 31-2. In this picture of the right lower quadrant, the lateral umbilical ligament (obliterated hypergastric artery) is seen coming from the left upper portion of the field. The inferior epigastric vessels are transversing the right upper portion of the field. The external iliac arteries are to the right in the right lower portion of the field. The uterus, right tube and ovary, and right round ligament are to the left and in the middle of the picture.

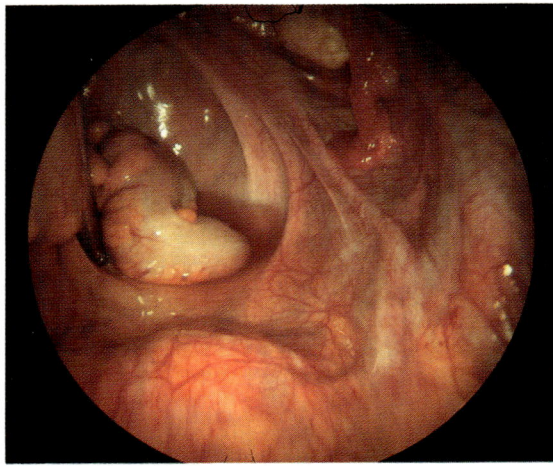

Figure 31-3. The rectosigmoid colon is to the left of the midline. The uterosacral ligament is immediately to the right and moving toward the sacrum. The ureter is lateral to the uterosacral ligament and courses up and over the pelvic brim in the lower right of the field. The right tube and ovary are seen in the upper portion of the picture.

retroperitoneal structure enters the pelvis over the sacroiliac joint; it crosses the external iliac vessels just after the bifurcation of the common iliac and runs downward and forward. The ureter crosses the base of the broad ligament below the uterine artery. After passing through the broad ligament, the ureter travels forward under the uterine artery and turns medial to reach the bladder. The trigone and bladder base rest on the anterior vaginal fornix and lower uterine segment. The remainder of the bladder is separated from the uterus by the anterior or uterovesical pouch.

UTERINE MASSES

Leiomyomas are the most common masses of uterine origin. They occur in one of every four to five premenopausal women.[1] Leiomyomas or fibroid tumors, as they are commonly referred to, are benign smooth muscle tumors arising from a single neoplastic cell. Estrogen is felt to have a role in tumor growth, but the etiology remains unclear.[2] Leiomyomas occur rarely prior to puberty and new myomas do not grow after menopause.

The appearance of the uterus can vary markedly as myomas can form in any site within the womb (Figs. 31-5 and 31-6). The tumors may be single or multiple and can be located in a subserosal, submucosal, or intramural location. Leiomyomas are solid tumors with a rubbery consistency. On sectioning, they have a whorled appearance, which on microscopic examination, reveals smooth muscle bundles mixed with strands of connective tissue.

It is estimated that 20 to 25 per cent of leiomyomas produce symptoms. These symptoms vary with the size and location of the

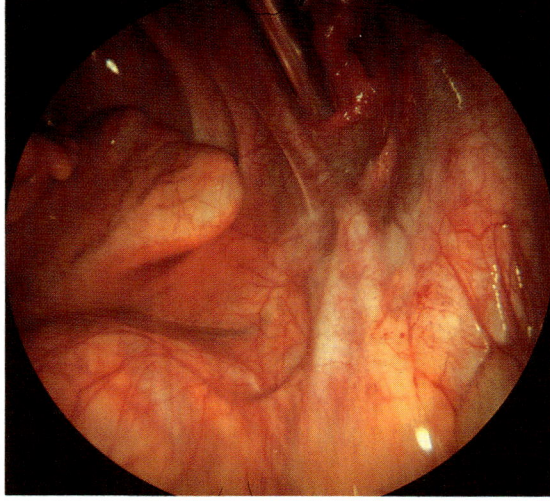

Figure 31-4. This picture of the right pelvic brim shows the ureter coursing over the right external and right internal iliac artery immediately adjacent to the bifurcation.

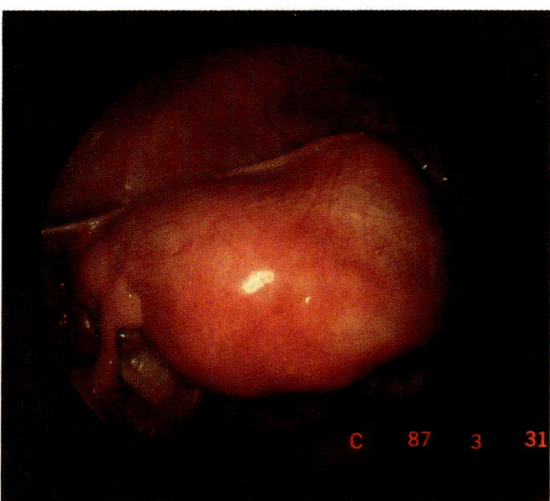

Figure 31-5. This uterus is distorted with intramural leiomyomas.

TUBAL DISORDERS

Pelvic inflammatory disease (PID) represents an ascending infection from the lower genital tract. Inciting agents such as *Chlamydia trachomatis* or *Neisseria gonorrhoeae* traverse the endocervix and enter the uterus and tubes causing endometritis and salpingitis. The infection in the upper genital tract and peritoneal cavity are, however, polymicrobial with an anaerobic predominance.[6] Further progression of the infection leads to tuboovarian abscess, a serious sequela.

Patients at risk for PID include sexually active women with multiple partners, women who have had previous sexually transmitted diseases, and women who use intrauterine devices. A patient who has had a previous episode of PID has a 23 per cent chance of having a further episode.[7] These patients typically are seen with abdominal pain, cervical and uterine motion pain, and adnexal tenderness. Purulent vaginal discharge may also be noted. In addition, fever and leukocytosis are generally present with gonorrhea but are commonly absent with chlamydia. Chlamydial infection is commonly an asymptomatic disease.

The clinical criteria for the diagnosis of PID developed by Hagar et al.[8] provide some standardization (Table 31-1), but often the diagnosis is uncertain and laparoscopy must be used. In a study by Jacobson and Westrom,[9] 815 women with a clinical diagnosis of

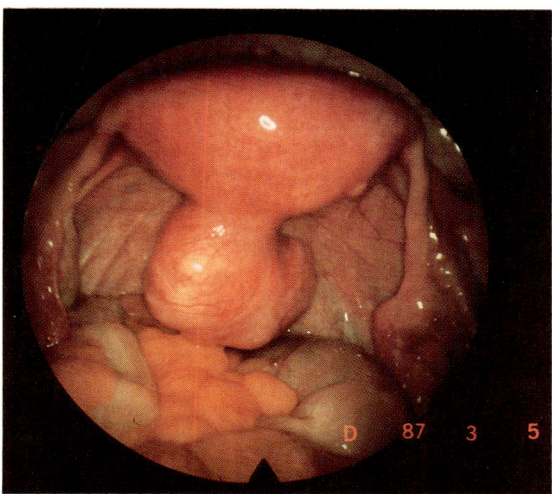

Figure 31-6. This pedunculated subserosal leiomyoma arises from the posterior uterine fundus.

tumors. Menstrual abnormalities are common. Uterine bleeding may be associated with an increased endometrial surface area as in the case of a submucous leiomyoma or with the compression of venous plexi of adjacent myometrium and endometrium as demonstrated by Farrer-Brown and associates.[3] Pressure or pelvic heaviness may be caused by the increased growth of a myoma. Compression of adjacent structures may lead to frequency or urinary retention or constipation with a posterior fibroid tumor. The ureters may also be compressed, leading to hydroureter and hydronephrosis. Leiomyomas can produce pain if they outgrow their blood supply and undergo degeneration. Pedunculated fibroid tumors can become infarcted by torsion. Leiomyomas have also been associated with decreased fertility, premature labour, and malpresentation. A rare complication is sarcomatous change which occurs at an estimated rate of less than 10 per cent or lower. Because of this rare occurrence, intact removal[4] or morsellation within a sack to avoid spill is recommended.

Congenital abnormalities of the female reproductive tract are relatively common. Many such anomalies are asymptomatic and therefore go undetected. Bicornate uteri, uterus didelphys and rudimentary uterine horn represent a spectrum of müllerian fusion defects. If such a defect is found, it is important to assess the urinary tract as these are frequently associated with genitourinary abnormalities.[5]

Table 31-1. Criteria for Clinical Diagnosis of Salpingitis

All of the following must be present
  Abdominal direct tenderness with or without rebound tenderness
  Cervical and uterine motion tenderness
  Adnexal tenderness

One of the following must be present
  Gram stain consistent with gonococcus
  Positive fluorescent antibody or culture for *Chlamydia trachomatis*
  Temperature >38°C
  Leukocytosis >10,000/mm³
  Leukocytes present in culdocentesis fluid
  Pelvic mass abscess or complex on bimanual or sonographic examination

Reproduced with permission from the American College of Obstetricians and Gynecologists (Obstet Gynecol 1983; 61:113–114).

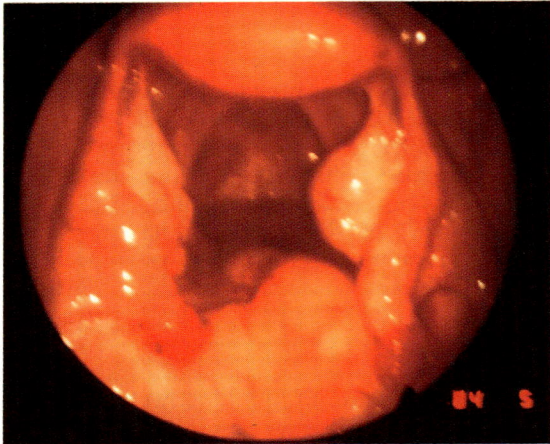

Figure 31-7. In acute pelvic inflammatory disease, the tubes are edematous and swollen and on occasion have exudate on the surface. (Reproduced with permission from Intra-Abdominal Laser Surgery, © 1986, Resurge Press, Memphis, TN.)

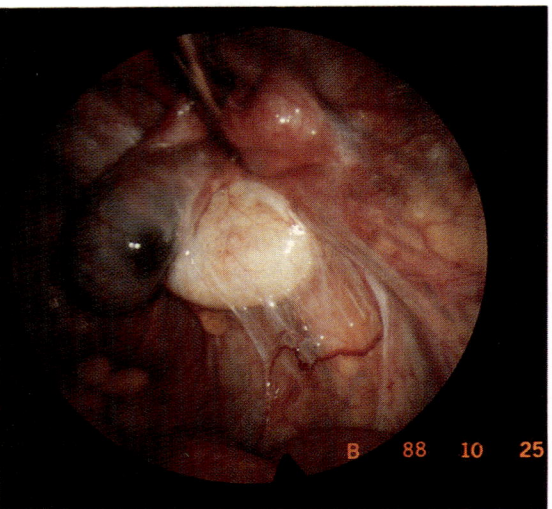

Figure 31-8. Filmy pelvic adhesions associated with a right hydrosalpinx have the ovary encased behind a cellophane-like barrier. Methylene blue dye has been injected into the right hydrosalpinx to check for tubal patency. The lumen of the right tube is open to the distal end but is closed in a complete hydrosalpinx.

salpingitis underwent laparoscopy. PID was confirmed in 512 (65 per cent). No pathologic condition was seen in 184 patients (22.6 per cent), and 98 (12 per cent) had other clinical entities. Unexpected salpingitis was found in 91 patients who did not have clinical evidence of PID. The other disease processes found included acute appendicitis, pelvic endometriosis, or intraperitoneal hemorrhage.

In acute salpingitis the tubes appear erythematous and slightly swollen (Fig. 31-7). A fibrinous or purulent exudate may be noted on the tubal serosa. Filmy adhesions (Fig. 31-8) from the tube to ovary or pelvic sidewall may also be seen. In Fitz-Hugh-Curtis syndrome the stigmata of pelvic infection will be seen as well as violin string adhesions between the liver and diaphragm (Fig. 31-9).

When the acute disease process is more advanced, a tuboovarian abscess may be noted (Fig. 31-10). The tubes are grossly dilated with pus and firmly adherent to the ovary in an inflammatory mass. Bowel and omentum may also be involved with adhesions. In the past, surgical treatment was required for tuboovarian abscesses but with improvements in antibiotics, such pelvic abscesses can be treated medically with broad spectrum coverage. Surgery is used if the patient fails to respond.

Infertility is the major sequela of PID today. By causing adhesions, tubal mobility is impaired. Hydrosalpinx can be thought of as the end stage of the tubal inflammatory process (Fig. 31-11). The fimbriated end of the tube is occluded. As a result the mucinous secretions of the tubal epithelium accumulates in the lumen producing dilatation. The tubes are enlarged and can be edematous and thick.

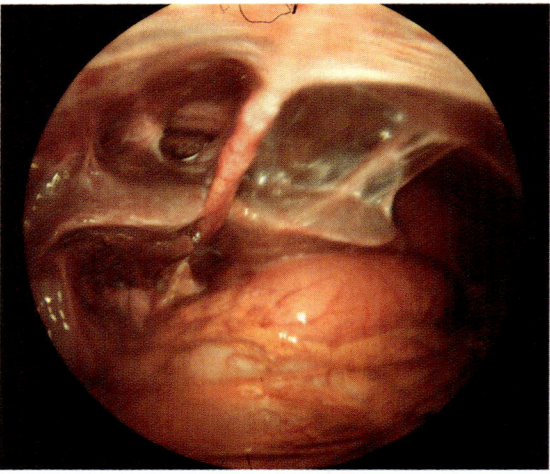

Figure 31-9. Fitz-Hugh-Curtis adhesions are seen between the liver and the diaphragm. Although these are most common to the right hemidiaphragm, occasionally they occur bilaterally as seen in this patient. The falciform ligament is in the middle of the field and the left and right lobes of the liver are noted.

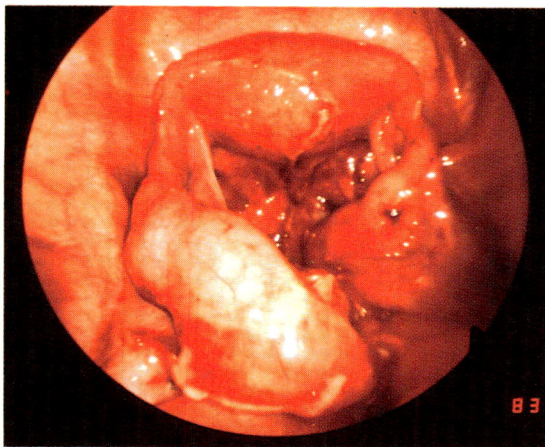

Figure 31-10. Acute bilateral tuboovarian abscesses with diffuse pelvic adhesions and organizing exudate are noted in this picture. (Reproduced with permission from Intra-Abdominal Laser Surgery, © 1986, Resurge Press, Memphis, TN.)

PARAOVARIAN CYSTS

Paraovarian cysts may also appear as tubal adnexal enlargements. These are mesonephric duct remnants that grow within the leaves of the broad ligament. Paraovarian cysts are usually simple thin-walled unilocular cysts, which do not have a pedicle. Symptoms, if any are present, are produced by displacement. Hydatid cysts of Morgagni, which are located on the distal end of the tube, are the most common variant and produce few if any sequelae (Fig. 31-12).

ADNEXAL TORSION

Torsion of the tube alone or in association with the ovary is a surgical emergency. It may occur whenever there is enlargement of the tube or ovary and the mass is relatively mobile. As the mass twists on its pedicle there is venous occlusion, which results in rapid engorgement. The ischemic tissue produces intense pain and signs of local peritoneal irritation. Leukocytosis and fever are also usually present. On examination, the mass is dusky or even black and the pedicle in torsion is clearly visible (Fig. 31-13). If the torsion is prolonged and the tissue is necrotic, excision is mandatory. This should be performed without untwisting the pedicle to decrease the risk of embolization.

ECTOPIC PREGNANCY

One of the most common and perhaps most serious tubal abnormality is an ectopic pregnancy. From 1970 to 1987 there was a 5-fold increase in the number of ectopic pregnancies, now accounting for approximately 1.7 per cent of all pregnancies.[10] This increase in tubal gestation is thought to be a result of the increase in PID, occurrence of

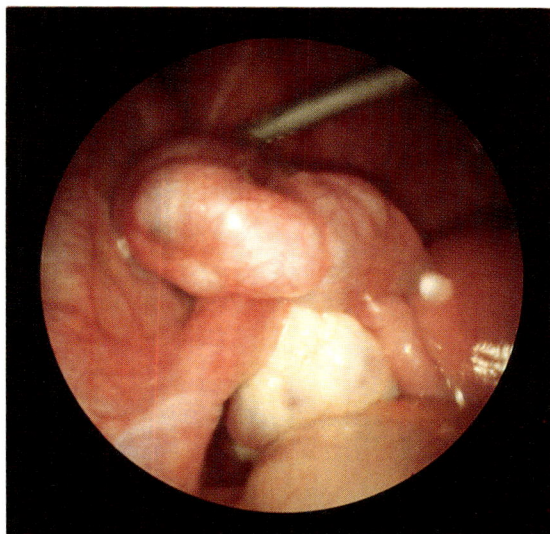

Figure 31-11. This chronic right hydrosalpinx is dilated and clubbed at the end. There are no fimbria. The right ovary is seen directly beneath the right hydrosalpinx.

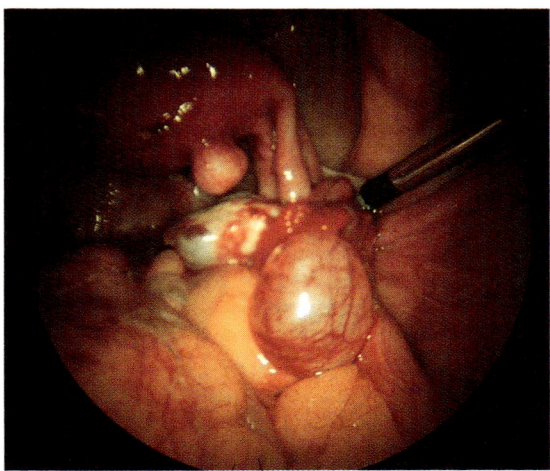

Figure 31-12. A hydatid cyst of Morgagni in a paratubal cyst, which is either congenital or is a dilated tubal frond.

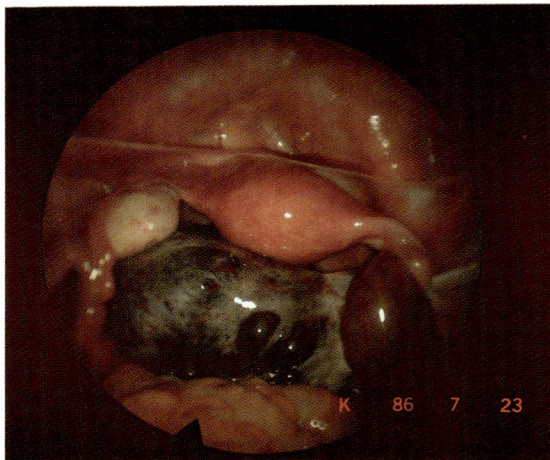

Figure 31-13. This adnexal torsion in a teenage patient was treated with salpingo-oophorectomy.

tubal surgery, presence of endometriosis, use of clomiphrene (Clomid), and history of previous abdominal surgery.[11] Ectopic pregnancies may occur anywhere outside the uterus, but the vast majority are found within the tube. These occur, in order of decreasing frequency, in the ampulla, isthmic region, and uncommonly in the fimbrial or interstitial portion of the tube.

Typically patients have pelvic pain and either abnormal uterine bleeding or amenorrhea. Diagnosis is not always straightforward as the differential diagnosis includes adnexal torsion, acute appendicitis, aborting intrauterine pregnancy, and a bleeding corpus luteum. Any woman of reproductive age seen with lower abdominal pain should be asked to give a menstrual and contraceptive history and a blood or urine human chorionic gonadotropin (HCG) test must be performed. Improvements in the sensitivity of HCG assays have made it possible to predict abnormal gestations. In a normal intrauterine pregnancy, the HCG level doubles every 2 to 3 days. In addition, once the HCG level is greater than 6500 mIU/ml, an intrauterine gestational sac should be seen on a pelvic ultrasound.[12,13] If the HCG is greater than 6500 mIU/ml and on the ultrasound the uterus is empty, there is strong grounds for the suspicion of an ectopic pregnancy. This discriminatory HCG zone is as low as 1500 mIU/ml with newer vaginal probe ultrasound.

If the pregnancy test is positive, management is generally based on clinical signs, vaginal sonography, and HCG titers. This management is covered in detail in other publications.[14,15] In summary, a laparoscopy is performed if clinical signs or sonograms suggest hemorrhage. If there is no suggestion of hemorrhage and the quantitative HCG titer is less than 1000 mIU/ml, the patient is reexamined in 48 to 72 hours. If the titer is more than 1000 mIU/ml, the sonogram shows no evidence of pregnancy, and the patient is asymptomatic, she is rechecked in 24 to 48 hours. As mentioned previously with a healthy pregnancy, the titer usually doubles every 2 to 3 days. These patients are rechecked every 1 to 4 days until a definitive diagnosis of healthy pregnancy, spontaneous abortion, or tubal pregnancy is made and appropriate therapy initiated.

Laparoscopy commonly reveals a localized swelling within the tube, often appearing bluish in color (Fig. 31-14). Bleeding from the distal portion of the tube may also be noted. The tube may also reveal evidence of rupture, which often results in profuse bleeding and subsequent hemoperitoneum. As a result, more conservative treatment such as methotrexate or salpingostomy with preservation of the tube can be used. With quantitative HCG titers of less than 500 mIU/ml, the tubal pregnancies can be small enough to escape detection at laparoscopy. The titer is rechecked in 24 to 48 hours and plans are made based on rising, stable, or falling titers.

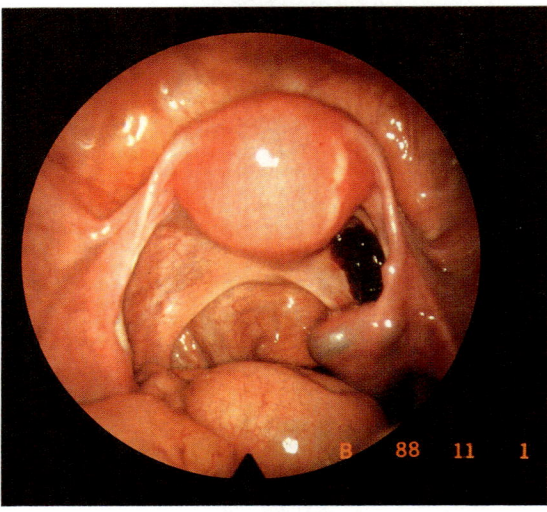

Figure 31-14. This right ampullary ectopic pregnancy is associated with clots in the right adnexa. Blood in the pelvis has been removed using an irrigation-aspiration system.

ENDOMETRIOSIS

Endometriosis is a condition in which functioning endometrium, glands, and stroma are located outside the uterus. The incidence of endometriosis is difficult to assess, but it is estimated to occur in 25 to 50 per cent of infertile women. Several theories of the etiology of endometriosis have been put forward. Sampson's theory[16] of retrograde menstruation with peritoneal seeding has survived the test of time. Evidence supporting this theory includes the occurrence of endometriosis in patients with outflow tract obstruction. On the other hand, endometriosis has also been found at distant sites such as the umbilicus, lymph nodes, brain, and kidney, giving support to the theory of hematogenous or lymphatic spread of endometriosis.[17] Meyer[18] proposed that chronic inflammation secondary to refluxed menstrual blood leads to celomic metaplasia, with peritoneal cells becoming endometriotic. Reflux menstruation occurs in most women to some degree, yet not all women develop endometriosis. Dmowski et al.[19] demonstrated that monkeys with endometriosis had decreased cellular-mediated immunity to endometrial tissue, suggesting that an immunologic defect may lead to endometriosis. A genetic component may also be responsible for endometriosis. Simpson et al.[20] reported an incidence of 6.9 per cent in first-degree relatives of patients with endometriosis compared to 1 per cent in a control group.

Classically the symptoms of endometriosis have included infertility, dysmenorrhea, and deep dyspareunia. Causes of infertility can be mechanical, such as adhesions, and biochemical, such as increased prostaglandins leading to interference with ovulation, ovum transport, or corpus luteum function.[21] Dysmenorrhea may be a result of peritoneal inflam-

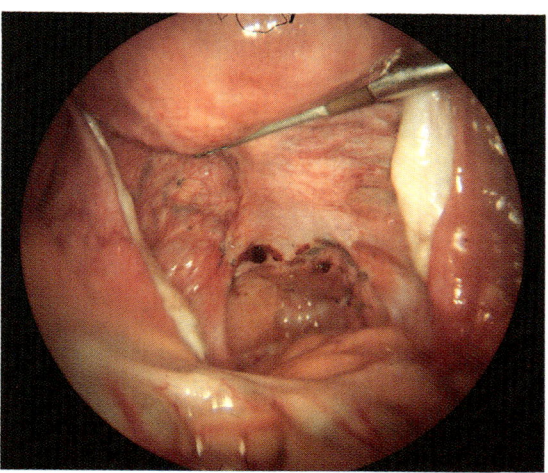

Figure 31-16. This diffuse endometriosis involves the entire cul-de-sac and is extending to the broad ligaments and toward the rectum.

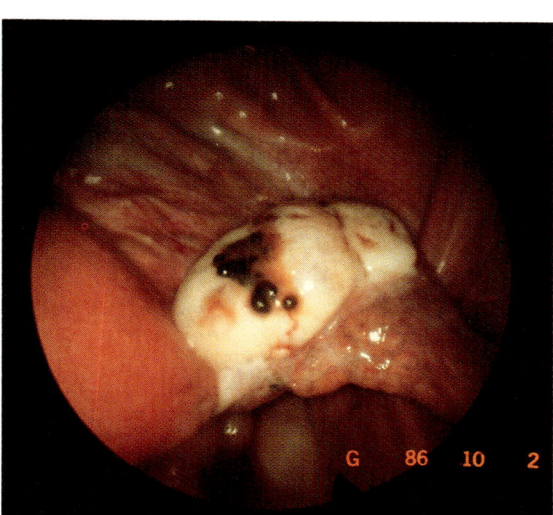

Figure 31-15. This right ovary has surface chocolate cysts, which are less than 15 mm in diameter. As these get progressively larger, their appearance may stay similar to this or, with deep encapsulation, they may appear whitish on the surface.

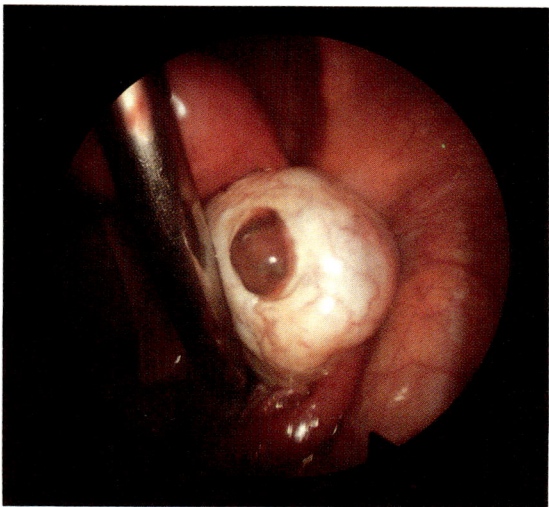

Figure 31-17. This hemorrhagic corpus luteum of the right ovary has an appearance very similar to the endometrioma of Figure 31-15. Histologic examination is needed to distinguish these two findings.

mation and irritation by the ectopic endometrium or increased prostaglandins leading to uterine hypercontractility. Deep dyspareunia may be a result of mechanical stretching of affected peritoneal surfaces.

Endometriosis has been described as black powder burn lesions and blebs on the peritoneum, chocolate cysts in the ovaries, and infiltrating fibromuscular nodules in the cul-de-sac[22] (Figs. 31-15 and 31-16). While dark, puckered, typical lesions are the easiest to recognize, subtle forms are more common and possibly more active than black lesions.[23-27] Indeed, endometriosis may be present in any peritoneal abnormality from clear vesicles to red blebs. Similarly, lesions that look like endometriosis may be granulation tissue, hemangiomas, and other pathologic conditions.[24-27] Histologic confirmation of the diagnosis is important. Endometriomas or chocolate cysts of the ovary result from the accumulation of blood and endometrial tissue in the ovary. Grossly, a cyst is seen which contains a viscous chocolate-like liquid. Histologic examination is needed to differentiate these cysts from hemorrhagic corpus lutea (Fig. 31-17).[28] Endometriosis can also be infiltrating, and this may be easier to palpate than to visualize.[29]

The bowel and bladder may also be involved with endometriosis (Figs. 31-18, 31-19, and 31-20). Urinary symptoms may include frequency/urgency or gross cyclic hematuria. Bowel symptoms range from pres-

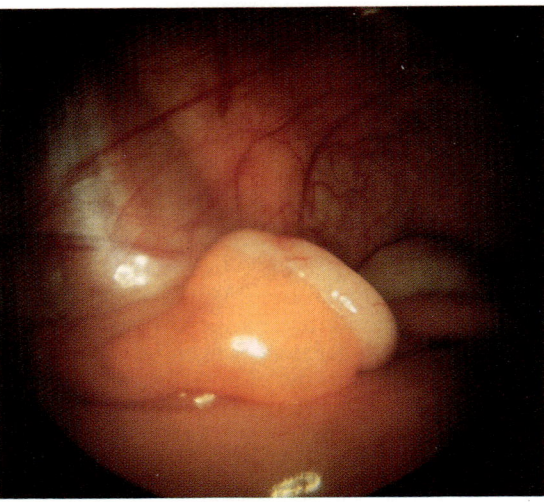

Figure 31-19. The fibrotic distortion of the appendix in this picture is caused by a small (3 mm) lesion of the tip of the appendix. With further involvement, the appendix may appear fibrotic but have no other evidence of endometriosis. Endometriosis can occlude the lumen and result in a mucocele. If the appendix proximal to the mucocele is not closely sectioned, the endometriosis may not be found.

sure, to cyclic hematochezia, to actual bowel obstruction.

Endometriosis can be found in the upper abdomen (Fig. 31-21) from disseminated intraperitoneal spread. Rare reports of pulmo-

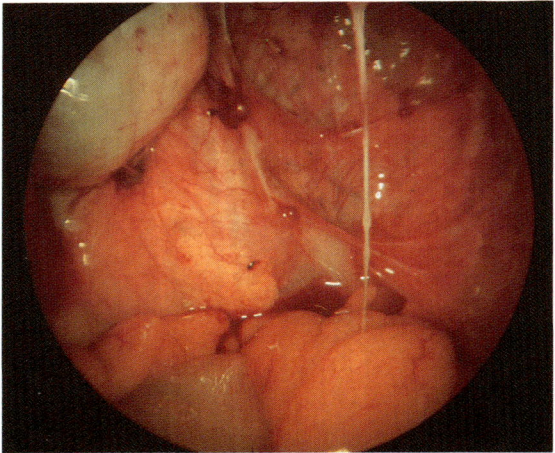

Figure 31-18. This patient has diffuse peritoneal endometriosis. In the middle of the field a red lesion is seen involving the rectum with distortion and puckering of the rectal serosa. This puckering implies that the muscularis is also involved.

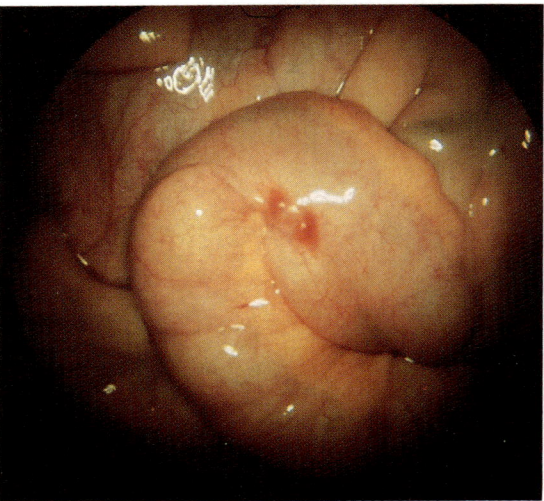

Figure 31-20. Endometriosis involving the serosa and superficial muscularis of the ilium. This was resected at laparotomy without entering the lumen.

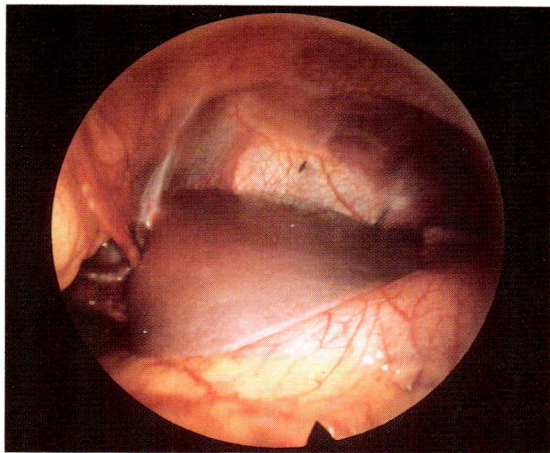

Figure 31-21. This picture of the left hemidiaphragm and left lobe of the liver shows endometriosis on the diaphragm immediately beneath the pericardium.

nary and occular involvement suggest that hematogenous spread occurs.

OVARIAN MASSES

The ovary is the most frequent site of pelvic masses. The differential diagnosis is greatly influenced by age (Table 31-2). For example, a palpable adnexal mass in a reproductive age woman would most often be benign, but an ovarian mass in a prepubertal child or postmenopausal female would be more worrisome. The size of the ovary itself varies through the periods of a woman's life, being nonpalpable in childhood and the postmenopausal period, to being 3.0 by 2.0 by 1.5 cm in the reproductive years.

FUNCTIONAL CYSTS

Functional cysts of the ovary represent exaggerations of the normal physiologic response of the ovary. They are very common and almost always have few clinical sequelae. Follicular cysts arise from a normal follicle that fails to ovulate or undergo atresia. These soft cystic structures are clear, thin-walled, and generally small (Fig. 31-22). Occasionally they will reach a diameter of 6 to 8 cm (Fig. 31-23). The fluid within a follicular cyst is serous and yellow in color and has a high concentration of estrogen. This may explain why these cysts may be associated with a menstrual disturbance. Follicular cysts usually disappear spontaneously during the subsequent menstrual cycle. If persistent, the cyst can be treated by ovarian suppression with an oral contraceptive pill.

Table 31-2. Ovarian Mass: Differential Diagnosis

Prepubertal	Reproductive	Menopausal
80% germ cell	Functional	95% derived
50% malignant	Unilateral	from germinal
	Mobile	epithelium
	Cystic	
	Less than	50% malignant
	8 cm	Always palpable
	Endometrioma	
	Neoplastic	
	Teratoma	
	Fibroma	
	Cystadenoma	
	Malignant	

Reproduced with permission from Kase NG, Weingold AB, Gerhenseon DM. Principles and Practice of Clinical Gynecology, 2nd ed. New York, Churchill Livingston, 1990, p 565.

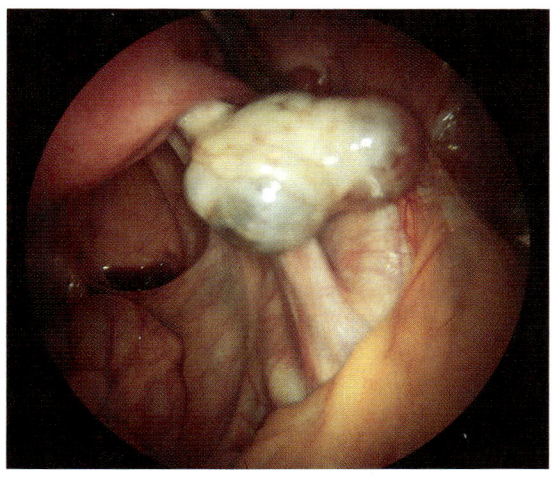

Figure 31-22. This right ovary has a simple follicular cyst medially and a corpus luteum cyst laterally. The simple follicular cyst contains clear fluid, but aspiration or drainage is needed to ensure that this is clear and not a chocolate cyst. The corpus luteum, which is lateral to the simple cyst, is generally avoided as significant bleeding occurs if these are explored. However, if the appearance is not typical of a corpus luteum, it is explored and bleeding is controlled if it occurs.

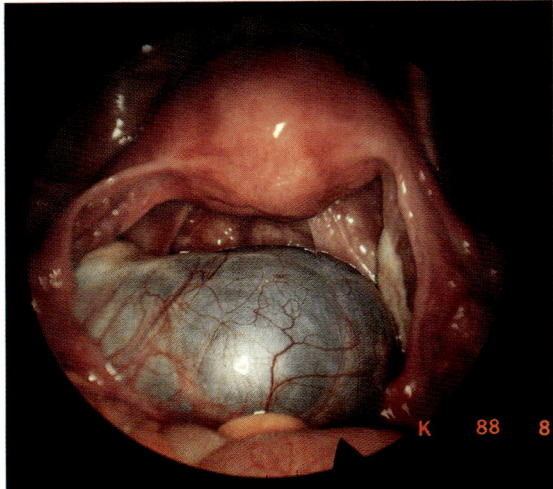

Figure 31-23. This is a large simple cyst which appears to be a large follicular cyst with old hemorrhage. The walls of these cysts can generally be resected at laparoscopy. Preoperative evaluation with sonography and CA-125 levels is useful in determining whether this patient should have the ovary removed intact or whether a conservative procedure can be performed at laparotomy or laparoscopy.

Corpus luteum cysts arise when a corpus luteum has intracavitary bleeding (Figs. 31-17 and 31-22). This leads to dilatation and cystic changes. These cysts are less common and usually larger than follicular cysts. They contain the yellow-orange steroid-producing cells for which the corpus luteum is named. Often a delay in the onset of menses is noted. Corpus luteum cysts usually resolve spontaneously but may rupture, leading to a hemoperitoneum. With resolution, hemosiderin accumulates in the wall and may leave a brown appearance. Because of internal hemorrhage and hemosiderin deposition, these cysts may be confused with endometriosis (see Chapter 32).[28]

Polycystic ovaries represent another functional change in the ovary associated with chronic anovulation. The ovaries are bilaterally enlarged and appear sclerotic. The surface does not reveal signs of recent ovulation (Fig. 31-24). On sectioning of multiple cysts, follicles that do not mature properly are noted, and there is thickening of the ovarian cortex. Treatment of this condition depends on the patient's desire for fertility. Induction of ovulation is used to increase fertility and ovarian suppression is used when fertility is to be avoided.

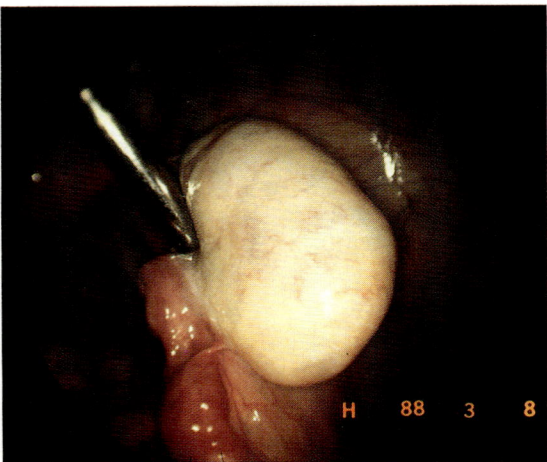

Figure 31-24. In polycystic ovarian syndrome, the ovary is enlarged with a smooth thickened capsule and no signs of recent ovulation.

OVARIAN NEOPLASMS

Ovarian neoplasms are the most worrisome of the ovarian pathologic conditions. About 20 per cent of all ovarian neoplasms are malignant.[30] The chance of a mass being malignant varies with the patient's age. Appearance at time of surgery also can be used to predict whether a tumor is benign or malignant (Table 31-3). The final diagnosis, however, is never certain before histopathologic examination of the tumor (Fig. 31-25).

Ovarian neoplasms are classified according to their histogenesis (Table 31-4). For each tissue type there are benign and malignant tumors. It is beyond the scope of this text to detail each type of ovarian tumor. Instead the difference between benign and malignant tumors will be stressed.

The differential diagnosis of an ovarian mass varies with the age of the patient. Prior

Table 31-3. Diagnostic Characteristics of Ovarian Lesions

Benign	Malignant
Cystic	Semicystic or solid
Unilateral	Bilateral
Mobile	Fixed
Smooth surfaces	External excrescence
Intact capsule	Capsule invaded
Normal peritoneal fluid	Hemorrhagic ascites
No internal papillations	Variable internal structure with necrosis

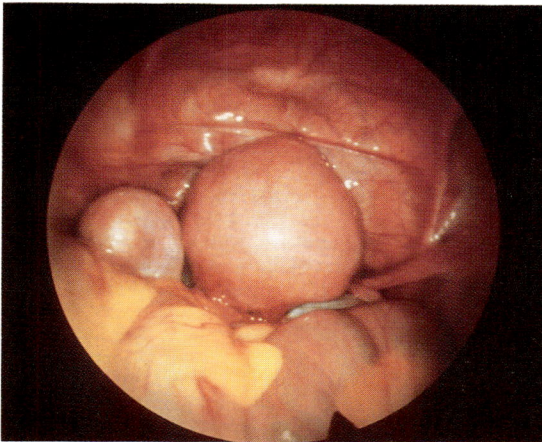

Figure 31-25. In this picture, the uterus is in the midline and what appears to be a corpus luteum is to the left of the uterus. However, this patient was receiving hormonal suppression for extensive endometriosis. The adhesion caused by the endometriosis is noted from the posterior uterine fundus to the bowel. In that this tumor persisted with hormonal suppression, it was excised intact. A small 1-cm well circumscribed malignant teratoma was found within an otherwise benign 3-cm dermoid cyst. In that this tumor was resected intact, the patient's prognosis is excellent. This case stresses the importance of histologic evaluation and avoiding spill when possible.

Table 31-4. Classification of Ovarian Tumors by Cell of Origin

Germinal epithelium
  Serous
  Mucinous
  Endometroid
  Brenner
  Clear-cell
  Solid undifferentiated
Germ cell
  Teratoma
    Benign
    Malignant
  Dysgerminoma
  Endodermal sinus tumor
  Primary choriocarcinoma
Mesenchymal cell
  Granulosa cell
  Theca cell
  Hilus cell
  Arrhenoblastoma
  Gonadblastoma
  Gynandroblastoma
Other stroma cells
  Fibroma
  Angioma
  Lipoma
  Lymphoma
  Sarcoma

to menarche, an ovarian enlargement is abnormal, and prompt surgical exploration is indicated. Germ cell tumors make up approximately 80 per cent of prepubertal neoplasms. In the reproductive years, ovarian masses are most often functional. In addition, endometriomas and benign neoplastic tumors such as teratomas are common. As the patient approaches menopause, malignant epithelial tumors predominate. Any ovarian enlargement in a peri- or postmenopausal patient is highly suspicious for a malignancy, and surgical exploration is indicated.

Benign tumors generally occur within the reproductive years. They are usually cystic and unilateral. The surface is smooth and intact without excrescences, and the ovary is mobile. On cutting, the cyst is unilocular and there are no internal papillations. Malignant tumors, on the other hand, tend to occur during the peri- and postmenopausal period. The tumor itself is often bilateral and fixed with cystic solid or solid appearance. Excrescences are noted on its surface and internally there are papillations. Ascites with peritoneal seeding is also common (Fig. 31-26).

The prior diagnostic criteria may give a general idea of the nature of the ovarian lesion, but histologic examination must be performed. A frozen section at the time of oo-

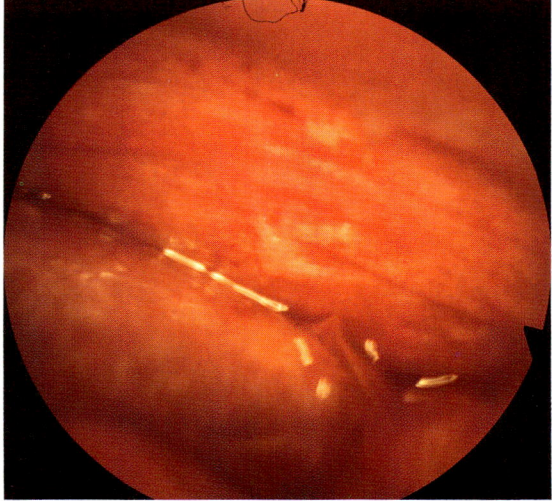

Figure 31-26. These diaphragmatic metastasis are from a Stage M ovarian carcinoma.

phorectomy or cystectomy will aid in making the proper therapeutic decisions.

REFERENCES

1. Stevenson DS. Myomectomy for improvement of fertility. Fertil Steril 1964; 15:367–384.
2. Robbins SL, Cotran RS, eds. Leiomyoma. The Pathogenic Basis of Disease, 3rd ed. Philadelphia, WB Saunders Company, 1984, p 1136.
3. Farrer-Brown G, Beilby JOW, Tarbit MH. The vascular patterns in myomatous uteri. J Obstet Gynaecol Br Commonw 1970; 77:967–975.
4. Stewart EA, Liau AS, Friedman AJ. Operative laparoscopy followed by colpotomy for resecting a colonic leiomyosarcoma. A case report. J Reprod Med 1991; 36:883–884.
5. Griffin JE, Edwards C, Ladden JD, et al. Congenital absence of the vagina. Ann Intern Med 1976; 85:224–236.
6. Sweet RL, Draper DL, Schaeter J, et al. Microbiology and pathogenesis of acute salpingitis as determined by laparoscopy: What is the appropriate site to sample? Am J Obstet Gynecol 1980; 138:985–989.
7. Westrom L. Effect of acute pelvic inflammatory disease on fertility. Am J Obstet Gynecol 1975; 122:707–713.
8. Hagar WD, Eschenbach DA, Spence MR, Sweet RL. Criteria for diagnosis and grading of salpingitis. Obstet Gynecol 1983; 61:113–114.
9. Jacobson L, Westrom L. Objective diagnosis of acute pelvic inflammatory disease: Diagnostic and prognostic value of routine laparoscopy. Am J Obstet Gynecol 1969; 105:1088–1098.
10. Ectopic pregnancy surveillance, United States, 1970–1987. MMWR 1988; 39:9.
11. Beral V. An epidemiological study of recent trends in ectopic pregnancy. Br J Obstet Gynaecol 1975; 82:775–782.
12. Kadar N, Caldwell BV, Romero R. A method of screening for ectopic pregnancy and its indications. Obstet Gynecol 1981; 58:162–166.
13. Kadar N, DeVore G, Romero R. The discriminatory zone: Its use in the sonographic evaluation for ectopic pregnancy. Obstet Gynecol 1981; 58:156–161.
14. Cartwright PS: Diagnosis of ectopic pregnancy. Obstet Gynecol Clin North Am 1991; 18:19–38.
15. Wheeler JM, Polan ML. Ectopic pregnancy: Diagnosis. In DeCherney AH, Polan ML, Lee RD, Boyers SP, eds. Decision Making in Infertility. Philadelphia, BC Decker, 1988, pp 102–103.
16. Sampson JA. The development of the implantation theory for the origin of peritoneal endometriosis. Am J Obstet Gynecol 1940; 40:549–557.
17. Halban J. Hysteroadenosis Mestastatica. Die Lymphogene Genese der Sog. Adenofibromatosis Heterotoaca Archiv Fur Gynecol 1925; 124:457–482.
18. Meyer R. Metaplasia theory with inflammation as the primary inducing factor. In Von Walter H, ed. Veit-Stockel Handbuch der Gynaekologic. München, Berguann, 1930.
19. Dmowski WP, Steele RN, Baker GF. Deficient cellular immunity in endometriosis. Am J Obstet Gynecol 1981; 141:377–383.
20. Simpson JL, Elias S, Malinak LR, Buttram VC Jr. Heritable aspects of endometriosis: I. Genetic studies. Am J Obstet Gynecol 1980; 137:327–331.
21. Weed JC. Prostaglandins as related to endometriosis. Clin Obstet Gynecol 1980; 23:895–900.
22. Sampson JA. Perforating hemorrhagic (chocolate) cysts of the ovary. Arch Surg 1921; 3:245–251.
23. Stripling MC, Martin DC, Poston WM. Does endometriosis have a typical appearance? J Reprod Med 1988; 33:879–884.
24. Martin DC, Hubert GD, Vander Zwaag R, El-Zeky FA. Laparoscopic appearance of peritoneal endometriosis. Fertil Steril 1989; 51:63–67.
25. Redwine DB. Age-related evolution in color appearance of endometriosis. Fertil Steril 1987; 8:1062–1063.
26. Vernon MW, Beard JS, Graves K, Wilson EA. Classification of endometriotic implants by morphologic appearance and capacity to synthesize prostaglandin F. Fertil Steril 1986; 46:801–806.
27. Martin DC, Vander Zwaag R. Excisional techniques with the CO_2 laser laparoscope. J Reprod Med 1987; 32:753–758.
28. Martin DC, Berry JD. Histology of chocolate cysts. J Gynecol Surg 1990; 6:43.
29. Martin DC, Hubert GD, Levy GS. Depth of infiltration of endometriosis. J Gynecol Surg 1989; 5:55–60.
30. Disaia PJ, Creasman WT. The adnexal mass and early ovarian cancer. In Disaia PJ, Creasman WT, eds. Clinical Gynecologic Oncology, 2nd ed. St. Louis, CV Mosby, 1984, p 258.

Chapter 32
Endometriosis

Michael P. Diamond
D. Alan Johns

Endometriosis is the presence of endometrial tissue, both glands and stroma, outside the uterine cavity. Its most common location is the dependent portion of the female pelvis, including the peritoneum and ovary, but it may be located anywhere throughout the body. Histologically, endometriosis shares characteristics with adenomyosis, but the latter is located specifically within the uterine myometrium. Interestingly, although endometriosis and adenomyosis share histologic criteria, there has been no identification of a propensity for them to occur concomitantly.

ETIOLOGY

The etiology of endometriosis remains unclear; no single hypothesis explains all of the locations at which it has been identified. The most common theory is that of retrograde menstruation, often called Sampson's theory. This hypothesis states that endometriosis results from the flow of menstrual discharge from the uterine cavity through the fallopian tubes into the peritoneal cavity. Once in the peritoneal cavity, the endometrial tissue implants on surfaces it contacts.

It would be expected that the retrograde flow would collect in the posterior cul-de-sac, which is precisely the location at which endometriosis is most frequently identified. Further support for Sampson's theory is the high frequency with which endometriosis is identified in women with obstruction of the uterine outflow tract (e.g., rudimentary uterine horn, cervical agenesis, or transverse vaginal septum). Additionally, endometriosis is frequently identified in women who have delayed childbearing until their thirties and less commonly in women who have a child at an early age. Potentially, the dilatation of the cervix during childbirth allows for future menstruations to flow more easily through the cervix, thereby decreasing the frequency and volume of retrograde menstrual flow, and consequently decreasing the development of endometriosis.

While retrograde menstruation could account for implants of endometriosis throughout the abdominal cavity (Fig. 32-1), it does not explain many locations at which endometriotic implants have been identified. Reports of catamenial hemoptysis have led to the identification of endometriosis in the lungs; it has also been identified in many other sites including the brain. Endometriosis in these distant locations is best explained by dissemination through vascular or lymphatic channels. Masses subsequently identified to be endometriosis have also been found in episiotomy incisions following a vaginal delivery and in the abdominal wall in a Pfannenstiel incision following a cesarean section. These locations suggest that endometriosis may also spread by direct extension.

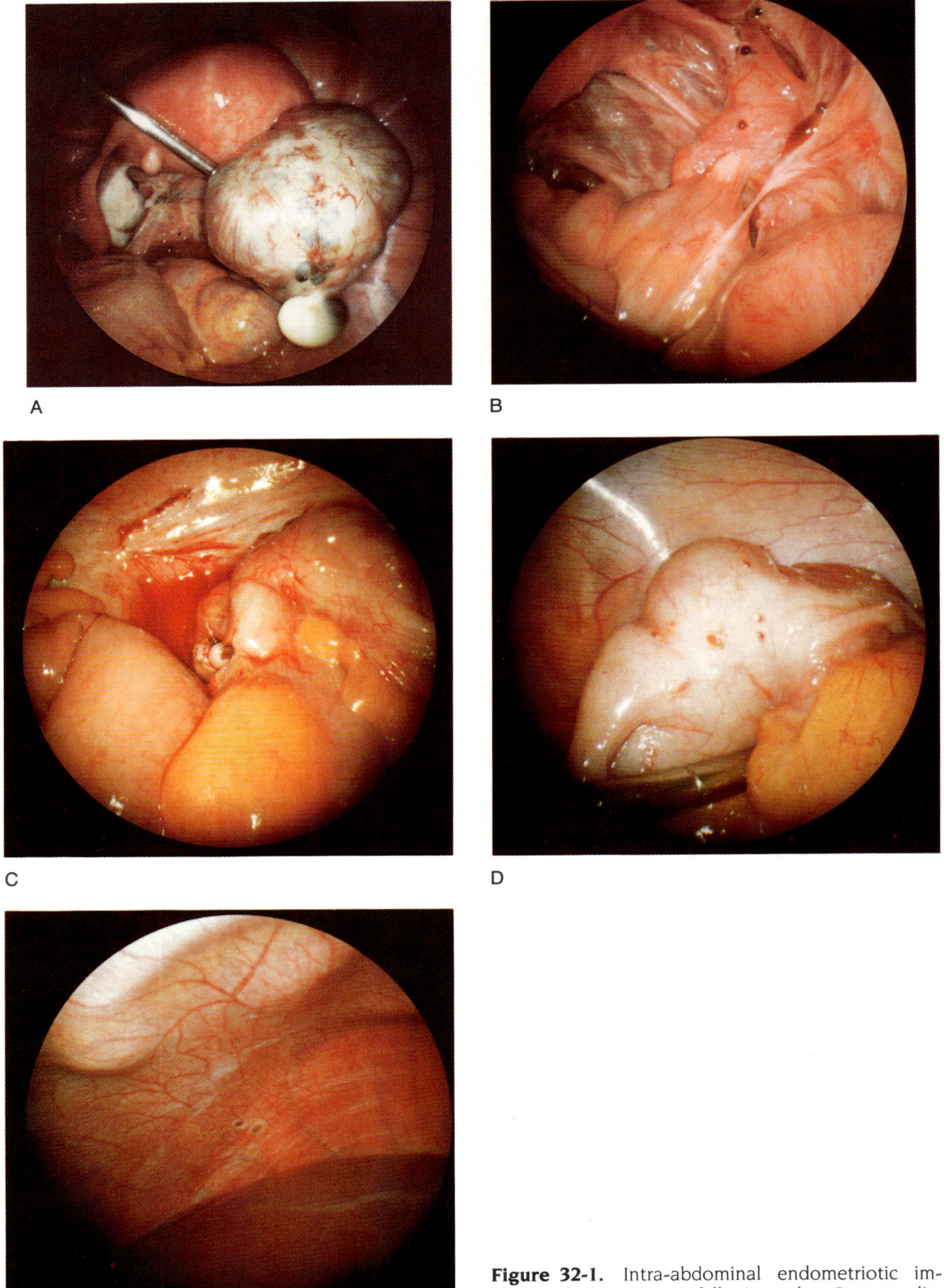

Figure 32-1. Intra-abdominal endometriotic implants of: A, ovary; B, fallopian tube; C, appendix; D, cecum; and E, diaphragm.

One additional theory of the etiology of endometriosis is that of celomic metaplasia. This theory says that tissue of the female reproductive tract and its surrounding peritoneum may be totipotent and able to differentiate along many lines, including the development of endometriosis. Support for this hypothesis is suggested by the ability of ovarian epithelial neoplasms to have characteristics of cells from throughout the female reproductive tract (e.g., endometrial and serous tumors).

Regardless of the etiology, endometriosis is a common cause of pelvic pain and infertility in women. Characteristically, patients with endometriosis frequently are seen with dyspareunia and dysmenorrhea and have difficulty conceiving. However, it may present with many symptoms including perimenstrual pain, hematochezia, hematuria, hemoptysis, bowel obstruction, and/or pelvic masses. It is often called the great impersonator because of the variation in presenting symptoms, as well as the difficulty in distinguishing the extent of disease prior to surgery. In contrast to expectations, some individuals with extensive endometriosis occasionally have no symptoms, whereas women with incapacitating pain may have only a minimal number of implants.

DIAGNOSIS

The diagnosis of endometriosis is often highly predicted by symptoms. The history can be complemented by pelvic examination, by the identification of adnexal masses (suggestive of ovarian masses or endometriomas), fixation of pelvic structures (suggestive of adhesions), and nodularity in the posterior cul-de-sac, particularly the uterosacral ligaments (suggestive of peritoneal endometriotic implants in the posterior cul-de-sac). Serum markers such as CA-125 may be present; however, this marker may be present in a wide variety of conditions, including many ovarian cancers. Recently, imaging studies have been increasingly used to help make a diagnosis, including ultrasound (particular transvaginal scanning), computed tomographic scanning, and magnetic resonance imaging. In the experience of one of the authors (M.P.D.), the latter has been particularly useful because of its ability to both identify and measure pelvic masses and to assess whether the contents of the cyst are hemorrhagic. Hemorrhagic cysts frequently represent endometriomas (in which contents represent old blood that has originated from the endometriotic cyst wall); however, a hemorrhagic corpus luteum can have the same appearance and be difficult to differentiate. (A hemorrhagic corpus luteum would not be expected to persist into subsequent menstrual cycles, as would an endometrioma.)

Despite the increasing preoperative accuracy in the diagnosis of endometriosis at the present time, still the initial diagnosis of endometriosis in a woman may be made at the time of surgery. The intra-abdominal operative procedure may be conducted either by laparotomy or laparoscopy, with diagnosis established by biopsy of the lesion or visual identification. Classically, endometriotic implants have a purplish-black appearance (Fig. 32-2). However, several recent studies have highlighted the observation that endometriosis can have diverse appearances (Fig. 32-3).[1,2] Endometriosis can be many different colors such as yellow, red, white, blue, and black. Additionally, endometriosis can be represented by clear vesicles, radiating vascular patterns, or cysts of endometriosis composed of thick brownish fluid. Unless a surgeon is aware of the wide variety of presentations possible, the diagnosis of endometriosis may be missed and in many patients therefore it remains untreated.

TREATMENT

Surgical treatment of endometriosis is increasingly being performed laparoscopically.[3] While a review of series in the literature

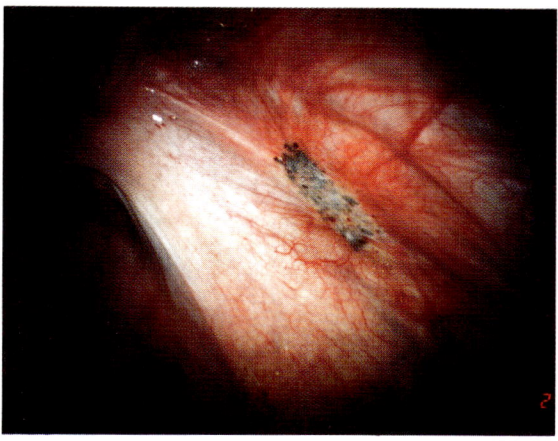

Figure 32-2. Classical appearing purplish-black implant of endometriosis.

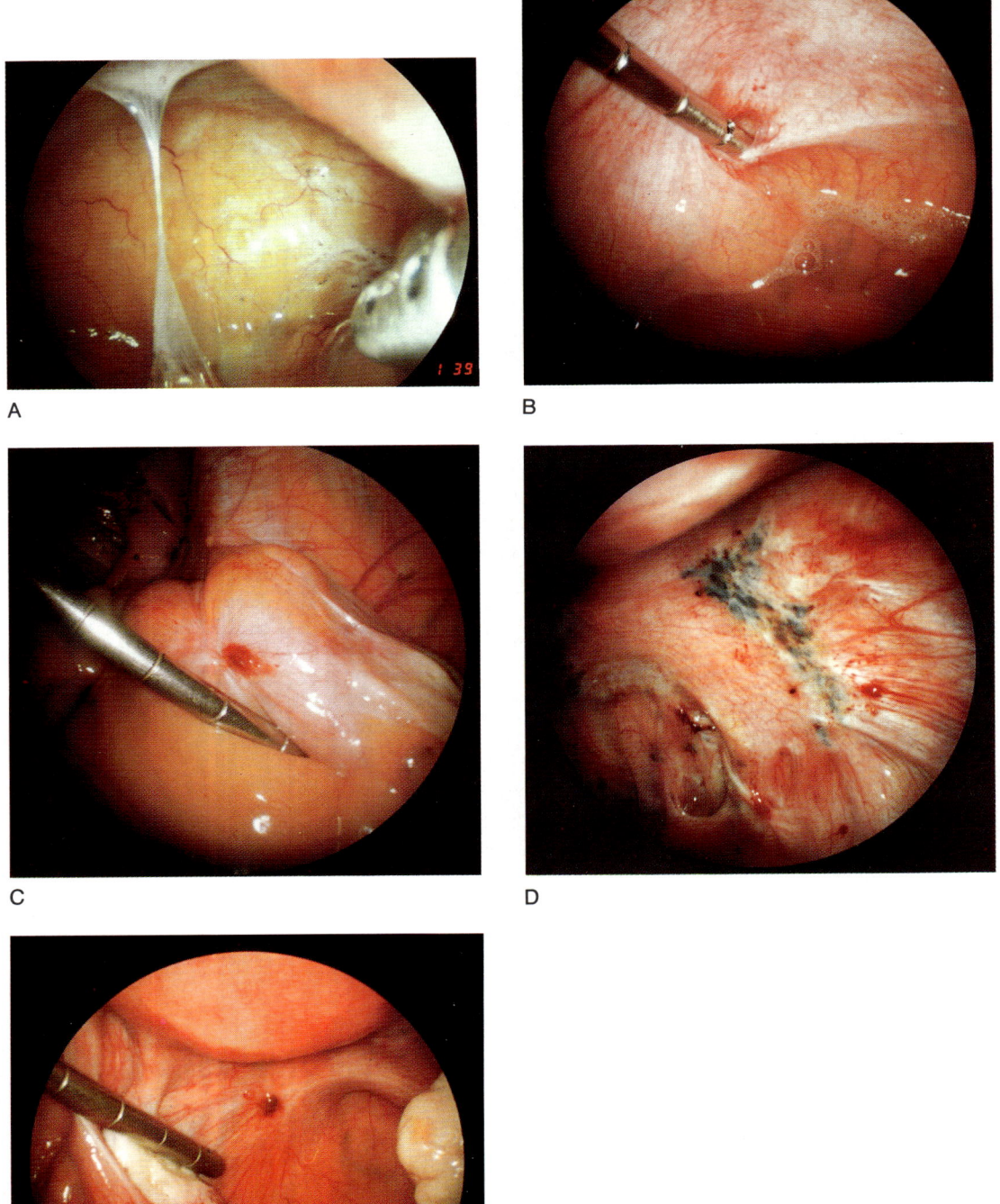

Figure 32-3. Other appearances of endometriosis: A, "black", clear, and scarred endometriosis implants; B, cul-de-sac pocket of endometriosis; C, reddish endometriosis implant; D, purplish lesions of endometriosis surrounded by scarring and accentuated vascular patterns; and E, reddish and clear endometriosis implants with prominent surrounding vascular pattern.

would suggest that pregnancy outcome following endometriosis therapy in procedures performed by laparoscopy or laparotomy may be equivalent (Table 32-1), in fact, appropriately designed studies comparing these two methods of entry into the abdominal cavity have not been conducted. Nonetheless, until such clinical trials are available, we must utilize the available literature to counsel and treat our patients.

Endoscopic surgery has many potential advantages for patients, the foremost of which is reduction in postoperative morbidity as assessed both by length of hospital stay and by time to return to work as compared with procedures performed at laparotomy. These endoscopic surgical procedures can be conducted by experienced surgeons with rates of complication no greater than those anticipated for procedures performed by laparotomy. Additionally, there is a potential for a cost savings when procedures are performed endoscopically. This results not from a savings during the operative procedure per se, but rather from a decrease in the length of hospitalization. However, this advantage is lost (or actually may be reversed so that laparoscopic procedures become more expensive) if there is extensive use of disposable instruments and trocar sleeves.

In the not too distant past, peritoneal endometriotic implants were treated by electrosurgical coagulation or laser vaporization. Either unipolar or bipolar instruments can be used for electrosurgical treatment. The former are associated with a more diffuse tissue effect with greater spread of energy and therefore a greater propensity for damage to surrounding tissues, such as bowel, bladder, ureter, and blood vessels.[18-20] This risk of electrosurgery can be greatly reduced by use of bipolar instruments, in which the flow of energy remains within a much more restricted area between the two electrodes. In addition to coagulation of implants, electrosurgery can be used in conjunction with endosurgical scissors to minimize bleeding and facilitate tissue dissection.

A variety of lasers are also now available for endoscopic use including the carbon dioxide (CO_2) laser, argon laser, potassium-titanyl-phosphate-532 (KTP-532) laser, and the neodymium-yttrium-aluminum-garnet (Nd:YAG) laser.[21] Of these lasers, the CO_2 laser has the least depth of penetration per unit of time and can be used for vaporization or excision of lesions. While a short depth of penetration facilitates application of this laser to implants on vital structures, it must be remembered that continued use of the laser (even with a small depth of penetration) can injure the underlying structure. Additionally, the CO_2 laser is not useful for establishing hemostasis from bleeding vessels, and thus other methods (e.g., electrosurgery, staples, or suture) must be available. The argon and KTP-532 lasers possess very similar characteristics and may also be used to vaporize or excise implants; they also possess slight hemostatic capabilities.[22,23] While they are preferentially absorbed by tissues with red pigment, they may be used on structures throughout the abdominal cavity. The Nd:YAG laser (when used as a bare fiber) primarily coagulates with a depth of penetration of approximately 4-mm. (For this reason, the Nd:YAG laser is frequently chosen for endometrial ablations or liver resections.) The characteristics of the bare Nd:YAG fiber may be modified in several ways (including the use of sapphire tips or sculptured fibers) to impart tissue action approaching that of the CO_2 laser.

Regardless of the particular modality used, controversy exists as to whether excision of implants provides more complete therapy than implant vaporization. While in practice more complete treatment by excision of the implant may tend to be true, this observation probably does not reflect the mode of therapy per se, but rather the more extensive treatment (particular depth of treatment) that is likely to be achieved by a surgeon excising implants.

Endometriosis is said to frequently "recur," with the likelihood positively correlated with the extent of the initial disease. In mild endometriosis, recurrence is found in approximately 20 to 30 per cent of women, increasing to approximately 40 to 60 per cent in women with severe and extensive disease. However, recent observations suggest that many of these recurrences may actually be persistence of disease untreated at the time of the initial operative procedure. For example, at the time of an early second-look procedure (performed in some patients with infertility), recurrent lesions are often found at the initial surgical sites, therefore suggesting that the initial surgical therapy was incomplete. For this reason, some surgeons advocate relatively deep treatment until normal tissue is identified, as well as extension of treatment circumferentially in an attempt to achieve complete eradication of the lesion.

When tissue diagnosis is desired, biopsies

Table 32-1. Pregnancy Outcome after Surgical Treatment of Endometriosis

	Laparotomy/ Laparoscopy	Laser	Class[a]	Total		Minimal-Mild		Moderate		Severe-Extensive	
				No. Patients	No. Pregnant (%)	No. Patients	No. Pregnant (%)	No. Patients	No. Pregnant (%)	No. Patients	No. Pregnant (%)
Acosta and co-workers[4]	Laparotomy	−	†	107	49 (46)	8	6 (75)	60	30 (50)	39	13 (33)
Rock and co-workers[5]	Laparotomy	−	*	214	115 (54)	45	28 (62)	88	48 (55)	81	39 (48)
Buttram[6]	Laparotomy	−	†	245	148 (60)	69	56 (81)	92	54 (59)	84	38 (45)
Gordts and co-workers[7]	Laparotomy	−	*	176	70 (40)	20	8 (40)	99	42 (42)	57	20 (35)
Garcia and David[8]	Laparotomy	−	†	71	23 (32)	3	2 (66)	19	7 (37)	49	14 (28)
Diamond and co-workers[9]	Laparotomy	+	*	82	28 (34)	8	1 (13)	35	10 (29)	39	17 (44)
Daniell[10]	Laparoscopy	−		60	34 (57)	35	20 (57)	25	14 (56)		
Kelly and Roberts[11]	Laparoscopy	+	*	10	6 (60)	3	3 (100)	7	3 (43)		
Martin[12]	Laparoscopy	+	*	115	55 (48)	56	23 (41)	45	22 (49)	14	9 (64)
Paulson and Asmar[13]	Laparoscopy	+	*	282	150 (53)	170	97 (57)	112	53 (47)		
Feste[14]	Laparoscopy	+	**	140	82 (59)	106	62 (58)	31	18 (58)	3	2 (67)
Davis[15]	Laparoscopy	+	**	65	37 (57)	31	20 (65)	26	15 (58)	7	2 (29)
Nezhat and co-workers[16]	Laparoscopy	+	*	102	62 (61)	24	18 (75)	51	32 (63)	27	12 (44)
Reich and McGlynn[17]	Laparoscopy	−	†	20	12 (60)						

[a] Reproduced with permission from Diamond MP. Surgical aspects of infertility. *In* Sciarra JJ, ed. *Gynecology and Obstetrics*. Philadelphia, Harper and Row, 1988, Vol 5, Chap 61, pp 1–23.
† Acosta; * American Fertility Society; ** Revised American Fertility Society.

of the lesions (or excision) can be performed. Pathologic identification of endometriosis has been facilitated by use of small biopsies so that the pathologist can section the tissue at the site the surgeon believes to represent endometriosis.

Ovarian implants of endometriosis can be superficial, in which case they may be treated in a fashion similar to that used for peritoneal implants. Alternatively, ovarian endometriosis may be characterized by endometriotic cysts, e.g., endometriomas (Fig. 32-4). Differentiation of endometriomas from other ovarian cysts and malignant ovarian neoplasms is of utmost importance, but is often extremely difficult. Laparoscopic treatment of ovarian neoplasms is an extremely controversial topic because of the concern for potential dissemination of an ovarian malignancy. This topic is beyond the scope of this chapter; for an extensive discussion of this important issue the reader is referred to recent chapters by Schwartz.[24,25]

Ovarian endometriomas can be treated by either excision or by drainage followed by treatment of the endometriotic cyst wall by either vaporization (which produces a great deal of smoke and is not advocated for larger endometriomas), coagulation, or stripping of the capsule. However, because of the dense adherence of the capsule to the cyst wall, a combination of these techniques is usually required for each endometrioma. If a woman desires future fertility, attempts to conserve ovarian tissue and avoid oophorectomy should be made, if possible. If an endometrioma is opened, the abdominal cavity should be copiously irrigated to remove the old hemorrhagic fluid. An irrigator can be placed inside the endometrioma, with subsequent irrigation to allow visualization of the capsule. If stripping is to be attempted, this can be facilitated by placement of a "relaxing" incision lateral to the initial incision. Any sections of the cyst wall that do not strip out can be coagulated or vaporized. At the completion of treatment of the endometrioma, hemostasis should be assessed and achieved, if necessary. Currently, controversy also exists as to whether the edges of the ovarian incision should be sutured closed. While ovarian closure has been the classical teaching, recent animal studies[26,27] suggesting that ovarian suturing increases postoperative ovarian adhesions have resulted in questioning of this practice.

In patients with hematochezia or gastrointestinal symptoms, endometriotic involvement of the bowel should be suspected. Examples of endometriotic involvement of the bowel are shown in Figure 32-5. These patients often benefit from preoperative evaluation of the intestines including sigmoidoscopy and barium enema. In such patients, preoperative preparations should include a bowel preparation (e.g., GoLITELY) in case intestinal surgery is found to be indicated. While superficial bowel lesions may be treated by vaporization, deeper lesions will require resection, sometimes necessitating entry into the bowel lumen. At the current time, in patients requiring entry into the bowel, most surgeons would convert a laparoscopic procedure to a laparotomy. However, some individuals have begun to treat such lesions laparoscopically with reasonable success even when segmental resection and anastomosis are performed. Clearly, while it is now readily possible to perform laparoscopic bowel surgery, its relative efficacy compared to treatment at laparotomy requires investigation.

Like lesions of the bowel, endometriotic implants overlying or invading the bladder can be treated laparoscopically (see Fig. 32-6 for examples). Involvement of the bladder mucosa often presents with hematuria and can be diagnosed by cystoscopy. Again, clinical trials comparing efficacy of procedures performed laparoscopically and by laparotomy are warranted.

As previously mentioned, the area most frequently involved by endometriosis is the posterior cul-de-sac. Disease in this area, while sometimes superficial, is often extensive and deeply infiltrating, requiring extensive dissection for complete treatment. Pre- and postoperative views are shown in Figure 32-7.

OUTCOME

In assessing the outcome of surgical procedures, it has frequently been claimed that performance of procedures laparoscopically or with the use of lasers will prevent the development of postoperative adhesions. Unfortunately, there have been relatively few circumstances in which patients undergo a second operative procedure shortly after the initial procedure to assess the validity of these claims. However, many infertility surgeons believe that an early second-look laparoscopy may improve pregnancy outcome in infertility patients.[28] Consequently, we have had the opportunity to assess whether adhesions develop postoperatively.

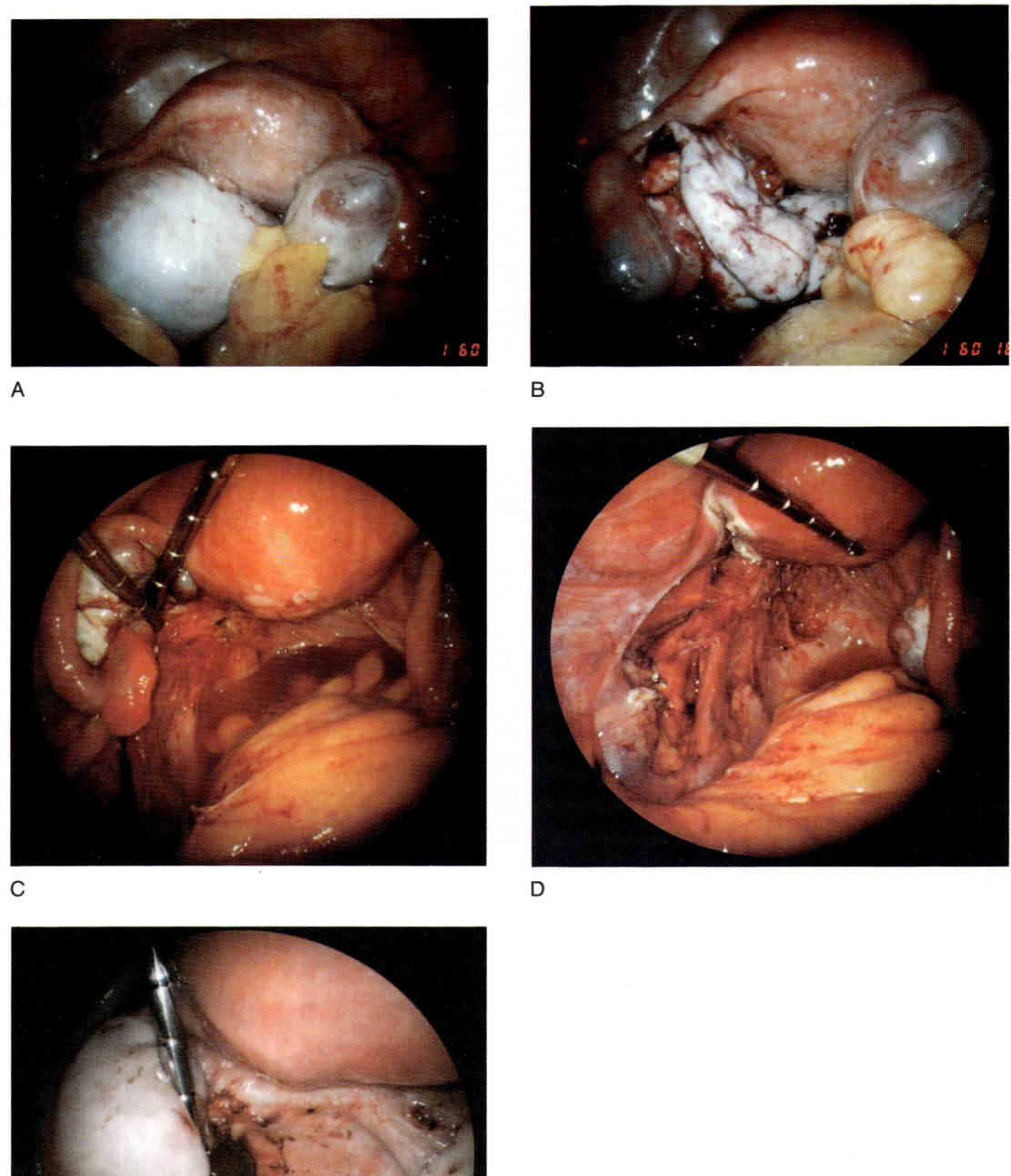

Figure 32-4. Ovarian endometriosis: A, left ovarian endometrioma preoperatively; B, same patient as A after treatment of endometriosis; C, endometriosis of left ovary and left pelvic sidewall; D, patient in C after laparoscopic excision of left ovary and tube; E and F, left and right endometrioma preoperatively; and G, same patient as E and F postoperatively.

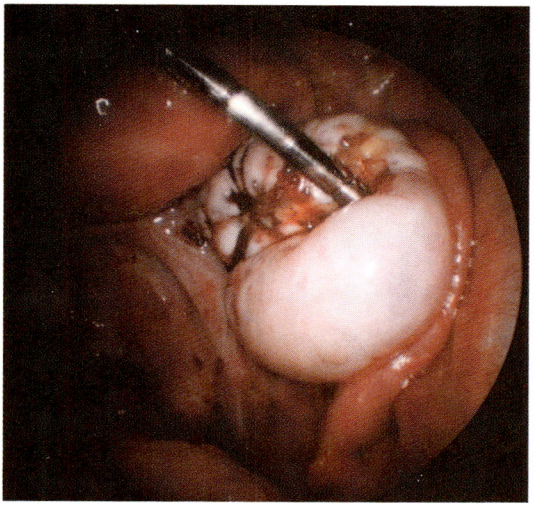 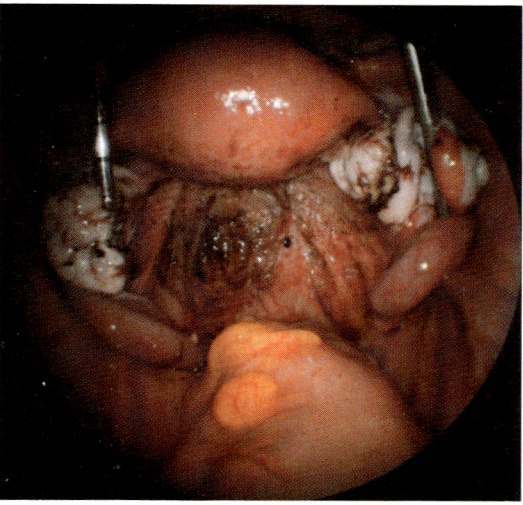

F G

Figure 32-4 *Continued*

In an early study nearly a decade ago, we investigated the frequency with which adhesions developed after adhesiolysis using a CO_2 laser in procedures performed at laparotomy. In the preliminary report, we found that 91 of 106 women (86 per cent) had adhesion reformation at sites at which adhesiolysis was performed at the initial operative procedure.[29] Subsequently, we found that of 121 women undergoing adhesiolysis at the initial procedure, at the time of the early second-look laparoscopy, adhesion scores were noted to be reduced in 91 subjects, unchanged in 14 women, and increased (i.e., worsened) in 16 women.[30] Additionally, adhesion reformation occurred with similar frequency (approximately 60 to 70 per cent) if the adhesions were dense and vascular or fine and filmy (i.e., "Saran-wrap"-like). Thus, adhesion reformation was a frequent occurrence following adhesiolysis at laparotomy.

Surprisingly, we found that these surgical procedures were complicated not only by adhesion reformation, but also by what we have come to call "de novo" adhesion formation.[30] We defined de novo adhesion formation as the development of adhesions at sites that did not undergo adhesiolysis at the time of the initial operative procedure. We were disheartened to find that such de novo adhesion formation occurred in 81 of 160 (51 per cent) of women in our study group, and at 31 per cent of available sites for de novo adhesion formation in these 81 women. Thus, these operative procedures performed using the CO_2 laser at laparotomy were frequently complicated by both adhesion reformation and de novo adhesion formation. Similar findings regarding the frequency of adhesion reformation have also been observed by other groups (see Ref. 28 for review).

Recently, we completed another multicenter study which examined whether postoperative adhesion development occurs after laparoscopic surgical procedures.[31] Among the 68 women enrolled into this laparoscopic adhesiolysis trial, adhesion scores were reduced 50 per cent following endoscopic lysis of adhesions. However, 66 of the 68 women (97 per cent of subjects) had adhesion reformation after laparoscopic adhesiolysis. De novo adhesion formation was identified in 8 women (12 per cent) and occurred at 23 per cent of available sites. While this may suggest that de novo adhesion formation may be less after laparoscopic procedures as opposed to operations performed at laparotomy, direct clinical evaluation will be necessary to prove this issue. Regardless, endoscopic surgery is not a panacea for the reduction of postoperative adhesion development. (The issue of reduction of postoperative adhesion development is beyond the scope of this chapter; the reader is referred to several recent reports on this important issue.[32-34])

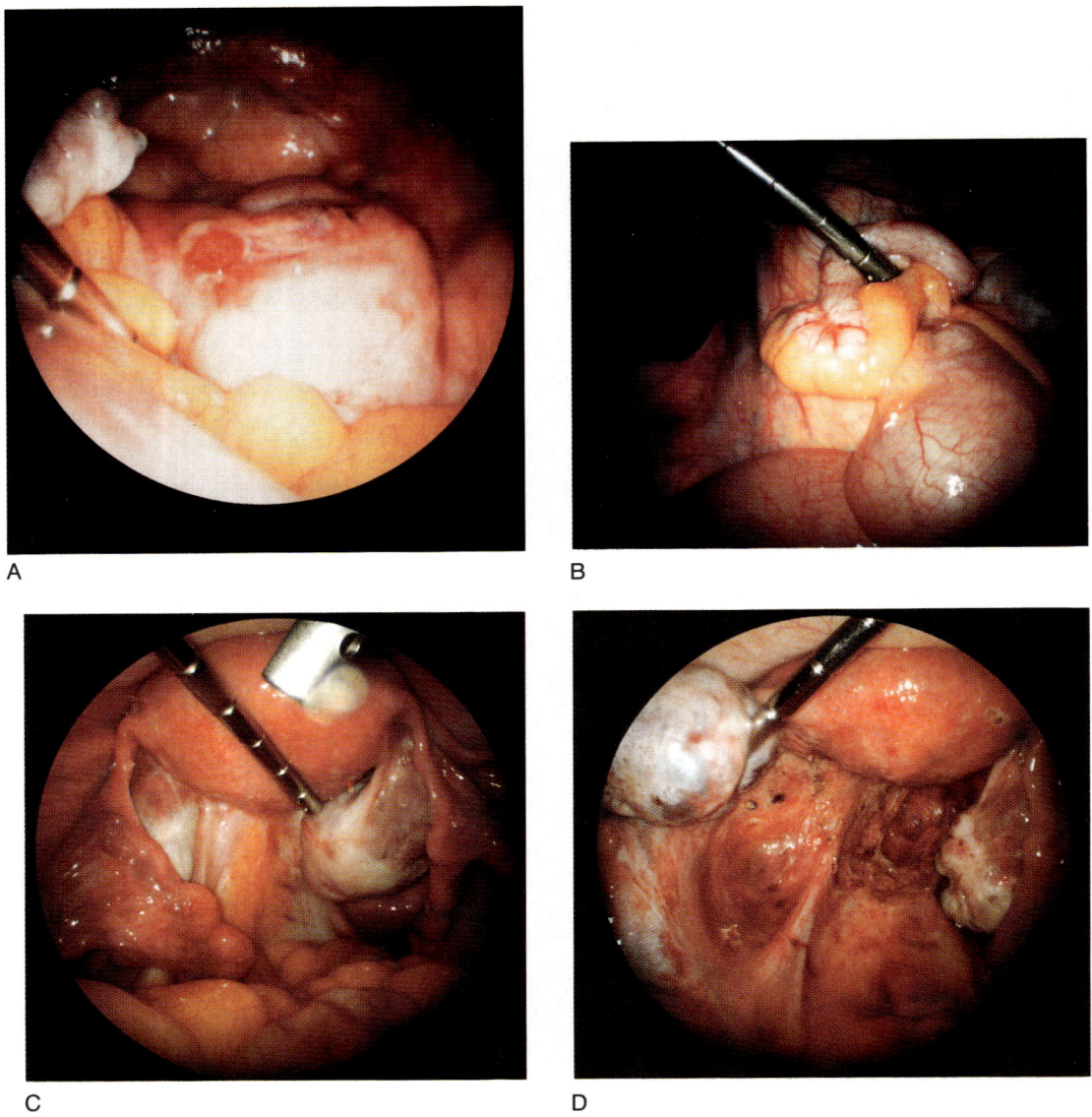

Figure 32-5. Bowel involvement by endometriosis: A, nodule on the bowel; B, obliteration of the posterior cul-de-sac by sigmoid colon preoperatively; and C and D, same patient as B after laparoscopic treatment.

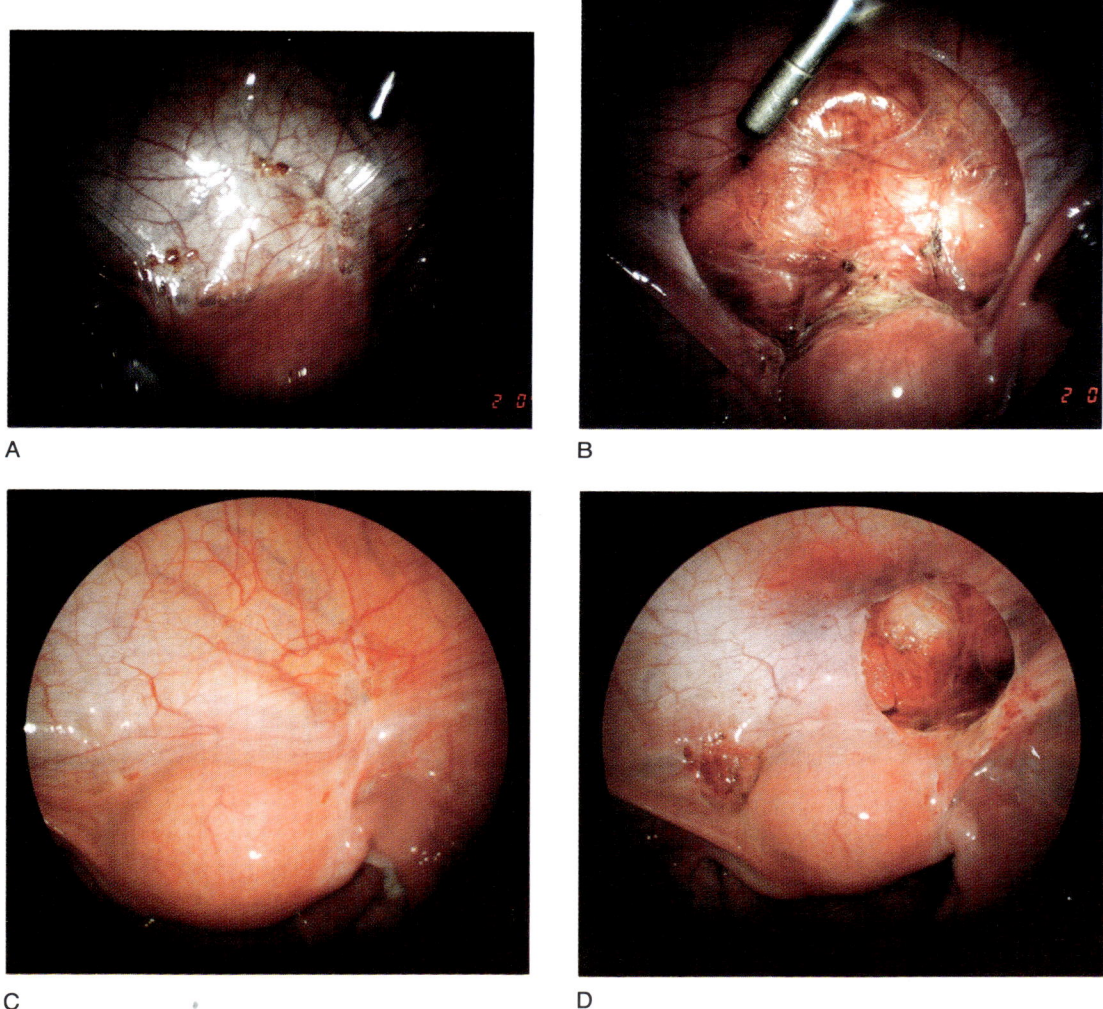

Figure 32-6. Involvement of the bladder by endometriosis: A, endometriosis of the anterior cul-de-sac peritoneum overlying the bladder, subsequently found to be penetrating to the bladder wall; B, postoperative view of the anterior cul-de-sac of A; C, endometriotic nodule penetrating to bladder muscularis; and D, postoperative view of nodule seen in C.

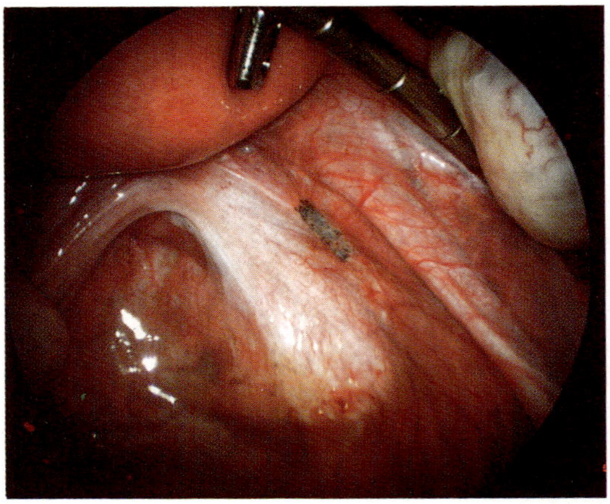

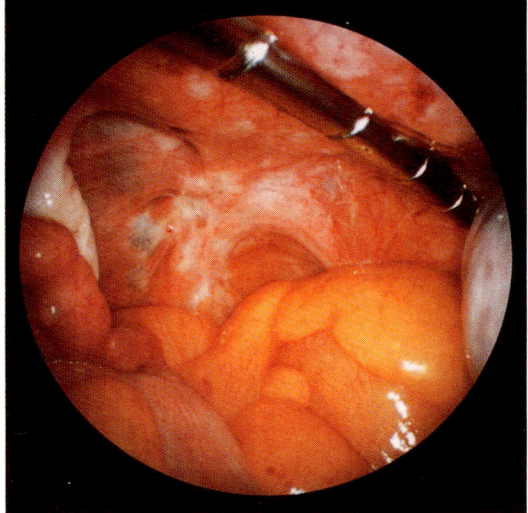

Figure 32-7. Posterior cul-de-sac involvement by endometriosis: A, implant medial and lateral to the right uterosacral ligament (note the prominence of the right ureter); B, postoperative view of A; C, extensive involvement of the posterior cul-de-sac by endometriosis and adhesions; D, postoperative view of C; E, deep uterosacral nodules; F, postoperative view after excision of nodules from E; G, deep posterior cul-de-sac nodules; and H, postoperative view of G; I, endometriosis of the right pelvic sidewall overlying the ureter; J, postoperative view of I; K, endometriosis penetrating from the posterior cul-de-sac into the vagina viewed preoperatively; L, patient in K after excision of endometriosis with entry into the vagina prior to vaginal closure; and M, patient in L after vaginal closure.

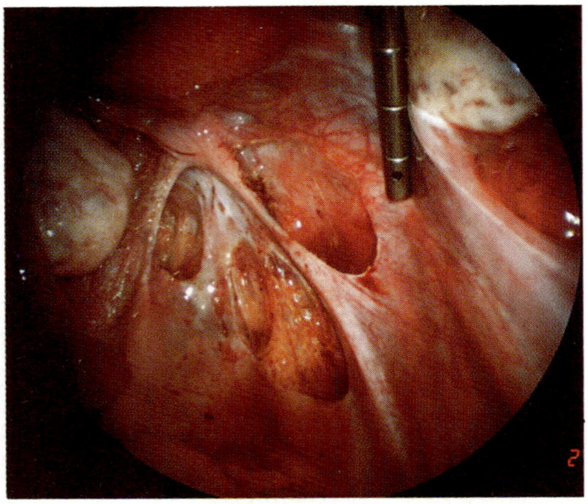

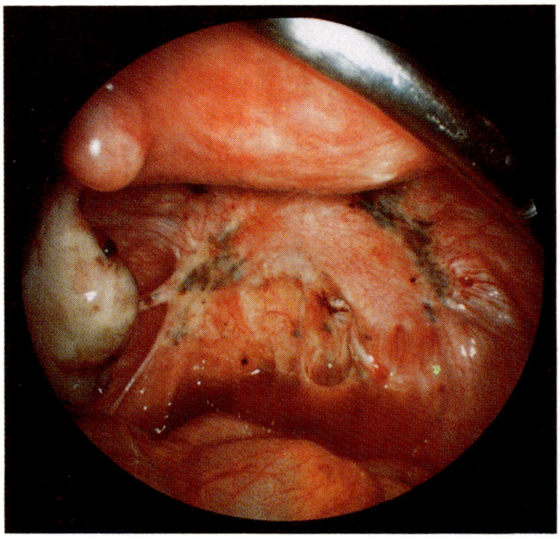

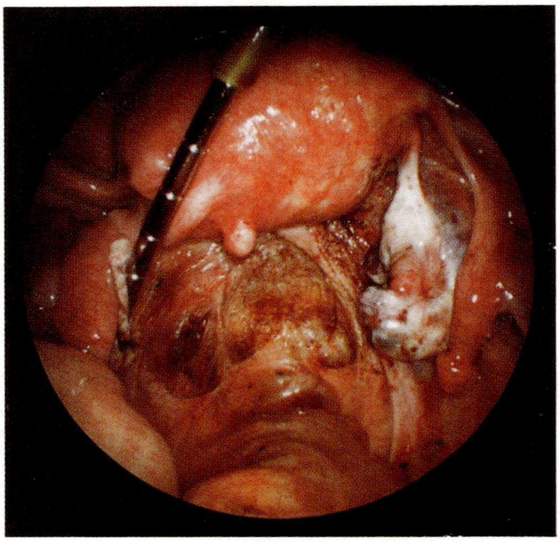

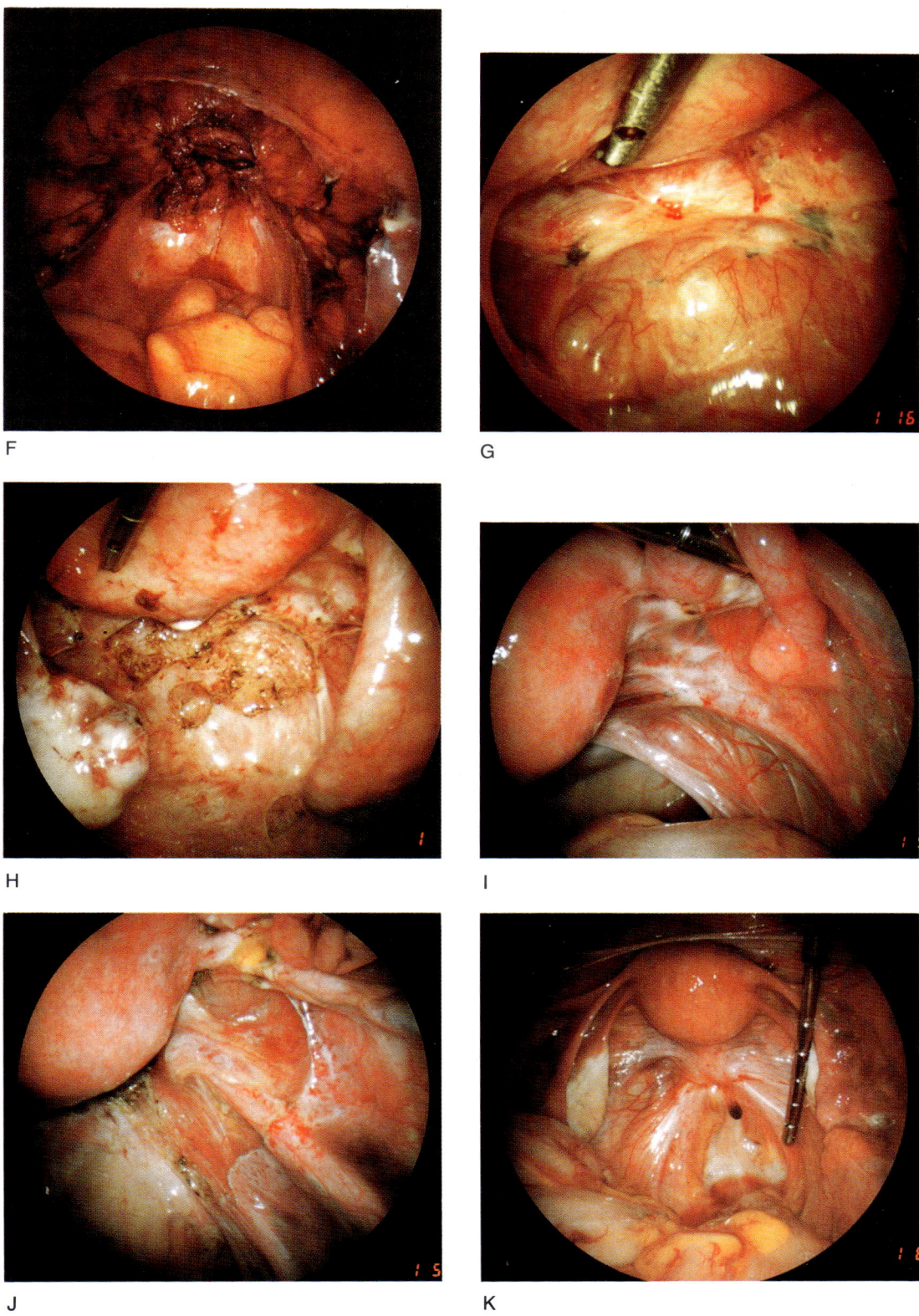

Illustration continued on following page

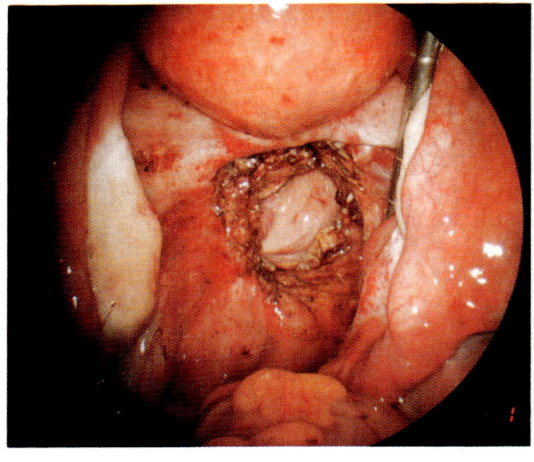 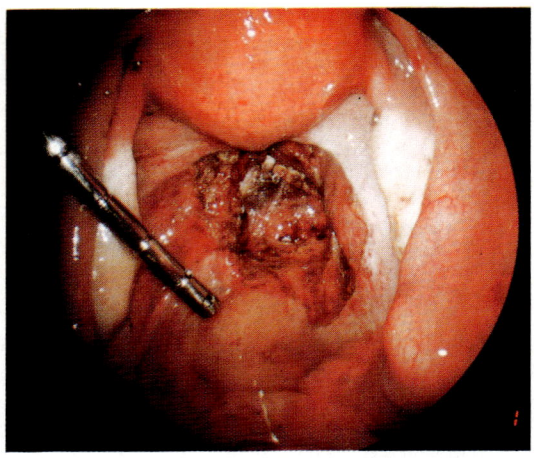

L   M

Figure 32-7 Continued

REFERENCES

1. Redwine DB. The distribution of endometriosis in the pelvis by age groups and fertility. Fertil Steril 1987; 47:173.
2. Stripling MC, Martin DC, Chatman D, et al. Subtle appearances of pelvic endometriosis. Fertil Steril 1988; 49:427.
3. Diamond MP. Review of endoscopic procedures in the treatment of the infertile woman. In Mishell DR, Paulsen CA, Lobo RA, eds, 1991 Yearbook of Infertility, Chicago, Mosby-Yearbook, 1991, pp 45–64.
4. Acosta AA, Buttram VC, Besch PK, et al. A proposed classification of pelvic endometriosis. Fertil Steril 1973; 42:19.
5. Rock JA, Guzick DS, Sengos C, et al. The conservative surgical treatment of endometriosis: Evaluation of pregnancy success with respect to the extent of disease as categorized using contemporary classification systems. Fertil Steril 1981; 35:131.
6. Buttram VC. Surgical treatment of endometriosis in the infertile female: A modified approach. Fertil Steril 1979; 32:635.
7. Gordts S, Boeckx W, Brosens I. Microsurgery of endometriosis in infertile patients. Fertil Steril 1984; 42:520.
8. Garcia CR, David SS. Pelvic endometriosis; infertility and pelvic pain. Am J Obstet Gynecol 1977; 129:740.
9. Diamond MP, Daniell JD, Martin DC, et al. Unpublished data.
10. Daniell JF. Combined laparoscopic surgery and danazol therapy for pelvic endometriosis. Fertil Steril 1981; 35:521–525.
11. Kelly RW, Roberts DK. CO_2 laser laparoscopy: A potential alternative to danazol in the treatment of stage I and II endometriosis. J Reprod Med 1983; 28:638.
12. Martin DC. CO_2 laser laparoscopy for endometriosis associated with infertility. J Reprod Med 1983; 28:638.
13. Paulson JD, Asmar P. Personal communication, 1986.
14. Feste JR. Endoscopic laser surgery in gynecology. In Reproductive Surgery. Postgraduate Course Syllabus, American Fertility Society, Chicago, 1985.
15. Davis GD. Instruments and methods: Management of endometriosis and its associated adhesions with the CO_2 laser laparoscope. Obstet Gynecol 1986; 68:422.
16. Nezhat C, Crowgey SR, Garrison CP. Surgical treatment of endometriosis via laser laparoscopic surgery techniques. Fertil Steril 1986; 45:778.
17. Reich H, McGlynn F. Treatment of ovarian endometriomas using laparoscopic surgical techniques. J Reprod Med 1986; 31:577.
18. Corfman RS, Diamond MP. Laser, cautery, or scalpel: Which is best? In McLaughlin DS, ed. Lasers in Gynecology. Philadelphia, JB Lippencott, 1990.
19. Martin DC, Diamond MP, Yussman, MA. Laser laparoscopy for infertility surgery. In Sanfilippo J, Levine R, eds. Operative Gynecologic Endoscopy. New York, Springer-Verlag, 1989, pp 211–235.
20. Grainger D, Soderstrom R, Schiff S, et al. Ureteral injuries at laparoscopy: Insights into diagnosis and management. Obstetr Gynecol 1990; 75:839–843.
21. Diamond MP, Daniell JD, Feste J, et al. Initial report of the carbon dioxide laser laparoscopy study group: Complications. J Gynecol Surg 1989; 5:269–272.
22. Diamond MP, Hill GA, Webster BW, et al. Comparison of human menopausal gonadotropin, clomiphene citrate, and combined human menopausal gonadotropin—Clomiphene citrate stimulation protocols for in vitro fertilization. Fertil Steril 1986; 46:1108–1112.
23. Diamond MP, Boyers SP, Lavy G, et al. Endoscopic use of the potassium-titanyl-phosphate 532 (KTP/532) laser in gynecologic surgery. Colposc Gynecol Laser Surg 1987; 3:213–216.
24. Schwartz P. Ovarian masses: Serologic markers. In Diamond MP, ed. "Pelviscopy," Clinical Obstetrics and Gynecology. 1991; 34:423–432.
25. Schwartz P. An oncologic view of when to perform endoscopic surgery. In Diamond MP, ed. "Pelviscopy," Clinical Obstetrics and Gynecology. 1991; 34:467–472.
26. Meyer WR, Grainger D, DeCherney AH, et al. Ovarian surgery on the rabbit: Effect of cortex closure on adhesion formation and ovarian function. J Reprod Med 1991; 36:639–643.
27. Brumsted JR, Deaton J, Lavigne L, et al. Postoperative adhesion formation after ovarian wedge resection with and without ovarian reconstruction in the rabbit. Fertil Steril 1990; 53:723–727.

28. Diamond MP. Surgical aspects of infertility. *In* Sciarra JJ, ed. Gynecology and Obstetrics, Philadelphia, Harper and Row, 1988, Vol 5, Chap 61, pp 1–23.
29. Diamond MP, Feste J, McLaughlin DS, et al. Pelvic adhesions at early second-look laparoscopy following carbon dioxide laser surgery. Infertility 1984; 7:39–44.
30. Diamond MP, Daniell JF, Feste J, et al. Adhesion reformation and de novo adhesion formation following reproductive pelvic surgery. Fertil Steril 1987; 47:864–866.
31. Diamond MP, Daniell JF, Johns DA, et al. Postoperative adhesion development following operative laparoscopy: Evaluation of early second-look procedures. Fertil Steril 1991; 55:700–704.
32. Diamond MP, DeCherney AH. Pathogenesis of adhesion formation/reformation: Application to reproductive pelvic surgery. Microsurgery 1987; 8:103–107.
33. Diamond MP. Adhesion Prevention. *In* Gershenson DM, DeCherney AH, Curry SL, eds. Operative Gynecology, Philadelphia, WB Saunders Company, 1993, pp. 147–158.
34. Gutmann JN, Diamond MP. Principles of laparoscopic microsurgery and adhesion prevention. *In* Azziz R, Murphy AA, eds. Practical Manual of Operative Laparoscopy and Hysteroscopy, Springer-Verlag, New York, 1992, pp. 55–72.

Section VII
Techniques of Laparoscopic Surgery

Chapter 33
Esophagogastrectomy

Patrick F. Leahy

Carcinoma of the esophagus is a major cause of mortality in Western civilization. The prognosis for patients with esophageal carcinoma remains poor, and despite innovative techniques surgery has not offered a realistic curative possibility. As most operations are performed to palliate the condition, the development of a minimally invasive technique would seem to be a logical progression.

The technique of endoscopic esophagogastrectomy is an arduous procedure, which requires the participation of both a thoracic team and an upper digestive surgical team.

PREOPERATIVE EVALUATION

Esophageal carcinomas are staged by endoscopic examination and biopsy. Routine investigations include chest radiograph and ultrasound examination of the liver. In some cases a laparoscopy is indicated to definitively rule out metastatic lesions in the liver.

Barium examinations of the esophagus remain a popular mode of examination. Incidental diagnosis is often made on routine upper GI investigations.

EQUIPMENT

For the thoracic approach four trocars (one 12-mm, two 10-mm, and one 5-mm), two Babcock clamps, and an ENDO GIA* stapling device are used. For the abdominal approach, a five-puncture technique is used (two 10-mm trocars, two 12-mm trocars, and one 5-mm trocar).

POSITION OF THE PATIENT

The patient is placed in a right lateral position with the thorax resting back against a chest comforter. The abdomen should be in a position as supine as is possible in this rotated position.

PLACEMENT OF EQUIPMENT

The thoracic monitor is placed toward a caudad position. The endoscopic monitor for the upper gastrointestinal surgical team is placed in a cephalad position.

TROCAR PLACEMENT

An open approach is used to insert short blunt trocars into the chest cavity. The trocars are placed in the sixth, fifth, fourth, and sixth position. This port is placed posterior to mid axillary line.

A five-puncture technique is used in the abdomen. The trocars are placed in a gentle

U shape. The initial 10-mm port for the laparoscope is placed two fingerbreadths above the umbilicus to the patient's left-hand side. The alternative 10-mm port is placed in the patient's right subcostal area. This is used for the retraction of the liver using a fan retractor. The remaining trocars can be either 10- or 12-mm ports at the surgeon's discretion. The 10-mm port is necessary for the ENDO CLIP* application. The 12-mm port is necessary for the ENDO GIA* stapling device used to transect the stomach and in some cases to divide the short gastric vessels.

PROCEDURE

Thoracic Approach

The surgeon first reflects the lung to identify the aorta; this is the landmark for esophageal dissection. Anterior to the aorta the esophagus is identified with the overlying vagus. Care is taken not to traumatize the pericardium and after gentle retraction of the lung and heart the esophageal dissection is commenced, separating the esophagus from the aorta. It is imperative to avoid entry into the right side of the chest. The esophageal mobilization is continued to the hilum of the lung. The phrenic nerve is identified as it innervates the diaphragm and great care is taken not to damage this nerve. The diaphragm is opened using electrocautery; this step should not be performed until the upper GI team has performed their gastric mobilization.

Gastric Resection

A Babcock clamp is introduced on the right-hand side of the patient to grasp the greater curve of the stomach, and tension is placed upon the body of the stomach. The liver retractor is placed below the liver, and the left lobe of the liver is retracted to identify the inferior phrenic veins and the hiatus and the diaphragm. The esophagus is identified. In palliative procedures the spleen is left in position; however, in more radical excisions the spleen must, of course, be removed. The short gastric arteries are individually identified and ligated using an 11-mm ENDO CLIP*. It is preferential to use three clips on both sides of these pedicles. The epiploic vessels are similarly identified and ligated. Alternatively the ENDO GIA* stapling device can be used to transect these vessels. The mobilization of the stomach is continued to the duodenum and a similar mobilization is performed in the lesser curve. Once the stomach has been fully mobilized and once the posterior adhesions have been divided, attention is now drawn to the hiatus in preparation for division of the diaphragm. Any major inferior phrenic veins must be ligated and divided. The diaphragm is divided in unison by the gastric team and the thoracic team. In this way great care is taken to avoid injury to any viscera that may be obscured from vision. The opening in the diaphragm is appropriate for the size of the tumor and allows easy entry of the gastric tube for esophagogastric anastomosis. The proximal body of the stomach is transected with several applications of the ENDO GIA*. The gastric tube is then placed alongside the esophagus at the site for division of the esophagus by the thoracic surgeon.

Anastomosis

The best anastomosis that can be fashioned at present is a side-to-side anastomosis using the ENDO GIA* stapling device. Alternatively the anastomosis can be fashioned using an EEA device introduced from a small incision below the xiphisternum.

SIDE-TO-SIDE ANASTOMOSIS

The ENDO GIA* stapling device is introduced into the lowest port in the thoracic cavity. A small gastrotomy is fashioned in the anterior wall of the stomach remnant. A similar esophagotomy is fashioned proximal to the lesion in the esophagus and both blades of the ENDO GIA* are inserted into these small openings. The ENDO GIA* is closed and fired and in certain cases it is preferential to use two sequential firings. This will prevent any future stricture or anastomosis. The distal esophagus is then removed, and the openings are closed by the application of an ENDO TA* 55. The esophageal-gastric remnant containing the carcinoma is removed through a small intercostal opening. If the tumor is large with serosal involvement, then it should be placed in an impermeable bag and removed through the abdomen or thoracic cavity.

In carcinoma patients with the potential for curative resection, extensive dissection of the nodal involvement of the esophagus is obviously required. This requires great patience and skill and should not be undertaken by surgeons who are not familiar with this form of extensive dissection.

The diaphragm is closed by the thoracic surgeon using a continuous running suture. The remnant of the stomach is anchored to the diaphragm with a suture technique or alternatively with a stapling technique using the ENDO HERNIA* stapler. The wounds are closed with 40 maxon to the subcuticular layer.

ANASTOMOSIS WITH CIRCULAR STAPLERS

This anastomosis can be fashioned by placing the anvil of the circular stapler PCEEA* into the proximal esophagus. This anvil has a suture material attached to it thus, the esophagus can be closed with the TA* device and the anvil shaft pulled through a small esophagotomy. The circular stapling device is introduced into the distal stump of the stomach and the anastomosis is fashioned under direct vision within the thoracic cavity. The opening in the stomach can be closed with a TA* stapling device.

COMMENTS

Esophagogastrectomy is an arduous procedure that should be approached by two teams of surgeons. The question that must be faced is the extent of dissection that can be performed using the endoscopic technique. Fashioning anastomoses in the thoracic cavity using endoscopic techniques requires careful forethought.

Nonetheless, with the improvement in technology and technique, this palliative procedure will become more common within the next few years.

Chapter 34
Cardiomyotomy

John Spencer

The treatment of achalasia has remained controversial for much of this century, with most of the debate relating to the choice between balloon dilatation of the cardia on the one hand, and surgical myotomy on the other. Because the disease is rare, affecting about 1 in 100,000 people across the world, most reports consist of random small series of patients. There are reports of large series, which show that good results can be obtained whatever method is used, but they do not allow valid comparisons to be made. In the only prospective randomized study comparing the two techniques, the use of myotomy gave superior results, the outcome being successful in 95 per cent of patients as opposed to 65 per cent with dilatation.[1]

Balloon dilatation is often considered by gastroenterologists to be "conservative" treatment when compared with "invasive" surgery. The implication that it is therefore safer has never been documented. Indeed, dilatation is essentially imprecise, often needing to be repeated when not enough sphincter fibers are ruptured or carrying the risk of perforation if too vigorous. Surgery is precise, but its major disadvantage has been the need for a major thoracic or abdominal incision. Apart from the residual scar, these wounds are painful and contribute to postoperative complications. An ideal treatment for achalasia would provide the precision and effectiveness of myotomy without the need for major wounds. Laparoscopic cardiomyotomy offers just such an option.

PATIENT SELECTION

Early in the disease simple medical therapy may give some relief of symptoms, but when dysphagia becomes a prominent feature myotomy should be considered. Stasis in the esophagus is not only hazardous in terms of overspill into the respiratory tract. It is likely that this stasis contributes to the high incidence of carcinoma of the esophagus seen in patients with this disease because of the contact time for ingested carcinogens and high cell turnover associated with secondary esophagitis.

There are no specific contraindications for laparoscopic treatment.

PREOPERATIVE EVALUATION

Diagnostic workup includes esophageal manometry to assess sphincter function. A chest radiograph excludes basal chest infection, which so commonly follows overspill, particularly in the elderly. General routine assessment of fitness for anaesthesia is performed.

An endoscopic examination is mandatory and is performed for diagnostic purposes in every patient. Carcinomas at the cardia can mimic achalasia, and carcinoma elsewhere in the esophagus can occur secondary to the disease. The presence of such tumors must be excluded.

PREOPERATIVE PREPARATION

In patients with severe stasis, a liquids-only diet for several days before the operation may reduce the dangers of spillover or of intraoperative leakage of infected contents. As the gut is not entered during the operation, there is no indication for perioperative antibiotics. If there is inadvertent breaching of the mucosa during the operation, then intravenous antibiotics may be given at that time.

EQUIPMENT

1. Laparoscope: A 30° forward-oblique telescope is essential to obtain good visualization of the cardiac area, and a full-size (10-mm) instrument ensures adequate illumination.
2. Trocars: Two 5-mm and two 10/11-mm trocars are required.
3. Instruments: (a) Grasping forceps are needed to retract the cardia downwards. (b) A 5-mm steel rod retractor is adequate, but ideally a spreading retractor should be available to retract the left lobe of the liver. (c) A simple suture should be available in case the mucosa is breached. Inability to suture will necessitate conversion to an open operation. Sutures are also necessary if a fundoplasty is added to the simple myotomy. Loop ligatures may be held in reserve but should not be essential. (d) A clip applier is necessary for dividing vessels encountered at the cardia.

POSITIONING OF THE PATIENT

The patient lies supine for this procedure. The first trocar, which is inserted above and to the left of the umbilicus, may be introduced with the patient horizontal, after the induction of the pneumoperitoneum. If the surgeon has any misgivings about this insertion, it is advised that a 5-mm trocar and telescope be introduced first at the umbilicus, and the other ports then introduced under vision. Once the ports are placed, a head-up tilt displaces organs away from the diaphragm, facilitating exposure of the esophagus.

A nasogastric tube is passed and the stomach is aspirated, having aspirated the esophagus thoroughly during passage of this tube. Frequent aspiration of the stomach facilitates good visualization.

POSITIONING OF THE VIDEO EQUIPMENT

This should be positioned on each side of the patient at the head end of the table, so that the surgeon and assistant can see clearly. The surgeon stands on the right of the patient, so as to face the left costal margin during dissection.

TROCAR PLACEMENT AND SIZE SELECTION

The laparoscopic ports used are illustrated in Figure 34-1 and are based on the method described by Cuschieri and his co-workers.[2] After induction of the pneumoperitoneum in the usual way an 11-mm port is inserted 25 mm above and to the left of the umbilicus. Because of its position I consider a disposable cannula, with a safety shield, to be essential for this particular port. The other cannulas can then be inserted under vision.

METHODS OF EXPOSURE AND RETRACTION

A retractor placed through the para-xiphisternal port lifts the left lobe of the liver. Identification of the caudate lobe of the liver, with the hepatic branches of the anterior vagus nerve crossing in front of it, gives an easy landmark, very familiar to surgeons who perform vagotomy (Fig. 34-2). Following those nerves to the left leads inevitably to the cardia, where the anterior cardiac branches of the left gastric artery can readily be seen, albeit often in fat, crossing towards the angle of His. Moving up from these familiar landmarks the diaphragm is clearly seen and the position of the hiatus visualized.

METHODS OF DISSECTION

The peritoneum is divided transversely with scissors over the anterior border of the

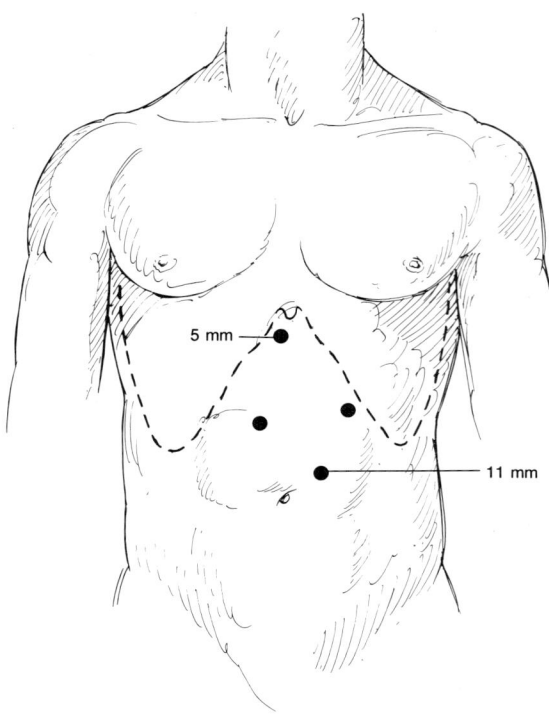

Figure 34-1. Position of the four ports used.

hiatus. A forceps can then be placed on the stomach immediately below the cardiac vessels to draw the cardia caudally. After this a combination of sharp and blunt dissection readily reveals the anterior wall of the esophagus and lengthens the abdominal component appropriately. If the esophagus cannot be seen readily, the insertion of a gastroscope gives a useful guide, as its light will transilluminate it—though not very brightly. If this is done, air should not be insufflated through the endoscope, for a distended stomach will obscure the view. Aspiration of air from the stomach only partly solves that problem, because the proximal small bowel may become distended.

Attention must now be given to the cardiac vessels mentioned earlier. As every surgeon who performs vagotomy or open myotomy knows, these can be quite substantial. Diathermy alone should not be relied on, as bleeding may obscure the view. Clipping is not difficult, and the vessels can then be divided. These vessels are an important landmark, as they indicate where the esophagus is likely to end and the stomach begin.

The myotomy is initiated to the left of the

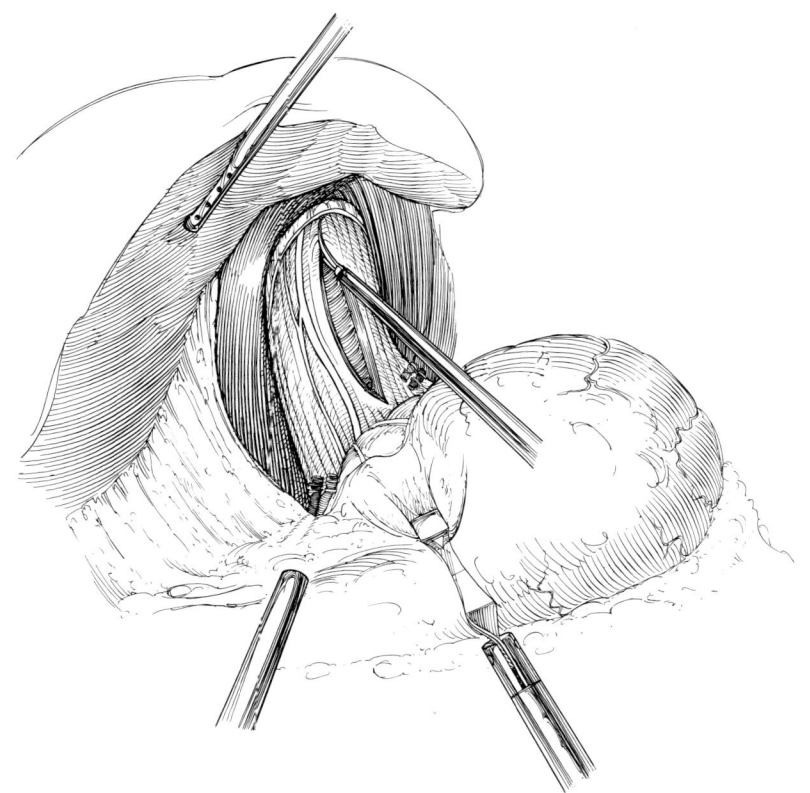

Figure 34-2. The myotomy is initiated to the left anterior vagus nerve.

anterior vagus nerve, which is clearly visible on the esophageal wall. A longitudinal incision is made with the diathermy hook, and this incision is widened and deepened with scissors exactly as in an open operation. Once circular fibers come into view they can be raised off the submucosa with the diathermy hook and divided. Initiating this division reveals at once a clear muscle edge from which the myotomy can be readily extended up and down.

At the upper end the incision must go beyond the sphincter. In patients with a dilated esophagus this is readily ascertained, as distention must represent suprasphincteral esophagus. Thus, extension for a short distance on to the dilated esophagus is adequate. If there is little or no dilatation, upward extension should be carried out so that about 5 cm of sphincter from the cardia has been divided.

At the lower end, the previously divided cardiac vessels form a valuable landmark. At that level the mucosa becomes bluish rather than white in color, is dimpled rather than smooth in appearance, and is more adherent to the muscle. Once it is certain that the incision is on to the stomach rather than the esophagus, there is no value in lengthening the incision further. For dissection of this lower end Cuschieri has recommended the use of a hook-knife microscalpel, as being less likely to damage the gastric mucosa.

Buess in Tubingen, Germany (personal communication), has performed intraoperative manometry to measure reduction of sphincter pressure. The value of this is rather doubtful, particularly because nothing more than complete sphincter section can be achieved.

As with the open procedure, the dissection should proceed outward around the esophagus until a good bulge of mucosa has been obtained.

SPECIFIC DETAILS OF THE PROCEDURE

If an antireflux procedure is to be added, it is helpful to place a sling around the cardia. As an alternative, a fiberoptic gastroduodenoscope (which has been disinfected, including the instrument channel) can be passed through the 11-mm operating port. Once sufficient blunt dissection has been carried out on each side of the esophagus, it is not difficult to negotiate the tip of the endoscope around the esophagus. It does not necessarily need to pass all the way around, but it is helpful if it does so. A grasper (biopsy or foreign body forceps) can then be passed through the endoscope and used to withdraw

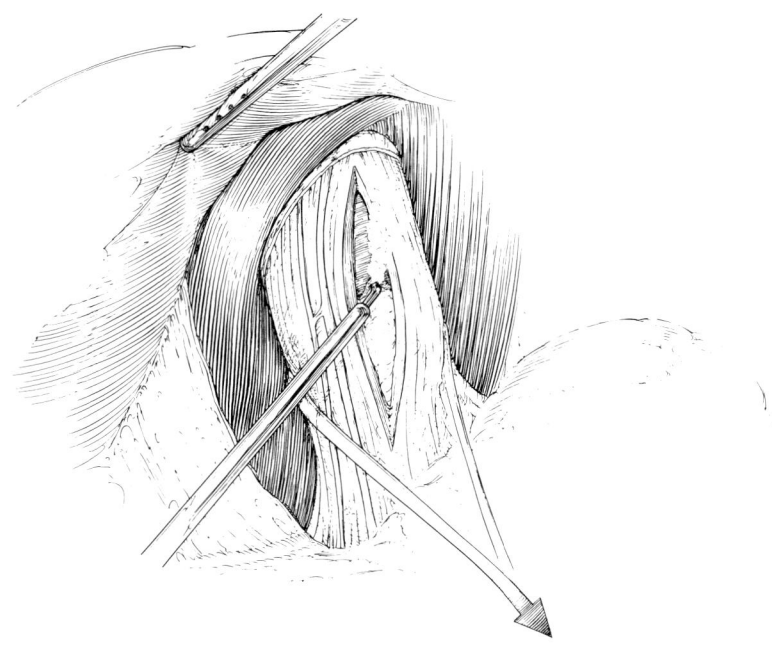

Figure 34-3. Circular muscle being divided with diathermy.

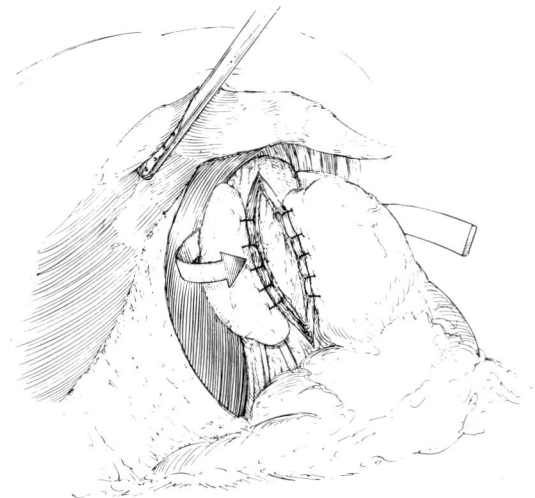

Figure 34-4. Cardioplasty modified from Johnston and colleagues.[5]

a plastic tube sling around the esophagus. The endoscope is withdrawn. Traction on the sling indicates the position in which exposure of the esophagus is optimal. If desired, the ends of the sling can then be exteriorized, and artery forceps may be applied to it against the skin and used to provide and adjust tension (Fig. 34-3).

Buess has demonstrated the feasibility of inserting a fundal patch into the muscular defect created by the myotomy. This procedure, originally described in France by Dor et al.[3] has value as an antireflux procedure and also prevents reapposition of the severed sphincter muscle.[4] An easier and equally effective option at laparoscopy is to adopt the procedure described by Johnston and his colleagues[5] as illustrated in Fig. 34-4. The fundus in this case is drawn from left to right behind the esophagus. Sutures then attach the fundus to the cut muscle edge, as illustrated, on each side of the myotomy.

At the completion of the myotomy, passage of an endoscope by mouth illuminates the protruding mucosa at the myotomy site and illustrates completion of the sphincter division.

CLOSURE

The closure of the port entry wounds is done in a standard manner with single sutures for the 10/11-mm ports and Steri-Strips to the skin of all port wounds.

POSTOPERATIVE MANAGEMENT

The nasogastric tube may be withdrawn at the end of the procedure, aspirating the stomach and esophagus again as this is done. If there has been no mucosal breach during the operation, the patient may take oral fluids as soon as desired, and solid foods within 24 hours. Early resumption of feeding may be advantageous to open up the myotomy.

CRITERIA FOR PATIENT DISCHARGE

The patient may be discharged as soon as general condition permits. Usually this is the following day, but general factors, such as age and social background, are more important than the specifics of this operation.

COMPLICATIONS

All operations for achalasia may be complicated by chest infection secondary to overspill from the esophagus, although with care this can be avoided. The only specific complication is breach of the mucosa during the procedure. This is sutured at the time of occurrence, and the integrity is checked by washing the lumen with sterile saline. If this complication has occurred, then oral liquids may be delayed for 24 hours. Some would take the precaution of a radiologic contrast study (e.g., with Gastrografin) before allowing the patient resume an oral diet.

REFERENCES

1. Csendes A, Braghetto I, Henriquez A, Cortes C. Late results of a prospective randomised study comparing forceful dilatation and oesophagotomy in patients with achalasia. Gut 1989; 30:299–304.
2. Shimi S, Nathanson LK, Cuschieri A. Laparoscopic cardiomyotomy fox achalasia. J R Coll Surg Edinb 1991; 36:152–154.
3. Dor J, Humbert P, Paoli J-M, et al. Traitment du reflux par la technique dite Heller-Nissen modifie. Presse Med 1967; 50:2563–2565.
4. Desa LA, Spencer J, McPherson S. Surgery for achalasia cardiae: The Dor operation. Ann R Coll Surg 1990; 72:128–131.
5. Crookes PF, Wilkinson AJ, Johnston GW. Heller's myotomy with partial fundoplication. Br J Surg 1989; 76:99–100.

Chapter 35
Vagotomy

Robert W. Bailey
Karl A. Zucker
John L. Flowers

Recently published studies have demonstrated the distinct advantages of laparoscopic cholecystectomy for the treatment of symptomatic cholelithiasis.[1,2] This realization has stimulated the development and adaptation of other routine surgical procedures to a "videoscopic" approach. Procedures such as appendectomy,[3] and, more recently, herniorrhaphy,[4] colectomy,[5] pelvic lymphadenectomy,[6] Nissen fundoplication,[7] and vagotomy[8,9] have all been successfully performed under laparoscopic guidance.

Among these new advances, laparoscopic vagotomy appears to offer a safe, feasible, and effective alternative to conventional ulcer surgery. It retains all of the advantages associated with traditional vagotomy while avoiding many of the disadvantages of a laparotomy. A procedure that provides definitive treatment of peptic ulcer disease while, at the same time, is associated with a relatively short hospital stay, minimal postoperative discomfort, and early return to work might prove to be a viable alternative to lifelong medical therapy.

SURGICAL OPTIONS

Several options are currently available for a minimally invasive approach to the treatment of peptic ulcer disease. Bilateral truncal vagotomy,[10] performed via a thoracoscopic or laparoscopic approach, may be safely and quickly accomplished. However, it requires a drainage procedure and is associated with all of the disadvantages (dumping, diarrhea) of a conventional truncal vagotomy. It is also possible to perform a conventional highly selective vagotomy under laparoscopic guidance, however, initial experience has revealed that access to the posterior leaflet is difficult. Because of the disadvantages of a bilateral truncal vagotomy and because a laparoscopic highly selective vagotomy leads to operatives times in excess of 4 to 5 hours, several modifications of standard ulcer operations have been developed.

The most commonly performed laparoscopic approach to ulcer disease consists of a posterior truncal vagotomy combined with some form of highly selective denervation of the anterior aspect of the stomach. It appears that leaving the anterior nerve supply to the antrum intact is sufficient to allow for normal gastric emptying.[11] This obviates the need for a drainage procedure and decreases the risk of postoperative diarrhea and dumping. The anterior denervation may be accomplished by individual ligation of the neurovascular bundles along the lesser curve of the stomach,[8] by a seromyotomy,[9] or by interruption of the nerve fibers with an endoscopic stapling device.[12]

Surgeons from the University of Nice were the first group to be recognized for the successful performance of a posterior truncal vagotomy and an anterior seromyotomy under laparoscopic guidance.[9] The seromyotomy along the lesser curve interrupts the small vagal fibers traveling through the gastric wall on their way to the gastric mucosa, thereby accomplishing effective vagotomy. The clinical basis for this operation stems, for the most part, from the work of Taylor and colleagues,[13-15] who have completed more than 700 of these procedures via laparotomy with excellent results.

The authors' institution, following observation with the group at the University of Nice, has developed a modified vagotomy, which can be performed under laparoscopic guidance. The technique consists of a posterior truncal vagotomy combined with an anterior highly selective vagotomy, performed in the standard fashion by individual ligation of the neurovascular bundles along the lesser curve of the stomach.

The choice of operative approach, however, remains controversial. The posterior vagotomy/anterior seromyotomy is commonly performed in Europe as an open procedure. It was quite logical, therefore, for surgeons in Europe to adapt the seromyotomy procedure to a laparoscopic approach. In the United States the use of an anterior seromyotomy for the treatment of peptic ulcer disease is minimal, at best. For this reason, anterior denervation is most often accomplished by individual ligation of the neurovascular bundles along the lesser curvature of the stomach. Although clinical experience with posterior truncal vagotomy/anterior highly selective vagotomy, performed via a laparotomy,[16] is limited, on a theoretical basis it should produce results similar to a conventional highly selective vagotomy. Experience with conventional highly selective vagotomy is extensive and widespread.[17-19] Modifying a conventional highly selective vagotomy to include a posterior truncal vagotomy should, if anything, improve the postoperative results. The posterior truncal/anterior highly selective procedure also shares similarities to the seromyotomy technique. Both procedures involve a posterior vagotomy (confirmed by histologic evaluation) and an anterior highly selective denervation of the stomach.

Regardless of each surgeon's preference, the preliminary reports on these techniques have been encouraging and in the near future a minimally invasive approach may become the preferred modality for the management of patients with peptic ulcer disease. The rest of this chapter describes the operative technique of posterior truncal vagotomy and highly selective denervation of the anterior gastric wall.

PATIENT SELECTION

Laparoscopic (or thoracoscopic) management of peptic ulcer disease is reserved, for the most part, for those individuals in whom medical management has failed or who require indefinite drug therapy to control their symptoms. A laparoscopic approach to patients seen with bleeding or gastric outlet obstruction has been successfully completed, but only in a few isolated situations (e.g., Reddick, personal communication, 1991). Laparoscopic closure of acute duodenal perforations has also been reported, but a simultaneous antiulcer operation (vagotomy) is usually not performed. With further experience and refinement of surgical technique, perhaps such conditions may be routinely managed via a minimal approach.

Patients with prepyloric or gastric ulcers are not considered ideal candidates for selective vagotomy. Previous studies with open highly selective vagotomy[17-19] as well as our own initial experience has shown that these individuals have a much higher risk for recurrence. Other contraindications to the performance of a laparoscopic vagotomy include pregnancy, extensive prior upper abdominal surgery, and irreversible coagulopathies.

PREOPERATIVE EVALUATION

The preoperative evaluation is very similar to that for patients scheduled for conventional ulcer surgery. A routine history, physical examination, and laboratory evaluation are done for all patients. Patients with atypical presentations of ulcer diathesis should also undergo a workup to exclude gastrinoma. All patients should undergo upper gastrointestinal endoscopy as well as contrast studies to determine the extent and severity of disease. In addition, to evaluate the effectiveness of this procedure, patients' acid secretion (basal and pentagastrin stimulation) and gastric emptying capacity should be determined. Repeat studies are performed at 3 to 6 months after surgery to confirm the effectiveness of the procedure. A thorough assessment of the patient's operative risk is made, similar to patients undergoing any major abdominal operation.

PATIENT PREPARATION AND POSITIONING

A single dose of a first-generation cephalosporin antibiotic is given just prior to surgery followed by two to three additional doses during the immediate postoperative period. A bowel preparation is not necessary for a laparoscopic vagotomy.

The operating room setup is quite similar to that for laparoscopic cholecystectomy. Two video monitors are placed on either side of the patient, near the head of the operating table.

The entire abdominal region is prepared and draped as for a standard ulcer operation. General anesthesia with endotracheal intubation is used in all patients. The patient may be positioned in the supine (with the primary surgeon standing on the right) or modified lithotomy position (with the surgeon or camera operator standing between the patient's legs). The use of the lithotomy procedure will allow the surgeon and first assistant to stand on either side of the patient while the camera operator is in an excellent position to direct the operative visualization during the procedure (Fig. 35-1).

Both of the patient's arms should be "tucked-in" at the sides. A nasogastric tube and urinary catheter tube are inserted to decompress the stomach and bladder. The gastric tube is subsequently replaced with a large esophageal tube (Maloney dilator) or a flexible gastroscope to distend the distal esophagus and facilitate its identification during the early stages of the operative dissection.

TROCAR PLACEMENT

A total of at least four primary laparoscopic cannulas are used in most patients (Fig. 35-2). The laparoscope is inserted through the umbilical port, and the right subcostal port will provide access for the liver retractor. The operating port is placed midway between the right costal margin and the umbilicus. Retraction of the stomach and esophagus is accomplished through the left

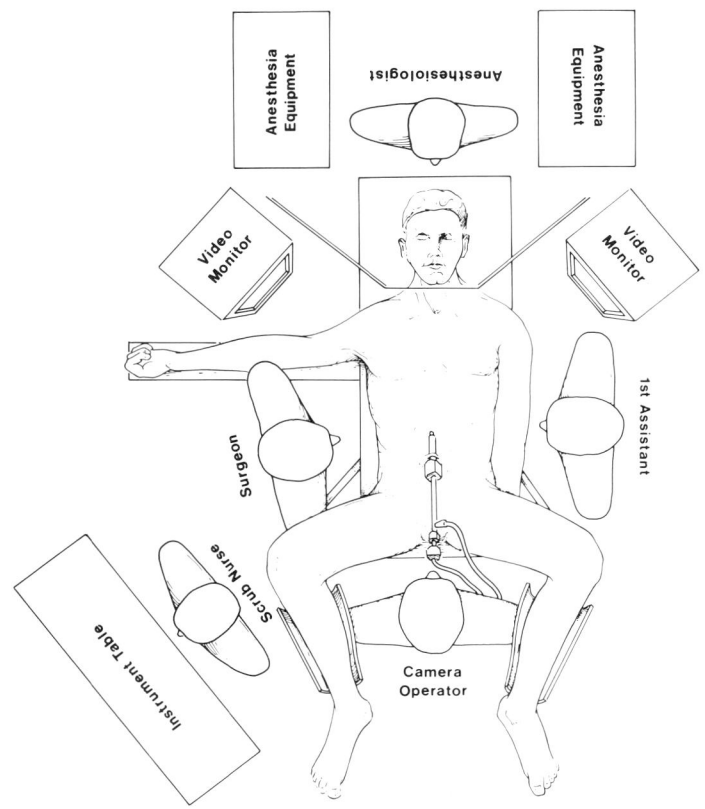

Figure 35-1.

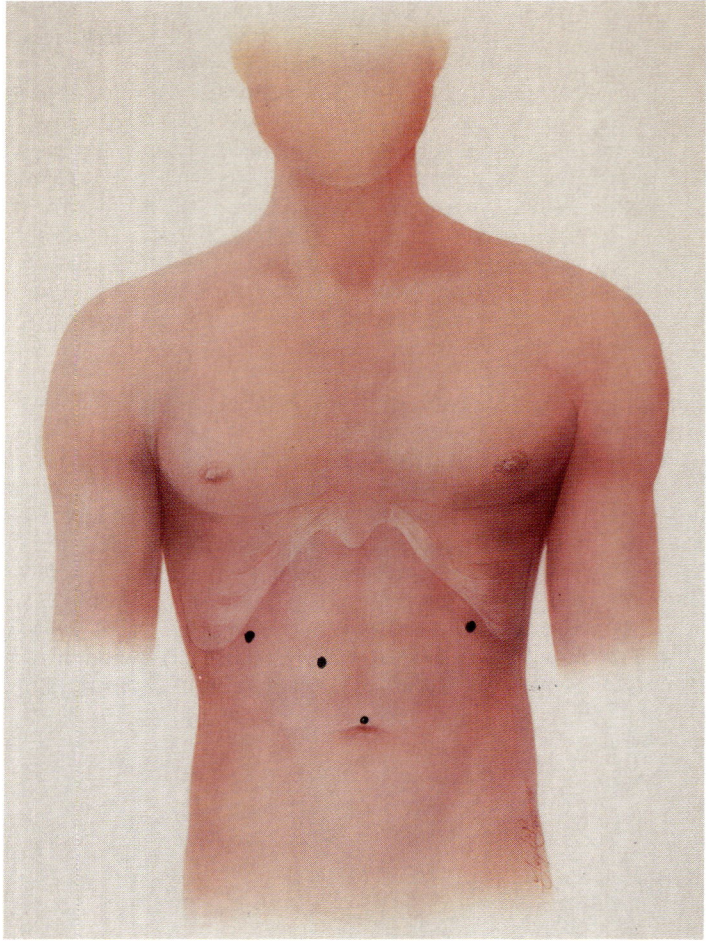

Figure 35-2.

subcostal port. An optional fifth or sixth puncture should be considered if additional retraction of the stomach or surrounding viscera is necessary.

The size of the individual laparoscopic trocars will depend on the choice and availability of instrumentation. Currently, we use 10.0- or 11.0-mm trocars for the four primary ports. This gives the surgeon greater versatility during the operation to exchange instruments (e.g., clip applier or laparoscope) from one port to another. The clip applier or laparoscope may then be inserted through whatever port is deemed most appropriate by the operating surgeon, thereby facilitating the operative dissection. Furthermore, converters are easily attached to the larger cannulas if a smaller (5-mm) instrument is desired. The size of any additional cannulas will depend largely upon the operative findings. In general, a 5.0-mm sheath will suffice for most situations.

INSUFFLATION AND INITIAL ASSESSMENT

Pneumoperitoneum is established in the standard fashion with carbon dioxide being used to distend the abdominal cavity until a pressure of 12 to 14 mm Hg is achieved. The laparoscope, with attached video camera, is introduced, and the peritoneal cavity is carefully examined. A 30- to 50-degree angled-viewing laparoscope will facilitate examination of the distal esophagus and hiatal region. The patient may also be placed in a 15- to 20-degree reverse Trendelenburg position to improve the visualization of the upper abdomen.

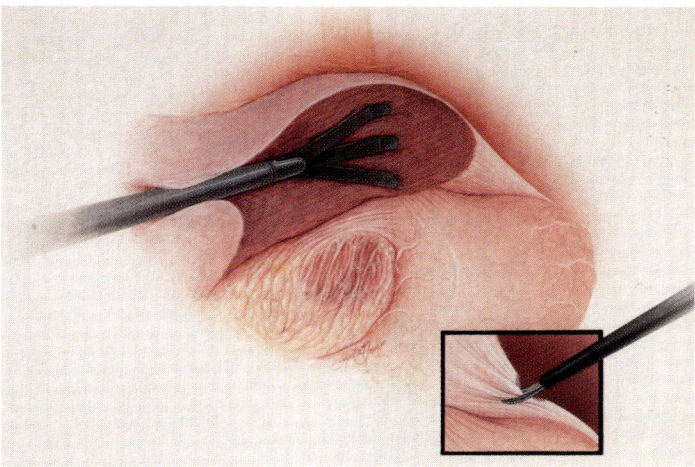

Figure 35-3.

RETRACTION OF THE LEFT LOBE OF THE LIVER

To provide adequate visualization of the distal esophagus, the left lobe of the liver must be retracted away from the hiatus. A 10-mm, fan-like liver retractor is inserted through the right subcostal cannula and opened within the abdomen. The atraumatic blades of this device allow the surgeon to elevate and retract the left lobe of the liver toward the right side of the patient (Fig. 35-3). If such a retractor is not available, it may be necessary to divide the left triangular ligament to gain adequate exposure of the gastroesophageal junction (Fig. 35-3, *inset*). Curved laparoscopic Metzenbaum scissors are used to divide the peritoneal attachments.

IDENTIFICATION AND DIVISION OF THE POSTERIOR VAGUS NERVE

The posterior aspect of the distal esophagus is approached through a window made in the lesser omentum, near the gastrohepatic ligament. A large esophageal tube or gastroscope is inserted into the stomach to facilitate visual identification of the distal esophagus. The greater curvature of the stomach is pulled to the patient's left with either an atraumatic grasping forceps or a Babcock retractor. This maneuver facilitates the initial approach to the esophagus. The opening into the lesser sac may be created with a "hook-spatula" electrocautery probe, scissors, or dissecting forceps (Fig. 35-4).

The right crus of the diaphragm is visual-

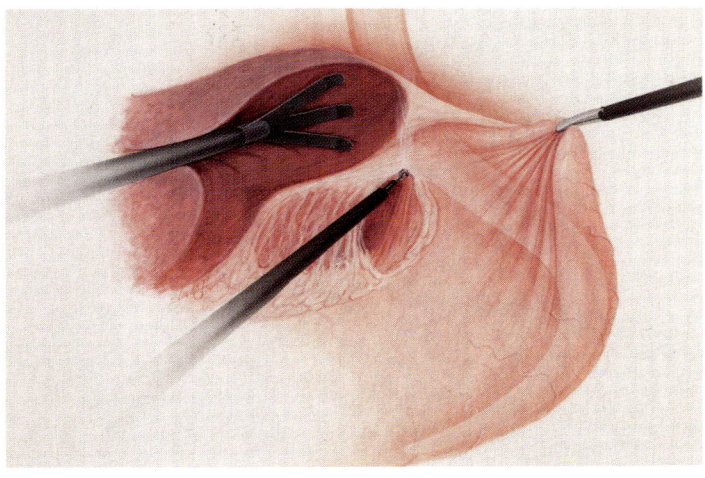

Figure 35-4.

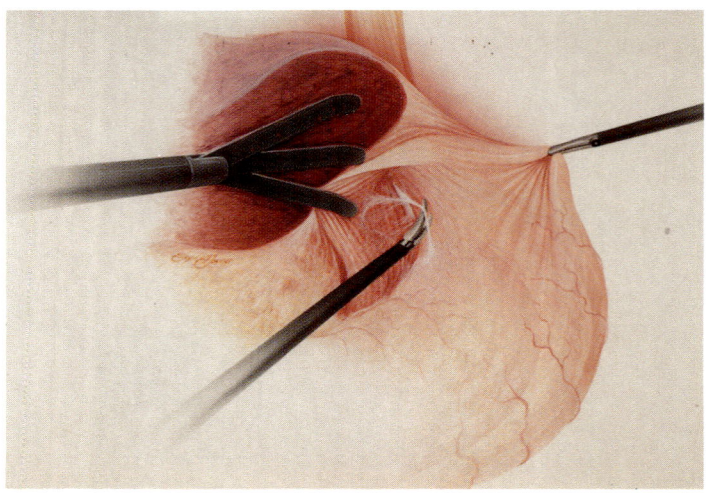

Figure 35-5.

ized and may be retracted away from the esophagus with one blade of the liver retractor (Fig. 35-5). A plane is then developed between the right crus and distal esophagus and continued in a posterior direction, behind the esophagus.

The posterior trunk of the vagus nerve is usually found along the right posterior aspect of the esophagus. It may be necessary to elevate the distal esophagus anteriorly and to rotate it to the patient's left side in order to visualize the main trunk. The previously placed esophageal dilator or gastroscope must be withdrawn from the gastroesophageal junction to permit this rotation of the esophagus. Atraumatic grasping forceps or a Babcock-like clamp, inserted through an optional fifth port, will assist in this maneuver. It may be necessary to ligate small branches of the posterior vagus nerve during this initial dissection (Fig. 35-6).

Continued dissection along the wall of the esophagus will identify the main posterior vagal trunk. The main trunk of the posterior vagus nerve is then ligated between clips and divided (Figs. 35-7 and 35-8). It is important to identify and transect this nerve as close to the crus of the diaphragm as possible. A short segment of nerve is excised and sent for histologic confirmation (Fig. 35-9). The posterior

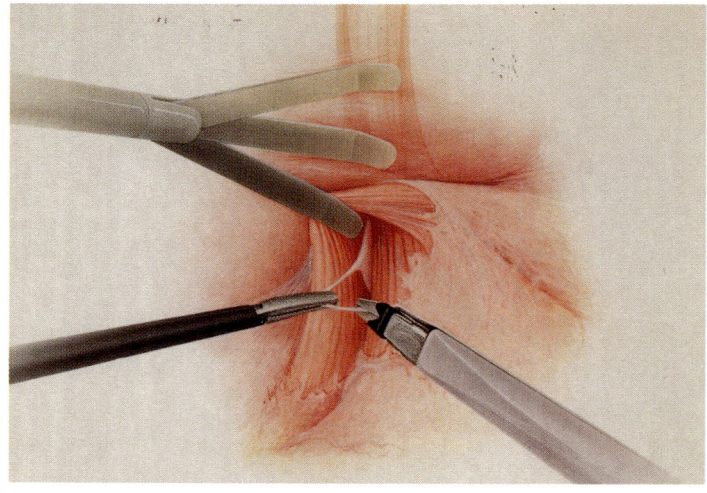

Figure 35-6.

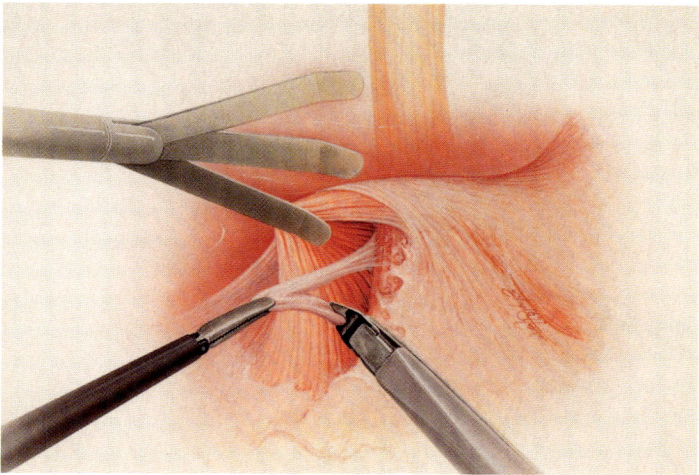

Figure 35-7.

aspect of the distal esophagus is irrigated and carefully inspected to confirm completeness of vagotomy and adequate hemostasis.

Following completion of the posterior truncal vagotomy, the next step is to identify the anterior vagus nerve. The opening in the phrenoesophageal membrane is carefully extended toward the patient's left side using blunt dissection with scissors or dissecting forceps. The anterior vagus nerve is usually smaller than the posterior trunk, and care must be taken to avoid inadvertent injury. The anterior vagus nerve may be found within the loose connective and adipose tissue overlying the distal esophagus. It is not unusual for the nerve trunk to be partially embedded within the muscle fibers of the esophageal wall (Fig. 35-10) or to be found on the left posterior aspect of the distal esophagus. A bilateral truncal vagotomy may then be easily accomplished at this juncture, if so desired (Fig. 35-11). Effective drainage may also be readily accomplished by endoscopic balloon dilatation of the pylorus (Fig. 35-12). In our experience, however, a highly selective vagotomy of the anterior leaflet can be quickly performed and thereby obviates the need for a drainage procedure.

The anterior vagus nerve is gently elevated away from the underlying esophagus with a curved dissecting forceps. Small branches of the anterior vagus, which are identified in

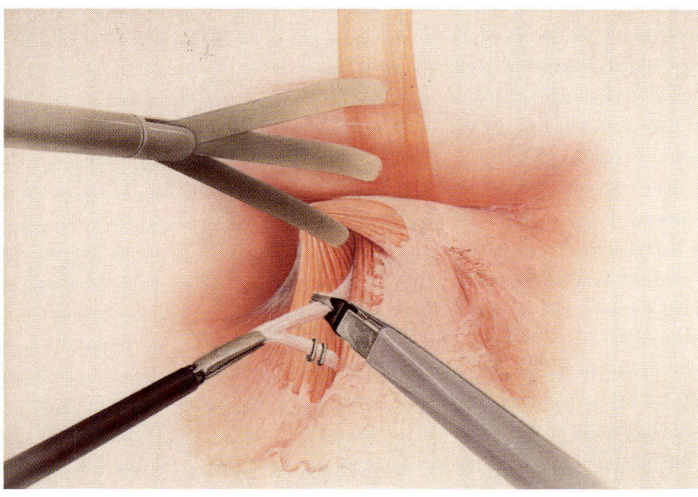

Figure 35-8.

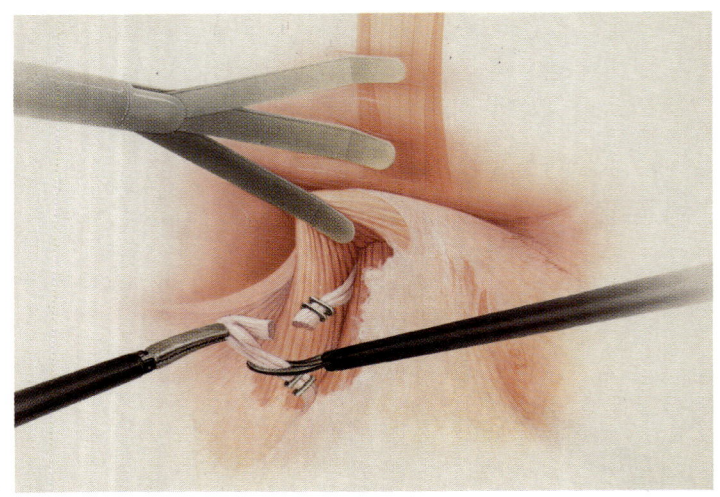

Figure 35-9.

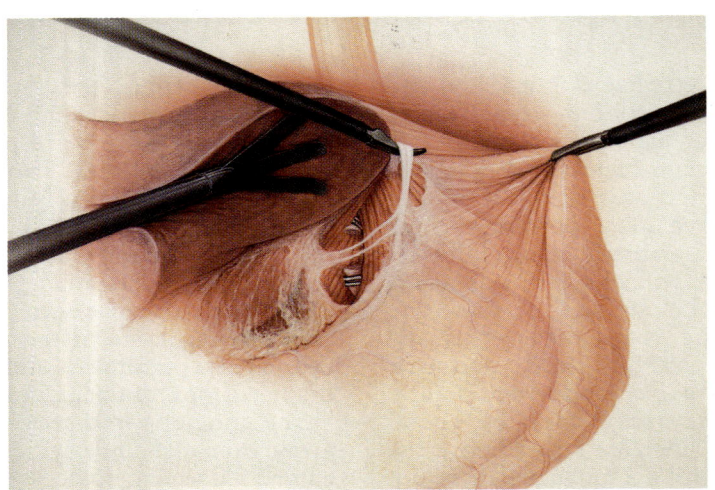

Figure 35-10.

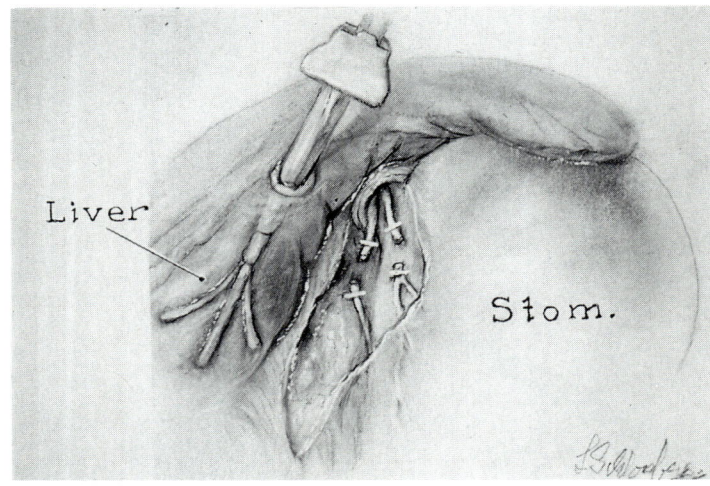

Figure 35-11.

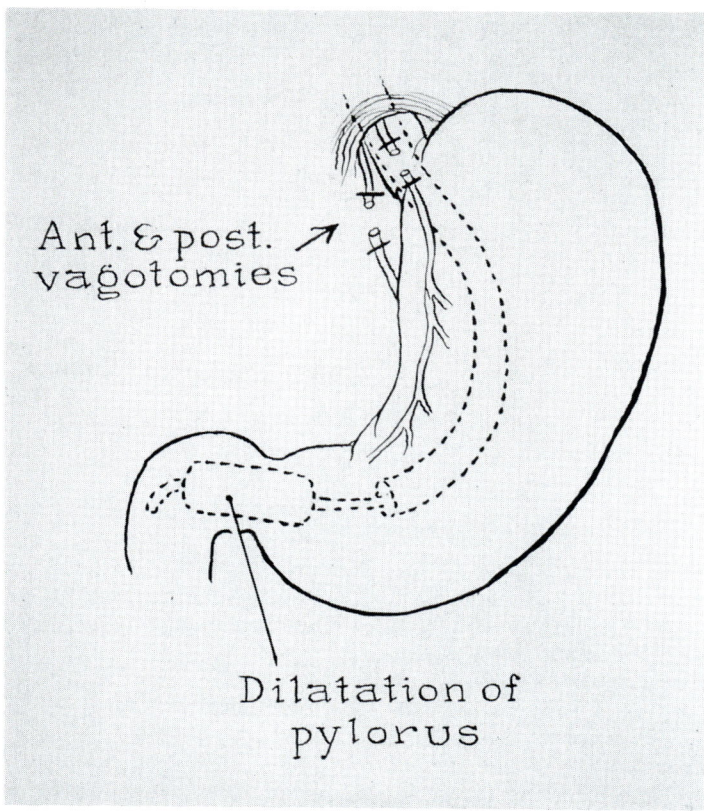

Figure 35-12.

this region, are ligated with clips and divided (Fig. 35-13).

Approximately 5 to 7 cm of intra-abdominal esophagus is eventually dissected free of surrounding tissues to ensure that any proximal branches from the anterior vagal trunk have been divided. The gastric antrum and pylorus serve as landmarks to help identify the "crow's foot" branches of the nerve of Latarget. A highly selective vagotomy of the anterior stomach is then begun 5 to 7 cm proximal to the pylorus. Usually, the most proximal branch of the crow's foot is identified and the dissection is begun at this loca-

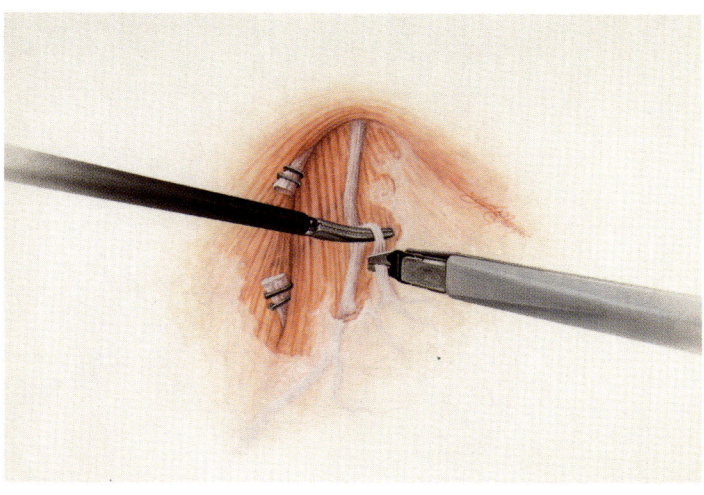

Figure 35-13.

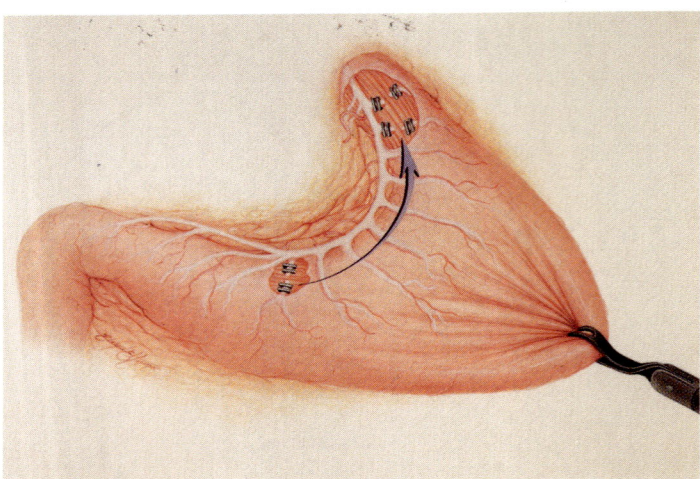

Figure 35-14.

tion. The first branch of the crow's foot, along with the accompanying artery and vein, is dissected away from the underlying gastric wall and ligated with clips (Fig. 35-14).

The entire neurovascular bundle is then divided with scissors. Electrocautery is avoided in this area for fear of injury to the gastric wall or anterior nerve trunk by the transmission of thermal energy. Continued retraction of the greater curvature of the stomach with the laparoscopic Babcock forceps facilitates identification of the branches of the anterior vagus nerve as they traverse the lesser curvature. The operative dissection continues along the lesser curvature in a cephalad manner, from the crow's foot toward the gastroesophageal junction. Each neurovascular bundle entering the fundus is ligated with surgical clips and sharply divided (Fig. 35-15).

CLOSURE

After the highly selective vagotomy is completed, the operative field is copiously irrigated with saline and carefully inspected to ensure adequate hemostasis. The laparoscopic cannulas are removed, and the carbon dioxide is evacuated from the abdomen. An attempt is made to close all of the larger (10 mm) fascial defects with interrupted sutures. The smaller (5 mm) fascial defects are not routinely closed as herniation through such punctures would be extremely unlikely. The

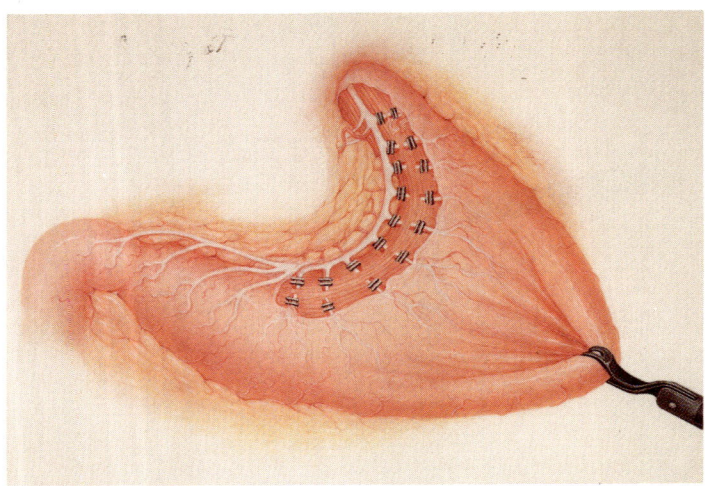

Figure 35-15.

skin edges are reapproximated with skin staples, sterile dressings are applied, and the patient is taken to the recovery room.

POSTOPERATIVE MANAGEMENT

The urinary catheter is usually removed when the patient is discharged from the recovery room. The nasogastric tube is left in place on low, intermittent suction for 6 to 12 hours. The tube may be removed the night of surgery (or the following morning if the operation was finished late in the day). Most patients are able to tolerate a liquid diet the morning after surgery, which may then be advanced to a regular diet as tolerated. The patient may be discharged in the afternoon of the first postoperative day or in the morning of the second postoperative day. Criteria for discharge are similar to those for patients undergoing laparoscopic cholecystectomy. Patients must be tolerating a regular diet, voiding well, and ambulating without assistance and be hemodynamically stable. Most patients are able to return to normal activity within 7 to 14 days.

COMPLICATIONS

Anticipated complications of laparoscopic vagotomy are similar to those for open vagotomy. Any of the potential complications associated with establishment of pneumoperitoneum are, of course, possible. These issues have been addressed in Chapters 8 and 12. Intraoperative injuries to the esophagus, stomach, liver, or colon are also possible during the laparoscopic procedure, as are major vascular injuries to the large vessels in close proximity to the operative dissection (e.g., left gastric artery and vein).

Postoperative complications include, among others, hemorrhage, infection, and gastric outlet obstruction. With careful surgical technique most of these difficulties should be avoided. Necrosis of the lesser curve of the stomach has been reported in rare situations after standard highly selective vagotomy.[17] This complication should be even more uncommon during posterior truncal vagotomy/anterior highly selective vagotomy because the posterior blood supply to the lesser curvature is not interrupted.

Of greatest concern is the incidence of recurrent ulcer disease. Initial anecdotal reports indicate that the recurrence rate is within an acceptable range (5 to 15 per cent) for a highly selective vagotomy. Careful patient selection (i.e., avoidance of patients with antral, prepyloric, and pyloric ulcers) should help to keep the recurrence rate at an acceptable level. The incidence of postoperative dumping and diarrhea should be low, in the range of 1 to 2 per cent. Obviously, definitive statements regarding the incidence of complications during laparoscopic vagotomy must await further published reports.

DISCUSSION AND EVOLVING TECHNIQUES

An operation to treat patients with intractable ulcer disease, which has been popular in Europe for the past two decades, is a posterior truncal vagotomy combined with anterior seromyotomy. This procedure has been popularized by the work of Taylor and colleagues from the United Kingdom.[11,13–15] The anterior seromyotomy is based in theory on the anatomic observation that the small gastric branches of the anterior vagus nerve course obliquely through the seromuscular layer of the stomach before reaching the acid-secreting mucosal layer (Fig. 35-16, *lower inset*). Dividing the seromuscular layer interrupts these small branches, thereby accomplishing a highly selective vagotomy of the anterior aspect of the stomach.

According to Taylor's original description,[13] the myotomy is begun 6.0 cm proximal to the pylorus and at a point that is approximately 1.5 cm from the edge of the lesser curve. The circular muscle is incised, and scissors are used to continue the dissection of the circular muscle in a cephalad manner. Any blood vessels encountered are ligated and divided. The myotomy is continued until the gastroesophageal junction is reached. Ongoing clinical investigation by Taylor and others has shown that posterior truncal vagotomy and anterior seromyotomy do not significantly alter gastric motility or emptying, and therefore a gastric-emptying procedure is usually not necessary.[11] Also according to Taylor's original description, a critical step in the operation is an extensive skeletonization of the anterior nerve trunk and distal esophagus.

Subsequent to their initial description, the group in France now extends the proximal extent of the laparoscopic myotomy to include the gastric cardia. This may stem from the fact that a complete dissection of the anterior nerve trunk is not routinely performed

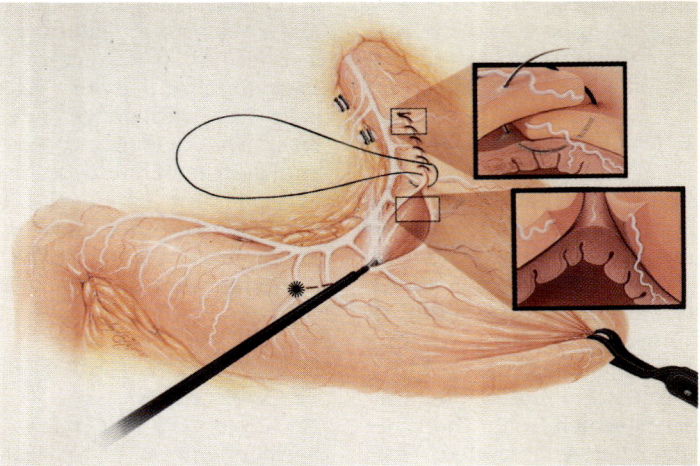

Figure 35-16.

with their laparoscopic approach. Their procedure therefore differs from that described by Taylor and colleagues, making extrapolation of the rationale for the laparoscopic modification somewhat difficult. Details of the technique of laparoscopic anterior seromyotomy will be presented in Chapter 36.

Recently a group of surgeons in Mobile, Alabama,[12] have developed a modification of the anterior seromyotomy technique, which uses a laparoscopic stapling instrument. In this procedure, Hannon, Snow, and Weinstein perform a posterior truncal vagotomy as previously described but divide the fundic branches of the anterior vagus nerve with a laparoscopic stapling device.

This instrument fires six rows of staples and houses a cutting blade, which simultaneously divides the tissue in between these rows of staples. This device allows the surgeon to rapidly interrupt the intramural vagal branches without risk of inadvertent gastric perforation.

Following ligation and division of the posterior vagus nerve (as previously described) the remainder of the distal esophagus is carefully dissected to assure completeness of vagotomy. The course of the anterior vagus nerve is then identified to avoid subsequent injury with the stapler. The pylorus and the branches of the Nerve of Latarget to the antrum (crow's foot) are visualized. A site

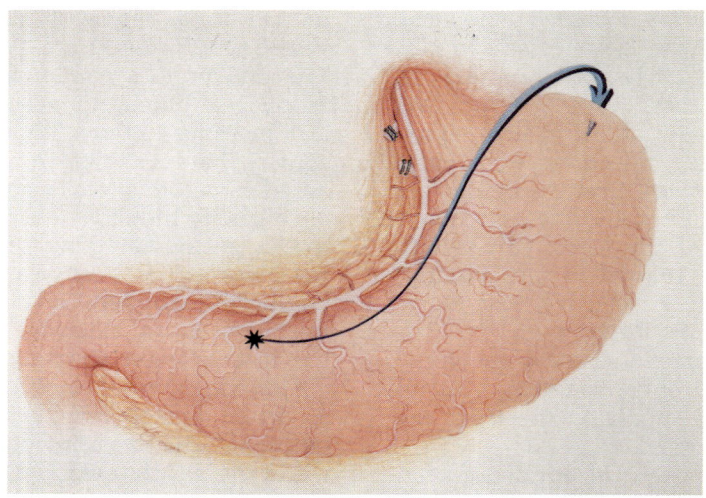

Figure 35-17.

Vagotomy 417

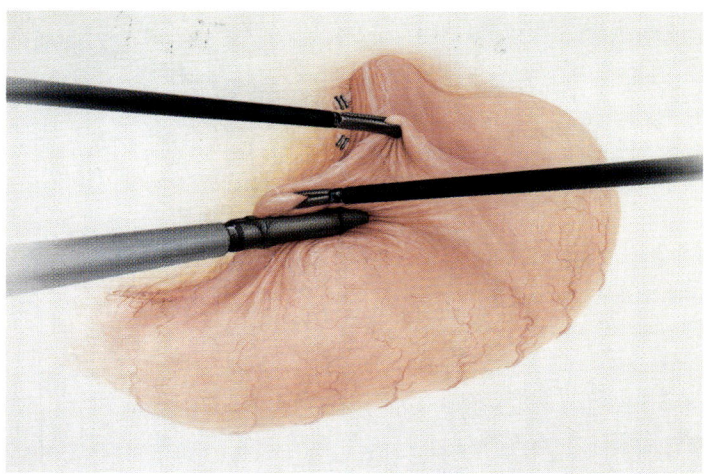

Figure 35-18.

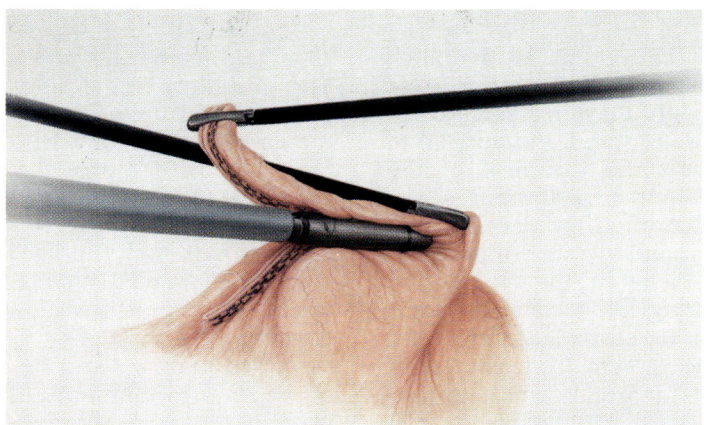

Figure 35-19.

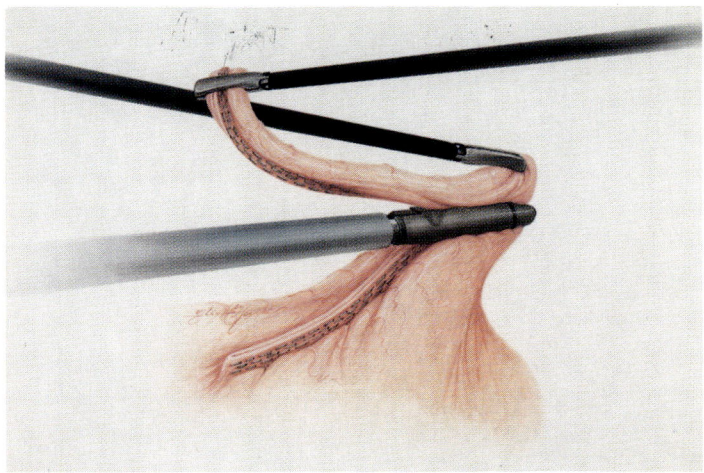

Figure 35-20.

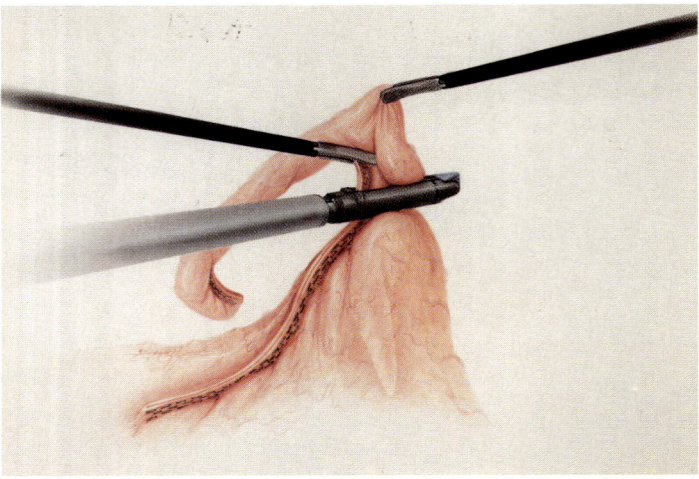

Figure 35-21.

7.0 cm proximal to the pylorus is identified, and the edge of the stomach along the lesser curve is elevated with grasping forceps. A specialized gauge is introduced and applied to the stomach to assess the thickness of the wall. This will determine the proper staple cartridge (2.4 or 3.5 mm) to be used. A stapled division (and simultaneous reanastomosis) of the anterior wall of the stomach is accomplished by firing of the laparoscopic stapling device. A long strip of gastric wall, approximately 1.5 to 3.0 cm from the lesser curvature, is then divided with serial applications of the laparoscopic stapling device in a cephalad manner (Figs. 35-17 through 35-22). The resulting staple line extends from the proximal antrum in a cephalad direction to the gastric cardia and then continues over the top of the cardia, onto the posterior aspect of the stomach (Fig. 35-22).

Although clinical experience with this technique is extremely limited, early results have been encouraging. The use of the laparoscopic stapling device allows the procedure to be completed in far less time then previously described methods and the stapled anastomosis appears to eliminate the risk of unrecognized gastric perforation.

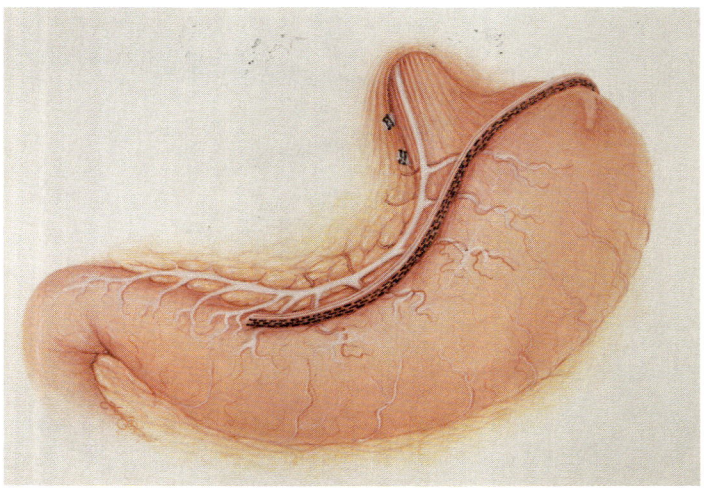

Figure 35-22.

ACKNOWLEDGMENTS

Sincere gratitude is expressed to all of the surgeons and operating room personnel in Europe and the United States who have assisted with our early clinical experience. Special thanks is also given to the nursing staff at the University of Maryland Medical Center.

REFERENCES

1. Bailey RW, Zucker KA, Flowers JL, et al. Laparoscopic cholecystectomy: Experience with 375 consecutive patients. Ann Surg 1991; 214:531–541.
2. Spaw AT, Reddick EJ, Olsen DO. Laparoscopic laser cholecystectomy: Analysis of 500 procedures. Surg Laparosc Endosc 1991; 1:2–7.
3. Pier A, Gotz F, Bacher C. Laparoscopic appendectomy in 625 cases: From innovation to routine. Surg Laparosc Endosc 1991; 1:8–13.
4. Spaw AT, Ennis BW, Spaw LP. Laparoscopic hernia repair: The anatomic basis. J Laparoendosc Surg 1991; 1:269–277.
5. Fowler DL, White SA. Laparoscopy-assisted sigmoid resection. Surg Laparosc Endosc 1991; 1:183–188.
6. Flowers JL, Feldman J, Jacobs SC. Laparoscopic pelvic lymphadenectomy. Surg Laparosc Endosc 1991; 1:62–70.
7. Dallemagne B, Weerts JM, Jehaes C, et al. Laparoscopic Nissen fundoplication: Preliminary report. Surg Laparosc Endosc 1991; 1:138–143.
8. Bailey RW, Flowers JL, Graham SM, Zucker KA. Combined laparoscopic cholecystectomy and selective vagotomy. Surg Laparosc Endosc 1991; 1:45–49.
9. Mouiel J, Katkhouda N. Laparoscopic truncal and selective vagotomy. In Zucker KA, Bailey RW, Reddick EJ, eds. Surgical Laparoscopy. St. Louis: Quality Medical Publishing, Inc, 1991; pp 263–279.
10. DuBois F. Invited presentation. Society of American Gastrointestinal Endoscopic Surgeons Postgraduate Course, Monterey, CA, 1991.
11. Taylor TV, Holt S, Heading RC. Gastric emptying after anterior lesser curve seromyotomy and posterior truncal vagotomy. Br J Surg 1985; 72:620–622.
12. Hannon JK, Snow LL, Weinstein LS. Endoscopic staple assisted anterior highly selective vagotomy combined with posterior truncal vagotomy for treatment of peptic ulcer disease. Surg Laparosc Endosc In press.
13. Taylor TV, Gunn AA, Macleod DAD, MacLennan I. Anterior lesser curve seromyotomy and posterior truncal vagotomy in the treatment of chronic duodenal ulcer. Lancet 1982; 2:846–848.
14. Taylor TV, Gunn AA, Macleod DAD, et al. Mortality and morbidity after anterior lesser curve seromyotomy with posterior truncal vagotomy for the treatment of duodenal ulcer. Br J Surg 1985; 72:950–951.
15. Taylor TV, Lythgoe JP, McFarland JB, et al. Anterior lesser curve seromyotomy and posterior truncal vagotomy versus truncal vagotomy and pyloroplasty in the treatment of chronic duodenal ulcer. Br J Surg 1990; 77:1007–1009.
16. Hill GL, Barker CJ. Anterior highly selective vagotomy with posterior truncal vagotomy: A simple technique for denervating the parietal cell mass. Br J Surg 1978; 65:702–705.
17. Jordan PH, Jr. Surgery for peptic ulcer disease. Curr Probl Surg 1991; 28:265–330.
18. Johnston D. Operative mortality and postoperative morbidity of highly selective vagotomy. Br Med J 1975; 4:545–547.
19. Hoffmann J, Olesen A, Jensen HE. Prospective 14- to 18-year follow-up study after parietal cell vagotomy. Br J Surg 1987; 74:1056–1059.

Chapter 36
Laparoscopic Treatment of Peptic Ulcer Disease

Namir Katkhouda
Jean Mouiel*

Few patients now require operative treatment for duodenal ulcer disease because of the availability of effective pharmacotherapeutic probes. Nonetheless, there still remain many patients who endure symptomatic and chronic duodenal ulcers despite well managed medical care. Indeed, the advent of laparoscopic surgery has not changed the indications for operative intervention in patients with duodenal ulcers, but rather has offered these patients an alternative and perhaps more effective therapy with very few sequelae. The first vagotomy by videolaparoscopy was accomplished in Nice in October 1989. Since then, more than 80 procedures have been done here with good initial results, and many centers have started to record their own experience. Although right truncal vagotomy with anterior fundic seromyotomy is our operation of choice, two other technical possibilities will be described in this chapter: bilateral truncal vagotomy with pyloric dilatation and right truncal vagotomy with anterior highly selective vagotomy suggested recently in Baltimore (see Chap. 35).

RIGHT TRUNCAL VAGOTOMY WITH ANTERIOR FUNDIC SEROMYOTOMY

Selection of Patients

This procedure is indicated for patients whose symptomatic chronic duodenal ulcer has not responded to appropriate medical treatment (i.e., type of medications as well as dosage and duration of treatment). All patients should be informed about the details of the operation. The patient must undergo certain tests before the decision for surgery is made. In particular, an endoscopic examination and gastric acidity test are necessary to select patients in whom a good result may be obtained.

Preoperative Evaluation

All preoperative tests can be obtained on an outpatient basis. These include routine ultrasonography of the liver and gallbladder to rule out or diagnose another condition, a complete esophagogastroduodenal endoscopic

---
* Francis Abihanna, M.D., Translator

examination to confirm the presence of the duodenal ulcer and to rule out other possible conditions such as pyloric stenosis or a hiatal hernia, an esophagogastroduodenal barium series to evaluate the morphology of the esophagocardiofundic area as well as the antropyloric channel, and baseline acidity and maximal acidity (stimulated with insulin or pentagastrin) tests. In addition, the presence of a gastrinoma associated with Zollinger-Ellison syndrome should be excluded.

Preoperative Care

The patient is admitted to the hospital on the night before surgery. The patient should be instructed not to smoke on the day before surgery and consume only light meals. Nothing by mouth will be given to the patient after midnight. A bowel preparation and perioperative antibiotics are not required.

Equipment

Usually we use a 10-mm laparoscope (Karl Storz GmbH & Co, Tuttlingen, Germany) and in our experience we have not needed to use a 5-mm laparoscope. We routinely use a 0-degree laparoscope. However, a 30-degree laparoscope is always available because it can help in some difficult cases to see the lateral view at the left side of the esophagus and the anterior aspect of the stomach.

Five trocars are used for this procedure. A 10-mm trocar is used to introduce the videoendoscope (Karl Storz GmbH & Co), and another 10-mm trocar is used to introduce the instruments for dissection. A 12-mm trocar can be substituted for a 10-mm trocar if the stapler is to be used to close the seromyotomy. Three 5-mm trocars are also used: two to introduce the grasping forceps and a third for the palpator or the irrigation-suction system.

Only a few good laparoscopic instruments which are used expertly by the surgeon are required for this procedure. In addition, instruments for traditional (open) surgery must be available in the operating room in case it becomes necessary to perform an open laparotomy. The grasping forceps should all be atraumatic; in visceral surgery and especially in esogastric surgery, the use of forceps with big teeth is prohibited because of the danger of injury during the grasping maneuvers. Two forceps with small atraumatic teeth, one forceps without claws and without teeth, and an endoscopic dissector are needed. The use of forceps without a ratchet is highly recommended; in fact, the ratchet prevents free movement, and it is not necessary in this type of surgery to have the instruments locked. For dissection instruments, we regularly use an unipolar coagulant hook, which is insulated down to its tip, leaving the horizontal portion denuded. Electrocautery scissors, both straight and curved, are essential. Two good needle holders of 5 and 3 mm are used to accomplish the suturing through the endoscope. For suturing we prefer nonabsorbable polypropylene material threaded on a needle (18 mm maximum) with a curved end. The suture material will be cut short at 15 or 20 cm maximum to prevent the formation of any undesirable loops inside the abdomen. To accomplish hemostasis, it is mandatory to have an automatic clip applier (Ethicon Inc., Cincinnati, Ohio). A stapler (Ethicon) can be used to close the seromyotomy.

Positioning of the Patient

The patient is positioned in the supine position with the lower limbs pushed aside ("French position") (Fig. 36-1). The surgeon stands between the lower limbs and looks at the monitor placed in front and on his or her left side. The first assistant holding the camera is on the right side of the surgeon, and the second assistant retracting the liver is on the left side of the surgeon. A small nasogastric tube is placed to suction the stomach and locate the esophagus. A Foley catheter is not needed if the patient urinated before surgery.

Positioning of the Video Equipment

The rolling table that holds the main monitor, the inflator, the source of light, and the recording machines is placed in front and on the left side of the surgeon, near the right shoulder of the patient. A second monitor placed on the left, for the second assistant, is helpful.

Placement of Trocars

If the pneumoperitoneum needle is usually placed in the umbilicus, we think it is impor-

422 Techniques of Laparoscopic Surgery

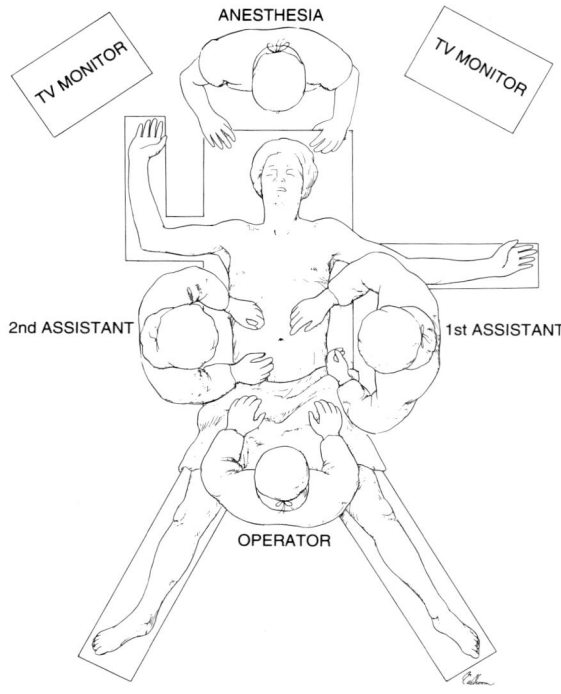

Figure 36-1.

Technical Principles of Dissection

Among the different techniques of dissection, our preference is for the one that is closest to open surgery, which we call "discision." This operation is done with bimanual dissection with the left hand stretching the tissues and the right hand manipulating alternatively the hook dissector or the scissors, dissecting the tissues free before cutting them with electrocautery. We rarely use blunt dissection, which in this highly vascularized area, may lead to hemorrhage that may prevent completion of the procedure.

Technique

First, the left lobe of the liver is elevated with the xiphoid palpator, because the procedure will be done under the left lobe of the liver. Then the surgeon should proceed step by step, following the important landmarks of

tant to place the other trocars above the umbilicus. Indeed, the videoendoscope will be introduced 3 fingers above and on the right side of the umbilicus where it will go through a 10-mm trocar. A 5-mm trocar is placed near the xiphoid. This trocar is used for retraction of the liver. A 5-mm trocar is placed in the left upper quadrant for use with grasping forceps. An additional 5-mm trocar is inserted in the right upper quadrant also for use with grasping forceps. Finally, a 10-mm trocar is positioned symmetrically with the videoendoscope trocar, 3 fingers above and on the left of the umbilicus. Dissection instruments are used by the surgeon through this trocar. The position of these trocars approximates a geometrical design (Fig. 36-2).

Accomplishing the Pneumoperitoneum

The pneumoperitoneum is insufflated through an umbilical puncture, after all security tests are done. The stomach must be empty before puncture. The pneumoperitoneum is maintained electronically at about 13 mm Hg.

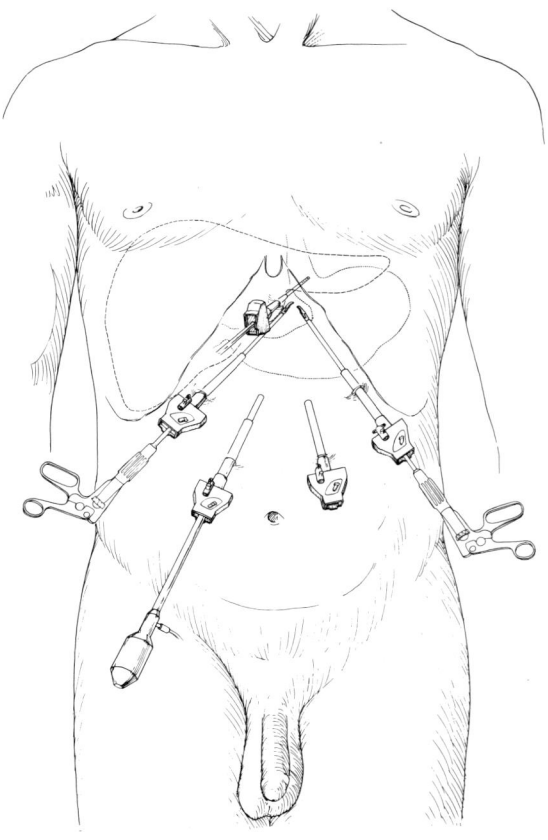

Figure 36-2.

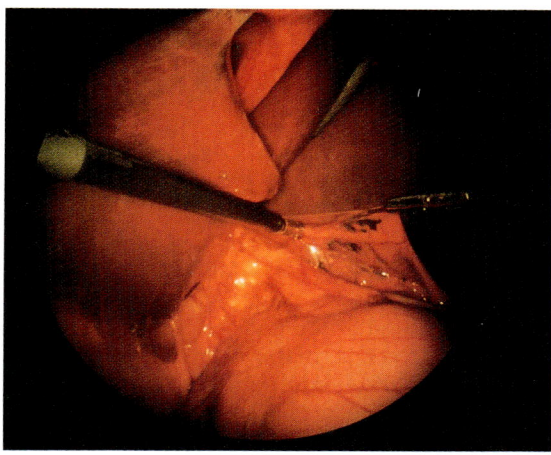

Figure 36-3.

the dissection. The first landmark is the avascular window of the lesser omentum, under which the quadrate lobe is seen. This window is gripped and divided with the coagulant hook above the hepatic branch of the left vagus (Fig. 36-3). This opening in the lesser omentum leads automatically to the right crus of the diaphragm. This is the second important landmark with the quadrate lobe on its right. Once the right crus of the diaphragm is identified, the gastric tube can be mobilized slightly so that the esophagus can be identified by its back and forth movements. A small opening of the peritoneum covering the abdominal esophagus is made at its junction with the right crus because a larger opening of the peritoneum on the anterior aspect of the esophagus may damage the anterior branch of the vagus nerve. After the peritoneum is opened the hook is introduced inside the angle formed by the right crus on the right and the right side of the esophagus on the left. The surgeon uses the grasping forceps in the left hand to seize the right crus of the diaphragm and to pull on it, while the first assistant with the left hand slightly retracts the grasping forceps, which are closed on the right side of the esophagus (Fig. 36-4). A cellular tissue layer appears in which the right vagus nerve is found posteriorly. Another secondary trunk is sought although this has been found only rarely in our experience. Once the right vagus nerve is dissected free with the hook, it is resected and the vagotomy done between two clips to assure hemostasis. A specimen is sent for histologic studies (Fig. 36-5).

Anterior Fundic Seromyotomy

The aim of the anterior fundic seromyotomy is to section the fundic branches of the left or anterior vagus nerve in their gastric

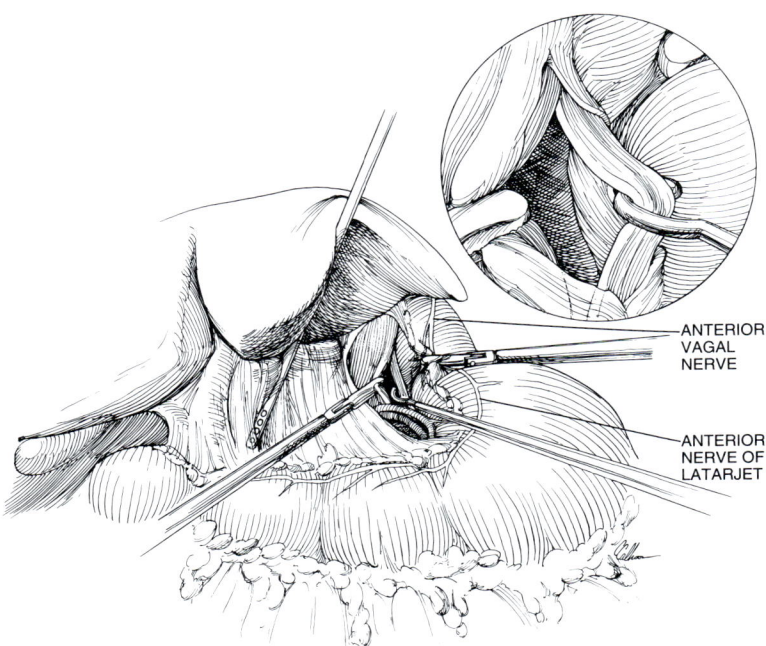

Figure 36-4.

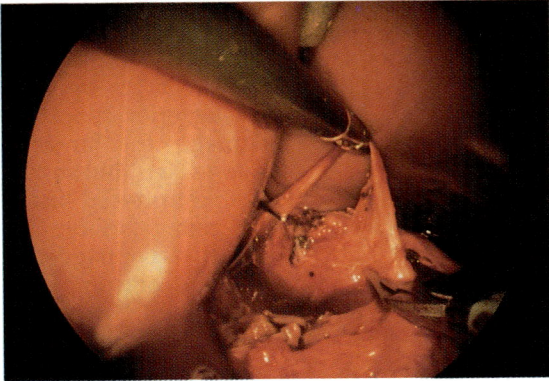

Figure 36-5.

intramural course while preserving the last two or three branches ("branches de la patte d'oie"), preservation of these three branches preserves antropyloric motility (Fig. 36-6). We have modified the initial technique described by Taylor—instead of starting the seromyotomy on the anterior aspect of the esophagus, we start it on the posterior side of the angle of Hiss. We continue in an "S" shape 1.5 cm from the lesser curve and end 6 cm from the pyloric muscle, thus taking the first branch of the last ones ("branches de la patte d'oie"), terminating in the anterior gastric nerve of Latarjet. Usually there are a few vessels on the anterior aspect of the stomach that should be secured for hemostasis prior to the seromyotomy. It is important at this stage of the procedure to introduce a small sized nasogastric tube down almost to the pylorus; this can be checked by laparoscopy. Slight tension can be placed on the greater curve with the tube to facilitate the exposure. The stomach is grasped by two atraumatic forceps, and the seromyotomy is "marked" with the unipolar coagulant hook to determine the path to follow. This is done with the help of an electrocoagulation device (Valleylab Force 2), allowing delivery of a unipolar electric source blending coagulation and section (for example, 50 W for coagulation and 15 W for section). Once the "landmarking" of the seromyotomy is accomplished, the few vessels running on the anterior aspect of the stomach are dissected free; usually there is one on the anterior side that is the largest.

The dissection is accomplished with curved scissors, and the section between two clips. The seromyotomy then begins. The edges of the planned seromyotomy are retracted apart. The hook cautery divides the seromuscular fibers. The magnification of the videolaparoscope displays beautifully the dissociating fibers. The tissue is divided down in the stomach wall until the bluish aspect of the boundary between the mucosa and submucosa becomes visible. The surgeon should stop at this level since if this limiting layer is divided, a gastric perforation will certainly ensue. If a gastric perforation is suspected, which did not happen in our experience, the stomach should be inflated with water mixed with methylene blue. Extravasation of the dye

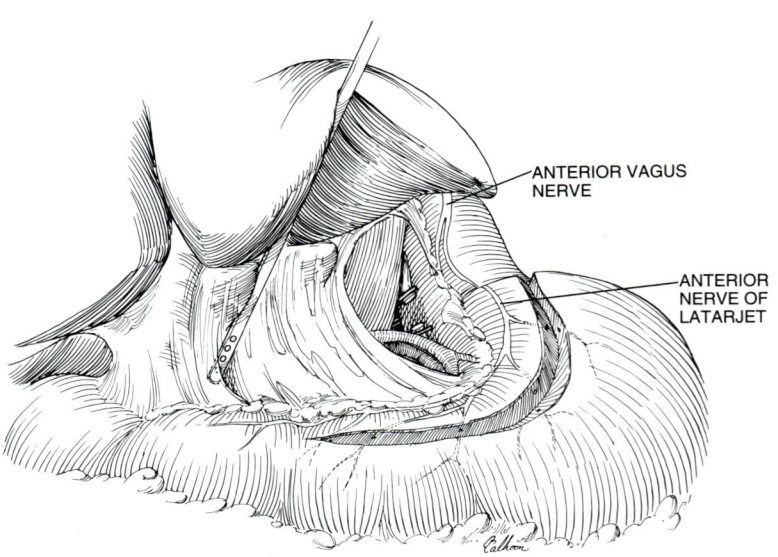

Figure 36-6.

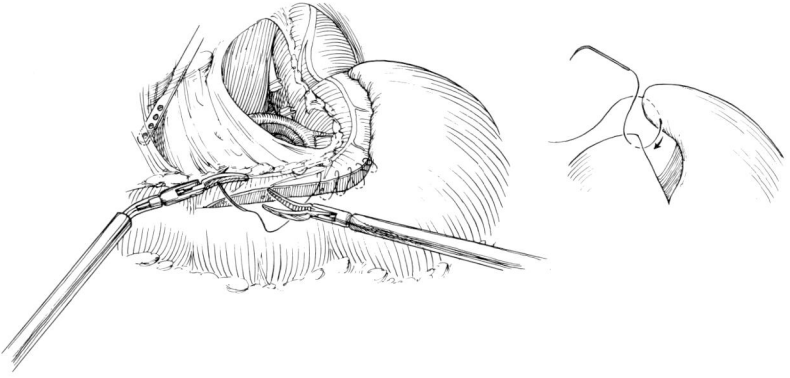

Figure 36-7.

reveals the perforation which is then sutured closed. The seromyotomy is terminated at the level of the first terminal branch of the nerve of Latarjet (branch of "la patte d'oie"). The two or three remaining branches of the anterior nerve of Latarjet should be left intact. This will preserve antral motility and through connections and circuit reflexes gastric motility as a whole. Taylor's studies did not show any significant modification of gastric motility and the emptying of the stomach after seromyotomy. The seromyotomy is then inspected centimeter by centimeter. The overlap repair of the two edges of the stomach is the final step of the procedure (Figs. 36-7 and 36-8). Actually the repair described by Taylor theoretically prevents nerve regeneration, although this was not proven, and it gives excellent hemostasis. The repair can be done in two ways: either laparoscopically sutured or with the help of an automatic stapler (Ethicon). We have found that the stapled closure shortens considerably the duration of the procedure. If the suturing technique is selected, the seromyotomy is closed with two or three running sutures. A straight needle (18 mm maximum) with a curved end holding a suture (15 cm in length) is introduced into the abdomen. We recommend locking the running suture at its beginning with two surgeon knots, because locking it with clips presents a risk of sliding. The running suture is accomplished by widely overlapping the left edge of the seromyotomy over the right edge with the suture running in staggered rows. At the middle of the seromyotomy, another suture is introduced and used to lock the first running suture. The second running suture finishes the seromyotomy. In the second technique, the seromyotomy is closed with "U" shaped staples. This obtains a result identical to that accomplished with sutures but in less time. The two grasping forceps overlap the edges of the seromyotomy so that the staple can fix one side of the gastric wall to the other. Approximately 15 staples are required for the closure.

The operative field is irrigated at the end of the procedure. During the procedure, however, we prefer to use only suction unless there is a major hemorrhage. The irrigation

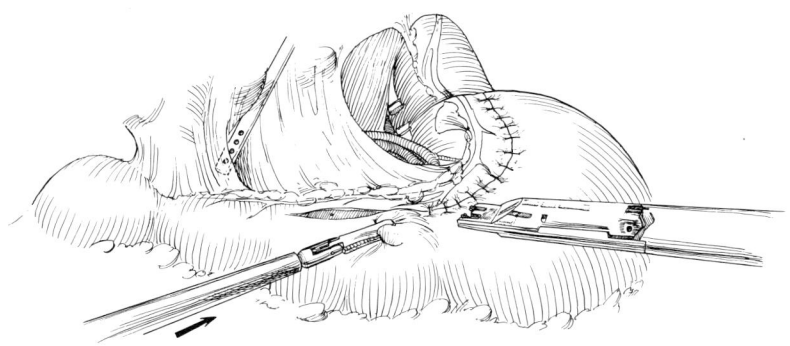

Figure 36-8.

leaves residual fluid that may hinder the operation. The fluid tends to pool in the left upper quadrant because of the negative pressure. Movement of the diaphragm during ventilation pushes the fluid back into the operative field. Thus, the peritoneal lavage is done at the end of the procedure.

Parietal Closure

When the procedure is completed, the instruments are taken out from the trocars. All the trocar valves are wide open because the balloon ventilation done manually by the anesthesiologist will help deflation of the remaining gas. In our experience this decreases postoperative pain significantly, thus improving the comfort of the patient and allowing earlier ambulation and then discharge. Once deflation is accomplished, the different skin incisions are closed with simple sutures or with skin Steri-Strips (3M Corp, Minn. MN).

Postoperative Care

We leave the nasogastric tube in place for 1 day, to suction the air in the stomach and to decrease sensations of nausea by emptying the stomach. However, it is always removed on the day after surgery. Generally the patient is allowed to get out of bed on the next day. The patient is given first a liquid diet followed by a solid diet as soon as the nasogastric tube is removed. Beside prophylactic intraoperative antibiotic treatment (cephalosporin, 2 g intravenously), no postoperative antibiotic is prescribed. Intravenous fluids are usually stopped on postoperative day 2, with discharge on postoperative day 3. Criteria for discharge include bowel movements, patient ambulation, and absence of distention and epigastric pain.

Specific Complications

Three types of specific complications follow this procedure: two are technical and encountered intraoperatively and one is encountered postoperatively.

The first complication during the procedure is hemorrhage from the gastric vessels which run on the anterior aspect of the stomach. This occurs if the vessels are coagulated and not clipped. This is why we recommend for all esophagogastric procedures that hemostasis be achieved with clips. These vessels (arteries and veins) supply an organ that is highly vascularized and do not have a tendency for rapid and spontaneous hemostasis. Thus, meticulous hemostasis should be secured before the seromyotomy is cut.

The second complication related to the seromyotomy is the possibility of perforation of the gastric mucosa. We think that surgeons who perform esophagogastric surgery should have experience in laparoscopic suturing. A surgeon should not perform advanced laparoscopic surgery without prior experience in suturing. If perforation occurs, the surgeon should be able to accomplish what is done in open surgery, i.e., closure of the perforation by interrupted extramucosal sutures with 4-0 nonabsorbable suture material. In the cases of perforation it is preferable to leave the gastric tube in place 1 extra day.

The third potential complication is the occurrence of bezoars causing gastric discomfort. These bezoars result from postvagotomy relative and temporary gastric atony. The diagnosis is made by upper endoscopy, and the treatment is generally medical and very efficient; the administration of papain by mouth solves the problem.

Results

We have operated on 87 patients so far. The follow-up of these patients consists of routine office visits during the first 3 months: after a month for a test of gastric acidity and an endoscopic examination, a second examination in the second month, and then an examination annually. At the second month's visit we have documented the healing of duodenal ulcers in 82 patients and the persistance of an asymptomatic linear scar in 5 patients, with the absence of the inflammatory reaction around the ulcer. Acidity measurement in the first month showed significant decreases in basal (79 per cent) and maximal acid output (82 per cent). Among the complications noted, we have performed another operation on a patient for esophagogastric reflux, probably misdiagnosed before surgery. Three patients had gastric bezoars, which needed medical treatment. One other patient had an umbilical inflammation. At the 2 months to 2 years followup, 2 recurrences were noted. Those early results are very encouraging and the 5 years follow-up will be subject to a scientific publication.

BILATERAL TRUNCAL VAGOTOMY AND PYLORIC DILATATION WITH BALLOON

For this technique patient selection, preoperative evaluation, equipment, and placement of trocars are the same as for the right truncal vagotomy with anterior fundic seromyotomy. This procedure begins just as the first. By adding the left truncal vagotomy to the right truncal vagotomy, a total vagotomy is accomplished.

Right Truncal Vagotomy

This is performed as described earlier.

Left Truncal Vagotomy

Once the right truncal vagotomy is performed, the anterior aspect of the esophagus as well as the posterior aspect is entirely denuded so as to accomplish an efficient bilateral vagotomy (Fig. 36-9). This can be done easily by stripping the anterior aspect of the esophagus with the coagulant hook. With an atraumatic grasping forceps the peritoneal layer covering the anterior aspect of the esophagus is gripped and then resected with the curved scissors. Hemostasis is maintained with clips for large vessels. The surgeon should be sure that the anterior aspect of the esophagus is denuded over at least 6 cm. Optical magnification produced by bringing the videoendoscope closer will allow refining of the dissection and the hooking of the different nerve branches sometimes closely related to the muscular layer of the esophagus. The residual branches found sometimes at the level of the angle of Hiss, which used to be called the criminal nerves of Grassi, are carefully removed. Once this nerve denudation on the anterior aspect is accomplished, the posterior aspect is denuded by rolling the esophagus with the help of closed grasping forceps.

Pyloric Dilatation

A balloon dilatator (Microinvasive Rigiflex OTW 5135) is used (Fig. 36-10). The balloon is placed under double guidance with an esophagogastroduodenal endoscope and laparoscope, allowing the dilatation of the pylorus to be seen. Once the pylorus is passed, the balloon is installed, inflated, and maintained in place inflated for 45 seconds. With the videoendoscope the positioning of the balloon and its inflation are controlled, theoretically permitting laceration of the pyloric to obtain an effect similar to pyloroplasty. Nevertheless, in our experience with three patients, we had to repeat this maneuver. Other authors in the literature have reported a similar experience.

RIGHT TRUNCAL VAGOTOMY COMBINED WITH ANTERIOR HIGHLY SELECTIVE VAGOTOMY

This technique was described by our collegues and friends Zucker and Bailey in Balti-

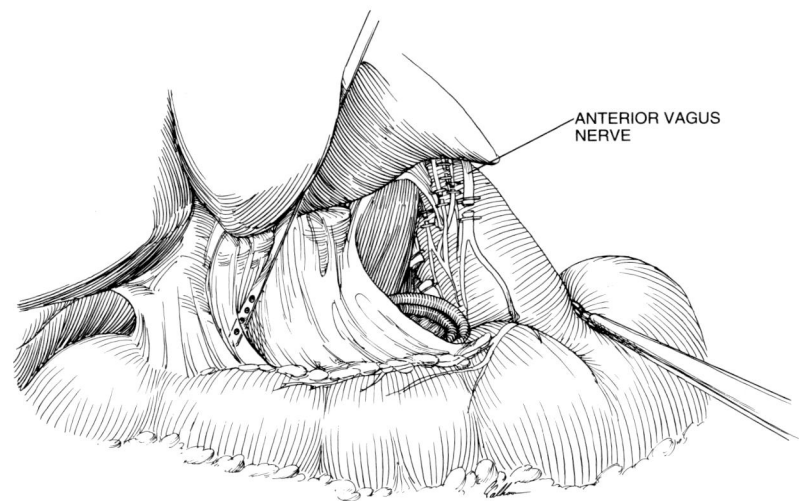

Figure 36-9.

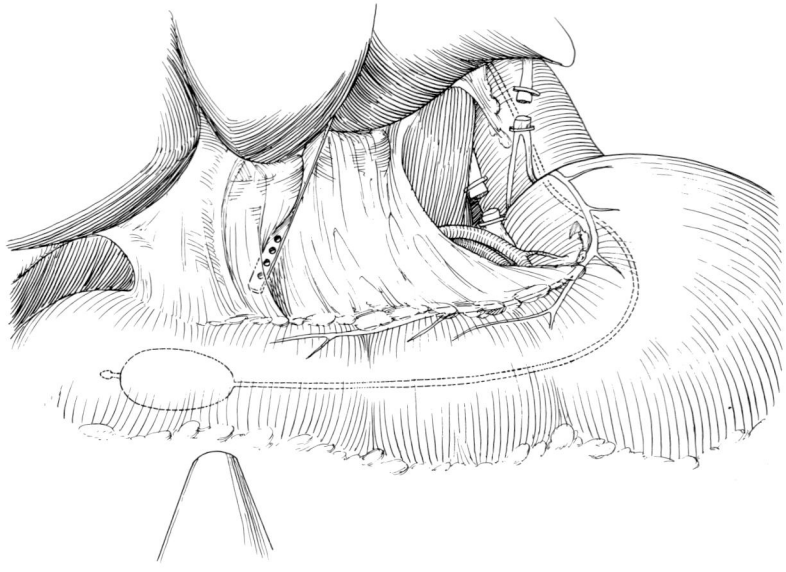

Figure 36-10.

more and consists of combining a right truncal vagotomy described earlier with an anterior highly selective vagotomy (Fig. 36-11). Theoretically, the procedure should preserve the anterior gastric branch of the anterior vagus nerve, denervating the lesser curve and thus accomplishing the first step in the total highly selective vagotomy. This is done step by step while the vessel satellites of the nerve branches are clipped. To obtain good results, the vagus nerve on the anterior aspect of the esophagus is dissected free for the last 3 cm over to the left side of the esophagus and even extending slightly over the posterior aspect of the left side of the esophagus. This technique was described for the first time by Hill and Baker in 1978, who reported on 20 cases; however, multicenter studies in open surgery are needed to confirm these initial good results.

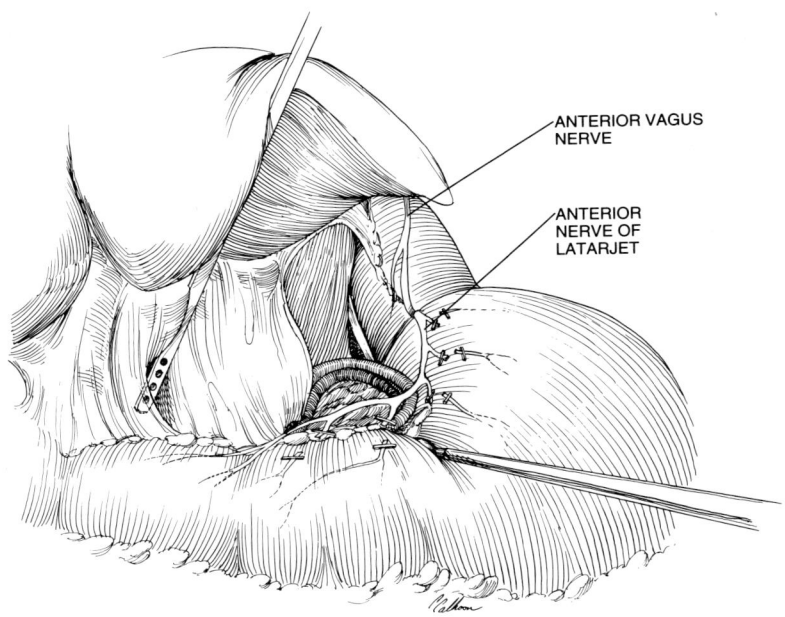

Figure 36-11.

BIBLIOGRAPHY

Bailey RW, Flowers JL, Graham SM, Zucker KA. Surg Laparosc Endosc 1991; 1:45–49.

Bemelman WA, Brummelkamp WH, Bartesman JFWM. Endoscopic balloon dilatation of the pylorus after esophagogastrostomy without a drainage procedure. Surg Gynecol Obstet 1990; 170:424–426.

Daniel EE, Sarna SK. Distribution of excitatory vagal fibres in canine gastric wall to central motility. Gastroenterology 1986; XX:295–420.

Dragstedt LR, Camp EH. Follow-up of gastric vagotomy alone in the treatment of peptic ulcer. Gastroenterology 1948; 11:460–465.

Dubois F, Icard P, Berthelot G, Levard H. Coelioscopic cholecystectomy. Preliminary report of 36 cases. Ann Surg 1990; 211:60–62.

Katkhouda N, Mouiel J. A new surgical technique of treatment of chronic duodenal ulcer without laparotomy by videocoelioscopy. Am J Surg 1991; 161:361–364.

Oost Vogel HJM, Van Vroonhoven TJMV. Anterior seromyotomy and posterior truncal vagotomy. Technic and early results of a randomized trial. Neth J Surg 1985; 37:69–74.

Pringle R, Irving AD, Longrigg JN, Wisbey M. Randomized trial of truncal vagotomy with either pyloroplasty or pyloric dilatation in the superficial management of chronic duodenal ulcer. Br J Surg 1983; 70:482–484.

Taylor TV. Lesser curve superficial seromyotomy. An operation for chronic duodenal ulcer. Br J Surg 1979; 66:733–737.

Taylor TV. Experience with the Lunderquist Ownman dilatator in the upper gastro-intestinal tract. Br J Surg 1983; 70:445.

Taylor TV, Gunn AA, McLeod DAD, et al. Morbidity and mortality after anterior lesser curve seromyotomy and posterior truncal vagotomy for duodenal ulcer. Br J Surg 1985; 72:950–951.

Taylor TV, Lythgoe JP, McFarland JB, et al. Anterior lesser curve seromyotomy and posterior truncal vagotomy versus truncal vagotomy and pyloroplasty in the treatment of chronic duodenal ulcer. Br J Surg 1990; 77:1007–1009.

Chapter 37
Nissen Fundoplication

Bernard Dallemagne

The concept of pathologic gastroesophageal reflux is relatively recent. During the first half of the twentieth century, radiologically documented hiatal hernia was thought to be responsible for symptoms such as retrosternal pain, acid regurgitation, and heartburn. Acid gastric reflux was never mentioned. In 1879, Quinck[1] described pathologic ulceration of the esophagus, but did not relate this phenomenon to reflux of acid gastric contents. It was only in the 1930s when Hamperl[2] and Winkenstein[3] discussed the concept of esophagitis caused by acid gastroesophageal reflux. The first attempt to treat this problem was presented by Allison in 1951:[4] he emphasized the need to place the gastroesophageal junction in its normal intra-abdominal position to restore its proper function. The early results of this procedure stimulated the imaginations of other surgeons (Sweet and Lortat-Jacob, for example).[5,6] It was rapidly observed, however, that simple anatomic reconstruction of the hiatal orifice to reestablish normal positioning of the cardioesophageal junction and its valvular function had a high rate of failure and recurrences of symptoms because of the lack of gastric anchorage.[7] With the exception of Hill's procedure, which anchors the gastroesophageal junction posterior to the median arcuate ligament,[8] the operations were progressively abandoned.

This led to the development of techniques aimed at improving valvular function of the cardioesophageal junction, such as reconstruction of the angle of Hiss, angulation of the junction with the ligamentum teres, and anterior or posterior valvuloplasty (partial, complete) using either abdominal or thoracic approaches.[9-15] Although each of these techniques gave good results in the hands of those who described them (or who performed them frequently), a gradual consensus developed, recognizing the advantages of the techniques described by Belsey and Nissen.[16]

Both of these procedures incorporate a portion of the distal esophagus into the stomach to ensure that it will be affected by changes in intra-abdominal pressure through the intragastric pressure. In 1955 Belsey (Fig. 37-1A) in Bristol and Nissen (Fig. 37-1B) in Basil described the valve repairs which created the basis of treatment of gastroesophageal reflux.[17-19] Their first aim was to treat the reflux and second the hiatal hernia. Nissen's technique initially consisted of the invagination of the esophagus into a sleeve of the gastric wall obtained from the upper portion of the stomach and the great tuberosity. The gastrosplenic vessels and the diaphragmatic hiatus were untouched. Numerous adaptations were subsequently made to the original technique, such as closure of the hiatal orifice, more or less extensive mobilization of the fundus, modifications of the valve, and variations of the length of the valve.[20,21]

The technique presented here is Nissen's,

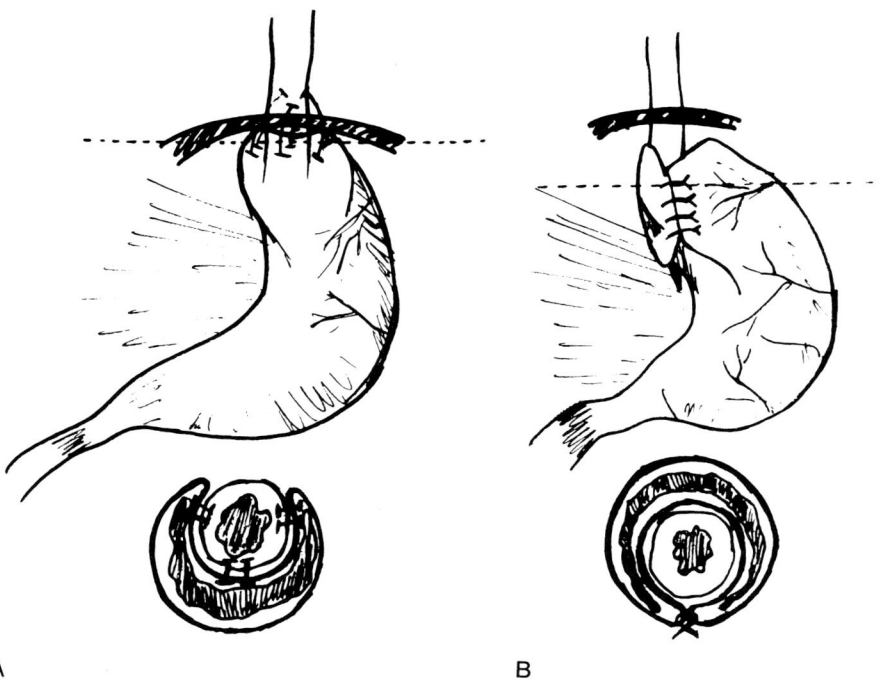

Figure 37-1.

which involves the construction of a 2- to 3-cm long valve after mobilization of the great curvature of the stomach by section of several short gastric vessels. Reduction in the caliber of the hiatus orifice is accomplished with sutures through the two crura muscles.

PATIENT SELECTION

Candidates for Nissen fundoplication suffer from documented pathologic gastroesophageal reflux, with or without hiatal hernia.[22,23] All patients have had at least 6 months of medical/dietetic/postural treatment. Either their symptoms recur when treatment is stopped, or symptoms or esophageal lesions do not resolve despite treatment. In these patients, esophageal function studies are done, including endoscopy and biopsy, barium studies, esophageal manometry, and 24-hour pH monitoring.[24–26] Figure 37-2 shows a patient with hiatal hernia and esophageal reflux.

PATIENT EVALUATION

The indications to proceed with antireflux surgery are: documentation of a mechanically defective lower esophageal sphincter (LES) and increased exposure to gastric juice. Patients with Barrett esophagus are candidates

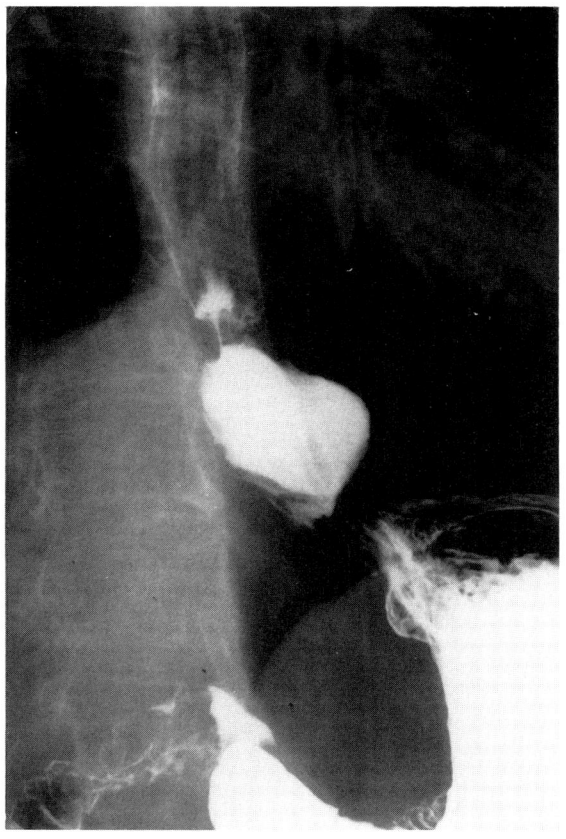

Figure 37-2.

for antireflux surgery. If, on biopsy specimens, severe dysplasia or intramucosal carcinoma is found, an esophageal resection should be done. Patients with a manometrically normal LES must be studied by 24-hour pH monitoring to assess the increased esophageal exposure to gastric juice. This increment can be related to gastric or esophageal causes. If results of the pH monitoring of a patient are normal, despite a defective LES, the possibilities of alkaline, drug-induced, or retention esophagitis must be considered. On the other hand, some patients do have large paraesophageal hiatal hernias or small hiatal hernias with a Schatzki ring. They complain mainly of dysphagia, chest pain, and sometimes of heartburn.[27] The LES is often normal. A surgical repair will relieve the symptoms, but must be associated with an antireflux procedure because of the potential destruction of the competency of the cardioesophageal junction during the reduction of the hernia.

Criteria for acceptability for surgery are the same as for all abdominal surgery. A standard preanesthetic workup is done. The only relative contraindications for surgery relate to previous gastric or hiatal surgery.

EQUIPMENT

Standard instruments are used: dissecting scissors, atraumatic grasping forceps, Babcock forceps, clip applier, needle holder, dissecting forceps, and palpators. A monopolar cautery device is attached to either the hook or the scissors. A wide angle viewing 0-degree laparoscope is used.

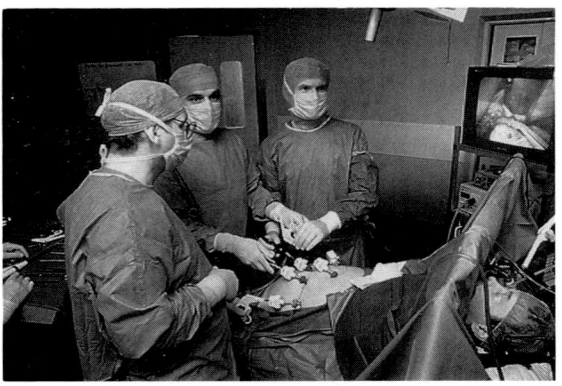

Figure 37-4.

POSITIONING OF THE PATIENT

The operation is performed under general anesthesia with endotracheal intubation; the patient is placed in the lithotomy position (Fig. 37-3). The surgeon stands between the legs of the patient with, at his right, the surgical assistant and on his left, the scrub nurse, or another assistant (Fig. 37-4). The videolaparoscopy column is placed either on the right or the left of the surgeon. At the beginning of the procedure a large bore (36- to 60-French) gastric tube is placed in the proximal esophagus, above the cardioesophageal junction.

PLACEMENT OF TROCARS

Pneumoperitoneum is established in the normal fashion, with the usual precautions. A maximal intraperitoneal pressure of 15 mm Hg is allowed.

The first trocar, 10 mm, is placed in the supraumbilical midline, at the junction of the upper two-thirds and lower one-third between the umbilicus and the xyphoid process. The laparoscope is introduced via this port. Visual inspection of the entire peritoneal cavity is carried out. Under direct vision, four other trocars are inserted: one 10-mm in the midline under the xyphoid process; another 10-mm at the left upper quadrant at the midclavicular line, at a left paraumbilical position; one 5-mm under the right costal margin in the midclavicular line; and another 5-mm, laterally under the left costal margin on the anterior axillary line (Fig. 37-5). The use of

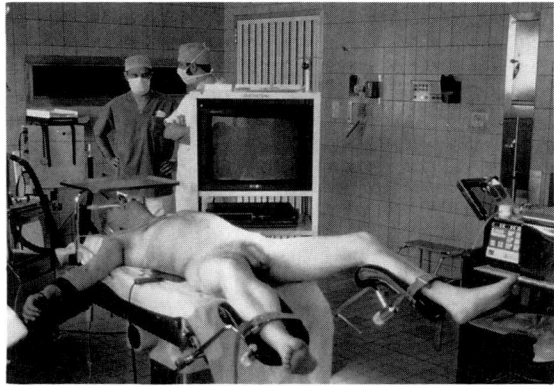

Figure 37-3.

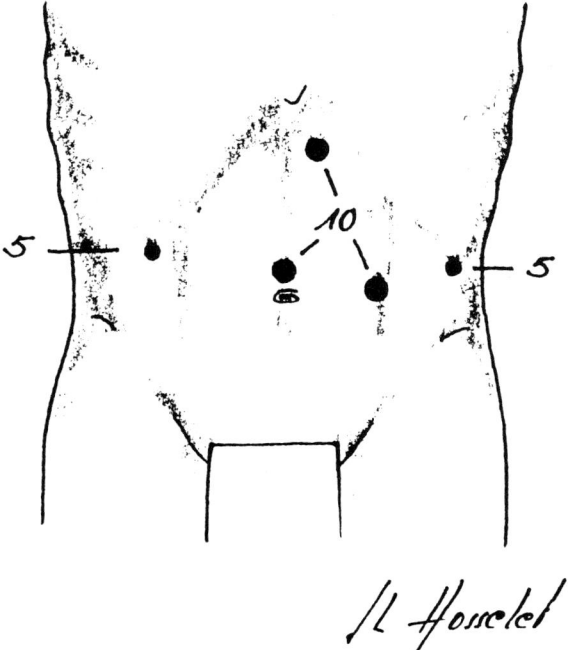

Figure 37-5.

10-mm trocars allows maximal freedom to change position of the laparoscope during the procedure, as well as the use of 10-mm instruments, such as the clip applier and certain needle holders and graspers.

METHODS OF EXPOSURE AND RETRACTION

The operation begins with retraction of the left lobe of the liver using either an atraumatic forceps or a liver retractor introduced through the 5-mm right trocar. This forceps is fixed to the suprahiatal diaphragm and lifts the left lobe allowing access to the hiatus. The remainder of the procedure follows the classical sequence of the operation done via laparotomy.

SPECIFIC DETAILS OF THE PROCEDURE

The phrenoesophageal membrane is divided on the anterior aspect of the hiatal orifice (Fig. 37-6). This incision is extended to the right to allow identification of the right crus. Then, along the inner side of this crus, the right esophageal wall is freed by dissecting the clivage plane. This dissection is carried out with either the coagulating scissors or with the dissecting hook.

The liberation of the posterior aspect of the esophagus is started by extending the dissection the length of the right diaphragmatic crus. The pars flaccida of the lesser omentum is opened, preserving the hepatic branches of the vagus nerve. This allows access to the

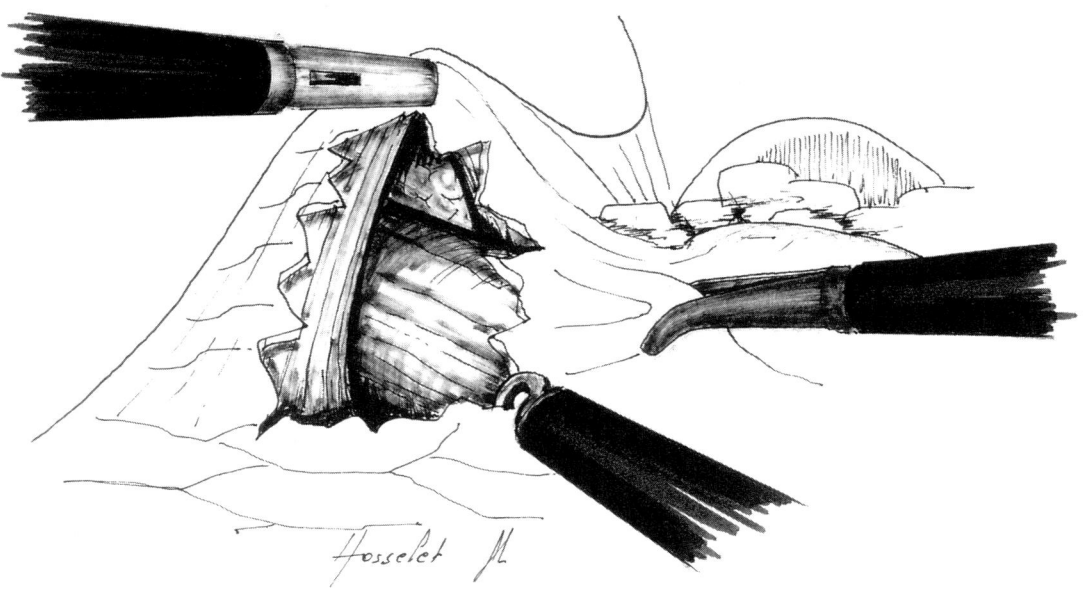

Figure 37-6.

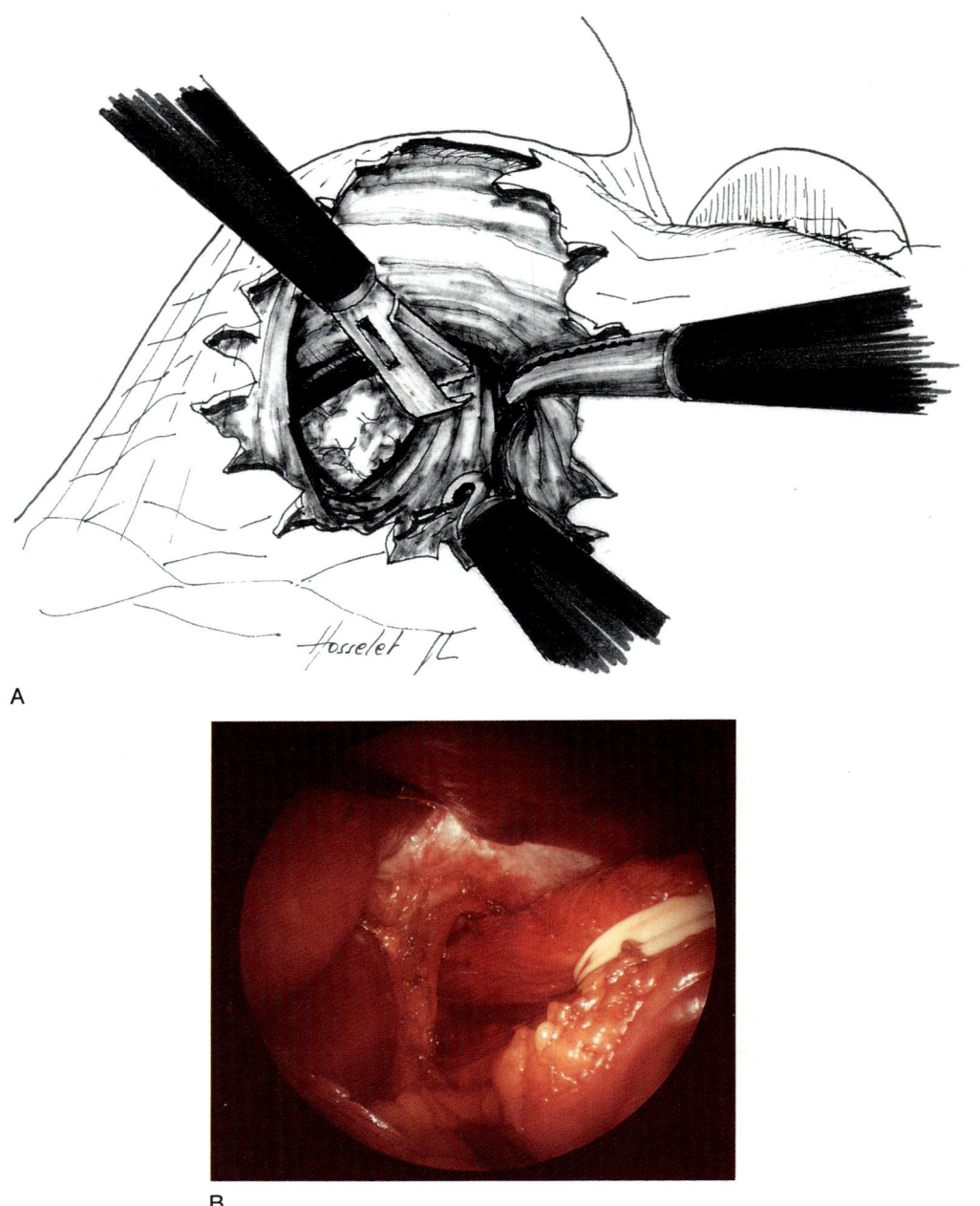

Figure 37-7.

crura, left and right, the right posterior aspect of the esophagus, and the posterior vagus nerve (Fig. 37-7).

Attention is next turned to the left anterolateral aspect of the esophagus. At its left border, the left crus is identified (Fig. 37-8). The dissection plane between it and the left aspect of the esophagus is freed. The gastrophrenic ligament is incised, beginning the mobilization of the gastric pouch. At this point, with the intramediastinal dissection of the esophagus, one obtains an elongation of its intra-abdominal segment and a reduction of the hiatal hernia if it exists.

The next step consists of the mobilization of the gastric pouch. This requires ligation and division of the gastrosplenic ligament and several short gastric vessels; two or three are clipped and divided, as required by the size of the fundus. This dissection starts on the

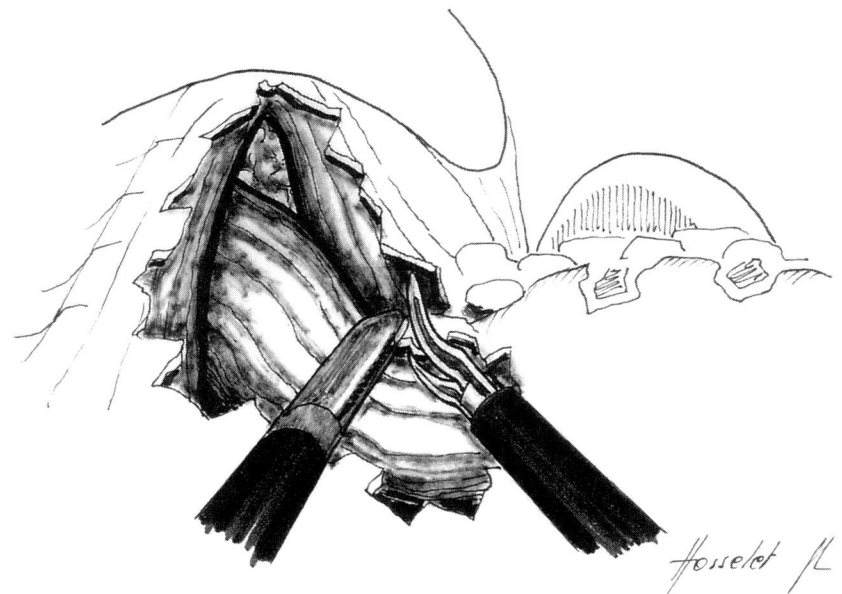

Figure 37-8.

stomach at the point where the vessels of the greater curvature turn toward the spleen, away from the gastroepiploic arcade (Fig. 37-9).

One now turns to the retroesophageal hiatal orifice. The esophagus is lifted by a forceps inserted through the left upper quadrant port. Careful dissection of the mesoesophagus and the left crus reveals a clivage plane between this crus and the posterior gastric wall. Confirmation of having opened the correct plane is obtained by visualizing the fatty tissue of the gastrosplenic ligament or the spleen itself, when looking behind the esophagus. This retroesophageal channel is enlarged to allow easy passage of the antireflux valve (Fig. 37-9B).

The next step involves repair of the hiatal orifice: two or three interrupted sutures, using nonabsorbable material (silk), are placed on the diaphragmatic crura to close the orifice. A distance of approximately 1 cm must be maintained between the highest suture and the esophagus (Fig. 37-10).

The last part of the operation consists of the passage and fixation of the antireflux valve. An atraumatic forceps is passed behind the esophagus, from right to left. It is used to grab the gastric pouch to the left of the esophagus and to pull it behind, forming the wrap (Fig. 37-11). At this point, the gastric tube placed at the beginning of the operation is passed down the cardia. It is used to calibrate the fundoplication. Three to four interrupted stitches form and secure the sleeve. They are passed into the sero-muscular layer of the anterior wall of the gastric pouch to the left of the esophagus, through the seromuscular layer of the anterior esophagus and, finally, to the right of the esophagus, through the seromuscular layer of the stomach which had been passed behind the esophagus. A 2- to 3-cm sleeve is thus constructed (Fig. 37-12). The passage of a forceps through the sleeve assures that the valve does not create a stenosis.

CLOSURE

The large gastric tube is then replaced by a standard nasogastric tube. The peritoneum is rinsed with warm normal saline. No drains are placed. The trocars are removed, and the wounds are stapled closed.

POSTOPERATIVE MANAGEMENT

An intravenous line is left in place until the morning of the first postoperative day at the latest. The nasogastric tube is removed at the same time; the patient is then allowed to eat and drink. On the second postoperative day,

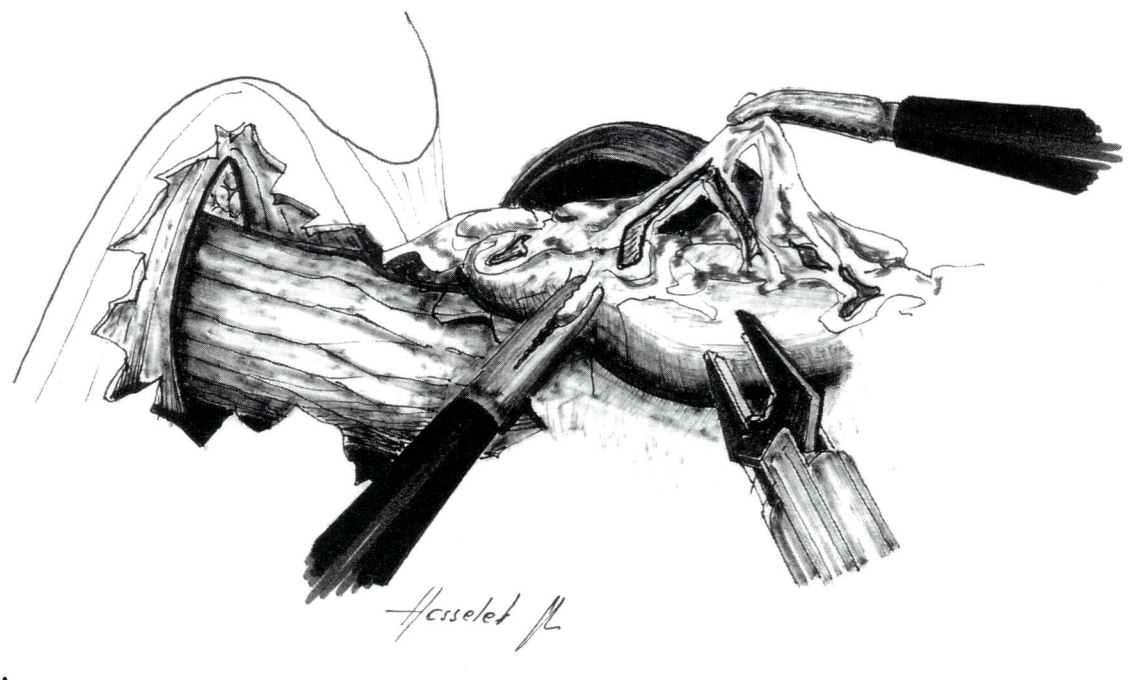

Figure 37-9.

a barium study of the esophagus, stomach, and duodenum is carried out to verify the position and the function of the antireflux valve, as well as to confirm the absence of significant stenosis. Figure 37-13 shows a patient after successful laparoscopic construction of a Nissen fundoplication.

CRITERIA FOR PATIENT DISCHARGE

The patient is discharged after the barium examination. Dietary instructions are given to avoid the risk of impaction at the sleeve in the early postoperative period. The patient is seen after 1 month: a history allows evaluation of the result and assessment of any secondary effects. At the end of 3 months, those patients who agree undergo a full evaluation including endoscopy, esophageal manometry, and pH-monitoring. A new clinical history concerning results is taken.

Conclusions

The operative technique presented is directly inspired by Nissen's original procedure.[28] The

Nissen Fundoplication

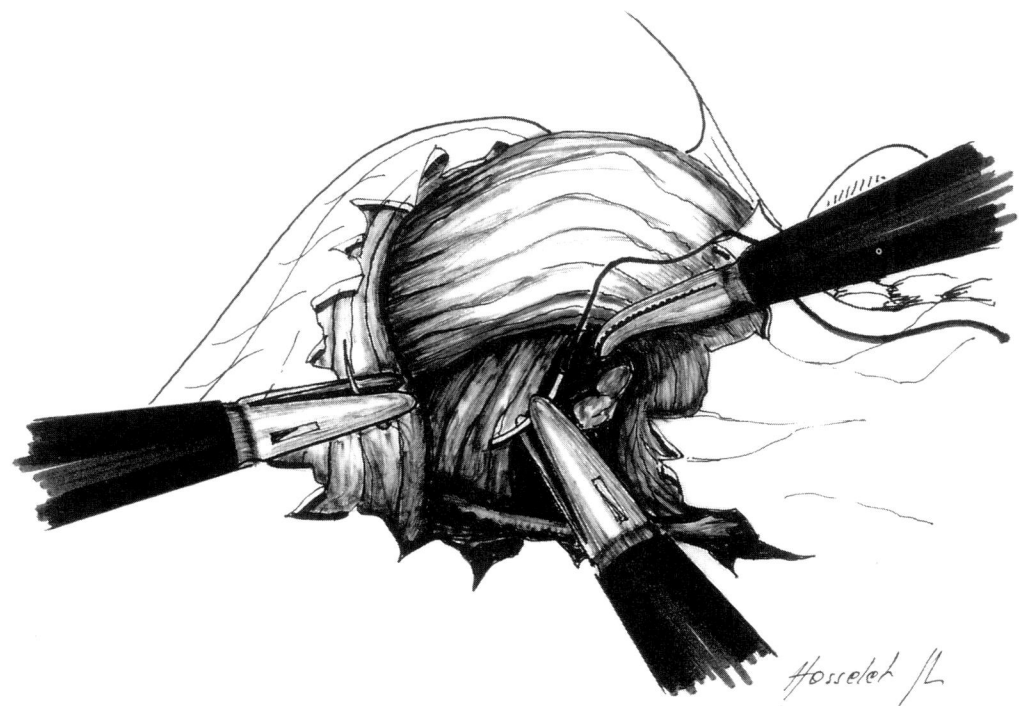

Figure 37-10.

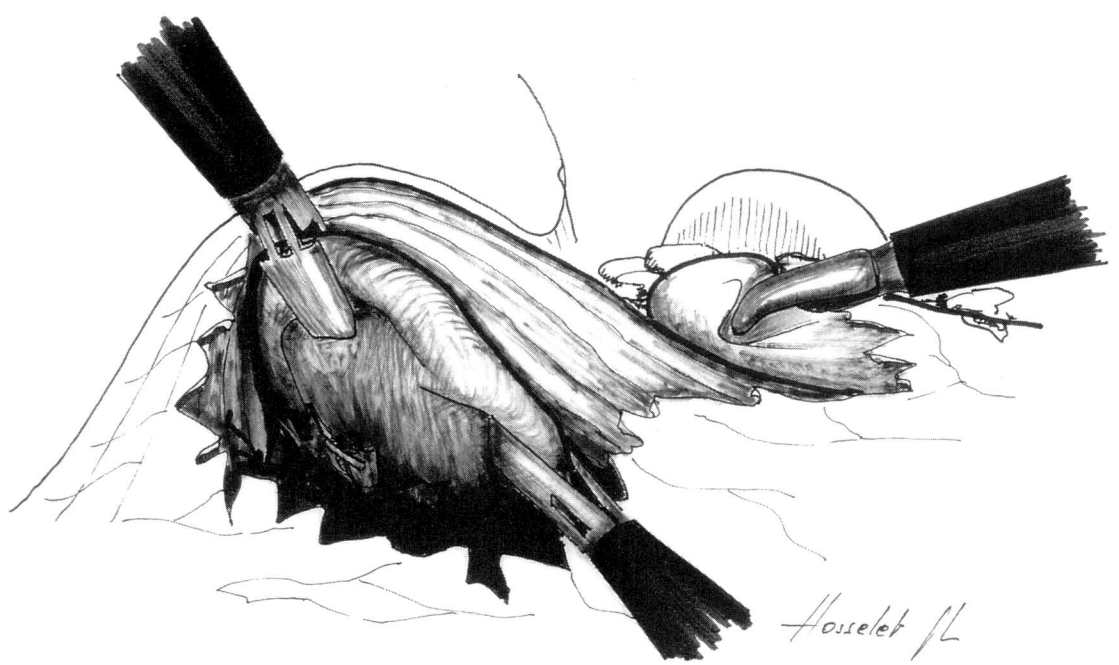

Figure 37-11.

438 Techniques of Laparoscopic Surgery

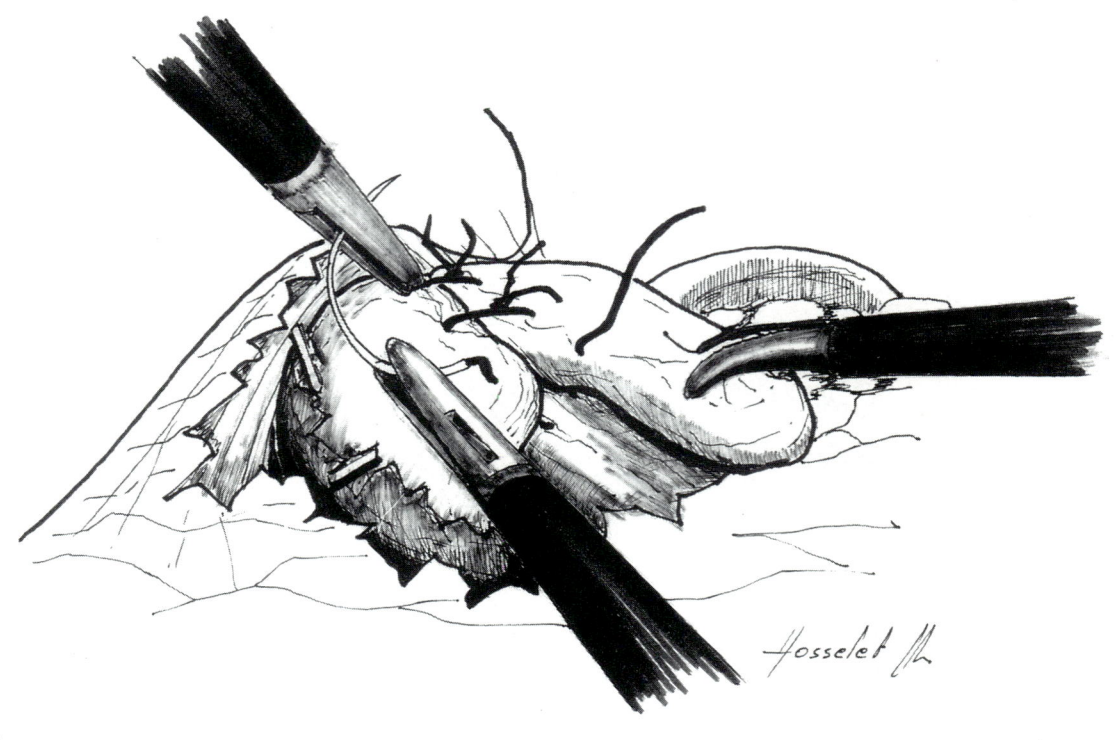

A

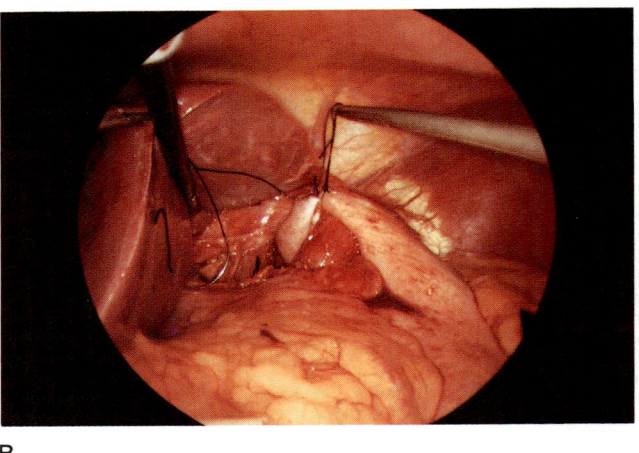

B

Figure 37-12.

same maneuvers used in an open procedure are reproduced with modifications for adaptation to laparoscopy. The results obtained are similar, from both clinical (symptom reduction) as well as objective (manometry, endoscopy, radiology, and pH-monitoring) standpoints, to those of the classical procedure. Postoperative recovery is easier after the laparoscopic approach just as with cholecystectomy.[29]

The initial long term evaluations suggest a clear reduction in the classically described secondary effects of this operation, i.e., the gas bloat syndrome and dysphagia. Problems related to scar pain and to the abdominal wall, which handicap a certain number of patients, after the open procedure are eliminated. The significant reduction in hospital stay and the early return to professional or domestic life are the classical advantages of laparoscopic surgery.[28–31]

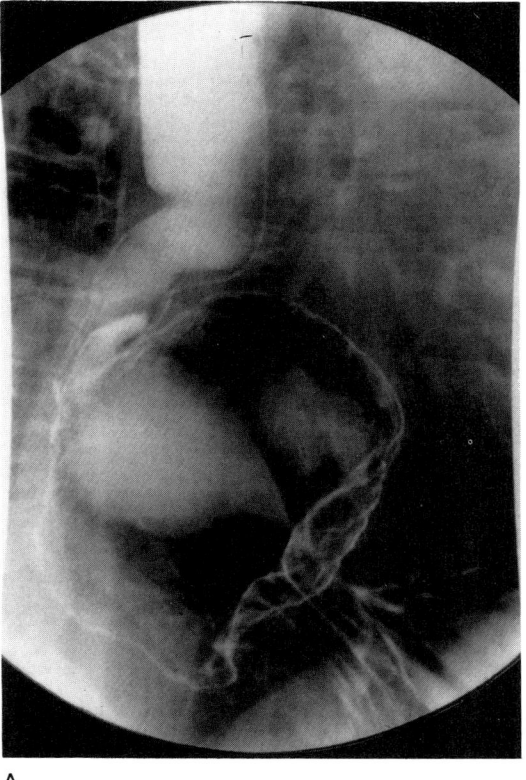 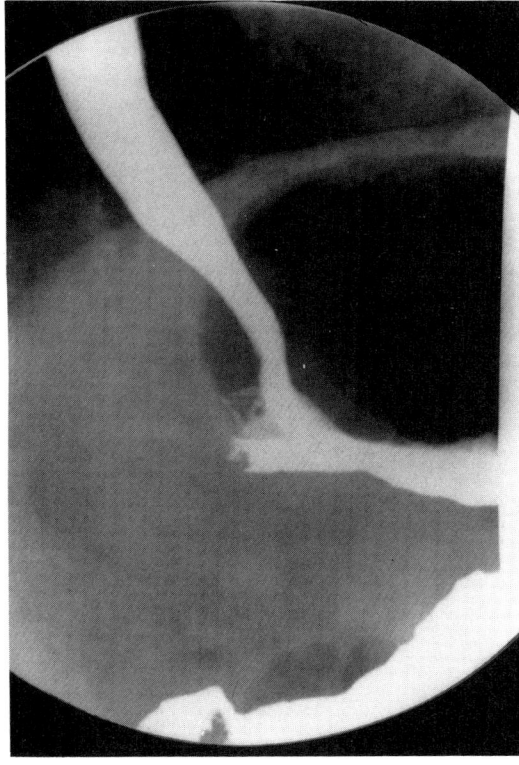

A B

Figure 37-13.

REFERENCES

1. Quincke H. Ulcus Oesophagi ex digestione. Dtsch Arch Clin Med 1879; 24:72.
2. Hamperl H. Peptische esophagitis. Verh Dtsch Pathol 1934; 27:208–215.
3. Winkelstein A. Peptic esophagitis: A new clinical entity. JAMA 1935; 104:906.
4. Allison PR. Reflux oesophagitis, sliding hiatus hernia and the anatomy of repair. Surg Gynecol Obstet 1951; 92:419–431.
5. Sweet RH. Esophageal hiatus of the diaphragm. Ann Surg 1952; 135:1–13.
6. Lortat-Jacob JL, Robert F. Les malpositions cardio-tuberositaires. Arch Mala Appar Dig 1953; 42:750–774.
7. Boerema I, Germs R. Fixation of the lesser curve of the stomach to the anterior wall of the abdomen after reposition of the hernia through the oesophageal hiatus. Arch Chir Neerl 1955; 7:351–359.
8. Hill LD. An effective operation for hiatal hernia: An eight year appraisal. Ann Surg 1967; 166:681–692.
9. Toupet A. Technique d'oesophago-gastroplastie avec phrenogastropexie appliquee dans la cure radicale des hernies hiatales et comme complement de l'operation de Heller dans les cardiospasmes. Mem Acad Chir 1963; 89:394–397.
10. Narbona-Arnau B, Molina E, Ancho-Fornos S, et al. Hernia diaphragmatica hiatal. Pexia cardio-gastrica con el ligamento redondo. Med Esp 1965; 2:25.
11. Thal AP, Hatafuku T, Kurtzman A. A new method for reconstruction of the esophagogastric junction. Surg Gynecol Obstet 1965; 120:1225–1231.
12. Pearson FG, Cooper JD, Patterson GA, et al. Gastroplasty and fundoplication for complex reflux problems. Ann Surg 1987; 206:473–481.
13. Watson A, Jenkinson LR, Ball CS, et al. A more physiological alternative to total fundoplication for the surgical correction of resistant gastro-oesophageal reflux. Br J Surg 1991; 78:1088–1094.
14. Woodward ER, Thomas HF, McAlhany JC. Comparison of crural repair and Nissen fundoplication in the treatment of gastroesophageal reflux. Ann Surg 1971; 173:782–792.
15. Thor KB, Silander T. A long term randomized prospective trial of the Nissen procedure versus a modified Toupet technique. Ann Surg 1989; 210:719–724.
16. DeMeester TR, Johnson LF, Kent AH. Evaluation of current operations for the prevention of gastroesophageal reflux. Ann Surg 1974; 180:511–522.
17. Belsey R. Surgical treatment of hiatus hernia and reflux esophagitis. World J Surg 1977; 1:421–423.
18. Belsey R. Mark IV repair of hiatal hernia by the transthoracic approach. World J Surg 1977; 1:475–483.
19. Nissen R. Eine einfache operation zur beeinflussung der refluxoesophagitis. Schweiz Med Wochenschr 1956; 86:590–592.
20. Rossetti M, Hell K. Fundoplication for the treatment of gastroesophageal reflux in hiatal hernia. World J Surg 1977; 1:439–444.
21. DeMeester TR, Bonavina L, Albertucci M. Nissen

fundoplication for gastroesophageal reflux disease. Evaluation of primary repair in 100 consecutive patients. Ann Surg 1986; 204:9-20.
22. Klinkenberg-Knol E, Castell DO. Clinical spectrum and diagnosis of gastroesophageal reflux disease. *In* Castell DO, ed. The Esophagus. Boston, Little, Brown and Co, 1992, pp 441-448.
23. Skinner BD: Pathophysiology of gastroesophageal reflux. Ann Surg 1985; 206:546-556.
24. DeMeester TR, Wang CI, Wernly JA, et al. Technique, indications and clinical use of a 24-hour esophageal monitoring. J Thorac Cardiovasc Surg 1980; 79:656-670.
25. Stein HJ, DeMeester TR, Naspetti R, et al. Three dimensional imaging of the lower esophageal sphincter in gastroesophageal reflux disease. Ann Surg 1991; 214:374-384.
26. DeMeester TR, Stein HJ. Surgical treatment of gastroesophageal reflux disease. *In* Castell DO, ed. The Esophagus. Boston, Little, Brown and Co, 1992, pp 579-625.
27. Kaul BK, DeMeester TR, Oka M. The cause of dysphagia in uncomplicated sliding hiatal hernia and its relief by hiatal herniorrhaphy. A roentgenographic, manometric and clinical study. Ann Surg 1990; 211:410-415.
28. Dallemagne B, Weerts JM, Jehaes C, et al. Laparoscopic Nissen fundoplication. Preliminary report. Surg Laparosc Surg 1991; 1:138-143.
29. Dallemagne B, Weerts JM, Jehaes C, et al. Cholecystectomie sous coelioscopie: Analyse de 368 interventions. Acta Gastro-Enterol Belg 1992; 55:4-10.
30. Dallemagne B, Weerts JM, Jehaes C, et al. Case report: Subtotal esophagectomy by thoracoscopy and laparoscopy. Minimally Invas Ther 1992; 1:183-185.
31. Dallemagne B, Weerts JM, Jehaes C, et al. Douleurs abdominales: Coelioscopie et chirurgie percoelioscopique. Rev Med Liege 1990; 45:152-156.

Chapter 38
Gastric Resection

Dennis L. Fowler

With the availability of laparoscopically deployed linear stapling devices, even more difficult laparoscopic gastrointestinal tract surgical procedures can now be contemplated. A few gastric resections have been performed,[1,2] using the videolaparoscope for visualization. Certainly laparoscopic suturing techniques can be used for surgery on the stomach, but the amount of suturing required for a hemigastrectomy would prevent all but the most persistent and skilled laparoscopic surgeon from completing both resection and anastomosis using sutures. Even with the linear stapler, the task is lengthy, but a few surgeons have now reported completing a partial gastric resection using a minimally invasive technique with the laparoscope.

The least technically demanding resection might be the excision of a benign lesion from the anterior wall of the stomach with immediate closure of the gastrotomy. Excision of a benign submucosal lipoma has been reported.[3] Antrectomy, with or without truncal vagotomy, is more difficult, but technique and instruments are available. Total gastrectomy has not been reported. Although it would certainly seem feasible and almost certainly will be performed laparoscopically in the future, improvements in technique, improved or newer instruments, and more experienced laparoscopic surgeons will all contribute to making it a more commonly performed procedure.

GENERAL TECHNICAL CONSIDERATIONS FOR LAPAROSCOPIC GASTRIC RESECTION

The patient is initially placed in the supine position, although during the procedure, particularly when the surgeon is working around the gastroesophageal junction, the Trendelenberg position may be helpful. A nasogastric tube and a Foley catheter are routinely placed before pneumoperitoneum is established. Video monitors are placed on either side of the head of the patient. For most of the time during the majority of procedures, the surgeon will stand on the patient's left side.

Four incisions for laparoscopic ports are usually sufficient and can be placed according to the location of the pathologic condition. The scope is usually inserted through an incision in the umbilicus. A 12-mm port is usually placed in each hypochondrium near the midclavicular line, and a fourth port is placed in the upper midline. By placing the 12-mm ports on each side, the stapler can be introduced from either side, and the best angle for stapling can be used.

Postoperatively, the nasogastric tube is left in the stomach overnight, but it can usually be removed the following morning. Patients can begin taking oral alimentation on the first postoperative day and often can be dismissed from the hospital on the third postoperative day. Although no series is available to document long term results, it is reasonable to follow these patients for many of the same potential complications that occur after open antrectomy. Anastomotic leak, duodenal stump leak, and recurrence of disease (e.g., ulcer or benign tumor) are all complications that could occur after laparoscopic gastrectomy. Additionally, there is no reason to think that there would be any lower incidence of dumping or alkaline reflux in these patients when compared with patients undergoing open resection.

LOCAL EXCISION OF BENIGN GASTRIC LESION

Although the easiest lesions to remove are located on the anterior wall, posterior lesions can also be approached through the lesser sac. If the lesion cannot be readily seen on the serosal surface, a gastroscope (flexible) can be passed into the stomach and the lesion can be localized by transilluminating the gastric wall with the light of the gastroscope. It may be helpful to use carbon dioxide for insufflation of the stomach, so that any of the gas that moves down into the small intestine during gastroscopy will be absorbed in a few minutes to avoid significant distention of the small bowel and stomach after the gastroscopy.

Once the lesion has been localized, it can be excised with scissors, electrocautery, laser, harmonic scalpel, or a combination of these. The full thickness of the gastric wall can be incised to circumferentially excise the lesion. The remaining gastrotomy can be closed with laparoscopic suturing techniques if necessary, but it can be closed more quickly with a linear stapler, such as the ENDO TA 30* or ENDO TA 60* (United States Surgical, Norwalk, CT). Depending on the size of the lesion, one of the incisions may need to be extended to allow for easy removal of the specimen from the abdominal cavity.

LAPAROSCOPIC ANTRECTOMY

Laparoscopic antrectomy or distal hemigastrectomy can be performed through the same four ports as previously described. It may or may not be combined with a truncal vagotomy according to the disease being treated. If a vagotomy is performed, an additional port may be necessary to accommodate an instrument to retract the liver.

Although laparoscopic gastrectomy for malignant disease seems technically possible, it is premature to address the issue at this time. Feasibility studies and long term outcome studies will be needed before cancer of the stomach can be routinely approached with the laparoscope. However, antrectomy for essentially any benign disease could conceivably be approached laparoscopically.

Antrectomy is started by making a window through the gastrocolic omentum to enter the lesser sac. Once this is done near the proximal line of resection on the greater curvature of the stomach, the small branch arteries from the left and then right gastroepiploic arteries can be exposed, clipped, and then divided. Alternatively the greater omentum can be divided parallel to the greater curvature with the linear stapler (ENDO GIA*, United States Surgical). The stomach can be divided at the proximal line of resection by the linear stapler as well. Once the stomach is divided and stapled here, the gastric vessels on the lesser curvature can be divided. Although the modalities used in open surgery for control of vessels can be utilized in laparoscopic surgery (ligatures and clips), the quickest and most secure way to divide these vessels is with the linear stapler.

At this point the greater and lesser curvatures can be cleaned down onto the duodenum, and the posterior wall of the duodenal bulb can be separated from the pancreas. Usually this can be done with blunt and sharp dissection. The duodenum can then be divided with the linear stapler. Depending on the nature of the disease, the specimen can be placed in a bag and cut into smaller pieces, or it can be brought out through a minilaparotomy incision.

An antecolic gastrojejunostomy is made with the linear stapler to create a Billroth II anastomosis. A small gastrotomy is made in the gastric remnant using cautery. This gastrotomy is placed through the anterior wall of the stomach near the greater curvature, just proximal to the staple line. Likewise, a small enterotomy is made through the antimesenteric border of the jejunum with cautery. Once these two holes have been made, the linear stapler is again introduced into the abdomen. The anvil of the stapler is placed through the enterotomy into the jejunum, and the cartridge containing the staples is placed through the gastrotomy into the stomach. The stapler is closed and fired, creating the anastomosis. The remaining defect can then be closed with the linear stapler that does not cut (ENDO TA*).

REFERENCES

1. Goh P. Laparoscopic antrectomy. Video Presentation at the meeting of the Society of American Gastrointestinal Endoscopic Surgeons meeting, Washington, DC, April 1992.
2. Fowler DL, White SA. Laparoscopic vagotomy and antrectomy. Oral Presentation at Minimal Access Surgery Symposium, Saskatoon, Saskatchewan, August 1992.
3. Fowler DL, White SA. Laparoscopic resection of a submucosal gastric lipoma: A case report. J Laparoendosc Surg 1991; 1:303–306.

Chapter 39
Antrectomy with Billroth II Anastomosis

Joseph F. Uddo, Jr.

As with other new advanced laparoscopic procedures, the laparoscopic approach to gastric surgery is evolving. Limited experience is available at this time. However, it seems that the stomach can be safely approached with current laparoscopic technology, tools, and techniques. In this chapter, laparoscopic antrectomy with Billroth II anastomosis will be discussed. The technique for this procedure will be detailed.

PATIENT SELECTION

The indications for laparoscopic gastric surgery have not been fully defined yet. The laparoscopic approach can be used for benign disease of the stomach. Gastric lipomas, leiomyomas, polyps, and angiodysplasia seem to be acceptable applications for laparoscopic gastric surgery.

The laparoscopic approach to gastric cancer requires continued investigation.

PREOPERATIVE EVALUATION

The preoperative evaluation for the laparoscopic approach to gastric surgery should be the same as that for open resection. Routine preoperative testing is performed. The patient's build and previous abdominal surgery should be assessed while the procedure is planned. The gastric lesion may require intraoperative identification. This can be expedited with intraoperative gastroscopy.

PREOPERATIVE PREPARATION

The patient is admitted on the morning of surgery. Preoperative antibiotics are administered. Deep venous thrombosis prophylaxis is used. General anesthesia is required. A nasal gastric tube and Foley catheter are placed when the patient is asleep.

EQUIPMENT

The following equipment is used during laparoscopic antrectomy with Billroth II anastomosis:

1. Laparoscopes: 10-mm 0-degree laparoscopes are used. A 10-mm 30-degree laparoscope and a 5-mm laparoscope should be available.
2. Video equipment: Two full camera sys-

tems with individual lights sources and two monitors are used.

3. Insufflation device: A rapid insufflation device with a smoke evacuator is preferred.
4. Electrocautery: A monopolar electrocautery device with an assortment of wands is needed.
5. Instruments
   A. Four noncrushing bowel graspers
   B. Probes and retractors
   C. Endoscopic clip applier (large)
   D. Endoscopic loop ties
   E. Endoscopic needle holder, knot pusher, and suture material
   F. Curved endoscopic scissors capable of conducting electrocautery
   G. An assortment of endoscopic dissectors capable of conducting electrocautery.
6. Endoscopic stapling devices
   A. ENDO GIA 60* and ENDO GIA 30*
   B. ENDO TA 60*

POSITIONING OF THE PATIENT

The patient is placed supine on the operating room table with both arms secured at the patient's side. Use of an electric table facilitates positioning of the patient and bowel retraction.

POSITIONING OF THE VIDEO EQUIPMENT

Two monitors are used. One is placed on either side of the head of the patient. Care should be taken not to place instrumentation in a way that would impede movement around the operating room table.

TROCAR PLACEMENT AND SIZES

Laparoscopic gastric surgery is similar to laparoscopic cholecystectomy in that the operative site is relatively fixed. The exact placement of laparoscopic trocars for this procedure is in evolution; however, it has been most useful to place a 10-mm port through the umbilicus for the laparoscope (Fig. 39-1). Two additional ports are placed in the right upper quadrant and two in the left upper quadrant. A lower midline 15-mm port has been used for introduction of the endoscopic 60-mm stapling device. This lower

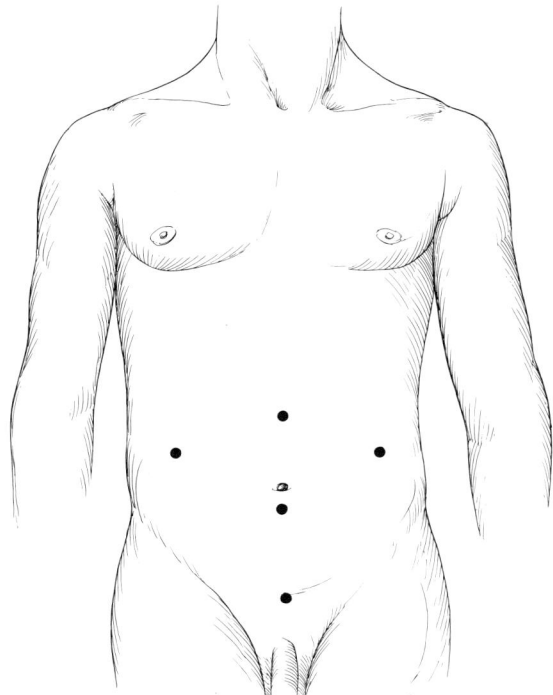

Figure 39-1.

midline placement allows adequate maneuverability of the 60-mm device. Use of closer ports hinders proper positioning of the stapler.

SPECIFIC DETAILS OF THE PROCEDURE

The abdomen is insufflated using an open or a closed technique. A 10-mm trocar is then placed through the umbilicus. Additional ports are placed as described.

After the abdomen is thoroughly explored laparoscopically, the stomach is grasped and held cephalad while the colon is retracted caudally. The gastrocolic ligament is then taken down and the lesser sac is entered. The vessels in the gastrocolic ligament are clipped proximally and distally and divided. Alternatively, this structure can be divided using an endoscopic stapling device. The lesser omentum is then taken down. This can be accomplished, for the most part, with electrocautery. The stomach and duodenum are transilluminated using an intraoperatively placed gastroscope to be certain that the pylorus (Fig. 39-2) is included in the distal extent of resection and that the lesion is clearly

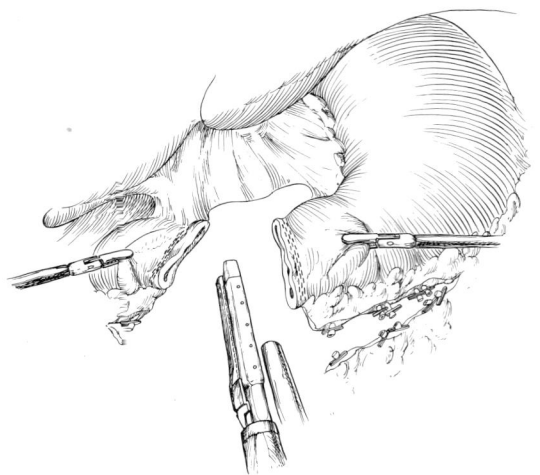

Figure 39-2.

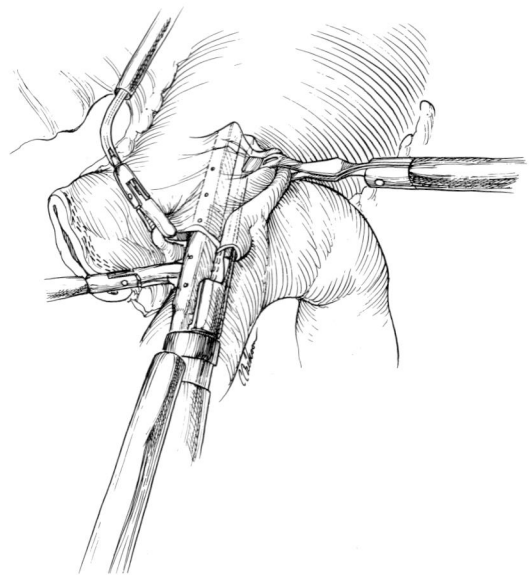

Figure 39-3.

identified. These points are marked with endoscopic clips. The duodenum is mobilized distally. An endoscopic 60-mm stapling device is used to divide the duodenum just distal to the pylorus. One application of this instrument is adequate to completely divide the duodenum. The proximal line of transection is then identified. A 60-mm stapling device is used to transect the stomach. Two applications of this device may be required; however, one application of the 60-mm device followed by a 30-mm device to complete transection may be adequate. At this point, all attachments to the specimen have been divided. The specimen is then placed in the right upper quadrant to be retrieved after completion of the anastomosis.

The ligament of Treitz is identified, and a loop of small bowel is brought into approximation with the gastric remnant in an anticolic fashion. The two limbs to be anastomosed can be kept in secure approximation using an endoscopic atraumatic Babcock clamp (Fig. 39-3). A gastrotomy is fashioned in the stomach and enterotomy in the small bowel. The 60-mm stapling device is introduced through the lower midline incision. The forks of the device are placed through the previously fashioned openings and, once proper positioning of the device is confirmed, the instrument is closed and then fired. The anastomosis can be easily inspected with the laparoscope. The remaining enterotomy is closed using an ENDO TA* stapling device, introduced through the lower midline 15-mm port (Fig. 39-4). Care should be taken to identify the full extent of the enterotomy to be certain it is fully and securely closed.

The specimen is then removed through the lower midline port site. Minimal extension of the excision may be required. Choosing the lower midline port site for extraction of the specimen yields better cosmesis as well as less postoperative pain.

CLOSURE

All fascial incisions for ports 10-mm or greater are closed with interrupted absorbable

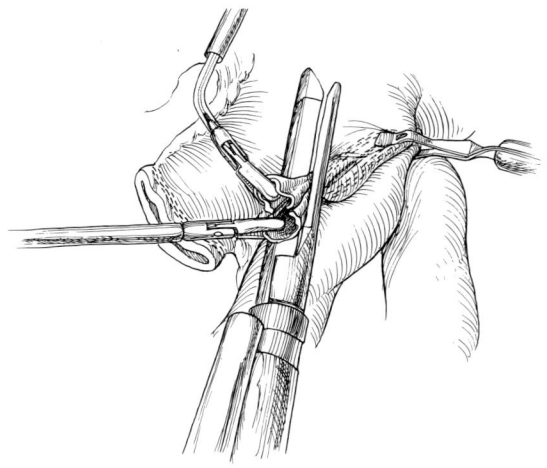

Figure 39-4.

sutures. Skin incisions are closed with staples or subcutaneous stitches.

POSTOPERATIVE MANAGEMENT

The Foley catheter is removed in the recovery room. The nasogastric tube is left in place until the first signs of recovery of bowel function. Liquids are started shortly after the nasogastric tube is removed (48 to 72 hours). Clear liquids continue until the patient has a strong desire to advance to a solid diet. Ambulation is encouraged on the first postoperative day. Minimal postoperative pain control is required. Discharge takes place within 3 to 5 days. The patient returns to unrestricted activity shortly after discharge.

Conclusion

Laparoscopic gastric surgery can be performed safely. There appears to be a significant decrease in postoperative pain and disability. There is little information available regarding the use of the laparoscopic approach at this time.

Chapter 40
Cholecystectomy

Eddie Joe Reddick

Minimally invasive surgery is quickly replacing laparotomy as the treatment for numerous surgical diseases. It has been projected that over 90 per cent of all general surgical operations will be performed by minimally invasive techniques by the turn of the century. The key that opened the door to this explosion was laparoscopic cholecystectomy.

Developed in the United States in 1988, laparoscopic cholecystectomy filled two needs for general surgeons: it allowed them to apply technology to their surgical practice and it allowed them to reestablish control over a speciality that was becoming fragmented. Many other specialities, including orthopedics, urology, radiology, gynecology, and gastroenterology, had benefited greatly from the technologic advances of the space program and computer revolution of the 1970s and 1980s. Minimally invasive techniques such as arthroscopy, extracorporeal shock wave lithotripsy (ESWL), computerized scanning, pelviscopy, and fiberoptic endoscopy had firmly established a market share for these specialities.

General surgeons, on the other hand, had seen their speciality splinter over the previous few years. Subspecialities in thoracic, vascular, pediatric, and colon and rectal surgery had nibbled away at the once vast expanse of general surgery. With the patient-driven emphasis on noninvasive techniques, general surgeons were beginning to see their "bread and butter operation," cholecystectomy, being challenged by the radiologists and gastroenterologists. Although the techniques were far from perfect, ESWL, chemical dissolution, and percutaneous removal of stones were being evaluated seriously as a replacement for cholecystectomy.

The problem with these noninvasive techniques was that they left the diseased gallbladder behind, making recurrence of gallstones likely. They also could not be used for most patients with gallstone disease. The obvious answer was to design an operation that had all the benefits of a standard cholecystectomy with few or none of the side effects.

Standard cholecystectomy was performed through a large abdominal incision. Despite the surgical manipulations performed internally, the offending trauma seemed to be the abdominal incision. Since the rectus muscle was transected, the incision caused extreme pain when the patient walked, talked, or even breathed, necessitating prolonged hospitalization for pain control. Making the incision smaller with a minilaparotomy incision helped some, but most patients still felt considerable pain.

The large incision also took time to heal. The fear of secondary herniation forced most surgeons and employers to require the patient to refrain from all but light activity for 6 weeks. Laparoscopy overcame these problems. The gallbladder was completely removed, giving the same long term cure as with standard cholecystectomy. Only the incision was changed. The four small puncture wounds caused minimal muscle trauma, and therefore, minimal pain. The lack of pain allowed patients to leave the hospital quickly. Because the incisions were small, the chance of herniation was decreased; therefore, patients could return to full activities at will.

Despite its obvious advantages, it was not welcomed with open arms by general surgical specialists. The first case report appeared in *Current Laser Monthly* in October 1988, documenting the initial laparoscopic cholecystectomy performed by Eddie Joe Reddick, M.D., earlier the same year. A compilation article appeared in February 1990, reporting the first four procedures performed by Dr. Reddick in Nashville, TN, and the first two performed by William Saye, M.D., and his group in Marietta, GA.[1,2,3,4]

These reports were met with skepticism by most general surgeons. However, when the first 16 cases were presented at the annual meeting of the American Society for Lasers in Medicine and Surgery in April 1989, there was standing room only and the new procedure gained a foothold among a small cadre of general surgeons. After Dr. Reddick presented a representative videotape of the first 100 cases at the 1989 annual meeting of the American College of Surgeons in Atlanta, GA, thousands of surgeons began searching for courses and preceptorships to learn this new technology.

Print and television media quickly recognized the value of laparoscopic surgery and gave heavy coverage. This, in turn, stimulated more patient interest. The few surgeons who had learned the technique early saw their practices explode, while those who were unable to get into courses, saw a quick decline in the number of cholecystectomies being performed in their practices. This economic crunch made surgeons even more frantic to get into courses and master laparoscopic cholecystectomy.

This "rush to the laparoscope," as ABC's *World News Tonight* dubbed it, led to incomplete training of some surgeons. It was recommended by most teachers that surgeons take a course, then attend a preceptorship or be proctored on a number of cases prior to performing the operation alone. Many surgeons performed the operation prior to completion of the suggested training. This led to many major complications during the steep learning curve. Many injuries occurred during the ensuing year with most occurring during the first 10 procedures performed by any given surgeon. As surgeons progressed past the learning curve, injuries became rare and laparoscopic cholecystectomy evolved into an extremely safe operation when performed correctly by properly trained surgeons.

To be historically correct, credit must be given to the French surgeons for performing laparoscopic cholecystectomy first. Phillipe Mouret did the first one in Lyon in late 1987. The initial international publication by the French was in the *Annals of Surgery* in January 1990 by Professor Francois Dubois of Paris.[2] The trocar positions and gallbladder retraction techniques differ significantly from the Reddick procedure, and, except for an occasional surgeon, the French technique is used infrequently outside of France.

PATIENT SELECTION

Although initially reserved for only the easiest procedures, laparoscopic cholecystectomy is now routinely performed on patients with obesity, previous surgery, common bile duct stones. and even acute cholecystitis.

PREOPERATIVE EVALUATION

Gallbladder disease should be diagnosed with a careful history documenting right upper quadrant pain, dyspepsia, gas/bloat syndrome, or fatty food intolerance. The diagnosis can be confirmed with radiographic contrast studies, radioisotope scans, or ultrasound, with ultrasound being the most common and least invasive. In the patient with gallbladder symptoms, but otherwise normal findings, in whom diagnosis is difficult, biliary drainage and ERCP may be used to support the clinical impression. Occasionally, a patient will have significant symptoms with totally normal findings, and the decision to operate becomes less clear. It has been the author's experience that the majority, but not all, of these patients fare better after their gallbladders have been removed.

With the growing popularity of laparoscopic surgery, some patients have been scheduled for surgery without a complete preoperative evaluation. Care should be taken to give the patient a thorough examination to rule out concurrent intestinal cancer, ulcer disease, or myocardial infarction. It is difficult to examine the large intestine laparoscopically; therefore, a rectal examination and an examination for occult blood should be performed prior to surgery. The stomach should be evaluated endoscopically preoperatively if any ulcer disease is suspected. Careful history can rule out myocardial disease.

PREOPERATIVE PREPARATION

The patient receives perioperative antibiotics. A 1.5-mg scopolamine patch is applied on the patient prior to surgery. This keeps postoperative nausea to a minimum after surgery. No other special preparation is required.

POSITIONING OF THE PATIENT

The patient is placed in a supine position under general anesthesia. Local and epidural anesthesia has been used sparingly and is not the anesthesia of choice. The abdomen is prepared and draped in a standard manner. The patient is dropped into the Trendelenburg position during establishment of the pneumoperitoneum. During the procedure the foot of the operating table is dropped down into a reverse Trendelenberg position. The right shoulder of the patient is rolled up. This allows the weight of the colon and omentum to retract tissue away from the porta hepatis area.

TROCAR PLACEMENT AND SIZE SELECTION

An insufflation needle is inserted into the umbilicus using standard technique. The abdomen is insufflated to a pressure of 15 mm Hg (Fig. 40-1). A 10-mm trocar is placed in the umbilicus. Under laparoscopic guidance, three other trocars are placed: a 10-mm trocar in the midline 5 cm below the xiphoid process, a 5-mm trocar in the midclavicular line 2 cm below the right costal margin, and a 5-mm trocar in the anterior axillary line at the level of the umbilicus. In obese patients or patients with a long torso, the anterior axillary trocar should be raised to just below the costal margin.

The obese patient is difficult to intubate with normal-sized trocars. It is frequently necessary to rely on long insufflation needles and long trocars to navigate through the large panniculus on the obese patient. Care should always be taken to insert only as much in-

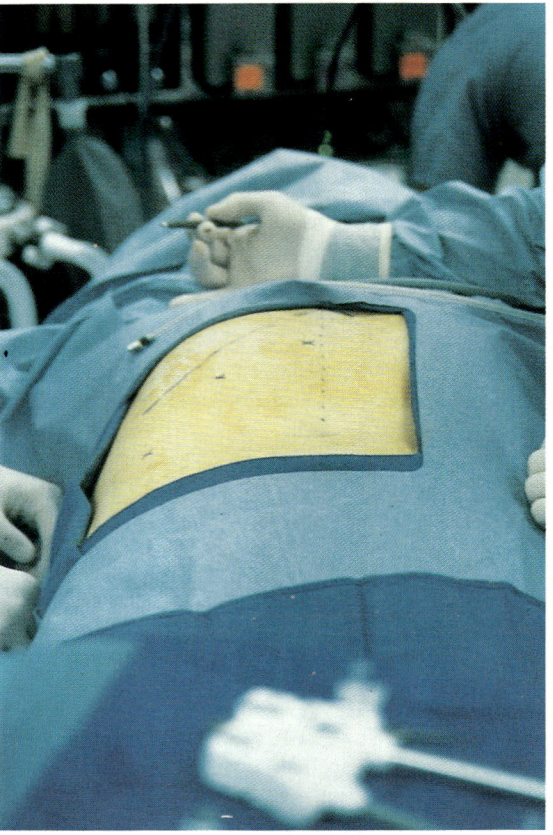

Figure 40-1.

strument as needed to penetrate the peritoneal cavity. If the needle or trocar is advanced too far, retroperitoneal vascular injury may occur or intestine may be pinned to the retroperitoneal space, causing an intestinal laceration.

METHODS OF EXPOSURE AND RETRACTION

After establishment of the pneumoperitoneum, the patient is rotated to the left and put in a foot-down position. The fundus of the gallbladder is grasped with the lateral trocar and pushed superiorly (Fig. 40-2). This retracts the liver superiorly and puts the gallbladder on longitudinal stretch. Hartmann's pouch is grasped by the midclavicular instrument and pulled inferiorly and laterally, stretching out the triangle of Calot and exposing the cystic and common ducts and the cystic artery.

If it is difficult to identify the anatomical structures, the retraction is probably incorrect.

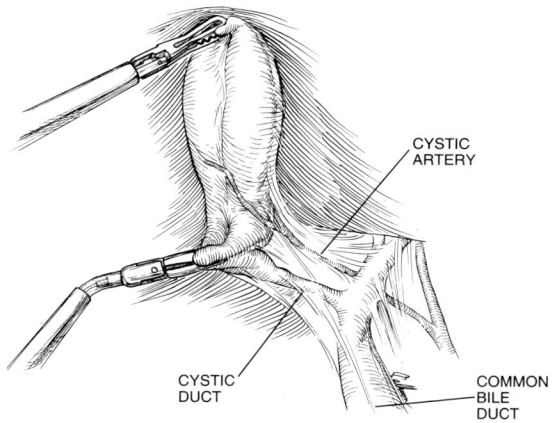

Figure 40-2.

The camera should be pulled back to visualize the retractors. Hartmann's pouch should be pulled away from the liver. Pushing the pouch into the liver collapses the triangle and makes anatomic visualization impossible. The fundus retractor should be pushing superiorly and laterally. If the fundus is pushed medially, the lateral aspect of the gallbladder and cystic duct will be seen; if pushed laterally, the medial-superior aspect of the triangle will be seen.

METHODS OF DISSECTION

Laparoscopic cholecystectomy can be accomplished with either laser or electrocautery dissection. Laser is the more precise instrument, allowing both cutting and coagulation with minimal tissue damage. Electrocautery is less precise and causes a wider band of tissue damage. Both modalites have their limitations and advantages. It is the duty of the surgeon to become skilled with his or her particular choice and use it safely.

SPECIFIC DETAILS OF THE PROCEDURE

The abdominal wall should always be elevated during trocar insertion to pull the wall away from the bowel. With the obese patient this may be impossible. Stabilization of the anterior abdominal wall is usually greatest where it inserts into the rib cage. If the initial puncture is made in the midclavicular line, 2 cm below the right costal margin, the abdominal wall will have minimal movement during intubation, thereby making insertion safer (Fig. 40-3). Once the abdomen is insufflated, a 5-mm trocar may be placed in the same spot, a 5-mm scope may be inserted, and the secondary trocars introduced under visual guidance. This insufflation and insertion technique has been used in more than 600 patients in the author's series without injury.

Previous surgery usually causes adhesions, which attach the intestine to the abdominal wall. This makes blind trocar insertion dangerous. In patients with previous lower abdominal surgery, especially pelvic surgery, adhesions will be prominent in the lower abdomen, but should be absent in the upper abdomen. Utilizing the alternate site technique in the right upper quadrant (described above), the surgeon should be able to enter most abdominal cavities safely. If the patient has had previous upper abdominal surgery or has acute cholecystitis, the alternate entry technique is not indicated.

Abdominal cavities in these patients can be entered using a cutdown technique at the umbilicus, much like one would perform a peritoneal lavage. A 2-cm incision is made in

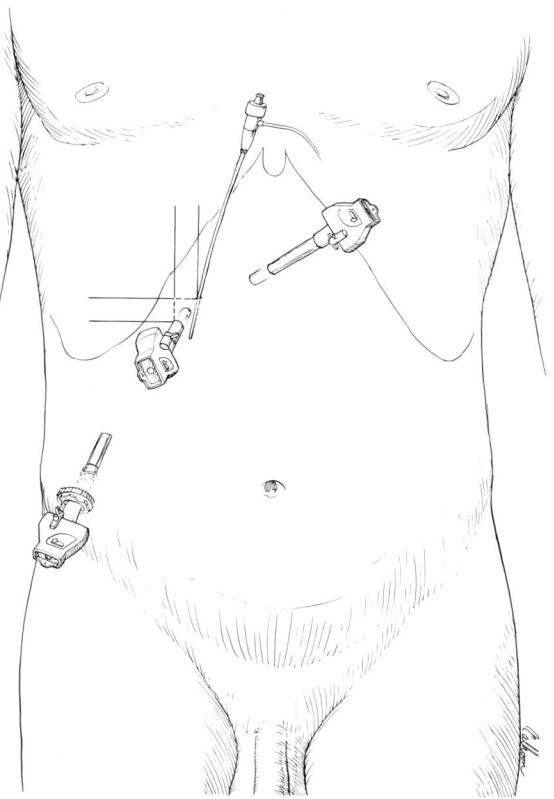

Figure 40-3.

the umbilicus and carried down sharply until the peritoneum is exposed. The peritoneum is opened under direct vision, and any underlying adhesions are sharply dissected away until a small cavity is created. Since the hole created is too large to be sealed with a regular trocar, a Hasson trocar or its equivalent is used to fill the incision. The Hasson trocar is designed with a movable "olive" used to seal the incision. A SURGIPORT* trocar (United States Surgical Corporation, Norwalk, CT) with attached SURGIGRIP* device (United States Surgical Corporation) or a disposable expanding trocar may be used in lieu of a Hasson trocar.

Once the trocar is placed, the camera is advanced and adhesions are dissected in a fashion similar to that in a laparotomy. Dissection is begun bluntly at the neck of the gallbladder and carried inferiorly and medially toward the cystic duct. When the duct is identified, dissection is continued around the cystic duct until it is circumferentially cleaned of its attachments. Dissection is continued medially on top of the cystic duct until the cystic-common duct junction is identified.

The cystic artery is dissected from the gallbladder to the right hepatic artery. It should be circumferentially cleared of its attachments. An automatic clip applier is placed through the xiphoid port, and the cystic artery is doubly clipped (Fig. 40-4). Care should be taken to visualize both jaws of the clip applier to assure that the clip will not injure the underlying right hepatic duct. The cystic duct is clipped at the neck of the gallbladder.

Cholangiography is routinely performed. The fundus of the gallbladder is grasped with the xiphoid grasper, leaving the lateral port free for insertion of the catheter. The surgeon moves to the right side of the table and introduces a pair of scissors into the lateral port. The scissors should always be introduced through the same port that the catheter will be introduced through. This will assure that the cut in the cystic duct will align with the catheter. The incision should be through the lateral one-fourth of the cystic duct. Cutting too far through the duct will hinder catheter insertion.

The scissors are removed, and the balloon catheter is introduced through the later port and inserted into the cystic duct. The balloon is inflated in the cystic duct with 0.2 ml of fluid or until the balloon can be seen dilating the cystic duct. Cholangiography is performed with full strength dye. In situations in which the duct is difficult to cannulate, retraction should be checked. Hartmann's pouch can be manipulated laterally until the cystic duct aligns with the catheter, making insertion easier. If valves are obstructing, they can be broken open with a pair of microscissors or with a Hall valvulotome prior to insertion of the catheter.

Another option for performing cholangiography involves percutaneously placing a sheathed 14-gauge needle into the right upper quadrant, superior and medial to the midclavicular trocar. The needle can be removed and a balloon catheter placed through the sheath into the cystic duct. The surgeon and assistant can maintain standard retraction utilizing this technique.

Recent advances in intraoperative ultrasonography may obviate the need for cholangiography. The side-viewing rectal probe has been used for scanning the common bile duct in over 400 patients in the Netherlands; however, the probe requires placing a larger trocar in the epigastrium than is currently used. The LaproScan (Baxter, McGaw Park, IL) allows for insertion of a 10-mm probe through the existing xiphoid port to scan the cystic and common ducts for stones and anatomy.

After cholangiography, the catheter is removed and double clips are placed on the cystic duct. The duct and artery are transected with the scissors. By applying traction to Hartmann's pouch laterally, a plane between the gallbladder and liver is easily identified and dissection can begin with either laser or cautery.

Dissection of the gallbladder bed is facili-

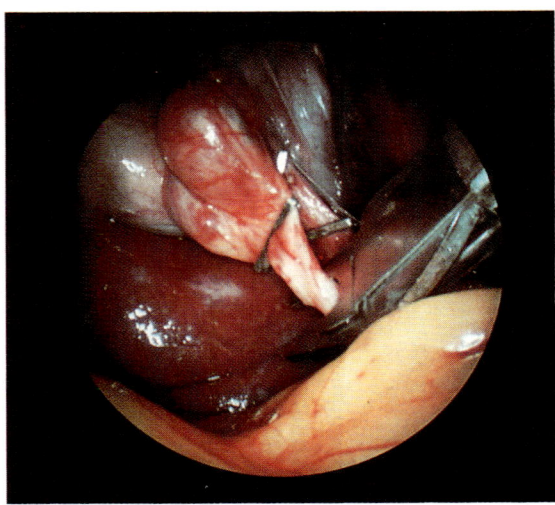

Figure 40-4.

tated by applying tension to either side of the peritoneal reflection. The medial reflection is exposed by pulling Hartmann's pouch inferiorly and pushing the fundus superiorly. The lateral reflection is exposed by pushing Hartmann's pouch superiorly and pulling the fundus slightly inferior (Fig. 40-5). The medial reflection should be transected until tension is no longer maintained; then the lateral reflection should be exposed and dissected until tension can no longer be maintained. With a gentle twisting motion on the gallbladder to maintain tension on the line of dissection, the gallbladder is removed from the neck to the fundus.

Near the end of the dissection, the bed should be examined for leaks and bleeding (Fig. 40-6). Since the pneumoperitoneum might mask a leak, the pressure should be reduced to 9 mm Hg and tension released on the liver. The bed should be irrigated during inspection. If no leaks are seen, the gallbladder is completely removed from the liver.

The camera is placed in the xiphoid port, and a grasper is placed through the umbilicus. The neck of the gallbladder is grasped and pulled into the neck of the umbilical trocar (Fig. 40-7). The clips on the neck of the gallbladder should not be grasped since they might dislodge during removal and cause the surgeon to drop the gallbladder. The trocar and gallbladder are pulled out of the umbilicus. The neck of the gallbladder is visualized on the exterior of the abdominal wall. The fundus remains inside. The neck can be opened and suction applied to remove the

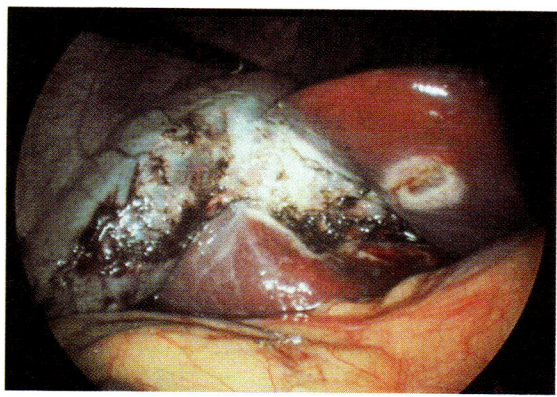

Figure 40-6.

bile, facilitating removal. At times, the gallstones must be removed individually through the neck. In more difficult cases, crushing the stones may be desirable. A high speed blender, the Laprolith (Baxter), is available for crushing large stones, either within the gallbladder or in a separate plastic bag. The instrument can be placed through the neck of the gallbladder. The spinning blade creates a vortex, which pulls the stones into its path. The stones are liquefied, assisting removal.

CLOSURE

Trocars are removed under visual guidance to assure hemostasis. The umbilical puncture site is closed with interrupted sutures. The skin is closed with Steri-Strips.

POSTOPERATIVE MANAGEMENT

Most patients require minimal pain medications. Nonsteroidal analgesics are given intramuscularly during surgery, so narcotic use is unusual. Full liquids are begun after nausea has subsided. Nausea is kept to a minimum by applying a 1.5-mg scopolamine patch prior to surgery. A regular diet is begun on postoperative Day 1. No physical restrictions are given.

CRITERIA FOR PATIENT DISCHARGE

Patients are discharged on the day of surgery or the following day. This is determined by their ability to tolerate a regular diet. Most patients return to work within 1 week of surgery.

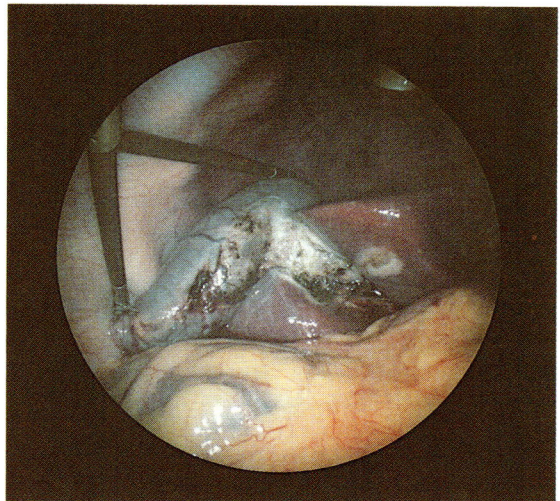

Figure 40-5.

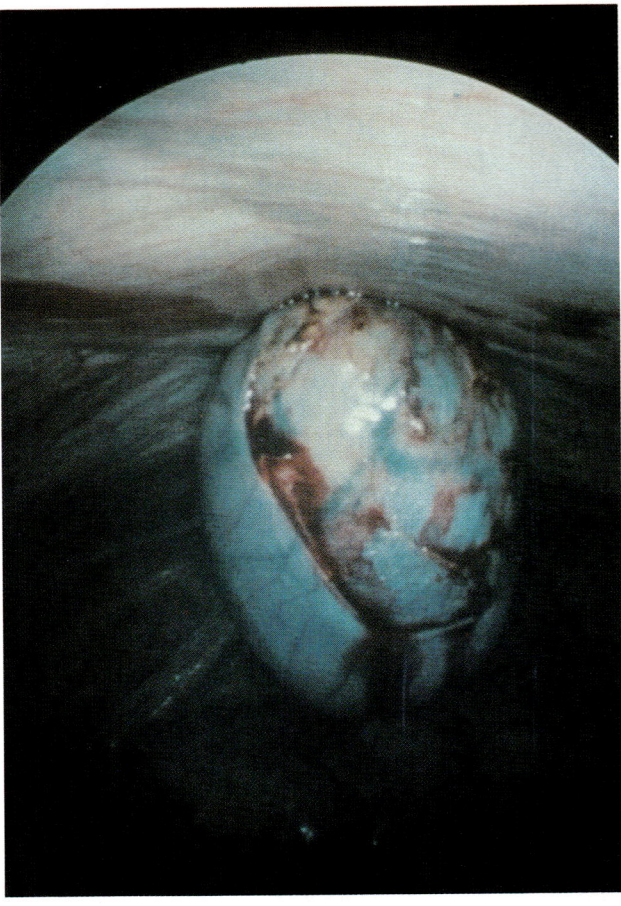

Figure 40-7.

COMPLICATIONS SPECIFIC TO THIS PROCEDURE

There has been an increase in morbidity over standard cholecystectomy, primarily from common bile duct injuries. Most of these injuries have occurred in the first 10 procedures of a surgeon's experience. After the surgeon becomes acquainted with the retraction techniques required to perform laparoscopic cholecystetomy, the incidence of injury decreases to that of open cholecystectomy.

There is still concern about relative contraindications to laparoscopic cholecystectomy. However, after the learning curve has been mastered, this operation appears to be safe in any situation. Pregnancy was an initial contraindication. The effect of increased intra-abdominal pressure on blood return from the uterus and the effect of a high carbon dioxide level on the developing fetus are not known. Less than 100 laparoscopic cholecystectomies have been performed on pregnant patients. Of the babies that have delivered, all reported have done well. From a technical standpoint, all procedures should be done with minimal intra-abdominal pressure, usually 10 to 12 mm Hg, and the initial entry into the abdomen should be performed with the open technique to decrease the chance of uterine injury. The family should be counseled that any operative intervention, whether open or laparoscopic, is associated with a chance of premature delivery.

The patient with cirrhosis should not have surgery unless absolutely necessary. Large vessels in the abdominal wall can cause profuse bleeding during trocar insertion and bleeding from the liver can impair laparoscopic visualization. With special attention to hemostasis, procedures in these patients can be done safely through the laparoscope. The large vessels that traverse the peritoneal covering of the gallbladder should be grasped and coagulated before any dissection. With careful attention to anatomic planes, the gallbladder can be removed from the gallbladder bed with the laser or cautery; however, if any excess bleeding is encountered, the posterior wall of the gallbladder can be left on the liver bed and the remaining mucosa can be cauterized with the laser or electrocautery. All trocar sites should be inspected after removal of the trocar to assure there is excellent hemostasis.

SPECIAL CONSIDERATIONS—COMMON BILE DUCT STONES

Common duct stones only occur in 10 per cent of patients with cholelithiasis. An open common duct exploration can always be performed if necessary; however, most stones can be managed with minimally invasive techniques. A detailed description of the laparoscopic technique of common bile duct exporation is given in Chapter 41.

The least invasive laparoscopic exploration of the common duct is cystic duct choledochoscopy. It can be performed laparoscopically through the cholangiogram incision, and, if unsuccessful, the cystic duct can simply be clipped and other methods of removal may be used. In short, no bridges are burned by this technique. The procedure requires a scope with a working channel of 1 mm or greater for irrigation and manipulation and a single-direction deflectable tip of 90 degrees. Although the cystic duct can be dilated in some cases, a scope of no greater than 3 mm (10 French) is required to facilitate introduction through the cystic duct. There are several new disposable or reusuable disposable scopes on the market that have all the needed characteristics and are as small as 2.4 mm in diameter.

The choledochoscope is passed through the lateral portal. Upward traction on the fundus of the gallbladder is provided by the xiphoid grasper and Hartmann's pouch is held with the midclavicular grasper. The scope should be passed through an introducer to keep it stiff and prevent the trocar valve from injuring the fiberoptic bundles. Entry into the cystic duct is facilitated by passing the scope over a 0.025-mm flexible tipped guide wire.

Once inside the common duct, a stone basket may be used for removal of stones, or they may be shattered with intraductal lithotripsy. Use of the pulsed dye laser is most efflcient. The rapid pulsations prevent heat buildup, thus making the instrument safe to soft tissue; however, the stones are shattered into small pieces that can be irrigated through into the duodenum after injection of 1 ml of intravenous glucagon. An electromechanical lithotriptor may also be used, but care should be taken to keep the fiber off the common duct wall since this instrument can potentially harm the soft tissue of the common duct.

The common bile duct may also be explored laparoscopically by introducing a laparoscopic knife through the xiphoid port and incising the common duct longitudinally. The stones are removed with a basket, balloon catheter, or lithotripsy. A T-tube is introduced into the abdomen, the wings are inserted into the choledochotomy, and the incision is closed with interrupted absorbable suture using any of a variety of suturing techniques.

A final option is ERCP. It is preferably performed on the day after surgery. If performed in the operating theater, valuable operating and anesthesia time is wasted setting up for the procedure and, frequently, operating room radiology equipment is not adequate for such a procedure. The procedure may also fill the intestine with gas, thereby inhibiting visualization.

Conclusions

Results of laparoscopic cholecystectomy have shown great improvement over those of standard cholecystectomy. Reduction in hospital costs and reduction in time lost from work have made insurance companies, third party payers, employers, and patients favor this operation. Laparoscopic cholecystectomy has become the accepted method of treatment of gallbladder disease in the United States and is quickly encompassing the world of general surgery. It is safe and effective and has distinct advantages for all concerned, especially the patient and the surgeon. It has opened the eyes of the once conservative general surgical community to the world of "high tech" minimally invasive surgery.

REFERENCES

1. Reddick EJ, Olsen DO, Daniell JF, et al. Laparoscopic laser cholecystectomy. Laser Medicine and Surgery News and Advances 1989; 7:38–40.
2. Reddick EJ, Olsen DO. Laparoscopic laser cholecystectomy. Surg Endosc 1989; 3:131–133.
3. Reddick EJ, Olsen DO. Outpatient laparoscopic laser cholecystectomy. Am J Surg 1990; 160:485–487.
4. Reddick EJ, Olsen DO, Spaw A, et al. Safe performance of difficult laparoscopic cholecystectomies. Am J Surg 1991; 161:377–387.

Chapter 41
Exploration of the Common Bile Duct

Stephen J. Shapiro
Leo A. Gordon
Leon Daykhovsky

Do not expect that I should make this letter, which is already too long, still longer, by adding many things in regard to the cure of this disease. Of which it will be sufficient to hint a few things. I have already said that this disorder often recurs, nor is certainly known, unless when some calculus has been discharged, which previous pains about the region of the liver, have proved to have proceeded from thence. Therefore, one part of the cure will be to endeavor, when very sharp pains of this kind shall return, that the calculus may be dislodged from these straights. A second part, that if any other calculus remains, after this has been dislodged, it may, if possible, be dissolved. A third, to prevent the generation of new calculi. And each of these parts of the cure are to be attended to separately, and distinguished according to our position, nor ought the times, which belong to every one of them, be rashly confounded, as some seem to do, who heap up remedies promiscuously upon their patients. (From Morgagni, John Baptist. *The Seats and Causes of Diseases Investigated by Anatomy*, Vol. II, Letter XXXVII "Of the Jaundice; and of Bilious Calculi," Book III, "Of Diseases of the Belly." Translated from the Latin by Benjamin Alexander, M.D. London, 1769.)

Morgagni's clear and precise description of common duct calculi and their effects hits at the heart of the dilemma raised by the discovery of common bile duct stones during laparoscopic cholecystectomy. Such stones are a separate entity within the sphere of laparoscopic surgery—an entity requiring a singularly well planned approach for effective treatment.

The goal of this chapter is to describe how we, as surgical laparoscopists, dislodge such calculi from their "straights" as described by Morgagni. He cautions us to attend to this problem separately from gallbladder calculi, which we will do. Whether we distinguish ourselves by relating our position will be left to the reader to decide.

OVERVIEW OF LAPAROSCOPIC EXPLORATION OF THE COMMON BILE DUCT

Patient Selection

Most patients are referred for laparoscopic exploration of the common bile duct as a subgroup of patients for laparoscopic cholecystectomy. The majority of patients will have the signs and symptoms of biliary tract disease, and common duct stones will be discovered during surgery.

Routine intraoperative cholangiography during laparoscopic cholecystectomy has led to increasing detection of common bile duct stones. There is little correlation between preoperative testing and the presence of such stones. In our own experience, half of the patients with common bile duct stones had no preoperative indication of their presence. Consequently, the intraoperative cholangiogram assumes a central role both in the performance of laparoscopic cholecystectomy and in the planning for laparoscopic common bile duct exploration. Some surgeons feel that such a study is essential to a safely performed laparoscopic cholecystectomy.

What is a good cholangiogram and how should it be viewed? The ideal cholangiogram is a dynamic cinefluorocholangiographic study. It is a roentgenogram performed by the surgeon, reviewed by an experienced biliary radiologist, and interpreted jointly in the context of the patient. There are two aspects to cholangiography: its performance and its interpretation. Laparoscopic cholecystectomy, with its new views of the porta hepatis and adjacent structures, has led to increased emphasis on the interpretation of such cholangiograms.

Specifically, the study evolves in the following manner. The porta hepatis is centered on the x-ray screen. The C-arm is then rotated, shifting the spine away from the area of the common bile duct, and 50 per cent contrast medium is then slowly injected under fluoroscopic control. The following sequential events are observed: (1) filling of the cystic duct; (2) filling of the common bile duct; (3) filling of the distal duct; (4) viewing of the ampullary anatomy; and (5) filling of the intrahepatic ducts. Each of these five phases must be viewed dynamically. If a concern arises during the study, further exposures of the area in question are obtained. After development of the films, each of these five areas is assessed.

1. *Filling of the cystic duct.* How long is the cystic duct? Are there filling defects in the cystic duct? What is the relationship of the cystic duct to the common bile duct? Does the anatomy lend itself to transcystic duct laparoscopic exploration of the common bile duct?

2. *Filling of the common bile duct.* Is the lumen compromised? What is the proximity of the cystic duct to the common bile duct? Are there filling defects, and if so are further films needed for definition? Is there extravasation?

3. *Filling of the distal duct.* Does the distal duct fill? Are there defects, and if so are further films needed for better definition? What are the size and location of the defects, and if there are stones, can they be extracted laparoscopically?

4. *Viewing of the ampullary area.* Does the distal duct empty? Are there exposures of the ampullary mechanism? Is the transduodenal portion of the sphincter mechanism seen?

5. *Filling of the intrahepatic ducts.* Do the intrahepatic ducts fill? Are there anomalies? Is the ductal anatomy such that manipulation of the cystic duct will injure a duct in close proximity?

Assessment of the cholangiogram by these guidelines allows safe laparoscopic cholecystectomy as well as a well planned laparoscopic common bile duct exploration. At this point in the procedure, if stones have been detected, the decision is made regarding the proper laparoscopic approach.

A select group of patients, however, may be referred for laparoscopy with a known preoperative diagnosis of a common duct pathologic condition. Procedures such as endoscopic retrograde cholangiopancreatography, transhepatic cholangiography, or ultrasonography that show ductal stones are usually quite sensitive and specific. These patients, however, are in the minority and the referral usually is the result of a workup for atypical upper abdominal pain.

Preoperative Evaluation

The patient is prepared for administration of a general anesthetic. A cardiogram, chest film, blood count, urinalysis, and a set of liver function tests, including amylase and lipase levels, are reviewed. Although abnormal liver function tests may be associated with common duct stones, there is wide variability. The amylase and lipase levels are routinely measured as screening tools for unsuspected biliary pancreatitis. Clotting studies have also become part of our preoperative assessment. Because many patients are taking baby aspirin or Persantine, we measure preoperative bleeding time.

Preoperative Preparation

Preoperatively, we spend a great deal of time informing our patients about the potential for finding a common duct pathologic condition during laparoscopic cholecystectomy. In today's medical environment, it is essential that the patient understand the following:

1. Common duct problems may be present even if results of blood tests are normal.
2. Although the tools are available to image the common duct preoperatively, they are not usually used because they are expensive, have a slight degree of risk, and will not answer any questions that the intraoperative cholangiogram, a routine part of the procedure, will answer.
3. Experience with laparoscopic common bile duct exploration is in its early stages. It is effective. It appears to be safe. It has definite benefits for the patient. Nevertheless, compared to 75 years of open surgical common bile duct exploration, laparoscopic common bile duct exploration is in its infancy.
4. An open laparotomy may be performed if there are intraoperative injuries or obscured anatomical features, or if in the judgment of the surgeon that is simply the safest thing to do. No surgeon can promise a patient a 100 per cent success rate with laparoscopic cholecystectomy or laparoscopic common duct exploration.
5. Stones may be left behind for expectant treatment if they are small or for endoscopic intervention at a later date. The patient must understand the limitations of the procedure and the thinking behind intraoperative decisions. The patient must be an active participant in any medical decision.
6. There are risks and complications with laparoscopic common bile duct exploration that are specific to the procedure. Perforation of the common duct by guide wires, tearing of the cystic duct, and injury to the ampulla causing postoperative pancreatitis are potential problems.

Once the patient's case has been reviewed and the patient has been prepared for surgery, the operation is usually scheduled for the morning. The patient reports to the hospital on the morning of surgery, having had nothing by mouth since midnight the day before. We use perioperative antibiotics. A dose is given 30 minutes prior to the procedure. Two additional doses are given postoperatively at 8-hour intervals.

Equipment

As soon as the decision has been made to perform a laparoscopic common duct exploration, the following equipment should be assembled:

1. A guide wire 150 cm long and 0.035 inch (0.89 mm) in diameter coated with hydrophilic gel. The 3-cm distal end of the guide wire may be straight or angulated.
2. A torque device, which when attached to the wire allows rotation of the distal end of the guide wire. This aids cannulation of the cystic duct and passage into the common bile duct.
3. A dilatation balloon catheter 70 cm long with a 5-French shaft diameter. This catheter is equipped with a 4- or 6-cm long balloon at its tip. The balloon is inflatable to 7 mm in diameter.
4. A LeVeen syringe with a pressure gauge. This has a 10-ml capacity and can easily be attached to the dilating balloon catheter. It allows sequential and controlled dilatation of the balloon.
5. A Segura wire basket, three- or four-pronged retrieving graspers, or a Fogarty balloon catheter. These tools are available in 2.5- or 3-French sizes. All tools should be 90 cm long and should pass through the working channel of the minicholedochoscope.
6. A flexible two-way deflecting fiberoptic endoscope 2.7 or 3.3 mm in diameter. These miniature endoscopes have a 1.0- or 1.2-mm diameter working channel and deflection capabilities of 90 to 120 degrees.

The surgeon and surgical team must be well trained in the manipulation of this equipment under video and fluoroscopic control. In our practice, after extensive laboratory experience we have chosen guide wires and dilatation balloon catheters manufactured by the Microvasive Boston Scientific Corporation.

Initially, laparoscopic duct exploration is labor and technology intensive. It is prudent to alert the nursing endoscopy team that a duct exploration is imminent. The establishment of a "common duct tray" for laparoscopy has streamlined the process. Such a prepared tray fosters a smooth transition from laparoscopic cholecystectomy to laparoscopic common bile duct exploration.

The flexible choledochoscope has a central role. Several choledochoscopes are available. We use a 3.3-mm outer diameter flexible pediatric ureteroscope (Olympus, Lake Success, NY) and a specifically designed 2.7-mm outer diameter miniature choledochoscope, the CBD-11 (Intramed, San Diego, CA). We feel that these are the safest and most reliable instruments for common bile duct exploration. The choledochoscopes with 1.2-mm diameter working channels allow placement of baskets and maintenance of adequate irrigation during choledochoscopic stone manipulation.

For large stones discovered by choledochoscopy, the 4-mm tunable pulse dye laser lithotriptor is used. The calculi are fragmented within the common bile duct.

Irrigation is an essential part of the choledochoscopy and should be obtained through specially designed endopumps. The solution used for irrigation must be prewarmed to body temperature.

Positioning of the Patient

In the operating room, the patient is prepared for a laparoscopic cholecystectomy. A nasogastric or orogastric tube is placed. The patient's head is raised, and the right side is elevated approximately 15 degrees. If a duct exploration is anticipated, we usually place a Foley catheter. The pneumoperitoneum is instilled, and trocars are placed as for laparoscopic cholecystectomy.

The position for laparoscopic common bile duct exploration is the same position used for routine laparoscopic cholecystectomy. An orogastric tube has been placed, and the patient's stomach has been completely decompressed. The head of the table is raised approximately 20 degrees, and the patient's right side is elevated another 10 to 15 degrees.

Positioning of the Video Equipment

The video equipment is set up exactly as for a routine laparoscopic cholecystectomy. However, an additional cart and video camera should be available for the choledochoscope. A number of manufacturers are now combining the choledochoscopic image into the main imaging system so that the operator can look at one screen and see both the laparoscopic image and the choledochoscopic image. This split screen approach will facilitate the performance of the procedure. It will also eliminate the need for a second camera cart.

In addition to the tools listed above, the following are needed:

1. A high resolution television monitor (13 or 19 inches in diameter) displacing over 700 lines of horizontal resolution.
2. A color miniature camera with a builtin zoom and focal lens that can easily be sterilized before each case. This is connected to the choledochoscope. These microchip cameras provide superb quality images.
3. A 300-watt xenon high intensity light source. This gives reliable illumination during choledochoscopy.
4. A 1/2- or 3/4-inch video recording system. This is necessary for proper education, training, and recording of procedures in patients with common bile duct stones. We have found the critical review of laparoscopic procedures to be a valuable teaching tool.

Trocar Placement and Size Selection

The trocars used are the same as those for routine laparoscopic cholecystectomy. We use a 10-mm SURGIPORT* in the subumbilical position, a subxiphoid 10-mm trocar, and two lateral 5-mm trocars. If a laparoscopic direct choledochotomy is to be carried out, we put an accessory trocar in the left upper quadrant at the midclavicular line.

Methods of Exposure and Retraction and Methods of Dissection

The laparoscopic cholecystectomy proceeds in the usual fashion. The techniques of safe dissection, the principles of retraction and assistance, and the many technical caveats that have evolved are described in Chapter 11. Review and assessment of the intraoperative cholangiogram is the first step in planning and performance of the laparoscopic bile duct exploration.

THE TRANSCYSTIC DUCT APPROACH TO EXPLORATION OF THE COMMON BILE DUCT

Specific Details of the Procedure

Most laparoscopic common bile duct explorations will be performed transcystically. Initially, a 0.035 Terumo guide wire is placed into a 5-French dilating catheter. The guide wire is threaded into the cystic duct and the common bile duct. Its position is verified fluoroscopically. The dilating balloon is then

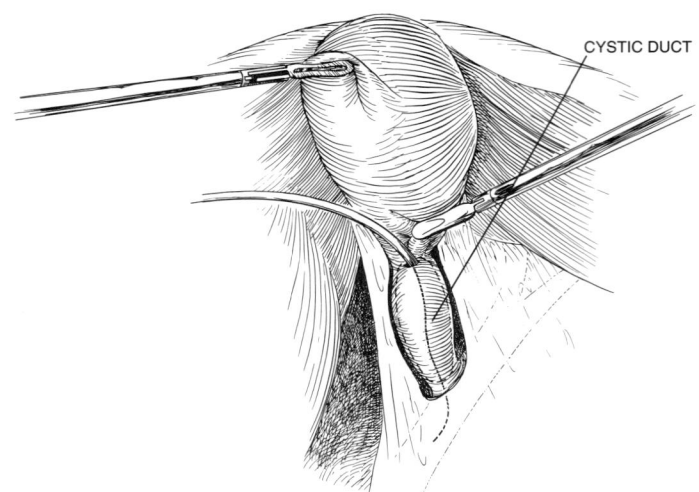

Figure 41-1.

threaded over the guide wire. The length of the dilating balloon should be judged by the length of the cystic duct; the dilating balloon should encompass the entire length of the cystic duct. The catheter is then placed at the level of the cystic duct opening, the balloon catheter is placed into the cystic duct and, using image amplification, the second radiopaque marker should be positioned just exiting the cystotomy.

The balloon dilating catheter is then inflated slowly to 10 atm of pressure using a LeVeen syringe (Fig. 41-1). This pressure is held for 3 to 5 minutes. The guide wire is kept in place, and the balloon catheter is then withdrawn.

For transcystic choledochoscopy, we use the Intramed 9-French disposable choledochoscope. This endoscope has two-way deflection, excellent optics, and a 1.2-mm working channel (Fig. 41-2).

The guide wire is threaded through the endoscope, and the choledochoscope is negotiated through the cystic duct into the com-

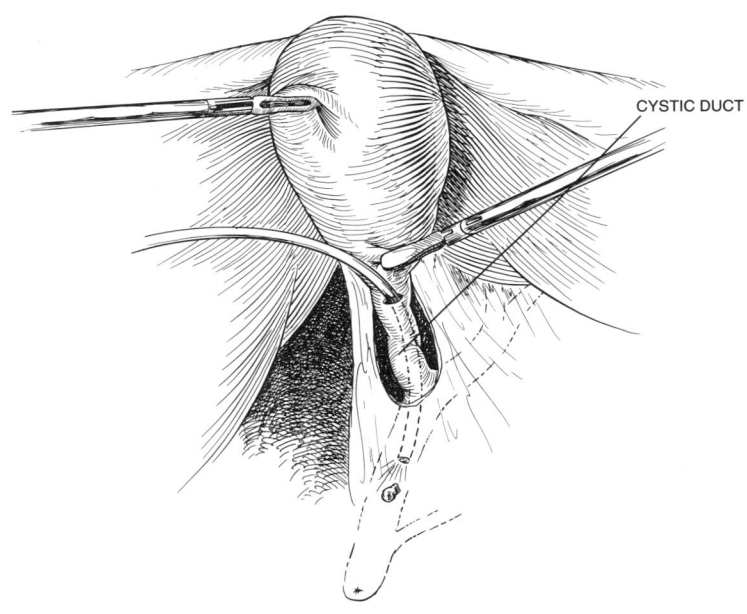

Figure 41-2.

mon duct over the guide wire. Once the choledochoscope is in the common duct, the guide wire is removed. The operating team visualizes both the choledochoscopic image and the laparoscopic image. It is important that the laparoscopic image is visualized at all times to avoid torsion injury of the cystic duct.

When a stone is visualized, a 3-French Segura basket is placed through the working channel and is negotiated to just beyond the stone. The basket is opened, and the stone is grasped and brought close to the endoscope (Fig. 41-3). The endoscope and stone are then removed in unison. The stone is placed into Hartmann's pouch, to be retrieved at a later time. The choledochoscope is then placed back into the common duct. This procedure is repeated until all stones are removed.

The other instruments that can be used through the choledochoscope include three- and four-prong graspers. These are easily placed through the working channel of the choledochoscope.

If the common duct stone is larger than 7 mm, it will usually not negotiate the cystic duct. In this circumstance, a tunable pulse dye laser is brought into the operating room. Through a 1-mm channel, a 200-micron laser fiber is placed in through the working channel of the choledochoscope. The choledochoscope is then negotiated to the region of the stone at which point the laser fiber is brought into contact with the stone (Fig. 41-4). The stone can then be pulverized or fractured. When we use this laser, we start with a setting of 10 Hz (pulses per second) at 60 mJ. If necessary for stone fragmentation, those settings are increased. We like to break large stones into three to four major fragments, so they can be retrieved by baskets or graspers after the laser has been withdrawn.

Another option using the laser is to try to pulverize the stone into very small fragments to be later irrigated through the ampulla of Vater. Fragments smaller than 2 mm will usually pass through the ampulla without difficulty.

If, after fragmentation, morcellation, and pulverization of common duct stones, debris remains, ampullary dilatation may be performed. The ampulla of Vater can be dilated safely with the same 5-French shaft dilating balloon used to dilate the cystic duct. Using image amplification, the guide wire is placed into the duodenum. The dilating balloon is

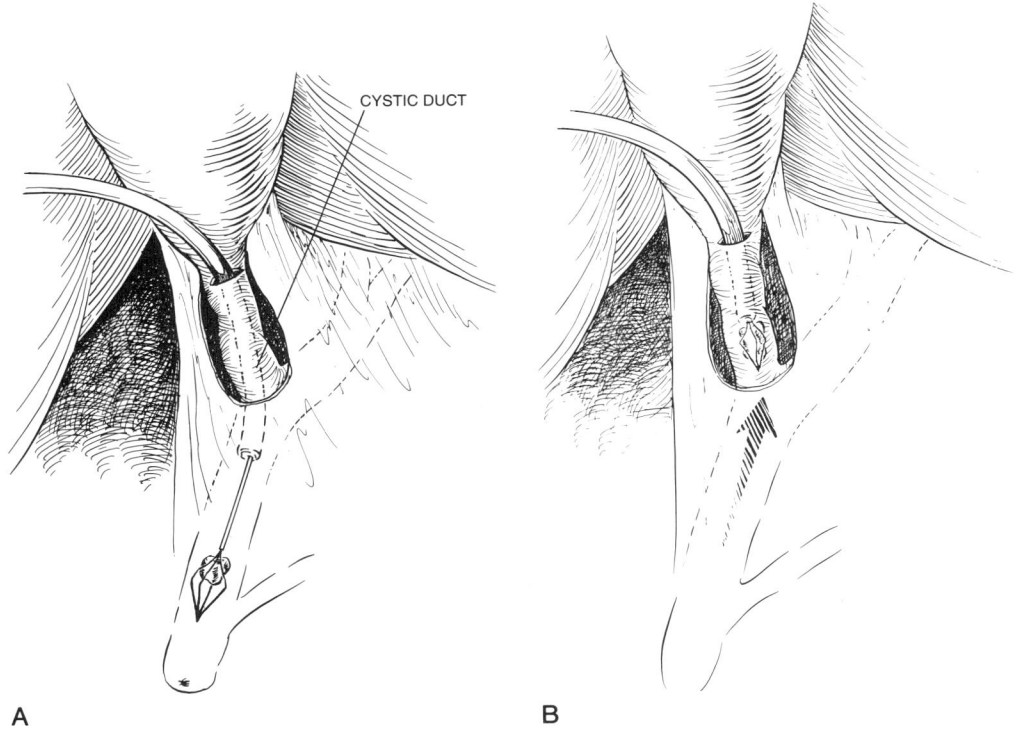

Figure 41-3.

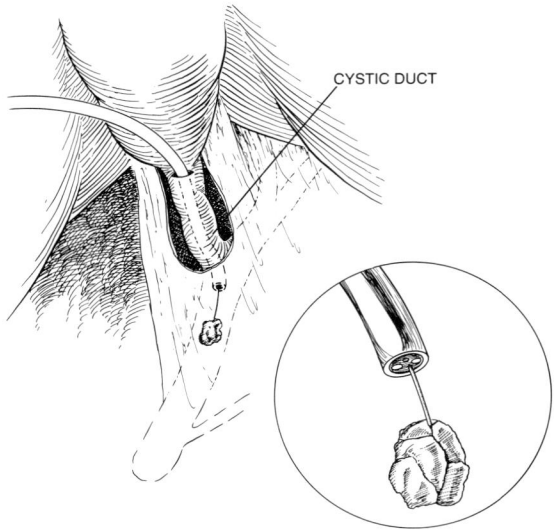

Figure 41-4.

then placed into the common duct. A cholangiogram is obtained using the image amplifier. The shaft of the dilating balloon is placed through the ampulla, noting the radiopaque marks in both common duct and duodenum. The catheter is again dilated to 6 to 10 atm of pressure for 3 to 5 minutes. The balloon is then deflated and withdrawn into the common duct. Residual stone fragments and primary stones smaller than 2 mm can then be irrigated safely into the duodenum.

The common bile duct may not be able to be dilatated. In those patients, a 1.5-mm, nonsteerable disposable choledochoscope can be placed through the cystic duct directly into the common duct so it can be visualized. A 200-micron laser wire can then be placed through the small choledochoscope, and, again, stones can be pulverized to less than 2 mm in size. The ampulla of Vater can then be dilated, as described above, and the small stones and fragments can be irrigated through. This technique can be used even in the absence of adequate dilatation of the cystic duct and should be kept in mind by the experienced endoscopic surgeon.

Stones that are seen in the common hepatic duct and the left and right hepatic ducts can also be retrieved, at times through a cystic duct approach. By using steerable guide wires and image amplification, a guide wire can be placed into the proximal ducts. The choledochoscope is then negotiated to adequately visualize the upper ducts. This can be accomplished approximately 50 per cent of the time. Patients in whom the cystic duct cannot be negotiated become candidates for direct laparoscopic common bile duct exploration.

After transcystic duct laparoscopic common bile duct exploration, a final cystic duct cholangiogram is performed. The duct should be free of calculi and should demonstrate free emptying into the duodenum. Attention should be paid to the integrity of the duct, looking for subtle signs of extravasation resulting from injury during manipulation. As of this writing, we have not seen any perforation of the common duct.

Once transcystic duct common bile duct exploration has been completed, the cystic duct is transected. We advocate the use of a PDS (Poly Diaxonone Ethicon®) endoloop for cystic duct closure. We use two ligatures for adequate control of the cystic duct. The gallbladder is then removed in the usual laparoscopic fashion.

Closure

Each laparoscopic common bile duct exploration is drained with a 19-French round Jackson-Pratt catheter placed into Morison's pouch. After the drain is shortened, it is placed under laparoscopic control through the subxiphoid trocar. The assistant grasps the drain and brings it entirely within the abdominal cavity. Using this technique, the pneumoperitoneum is sustained, and direct visualization of the drain placement is easily accomplished. The lateral trocar is then removed, and a hemostat is placed through the trocar hole in the abdominal wall, grasping the end of the drain. The assistant withdraws the end of the drain through the body wall, and the drain is immediately sewn to the skin. The surgeon then places the drain into Morison's pouch under direct laparoscopic control.

At this point, a 0.5 per cent Marcaine solution is used to inject all trocar sites. The pneumoperitoneum is withdrawn slowly. The orogastric tube is then removed prior to the patient's going to the recovery room.

Postoperative Management

The postoperative course for laparoscopic transcystic duct exploration is the same as that for laparoscopic cholecystectomy. A liquid diet is started within 2 to 3 hours of the operation. The diet is rapidly advanced to a soft diet by the following day. Most patients require only oral analgesics. If there is no evidence of a bile leak, the drain is removed on the first or second postoperative day.

Criteria for Patient Discharge

The average length of stay for our 25 patients who underwent transcystic common bile duct exploration was 2.6 days. Recently, patients have been leaving on the first postoperative day. The patient is discharged when a regular diet can be tolerated.

THE DIRECT LAPAROSCOPIC APPROACH TO EXPLORATION OF THE COMMON BILE DUCT

Specific Details of the Procedure

In 12 to 15 per cent of patients the transcystic duct approach cannot be used. There are several anatomic reasons for this. Stones that are in the common hepatic or left or right hepatic ducts usually cannot be accessed through the cystic duct. Cystic duct anatomy may make transcystic exploration impossible. Examples include a low insertion of the cystic duct, a spiral cystic duct, a small cystic duct that will not allow negotiation of either a guide wire or a balloon dilating catheter, and obliteration of the cystic duct. In these patients direct laparoscopic common bile duct exploration should be considered.

For direct laparoscopic common bile duct exploration, we use at least one additional trocar site in the left upper outer quadrant at the level of the midclavicular line. The cystic duct is held laterally, and the peritoneum overlying the anterior common duct wall is dissected. We visualize at least 2 cm of common duct for adequate exposure (Fig. 41-5). Small vessels coursing over the top of the common duct are coagulated with a bipolar electrocautery hook. Additional retractors, such as the Solos fan retractor, can be used to improve exposure of the porta hepatis. With the cystic duct being held laterally, the needle electrocautery is placed through the subxiphoid trocar, and a small incision is made along the anterior common duct wall with the cutting current. Once a 1- to 2-mm hole is made in the common duct, a Potts scissors is placed through the subxiphoid trocar, and the choledochotomy is lengthened to 7 to 10 mm.

With the initial opening of the common duct, the laparoscopic team should be able to retrieve common bile duct stones. Frequently a number of stones will percolate out of the choledochotomy; a grasping forceps should be ready to retrieve them. A 9-French choledochoscope can then be used for choledochoscopy. If the duct is over 1 cm in width, one should consider using the larger, 4.5-mm choledochoscope, which has a large, 2-mm working channel.

The choledochoscopic evaluation is then performed. Initially the distal duct is examined. Following that examination, the proximal duct is visualized. If large stones are present a 4.5-French Segura basket is used for stone withdrawal. The 4.0- and 4.5-mm three- and four-prong graspers are also used. If necessary, the ampulla of Vater can be dilated as was described for transcystic duct exploration.

Closure

At the conclusion of the common bile duct exploration a 12- or 14-French T-tube is fashioned. It is then placed through the subxiphoid trocar. The entire T-tube is placed into the abdominal cavity. Using the additional left upper quadrant trocar, the T-tube is seated into the common duct. We use 3-0 or 4-0 suture, which is placed through the subxiphoid trocar. The common duct is then sutured using intracorporeal suturing techniques. The T-tube is sutured securely, so that the choledochotomy is completely closed around this tube. The end of the T-tube is then temporarily clipped. The cystic duct is transected, and the gallbladder is removed through the subumbilical trocar (Fig. 41-6). A 19-French Jackson-Pratt drain is placed through the subxiphoid trocar into Morison's pouch, as was described for the transcystic technique (Fig. 41-7). The T-tube is then grasped through the midclavicular trocar and sutured to the skin. A gentle curve is allowed on the inside of the abdomen to make sure there is no tension against the choledochotomy.

A final T-tube cholangiogram is then performed. This study ensures that there are no additional common bile duct stones and that there has been no trauma or perforation of the common bile duct and shows that the choledochotomy has been closed adequately without evidence of extravasation. The pneumoperitoneum is evacuated.

464 Techniques of Laparoscopic Surgery

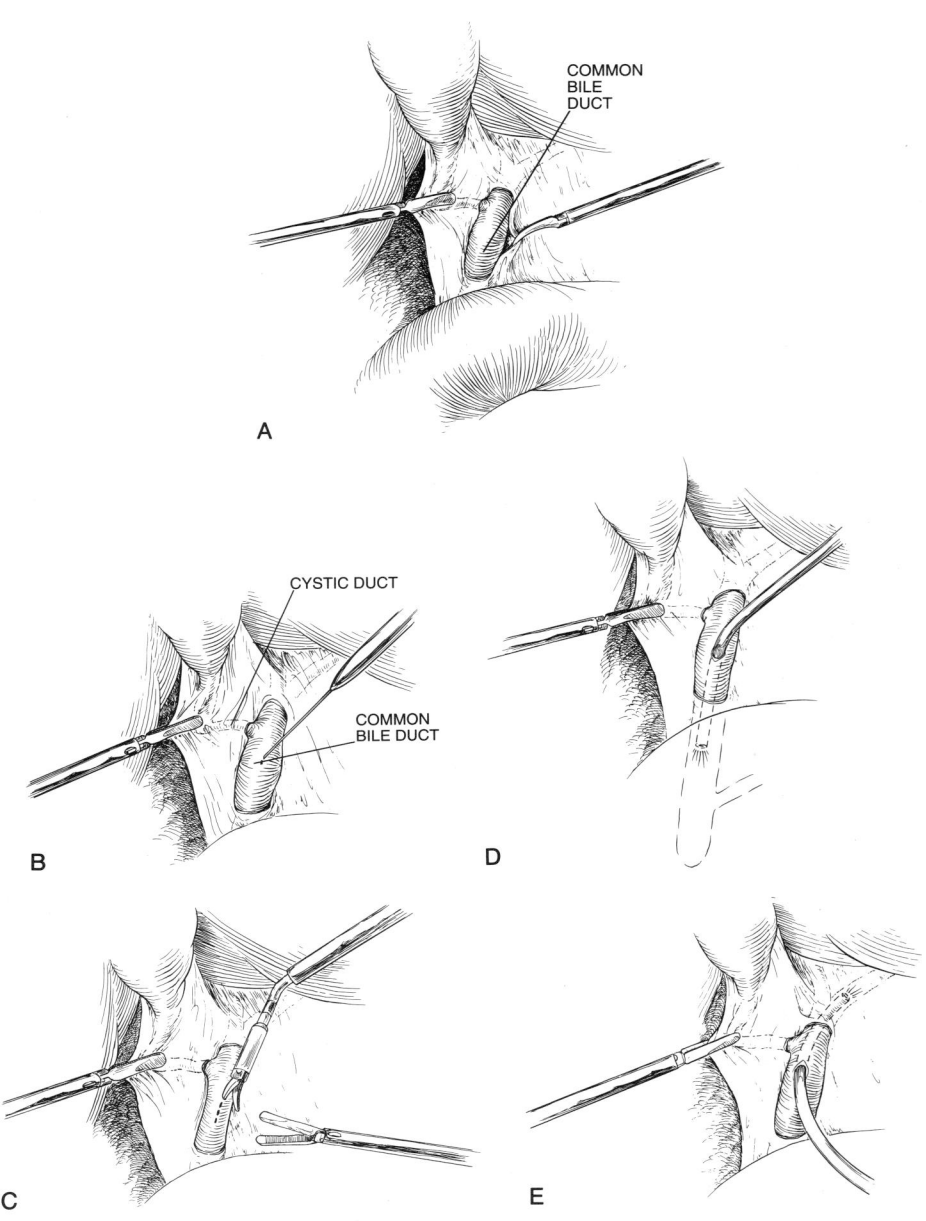

Figure 41-5.

Exploration of the Common Bile Duct 465

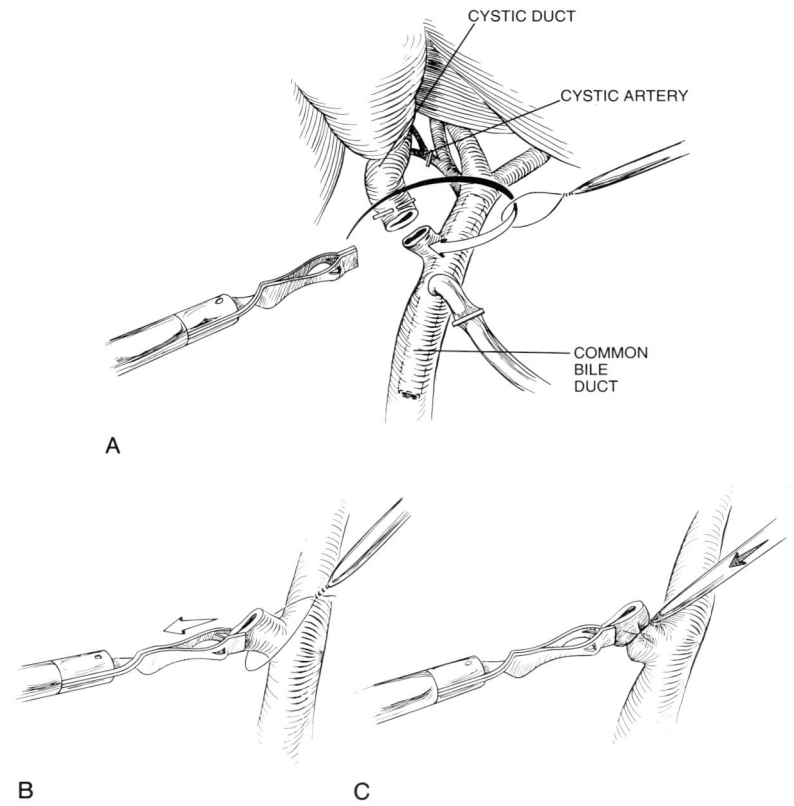

Figure 41-6.

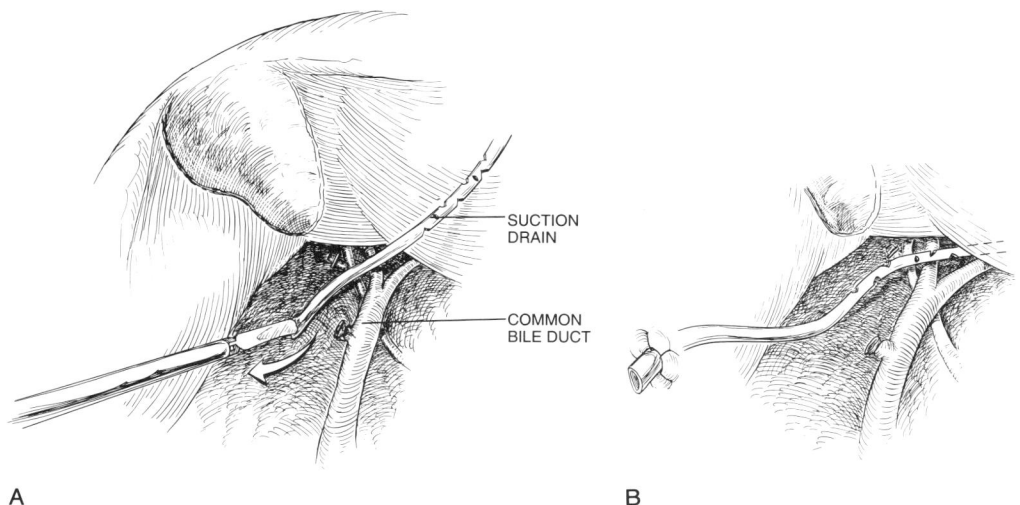

Figure 41-7.

Post-operative Management

The patient is transferred to the ward. A liquid diet is begun in 12 to 24 hours. These patients also require additional pain medication and their recoveries are more prolonged than for those patients who have undergone laparoscopic cholecystectomy only.

Criteria for Patient Discharge

The patients who have had direct laparoscopic common bile duct exploration require additional hospitalization. The patient is discharged on the 3 to 5 postoperative day, after a T-tube cholangiogram. If results of the cholangiogram are satisfactory, the Jackson-Pratt catheter is removed.

Summary

Laparoscopic common bile duct exploration is a safe and effective method of dealing with common bile duct stones discovered during laparoscopic cholecystectomy. Most patients with these stones will have no preoperative evidence of their presence. A careful review of a well performed cholangiogram dictates the approach—transcystic or direct. Alternative treatments include open surgical bile duct exploration, expectant treatment, and treatment by postoperative endoscopic retrograde cholangiopancreatography. We feel these are becoming less desirable as the experience with laparoscopic duct exploration increases. As with any new procedure, the judgment, skill, and limitations of the operative team viewed in the context of patient safety are the guiding principles.

BIBLIOGRAPHY

Berci G, Hamlin JA, Daykhovsky L, et al. Common bile duct laser lithotripsy. GI Endosc 1990; 36:137–139.

Braghetto A, et al. Treatment of residual common bile duct stones after cholecystectomy. Hepato-gastroenterology 1989; 36:123–127.

Cuscllieri A. Results of transcystic common bile duct exploration: The European experience. Presented at the Royal College of Surgeons, London, March 16, 1991.

Gadacz TR. Reoperation versus alternatives in retained biliary calculi. Surg Clin North Am 1991; 71:93–108.

Hart R, Classen M. Complications of diagnostic gastrointestinal endoscopy. Endoscopy 1990; 22:229–233.

Heinerman MP, Pimpl W. Selective ERCP and preoperative stone removal in bile duct surgery. Ann Surg 1989; 209:267–272.

Meador JH, Nowzaradan Y, Matzelle W. Laparoscopic cholecystectomy. South Med J 1991; 84:186–189.

Petelin JB. Laparoscopic approach to common duct pathology. Surg Laparosc Endosc 1991; 1:33–41.

Ponchon T, Bory R, Chavaillon A. Biliary lithiasis: Combined endoscopic and surgical treatment. Endoscopy 1989; 21:15–18.

Ponsky JL, et al. Endoscopic retrograde cholangiography: An adjunct to endoscopic exploration of the common bile duct. Am Surg 1990; 56:235–237.

Sackier J, Berci G, Phillips E, et al. The role of cholangiography in laparoscopic cholecystectomy. Arch Surg 1991; 126:1021–1026.

Scheeres DE. Endoscopic retrograde cholangiopancreatography in a general surgery practice. Am Surg 1990; 56:185–191.

Spaw AT, Reddick EJ, Olsen DO. Laparoscopic laser cholecystectomy: Analysis of 500 procedures. Surg Laparosc Endosc 1991; 1;2–7.

Swanstrom L, Sangster W. Laparoscopic management of common bile duct stones. Presented at the British Columbia Surgical Society, Vancouver, BC, May 10, 1991.

Chapter 42
Placement of a Feeding Jejunostomy

David M. Ota
Douglas B. Evans
Paul F. Mansfield

The enteral route is the most cost effective and least complicated method to provide nutrition to a patient who has a functional intestinal tract but cannot be adequately nourished by mouth.[1] Access for enteral nutrition can be achieved by placing a feeding tube in the stomach or proximal jejunum. This is usually done by passing a tube through the nose into the stomach. It can also be done by endoscopic techniques such as percutaneous endoscopic gastrostomy or under fluoroscopic guidance. These procedures are done with intravenous sedation and local anesthesia in an outpatient setting but are successful only if the upper gastrointestinal tract is open.

GENERAL CONSIDERATIONS FOR FEEDING TUBE PLACEMENT

Patient Selection

Obstruction of the esophagus, stomach, or duodenum can preclude placing feeding tubes with these methods. The strictures can be related to inflammatory or neoplastic processes. Inflammatory causes include corrosive esophagitis, radiation therapy, autoimmune diseases, and reflux. Neoplastic diseases include primary esophageal malignancies, locally invasive thoracic malignancies, and gastric, duodenal, and pancreatic malignancies. When significant strictures are present in the upper intestinal tract, endoscopic or fluoroscopic procedures to provide enteral access may not be feasible, and a laparotomy under general anesthesia may be necessary for placing a feeding tube into either the stomach or proximal jejunum.

The development of laparoscopic technology has significantly increased the capability of performing abdominal procedures with minimally invasive techniques and feeding tubes can now be placed into the upper gastrointestinal tract without a formal laparotomy. The advantages of the laparoscopic procedure over open laparotomy include (1) reduced patient discomfort, (2) faster recovery, (3) placement in an outpatient setting, and (4) reduced costs. Laparoscopic feeding gastrostomy and jejunostomy tubes can be used in patients who require palliative treatment for advanced malignancy or who were receiving preoperative therapy for locally advanced esophageal, gastric, duodenal, or pancreatic carcinomas. The gastrostomy tube is preferred if the duodenum and distal stomach are not involved with tumor.

Another advantage of laparoscopy in placing the feeding tubes is the ability to further stage gastric, duodenal, and pancreatic carcinomas. If there is no evidence of systemic or peritoneal metastasis, our current strategy for upper gastrointestinal-pancreatic tumors is to treat these patients preoperatively with chemotherapy or chemoradiation therapy.[2,3] Because these malignancies can spread to the peritoneal cavity, we routinely inspect the peritoneal surface laparoscopically before beginning preoperative therapy. If suspicious implants are seen, a biopsy is taken. If no implants are seen, peritoneal washings for cytologic examination are done. If there is a recent history of weight loss and early satiety, the appropriate feeding tube is placed during the laparoscopic procedure. This is necessary because systemic chemotherapy or chemoradiation therapy often accentuates nutritional problems, which can become a rate-limiting factor in completing a planned course of therapy.

Pre-operative Preparation

No specific preparations are required for this procedure.

Equipment

The instrumentation for this procedure is widely available. The laparoscopic instruments for a cholecystectomy, such as graspers, can be used for this procedure. A 16- or 18-French Silastic Foley catheter can be used for a gastrostomy tube. The tip of the catheter should be cut to create an end lumen. This should be done carefully such that the lumen to the balloon is not severed. The balloon is needed to secure the tube in the stomach. A feeding jejunostomy tube can be made from a 12-French Silastic nasogastric feeding tube. The tube is cut to a length of 40 cm.

Positioning of the Patient

The patient is placed supine on the operating table and dropped into the Trendelenburg position. A nasogastric tube and urinary catheter are inserted.

Positioning of the Video Equipment

Use of two video monitors facilitates the performance of these procedures. The two monitors are placed in the standard positions for laparoscopic cholecystectomy: one on the right side of the patient and one on the left. This allows easy observation of the monitors by both the surgeon and his assistant.

FEEDING JEJUNOSTOMY

Trocar Placement and Size Selection

After induction of general endotracheal anesthesia, a carbon dioxide pneumoperitoneum is established through a Veress needle inserted in the infraumbilical position. Once adequate pressure is generated, the needle is replaced with a 10-mm port for the videolaparoscope; 5-mm ports are placed in the right and left upper quadrants (Fig. 42-1). A third 5-mm trocar is eventually inserted in the midline half way between the xiphoid process and the umbilicus. This is used to assist in the delivery of the loop of jejunum.

Methods of Exposure and Retraction

The fundamental basis for placing a feeding jejunostomy tube laparoscopically is identifying the ligament of Treitz. Once this is done, the jejunostomy tube can be easily

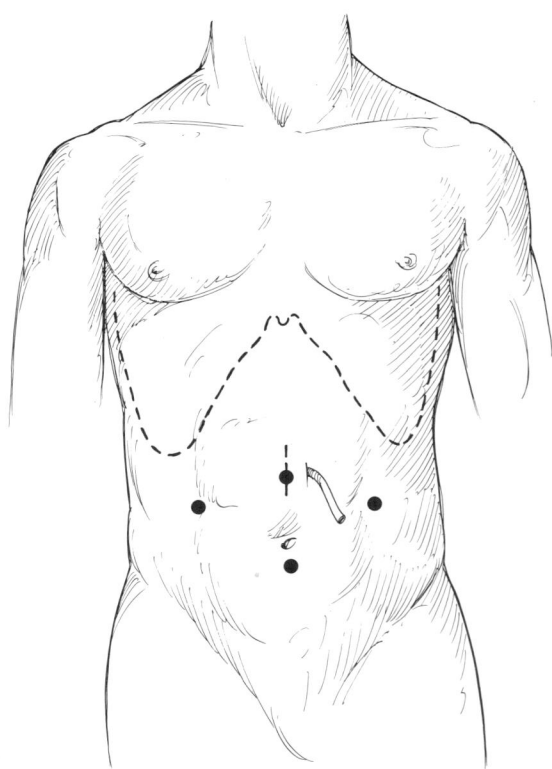

Figure 42-1.

placed in the proximal jejunum. Graspers are inserted into the abdomen through the 5-mm ports in the right and left upper quadrants (Fig. 42-1). The greater omentum is usually draped over the small bowel. If previous abdominal procedures have been done, the omentum may be adherent to the anterior parietal peritoneum or pelvis and with careful dissection, these adhesions can be taken down using laparoscopic dissecting scissors and electrocautery. The greater omentum is then grasped and moved cephalad over the transverse colon. This usually requires sequential grasping, retracting, and releasing with the two graspers.

Specific Details of the Procedure

The midtransverse colon is held up, exposing the inferior leaf of the mesocolon. The other grasper is used to trace the small intestine to the base of the transmesocolon. The ligament of Treitz is identified, and at approximately 15 cm from the ligament of Treitz a loop of jejunum is selected. Next the feeding tube is placed in the upper abdomen to the left of the midline (Fig. 42-2). This is accomplished by a modified Seldinger technique involving a needle, guide wire, dilators, and a peel-away sheath. The entry point of the tube should be 1 to 2 cm lateral to the midline.

A 3-cm midline upper abdominal skin incision is made. A 5-mm port is placed in the middle of this incision, and a grasper is introduced through this port. The feeding tube is brought out through the midline incision using the grasper. The 5-mm port and grasper are reintroduced into the abdomen, and the proximal jejunum is transferred to this mid-

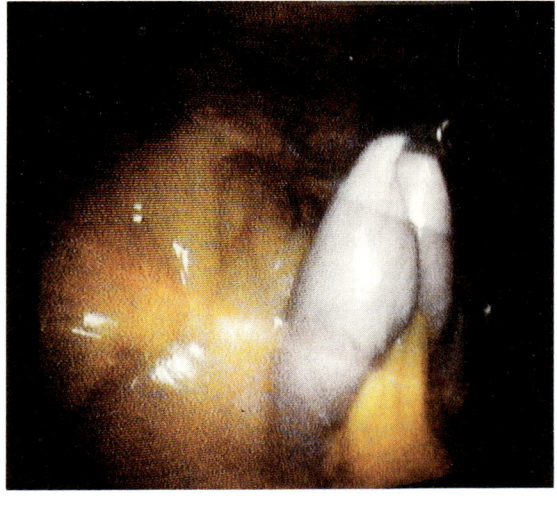

Figure 42-3.

line grasper (Fig. 42-3). The midline fascia is opened about 3-cm. The peritoneum is carefully opened releasing the carbon dioxide. The loop of jejunum is brought up with the grasper and a standard Babcock clamp is used to hold the jejunum. The loop is exteriorized, and a standard Witzel feeding jejunostomy tube is placed (Fig. 42-4). A 3-0 silk purse-string suture is placed on the antimesenteric side of the bowel. A small enterotomy is made, and 15 to 20 cm of the 12-French Silastic tube is gently placed into the distal limb. The purse-string is tied, and a serosal tunnel is created around the tube using interrupted 3-0 silk (Fig. 42-5). The tube is secured to the exit of the serosal tunnel with a 3-0 absorbable suture to prevent the tube from backing out. The jejunal loop is gently

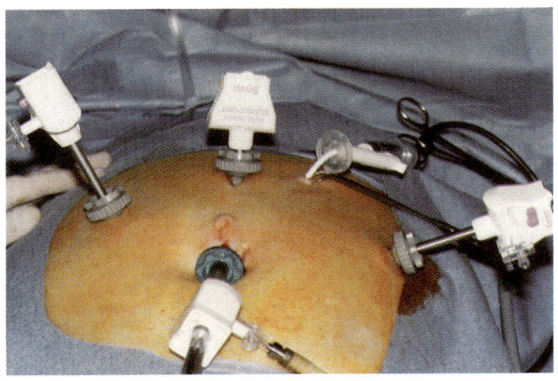

Figure 42-2.

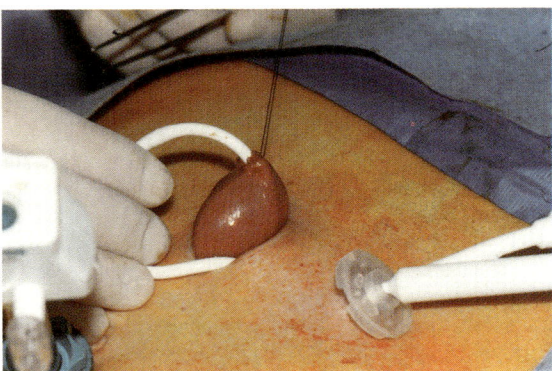

Figure 42-4.

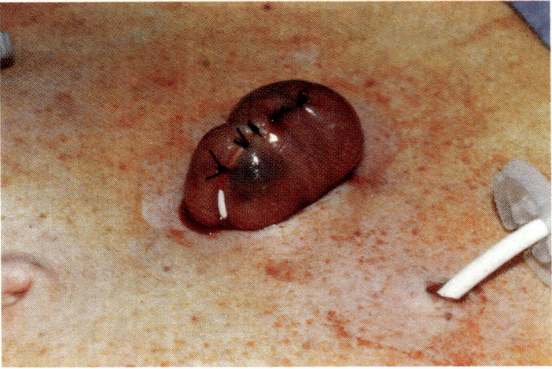

Figure 42-5.

pushed back into the abdominal cavity, and the jejunostomy tube is secured to the anterior abdominal wall. This is done through the small midline incision and can be done because the feeding tube enters the abdominal cavity adjacent to the incision.

Closure

The fascia is reapproximated with appropriate sutures. The skin edges are brought together, and the feeding tube is secured to the skin with a nonabsorbable suture. The other port sites are then closed.

Post-operative Management

The patient is taken to the recovery room and can be discharged from the recovery room with Tylenol-codeine elixir via the feeding tube for pain control. Tube feedings and care of the jejunostomy tube site can be done in the outpatient setting. Intermittent gravity feedings through a gastrostomy tube are usually well tolerated and much simpler than continuous feeding. A feeding jejunostomy usually requires an ambulatory feeding pump.

FEEDING GASTROSTOMY TUBE

Specifics of the Procedure

A feeding gastrostomy tube can be placed in a similar way. The patient is placed in a supine, flat position. After general anesthesia and carbon dioxide insufflation have been obtained, an infraumbilical port is placed for the videolaparoscope. Once the greater curvature of the stomach is identified, a 5-mm port is placed through a 3-cm upper midline incision (Fig. 42-6). A grasper is placed through this port, and the distal stomach along the greater curvature is held. The fascia and peritoneum are opened around the port, and the stomach is exteriorized in a manner similar to bringing the jejunum through a small incision for a feeding jejunostomy. Once the stomach has been brought up through the incision, a standard Babcock clamp is used to hold the stomach. A 3-0 silk purse-string suture is placed and the 16- or 18-French Silastic Foley catheter is inserted through a gastrotomy. The balloon is inflated, and the purse-string suture is secured. The gastrostomy tube is wrapped with a serosal tunnel using interrupted 3-0 silk sutures completing a Witzel gastrostomy tube. The gastrostomy tube is secured to the exit tunnel with a 3-0 absorbable suture. The gastrostomy site is secured to the anterior abdominal peritoneum.

It is likely that these procedures will undergo future modifications such that the Witzel jejunostomy and gastrostomy tube can be placed intracorporeally using laparoscopic suturing techniques.

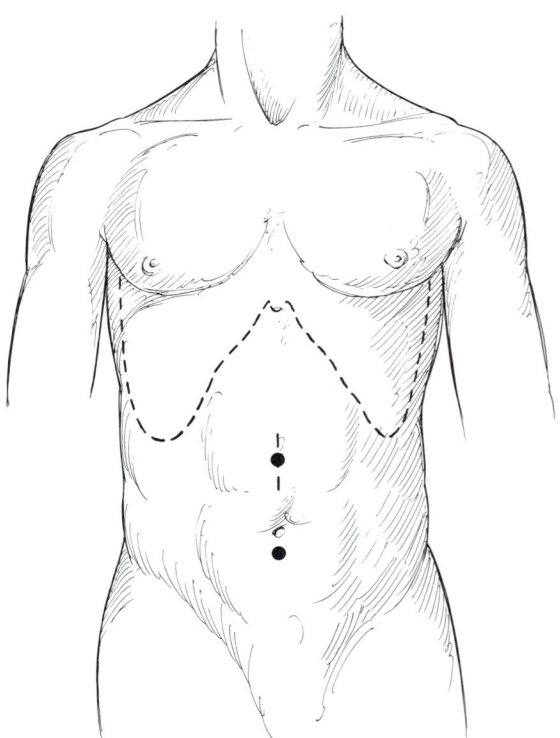

Figure 42-6.

Closure

The fascia and skin are reapproximated around the tube, which is then secured to the skin. The videolaparoscope port is removed, and the skin edge is closed. Recovery from this procedure is similar to that for the feeding jejunostomy tube.

Complications

We have placed these tubes in 15 patients laparoscopically with minimal complications perioperatively. Currently, the laparoscopic approach is used to place feeding jejunostomy and gastrostomy tubes, and if any difficulties are encountered with laparoscopy, an open laparotomy is performed.

ROUX-EN-Y FEEDING JEJUNOSTOMY

Patient Selection

Occasionally a permanent feeding stoma is needed for chronic strictures of the upper gastrointestinal tract. With the development of laparoscopic staplers a Roux-en-Y feeding jejunostomy can be made through small laparoscopic incisions.

Trocar Placement

Once the infraumbilical laparoscopic video port is placed, additional ports are placed in the left and right upper quadrants. A 12-mm SURGIPORT* is required in the left upper quadrant for passage of the ENDO GIA 30* stapling device.

Specific Details of the Procedure

The proximal jejunum at the ligament of Treitz is identified as previously described. A laparoscopic ENDO GIA 30* stapling device is introduced through the left port. The bowel is transected intracorporeally about 15 to 20 cm from the ligament of Treitz. The distal end is held by the right grasper while the left grasper is "walked" 50 cm down the distal limb. This point is identified and held by the left grasper while the incision around the left port is enlarged. The fascia, muscle, and peritoneum are opened, and the distal limb is exteriorized and grasped with a standard Babcock clamp. Then, the distal jejunum and Babcock clamp are dropped into the abdominal cavity.

The proximal jejunal end is located in the abdomen by closing the incision with two or three fingers and using the laparoscope. The pneumoperitoneum is reestablished. The proximal end is held by the right grasper and moved to the left abdominal incision. The distal end is transferred from the right grasper to another standard Babcock clamp introduced through the left incision. Both Babcock clamps with bowel are pulled out of the abdominal cavity. The forks of a GIA stapler are inserted into an enterostomy in the proximal end of the jejunum and the antimesenteric side of the distal loop of jejunum. An end-to-side anastomosis is constructed forming the Roux limb. The stapler is fired, and the common enterotomy is closed extracorporeally using a running 3-0 Vicryl suture. This Roux-en-Y anastomosis is dropped into the peritoneal cavity.

Closure

The incision may have to be closed momentarily with fingers or hand. The abdomen is reinsufflated with carbon dioxide to locate the distal end with the videolaparoscope. The distal end is brought out, and the incision is closed around the bowel. The stapled end is cut, and the stoma is matured. All ports are removed, and the skin is closed.

Post-operative Management

Feedings through the stoma can be started 24 hours after the operation.

Summary

Advances in laparoscopic instruments offer an opportunity to reduce the stress and postoperative recovery time associated with abdominal surgery. The feeding jejunostomy and gastrostomy tube placement and the Roux-en-Y feeding jejunostomy are procedures that can be done with laparoscopic technology and replaces the standard open laparotomy technique. As the instrumentation improves, the extracorporeal aspects of these procedures may be eliminated and the entire procedure will be done within the abdominal cavity.

REFERENCES

1. Ota DM, Kleman K, Diamond K. Practical considerations in the nutritional management of the cancer patient. Cur Probl Cancer 1986; 10:345–398
2. Ajani JA, Ota DM, Jessup JM, Ames FC, et al. Resectable gastric carcinoma: an evaluation of pre- and postoperative chemotherapy. Cancer 1991; 68:1501–1506.
3. Evans DB, Rich TA, Byrd DR, Ames FC. Adenocarcinoma of the pancreas: Current management of resectable and locally advanced disease. South Med J 1991; 84:566–570.

Chapter 43
Small Bowel Resection

Nathaniel J. Soper

Totally intracorporeal methods of laparoscopic resection of hollow viscera have been limited by the difficulty of extracting large organs through small incisions. This problem has recently been solved by application of a nylon entrapment sack and automatic electric tissue morcellator, which has been used for the removal of kidneys[1] and uterine fibromata. With the development of this technology, it became possible to remove segments of bowel through 1-cm incisions.

PATIENT SELECTION

Indications for small bowel resection are limited, but include benign and malignant tumors of the small bowel, small intestinal diverticula including Meckel's diverticulum, limited segments of inflammatory bowel disease (Crohn's), and arteriovenous malformations localized to the small bowel. All patients with these conditions would be potential candidates for laparoscopic small bowel resection except for those who would not be candidates for laparoscopy under general anesthesia. This group would include patients with multiple previous operations and a suspected "frozen abdomen," those who are not candidates for a general anesthetic, patients with generalized peritonitis, an uncorrectable coagulopathy, or severe portal hypertension with extensive collateralization within the abdominal cavity.

PREOPERATIVE EVALUATION

The patient should be evaluated using standard diagnostic techniques. In most cases this would include an abdominal computed tomogram and a barium small bowel follow-through or enteroclysis to obtain accurate information concerning the mucosal surface of the small intestine. For patients with lower gastrointestinal bleeding that is not localized by upper gastrointestinal endoscopy or colonoscopy, a radionuclide red blood cell scan or "Meckel's scan" may demonstrate a bleeding site in the small bowel or the presence of a Meckel's diverticulum. Further evaluation would include a mesenteric arteriogram and if this examination revealed a small intestinal arteriovenous malformation, the catheter could be advanced out into the specific vascular arcade just prior to surgery so the involved segment may be injected with methylene blue for accurate localization at the time of laparoscopy.

PREOPERATIVE PREPARATION

The patient may consume oral clear liquids on the day prior to surgery and nothing by mouth after midnight preceding the operation. To limit the possibility of intra-abdominal contamination from small intestinal chyme, a standard bowel preparation regimen should be administered. This may include the intake of 4 liters of polyethylene glycol solution or magnesium citrate and enemas, as well as nonabsorbed oral antibiotics such as erythromycin base and neomycin. Prophylactic antibiotics should be administered in the perioperative period, usually as a second generation cephalosporin with adequate anaerobic coverage (e.g., cefotetan).

EQUIPMENT

For adequate visualization of the peritoneal cavity, a standard 10-mm laparoscope with attached video camera should be utilized. The laparoscope itself may be either a 0-degree (end-viewing) or 30-degree (fore-oblique). A high intensity xenon light source and video camera with bayonet mount for the laparoscope must be available. A high flow pressure-triggered automatic carbon dioxide insufflator is mandatory. These electronic machines are placed on a cart with one of the video monitors so that they may be protected from damage in the operating room.

Five laparoscopic ports are used, including two 10-mm, one 12-mm, and two 5-mm trocars. Atraumatic grasping forceps should be used to manipulate the bowel. Many instrument companies are now manufacturing laparoscopic forceps with tips that are similar to standard DeBakey forceps, Allis clamps, Babcock clamps, and Glassman clamps. Laparoscopic sutures 3-0 and 4-0 gauge should be available for use during all operations involving the intestines. An automatic clip applier is used for ligation of mesenteric blood vessels. Pre-tied slip knots may also be useful for this purpose. For performance of the laparoscopic anastomosis, a 30-mm ENDO GIA* (United States Surgical Corporation, Norwalk, CT) has been used for rapid and effective creation of intestinal anastomoses.

For entrapment of resected tissue, an impermeable nylon sack with drawstrings at its neck should be available. If the lesion in question does not require accurate histologic tumor staging, an automatic electrical tissue morcellator (Cook Urological, Inc., Spencer, IN) can be used to reduce the resected tissue mass to a size that can easily be removed through an 11-mm incision.

POSITIONING OF THE PATIENT

The patient is placed in either the supine or lithotomy position, and general inhalational anesthesia is induced. A Foley catheter and orogastric tube are placed to decompress the bladder and stomach, respectively. The operating table must be adjustable such that it can be tilted to the patient's left or right and into head down (Trendelenburg) or head up (reverse Trendelenburg) positions.

POSITIONING OF THE VIDEO EQUIPMENT

Two video monitors are utilized, being placed on each side of the patient and angled toward the operating table such that the surgeon and assistant may view the procedure from each side of the operating table without strain. The location of the monitors depends on the anatomic site of the primary operative field. If the lesion is in the distal ileum, the monitors are placed at the foot of the bed, and if the lesion is in the proximal to mid small bowel, the monitors are positioned at the head of the operating table. In this way, the surgeons will be operating in line (coaxially) with their visual orientation; attempts to manipulate instruments toward the camera, thereby creating a mirror image, are usually frustrating.

TROCAR PLACEMENT AND SIZE SELECTION

The initial laparoscopic trocar is placed at the umbilicus for insertion of the videolaparoscope. The technique for insertion should be similar to that for other laparoscopic procedures, performed either in an "open" or "closed" fashion. When trocars are inserted by the open technique, a cut down is made on the peritoneum and a blunt laparoscopic sheath is placed into the peritoneal cavity under direct vision, either by using a Hasson cannula or by first placing fascial purse-string sutures to seal the pneumoperitoneum around a standard laparoscopic sheath. When the closed technique is used, a Veress needle is placed through a small periumbilical skin incision and a pneumoperitoneum is created using carbon dioxide to a pressure of 12 to 15 mm Hg. The needle is then removed and the initial 10/11-mm trocar is introduced using a steady controlled drilling action. After prewarming, the videolaparoscope is inserted into the abdominal cavity, and all subsequent trocars are placed under video guidance. The location of auxiliary trocars depends on the location of the intestinal lesion. For proximal small intestinal lesions, 5-mm trocars are placed in the left upper quadrant and left lower quadrant for tissue manipulation by the assistant, while an 11-mm trocar is placed in the right upper quadrant and a 12-mm incision placed in the right midabdomen (Fig. 43-1). The 5-mm ports are used for the placement of bowel grasping forceps, while the 11-mm trocar is used for the placement of various tissue forceps as well as for introduction of the nylon entrapment sack. The 12-mm trocar is used for insertion of operating instruments and the ENDO GIA* stapler. For lesions localized to the lower abdomen, the trocar positions are reversed.

METHODS OF EXPOSURE AND RETRACTION

The patient's position is varied to allow gravity to expose the segment of bowel in question. For upper abdominal lesions the reverse Trendelenburg position is employed, while lesions in the distal bowel are best exposed using Trendelenburg position. Atraumatic grasping forceps are used to "run" the bowel from the ligament of Treitz to the ileocecal valve. The segment of bowel to be resected is then isolated and pulled up to the anterior abdominal wall using two grasping forceps placed at an appropriate distance from each margin of the lesion (Fig. 43-2). The bowel proximal and distal to this area should be carefully manipulated to ensure that there is no tension interfering with free movement of these segments.

METHODS OF DISSECTION

After elevation of the segment of bowel to be removed between two atraumatic grasping forceps, the mesenteric arcades are examined. The peritoneum over the avascular portions from the bowel wall down to its base are divided using a thermal device. We have used monopolar "hot" cautery scissors (ENDO SHEARS*, United States Surgical Corporation) for this purpose, but bipolar cautery or laser energy may be used. The mesenteric blood vessels themselves are then doubly clipped and divided (Fig. 43-3). The segment of bowel is thus devascularized and isolated between the two grasping forceps.

Specific Details of the Procedure

The bowel is then stapled and divided using a linear cutting stapler, the ENDO GIA*. The stapler is introduced through the 12-mm port, its jaws are opened, and the stapler is placed across the bowel at one of the extremities of the devascularized portion. The jaws of the stapler are then closed and the instrument is fired. The ENDO GIA* is removed and a refill cartridge is loaded prior to insertion of the stapler back into the peritoneal cavity. Another application of the stapler ligates and divides the other end of the isolated segment (Fig. 43-4). The resected specimen is then placed into a remote area of the abdomen where it can be retrieved later, such as on the surface of the liver. Use of this stapling device prevents excessive contamination of the peritoneal cavity by intestinal chyme. If the lesion being removed is suspected to be a malignant tumor, it is placed within the nylon entrapment sack (see later section) prior to proceeding with the anastomosis.

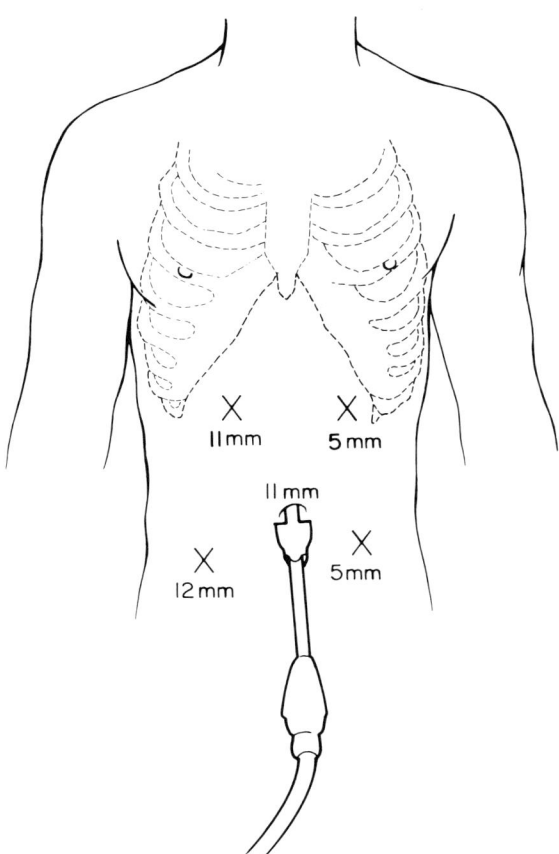

Figure 43-1.

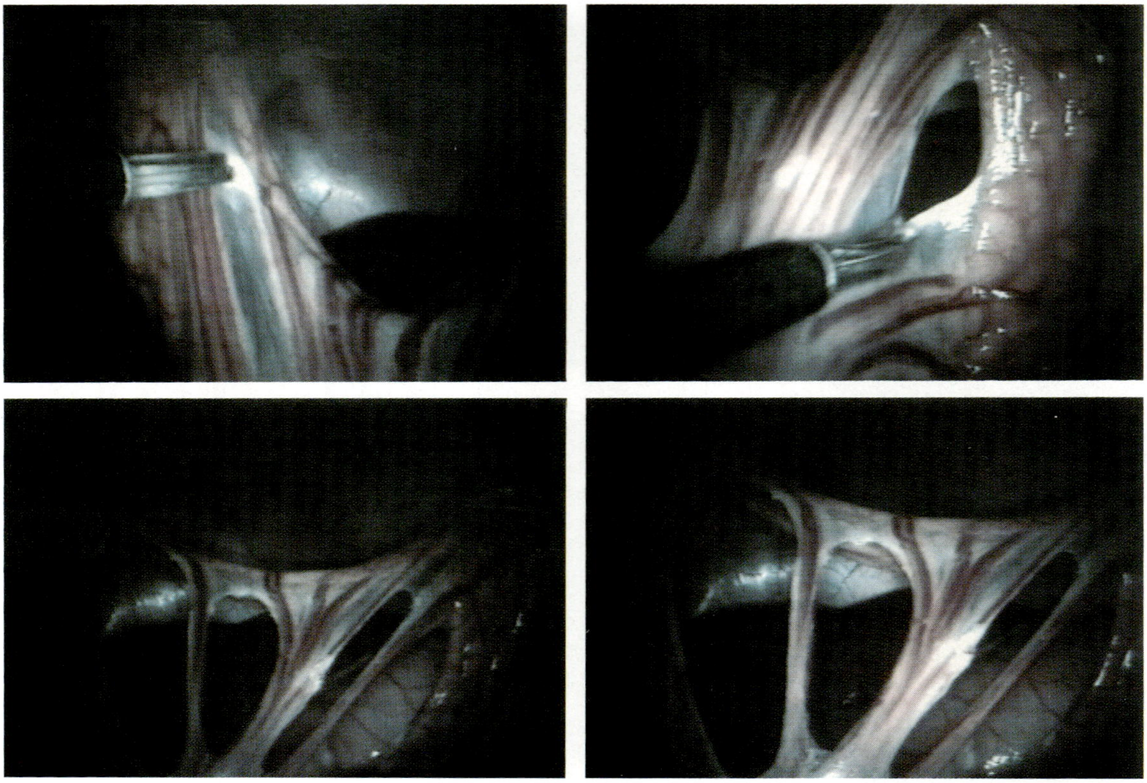

Figure 43-2.

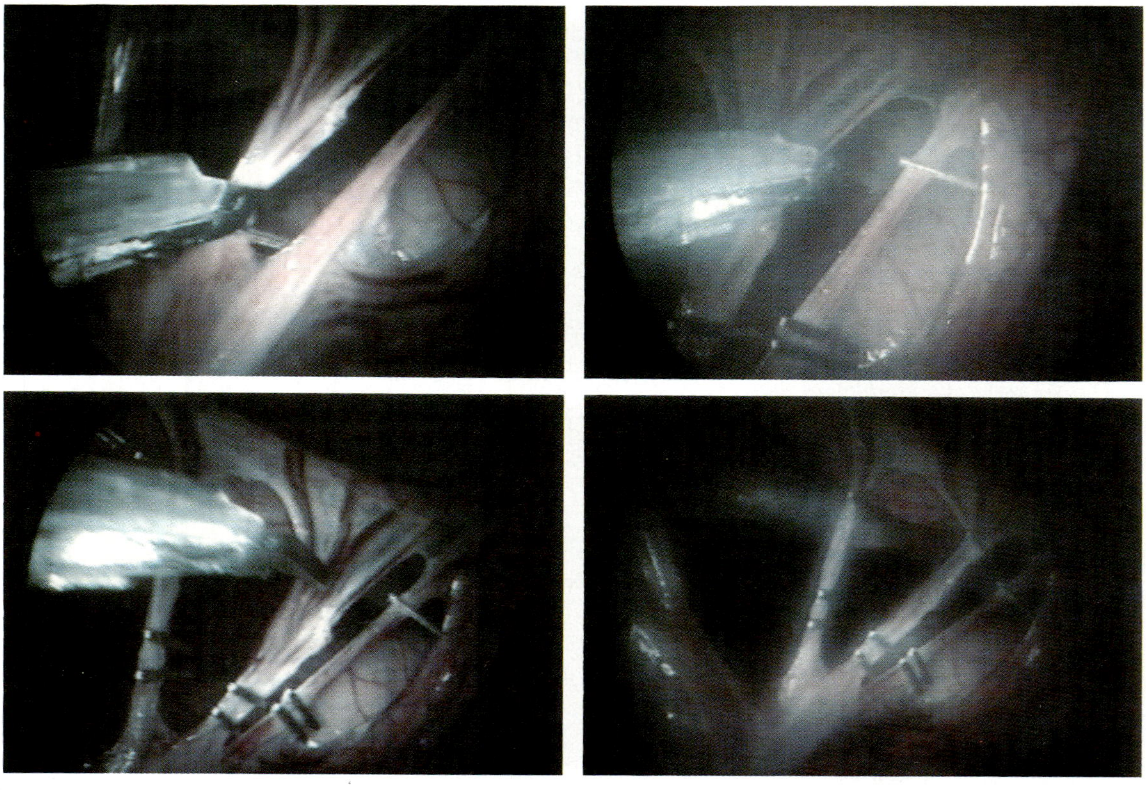

Figure 43-3.

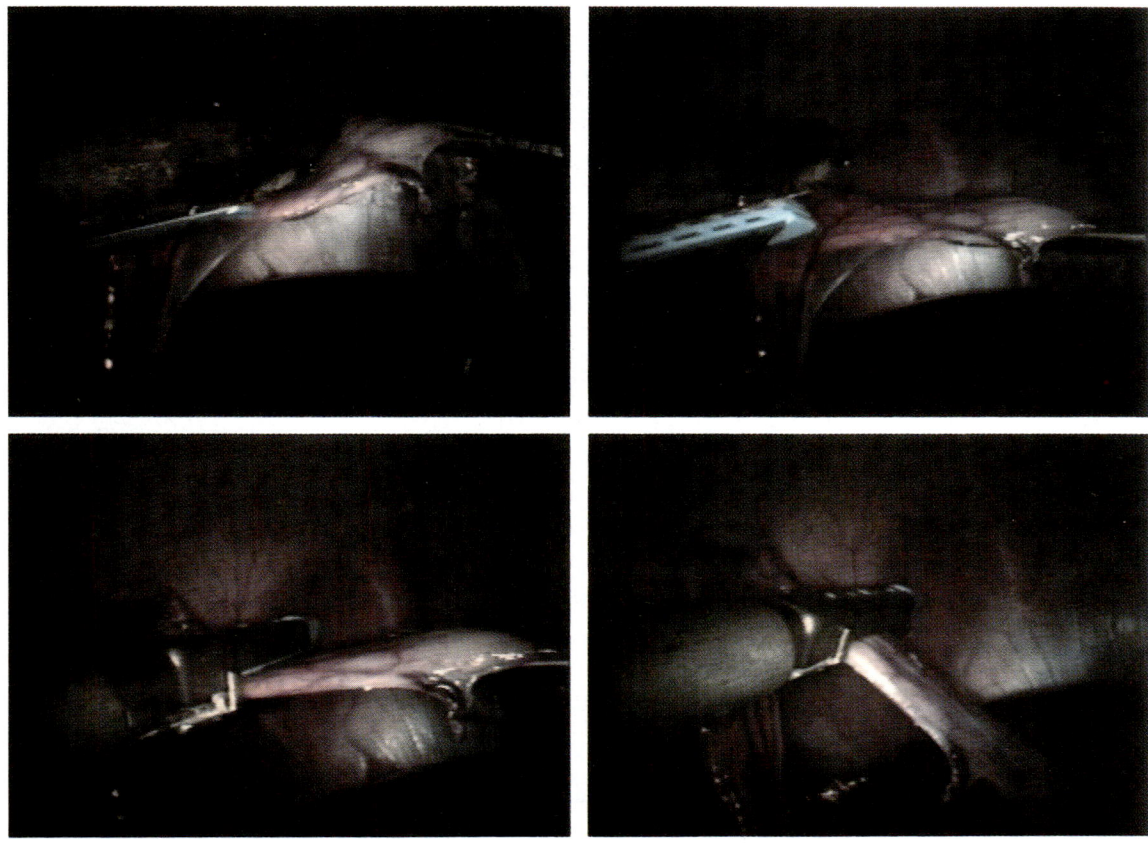

Figure 43-4.

The two bowel ends are then prepared for side-to-side, functional end-to-end anastomosis. The mesenteric corners of each segment of the bowel are brought together using a locking atraumatic bowel forceps, such as an Allis clamp. The antimesenteric corners of the staple lines on each of the segments of bowel are excised, and the piece of tissue is removed through the sheaths (Fig. 43-5). A grasping forceps is then placed into each bowel lumen, and the enterotomy is gently dilated and sized to assure that the stapler jaws will fit into the enterotomies without excessive force. At this point, the grasping forceps holding the mesenteric border of the segments of bowel is drawn posteriorly and toward the camera and the proximal and distal portions of bowel are gently elevated and drawn away from the videolaparoscope to position the intestinal segments for application of the stapler. The stapler is then reloaded and brought into the abdominal cavity. The jaws of the stapler are opened, and one jaw is inserted into each limb of the bowel. The edge of each enterotomy is grasped, and the bowel is gently pulled up over the anvils of the stapler. After the bowel has been brought up to the end of the stapling device, the ENDO GIA* device is closed (Fig. 43-6). The bowel segments are then closely examined to assure that the stapler resides near the antimesenteric borders, and a grasping forceps is placed between the leaves of mesentery to assure that the mesentery is not included within the stapler's jaws. When the surgeon is sure that the bowel is appropriately positioned for anastomosis, the stapler is fired and removed from the bowel segment. Both staple lines are then closely examined for hemostasis while the staple lines are gently everted. Because of concerns that the 30-mm ENDO GIA* device would not create an adequate anastomotic lumen, a second staple line is applied. The ENDO GIA* device is reinserted into the peritoneal cavity, the jaws are opened, and the stapler is inserted into the common enterotomy joining the two limbs of bowel. Each jaw of the

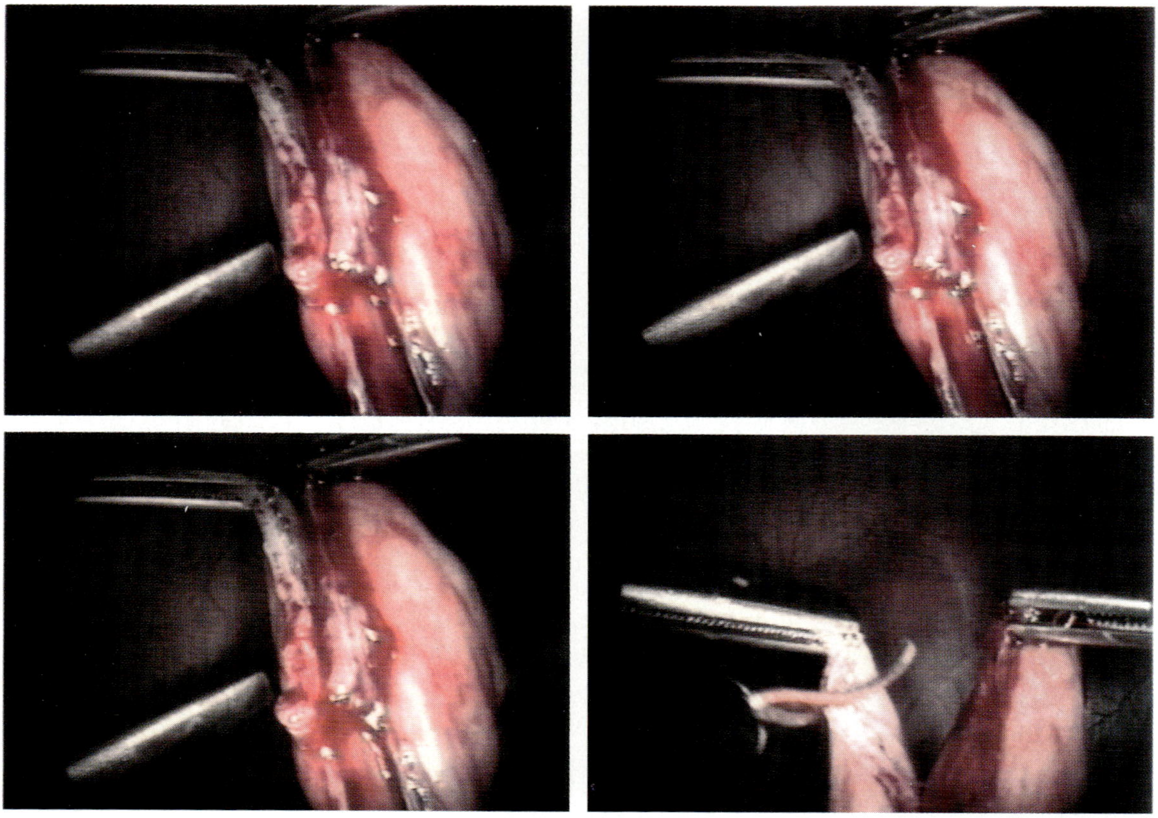

Figure 43-5.

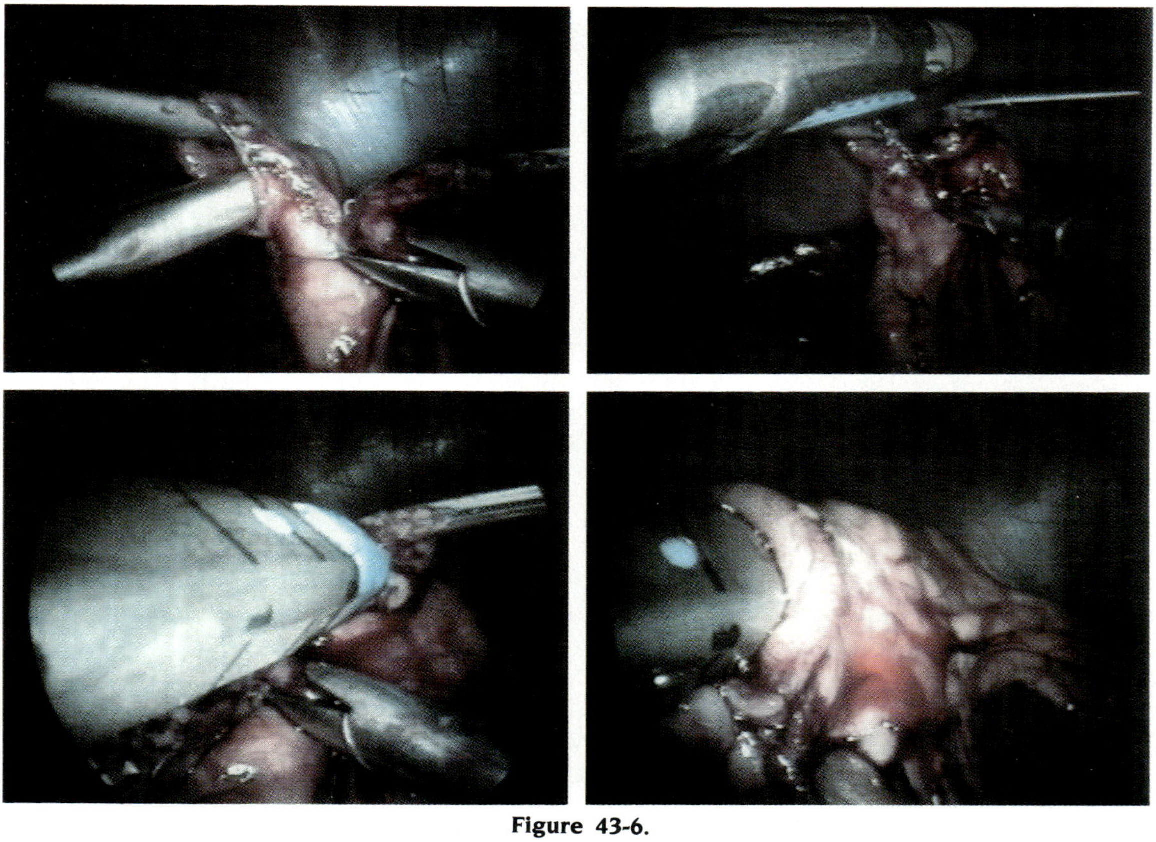

Figure 43-6.

Small Bowel Resection

ENDO GIA* device is inserted into the limbs of bowel, and the bowel is telescoped up over the stapler prior to closing the stapler and firing it for the second time (Fig. 43-7). The same precautions are taken to assure freedom of the mesenteric vasculature. The stapler is then opened and removed from the lumen of the bowel, and the interior aspect of the staple line is once again viewed for hemostasis.

The common enterotomy on the antimesenteric border of the bowel loop must now be closed. We have utilized two more applications of the ENDO GIA* device for this purpose, but the enterotomy could be closed with a single running suture of 3-0 polyglycolic acid suture. For the stapled closure, atraumatic grasping forceps are placed on the corner of each linear staple line so that the staple lines can be distracted to their maximal extent. Another grasping forceps is then placed with one jaw on each side of the enterotomy at its midpoint to approximate the edges with eversion. These forceps are then pulled up toward the anterior abdominal wall, and the ENDO GIA* stapler is brought back into the abdominal cavity, opened, and inserted across the bowel just below the forceps (Fig. 43-8). This usually requires two more applications of the stapler to ensure complete closure of the enterotomy. When the enterotomy is closed using this technique, there is a small amount of discarded tissue from the edges of the enterotomies; this tissue is placed in the upper abdomen with the resected segment of bowel.

Time is then taken to examine the staple lines carefully to assure absence of a defect. The antimesenteric staple line can be clearly viewed and a single absorbable suture may be placed to bridge the two bowel limbs at the end of the staple line for reinforcement. The mesenteric portion of the staple line is viewed by distracting the two limbs of bowel and inserting the laparoscope beneath the loop (Fig. 43-9).

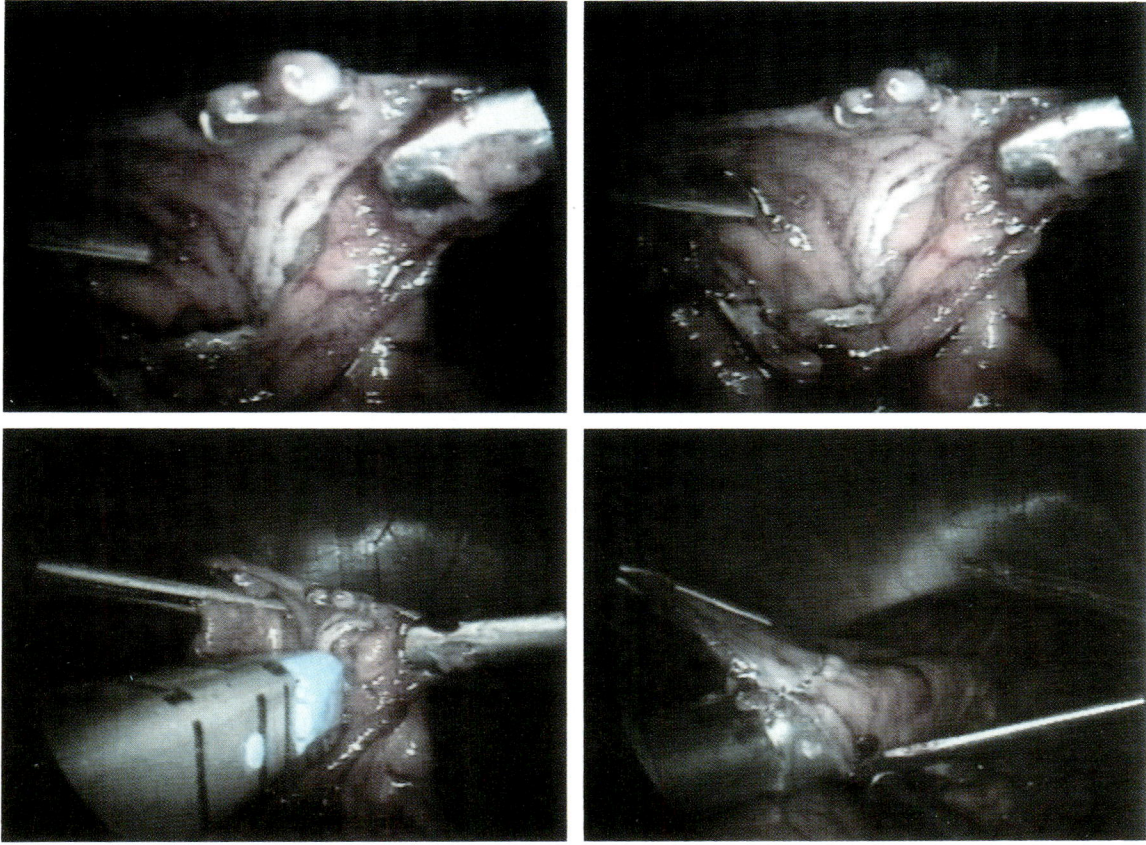

Figure 43-7.

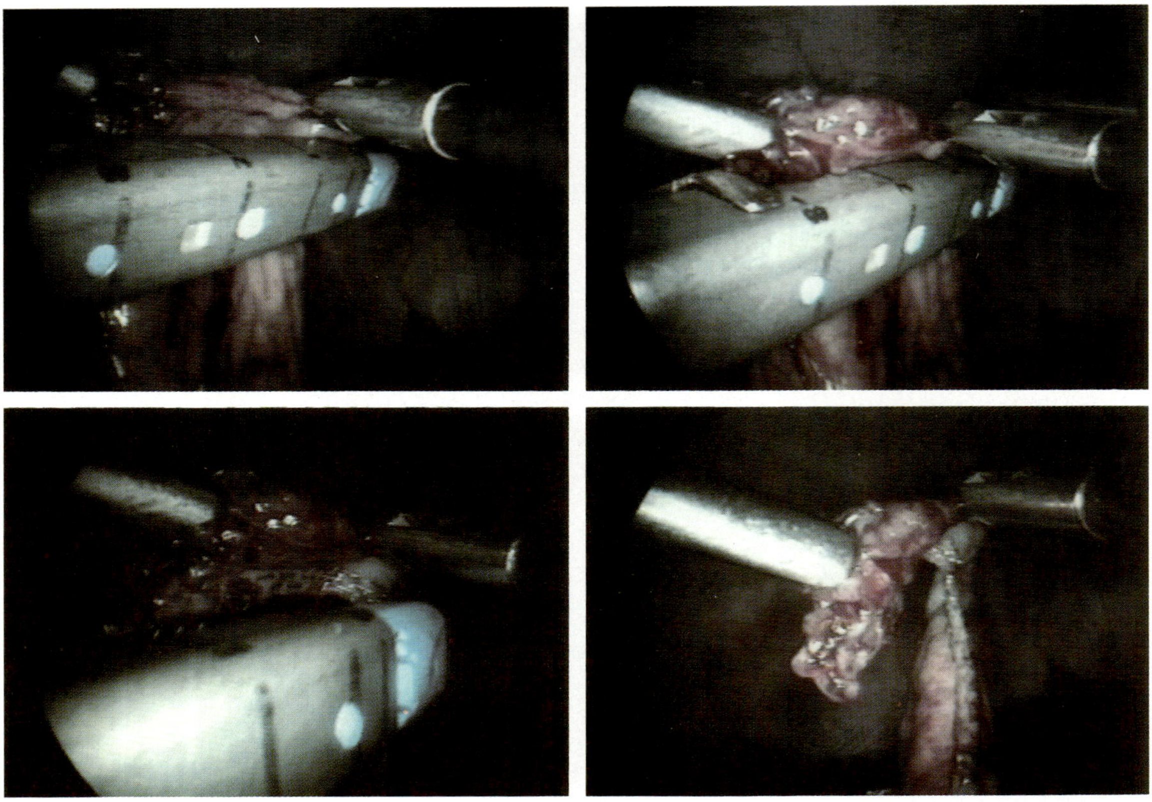

Figure 43-8.

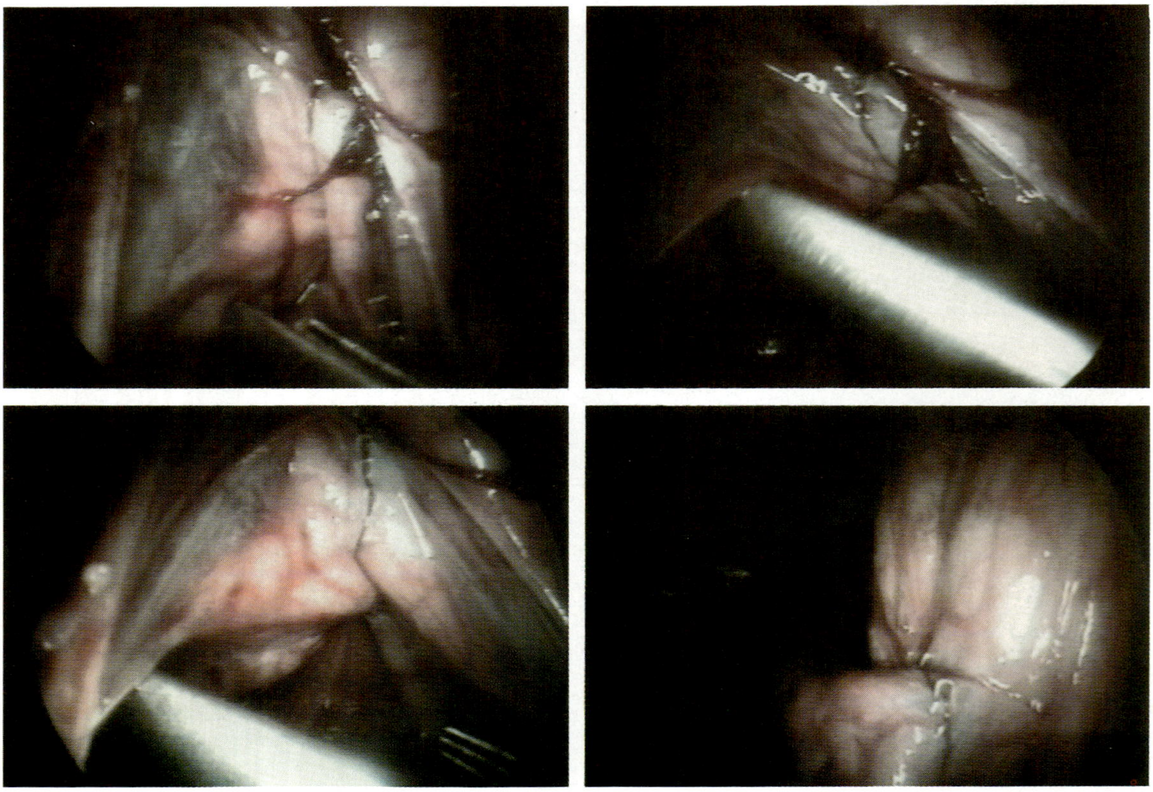

Figure 43-9.

The mesenteric defect is then closed. If there is adequate peritoneum adjacent to the mesenteric blood vessels, the defect may be simply clipped using the automatic clip applier. If the vessels have been skeletonized, great care must be taken while placing interrupted stitches of 3-0 absorbable suture to approximate the two edges of the mesentery.

The excised segment of bowel must now be removed from the peritoneal cavity. An impermeable nylon sack with a drawstring around its neck is prepared by twisting it diagonally into a sheath that fits into the 11-mm laparoscopic trocar. The nylon sack is then inserted into the peritoneal cavity, and the sack is unfolded and its mouth opened using dissecting forceps. The sack is designed with three tabs placed at equidistant points for orientation purposes. The resected specimen and the excess tissue from the enterotomy are then placed into the sack (Fig. 43-10) and the drawstrings are pulled closed. The closed neck of the sack is withdrawn into the 11-mm laparoscopic sheath, and the sheath and the neck of the sack are pulled as a unit onto the anterior abdominal wall. When staging of a resected tumor is important, the specimen is removed intact without morcellation by gently dilating or enlarging the incision around the laparoscopic sheath. With traction on the sack the specimen should be able to be removed through an incision of no more than 2 or 3 cm in length. When the lesion does not require pathologic staging, an automatic electrical tissue morcellator (see earlier) is used to reduce the specimen to small fragments, thereby allowing removal of the sack through the 11-mm incision. The morcellator has a strong vacuum running through it with a filter to catch tissue fragments at the port of egress. It consists of a 10-mm fixed outer sheath with a rotating bit in its center which is used to "drill" the tissue within the sack. With a segment of small bowel between 5 to 15 cm in length the tissue morcellation requires less than 5 minutes to perform. When the specimen has been reduced to a small enough size the sack can

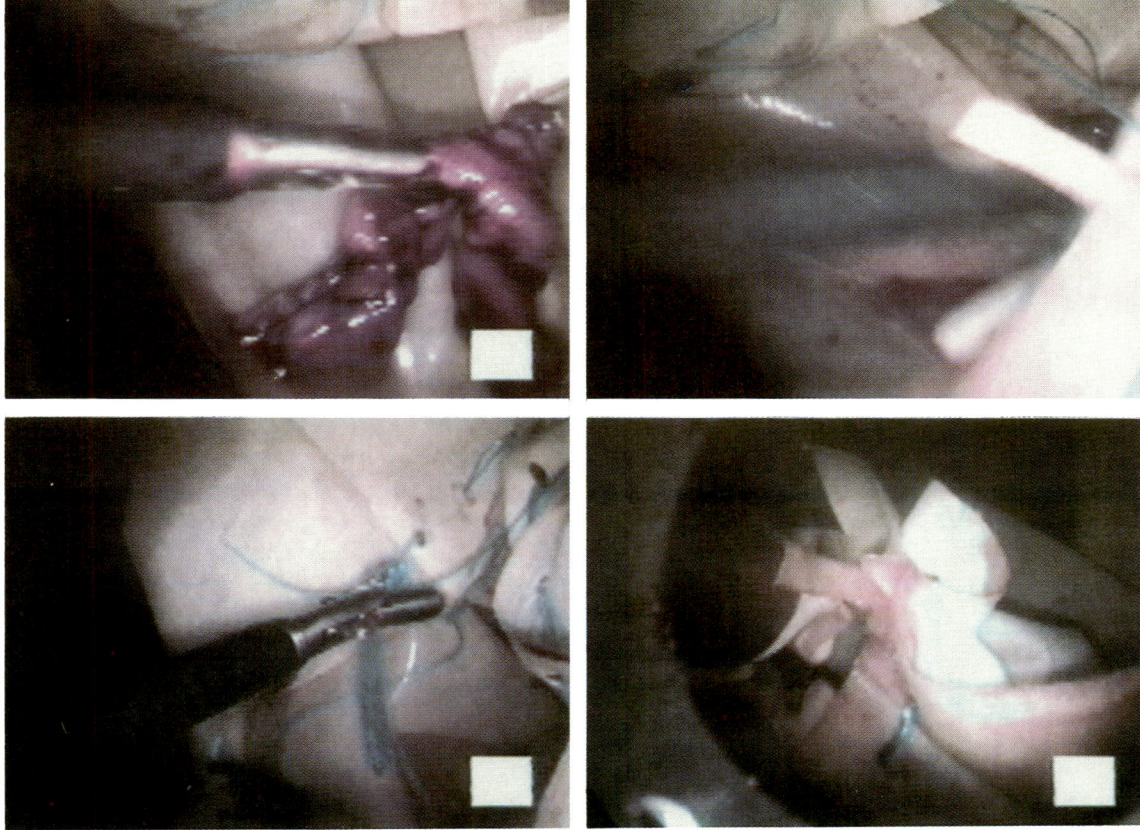

Figure 43-10.

simply be pulled through the abdominal wall (Fig. 43-11).

The entire operative field is then examined for hemostasis, the abdominal cavity is irrigated copiously with saline solution, and the irrigant is removed by aspirating. The external aspects of the staple lines are examined for hemostasis and any small bleeding points are lightly cauterized or ligated.

CLOSURE

After scanning the interior of the abdominal cavity, the entry points of the laparoscopic sheaths are then examined to rule out significant abdominal wall hemorrhage. The carbon dioxide is allowed to escape through the sheaths by opening their valves, and the laparoscope is withdrawn into the umbilical sheath. The sheath is then removed while the entry point under direct vision is evaluated during withdrawal. Each incision is infiltrated down to the peritoneal level with 0.5 per cent bupivacaine and irrigated with saline. The fascia of the large incisions is closed using a single stitch of heavy absorbable suture material, and the skin is reapproximated with adhesive tape.

POSTOPERATIVE MANAGEMENT

The gastric tube and bladder catheter are removed in the operating room prior to extubation. A second dose of intravenous cephalosporin antibiotic is administered on the evening following surgery and then discontinued unless the peritoneal cavity is heavily contaminated by intestinal contents during the operation. The patient is maintained without oral intake overnight and antiemetic agents are administered if necessary. On the morning after the operation, if bowel sounds are present, clear liquids are begun orally, and the diet is advanced to a regular one as tolerated.

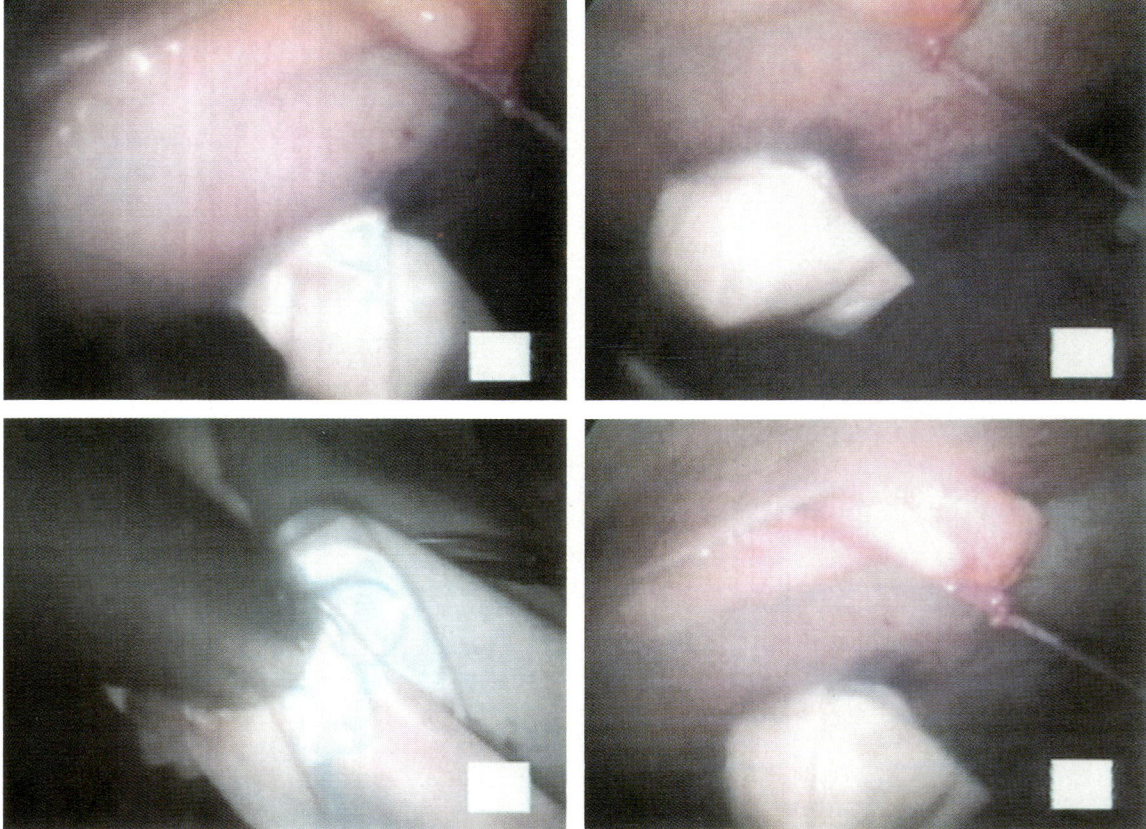

Figure 43-11.

CRITERIA FOR PATIENT DISCHARGE

The patient is discharged when he or she tolerates an oral diet and passes flatus per rectum. This should occur between 48 to 72 hours postoperatively. The patient's abdominal examination must be normal, and blood tests are obtained only if clinical indications exist. The patient is instructed to examine the incisions for evidence of infection and is counseled that he or she may return to full activity as soon as the incisional pain allows. Discharge medications include only oral analgesics as necessary. The patient is examined in the office at 1 week and 1 month postoperatively, and additional follow-up is undertaken if the clinical situation warrants.

COMPLICATIONS SPECIFIC FOR THIS PROCEDURE

As with any laparoscopic procedure, complications of the abdominal puncture and pneumoperitoneum may occur (injury to abdominal wall or intraperitoneal blood vessels, puncture of the bowel, cardiac arrhythmias, or carbon dioxide retention). Complications specific to small bowel resection may occur. Inadequate control of the mesenteric vessels may lead to postoperative hemorrhage. This may be avoided by assuring hemostasis intraoperatively, and if the hemoclips do not appear to control a vessel adequately, an additional ligature may be placed on the vessel, either using a pre-tied slipknot or a suture, which is placed and tied laparoscopically. Leakage of the anastomosis should manifest itself early postoperatively as increasing abdominal pain and signs of peritoneal irritation. A low threshold for repeat laparoscopy or laparotomy must be maintained because of this possibility. Ischemia of the anastomosis may be caused by occlusion of the blood vessels at the margins of the mesenteric arcade during closure of the mesenteric defect or by division of the bowel at a point remote from the site of mesenteric division. Intraoperatively, the edges of the site of bowel resection must be evaluated for appearance and for the presence of pinpoint hemorrhage at the staple lines. In the late postoperative interval, anastomotic stricture is a possibility and, should signs of bowel obstruction exist, a barium small bowel radiograph should be obtained to assess anastomotic patency.

Conclusions

Intracorporeal laparoscopic bowel resection and anastomosis is an operation that may be performed technically at the present time, but the indications for this procedure are not seen frequently. As instrument companies develop longer linear stapling devices, this procedure will be facilitated by allowing a single application of the stapler rather than two applications to ensure an adequate lumen. These techniques may be modified to perform resection of the intra-abdominal colon. Only individuals with broad experience in laparoscopic operations who have developed expertise in intracorporeal suturing or knot tying techniques should attempt these procedures, as failure of the stapled anastomosis may mandate more conventional surgical techniques. With care and patience, intracorporeal laparoscopic small bowel resection should lead to less postoperative discomfort, shorter duration of hospitalization, and more rapid return to full activity than its open counterpart.

REFERENCES

1. Clayman RV, Kavoussi LR, Long SR, et al. Laparoscopic nephrectomy: Initial report of pelviscopic organ ablation in the pig. J Endourol 1990; 4:247–252.
2. Soper NJ, Brunt LM, Fleshman J, Meininger TA, Dunnegan DL. Laparoscopic small bowel resection and anastomosis. Surg Laparosc and Endosc 1993; 3:6–12.

Chapter 44
Lysis of Adhesions

Phillippe Mouret
Charles Gelez[1]

The procedure described in this chapter is different from other procedures described in this book. A laparoscopic procedure is generally a copy of a well known surgical procedure, in its technical aspects as well as the indication for its use. This rule allows us to obtain a similar result after either laparoscopic surgery or after classical open surgery. Thus, we can focus on the laparoscopic technique. This is not true for bandolysis, which is not performed as a primary open surgical technique. Except for the treatment of obstruction and partial obstruction (and some caution in this last example), bandolysis is only an accessory technique for surgical exposure in the classical surgery for resection. In fact, the usual failure of bandolysis for treatment of abdominal pain prevents the use of this technique in most patients. The idea that adhesions could be the reason for abdominal pain is not well recognized by the majority of physicians and surgeons. Therefore, this chapter will present: 1) the definition and technique of bandolysis; 2) the justification for the performance of bandolysis as a therapeutic concept; and 3) methods for the accomplishment and evaluation of this technique.

DEFINITION OF BANDOLYSIS

Bandolysis is defined in relation to abnormal adhesions in the peritoneal cavity. The goal is to recreate the integrity of the peritoneal cavity. Consequently, what is inside the interface between the two peritoneal linings will be removed. Schematically, we can describe two types of adhesions. (1) A membranous adhesion is a vascular, simple filling of the peritoneal space with a neocellular tissue. It is really a sandwich type, however, without any alterations of the peritoneal structure. (2) A dense adhesion is a well organized fibrous tissue vascularized with orientation of the fibers (Fig. 44-1). Often the adhesions, however, have a complex structure, in which both types of adhesions are present (3 and 4). Frequently, large areas of membranous adhesion are found for which the "key of opening" is an adhesion which is well organized and dense. Manhes called this phenomenon "the key of the adhesion." This morphologic definition of adhesion allows us to understand that the surgical technique used for the liberation of the adhesion will be related to dissection and also to section.

TECHNIQUES OF BANDOLYSIS

Dissection

There is no need to explain this technique to the surgeon or to the anatomist for whom this represents the basis of surgical technique. The goal of dissection is to reestablish the anatomical planes. However, laparoscopic surgery presents several peculiarities. Digital dissection, which is the introduction of the tip of the finger inside the anatomical space, be-

---

[1] Bernard Vasseur, M.D., Translator

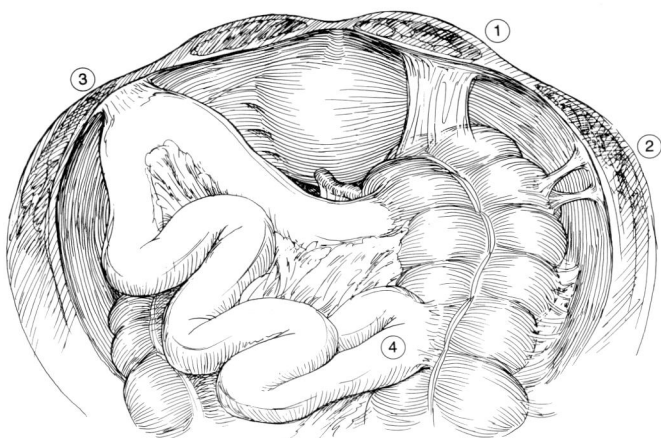

Figure 44-1.

comes instrumental. Any traumatic instrument can be used for dissection, if applied gently (e.g., palpator, tip of a closed scissors, suction cannula, tip of forceps). All the surgeon has to remember is that a space will open under pressure rather than by traction. This is why the opposite reaction of two forceps used to open anatomical space can only serve to open the route for another instrument to perform the actual separation. With the use of celioscopy, two techniques should be mentioned. First is pneumodissection, which is the penetration of insufflated gas inside the open space as soon as the key of adhesion is divided or when the mesothelial layer is pushed down. The simple weight of a small bowel loop attached to the anterior abdominal wall can demonstrate this phenomenon. Second is aquadissection using the device for washing and aspiration, which does the same thing by inserting a water jet on one side of the anatomical space. Water is used instead of gas in this case to create a true interstitial edema, which is very localized. It also offers the opportunity to visualize the smallest capillary and vascular structures with the help of a surgical optical device.

Section with Scissors

Section with scissors is again a basic technique in traditional surgery, and its use in celioscopic surgery would be easy if the laparoscopic scissors had exactly the same characteristics as the surgical scissors. Unfortunately, this is not the case. Each type of scissors (e.g., one moving part, two moving parts, straight scissors, curved scissors) is associated with a special technique. All can be used; however, they each have variable qualities depending upon the concept as well as on the manufacturer. We prefer, if possible, to use scissors with some degree of curvature, which will allow the constant pressure of one blade on the other, and to have the blades cutting perfectly well. Single use type of instruments fit these objectives well. This is particularly true if curved scissors can be rotated, allowing orientation of the plane of section parallel to the plane of dissection. In fact, the use of scissor dissectors, we believe, is the fundamental basis of bandolysis, combining the effect of laceration and section obtained by gentle penetration of the open space and allowing the laceration of cellular space as well as the sectioning of fiber tracts resistant to previous maneuvers. Sectioning with scissors also has the advantage of creating a clean cut. A disadvantage is that the cut is not hemostatic when the open anatomical space is not completely avascular. In most dissection, the operator is obliged to find the right open space, which most of the time is completely avascular. Several companies now offer scissors that also have the ability to coagulate. Personally, we try not to use them, because the area of coagulation is relatively large and because often this will damage the cutting blade of the instrument.

Monopolar Electrosurgery (Tip, Hook, or Spatula)

Cutting current that has little coagulation effect, or current that creates extensive tissue effect with a relatively small cutting effect, or a combination of both can be used. Electrosurgery is associated with certain adverse effects, e.g., tissue necrosis and secondary perforation. We have used electrocautery in more than 6000 procedures without electrical incident. The reported accidents are not usually a result of the technique itself, but often to imperfect knowledge of the use of electrosurgery. However, we agree that a potential danger exists, in particular for the operator in training, and we tend not to use this technique during operative demonstration. Today, we perform, if possible, a clean cut with a scissors, with hemostasis only being completed when it is necessary, either with a monopolar electrode or preferentially with bipolar coagulation.

The Laser Cut

The laser was hoped to be the universal instrument. It can be either an instrument for extremely precise cutting with its ability for focalization or an instrument for obtaining hemostasis. However, during bandolysis, the difficulty of presenting the tissue to the instrument where one wants to cut and the difficulty of knowing what is behind the cutting area may cause the laser to be more dangerous than useful in this procedure. It appears also to be more difficult to set up than electrosurgery. The problem with the laser is the nonmaterialized character of its beam. It can cut or coagulate but cannot be a dissector, and during bandolysis the combination of both is necessary. In summary, the choice between laser or electrosurgery is mostly a matter of habit and availability of equipment in the operating room.

The Stapling Section

Some times adhesions from viscera to viscera or from viscera to abdominal wall are so dense that it is practically impossible to dissect them. In these cases, after the dissection is completed as far as possible, the only way to proceed is section suture: either section or true resection with interruption of the continuity and reanastomosis with sutures or resection of a piece of the intestinal wall. The technique of section suture using manual suturing represents bandolysis in its most elaborate form. This was a relatively difficult procedure when performed through a traditional incision and is even more difficult to master now during laparoscopic operations. The use of laparoscopic stapling devices, however, facilitates section suture during laparoscopic bandolysis. These new stapling devices allow almost completely clean surgery (Fig. 44-2). The stapling device ligates and transects the adhesion simultaneously.

AVOIDING REOCCURRENCE OF ADHESIONS

The different ways to prevent adhesions result from an obvious reality, but these techniques should be considered new methods, which are, as yet, unproved. However, they are the consequences of logical research and should be familiar to surgeons. Hydroflota-

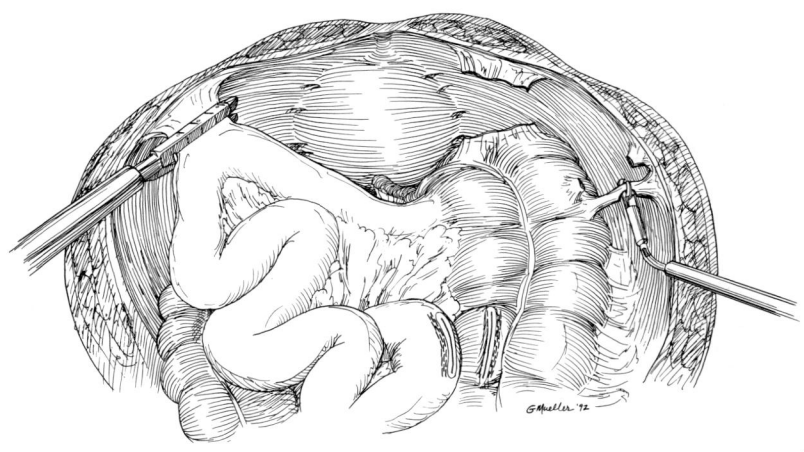

Figure 44-2.

tion consists of leaving inside the peritoneal cavity a certain amount of liquid: different investigators have used micromolecular solutions with the addition of steroids, antiseptics, antibiotics, or anti-inflammatory agents. Its efficacy was demonstrated in gynecology. It can be used when bandolysis is required for therapy. On the contrary, because of its probable efficacy, hydroflotation is not indicated when bandolysis is only used for exposure. In such cases hydroflotation with its risk of sepsis should not be used.

Fibrin glue has also been used to prevent the recurrence of adhesions. The glue is sprayed onto the lining of open spaces. It was hoped that this would prevent the formation of new adhesions but the efficacy of this technique has not been established. Also, application of the glue is difficult. As a result, the role of this method in the future is uncertain.

Mechanical mobilization of the abdominal viscera in the early postoperative period may also retard the recurrence of adhesions. Early movement of the viscera results from two mechanisms. Laparoscopic operations are minimally invasive and, consequently, bowel function returns almost immediately after the procedure. We believe that normal peristalsis helps prevent adhesion formation. The second element is the early mobilization of the patient allowed by the absence of postoperative pain. Ambulation by the patient increases mobilization of the peritoneal cavity content, resulting from the upright position and immediate activity of the patient with specific exercises (head down and knee flexion). We think it plays a very important role and one has to encourage it.

JUSTIFICATION OF BANDOLYSIS AS A THERAPEUTIC CONCEPT

The objectives, strategies and indications for the technique of bandolysis are based on its role as a therapeutic modality. In 1966, we started to use laparoscopy to explore the abdominal cavity, leading us to some observations. During that period our approach was more contemplative rather than active. Our findings can be summarized as follows.

1. Adhesions are a reality and their occurrence is common. They are, in fact, a sequelae of any inflammatory state of the peritoneal serosa.

2. Surgery, which initiates the process of wound healing and consequently an inflammatory state, frequently creates adhesions. The inspection of the right inguinal wall of patients who underwent an appendectomy showed the presence of adhesions in most patients. Some of these adhesions modified the anatomy and the position of organs. Because of this finding we have issued in France, where incidental appendectomy is frequently performed, a recommendation against the abusive performance of appendectomy.

3. Surgery, however, is not the only cause of adhesions. Any infection or inflammatory process has a tendency in its acute phase to cause formation of peritoneal walls around the initial lesion. This phenomenon is known to occur after cholecystitis, colitis, or pelvic peritonitis, and it is not necessary to describe it. However, we have found to our surprise that certain adhesions of the right iliac fossa, which are identical to the adhesions we described after appendectomy, may exist spontaneously without any previous surgery. This phenomenon is associated with a normal appendix away from the adhesions. This leads us to think that pathologic conditions of the right colon that are incompletely known, may lead to an inflammatory reaction of the peritoneum and subsequently to adhesions. Large bowel obstruction seems to play a role. We subsequently thought about the existence of a new pathologic condition for this area, which we called the adhesive syndrome of the right iliac fossa. In its acute phases this phenomenon simulates appendicitis clinically and leads to an operation. Appendectomy through the classical approach may include the destruction without realization, of these adhesions, however, this does not always happen. And, a comparison between laparoscopic and surgical findings when we undertake laparoscopic appendectomy convinces us that the classical right iliac fossa approach to the ileocecal appendix does not allow us to correctly identify these adhesions. It can simply be in some cases just as difficult to mobilize the cecum.

4. When the concept of laparoscopy was new and not common therapy, adhesions represented an obstacle to abdominal exploration. Thus, we have done lysis of adhesions with the exploration of the abdomen as a goal. In certain patients, we tried to interpret this finding in light of the anatomical-clinical correlation. Indeed, we have found that in some patients lysis of adhesions could lead to the decrease or even the disappearance of ab-

dominal pain, which was until then not understood and resistant to treatment.

5. With this laparoscopic approach and after having acquired enough experience with this technique, we performed for the first time in 1972, theraputic bandolysis for acute small bowel obstruction secondary to adhesions. The success of this technique led us to extend our indications. We have found that incomplete or complete bowel obstruction caused by mechanical straining of the bowel that is secondary to adhesions has consistent microscopic and anatomopathologic findings. We were then able to define the obstructive band, which is by nature pathologic, as always having fibrous as well as vascular protractile characteristics. This band can be compared to a cord or an elastic sheet, which exerts its mechanical effort upon the bowel through its attachment to a fixed portion of the abdomen. Hubert Manhes, in Vichy, working totally independently of us, reported similar findings in the gynecologic field. Extrapolating to the gastrointestinal field and interpreting data the same way we did, he called this phenomenon "intestinal straining from peritoneal origin." We think that this is an excellent definition.

6. We thought about widening even further this physiopathological concept to define the mechanism, the potential for evolution, and the therapeutic conclusion. We were able to formulate hypotheses. Despite the fact that they appear to be convincing, they are only hypotheses and as such need to be studied and confirmed.

However, at this stage these hypotheses appear to be strong enough to build a coherent argument for surgical therapy, which repairs the peritoneum by using bandolysis. (a) The pathologic peritoneal adhesion, which leads (sometimes after a long time) to the phenomenon of intestinal straining, is without question an evolving process. The first hypothesis is that its pathology and its appearance are to different degrees, characteristic of obstruction. Because of the evolving feature of this adhesion we are able to identify it. (b) The relative adhesion, even if it does not affect the abdominal wall or bowel function, can cause pain. This correlation between pain and adhesions is certain in some patients and can explain the therapeutic effect, initially unexpected, of some bandolysis procedures. We, however, do not know with certainty that all the evolving adhesions are symptomatic. We, in fact, believe the contrary after looking at some types of obstruction which occurred late in relation to the etiology, with an asymptomatic interval between the two. (c) The last hypothesis, and certainly the least demonstrated, is that if the obstructive adhesion causes symptoms by creating mechanical straining at the level of the viscera, we think that the repeated pressure of this adhesion creates reinforcements, and a vicious cycle of straining. With this hypothesis in mind we generated the concept of intestinal straining leading to the disease of peritoneal straining. Bandolysis treats both the symptoms as well as the pathology and thereby breaks the vicious cycle. This will result in the following consequences. We have said that the objective of bandolysis was to restore the normal anatomy of the peritoneal cavity. We think that the objective is more the suppression of straining than the return of mobility. In other words, we tried to suppress focal straining in order to have it redistributed over a larger area of tension. This led us to consider that the objective of bandolysis can be and to some extent paradoxically is the same objective that one is looking for with organopexia. The failure to accomplish this objective with open surgery could be partially a consequence of the inability to assess correctly whether the objective was achieved or not. We think with laparoscopy, where one looks at the viscera in a much more anatomical position, this objective is easier to reach.

From the point of view of therapeutic efficacy and permanent resolution of symptoms, the problem is not whether these adhesions will reoccur but to know if the removal of straining is definitive. Indeed, the intended goal will be the removal of a focal adhesion and its replacement by larger and permanent adhesions. This goal is almost equivalent to the reconstitution of normal anatomy. The definition of normal anatomy, however, deserves a more careful discussion. It has been defined by dissection on cadavers, but the pathologic alterations acquired during a long life are often ignored. Thus, surgeons may focus attention on some frequently found localized adhesions that we have a tendency to consider as normal. This is perhaps not always true, for example, the fixation of the omentum and of the right colon in the right lower quadrant. Thus, it was based on our hypothesis that straining is both a pathological as well as an evolving condition that has caused us to decide which patients to treat with bandolysis and which to leave untreated.

PROCEDURES FOR BANDOLYSIS

What we have said above was to show that the objectives of bandolysis are coherent, although they are not yet absolutely proven. Bandolysis uses techniques, which by conception are simple in principle, but can be very difficult to accomplish practically, and to arrange into a therapeutic strategy. We will look now at these different aspects.

Patient Selection

Although technical aspects in this book are dominant, the problem of indications appears to be a central concern. In our minds, when indications are discussed, there is a lot of ambiguity and two almost opposite tendencies.

On the one hand, we would like to push for the development of bandolysis because we believe in its value and we wish that all patients who need it could benefit from it. In this regard, we noticed in our teaching experience that surgeons refer patients to us for indications, which are difficult procedures. In our own practice we select the indication to alternate complex procedures with a large number of easy procedures. These latter indications, which may often end with good results, are evidently underestimated, particularly during the initial phase of training. The process of patient selection depends upon the ability to distinguish between functional and organic pathologic conditions. Organic pathologic conditions can be treated surgically. Functional pathologic conditions cannot. To recognize the difference, one has to be able to avoid prejudices and habits and understand that a pathologic process is very often called functional until one discovers the organicity. On the other hand, we would like our patient selection to be limited to those that will be benefited by the procedure. Insufficient indications would only lead to the discredit of this technique. Thus, indications for bandolysis remain in a period of evolution.

Symptoms That Might Be Treated by Bandolysis

The goal is to characterize the symptoms that represent peritoneal tension. Notionally, there are two types of criteria: problems with intestinal motility and problems with abdominal pain.

INTESTINAL MOTILITY

Complete bowel obstruction and partial bowel obstruction may produce similar symptoms. They both display clinically and radiologically the criteria for bowel obstruction. However, one should determine from this clinical and radiologic analysis the level of obstruction. The small bowel rather than the large bowel is usually obstructed although obstruction of the large bowel from adhesions is not rare. If the diagnosis is difficult, contrast studies, either anterograde or retrograde done with Hypaque rather then barium, can give useful information. Endoscopy of the lower gastrointestinal tract should also be considered. All these tests are used to differentiate between pathologic conditions of the bowel itself and peritoneal tension, which we are trying to identify. One has to realize, however, that an error of excessive evaluation does not usually have terrible consequences. Laparoscopy for an obstruction from an intraorgan pathologic condition is not ideal; however, usable information regarding the resectability of the lesion can be gained. On the contrary, an excessive delay before performing bandolysis in acute obstruction may be detrimental to the patient and could decrease the chance of success of laparoscopic bandolysis.

With more subtle types of obstruction, the same symptoms must be sought, but the labile character of the symptoms makes this task difficult. One often needs to follow a patient for several months to identify the syndrome of intestinal tension. It is often necessary to ask the patient to participate in this search for symptoms by checking on himself or herself. Also a radiograph of the abdomen during the phase of obstruction helps to make the diagnosis. This is not always easy when the crisis occurs far from home or during the night.

PAIN

The presence of pain is different from obstruction because of the absence of intestinal tension. However, all the transitional presentations or associations are possible. One should show the same care in defining the symptoms and trying to suspect the organic nature of these painful symptoms. This search is entirely directed toward the characterization of the mechanical origin of these symptoms. First, it can be useful to define how the pain starts—with special movement, with changes in position, or after intestinal intake, which results in increased tension of the peritoneal attachment from the weight of the organ. This is usually not caused by intestinal obstruction. The ways that the pain stops are also important. We have found that the patient knows what brings relief–either decubitus position or massage or any other maneuver to decrease the pain. We noticed the bothersome fact that the zone of tension is often more painful during the maneuver that was supposed to bring relief, and increased tension may relieve the pain. We do not have a good explanation for this phenomenon, but it occurs frequently enough to mention it.

In every patient, physical examination is fundamental to define the focal area of pain. The evolving lesions from peritoneal tension often are associated with inflammatory or pseudoinflammatory signs. They are translated into focal painful areas sometimes associated with abnormal laboratory values. This finding is especially important in what we called the syndrome of adhesion of the right lower quadrant. This syndrome is characterized by pain, a general inflammatory state (which is sometimes difficult to differentiate from subacute appendicitis in children and right-sided colitis in adults). The painful area is often located superior and lateral to McBurney's point. Also this finding of a painful area may be best elicited in left decubitus, which is called by some the "sensitive McBurney." This is considered by some surgeons a good sign of retrocecal appendicitis. It is, in our opinion, however, more characteristic of the pathologic syndrome of adhesion of the right lower quadrant. Finally, the presence in the patient's history, of multiple abdominal crises which resolve spontaneously is another sign that confirms this diagnosis.

With these clinical findings, laparoscopy can be justified either for exploration or for treatment and even more often for both because of two crucial elements, the repetition of the crisis and the intensity and the duration of the pain. These two elements deserve treatment when there is enough functional or social handicap. Also, another indication for laparoscopy is to rule out appendicitis.

We have already explained how to identify the syndrome of abnormal adhesions. We believe that this syndrome accounts for a large number of unnecessary appendectomies. A good number of these patients deserve exploration and therapeutic laparoscopy. Globally, however, the identification of this syndrome allowed us to decrease the number of procedures even when both appendectomy and bandolysis are considered. With the finding of a syndrome of adhesion of the right lower quadrant in its acute phase simulating an acute appendicitis, should we perform incidental appendectomy? We do not have a good answer to this question because there are good reasons on both sides.

OTHER CONSIDERATIONS

There are two different circumstances that can modify the strategy of laparoscopy: the presence or the absence of previous abdominal surgery. One has to remember that adhesions in the abdomen of a patient who has not undergone a previous operation are the result of a special pathologic process, which is precisely regulated even if it is not well defined. Adhesions, consequently, have some similarity and stereotypes.

We have discussed earlier the syndrome of adhesion of the right lower quadrant which is characterized by a kind of falciform ligament between the cecum and ascending colon, sometimes reaching far to the anterior abdominal wall and sometimes including the omentum. In other patients, it is an inflammatory and red membrane in front of the ascending colon and the cecum and fixed to the lateral peritoneum of Morison pouch and sometimes extending even to the right lobe of the liver. Similarly, we know the tendency of some gynecologic peritonitis to generate a syndrome of pelvic adhesion with multiple cords as well as forming an adhesive pillar in the space between the liver and diaphragm (Fitz-Hugh-Curtis syndrome). Another example is the tendency for recurrent salpingitis to form lesions that progressively circle the ovaries.

In contrast, adhesions after surgery are characterized by great variations in shape, positioning, and size. However, knowledge of the operative technique that was used, the postoperative course, and the complications is useful for the prediction of these adhesions.

The differences between uniform adhesions of spontaneous pathologic processes and the wild adhesions after surgery can also be found at the level of their evolution. Obstruction, for example, is only a complication of adhesion after surgery. In all patients, one has to know that the feasibility of the procedure and its magnitude can only be determined during the intervention. Even with a great deal of experience, one cannot predict for sure whether the procedure will be easy or difficult. In order to justify the surgical indication, the reasons needs to be convincing enough to start a procedure that could eventually be switched to an open procedure.

Preoperative Preparation

We do not recommend any special physical preparation before the procedure. However, we think that the active participation of the patient in defining the symptoms is an important part of the education of the patient to obtain an informed consent. Regarding the syndrome of adhesion leading to intestinal tension, i.e., changes in intestinal motility, we do not think it is useful to try to stop the syndrome of intestinal tension before performing the intervention. We even think that the presence of the syndrome of intestinal tension during the intervention will give direct signs to orient the surgeon toward the area of tension. This will facilitate greatly the identification of the lesions.

Methods of Exposure and Retraction

This is indeed the most difficult part of the procedure and there is no recipe for complete safety. The adhesion may trick the surgeon from the start and make this procedure dangerous. Also, we had to agree to operate on patients who had undergone previous surgery, which was going against classical contraindications.

The pneumoperitoneum is usually insufflated in the left upper quadrant in bandolysis (Fig. 44-3). It is the area of the abdomen in which adhesions are the least frequent. The jejunum is usually well covered with the omentum, and it is relatively preserved from adhesions because of its protection but also probably because of its important motility. Our habit of choosing the left upper quadrant for insufflation for bandolysis because it was safer led us to adopt this approach for all laparoscopic procedures. This approach has several advantages.

First, the penetration of the abdominal wall through the slightly oblique rectus sheet, defines easily the different planes. The relatively tight adhesion of the peritoneum to the deep rectus sheath makes this penetration easy. Also a single use device because of its

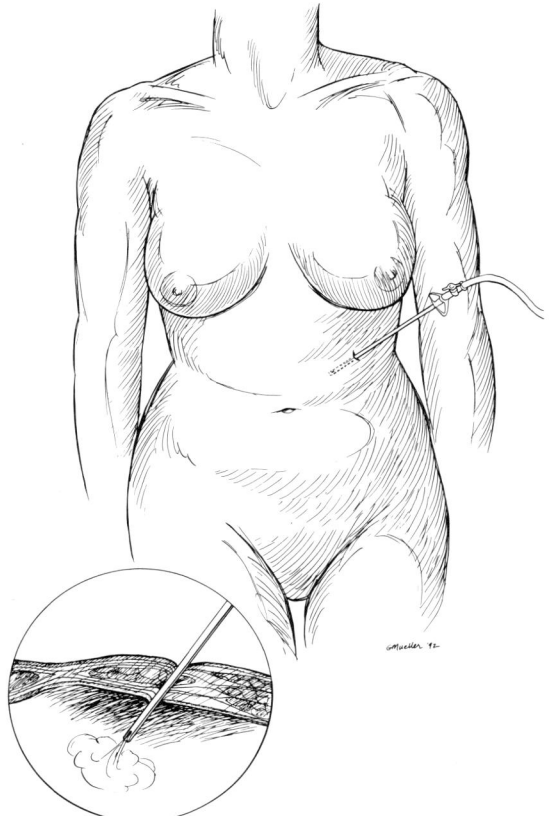

Figure 44-3.

quality of penetration and because of the safety of its mechanism is clearly superior to other types of devices.

Second, this approach allows the performance of the maneuver of "retroperitoneal sweeping." This is done by holding the insufflation needle against the abdominal wall to get a feeling for the presence of adhesions in the umbilical area in particular where the trocar for the camera will be introduced. Also placing this palpator inside the abdomen gives the opportunity to insert the trocar for the camera in a less blind fashion. This is sometimes very useful in patients with thick abdominal walls.

If, during this maneuver, a gas leak occurs, the risk of organ or vascular injury is high. In this circumstance, double entry in the abdomen allows the peritoneum to be reinsufflated to sufficient pressure.

Finally, if a visceral adhesion is present in this area, there is a good chance that it is either colon or stomach. The perforation with a fine needle in the area of the adhesion would not lead to any major problem. Only uncontrolled distention could be dangerous. The safety maneuver with the syringe is then essential and would avoid this complication.

Of course, depending upon whether the patient has undergone previous surgery and in particular, whether the patient has a scar in the left lower quadrant, another area of penetration would be chosen.

In some circumstances, one can expect penetration of the abdomen to be extremely difficult, but we think that by following the safety rules one can decrease the danger of penetration to almost nothing. In fact, although we have never stipulated an absolute contraindication for laparoscopy, we have encountered an occasional patient in whom laparoscopy was practically impossible. In these patients, if the indication for the procedure is real, we utilize open laparoscopy as a last resort.

Trocar Placement

Although at this stage it is still a blind procedure, the insertion of the needle of the pneumoperitoneum greatly facilitates the intervention. The needle can be used for palpation—the "white cane" of the surgeon.

In most patients, the camera is best positioned next to the umbilicus. Although this is not always the ideal position, it usually allows adequate visualization of the abdominal cavity and proves adequate for most procedures. However, in patients that have undergone previous abdominal operations, the umbilical area and, indeed, the entire midline is often stuck to numerous adhesions. These adhesions can often be palpated. Under these circumstances, the camera is best positioned for safety reasons away from the umbilicus. This also serves to improve exposure of these adhesions and facilitates their transection. Furthermore, this allows easier operative movement of the camera. A position lateral to the rectus sheath in the left lower quadrant is most commonly selected for an alternative camera site. This provides an ascending view of the midline. After this initial exploration, two common situations may be encountered. Adhesions may not limit visibility and the global strategy of the procedure may be determined. Alternatively, adhesions may limit the assessment of the pathologic process and bandolysis may be required prior to further exploration.

After the identification of the lesion, the trocars required for the procedure are inserted. Positions should be selected which avoid areas with a high risk of vascular injuries. We always try to insert trocars as far as possible away from the camera to avoid crossing of instruments. This facilitates the procedure and makes the control of the instruments much easier. The trocars should be placed so that they can be used in an arc that encompasses 70–90 degrees (Fig. 44-4).

Depending upon the way the operation is going, it is not unusual to change the area of insertion of the trocar as well as to change the position of the camera itself during the procedure (Fig. 44-5).

Positioning of the Patient

Positioning of the patient for the planned procedure is feasible only if wide exploration of the peritoneal cavity is possible at the beginning of the procedure. If adhesions obscure the pathology, we alternate between periods of dissection and exploration. Al-

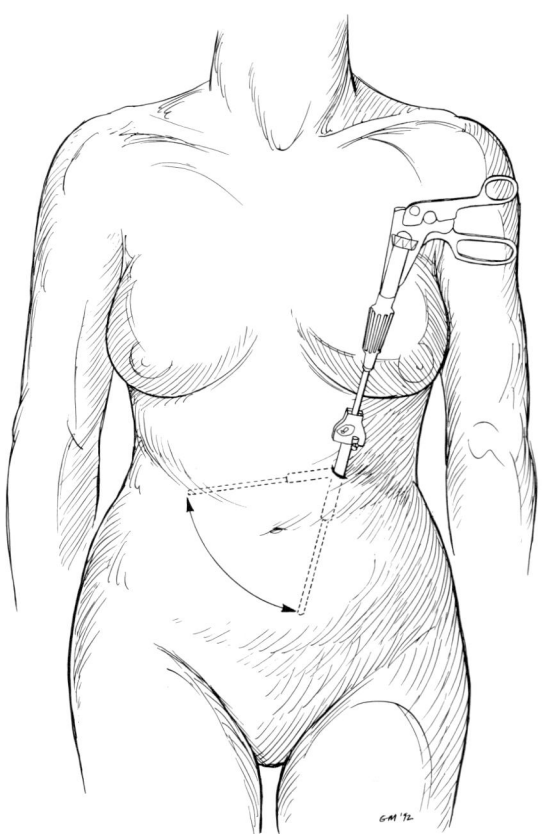

Figure 44-4.

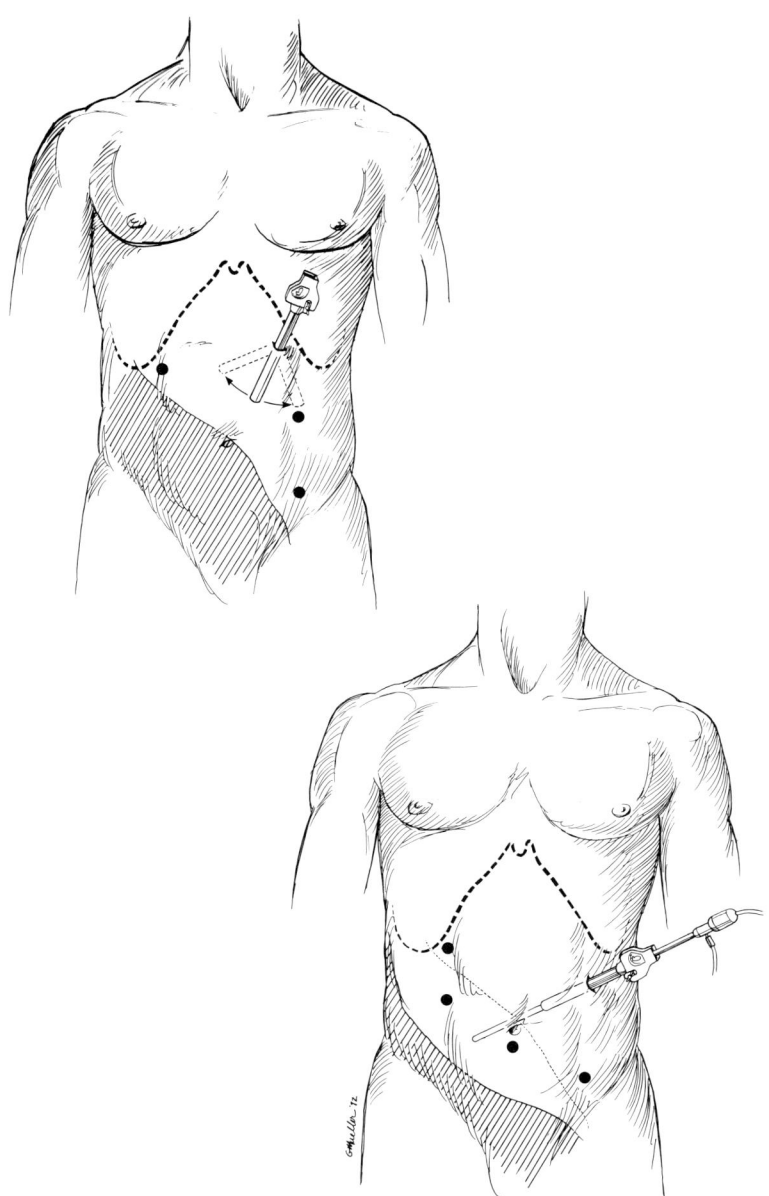

Figure 44-5.

though this may seem a disorganized approach, it allows us to adapt the operation to the pathology that we encounter. Indeed, in these difficult procedures, the operation may prove infeasible at any time. An unsurmountable obstacle may be encountered at any time, stopping the laparoscopic procedure. One of the fundamental characteristics of performing laparoscopic procedures in this difficult situation, is to mix the indication and the strategy during the procedure itself.

One has to remember that adhesions are not always found at the first inspection but may require careful study. Spontaneous adhesions follow rules that we have mentioned previously. The anatomy of these adhesions needs to be well known, particularly in the right lower quadrant.

A change in the position of the patient may help to identify the adhesion, which is producing the symptoms of the patient. Dropping the patient into Trendelenberg's position facilitates the exploration of the pelvis. Retroceal or rectosigmoid adhesions as well as ad-

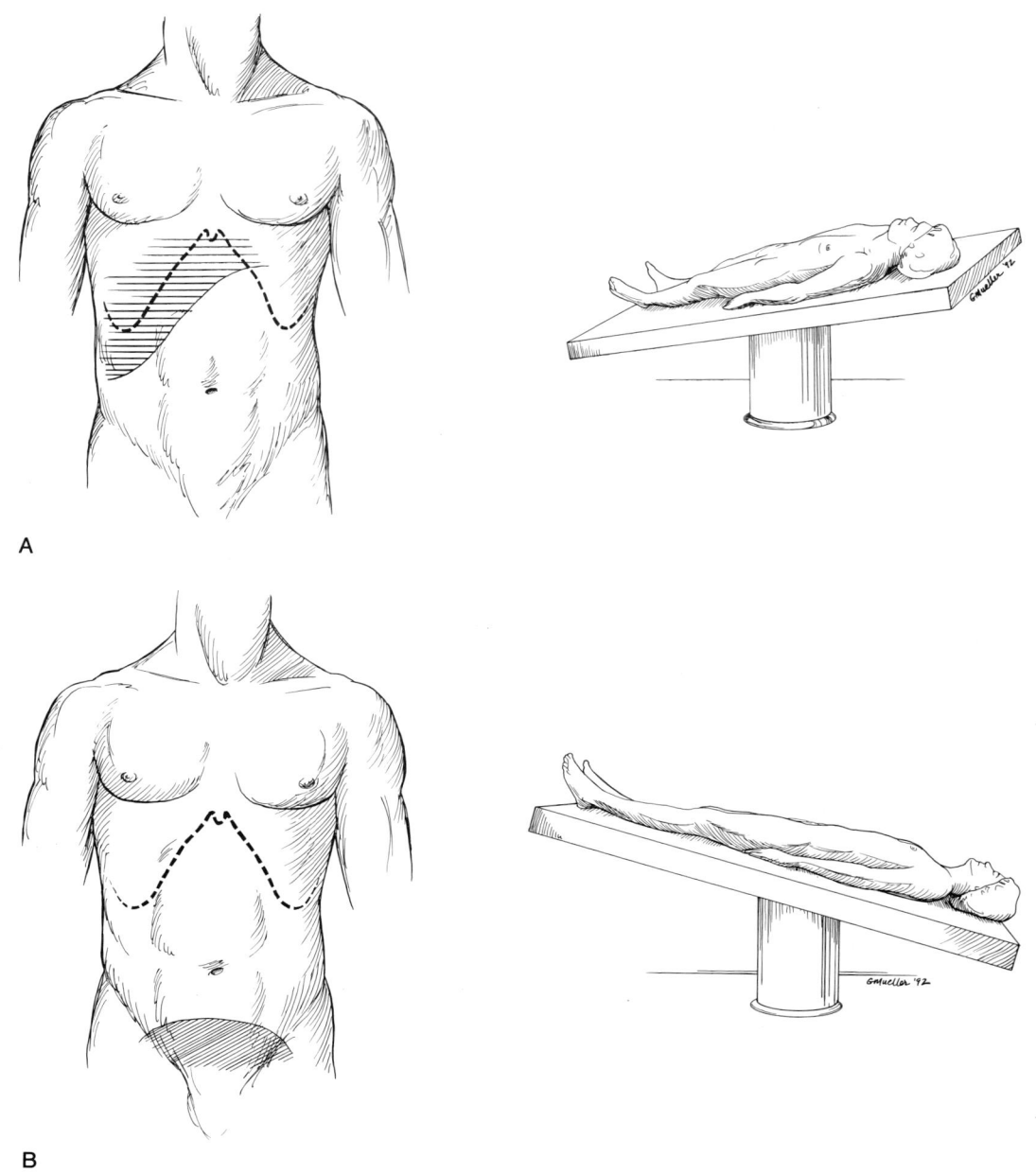

Figure 44-6.

hesions to the dome of the bladder are often exposed by this position (Fig. 44-6). In contrast, reverse Trendelenberg position aids the exploration of the subhepatic and subphrenic spaces (Fig. 44-6A). The parietocolic gutter is best explored with the patient in the left lateral decubitus position. A combination of longitudinal and rotational position changes may be required to expose completely complex adhesions.

In addition to these changes in patient position, the mobilization of organs with instruments such as grasping forceps is often necessary. The combination of several techniques is required to allow the exploration of the entire small bowel and in particular the proximal small bowel up to the angle at the connection between the duodenum and the jejunum, which is particularly difficult to visualize well. There are, however, often helpful guides to orient the surgeon toward the area of tension. We have already described the anatomic pathologic structure of the area of the peritoneum with tension and the characteristics, which are vascular, retractile, thick, and inserted on a fixed point. Consequently, the surgeon will look particularly for the area of limited mobility that is fixed during a change in position of the patient. Also dilated capillaries are often directed toward the point of tension. In particular, when dealing with obstruction, this observation will allow the surgeon to suspect the position of the band even before seeing it well.

Finally, in the case of intestinal tension obstructing the bowel, the rule is to follow the nondistended small bowel when this is possible or to follow the dilated small bowel in other cases to discover the area of stricture. This is why we have said that the operation during the acute phase is often easier.

Specific Details of the Procedure

We have emphasized earlier that the progression of the procedure depends on the field of vision and that often exploration and progression follow each other in a continuous manner. We will now discuss three different situations in which bandolysis may be indicated.

BANDOLYSIS FOR EXPOSURE

Bandolysis may be required to divide adhesions so that other procedures may be accomplished. The objective of this bandolysis is only to make the laparoscopic procedure possible. One has to remember, however, that the lysis of wide areas of membranous adhesion, which are not a pathologic process, may lead to the creation of areas of localized tension which could become a secondary pathologic process. Experience and judgment are the best guides to know where to stop the bandolysis.

COMPLEMENTARY BANDOLYSIS

In many procedures bandolysis may be indicated to complement another laparoscopic procedure. Adhesions with evolving morphologic or anatomopathologic characteristics may be encountered during laparoscopic procedures for other conditions. Similarly, adhesions which may suggest an increased risk of producing obstruction because of their position may be found. Under these circumstances it seems appropriate to perform bandolysis so that intestinal obstruction might be prevented in the future.

In all circumstances, bandolysis can be indicated to complement another procedure when the clinical symptoms of the patient are not totally explained by the main disease. We will cite two commonly encountered examples.

Frequently the indication for laparoscopic cholecystectomy is not only signs of gallbladder dysfunction but also signs of dyspepsia or abdominal pain in the right flank. These symptoms can be wrongly attributed to biliary dysfunction or the diagnosis of old colitis. These patients deserve a cholecystectomy as well as a therapeutic bandolysis. In our personal practice, we think we have reduced considerably the functional symptoms in the postoperative period—the so-called pseudopostcholecystectomy syndrome. This therapeutic complement is in our opinion so important that it is one of the major indications for laparoscopic cholecystectomy. Unfortunately, this is not commonly done yet.

The second example is in patients who are seen with a long history of duodenal ulcer disease, which has been treated medically. Frequently the symptoms worsen, loosing their characteristic of recurrence and onset. These episodes of abdominal pain very often do not have any correlation with the evolution of the ulcer as seen on endoscopy. We found that in a high number of patients this pain was due to a periduodenitis that was retractile and included the peritoneum. Periduodenal bandolysis has proven very beneficial for these symptoms.

THERAPEUTIC BANDOLYSIS

Therapeutic bandolysis is a procedure done specifically to treat the consequences of adhesions. Ideally these operations should address only the pathologic band. Unfortunately, this is often only a theoretical goal because of the need to visualize, to unfold intra-abdominal organs, and in general, to do a complete exploration. The strategy is to progress slowly until the best therapeutic approach is identified. Nevertheless, one has to try to follow a well organized plan and not to proceed in a random fashion. When there are many adhesions involving several organs or several organs and the omentum, one has to avoid freeing the adhesion in a block from the abdominal wall. On the contrary, one has to free one organ at a time to restore mobility. The best comparison we can offer is to free each plane of adhesion one after the other in the same way that one opens the pages of a book. In other cases of large pillars of adhesion one has to try to separate the organ from the periphery to the center in the same way one would peel a banana. It is important to realize, however, that some adhesions to the anterior abdominal wall help maintain exposure of associated adhesions. Indeed, these adhesions temporarily replace the need of an additional instrument used for retraction. The question of knowing how far this bandolysis has to be done is a difficult problem to solve. Everybody will use his or her own experience and will act depending upon faith in the pathogenic hypothesis that we talked about. It is through this thought process that one can determine if the objectives of the procedure were achieved. It is extremely important to clearly remember the symptoms, the intestinal tension, and other complaints of pain and to systematically look for anatomic-clinical correlations between the operative findings and the symptoms previously identified. It is useful to remember at this point that the objective to reach is less directed toward the return to normal anatomy than to an interruption of what we called intestinal tension.

Postoperative Management

Fortunately, in most patients, the extreme simplicity of the postoperative period compared to the complexity of the procedure is disappearance of the symptoms, particularly if they were precisely identified preoperatively, is the best proof of the efficacy of this procedure.

The immediate relief of the patient's pain is such that the pain of the postoperative period appears as a minor problem. The clinical success is even better if the patient suffered from intestinal obstruction. One has to remember that bandolysis of large areas is, however, followed in the postoperative period with complaints of pain, which are sometimes acute and relatively sustained. They can also be variable, capricious, and of short duration. The patient should be told of these phenomena and, if needed, be reassured.

Postoperative follow-up in the hospital may be a very short time. The problem for the surgeon is to deal with two possible complications: the first one is bleeding and the second one is the possible necrosis of organs after bandolysis. These two risks can be reduced to almost nothing as long as the surgical technique was good, the hemostasis secured precisely, and the plan of dissection followed. The duration of postoperative follow-up will consequently depend upon the confidence one has in the quality of the surgery.

The principal goal of postoperative follow-up is to detect as soon as possible any injury to organs that would have been missed by the surgeon. Abdominal pain may be relatively intense during the first few hours. However, it never reaches an alarming level and it is never followed by clinical peritonitis with abdominal guarding. The onset of such symptoms should lead immediately to a new exploratory laparoscopic procedure.

The evaluation of the postoperative results should be done, in our opinion, with at least two examinations of the patient. One should occur 1 month after the operation and the other 6 months later and should include a detailed questionnaire of symptoms. These should be compared to the preoperative complaints.

Acquisition of the Technique of Bandolysis

In this discussion of the different strategies of bandolysis we think it is useful to say a few words about the teaching of this technique. We hope that this detailed description that we have given of bandolysis will help the acquisition of the thought processes and of the surgical technique necessary to perform this procedure.

However, nothing can replace experience and particularly personal experience. We think the first thing to master is the surgical technique of dividing adhesions. This may be mastered while performing other laparoscopic procedures. The surgeon must often perform bandolysis to achieve exposure in patients that have undergone previous abdominal operations. This gives the surgeon an opportunity to learn the surgical technique of bandolysis and also to progressively decrease the need for conversion to open surgery.

The second step is to undertake bandolysis to complement another procedure. It is a technique that can be done according to the surgeon's own ability without bad consequences if the surgeon stops the bandolysis.

Finally, therapeutic bandolysis is the final step on the technical scale. It is easier and more justified to start with acute or critical obstruction because they require and otherwise justify the conversion to open surgery.

We have said in the past and we want to repeat here that the principal difficulty of using therapeutic bandolysis for pain outside of an acute phase is the recognition of the symptoms that could lead to its indications. Nonetheless, the mastery of both recognition of appropriate symptoms and of the surgical techniques of bandolysis are required to obtain good outcomes in these patients.

Result of Bandolysis

The results of bandolysis presented here are preliminary and have not been produced from rigorously designed randomized trials. Nonetheless, we are taking the risk of presenting to our American colleagues these results that are as yet incomplete and with our subjective interpretation, because we hope that our concept will be developed, criticized, and analyzed and that the future experience of different surgeons will allow some more definitive conclusions to be drawn.

The use of bandolysis started more than 20 years ago. We developed this procedure in complete "isolation." Consequently, our results were never compared to that of other groups. Indeed, our therapeutic concepts have evolved over the years as a result of the treatment of many patients. Thus, it is impossible for us to compare our current results with those obtained early in our experience.

However, we hope that this preliminary evaluation will serve as a baseline that will generate the desire among our colleagues to start their own experience without having to repeat what we have done. During the meeting of the Society of American Gastrointestinal Endoscopic Surgeons in Atlanta in 1990, we presented the statistical analysis of bandolysis as a therapeutic entity. We studied the population of patients in whom laparoscopic bandolysis was performed for repeated abdominal pain of precise location with identifiable mechanical onset. During the period from 1984 to 1989, 320 patients underwent operations: 240 patients had previous abdominal surgery (127 procedures), 198 patients had an appendectomy, 146 patients had a gynecology procedure, 72 patients had other types of operations, and 75 patients never had surgery before. In 293 patients, an exploratory laparotomy procedure confirmed the hypothesis of adhesions that were fibrous or large with pillars of adhesion, and hypervascular and consequently mechanically responsible for tension. Among these patients the procedure was performed as per plan (which represents over 90 per cent with correct diagnoses). Among these 293 patients, bandolysis was performed 261 times. In 7 patients exploratory laparotomy or "safety laparotomy" was necessary to complement bandolysis with resection or closure of a tear. Of note is the fact that if a laparoscopic bandolysis was not technically possible, an open bandolysis was usually also not possible and resection became necessary. In 1 patient laparotomy was required for organ perforation found during the laparoscopic procedure. We called this a second chance laparotomy. Two secondary laparotomies were necessary because of perforation 2 and 3 days after bandolysis.

Clinical evaluation was done at 1 month, 3 months, and after 6 months. Fifteen patients were lost to follow-up, 31 patients showed no improvement, 88 patients showed partial improvement, and 137 patients were cured or significantly improved. Among the group of patients with no improvement, 28 patients had to undergo another procedure. If bandolysis was again performed, the patient appeared in the above statistics because he or she fit the criteria of selection from a technical aspect. In summary the procedure confirmed the presence of the pathologic condition in 90 per cent of the patients and if it was done in a satisfactory manner, helped in more than 80 per cent of the patients with no mortality in this series.

Experience from the Second Look Operation

The second look operations are either reintervention done for adhesions previously treated or laparoscopy done for other reasons in patients having undergone a bandolysis by us previously. The number of second look operations we have performed, however, is not enough to draw definitive conclusions. Nonetheless, we offer the following preliminary observations.

Among patients who underwent a complementary bandolysis after an unsatisfactory initial result, the delay between those procedures was more than 4 months. In these patients we always found a different type of adhesion at reoperation. These adhesions were usually neglected during the first procedure either because they were considered not responsible for the symtoms, or because the length and the complexity of the procedure were thought to be excessive. In no patients did we find identical reoccurrence of adhesions after correct bandolysis. It was based on this observation that we decided to avoid long and difficult procedures with major peritoneal trauma. If necessary, we now prefer to accomplish these procedures in several stages.

Similar findings were noted when the laparoscopy was done for other type of pathologic conditions. The largest group was patients who had undergone bandolysis of the right lower quadrant performed for chronic pain. In most of these patients, we did not find a completely free ileocecal segment despite complete mobilization at the first operation. In general, what we found was uniform adhesions of the right colon. We did not encounter a recurrence of the thick and evolving adhesion typical of the initial symptoms. However, in a few cases we operated on the patient after more than 10 or 15 years for recurrence of the same painful symptoms in the right lower quadrant. In these few cases we did discover adhesions similar to those present at the initial procedure. This is not really amazing, knowing that adhesion formation is a spontaneous phenomenon in which disturbance of intestinal motility plays a major role. The same causes will lead to the same effects.

Extending the conclusions that we presented in Atlanta in 1990 with patients operated on before 1989, we think it is useful to add the following comments. Because of the publication of our research in the field of lysis of adhesions, patients who have more and more complex pathologic conditions are referred to us. As our experience increases, we are testing the limits of feasibility of bandolysis. It appears to us, and this will need to be more closely examined in the future, that when the length of the procedure or its complexity and difficulty increase, the results are not as good. This is in fact not a real surprise if you think that a complex laparoscopic procedure is really equivalent to open surgery from a surgical stress point of view. This reinforces our belief that lysis of adhesion should be done in several stages when the procedure is too complex. We finally hope that as others become more experienced, we will be able to compare our results with that of others and that we will be able to initiate multicenter trials. However, comparisons are extremely difficult for this type of procedure because of the nature of the indications and the way it is done.

In order to be able to compare results in our own patients, we now record systematically and completely the entire procedure. This task is difficult because of the amount of data and the storage is rapidly becoming problematic. However, we believe that this data collection is absolutely necessary to develop further the concept of lysis of adhesions, which has reached so far only an early stage of development. In addition to what we have said in the introductory comments of this chapter, we think it is useful to remind the reader that bandolysis is a technique entirely endoscopic by its concept, its justification, and the way it is performed. Whereas a comparison between open and closed surgery is usually required to prove the advantages of the new laparoscopic procedure, no such comparison is feasible for laparoscopic bandolysis. Open laparotomy for lysis of adhesions is inappropriate and consequently there is no open operation equivalent to laparoscopic bandolysis. Thus, laparoscopic bandolysis is a novel area of development unique to laparoscopic surgery in which the potential for progress is significant.

Chapter 45
Appendectomy

Lawrence E. Harrison
Thomas S. French
Philip F. Caushaj

Acute appendicitis is one of the most common conditions requiring surgical intervention, approaching almost 300,000 cases each year. This disease may occur at any age, but predominately presents in the second and third decades. Although the classic clinical picture is straightforward, the presentation of acute appendicitis takes on changeable manifestations, especially with patients in the extremes of age (Table 45-1). Presently there is no pathognomonic sign, symptom, or test for acute appendicitis and the disease has frustrated and fooled surgeons for many years.

The appendix was first depicted in 1492 by Leonardo da Vinci. Laurentine in 1600 likened the appendix to a "twisted worm," while later in 1710, Phillippe Verheyen coined the term "appendix vermiformis." Although the appendix was suggested to be the cause of "abdominal affections of the right side" by Parkinson and Melier in the early 1800s, the popular belief of the time was that "perityphlitis" or inflammation of the cecum was the cause of this common malady. This was supported by famous surgeons such as Duuytiens and Pachelt. It was not until Reginald H. Fitz presented his paper, "Perforating Inflammation of the Vermiform Appendix with Special Reference to Its Early Diagnosis and Treatment" in 1886 that the importance of this condition was recognized. It was Dr. Fitz who coined the term "appendectomy" and emphasized that appendicitis was a disease that required surgical treatment. Subsequently Charles McBurney and John B. Murphy championed the idea of early surgical treatment, thus improving the extraordinary mortality and morbidity associated with acute appendicitis.[1]

By the 1940s this soon became surgical dictum. In fact, surgeons who did not have a 10 per cent or more unnecessary appendectomy rate were accused of subjecting their patients to the possibility of complications from a ruptured appendix. For many years there has been an accepted unnecessary appendectomy rate of approximately 5 to 20 per cent with some series reporting unnecessary laparotomy rates of 40 per cent in women of childbearing age.[2-4]

The popular belief has been that an unnecessary appendectomy carries minimal morbidity, whereas a greater risk occurs with a ruptured appendix after a delay in treatment. Recent studies report, however, that an unnecessary appendectomy is not an innocuous procedure, with complication rates as high as 15 per cent.[5-7] These include wound infection, pneumonia, pelvic abscess, ileus, bowel obstruction, deep venous thrombosis, infertility, and even death.[8]

Early diagnosis and treatment of appendicitis has evolved with the recent enthusiasm for laparoscopy by the general surgeon. Diagnostic laparoscopy has been reported to be useful in the diagnosis of appendicitis,[9-12]

Table 45-1. Differential Diagnosis of Acute Appendicitis

Mesenteric lymphadenitis
Meckel's diverticulum
Intussusception typhlitis
Inflammatory bowel disease
Diverticular disease
Cholecystitis
Right inguinal hernia
Henoch-Schönlein purpura
Perforated duodenal/gastric ulcer
Pancreatitis
Cecal carcinoma perforation
Urinary tract infection
Pelvic inflammatory disease
Tubo-ovarian abscess
Ectopic pregnancy
Right renal calculus
Mittleschmerz
Endometriosis
Torsion of right ovary/testis
Ruptured ovarian cyst

---

suggesting that it may reduce the unnecessary appendectomy rate. With the advent and advances in optics and laparoscopic equipment, laparoscopic appendectomies have been added to the surgeon's therapeutic armamentarium.

Laparoscopic appendectomy for the noninflamed appendix was first reported by Semm in 1983.[13] Four years later in 1987, Schrieber reported his experience with laparoscopic appendectomy in patients with acute appendicitis.[14] Recent large series have been presented, indicating the reliability, practicality, and safety of this technique. Although not as universally accepted as laparoscopic cholecystectomy, a number of surgeons are becoming comfortable with laparoscopic appendectomy techniques.

PATIENT SELECTION

Patients who are seen with the typical picture of acute appendicitis or those who are seen with a confusing clinical picture with right lower quadrant pain should be considered candidates for laparoscopic appendectomy.

There are two groups of patients for whom laparoscopic evaluation of right lower quadrant pain offers specific advantages. Laparoscopy facilitates the evaluation of right lower quadrant pain in women during their childbearing years. The visualization of the pelvis, fallopian tubes, and ovaries obtained through a laparoscope is vastly superior to that obtained through a right lower quadrant incision.

The second group of patients is those over the age of 50 in whom right lower quadrant pain develops. Laparoscopic assessment in these patients will help distinguish between acute appendicitis, perforated cecal carcinoma, solitary cecal diverticulitis, and acute sigmoid diverticulitis. Once the correct diagnosis is established, the feasibility of treating the condition with laparoscopic techniques or the necessity for traditional operations can be judged. If it proves necessary to proceed with an open operation, the surgeon can use the incision that he of she favors for the appropriate operation rather than attempting to operate through a right lower quadrant incision.

PREOPERATIVE EVALUATION

Patients undergo the same preoperative evaluation as they would for the open procedure. Counseling as to the possibility of conversion to an open appendectomy as deemed necessary by the surgeon is important as well.

PREOPERATIVE PREPARATION

All patients receive a preoperative dose of a second generation cephalosporin.

POSITIONING OF THE PATIENT

The patient is placed in the supine position. After endotracheal intubation, all patients undergo bladder and gastric decompression with appropriate catheters. The abdomen is prepared and draped widely in case conversion to open laparotomy is required.

POSITIONING OF THE VIDEO EQUIPMENT

The positions of the video monitor, surgeon, assistant, and scrub nurse are shown in Figure 45-1. This setup allows the surgeon to operate in a comfortable position. In this setup, the movements of the assistant surgeon are generally reversed on the video monitor. This is slightly inconvenient, but once expo-

Appendectomy   501

vector for cecal retraction. These ports will allow manipulation and mobilization of the cecum and perhaps the right colon to visualize the appendix, especially if the appendix is retrocecal. If a normal appendix is noted, further inspection of other organs is required. This can generally be accomplished with the placement of a second 10-mm trocar in the suprapubic position.

METHODS OF EXPOSURE

Placing the patient right side up in the Trendelenburg position facilitates inspection of the right lower quadrant, including the appendix, cecum, distal small bowel, ovaries, fallopian tubes, and uterus. An atraumatic grasping instrument or simply a blunt probe is inserted through the suprapubic port. This is used to push the small bowel out of the pelvis. With the patient in a deep Trendelenberg position, the small bowel will generally slide up toward the stomach and remain out of the way. The sigmoid colon is displaced first toward the left side and then toward the right side. The grasping instrument or probe can be used to elevate the uterus anteriorly and thereby improve the exposure of the

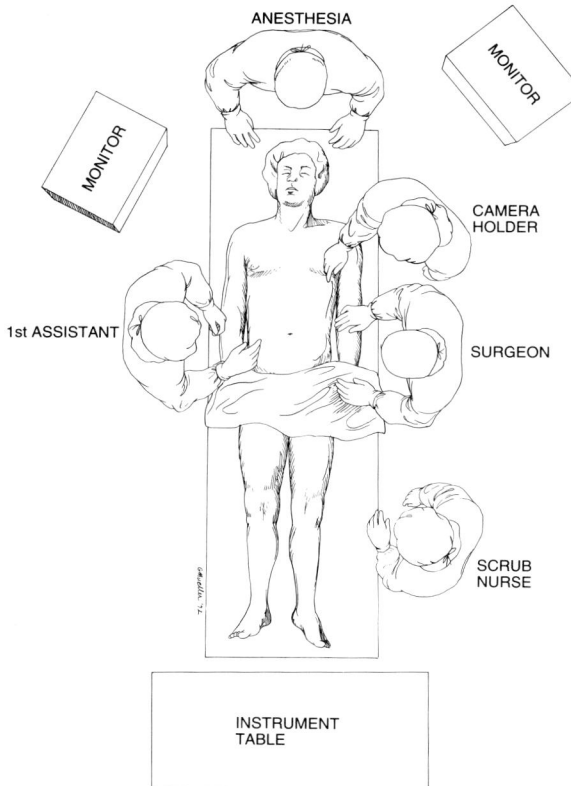

Figure 45-1.

sure of the appendix is established the position of the assistant remains relatively static. It is often easier for the surgeon to position the instruments of the assistant since the motions of the surgeon are not reversed on the monitor. Alternatively, some surgeons prefer to have the monitor placed at the feet of the patient.

TROCAR PLACEMENT AND SIZE SELECTION

The carbon dioxide pneumoperitoneum is insufflated. A 10-mm trocar is inserted into the abdomen in the umbilical position (Fig. 45-2). A 10-mm forward-viewing laparoscope is passed through the trocar, and inspection of the peritoneal cavity is performed. If acute appendicitis is noted or visualization of the appendix cannot be achieved, a 12-mm trocar is placed midline in the suprapubic region below the "bikini line" and a 10-mm trocar is placed either in the right upper or lower quadrant. The authors prefer the upper quadrant placement because it achieves a better

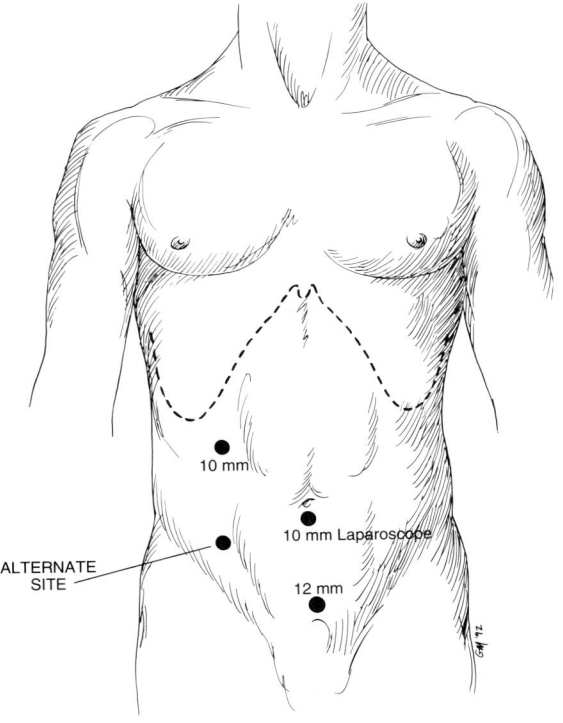

Figure 45-2.

pelvis, fallopian tubes, and ovaries. Alternatively, the uterus can be retracted anteriorly with the transvaginal placement of a uterine sound. The grasping instrument can be used to examine the small bowel. This is most easily accomplished by starting at the ileocecal valve and running the bowel back toward the ligament of Treitz. In some patients, it may prove necessary to insert a second trocar so that two grasping instruments can be used to sequentially grasp the bowel.

Laparoscopy also affords the opportunity to inspect the upper abdomen. This is best accomplished with the patient in the reverse Trendelenberg position. With the patient's head up, the liver, gallbladder, spleen, stomach, and proximal small bowel are readily visualized.

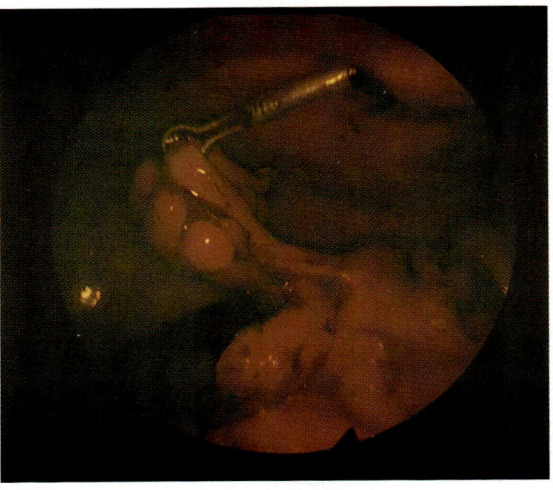

Figure 45-3.

SPECIFIC DETAILS OF THE PROCEDURE

After placing the patient in the Trendelenburg position, a 10-mm periumbilical skin incision is made. The Veress needle is placed through the incision into the abdominal cavity. Position is confirmed by the saline drop test and initially low pressures with insufflation. The peritoneal cavity is insufflated with carbon dioxide to 14 to 15 mm Hg. After adequate pneumoperitoneum is achieved, a 10-mm trocar is introduced. Then the appendix is mobilized and the diagnosis of acute appendicitis is made by direct inspection. Removal of the appendix begins with the exposure and ligation of the mesoappendix. The appendiceal tip is retracted with an atraumatic grasper or SURGITIE* ligating loop to "tent" the mesoappendix (Fig. 45-3). The mesoappendix can be ligated with the ENDO GIA 30* stapling device after a small fenestration is fashioned at the base of the appendix with a blunt instrument (Fig. 45-4). Alternatively, the mesoappendix may also be dissected with electrocautery or laser after titanium clip or SURGITIE* ligating loop of the appendiceal artery (Fig. 45-5). Dissection may start at the tip or base, depending on the position of the appendix and/or associated adhesions. Division of the mesoappendix should be done as close to the appendix as possible. This allows better hemostasis and less bulk on the appendix for easier extraction.

After the appendix is skeletonized, the base is exposed and two to three chromic SURGITIE* ligating loop are secured on the proximal cecal portion of the appendix. An additional SURGITIE* ligating loop is placed distally. The appendix can then be ligated with scissors, laser, or electrocautery (Fig. 45-6). Alternatively, the ENDO GIA 30* stapling device may be used to transect the appendix from the cecum (Fig. 45-7). After transection by either method, inspection of the appendiceal stump as well as the mesoappendix is mandatory. Titanium clips, electrocautery, or SURGITIE* ligating loop may be used to secure hemostasis. The appendiceal stump may be cauterized as well.

Invagination of the appendiceal stump is not routinely done. This is technically more challenging and has been shown to be unnecessary.[15] Occasionally, the base of the appendix or cecum is so inflamed that simple ligation of the appendiceal stump may not be secure. It is in this situation that stump invagination is useful. As described by Semm, a suture is used to invaginate the stump by either a purse-string or Z stitch. The suture is tied extracorporally, using an atraumatic grasper to "dunk" the base.

Occasionally an appendix may be so inflamed or gangrenous that a retrograde approach may be useful.[16] This approach begins with dissection, ligation, and division of the appendiceal base. By placing traction on it, the appendix is used as a retractor. The appendix is systematically dissected free from its mesentery and adhesions using laser or electrocautery or sharp and blunt dissection. If an appendiceal abscess is encountered and surrounding tissue is too inflamed and friable for a safe appendectomy, laparoscopic directed drainage and irrigation are performed. A closed suction drain is placed into the ab-

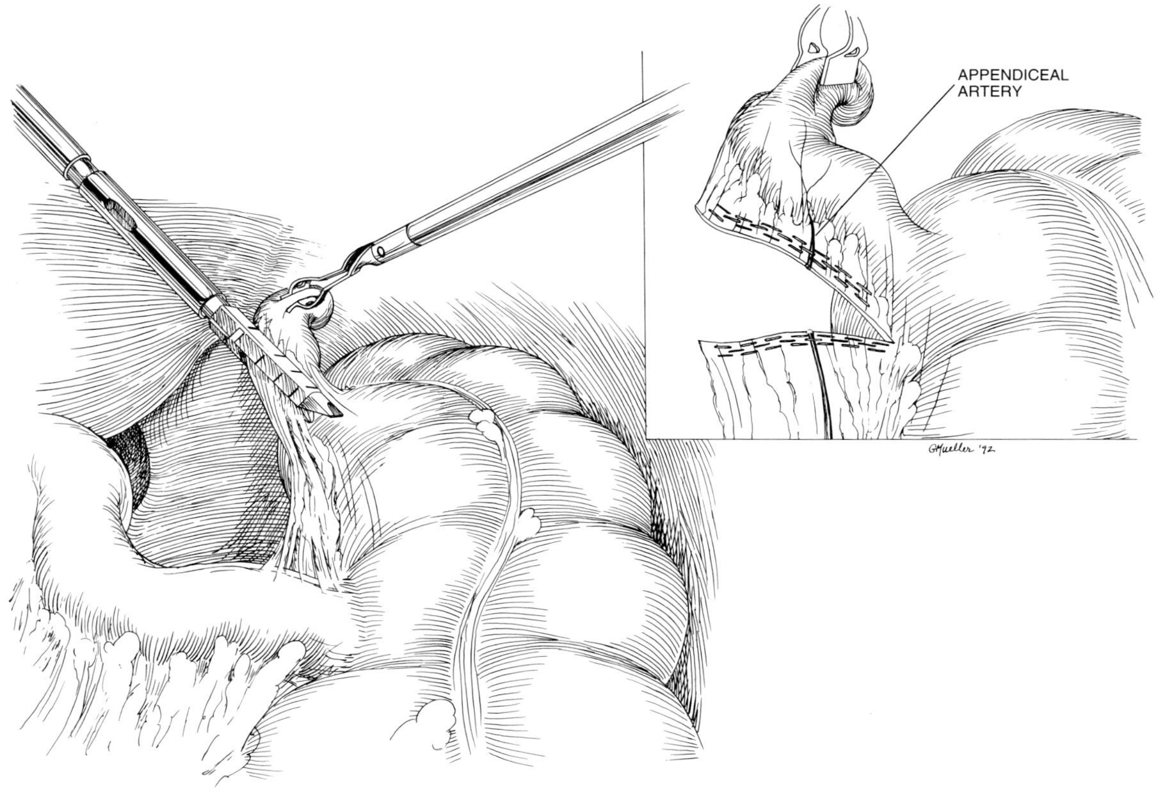

Figure 45-4.

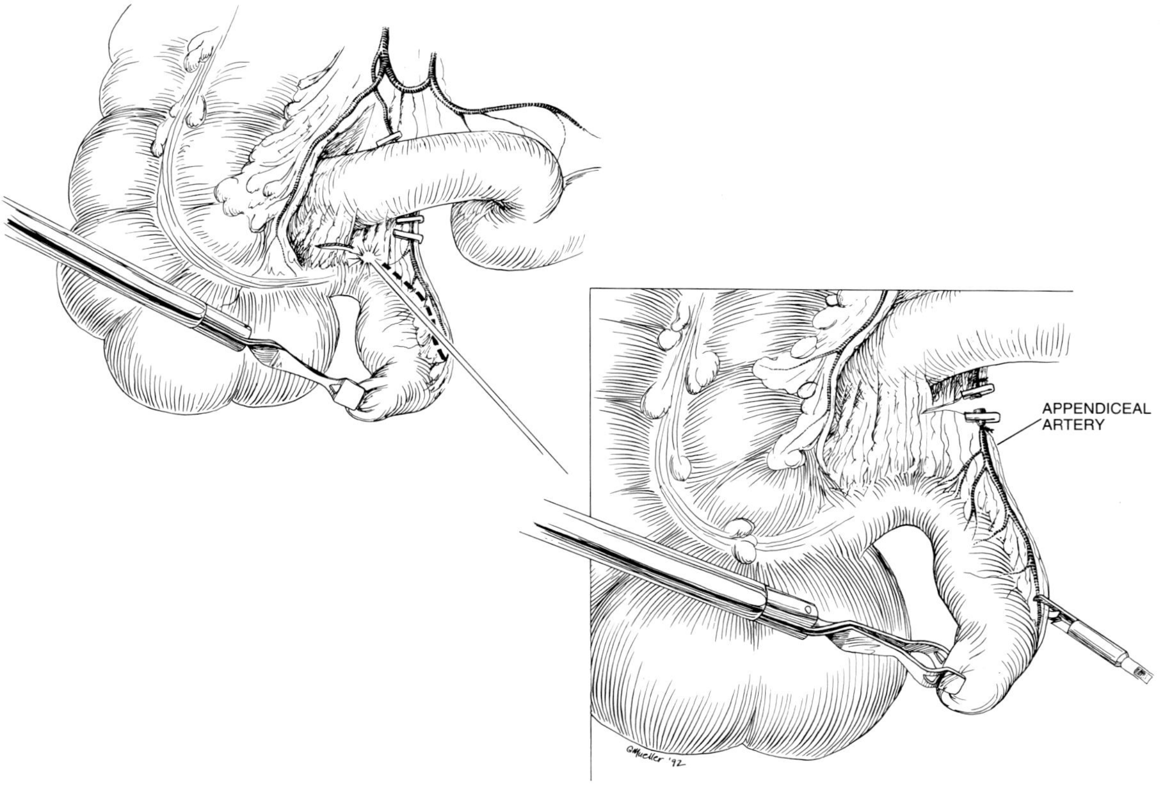

Figure 45-5.

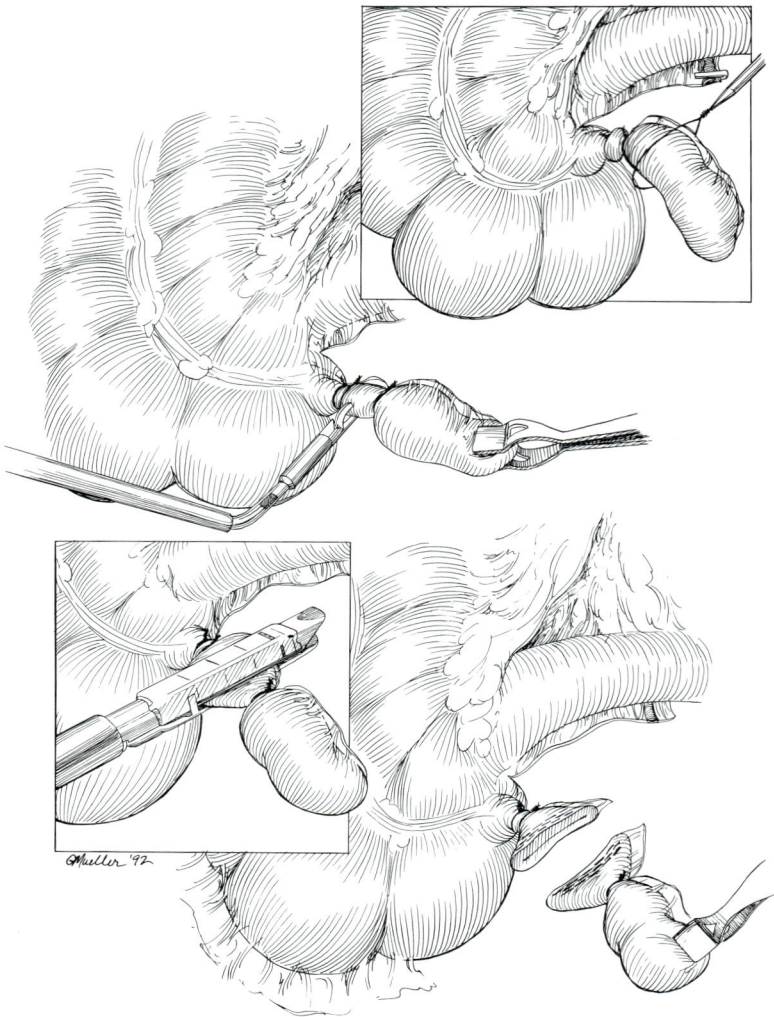

Figure 45-6.

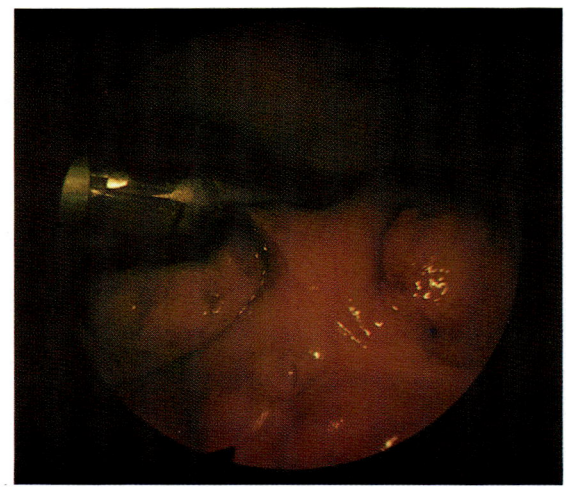

Figure 45-7.

scess cavity and brought out through the right sided trocar site. An interval appendectomy, either laparoscopically or open, is performed at a later date.

Once ligated, the appendix is removed via the 12-mm suprapubic trocar site (Fig. 45-8). If it is exceedingly inflamed or bulky, a 15-mm trocar can be placed. An alternative technique is to encase the appendix in a sterile condom or bag such as the ENDOCATCH* device prior to extraction (Figure 45-9). This prevents rupture of the appendix and contamination of the peritoneum and abdominal wall.

CLOSURE

After removal of the appendix, the patient is placed in the right side down, reverse

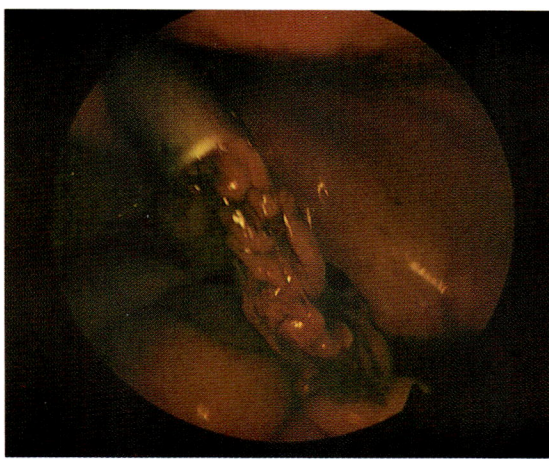

Figure 45-8.

Trendelenburg position, and the abdomen is irrigated with copious amounts of heparinized Ringer-lactate solution, which is subsequently aspirated. A drain may be left in the right-lower quadrant and brought out through the right-sided trocar site in the case of a localized collection or phlegmon. The cecum, mesoappendix, and stump are inspected once again for security of suturing and hemostasis. The trocars are removed under direct visualization, and the pneumoperitoneum is released. The wounds are irrigated and closed with either metal staples or a 4-0 Vicryl subcuticular suture and dressed with Steri-Strips. The Foley catheter and nasogastric tube are removed postoperatively in the operating room.

POSTOPERATIVE MANAGEMENT

Postoperatively, the patient may receive antibiotic therapy, depending upon the degree of inflammation or purulence as well as on the individual surgeon's preference. Most patients' diets can be advanced from liquid to solid after 8 to 12 hours, and patients can become ambulatory soon after surgery. Patients can be discharged as soon as 24 hours after surgery.

COMPLICATIONS

The diagnosis of acute appendicitis continues to be a dilemma for the clinical surgeon, with little progress being made over the last several decades. A diagnostic error rate of 20 per cent is often reported with rates as high as 40 per cent in women in their reproductive years. These figures have been described as a "necessary evil" to avoid the complications of a perforated appendix. In some groups, such as young healthy men, diagnostic accuracy is as high as 88 per cent.[17] However, in certain populations of patients, surgeons continue to fall short of the mark: namely, pediatric and elderly patients and women of childbearing age.[4] Perforation rates for these groups are high: for the pediatric population, 32 per cent[4,18]; for the elderly, up to 50 per cent[4,19]; and for ovulating women, 17 per cent.[4,17]

Recent studies report the use of laparoscopy as a diagnostic aid in patients with suspected acute appendicitis. Leape and Ramenofsky[12] studied 32 pediatric patients who were seen with atypical and equivocal clinical findings for acute appendicitis. The diagnosis of acute appendicitis was made in 17 patients. In 7 patients no pathologic condition was found, and 8 patients had another disease process. Twelve patients were spared an unnecessary appendectomy (38 per cent), and the unnecessary appendectomy rate was lowered from 40 per cent to 5 per cent in this group of patients and from 10 per cent to 1 per cent overall. In this study, there were two false negative and one false positive result.

Deutsch et al.[11] prospectively studied women aged 18 to 50 with suspected acute appendicitis. Appendicitis was diagnosed in 20 patients, while 12 patients (37 per cent) were spared an unnecessary laparotomy. The unnecessary appendectomy rate improved from 44 per cent to 16 per cent. No false negative or false positive results were reported.

Spirtos et al.[7] performed laparoscopy on 86 women between the ages of 16 and 42 with the presumed diagnosis of acute appendicitis. In 6 of these, the appendix could not be ade-

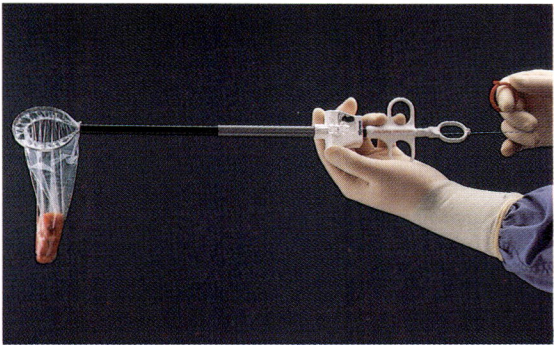

Figure 45-9.

quately visualized (93 per cent visualized). Acute appendicitis was found in 51. Laparoscopy prevented 22 patients (26 per cent) from undergoing an unnecessary appendectomy while the unnecessary appendectomy rate was improved from 41 per cent to 19 per cent.

The utility of laparoscopy in the evaluation of right lower quadrant pain has been well described by others also.[20-23] With adequate visualization of the appendix, laparoscopy is both sensitive and specific for acute appendicitis. If approximately 300,000 appendectomies are performed each year and laparoscopy could potentially lower the false positive rate from 20 per cent to 5 per cent, about 45,000 appendectomies with all their associated complications could be avoided.

Laparoscopic cholecystectomy revolutionized the treatment of cholelithiasis in a relatively short time and has been enthusiastically welcomed and adopted by the general surgeon. Laparoscopic appendectomy, first reported in 1983 by Prof. K. Semm, has not been as widely accepted, even though it is a safe and straightfoward operation. The argument against laparoscopic appendectomy includes the fact that an open appendectomy is an easy and quick operation and can be accomplished through a small incision, which unlike a Kocher incision for cholecystectomy, offers little postoperative disability.

In spite of the initial resistance to laparoscopic appendectomy, large series have now been reported. Pier et al.[24] reports a series of 625 laparoscopic appendectomies for acute appendicitis on patients ranging from age 2 to 80. Their conversion to open appendectomy rate was only 2 per cent (14 patients), and these were due to adhesions, extreme adiposity, bleeding abnormal appendiceal location, and abscess. Most conversions were done early in the series. Saye et al.[25] performed laparoscopic appendectomies on 109 patients, although only 10 per cent were for acute appendicitis. Like the findings from the Pier group, the average operative time was about 20 minutes. Patients undergoing incidental appendectomies were discharged home a mean of 23 hours postoperatively and the patients undergoing surgery for acute appendicitis were home within 36 hours. Valla et al.[26] reported on 465 pediatric patients, 3 to 16 years of age, undergoing laparoscopic appendectomy. Their conversion rate was 1 per cent (5 patients). They also report a 3.6 per cent (17 patients) intraoperative incident rate, including pneumoomentum, appendiceal rupture, and with visceral puncture (2 patients: 1 liver, 1 stomach). A 3 per cent postoperative complication rate was reported, and 1.3 per cent of patients either required another laparoscopy or open laparotomy later.

Summary

Many published reports confirm that laparoscopic appendectomy offers at least equivalent, if not better, treatment for acute appendicitis as open appendectomy. Laparoscopic appendectomy, in summary, offers the following advantages over an open appendectomy:[24-30]

1. Evaluation of the patient in whom diagnosis is clinically difficult
2. Reduction in the number of unnecessary laparotomies
3. Smaller incisions
4. Better exposure in obese patients
5. Easy and complete evaluation of the entire abdominal cavity
6. Better exposure for retrocecal appendix
7. Allowance for more complete intra-abdominal lavage
8. Possible lowering of the incidence of postoperative adhesions
9. Less postoperative pain
10. Possible shorter hospital stay (especially in patients with a normal appendix)

The role of laparoscopic appendectomy for removal of the normal appendix has not been defined. The situation in which this is a concern is its utilization in patients undergoing diagnostic laparoscopy for lower abdominal pain and performance of an incidental appendectomy during an unrelated procedure. Welch et al.[31] address this issue in their excellent editorial. Presently they are quantifying the complication rate for laparoscopic appendectomy, although recent series report complication rates of 1 to 3 per cent. Our preference is to remove the appendix in patients being evaluated for abdominal pain. We do not, however, perform incidental appendectomies during laparoscopic cholecystectomies or other procedures.

REFERENCES

1. Herrington JL. The vermiform appendix: Its surgical history, Contemp Surg, 1991; 39 (Oct):36–44.
2. Gilmore OJA, Browett JP, Williamson RCN, et al.

Appendicitis and mimicking conditions. Lancet 1975; 2:421–424.
3. Jess P, Bjerregard B, Brynitz S, et al. Acute appendicitis prospective trial concerning diagnostic accuracy and complications. Am J Surg 1981; 141:232–234.
4. Dunn EL, Moore EE, Elerding SC, et al. The unnecessary laparotomy for appendicitis—Can it be decreased? Am Surg 1982; 48:320–323.
5. O'Rourke M, Milton GW. The results of removing a "normal" appendix. Aust N Z J Surg 1963; 33:12–14.
6. Jersky J, Hoffman J, Kurgan A. Laparoscopy in patients with suspected acute appendicitis. South Afr J Surg 1980; 19:147–150.
7. Spirtos NM, Eisenkop SM, Spirtos TW, et al. Laparoscopy—A diagnostic aid in cases of suspected appendicitis. Am J Obstet Gynecol, 1987; 156:1–5.
8. Howie JGR. Death from appendicitis and appendectomy—An epidemiological survey. Lancet 1966; 4:72.
9. Horsch RF. Laparoscopy in the diagnosis of acute appendicitis. Contemp Surg 1989; 34–38.
10. Whitworth CM, Whitworth PW, Sanfillipo J, Polk HC. Value of diagnostic laparoscopy in young women with possible appendicitis. Surg Gynecol Obstet 1988; 167:187–190.
11. Deutsch AA, Zelikovsky A, Reiss R. Laparoscopy in the prevention of unnecessary appendectomies: A prospective study. Br J Surg 1982; 69;336–377.
12. Leape LL, Ramenofsky ML. Laparoscopy for questionable appendicitis—Can it reduce the appendectomy rate? Ann Surg 1980; 191:410–413.
13. Semm K. Endoscopic appendectomy. Endoscopy 1983; 15:59–64.
14. Schreiber J. Early experience with laparoscopic appendectomy in women. Surg Endosc 1987; 1:211–216.
15. Engstrom L, Fernyo G. Appendectomy: Assessment of stump invagination versus simple ligation: A prospective randomized trial. Br J Surg 1985; 72:971–972.
16. Schultz LS, Pietrafitta JJ, Graber JN, Hickock DF. Retrograde laparoscopic appendectomy: Report of a case. J Laparosc Endosc Surg 1991; 1:111–112.
17. Lewis FR, Holcroft JW, Boey J, Dunphy JE. Appendicitis—A critical review of diagnosis and treatment in 1000 cases. Arch Surg 1975; 110:677–684.
18. Marchildron MB, Dudgeon DL. Perforated appendicitis: Current experience in a children's hospital. Ann Surg 1977; 185:84–87.
19. Owens BJ, Hamit HF. Appendicitis in the elderly. Ann Surg 1978; 187:392–396.
20. Kleinhaus S, Hein K, Sheran M, et al. Laparoscopy for diagnosis and treatment of abdominal pain in adolescent girls. Arch Surg 1987; 112;1178–1189.
21. Diehl J, Eisenstat M, Gillinor S, Rao D. The role of peritoneoscopy in the diagnosis of acute abdominal conditions. Cleve Clin J Med 1981; 48:325–330.
22. Clarke P, Hands L, Gouch M, Kettlewell M. The use of laparoscopy in the management of right iliac fossa pain. Ann R Coll Surg 1986; 68:68–69.
23. Reiertsen O, Rosseland AR, Hiovik B, Solheim K. Laparoscopy in patients admitted for acute abdominal pain. Acta Chir Scand 1985; 151:521–524.
24. Pier A, Gotz F, Bacher C. Laparoscopic appendectomy in 625 cases: From innovation to routine, Surg Laparosc Endosc, 1991; 1:813.
25. Saye WB, Rives DA, Cochran EB. Laparoscopic appendectomy: Three years experience. Surg Laparosc Endosc, 1991; 1:109–115.
26. Valla JS, Limonne B, Valla V, et al. Laparoscopic appendectomy in children: Report of 465 cases. Surg Laparosc Endosc, 1991; 1:166–172.
27. Nowzaradan Y, Westmoreland J, McCarver CT, Harris RJ. Laparoscopic appendectomy for acute appendicitis: Indications for current use. J Laparoendosc Surg 1991; 1:247–258.
28. Olsen DO. Laparoscopic appendectomy using a linear stapling device. Surg Rounds 1991; 873–883.
29. Geis WP, Miller CE, Kokoszka JS, et al. Laparoscopic appendectomy for acute appendicitis: Rationale and technical aspects. Contemp Surg 1992; 40:13–19.
30. Cristalli BG, Izard V, Jacob D, Levarson M. Laparoscopic appendectomy using a clip applier. Surg Endosc, 1991; 5:176–178.
31. Welch NT, Hinder RA, Fitzgibbons RJ. Laparoscopic incidental appendectomy. Surg Laparosc Endosc, 1991; 1:116–118.

Chapter 46
Polypectomy

Garth H. Ballantyne

Most benign neoplasms of the colon and rectum less than 2 cm in diameter are easily removed during colonoscopy. As polyps increase in size to greater than 2 cm, the difficulty of colonoscopic polypectomy increases. Although it is possible to excise piecemeal some of these large polyps, this approach presents several disadvantages: pathologic staging of the lesion may be compromised, the risk of perforation may increase, and difficulties in hemostasis may be encountered.

Large polyps may be the harbinger of invasive carcinomas.[1] Piecemeal extraction may preclude accurate determination of the depth of penetration and the margins of resection for a cancer in a polyp. Indeed, all current recommendations on the subsequent treatment of an endoscopically excised cancer in a polyp are based on the histologic features of the cancer found on the whole mount of the sectioned polyp.[2]

The wall of the right colon is thinner than that of the left. Unfortunately, polyps in the right colon are generally sessile. Piecemeal extraction of large sessile lesions requires extensive use of electrocautery. The thin wall of the right colon may be perforated during the initial excision or shortly after the procedure because of tissue injury from the electrocautery. Thus, there may be a greater risk of perforation with aggressive colonoscopic polypectomy of a sessile polyp in the right colon than for a lesion in the left colon.

Polyps in the left colon tend to be pedunculated and to hang from long stalks. In addition, the wall of the left colon is thick. Thus, many large polyps in the left colon are easily and safely lassoed with a snare cautery and excised *in toto*. Unfortunately, the left colon is generally serpentine. Sometimes the base of the stalk is concealed by a sharp angulation of the sigmoid colon. Should hemostasis prove inadequate after division of the stalk with the snare cautery, control of hemorrhage from the poorly visualized stalk may prove problematic. In some polyps, the head of the polyp exceeds the diameter of the loop of the snare cautery despite the presence of a narrow stalk. In these cases, excision of the polyp in one piece is also precluded.

Laparoscopy and new stapling instruments offer several novel approaches that may facilitate the management of large polyps of the colon and rectum. These include: laparoscopically assisted colonscopic polypectomy, laparoscopically assisted colotomy and polypectomy, laparoscopic colotomy and polypectomy, and transanal polypectomy.

The purpose of this chapter is to offer some advice on the selection of patients and to describe the surgical technique of these procedures. The goal of these procedures is to treat benign lesions by techniques that minimize complications and patient discomfort. In addition, these procedures avoid colorectal resections and, thereby, avoid compromise of bowel function.

DEFINITIONS

Laparoscopically Assisted Colonoscopic Polypectomy

Colonoscopic polypectomy is performed under direct visualization by the laparoscopic surgeon. When necessary, colonoscopic polypectomy is facilitated by mobilization of portions of the bowel. Mobilization and retraction of the sigmoid colon, for example, may expose to the colonoscopist the previously concealed stalk of a pedunculated polyp. This procedure serves to improve exposure for the colonoscopist and allows immediate identification of perforation during aggressive colonoscopic polypectomies.

Laparoscopically Assisted Colotomy and Polypectomy

Portions of the colon are mobilized laparoscopically and withdrawn from the abdomen through a small incision. The location of the lesion is identified colonoscopically. The colotomy, polypectomy, and closure of the colotomy are achieved extracorporeally by traditional surgical techniques.

Laparoscopic Colotomy and Polypectomy

Portions of the colon are mobilized laparoscopically. The polyp is localized colonoscopically. The colotomy, polypectomy, and colotomy closure are accomplished intracorporeally by laparoscopic techniques. After excision the specimen is reinserted into the colon and retrieved through the colon with a colonoscope.

COLONIC POLYPS

Patient Selection

Laparoscopically assisted polypectomy and laparoscopic polypectomy are new procedures. Complication rates for these procedures are not documented yet. Long term rates of recurrence following these approaches also remain undefined. Consequently, hard and fast recommendations for patient selection would be premature at this time. Nonetheless, the advent of laparoscopic techniques has increased the options available to the surgeon for the care of patients with benign neoplasms of the colon and rectum.

All patients with colonic polyps undergo initial evaluation by an experienced colonoscopist. Whenever appropriate, benign neoplasms of the colon and rectum are removed by snare polypectomy. Laparoscopic approaches to treatment of colonic polyps are considered when:

1. Large (greater than 2 cm) sessile polyps are encountered.
2. The diameter of the head of the polyp exceeds the width of the loop of the snare cautery.
3. Problems with hemostasis are anticipated.
4. The base of the polyp's stalk is poorly visualized.

Patient selection will change as the surgeon's experience with laparoscopy increases. Several features will increase the difficulty of the procedure, including (1) previous abdominal operations, (2) polyps at the hepatic or splenic flexures, (3) obesity of the patient. The surgeon may wish to offer different modalities of therapy to patients with these characteristics early in his or her experience.

Patient Evaluation

Evaluation of patients prior to laparoscopic procedures for colonic neoplasms is the same as that for patients who are scheduled for open colorectal resections. Findings at the time of laparoscopy or complications encountered during the procedure may require immediate conversion to an open laparotomy. The pulmonary and cardiovascular status of patients require particular attention. The insufflation of the peritoneum with carbon dioxide generates a respiratory-type acidosis. This may lead to arrhythmias or otherwise impair myocardial function. Restrictive pulmonary disease may hamper the ability of the anesthesiologist to maintain the acid-base balance within physiologic limits through increases in ventilation.

Preoperative Preparation

All patients undergo standard bowel preparations prior to the operation. The patients drink two liters of GoLYTELY or NuLYTELY the night before or the morning of the procedure. In addition, the patient receives either oral or perioperative intravenous antibiotics.

Equipment

The full complement of laparoscopic instruments should be available within the operating room. Laparoscopically assisted procedures will require the following instruments:

1. 10-mm, 0-degree laparoscope,
2. five 10-mm ports,
3. one disposable scissors,
4. one grasping instrument, e.g., an ENDO DISSECT* instrument,
5. two Babcock clamps, and
6. one Multifire clip applier.

Laparoscopic colotomy, polypectomy and closure of the colotomy will require several additional instruments:

1. one 12- or 15-mm port,
2. two Allis clamps,
3. one needle driver, and
4. one ENDO GIA 30* or ENDO GIA 60* stapling device and additional cartridges.

An intraoperative colonoscopy is performed during each procedure. A videocolonoscope allows the laparoscopic surgeon simultaneous views of the lumen of the colon. An electrocautery snare is required if endoscopic polypectomy proves feasible.

Surgical instruments for open laparotomy and colectomy must be available within the operating room. Findings during laparoscopy or intraoperative complications may necessitate a rapid change to an open operation.

Positioning of the Patient

Patients are placed in a supine position with legs supported by Lloyd-Davies stirrups. The thighs are straight. Flexion of the hips causes the thighs to limit the excursions of the laparoscopic instruments. This position allows access to the anus for insertion of the colonoscope. At least one arm is tucked at the side of the patient. This makes additional room available at the side of the patient for the cameraman. Nasogastric tubes and urinary catheters are inserted in all patients. These decrease the risk of stomach or bladder injury during trochar insertion.

Video Equipment and Placement

The placement of the monitors varies with the location of the polyp. When lesions in the right colon, transverse colon, or descending colon are encoutered, the two monitors are positioned near the shoulders of the patient (Fig. 46-1, A and B). When the polyp is in the sigmoid colon, one monitor is placed between the legs of the patient and the second monitor by the left shoulder. The monitor of the videocolonoscope is situated lateral to the outstretched leg of the patient where it can be observed by both the endoscopist and the laparoscopist.

Trochar Placement

Trochar placement differs for polyps of the right colon and left colon. In both locations, the pneumoperitoneum is established through a supraumbilical port. Initial exploration of the abdomen is accomplished via a 10-mm port at this site. Mobilization of the cecum requires ports in the right lower quadrant and above the pubis (Fig. 46-2). This permits lateral access and visualization of the right gutter. The telescope is moved to the 10-mm suprapubic port. The surgeon frees the cecum and right colon of its retroperitoneal attachments with electrocautery scissors. The scissors and a grasping instrument are inserted through the two 5- or 10-mm ports placed in the right lower quadrant. The assistant retracts the cecum medially and anteriorly with a Babcock clamp admitted through the supraumbilical port. An additional 10-mm port, which is positioned in the left upper quadrant lateral to the rectus sheath, may facilitate mobilization of the ascending colon and hepatic flexure. This allows insertion of a second Babcock clamp for retraction. When an ENDO GIA* stapling device is used for a cecal polypectomy, a final 12- or 15-mm port is placed on the midline halfway between the umbilicus and pubis.

Trochar placement for removal of a polyp in the sigmoid colon is identical to that used for a left colon resection (Fig. 46-3). Five 10-mm ports are required: one is placed on the midline just cephalad to the umbilicus; two are placed in the right lower quadrant lateral to the rectus sheath; and two are placed in the left lower quadrant lateral to the rectus sheath. The telescope is inserted through the supraumbilical port. The surgeon accomplishes the dissection through the left lower ports. The assistant retracts the sigmoid colon medially and anteriorly with Babcock clamps introduced through the right lower quadrant ports. When an ENDO GIA* stapling device is used during the polypectomy, one of the

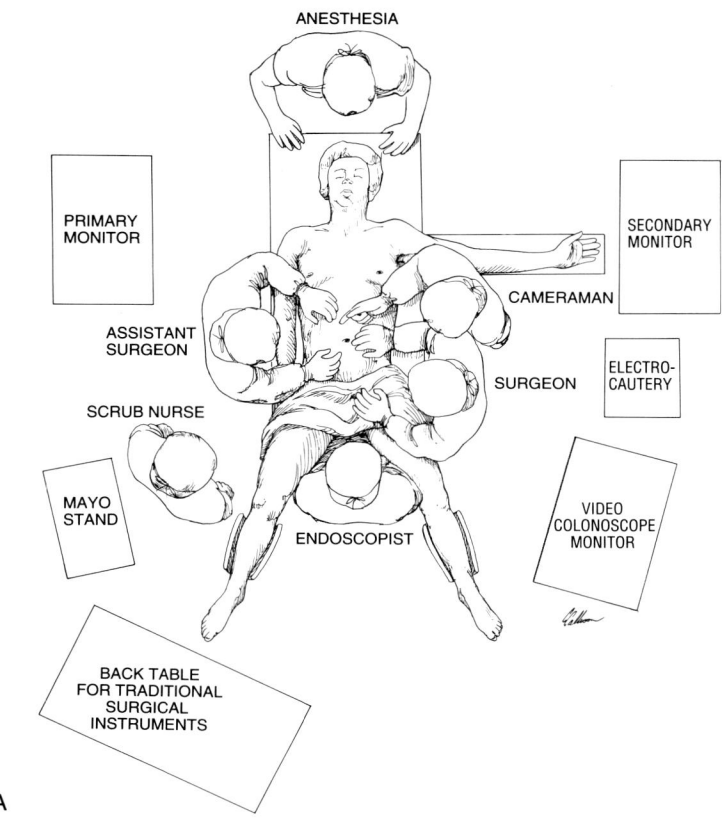
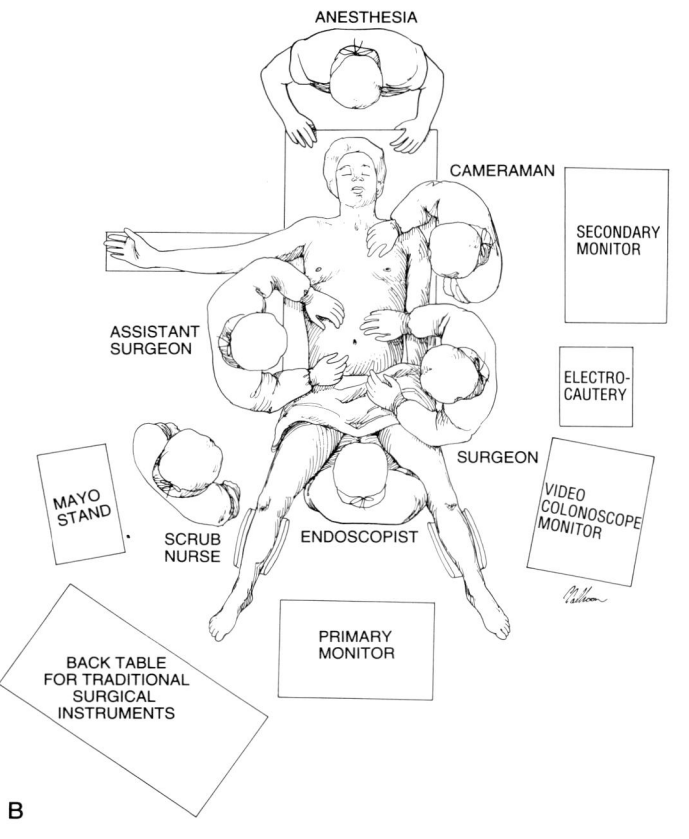

Figure 46-1.

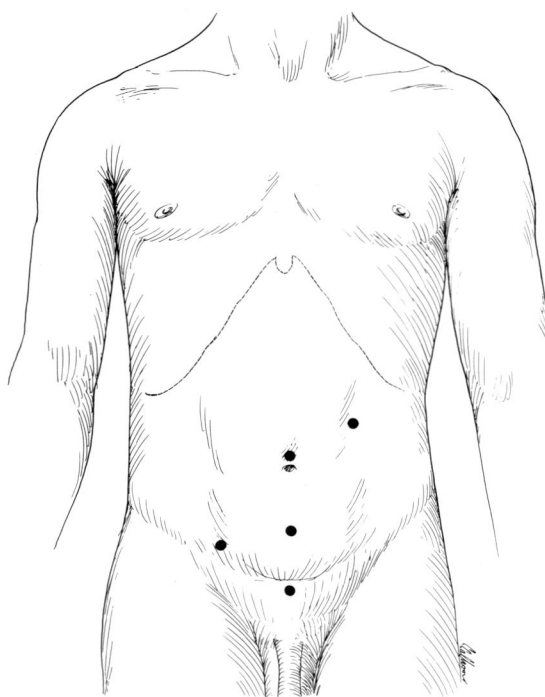

Figure 46-2.

right lower quadrant 10-mm ports is replaced by a 12- or 15-mm port.

Methods of Exposure and Retraction

RIGHT COLON

The patient is dropped into a deep Trendelenburg position. The right shoulder is rolled up. The small bowel slides out of the pelvis and away from the right colon. After exploration of the abdomen, the telescope is advanced into the abdomen through the suprapubic port. The dissection is observed on the video monitor, which is near the right shoulder of the patient. The cecum is grasped with a Babcock clamp passed into the abdomen through the supraumbilical port. This exposes the right gutter and the base of the cecum over the iliac vessels.

TRANSVERSE COLON AND FLEXURES

The telescope remains in the supraumbilical port. A 10-mm, 30-degree telescope improves visualization of the lateral aspects of the mobilization of the flexures. Parts of the dissection may be better visualized with the telescope inserted through a port in the left or right upper quadrant. The head of the patient is elevated into a reverse Trendelenberg position. The right side of the patient is rolled up for lesions of the hepatic flexure and proximal transverse colon. The left side is rotated up for lesions located in the distal transverse colon and splenic flexure. The omentum is pushed toward the head of the patient and anteriorly with Babcock clamps. The grasping instrument of the surgeon retracts the colon medially and posteriorly.

LEFT COLON

The telescope remains in the supraumbilical port. The head of the patient is lowered into a deep Trendelenburg positioned. The left shoulder is rolled up. The small bowel rolls away from the pelvis and sigmoid colon. The assistant surgeon on the right side of the patient retracts the sigmoid colon medially and anteriorly.

Methods of Dissection

All dissection is accomplished with electrocautery scissors. The assistant pulls the bowel

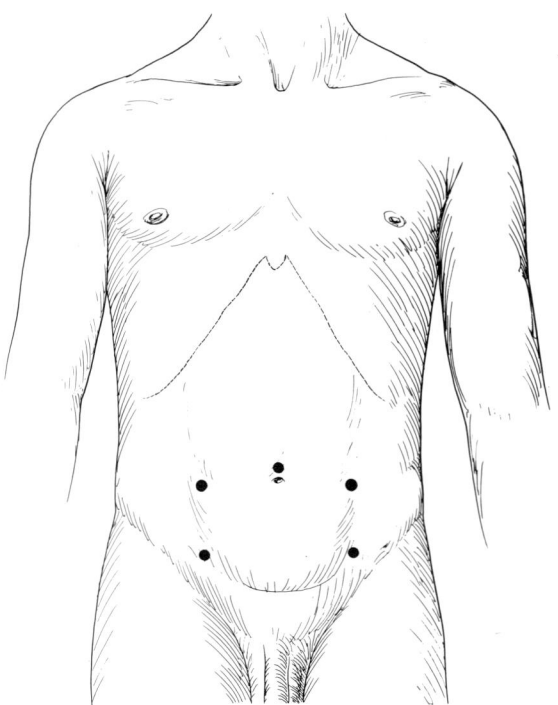

Figure 46-3.

medially and anteriorly with Babcock clamps. The surgeon maintains lateral countertraction with a grasping instrument such as an ENDO-GRASP*. Meticulous hemostasis greatly facilitates the dissection. Even small amounts of blood stain tissues and obscure tissue planes.

Specific Details of the Procedure

EXPLORATION OF THE ABDOMEN

After induction of anesthesia, the nasogastric tube and urinary catheter are inserted. The abdomen is prepared and draped in a sterile manner. The head of the patient is dropped into a deep Trendelenburg position. A small incision is made above the umbilicus. The Veress needle is inserted above the umbilicus. Its position is verified. The abdomen is insufflated with carbon dioxide. The Veress needle is removed, and a 10-mm trochar is inserted into the abdomen. The pneumoperitoneum is reestablished. The bowel directly below the insertion site is inspected for evidence of puncture by the trochar or Veress needle. The additional working ports are inserted under direct observation. The lower abdomen is explored. The small bowel is run from the ileocecal valve back to the ligament of Treitz. The small bowel is exposed by alternately grasping sections with Babcock or atraumatic bowel clamps. The head of the patient is elevated into a reverse Trendelenburg position. The upper abdomen is visualized. The diaphragmatic surfaces of the liver are more easiliy viewed through a 10-mm, 30-degree telescope.

LOCALIZATION OF THE POLYP

The position of the polyp can not be visualized through the laparoscope. After establishment of the pneumoperitoneum and initial exploration, a colonoscope is advanced into the colon via the anus. The light intensity of the laparoscope is decreased. The light of the colonoscope is observed as it advances around the colon (Fig. 46-4). The lumen of the colon is insufflated with as little air as possible. The colonoscopist locates the polyp. The laparoscopic surgeon marks the position of the polyp with clips (Fig. 46-5, A and B). The colonoscopist observes the indentation in the colonic wall caused by the clip applier and directs the placement of the clips in relation to the polyp.

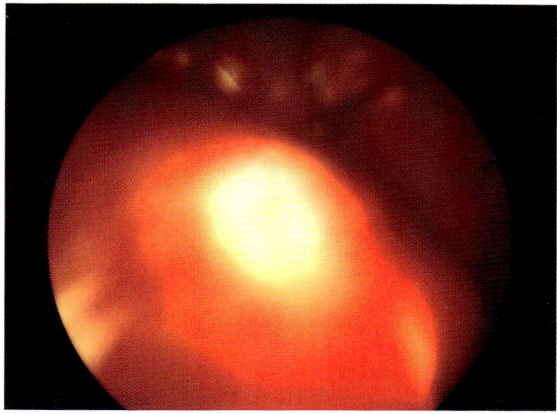

Figure 46-4.

During this procedure, the cecum may become excessively distended by air, which will significantly compromise exposure during the remainder of the procedure. When this occurs, the colonsocope is advanced into the cecum. The air is removed by suction. The entire colon is easily collapsed by applying nearly continuous suction as the colonoscope is withdrawn. Usually the small bowel is not distended by intraoperative colonoscopy. If insufflation of the small bowel is observed, the terminal ileum is obstructed with an atraumatic bowel clamp.

LAPAROSCOPICALLY ASSISTED COLONOSCOPIC POLYPECTOMY

The location of the polyp is identified and marked. If the polyp is well visualized through the colonoscope, endoscopic polypectomy with the snare cautery is attempted. The outside wall of the colon is observed by the laparoscopic surgeon during application of the snare. The wall is checked for evidence of cautery burn during the polypectomy. The advantage of this approach is immediate identification of perforation during an aggressive polypectomy. Additionally, hemorrhage precipitated by the polypectomy can be immediately treated by laparoscopic techniques.

When visualization of the polyp by the colonoscopist is inadequate, the laparoscopic surgeon mobilizes the appropriate segment of bowel. This generally occurs in the sigmoid colon where fixed angulations of the bowel may make visualization of the base of the polyp's stalk difficult. The 10-mm, 0-degree

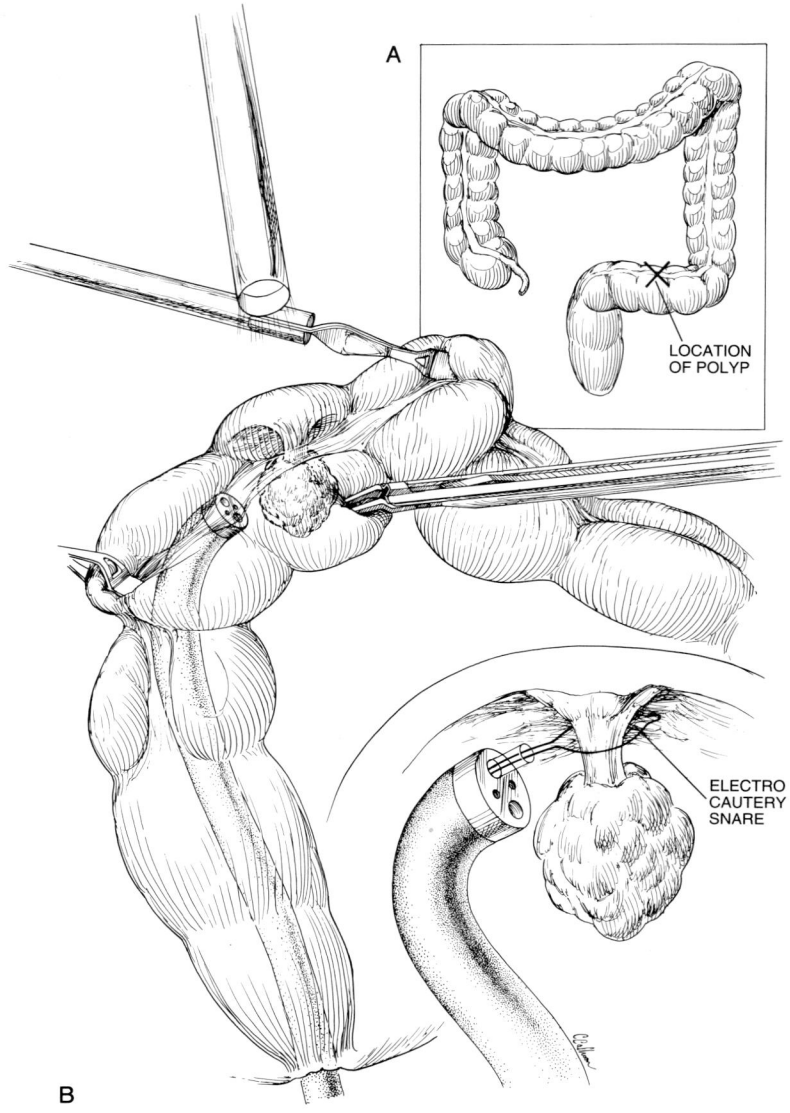

Figure 46-5.

telescope remains in the supraumbilical port. The patient is dropped into a Trendelenburg position. The left shoulder is rolled up. The assistant inserts two Babcock clamps through the right lower quadrant ports. These grasp the sigmoid colon and rectosigmoid junction and provide medial and anterior traction. The surgeon incises the lateral attachments of the sigmoid colon. The left ureter is identified as it traverses the left iliac vessels. The mesocolon is bluntly pushed medially off of the retroperitoneum with the shaft of the scissors. Mobilization continues until the angulation that is obscuring the base of the polyp is straightened. The colonoscope is reintroduced. The polyp is visualized by the endoscopist. Endoscopic polypectomy is attempted. The laparoscopic surgeon observes the serosal surface of the colon during the snare polypectomy for evidence of perforation (Fig. 46-6). The endoscopist retrieves the polyp. A surgical pathologist evaluates the polyp by frozen section for the presence of invasive carcinoma. If treatment by snare polypectomy is judged adequate based on the histologic findings, the procedure is terminated. The advantage of this procedure is that a colotomy or colonic resection is avoided.

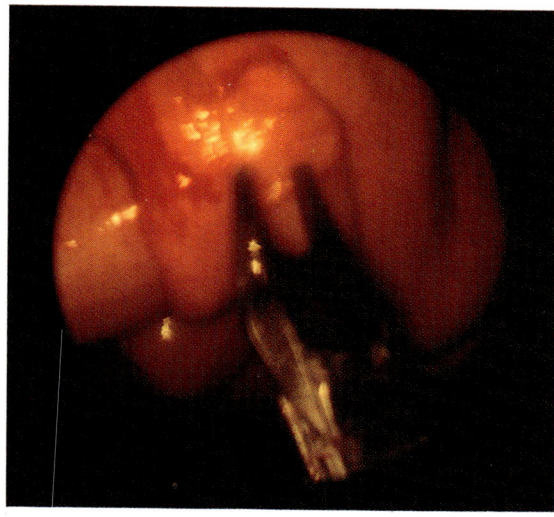

Figure 46-6.

LAPAROSCOPICALLY ASSISTED COLOTOMY AND POLYPECTOMY

Large sessile lesions, which are thought to be benign, can be removed by laparoscopically assisted mobilization of the segment of bowel and extracorporeal colotomy and polypectomy. If the polyp is found in the cecum, the patient is dropped into a Trendelenburg position. The right shoulder is rolled up. The telescope is repositioned in the suprapubic port. The assistant retracts the cecum medially and anteriorly with a Babcock clamp, which is introduced through the supraumbilical port. The surgeon stands between the legs of the patient. The dissection is viewed on the monitor, which is positioned by the patient's right shoulder. The posterior peritoneum is incised by the surgeon with electrocautery scissors near the appendix. The right ureter is identified. The areolar plane between the mesocolon and retroperitoneum is entered. The peritoneal reflection is incised along the right gutter. The retroperitoneum is bluntly swept off the mesocolon with the side of the long shaft of the scissors. The retroperitoneal attachments of the terminal ileum are also incised. The cecum and ascending colon are mobilized until the segment in which the polyp is located reaches easily up to the abdominal wall.

When lesions are situated in the left colon, the sigmoid and descending colon are mobilized as described above. This is most easily accomplished with lesions found in the sigmoid colon. Indeed, in some patients, the sigmoid colon is sufficiently mobile that the region of the polyp will reach up to the abdominal wall without any dissection. Similarly, the middle portion of the transverse colon may demand little or no mobilization. In contrast, exteriorization of the proximal descending colon or splenic flexure requires extensive mobilization.

The marked portion of colon, which contains the polyp, is lifted toward the abdominal wall with Babcock clamps (Fig. 46-7). A site for a small transverse incision is selected over the mobilized section of colon. If mobility is inadequate for exteriorization, further dissection is needed. The skin and subcutaneous tissues are incised down to the fascia. The fascia is incised. The muscles are separated along the direction of their fibers with a blunt clamp. The abdomen is entered through a small incision. The surgeon quickly plugs this hole with his or her index finger, maintaining the pneumoperitoneum. The surgeon slides a Babcock clamp along the finger into the abdomen. Under direct laparoscopic visualization, the mobilized segment of colon is grasped with the Babcock clamp. The colon is pulled into the wound. The pneumoperitoneum is released. This allows the abdominal wall to collapse. The incision is expanded to the minimal size that will allow exteriorization of the marked portion of colon.

The colon is entered through a longitudinal colotomy in the antimesenteric teniae coli. A sessile polyp is excised by a submucosal dissection similar to that commonly performed for rectal villous adenomas. The edges of the mucosa are approximated with a continuous suture of 000 chromic catgut. Pedunculated lesions are excised by firing a TA 30 or TA 55 stapling device across their pedicles (Fig. 46-8). The specimen is submitted for examination by a surgical pathologist and assessed by frozen section. The edges of the colotomy are grasped with Allis clamps. The longitudinal colotomy is closed transversely with a TA 55 stapling device.

LAPAROSCOPIC COLOTOMY AND POLYPECTOMY

The need for an abdominal incision is obviated by performing an intracorporeal colotomy and polypectomy. The quality of the bowel preparation is evaluated by the colonoscopist. If necessary, the colon is further irrigated through the colonoscope. The location of the polyp is marked and the bowel mobi-

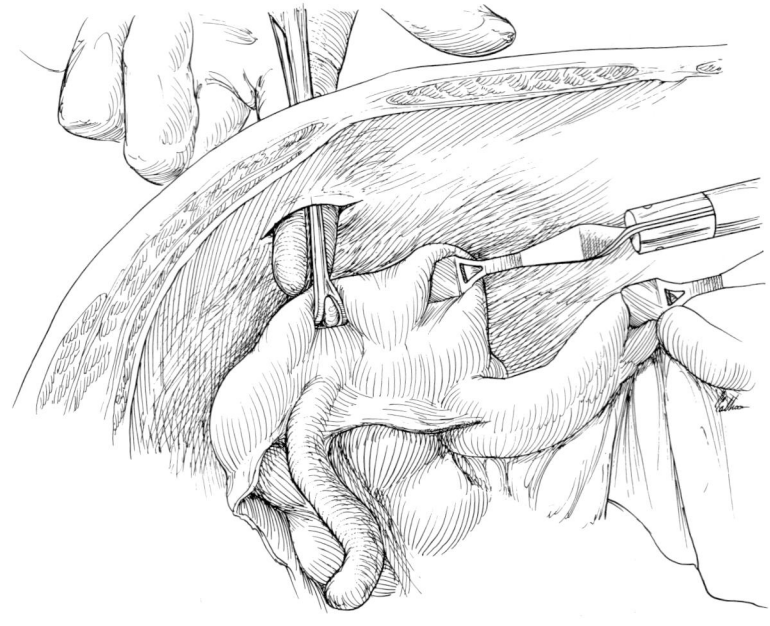

Figure 46-7.

lized as described above. A convenient point for the colotomy is selected on the antimesenteric teniae coli proximal to the polyp. For a sigmoid polyp, the colon is grasped with Allis clamps or Babcock clamps on either side of the teniae coli. These clamps are introduced through the two caudad ports in the left and right lower quadrants. The telescope remains in the supraumbilical port. The teniae is incised with the electrocautery scissors, which are introduced through the cephalad left lower quadrant port. The scissors are removed and replaced with a Babcock clamp. This is inserted into the colon and used to grasp the polyp. This maneuver is observed by the laparoscopic surgeon on the video monitor of the colonoscope. The polyp is extricated from the colon and elevated toward the abdominal wall (Fig. 46-9). The cephalad port in the right lower quadrant is replaced by a 12- or 15-mm port. The stalk of the polyp is sized with an ENDO GAUGE* in-

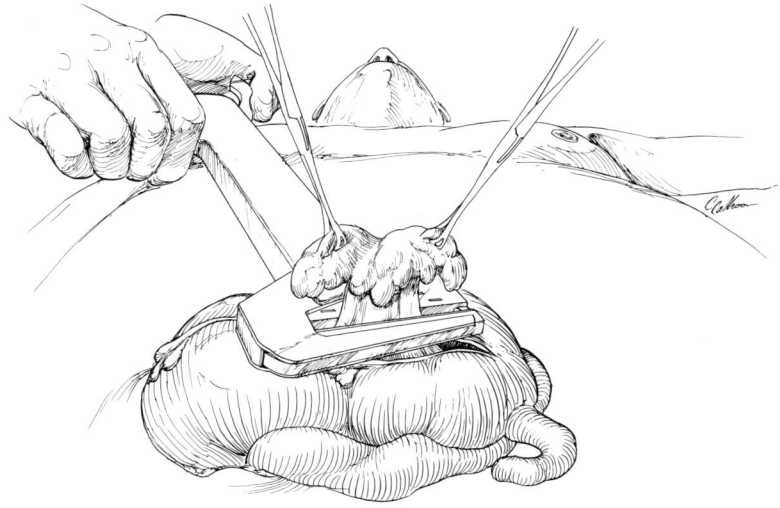

Figure 46-8.

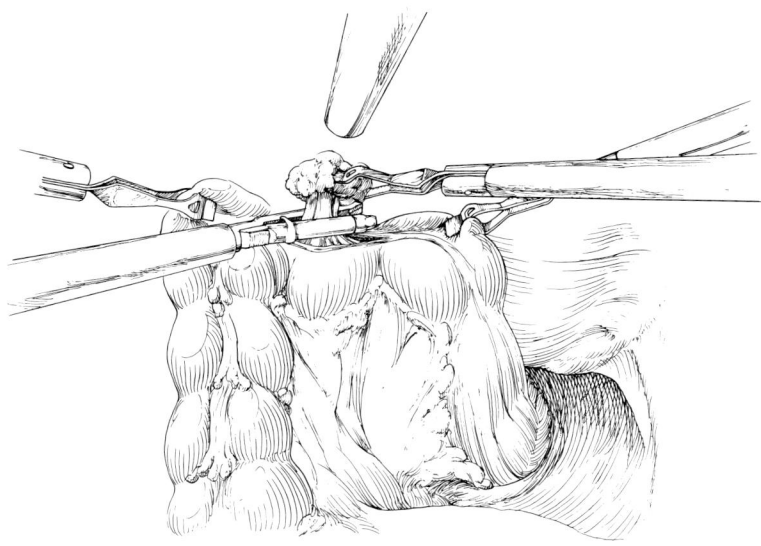

Figure 46-9.

strument. The white or blue cartridge is selected. The stalk of the polyp is divided with the ENDO GIA 30* or ENDO GIA 60* stapling device. The excised polyp is reinserted into the colon with the Babcock clamp. The polyp is retrieved with the colonoscope and submitted for pathologic assessment. The contaminated Babcock clamp is withdrawn from the abdomen.

During the polypectomy, the Allis clamps or Babcock clamps continue to elevate the edges of the colotomy. This diminishes the risk of spillage of luminal contents. The longitudinal colotomy is closed transversely. The Babcock clamps separate the middle portion of the colotomy (Fig. 46-10). A new Babcock or Allis clamp is inserted into the abdomen through the cephalad left lower quadrant port. It apposes the two corners of the colotomy in the center of the planned closure. If the colotomy is long, an additional Babcock or Allis clamp may be required to properly align the edges. The Babcock clamps must

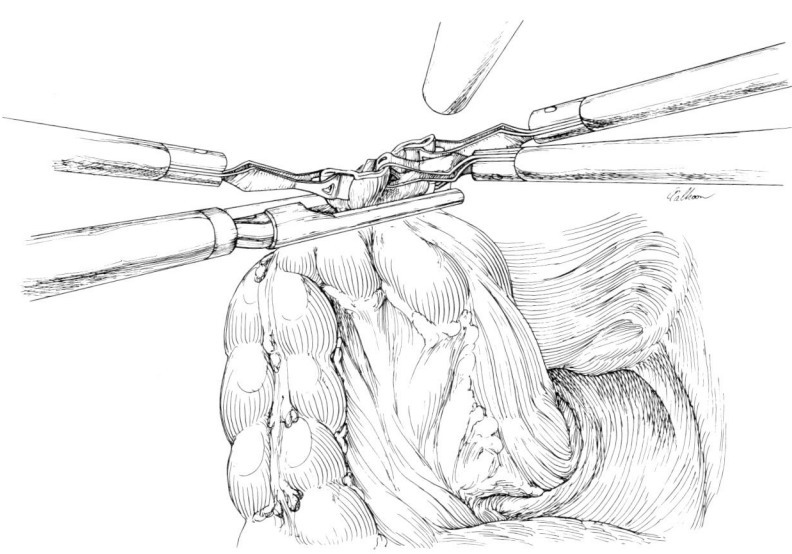

Figure 46-10.

grasp the full thickness of both edges of the bowel wall. On some occasions, sutures may facilitate closure of the colotomy. These are placed through the full thickness of the bowel wall on either side of the colotomy. A grasping instrument elevates the ends of the sutures up toward the abdominal wall. The edges of the colotomy are more closely apposed when a knot is tied in the suture. This may be tied either intracorporeally or extracorporeally. Alternatively, a pre-tied loop such as a SURGITIE* ligating loop is placed around the shaft of an Allis or Babcock clamp. After the clamp apposes the edges of the colon, the loop of the suture is dropped down onto the two edges of bowel below the clamp and tightened. Once the edges of the colotomy are aligned transversely, the ENDO GIA 30* or ENDO GIA 60* stapling device is inserted into the abdomen through the 12- or 15-mm port. These instruments fire six overlapping rows of staples, and the tissue is divided with a scalpel blade. In the near future, ENDO TA 30* and ENDO TA 60* stapling devices, which fire only three rows of staples, will become available. The stapling device is positioned near the colotomy, and its jaws are opened. The stapling device remains stationary. The colon is pushed and pulled by the Babcock and Allis clamps into the open jaws. The tips of the jaws are carefully observed since the tips can tear the bowel wall. The stapling device is closed below the clamps and sutures. The full thickness of the bowel wall edges should be visible above the jaws of the stapling device. The stapling device is fired. The edges of the closure are checked for hemostasis. Larger colotomies may required two applications of the ENDO GIA 30* stapling device for complete closure.

The colonoscope is inserted through the anus and advanced to the level of the colotomy closure. The colon is insufflated. The staple line should be airtight. The luminal side of the staple line is inspected for hemostasis. The colonoscope is passed through the closure to ensure that the lumen remains patient.

Closure

Once the colotomy is closed, the abdomen is liberally irrigated with warmed saline. If an incision is present, the saline is poured directly through the open wound and then suctioned out; otherwise, it is poured down the largest available port. The abdomen is inspected for hemostasis. The working ports are removed under direct observation through the laparoscope. This ensures that loops of bowel are not sucked into the fascial defect left by the port. The telescope is removed. The pneumoperitoneum is released through the remaining port, which is then removed. The anterior fascial defects created by ports 10 mm and larger are closed with interrupted sutures of 00 Dexon. The smaller skin incisions are apposed with Steri-Strips and the larger ones with subcuticular sutures of 0000 Dexon. Band-Aids cover the wounds.

Postoperative Management

The nasogastric tube is removed immediately after extubation on the first morning following the operation. The urinary catheter is removed when the patient is up and walking around. This is typically on the first or second day after the operation. The diet is advanced to clear liquids when the patient states that he or she is hungry. The patient receives a regular diet the next day. Often the patient can tolerate clear liquids on the first or second day following the procedure.

RECTAL POLYPS

Stapling devices can expedite transanal polypectomies performed with traditional techniques. Two techniques are shown below and are included in this chapter since they offer a minimally invasive technique, which is similar in concept to the laparoscopic techniques described above. Moreover, these procedures offer an opportunity for surgeons who are not accustomed to excision of polyps with stapling devices an opportunity to apply this technology under favorable circumstances.

Patient Selection

These procedures may prove helpful in the management of patients who have developed benign neoplasms of the distal two-thirds of the rectum. Smaller (less than 2 cm) polyps are excised endoscopically. These procedures are particularly suited for removal of sessile villous polyps. Posterior lesions are more easily excised, but there is no reason to exclude anterior lesions. There is no limit on the longitudinal size of the polyp. Application of the stapling devices to sessile polyps which extend around more than half of the circumference of the lumen, however, is difficult. Circumferential lesions cannot be excised by these stapling techniques. It may be possible to achieve a transanal excision of a polyp in the proximal third of the rectum. On occasion, the proximal rectum can be intussuscepted down toward the anus. A laparoscopic approach to these lesions, however, may prove to be easier.

Preoperative Evaluation

These patients will require regional or general anesthesia. Consequently, they should undergo standard preoperative pulmonary and cardiovascular evaluation. Larger polyps are evaluated by colonoscopic biopsy for the presence of invasive carcinoma before operation.

Preoperative Preparation

The preparation of these patients for operation is the same as described earlier for the laparoscopic procedures.

Equipment

The required number of instruments is small:

1. St. Mark's rectal retractor,
2. needle driver,
3. curved Mayo scissors,
4. TA 55 stapling device, and
5. ENDO GIA 30* or ENDO GIA 60* stapling device.
6. Babcock clamps

Positioning of the Patient

The patient is placed in lithotomy position. The table is tilted into the Trendelenburg position. An urinary catheter is inserted, but a nasogastric tube is not required.

Specific Details of the Procedure

The anus is slowly dilated until four fingers are easily inserted into the rectum. The St. Mark's rectal retractor or Buie anal retractor is positioned and opened. The polyp is grasped with two Babcock clamps. The mobility of the lesion is assessed.

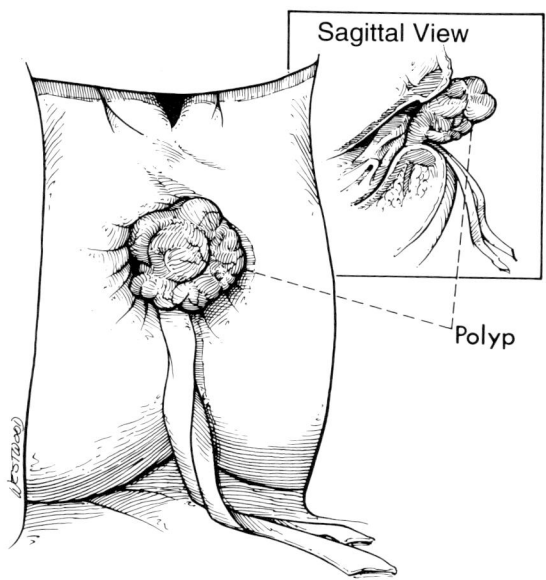

Figure 46-11.

POLYPS THAT PROLAPSE THROUGH THE ANUS

Polyps that protrude outside the anus are rapidly excised with a stapling device (Fig. 46-11). The St. Mark's retractor is removed since it may limit the mobility of a distal rectal polyp. The lesion is prolapsed out through the anus. Traction sutures of 000 chromic are placed through the lesion (Fig. 46-12). A TA 55 stapling device is closed around the base of the polyp proximal to the traction sutures. The margin of resection is checked. The stapling device is fired. The specimen is transected with curved Mayo scissors along the edge of the stapling device. The specimen is submitted for pathologic examination. The deep and lateral margins of resection are evaluated by frozen section. The Buie anal retractor is reinserted. The staple line is inspected for hemostasis (Fig. 46-13). Sometimes small bleeding arteries are visible along the staple line. These are ligated with 000 silk. The retractor is removed. A rigid proctosigmoidoscope is advanced up to the distal sigmoid. This ensures that the lumen of the rectum remains patent.

RECTAL POLYPS THAT DO NOT PROLAPSE

The ENDO GIA 30* and ENDO GIA 60* stapling devices facilitate the excision of sessile

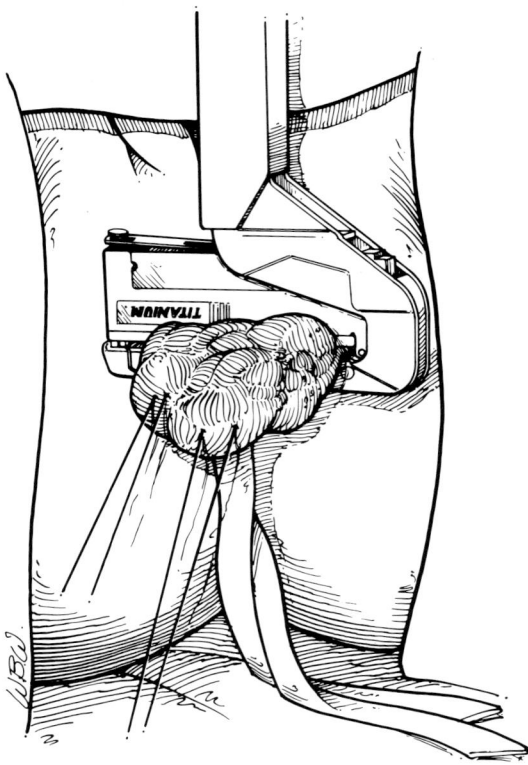

Figure 46-12.

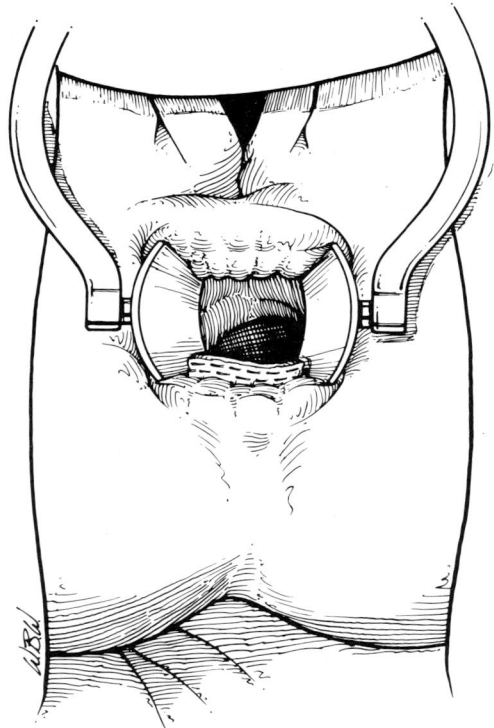

Figure 46-13.

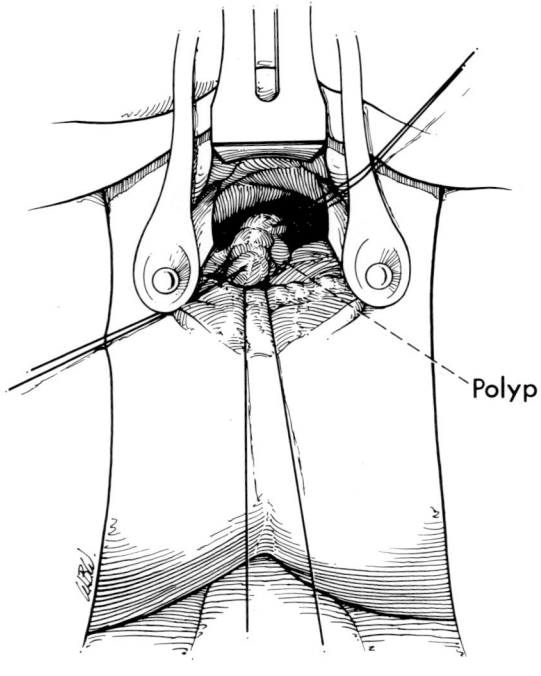

Figure 46-14.

rectal polyps that do not prolapse outside the anus. The polyp is exposed with the St. Mark's rectal retractor. Traction sutures of 000 chromic catgut are passed through the lesion transversely (Fig. 46-14). The sutures are placed first distally and then more proximally. The initial sutures are used to prolapse the lesion as much as possible and thereby improve the exposure of the more proximal portion of the lesion. The polyp is retracted

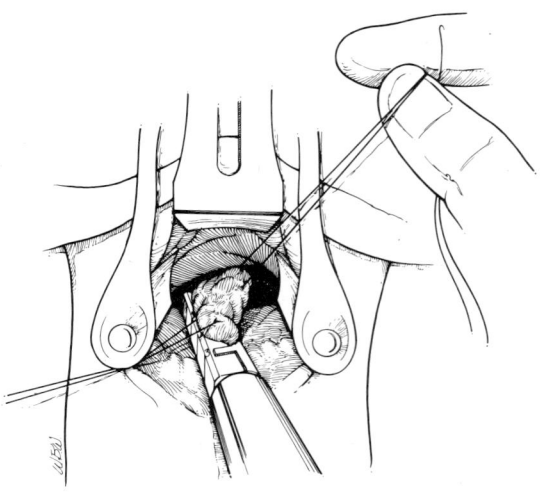

Figure 46-15.

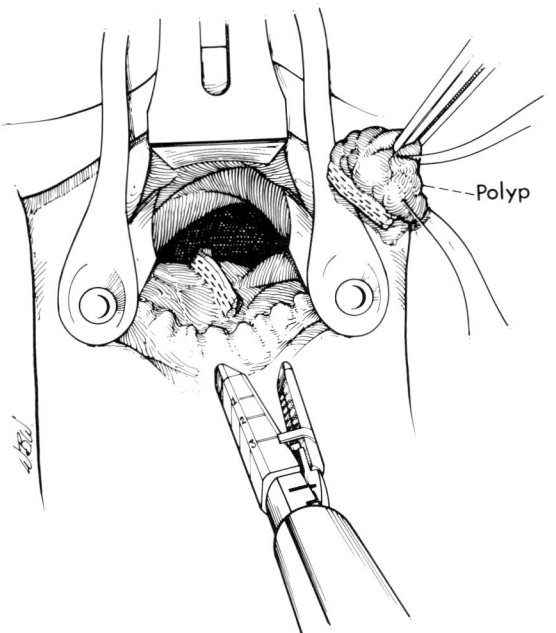

Figure 46-16.

away from the bowel wall with the sutures. In more proximal lesions, the sutures are clamped with a long straight clamp. Traction on the clamp exposes the base of the polyp. The thickness of the base of the polyp is measured with the ENDO GAUGE* instrument. The appropriate size of cartridge is selected. The jaws of the ENDO GIA 30* or ENDO GIA 60* stapling device are opened, and it is advanced over the base of the polyp (Fig. 46-15). The margin of resection is appraised by rolling the polyp from one side to the other. The stapling device is fired. It divides the tissue with a scapel blade between six rows of staples leaving three rows on the patient's side and three on the specimen side. The specimen is submitted to the pathologist. The presence of malignancy and the deep and lateral margins of resection are evaluated by frozen section. The staple line in the rectum is inspected (Fig. 46-16). Any bleeding arteries are suture ligated with 000 silk. The retractor is removed. A rigid proctosigmoidoscope is passed through the anus up to the distal sigmoid. The rectum is insufflated to make sure that its diameter has not been unduly compromised by the longitudinal closure.

Criteria for Discharge

Following laparoscopic procedures, the patient is discharged home when he or she is eating a regular diet and does not have a fever. The patient is followed closely as an outpatient and returns to the office 2 and 5 days after discharge. The patient monitors his or her temperature at home and returns to the office if a fever greater than 100 degrees F is seen. After transanal excisions, the patients are discharged home on the same day or the next morning after surgery.

Complications

Specific rates of complications are not known for these laparoscopic procedures at this time. It is anticipated, however, that for procedures which require a colotomy, rates of complications will be similar to those following open colotomies and polypectomies. Rates of wound complications may be decreased, but this remains uncertain.

The most frequent complication following transanal excision of polyps is urinary retention. An urinary catheter is inserted if the patient has not urinated within 12 hours of the completion of the procedure. Patients who are discharged home on the day of the procedure are instructed to return to the office or emergency room if they have not voided by the time they plan to go to bed.

REFERENCES

1. Tierney RP, Ballantyne GH, Modlin IM. The adenoma-carcinoma sequence: A review. Surg Gynecol Obstet 1990; 171:81–94.
2. Bilchik AJ, Ballantyne GH. Should malignant polyps of the colon and rectum be treated conservatively? *In* Gitnick G, ed. Debates in Medicine. Littleton, MA, Yearbook Medical Publishers, Inc, 1990. Vol 2, pp 254–287.

Chapter 47
Right Colectomy

Robert W. Beart

PATIENT SELECTION

The indications for laparoscopic colectomy are essentially the same as for traditional colectomies. The use of this technology should in no way alter traditional surgical judgments or compromise the traditional value of surgical techniques.

When utilizing this technology, the surgeon must adopt an appropriate philosophy. Patients should not be subjected to a procedure that compromises the effectiveness of the surgical procedure or unnecessarily subjects them to increased risks of a prolonged procedure. If, in the middle of a procedure, the surgeon feels that the efficacy or safety of the procedure is being affected, then it is appropriate to abandon laparoscopic surgery and return to traditional surgical techniques.

Of our initial 50 patients, laparoscopic colectomy was deemed inappropriate for 26 of them. Eleven of these patients were candidates for ileoanal or coloanal anastomosis, procedures which currently cannot be adequately performed with laparoscopic techniques. Five patients were not considered candidates because of the surgeon's preference, and 10 patients were not considered candidates for technical considerations. Technical considerations included multiple previous operations and unavailability of equipment. Laparoscopic colectomy was initiated in 24 patients. In 8 of these patients, the procedure could not be completed for various reasons. One had unacceptable bleeding during the procedure, and the procedure was terminated. In two patients, the anatomic landmarks were unclear, and the procedure was terminated. In five patients, the exposure was inadequate to resect the mesentery adequately, and the procedure was terminated.

PREOPERATIVE EVALUATION

Patients are evaluated in the same manner as when right colon resections using open surgical techniques are planned.

EQUIPMENT

The following instruments are used:

1. Laparoscope: 10-mm 0-degree laparoscope
2. Trocars: three 10- to 12-mm trocars and two 5-mm trocars
3. Instrumentation:
    A. Paddle electrocoagulation device
    B. Two graspers
    C. One endoscopic clip applier
    D. Two pre-tied endoscopic loop ligature devices

POSITIONING OF THE VIDEO EQUIPMENT

Patients are prepared and draped in the usual fashion, and the equipment is placed in a way that the video monitors can be adequately seen from both sides of the field. A recommended operating room configuration is seen in Figure 47-1.

TROCAR PLACEMENT AND SIZE SELECTION

The umbilicus is not an appropriate position to place a video camera, because it does not allow adequate visualization of the ileocolic vessel. For this reason, we routinely place the laparoscope in the left upper abdomen to the left of the midline, using a Hassan technique. Once the abdomen is entered and the intra-abdominal cavity is visualized, additional ports can be placed as shown in Figure 47-2. The 10- to 12-mm ports are placed at the site of camera placement and in the suprapubic area. When it is necessary to visualize either the hepatic flexure or the transverse colon, then the camera can be moved to the supraumbilical port. The 5-mm ports are placed in the right and left lower quadrants in the lateral third of the rectus sheath. This approximates the site of colostomy placement.

The operating surgeon uses the suprapubic port and the 5-mm port, which are on the left side of the abdomen. The assistant uses the operative port on the right side of the abdomen, and an additional operative port can be placed for the assistant if the assistant is capable of using the two-hand technique.

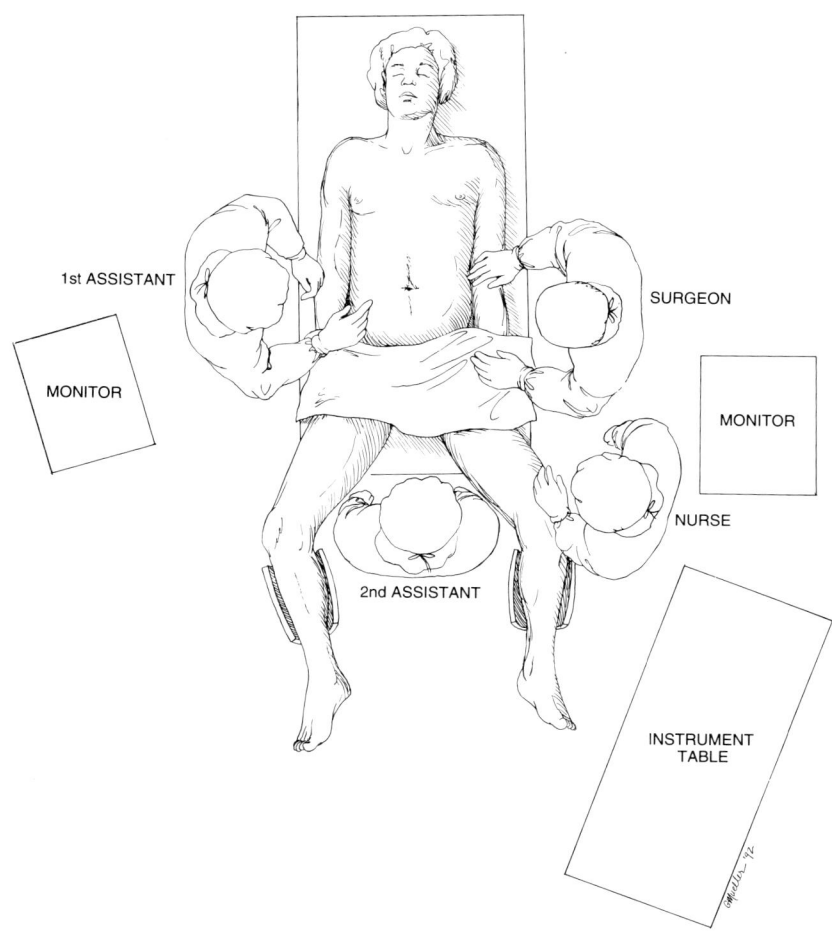

Figure 47-1.

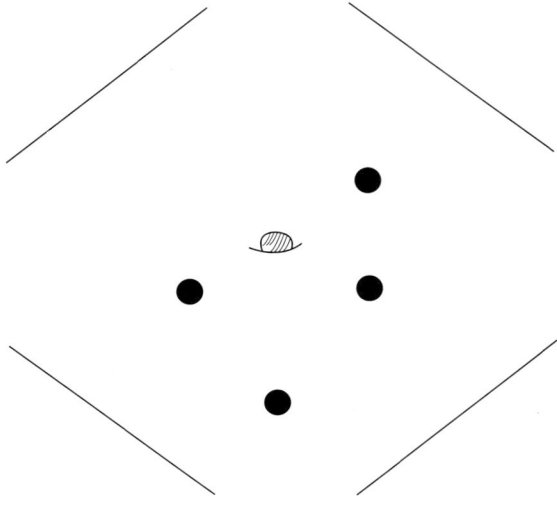

Figure 47-2.

POSITIONING OF THE PATIENT

The patient is placed in a steep Trendelenburg position and rotated sharply to the left. After the small bowel is pushed out of the way of the resected bowel, dissection can be initiated.

METHODS OF DISSECTION

We prefer electrocautery for the mobilization of the right colon and use a paddle electrocoagulation device as opposed to the hok. The hook tends to become entangled with mesenteric vessels and fat.

SPECIFIC DETAILS OF THE PROCEDURE

Dissection is initiated by retracting the segment of colon toward the midline and dividing the lateral perineal reflections. This should be carried out widely. Particular attention should be given to freeing the entire peritoneum, which is binding both the terminal ileum and right colon. Only when this attachment is transected can the retroperitoneum be fully exposed and the bowel mobilized.

The bowel is bluntly reflected toward the midline, until the ureter is identified, and the ureter is freed over the length of the involved segment of bowel. Once the bowel is fully mobilized, and the ureter identified, the bowel is placed laterally and the medial aspects of the mesentery are incised with electrocautery using blunt dissection. The mesentery is then placed on traction, so that the primary feeding vessel is placed on traction. Using the paddle dissector and alternating blunt dissection with electrocautery, the primary vessel can then be identified at its origin and ligated.

We ligate the ileocolic artery and vein separately, using double hemoclips, on the proximal and distal ends, and then divide the vessels. Proximal vessels are then ligated with the Endo loop. The avascular segment of mesentery, proximal and distal to the ligated vessel, is carefully dissected. It is usually not necessary to complete the mesenteric dissection to the bowel wall as this can be carried out extracorporally.

If an intracorporal anastomosis is to be done, then the mesentery must be dissected completely. At this time, however, we are not satisfied with techniques for intracorporeal anastomosis. For this reason and because of the need to remove an intact specimen, we generally favor a small incision through which the specimen is removed. Furthermore, this allows completion of the anastomosis extracorporally.

Once the mobilization is completed, the bowel is grasped through the right lower quadrant operative port. A small incision is made adjacent to this port. The bowel is visualized and then grabbed with a Babcock clamp and drawn into the wound. Generally, a 5-cm incision is large enough, unless the size of the lesion requires a larger incision for extraction. A finger of the surgeon is then inserted through this incision, and the window in the dissected mesentery is palpated. With traction on this window, the mobilized bowel could be drawn completely into the incision and the undissected mesentery identified. This mesentery can then be divided and ligated between clamps.

Once the mesenteric dissection is completed, noncrushing bowel clamps are placed on the bowel, crushing clamps are placed on the segment to be removed, and the bowel is divided. Once the pathologic segment has been removed, the anastomosis can be completed with the surgeon's preferred technique. The re-anastomosed bowel is then returned to the abdomen.

CLOSURE

The incision is closed in two layers, with running suture, and the abdomen is re-insufflated. The previously placed ports were all left *in situ,* but the port through which the bowel was removed has now been removed. The abdomen is then carefully inspected for adequate hemostasis and irrigated with saline, and all blood clots are removed. The ports are removed under direct visualization, and the port sites are closed. This completes the surgical dissection. Drains can be placed as indicated through the port sites.

POSTOPERATIVE MANAGEMENT

Following the patient's recovery from anesthesia, we feel comfortable in initiating a full liquid diet. The patients are then followed until they are passing flatus and stool, and pain control is adequate.

In 16 patients, the procedure was completed using laparoscopic techniques. In these patients, the average time to eating was 1.1 days; the average time for which narcotic pain control was required was 1.6 days. Flatus was passed on an average of 2.6 days following surgery, and stool was passed on an average of 2.9 days following surgery. These patients were discharged from the hospital on an average of 3.7 days following the operative procedure.

CRITERIA FOR PATIENT DISCHARGE

Discharge from the hospital is initiated by the usual clinical criteria.

COMPLICATIONS

Complications noted included one patient who had excessive blood loss during the procedure (800 ml) and two patients who developed laparoscopic port site infection in the postoperative period and were treated with oral antibiotics.

Only time will determine whether or not this is a technique which allows adequate cancer treatment. It is our impression, however, that the traditional margins of resection required to treat cancer of the colon and rectum can be preserved. We have documented the level of transection of the mesentery by placement of metallic clips. Postoperative radiographs confirm that the clips are clearly located high on the inferior mesenteric artery on left colic resections or near the course of the superior mesenteric artery on right colic resections.

Long term results of this procedure remain to be documented. Nevertheless, early experience suggests that adequate surgical resections are possible. In addition, the morbidity and mortality of a right colon resection with laparoscopic techniques appears acceptable. It is clear, however, that not every patient is a candidate for the use of this technique, but when it is successfully used, postoperative morbidity and mortality seem to be reduced.

BIBLIOGRAPHY

Cooperman AI, Katz V, Zimmon D, Botero G. Laparoscopic colon resection: A case report. J Laparoendosc Surg 1991; 1:221–224.

Fowler DL, White SA. Laparoscopy-assisted sigmoid resection. Surg Laparosc Endosc 1991; 1:183–188.

Jacobs M, Verdeja JC, Goldstein HS. Minimally invasive colon resection (laparoscopic colectomy). Surg Laparosc Endosc 1991; 1:144–150.

Lange V, Meyer G, Schardey HM, Scildberg FW. Laparoscopic creation of a loop colostomy. J Laparoendosc Surg 1991; 1:307–312.

Redwine DB, Sharpe DR. Laparoscopic segmental resection of the sigmoid colon for endometriosis. J Laparoendosc Surg 1991; 1:217–220.

Saclarides TJ, Ko ST, Airan M, et al. Laparoscopic removal of a large colonic lipoma: Report of a case. Dis Colon Rectum 1992; 34:1027–1029.

Schlinkert RT. Laparoscopic-assisted right hemicolectomy. Dis Colon Rectum 1992; 34:1030–1031.

Chapter 48
Right Hemicolectomy with Intracorporeal Anastomosis

Joseph F. Uddo, Jr.

With the widespread acceptance of laparoscopic cholecystectomy, the laparoscopic approach has been expanded to other abdominal procedures. Experience is rapidly being gained with laparoscopic colon surgery. In this chapter, laparoscopic right hemicolectomy with intracorporeal anastomosis will be discussed. The indications for the procedure as well as the procedure itself will be detailed.

PATIENT SELECTION

As with any new procedure, the indications for laparoscopic right hemicolectomy are not yet fully defined. It is possible that the laparoscopic approach may be used for any colon lesion requiring removal. It is generally accepted that benign mucosal lesions that cannot be removed colonoscopically can be approached with the laparoscope. Other benign colon problems such as diverticular disease and angiodysplasia also seem to be acceptable applications for laparoscopic colectomy.

Colon cancer with metastatic disease may be handled laparoscopically without fear of compromising the resection. However, not everyone agrees that confined colon cancer should be removed with the laparoscope. Concern that an "adequate cancer operation" cannot be performed successfully with the laparoscope keeps this disease process a debatable indication for laparoscopic colectomy. However, once the surgeon has become familiar with laparoscopic colon procedures, it becomes apparent that the same resection is performed laparoscopically as with the open technique. High ligation of the vessels is possible, and adequate margins and adequate mesenteric dissection can be obtained. Nevertheless, long term follow-up of patients with confined colon cancers treated laparoscopically will be the only way to put this issue to rest.

PREOPERATIVE EVALUATION

The preoperative evaluation for laparoscopic right colon resection should vary little from that for open colon resection. Routine preoperative testing is performed. In patients with cancer, a carcinoembryonic antigen level should be obtained. Patients with complex medical problems should have appropriate consultation.

Special attention should be given to the patient's body habitus in planning the operation. Of particular importance is the history of previous abdominal surgery and the location of old incisions. Extensive previous surgery can make it impossible to complete a laparoscopic procedure successfully. However, there is no way preoperatively to identify those patients who will not be good candidates for laparoscopic procedures either because of body build or because of previous surgery. Consequently, any patient who may be a candidate for laparoscopic colectomy should be evaluated at the time of laparoscopic exploration and a final decision made at that time as to proceeding with a laparoscopic procedure or converting to an open procedure. Successful laparoscopic procedures can be performed regardless of body build, and, with few exceptions, previous surgery. Freeing extensive adhesions can prolong the procedure considerably. Therefore, if extended anesthesia time may not be well tolerated by a particular patient, an early conversion to an open procedure is in order.

When the procedure is done for a mucosal lesion identified by colonoscopy, it is helpful to also obtain a preoperative barium enema. This confirms the relative position of the lesion and will facilitate planning of the procedure. Because the laparoscopic approach eliminates the ability of the surgeon to palpate, in patients with colon cancer, a preoperative computed tomographic scan of the abdomen is also helpful, particularly for evaluation of the liver and retroperitoneum.

Special attention should be given to the consent process because all patients must consent to an open procedure in the event that the laparoscopic procedure is not successful. It is not reasonable for a patient to limit consent to a laparoscopic procedure only.

PREOPERATIVE PREPARATION

A clear liquid diet is started on the day prior to surgery. The patient is given a bowel preparation of 1 gallon of a polyethylene glycol electrolyte solution over 4 hours on the day prior to surgery. Erythromycin base (1 g) and Neomycin (1 g) are given orally at 1:00, 2:00, and 11:00 p.m. on the day prior to surgery. A bisacodyl suppository is given on the evening prior to surgery.

Most patients are admitted the morning of surgery. Preoperative antibiotics are given intravenously. Some form of deep venous thrombosis prophylaxis is used (support hose, subcutaneous heparin, or intermittent compression devices). General anesthesia is used. A nasogastric tube and Foley catheter are placed once the patient is asleep.

EQUIPMENT

The following equipment is used for laparoscopic right hemicolectomy:

1. Laparoscopes: Two 10-mm 0-degree laparoscopes are used. A 10-mm 30-degree laparoscope and a 5-mm laparoscope should be available.
2. Video equipment: Two full camera systems with individual light sources and three or four monitors are used.
3. Insufflation device: A rapid automatic insufflation device with smoke evacuator is preferred.
4. Electrocautery: A monopolar electrocautery device with an assortment of wands is needed.
5. Instruments
    A. Four noncrushing bowel graspers
    B. Probes and retractors
    C. Endoscopic clip applier
    D. Endoscopic loop ties
    E. Endoscopic needle holder, knot pusher, and suture material
    F. Curved endoscopic scissors capable of conducting electrocautery
    G. An assortment of endoscopic dissectors capable of conducting electrocautery
6. Endoscopic stapling devices
    A. ENDO GIA 30* or ENDO GIA 60*
    B. ENDO HERNIA* stapler
    C. ENDO TA 60*

POSITIONING OF THE PATIENT

The patient's position depends on where the lesion is located and how the anastomosis is to be accomplished. For a laparoscopic right hemicolectomy with intracorporeal anastomosis, the supine position with both arms at the patient's side has been our position of choice.

If the lesion requires intraoperative localization with a colonoscope, the patient's legs are placed in a low stirrup position. However, if the lesion is confidently localized preoperatively, the supine position offers more latitude in manipulation of instrumentation.

Use of an electric table facilitates intraoperative positioning of the patient. During the procedure, it is helpful to lower one side or the other of the patient to allow the small intestines to fall away from the operative site.

POSITIONING OF THE VIDEO EQUIPMENT

The use of three or four video monitors help to decrease potential stress during these cases. A minimum of two monitors, placed at either side of the head of the patient, are required. A third and fourth monitor on either side of the patient's feet allows an adequate view of the operative field from almost any position around the table. If only three monitors are available, placing the third monitor at the end of the table will accomplish nearly the same effect as having four monitors.

Because laparoscopic colon resection may require frequent moves from one side of the table to the other, it is essential that the surgeon not get "roped in" by cables and tubing. All video cables and suction/irrigation tubing should be placed so that free movement is allowed around the table without having to disconnect and reconnect equipment. This is easy to accomplish with proper attention to placement of equipment. This room layout, seen in Figure 48-1, has been successful.

TROCAR PLACEMENT AND SIZES

Unlike laparoscopic cholecystectomy, which has well established approaches to trocar placement, there is no consensus on the number and location of trocars to be used in laparoscopic colon resection. In general, it is most useful to begin with an umbilical 10-mm port and a 10-mm port in each quadrant of the abdomen. This affords full access to abdominal contents and allows placement of a 10-mm scope and laparoscopic Babcock clamp from any direction. This is particularly important when two scopes are used.

Because the endoscopic stapling device requires large parts an additional 12-mm (ENDO GIA 30*) or 15-mm (ENDO GIA 60*

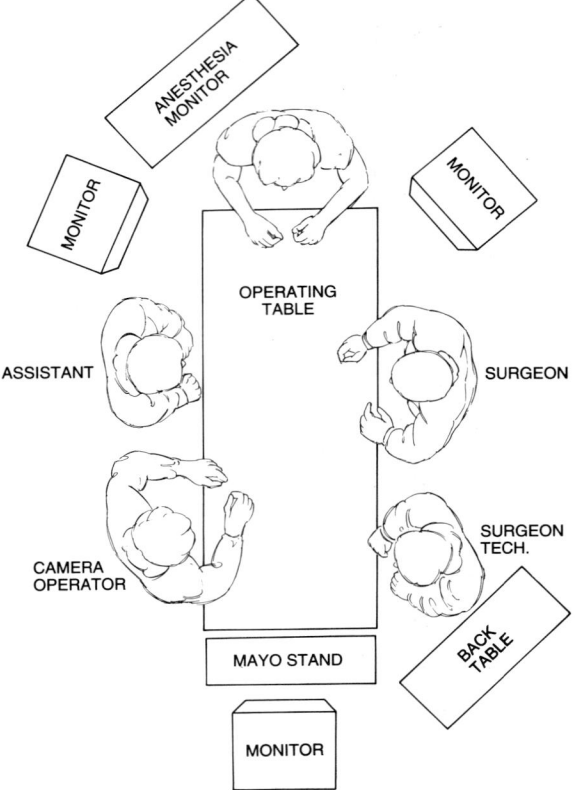

Figure 48-1.

or TA 60*) port is needed to accomplish the intracorporeal anastomosis. The placement of this port is crucial, and its position should be chosen just prior to anastomosis. After the positions of the colon and terminal ileum are evaluated, the most appropriate site for the large trocar can be determined (Fig. 48-2).

Once the 12- or 15-mm port site is determined, a videolaparoscope placed behind it and slightly to one side will provide the best visualization for the anastomosis. To complete the anastomosis, the umbilical 10-mm port should be changed to a 12- or 15-mm cannula. Alternatively, a 12- or 15-mm port can be placed in the umbilicus initially.

To perform a laparoscopic right hemicolectomy with intracorporeal anastomosis, at least five 10-mm trocars and two 12- or 15-mm trocars are needed. Additional 5-mm trocars should be used for retractors as needed. There is no evidence that the cumulative length of incisions for trocars or increasing the number of trocars leads to significantly increased postoperative pain or prolonged ileus.

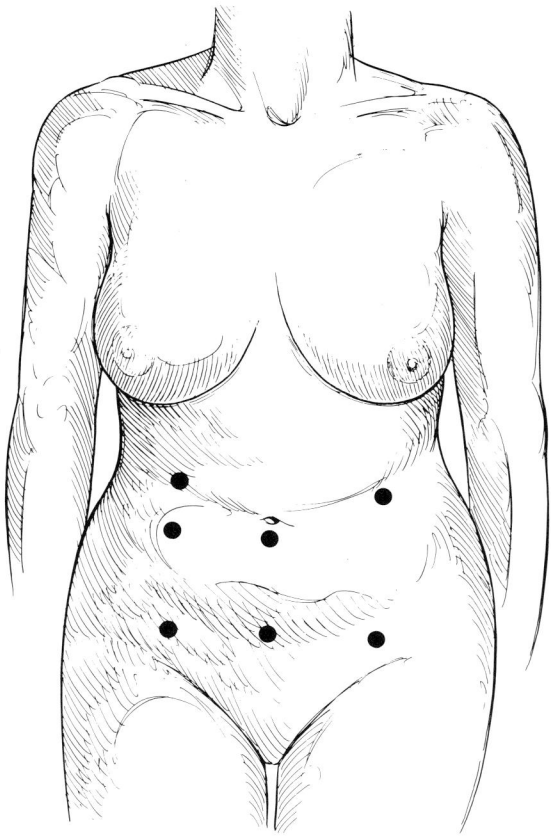

Figure 48-2.

SPECIFIC DETAILS OF THE PROCEDURE

The peritoneal cavity is insufflated using the surgeon's technique of choice. We prefer use of a Veress needle for insufflation of the pneumoperitoneum. If the patient has had prior surgery, an alternative site away from the old incision is chosen for the Veress needle insertion. The insufflator is preset to 15 mm Hg. Occasionally higher settings will be required. A 10-mm port is placed, and a videolaparoscope is introduced. A brief survey of the abdomen is made. If there is no obvious contraindication to continuation of the laparoscopic procedure, an additional 10-mm port is placed in each abdominal quadrant as noted. The abdomen is then fully explored. The small bowel, colon, omentum, peritoneum, and liver are inspected.

Because the surgeon's ability to palpate anatomical structures is lost, a thorough visual examination should be done. In patients with cancer the ability to thoroughly palpate the liver and retroperitoneum is the greatest loss. However, with preoperative computed tomographic scans, both the liver and retroperitoneum can be evaluated adequately.

Once the exploration is completed, attention is turned to the right colon, which is grasped proximally and distally with atraumatic bowel graspers and pulled to the left (Fig. 48-3). Even though laparoscopic bowel graspers are atraumatic, when not handled properly, most bowel clamps available at this time can still damage intestinal serosa and possibly cause full thickness tears. Consequently, when the bowel is manipulated, it is important to try to place graspers on the portion of bowel to be removed. The surgeon must be as gentle as possible when manipulating the remainder of the bowel.

With the colon retracted to the left, a dissector (scissors or electrocautery) is placed through a lower quadrant port. The attachment of the colon to the parietal peritoneum ("white line" of Toldt) is dissected. The colon is drawn to the left and the colon mesentery is dissected using blunt and sharp dissection. Use of electrocautery scissors and a laparoscopic Kittner facilitates the mobilization of the right colon. The right ureter is identified as mobilization of the mesentery is completed.

The hepatic flexure is then mobilized (Fig. 48-4). The hepatocolic ligament is divided. Division of the white line is continued around the hepatic flexure, and the gastrocolic ligament is dissected to the point of division of the transverse colon. The hepatic flexure can then be swept off the duodenum with blunt dissection. Occasionally, we have found "flipping" the opentum cephalad to be helpful at this point. Mobilization of the hepatic flexure is the most difficult phase of this operation.

The right colon, now fully mobilized, is grasped and held anterior and to the right. This exposes the medial side of the colic mesentery. Electrocautery scissors are used to score the mesentery along the line of dissection. The mesentery is then divided along this path. Blunt dissection and dissection with electrocautery aids in this process. A second videolaparoscope placed behind the mobilized right colon transilluminates the mesentery and helps to identify vessels (Fig. 48-5). The light source on the first camera will need to be dimmed to appreciate the transillumination of the mesentery. As small vessels are encountered, they can be clipped and divided (Fig. 48-5, *inset*). Larger vessels can be

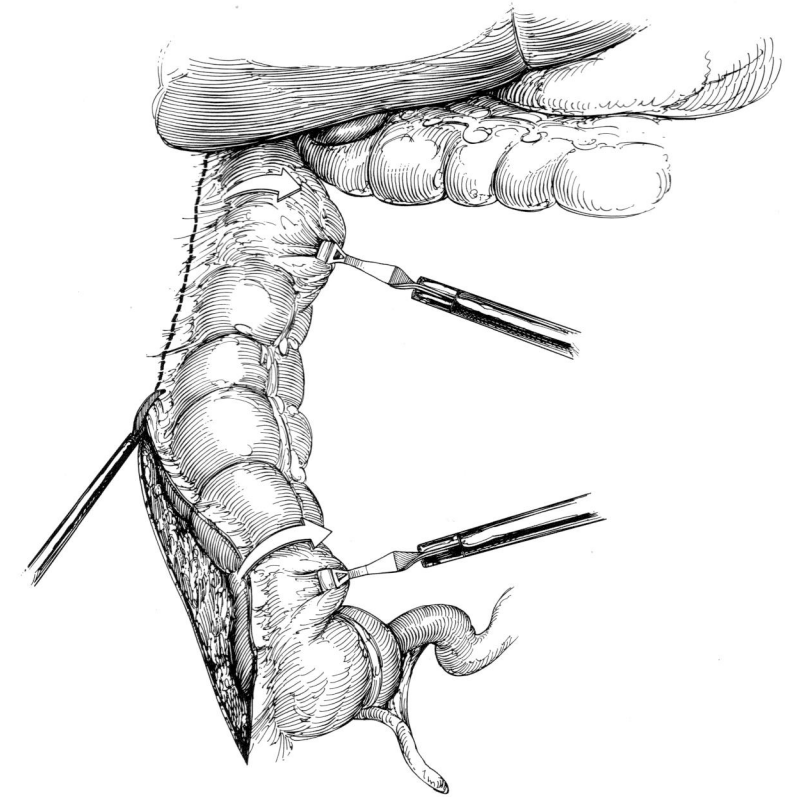

Figure 48-3.

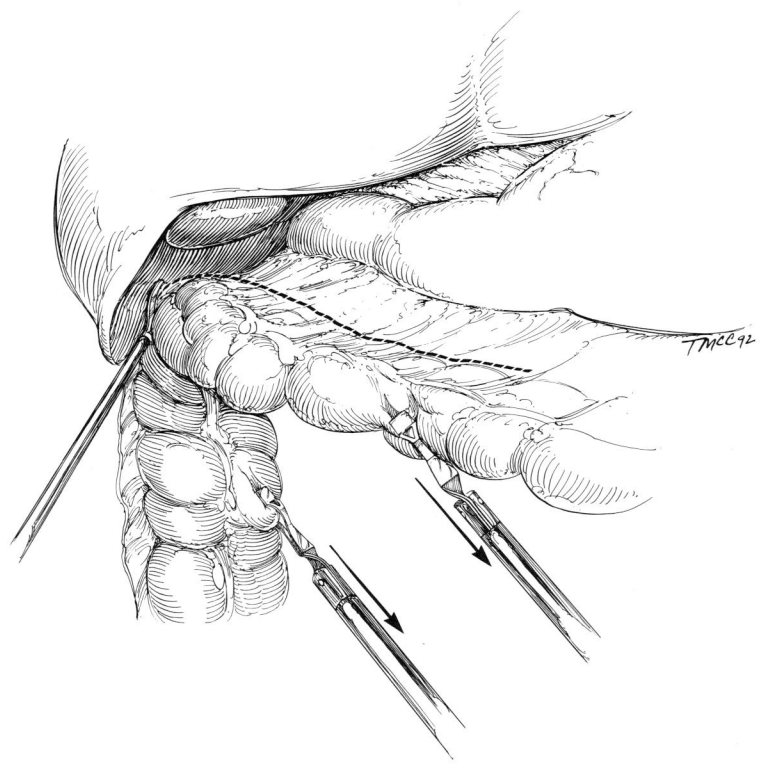

Figure 48-4.

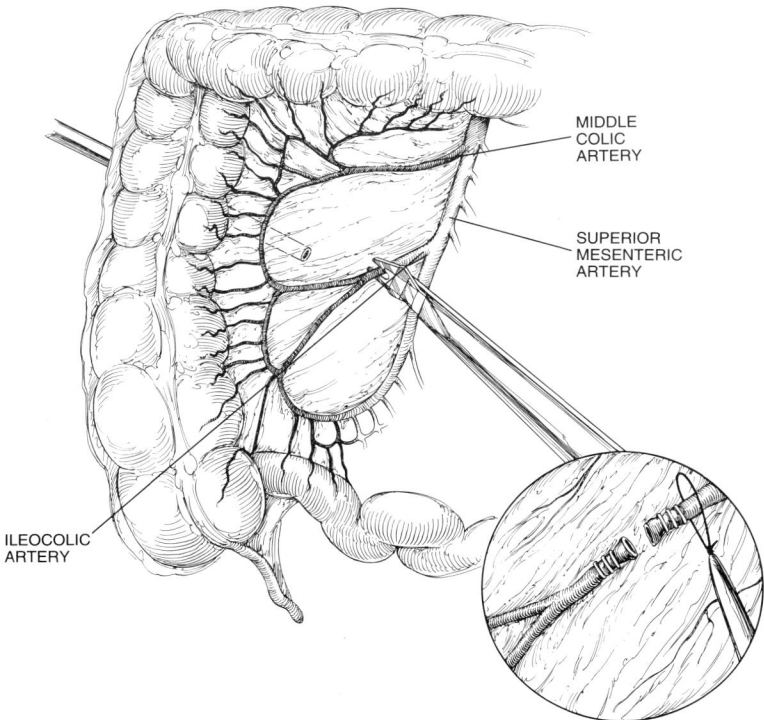

Figure 48-5.

clipped, ligated with endoscopic ties or divided using the ENDO GIA* stapling device with a vascular cartridge in place. A full mesenteric dissection can be accomplished laparoscopically with great precision and minimal blood loss owing to the enhanced visualization.

A window in the mesentery is created at the point of transection of the terminal ileum. The ENDO GIA* stapling device is then placed through the umbilical port and the ileum is divided (Fig. 48-6A). An opening in the transverse mesocolon is made at the site of transection. The omentum may be divided to this point. The gastrocolic ligament has previously been opened and should not pose a problem. The ENDO GIA* stapling device is again placed through the umbilical port and used to divide the transverse colon (Fig. 48-6B).

Each time the ENDO GIA* stapling device is used, it is helpful to place a second videolaparoscope 90 degrees to the first. This essentially adds depth perception to the otherwise two-dimensional perspective of one camera. The second scope affords complete visualization to the ends of the stapling device and confirms good positioning prior to firing with minimal manipulation of bowel.

Once the specimen has been completely freed from all attachments, it can be placed in the pelvis to be extracted at the completion of the procedure. Both ends of the specimen are securely stapled, and spillage from the specimen should not be a concern. The specimen is not removed at this point because the required enlargement of the umbilical incision makes retention of pneumoperitoneum difficult.

The midtransverse colon and distal ileum are then prepared for anastomosis. A functional end-to-end anastomosis using the ENDO GIA* stapling device is constructed. Each limb of bowel is controlled with two graspers. A small enterotomy using the electrocautery scissors is made in each limb. Alignment of the bowel for anastomosis is crucial. The bowel ends are placed side by side with the enterotomies aligned. At this point the second 12- or 15-mm port is placed. The position is determined by assessing the position of the limbs of bowel. Adequate distance from the bowel is required for manipulation of the stapling device. A second videolaparoscope behind and just to the side of the stapling device aids in introduction of the ENDO GIA* stapling device into the enterotomies by giving a "straight on" view (Fig.

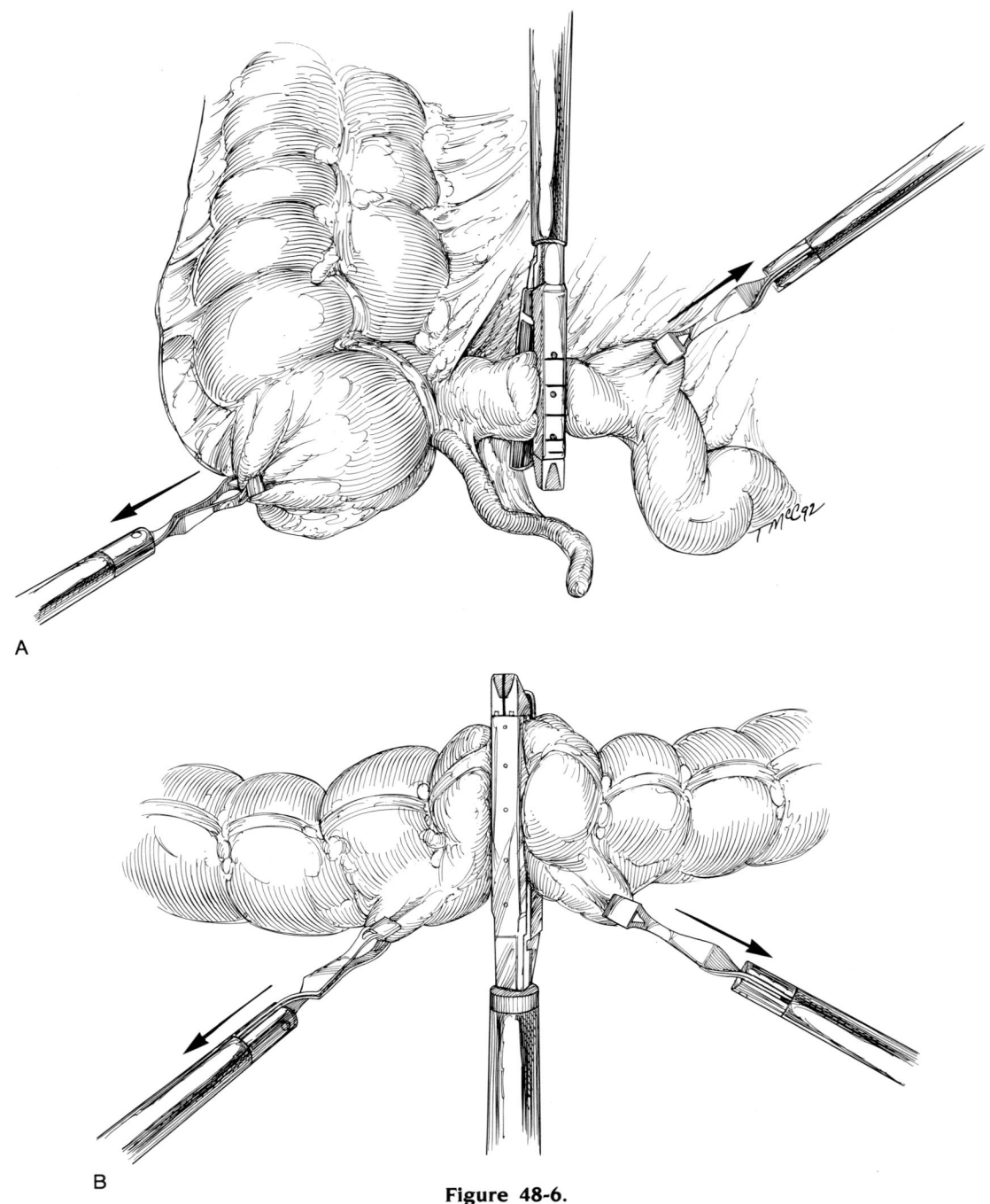

Figure 48-6.

48-7A). The first camera is placed through one of the lower abdominal ports for a 90-degree view of the introduction of an ENDO GIA* stapling device. The stapling device is placed in the abdomen, opened, and inserted into the enterotomies (Fig. 48-7B). Care must be taken to assure accurate placement. Confirmation that both limbs of the stapling device are in the bowel is essential (Fig. 48-7C). The stapler is closed and fired. If the 30-mm device is used, two or three firings will be required. However, with the availability of a 60-mm device, one firing should be adequate.

The anastomosis is inspected through the second videolaparoscope which looks directly into it. Both sides of the anastomosis and cost of open colectomy will need to be assessed cirtically.

In many patients a laparoscopically assisted right hemicolectomy with extracorporeal anastomosis may be faster and afford the same postoperative advantages. However, in the obese patient or the patient with a foreshortened mesentery, it may not be possible to safely perform an extracorporeal anastomosis. Consequently, the technique of laparoscopic right hemicolectomy with intracorporeal anastomosis will have a role in the evolution of laparoscopic colon surgery.

Chapter 49
Right Hemicolectomy with Extracorporeal Anastomosis

Garth H. Ballantyne

PATIENT SELECTION

Criteria for selection of patients for laparoscopically assisted right hemicolectomy will vary with the level of experience of the surgeon. Initial attempts to perform this procedure will be facilitated by the selection of a patient who is thin and who has not undergone previous abdominal operations. Initial experience might be best limited to patients with benign lesions or patients with incurable metastatic disease. In these patients, high ligation of the mesenteric vessels is less critical than in a patient afflicted with a curable early colorectal cancer. Patients with lesions in the cecum rather than in the more distal right colon may also be preferred during a surgeon's early experience. Hepatic flexure and proximal transverse colon lesions present the greatest challenge since the most difficult part of this operation is mobilization of the hepatic flexure and exposure of the middle colic vessels.

Previous abdominal operations may impede attempts at laparascopically assisted resection of the right colon. Hysterectomies, for example, often generate adhesions between loops of small bowel and the vaginal cuff, which are particularly difficult to visualize through a laparoscope. Similarly, a previous cholecystectomy through a subcostal (Kocher) incision may make mobilization of the hepatic flexure difficult. In contrast, adhesions to an appendectomy incision are generally easy to divide and may even improve exposure of the initial mobilization of the cecum by providing anterior traction. As the experience of the laparoscopic surgeon increases, lysis of adhesions from previous operations becomes as much of a routine portion of the operation as it is in many open operations.

The general condition of the patient is an important factor in criteria for selection for this operation. During the early experience of a laparoscopic surgeon the duration of the operation will be prolonged compared to an open resection. Consequently, patients in good health should be selected. The presence of arrhythmias or advanced chronic obstructive pulmonary disease might mitigate against performance of a laparoscopic procedure. The increased partial pressure of carbon dioxide in the serum associated with a carbon dioxide pneumoperitoneum may aggravate these conditions.

PREOPERATIVE EVALUATION

Patients undergo the same evaluation as obtained prior to open operations. Cardiac and pulmonary assessments require particular scrutiny because of the problems of hypercapnia generated by the carbon dioxide pneumoperitoneum.

Localization of the lesion demands careful consideration. Most lesions are not visible through a laparoscope. A barium enema air contrast study can achieve this requirement. Alternatively, some people have tattooed the location of the lesion with injections of India ink into the wall of the colon. A long sclerotherapy needle is used for the injection. Intraoperative colonoscopy with transillumination of the lesion offers a third method.

PREOPERATIVE PREPARATION

The patient is admitted on the night before the operation and takes nothing by mouth after midnight. On the afternoon before the operation, a standard polyethylene glycol mechanical bowel preparation is initiated. This is followed by a standard oral antibiotic dosage of neomycin and erythromycin. The patient also receives broad spectrum antibiotics intravenously in the perioperative period

EQUIPMENT

The following equipment is used:

1. Laparoscopes: 10-mm 0-degree telescope and 10-mm 30-degree telescope (optional).
2. Trocars: Five 10-mm and one 12- or 15-mm trocar
3. Instruments
    A. One disposable laparoscopic scissors
    B. One laparoscopic grasping instrument
    C. Two laparoscopic Babcock clamps
    D. One laparoscopic clip applier
    E. One three-finger laparoscopic retractor
    F. One ENDO GIA 30* (United States Surgical Corporation, Norwalk, CT) or ENDO GIA 60* (United States Surgical Corporation) stapling device with multiple cartridges
    G. Two GIA 60* (United States Surgical Corporation) and one TA 55* (United States Surgical Corporation) stapling devices

POSITIONING OF THE PATIENT

The patient is placed in a supine position on an electric operating room table. The legs are supported with Lloyd-Davies stirrups. The thighs are straight. Automatic pneumatic compression boots are wrapped around the calves. During the majority of the operation, the patient is dropped into a deep Trendelenberg position and the right shoulder is rolled up.

POSITIONING OF THE VIDEO EQUIPMENT

The principal video monitor is placed near the right shoulder of the patient. In this position, the surgeon, assistant surgeon, and camera operator can all easily observe the progress of the operation (Fig. 49-1). A second monitor on the left side of the patient facilitates establishment of the pneumoperitoneum and initial insertion of the trocars. Alternatively, the second monitor can be placed near the right knee of the patient. This may facilitate exposure of the right ureter.

TROCAR PLACEMENT AND SIZE SELECTION

The placement of trocars for a laparoscopic technique of right hemicolectomy has not as yet been standardized. Indeed, a wide variety of strategies have been used. This variation stems from two factors: some surgeons prefer to perform the dissection from the left side of the patient while others prefer to stand between the legs of the patient, and visualization of the right gutter and lateral attachment of the hepatic flexure through a centrally positioned rigid telescope is difficult. These limitations of rigid telescopes may be overcome with the introduction of flexible telescopes.

The initial 10-mm trocar is inserted in the supraumbilical position (Fig. 49-2). Four addi-

538 Techniques of Laparoscopic Surgery

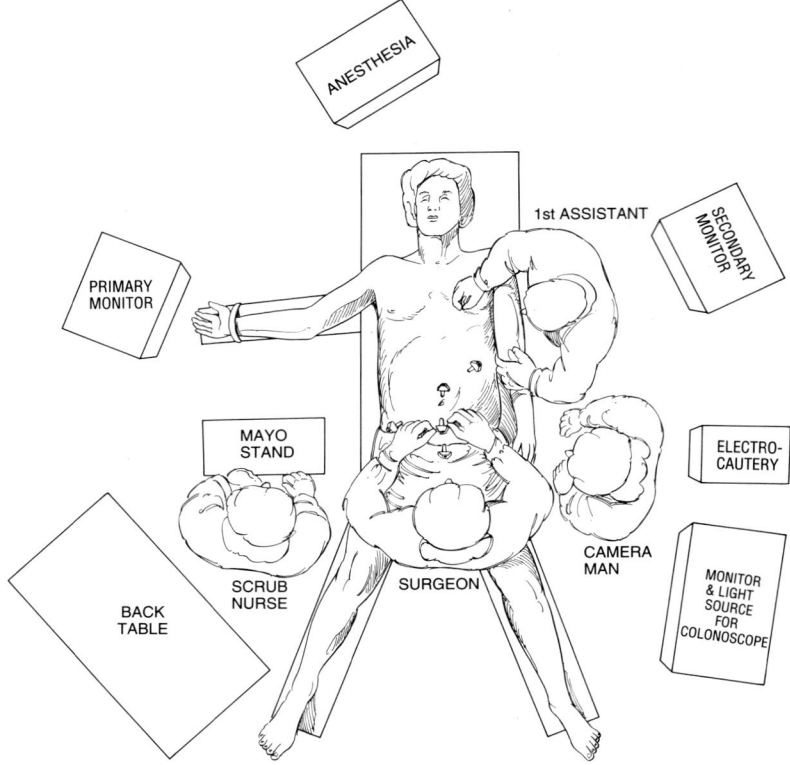

Figure 49-1.

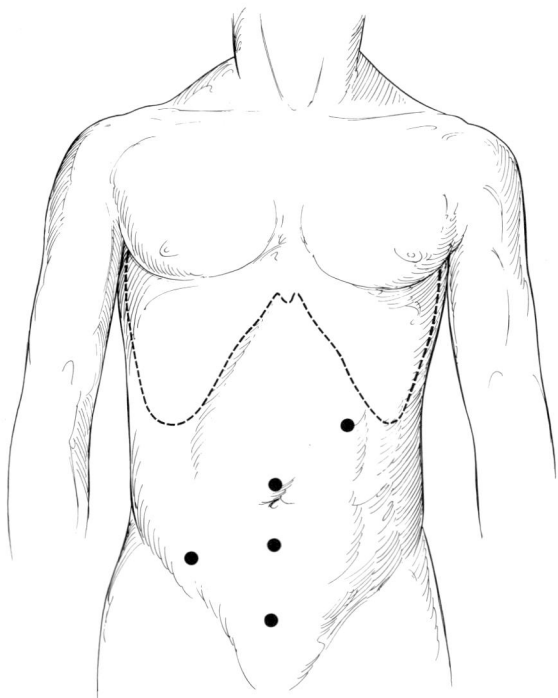

Figure 49-2.

tional 10-mm trocars are then introduced. This allows both the surgeon and assistant surgeon to use two instruments throughout the operation. One trocar is placed in the right lower quadrant lateral to the rectus sheath near McBurney's point. One trocar is inserted on the midline just above the pubis. Usually the edge of the bladder is visible through the laparoscope and can be easily avoided. One trocar is inserted on the midline halfway between the pubis and umbilicus. This trocar will eventually be converted to a 12- or 15-mm trocar and used for insertion of the ENDO GIA 30* or ENDO GIA 60* stapling device. One trocar is positioned in the left upper quadrant lateral to the rectus sheath.

METHODS OF EXPOSURE AND RETRACTION

The disposition of trocars outlined above is used when the surgeon performs the dissection and mobilization of the right colon while standing between the legs of the patient. The surgeon uses a grasping instrument inserted through the right lower quadrant trocar for countertraction. Alternatively, a three-finger retractor (ENDO RETRACT*, United States Surgical Corporation) is used for elevation and blunt mobilization of the right colon (Fig. 49-3). He uses a cautery scissors placed through the suprapubic port for dissection and mobilization of the cecum and ascending colon.

The assistant provides exposure by retraction of the bowel with two Babcock clamps inserted through the left upper quadrant and midhypogastric trocars. During mobilization of the cecum, Babcock clamps are used to retract the terminal ileum and cecum medially and anteriorly. During mobilization of the ascending colon, the two Babcock clamps are used to grasp the proximal and distal right colon. While taking down the hepatic flexure, one Babcock clamp is attached to the colon proximally to the hepatic flexure and one distally.

Movement of a rigid 0-degree telescope from one trocar to another may improve exposure. Mobilization of the cecum and hepatic flexure are telecast well with the videolaparoscope in the supraumbilcal trocar. Mobilzation of the right colon is better viewed with the telescope in the midhypogastric or suprapubic trocar. This allows advancement of the telescope up the right gutter, lateral to the colon. Alternatively, a 30-degree telescope broadcasts the entire operation well from the supraumbilical port. The angle of view allows the centrally placed telescope to view the dissection which is occurring lateral to the colon.

METHODS OF DISSECTION

The lateral attachments of the cecum and right colon are readily divided with electrocautery scissors (ENDO SHEARS*). Elevation and blunt mobilization of the ascending colon of the retroperitoneum are assisted with a three-finger retractor (ENDO RETRACT*). Division of the terminal ileum and mesenteric vessels is achieved with a laparoscopic stapling device (ENDO GIA 30* or ENDO GIA 60*).

SPECIFIC DETAILS OF THE PROCEDURE

After induction of general endotracheal anesthesia, a nasogastric tube and urinary catheter are inserted. The abdomen is prepared and draped. The patient is dropped into a deep Trendelenberg position. The pneumoperitoneum is insufflated with a Veress needle. The supraumbilical 10-mm trocar is inserted into the abdomen. The videolaparoscope is introduced and the abdomen is inspected for evidence of injury to the gut or blood vessels caused during placement of the first trocar. The other four 10-mm trocars are inserted.

The abdomen is explored. The small bowel is examined from the ligament of Treitz to the ileocecal valve. This is accomplished by sequential grasping of the small bowel with ENDO BABCOCK* clamps. The head of the patient is elevated into a reverse Trendelenberg position. This causes the liver to drop away from the diaphragm and improves exposure

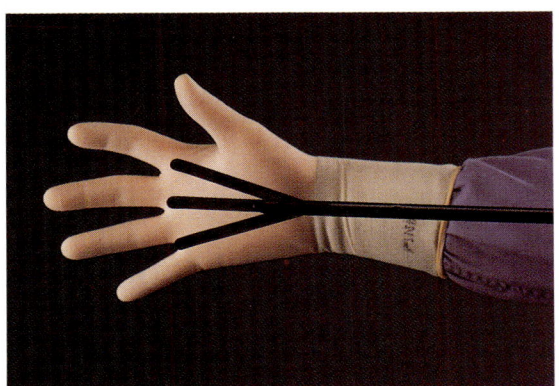
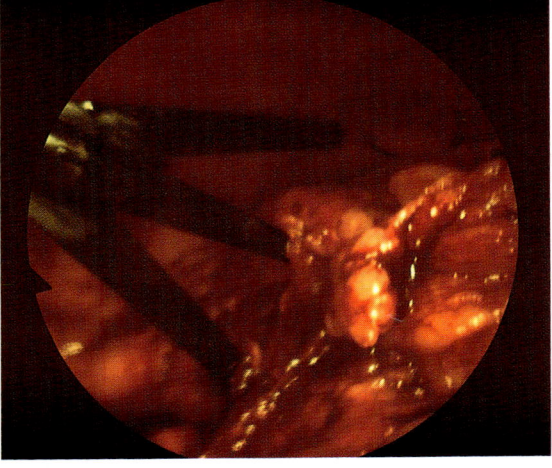

Figure 49-3.

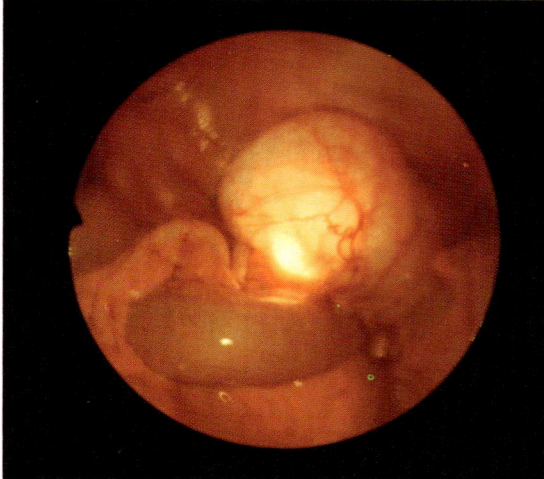

Figure 49-4.

of the lobes of the liver. The liver is inspected for evidence of metastatic disease. A laparoscopic ultrasound is used to identify metastases within the parenchyme of the liver.

If the position of the lesion is uncertain, an intraoperative colonoscopy is performed. The colonoscope is advanced to the level of the lesion. The light intensity of the laparoscope is turned down. This causes the light of the colonoscope to become visible through the colonic wall (Fig. 49-4). The laparoscopic surgeon marks the position of the lesion with surgical clips (Fig. 49-5A). The colonoscopist monitors the placement of the clips by observing the indentation of the colonic wall produced by the open jaws of the ENDO CLIP* device (Fig. 49-5B). Based on the position of the lesion, the scope of the operative resection is planned.

The cecum is mobilized first. The patient is dropped back into a deep Trendelenberg position. The right side of the table is rolled up. Any loops of small bowel that are sitting in the pelvis are pushed up toward the diaphragm. Unless the mesentery of the small bowel is foreshortened because of inflammatory disease or obesity, the small bowel will roll easily out of the pelvis and remain out of the operative field. The course of the iliac vessels is easily visualized (Fig. 49-6A). The assistant surgeon grasps the terminal ileum with one ENDO BABCOCK* clamp and the cecum with another (Fig. 49-6B). The operative field is irrigated with heparinized saline (3000 units/liter) before commencement of dissection. This retards clot formation and thereby facilitates aspiration of any small pools of blood.

The junction of the visceral peritoneum and the posterior parietal peritoneum is incised over the iliac vessels under the cecum. This incision is extended toward the sacral promontory and then along the right gutter. The cecum is pulled medially by the assistant while the surgeon bluntly pushes the flimsy retroperitoneal attachments off of the cecum and ileocolic mesentery. Once this fusion plane is entered, it is easily followed. Sweeping motions with the shafts of the laparoscopic scissors or with an ENDO RETRACT* device admirably accomplish this blunt dissection.

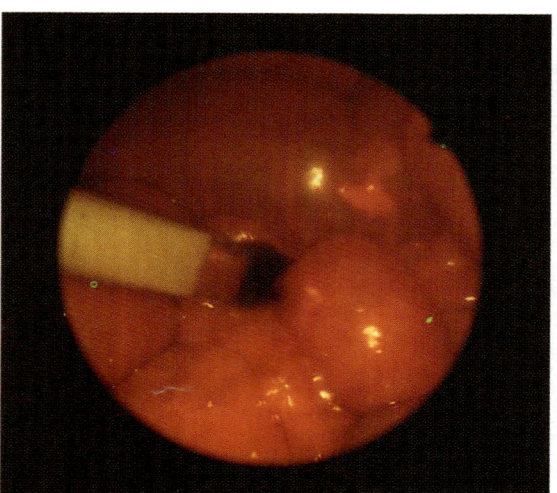

A

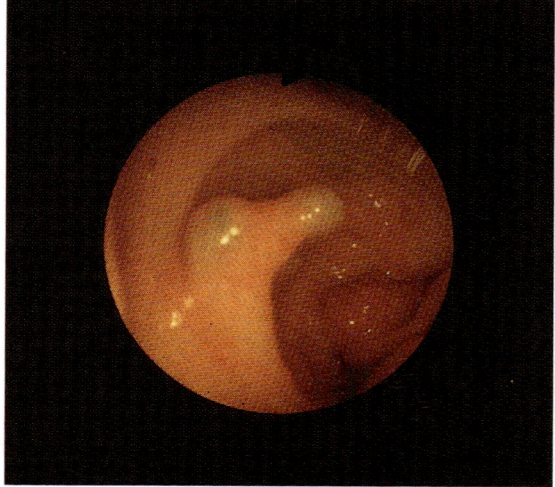

B

Figure 49-5.

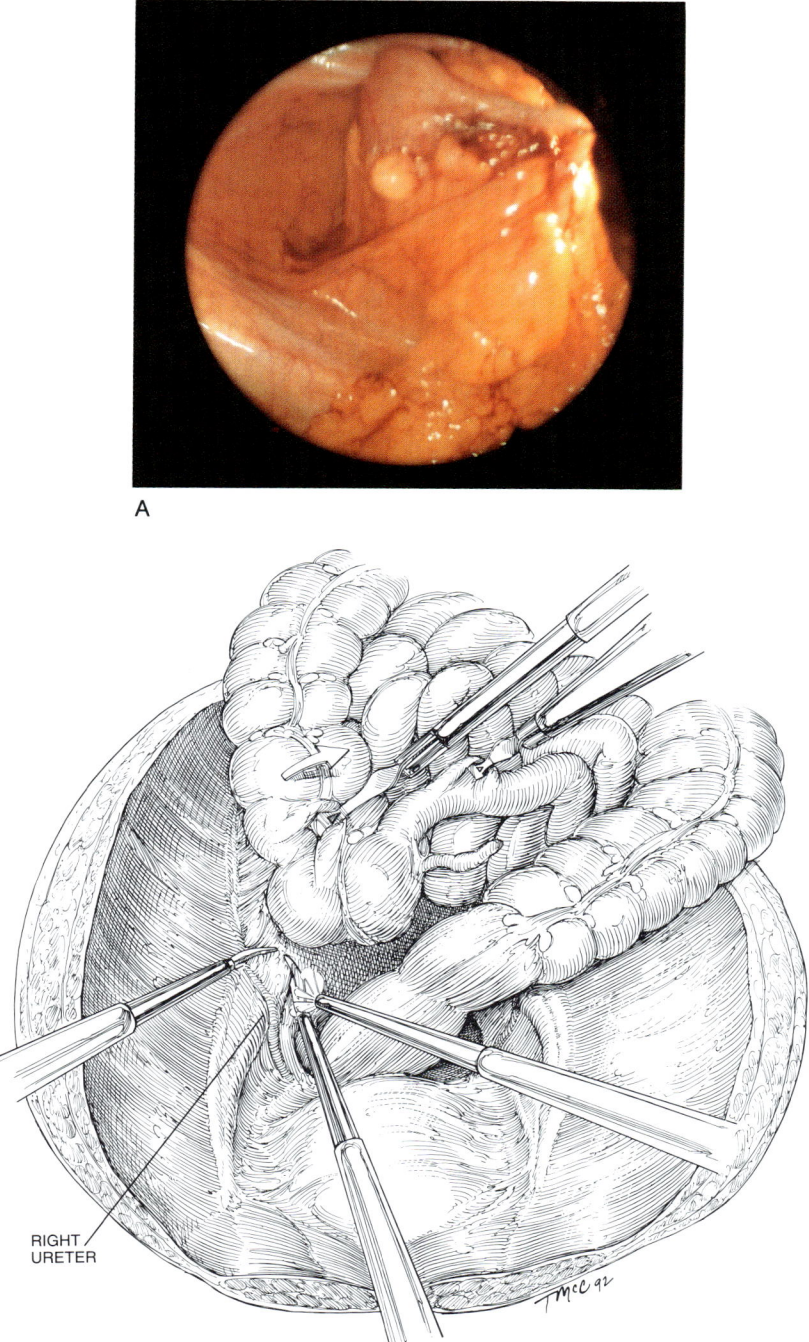

Figure 49-6.

After initial mobilization of the cecum, the 0-degree laparoscope is moved to the midhypogastric port. The assistant grasps the proximal and distal ascending colon with the two ENDO BABCOCK* clamps and elevates the colon and retracts it medially. The surgeon divides the peritoneal reflection along the right gutter with electrocautery scissors. The relationship of this incision to the wall of the colon should be checked frequently. It is easy to veer laterally and wind up behind the right kidney. Dissection continues toward the hepatic flexure and while the exposure remains satisfactory.

The proximal transverse colon is freed next. The lesser sac is entered through the avascular plane between the colon and omentum. The assistant surgeon pushes the edge of the omentum toward the liver and cephalad above the transverse colon. The two ENDO BABCOCK* clamps elevate the omentum. The grasping instrument in the nondominant hand of the surgeon pulls the transverse colon posteriorly. The adhesions between the omentum and colon are divided with the electrocautery scissors (Fig. 49-7). Dissection is initiated near the midtransverse colon and then advances toward the hepatic flexure. This is continued until the omentum is entirely freed from the hepatic flexure and proximal transverse colon.

Any omentum attached to the colon near the lesion is resected en bloc with the specimen. Under these circumstances, the omentum is divided with multiple applications of the ENDO GIA 30* or ENDO GIA 60* stapling device (Fig. 49-8A). The stapling devices provide effective hemostasis (Fig. 49-8B). In thin patients, division of the omental vessels between clips may be feasible.

With the ascending colon mobilized and the transverse colon freed of omental attachments, the lateral attachments of the hepatic flexure are more easily exposed. The assistant surgeon grasps the distal ascending colon and the proximal transverse colon with the two ENDO BABCOCK* clamps. The hepatic flexure is retracted toward the umbilicus. Electrocautery scissors divide the remaining peritoneal attachments of the hepatic flexure. Similarly, adhesions between the duodenum and the mesocolon are sharply cut.

The terminal ileum is next transected. The midhypogastric trocar is replaced with a 12-

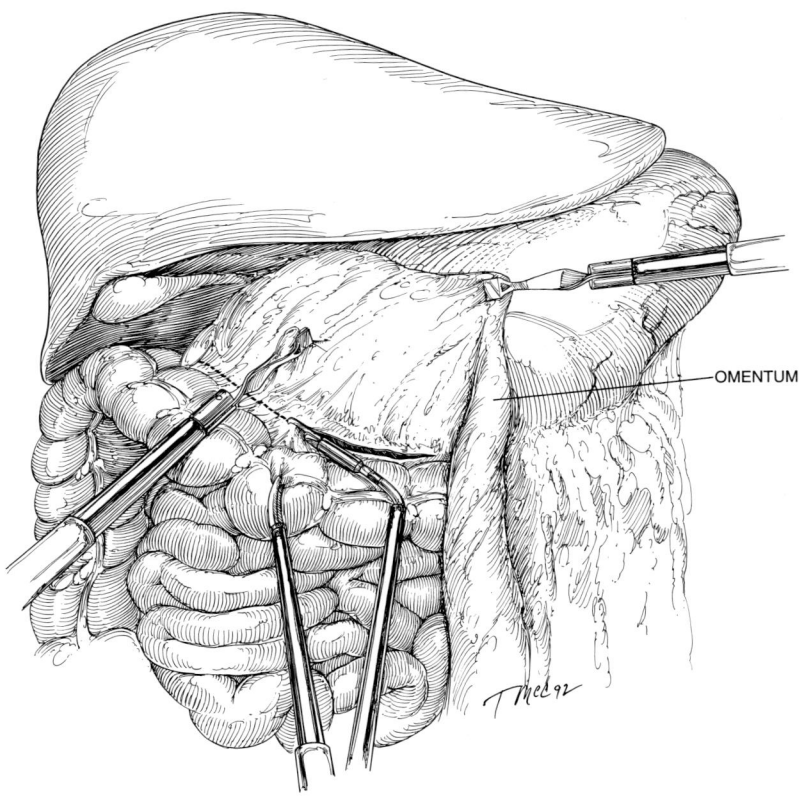

Figure 49-7.

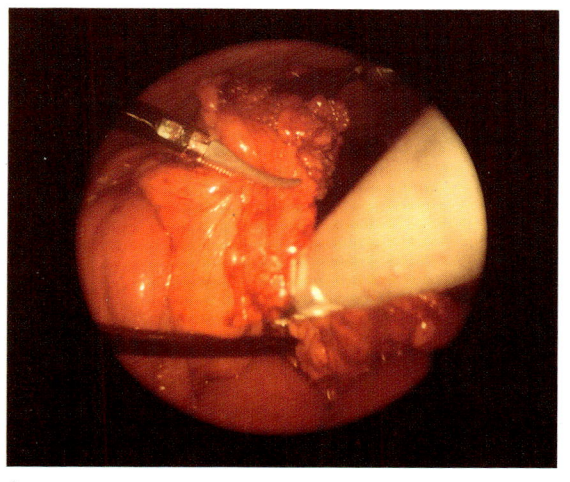 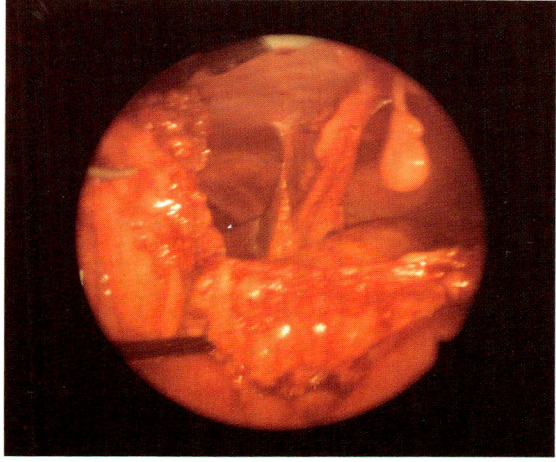

Figure 49-8.

or 15-mm trocar. The terminal ileum is elevated with two Babcock clamps: one placed through the suprapubic port and one through the left upper quadrant port. The terminal ileum is divided with two applications of the ENDO GIA 30* or one of the ENDO GIA 60* stapling device using the blue (3.5-mm) cartridge (Fig. 49-9). The arcades of the ileal mesentery are then divided with the ENDO GIA 30* stapling device using the vascular cartridge (Fig. 49-10).

The ileocolic vessels are traced to their origin. The avascular plane adjacent to the ileocolic vessels (avascular plane of Treves) is entered and followed to the origin of the ileocolic vessels. Any remaining retroperitoneal attachments of the mesocolon behind these vessels are divided. Elevation of the transected terminal ileum toward the anterior abdominal wall maintains exposure. The ileocolic vessels are ligated and transected with the ENDO GIA 30* stapling device using the vascular cartridge (Fig. 49-11). Often the right colic vessels can be divided at the same time. The avascular tissue between the right colic vessels and the origin of the middle colic vessels are divided with the electrocautery scissors. Any remaining attachments to the duodenum or retroperitoneum are severed.

Mobility of the terminal ileum is checked. It is necessary that the terminal ileum be able to reach easily to the planned incision site. Additional division of retroperitoneal attachments of the ileal mesentery may be required so that a tension-free anastomosis can be constructed.

The two terminal ileal staple lines are grasped with ENDO BABCOCK* clamps. The edge of the ileal mesentery is traced from the staple line back to the route of the mesentery. This ensures that the terminal ileum has not twisted. A transverse incision is made in the right upper quadrant over the hepatic flexure. Alternatively, a midline incision is made in the midepigastrium over the middle colic vessels. Initially, the incision is kept small. A finger is poked into the abdomen through the incision and is used to maintain the pneumoperitoneum (Fig. 49-12). A standard Babcock clamp is advanced along the finger into the abdomen. The staple line of the terminal ileum on the specimen is transferred from the ENDO BABCOCK* clamp to the traditional Babcock clamp. The incision is lengthened to a size that will allow retrieval of the specimen. In benign conditions, a 1.5-inch incision is usually adequate. In malignant afflictions, the size of the lesion will mandate the size of the incision. The specimen is pulled out of the abdomen (Fig. 49-13).

The remaining mesocolon is divided extracorporeally between clamps and tied with silk. The left branch of the middle colic artery is preserved. The proximal transverse colon is divided with a GIA 60 stapling device (Fig. 49-14). The specimen is given to a pathologist and opened within the operating room.

Prior to deflation of the pneumoperitoneum, the stapled closure of the terminal ileum is positioned near the incision. The mesentery of the ileum is traced back to its origin to make sure no volvulus has devel-

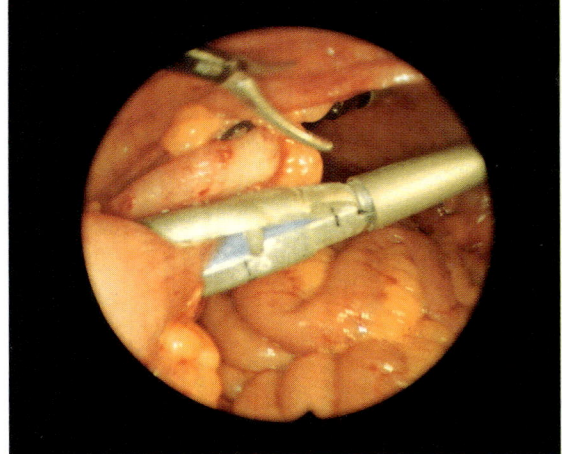

A

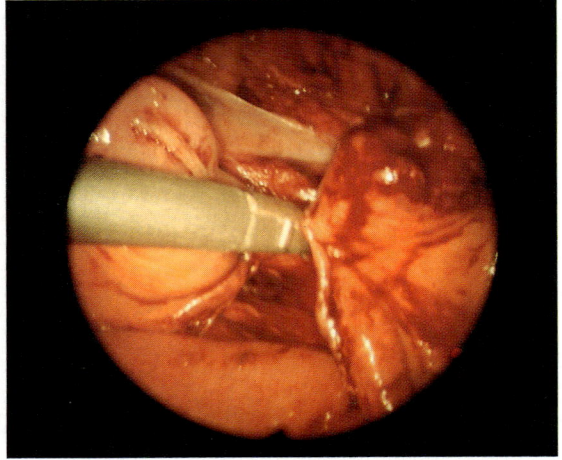

Figure 49-10.

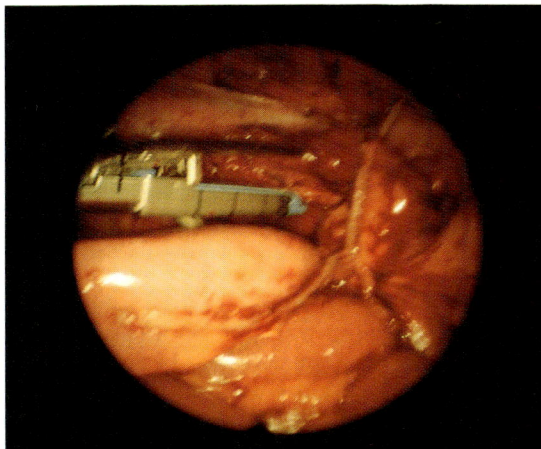

B

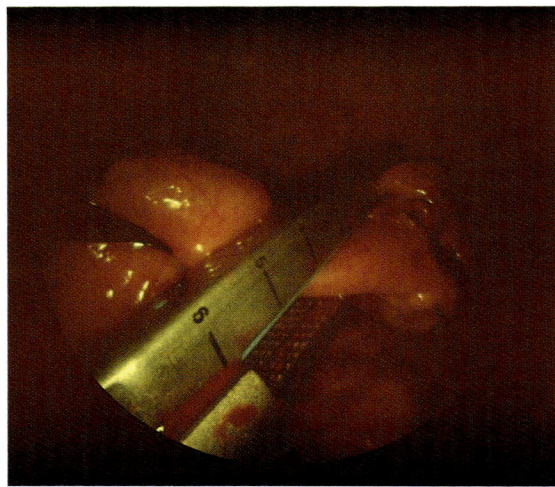

C

Figure 49-9.

oped. After resection of the specimen, the staple line on the terminal ileum is grasped with a standard Babcock clamp through the incision. If the terminal ileum has wandered away from the incision, traction on the abdominal wall with towel clips will usually provide enough visibility through the laparoscope for proper repositioning. The terminal ileum is delivered through the wound.

The antimesenteric borders of the terminal ileum and transverse colon are aligned and secured with two silk sutures. The corners of the staple lines of the ileum and colon are excised with curved Mayo scissors. The jaws of the GIA 60 stapling device are inserted through the two enterotomies and the side-to-side, functional end-to-end anastomosis is constructed by firing the stapling device. The staple line is inspected for hemostasis. The edges of the remaining enterotomy are apposed with four Allis clamps and stapled closed with a TA 55 stapling device using the green (4.8 mm) cartridge. A single silk Lembert suture is used to close the crotch of the anastomosis staple line. If desired, most of the mesenteric defect can be closed extracorporeally. The anastomosis is dropped back into the abdomen.

CLOSURE

The incision is used as a portal for irrigation of the abdomen. Any clots that have accumulated within the operative field are removed through the incision. A large pool sucker is used to aspirate as much of the

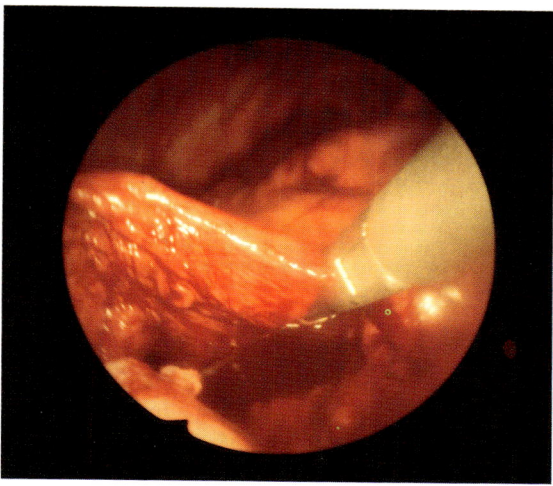

Figure 49-11.

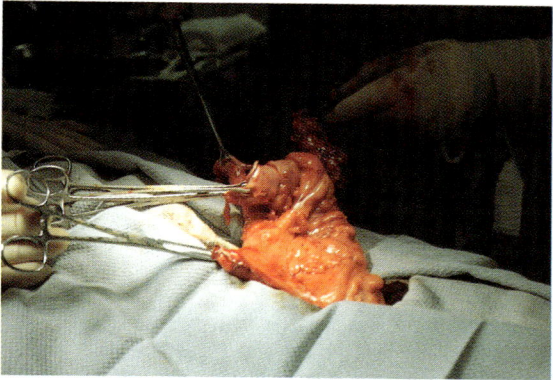

Figure 49-13.

irrigation as possible. The fascia of the incision is closed with interrupted stitches of an absorbable suture.

The pneumoperitoneum is re-inflated. The anastomosis is inspected. The antimesenteric border of the terminal ileum is followed proximally to ensure that a volvulus of the small bowel was not generated during construction of the anastomosis. The mesenteries of the terminal ileum and transverse colon are also examined for signs of torsion. If desired, any remaining rent in the mesentery is closed with the ENDO HERNIA* stapler. Each staple is pushed part way out so that the tips of the staple are exposed. One side of the defect is speared with an exposed staple leg and then dragged into apposition with the other side of the defect. The stapler is fired, and the two edges are secured together.

The abdomen is scrutinized for any persistent hemorrhage. Any remaining irrigation fluid is aspirated. The omentum is dragged back into proper position. The trocars are removed one at a time. The fascial defect of each puncture site is closed with interrupted sutures. Placement of the stitches is observed with the videolaparoscope to ensure that the bowel is not speared by the needle. The laparoscope is removed from the last trocar. The pneumoperitoneum is slowly deflated by opening the valve of the trocar. The trocar is withdrawn. The last fascial defect is closed. All of the incisions are irrigated with a solution which contains antibiotics. The skin edges are apposed with skin staples. Band-Aids (Johnson & Johnson, Inc., Skillman, NJ) cover each wound.

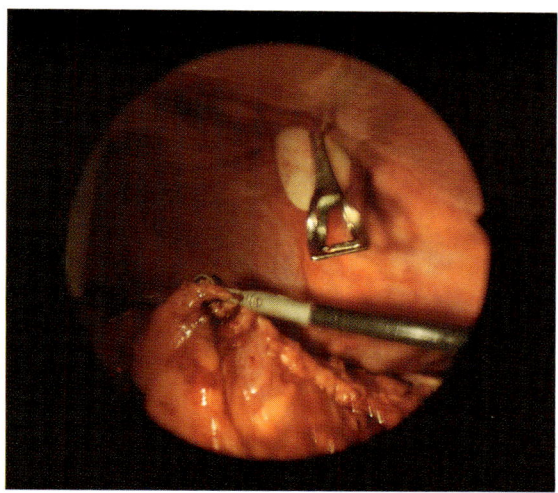

Figure 49-12.

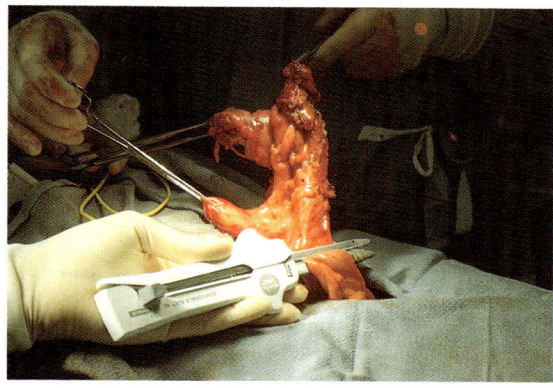

Figure 49-14.

POSTOPERATIVE MANAGEMENT

The nasogastric tube is removed in the recovery room on the morning after the operation. The urinary catheter and pneumatic compression boots are removed when the patient is alert and able to walk. The patient is given pain medicine intramuscularly as needed. Generally, the patient has so little pain that very few injections are requested. The patient is offered clear liquids on the morning after surgery and advanced to a regular diet the next day if the liquids are tolerated. The intravenous line is removed when the patient is taking liquids well.

CRITERIA FOR PATIENT DISCHARGE

When drinking an adequate volume of liquids and able to eat a regular diet, the patient can be discharged. Other considerations, however, must influence this decision. Early discharge on the third or fourth postoperative day is feasible if the patient lives near the hospital and has a spouse or children at home who can provide supportive care. If the patient lives alone, discharge should be delayed until at least the fifth postoperative day. Patients tend to move their bowels for the first time after the operation between the second and fourth postoperative day. Although defecation is not a prerequisite for discharge, it is one of the factors that should enter into the final decision.

COMPLICATIONS SPECIFIC FOR THIS PROCEDURE

During construction of the anastomosis, it is very easy to twist the terminal ileum. The antimesenteric border of the ileum and its mesentery must be carefully examined before the abdominal wall is incised and the pneumoperitoneum is lost. Similarly, after the anastomosis is returned to the abdominal cavity and the pneumoperitoneum is reinflated, the terminal ileum and its mesentery must be inspected for evidence of a volvulus.

Rates of other complications for this procedure remain undetermined at this time. The frequency of anastomotic leaks, however, should be the same as has been previously published for stapled side-to-side, functional end-to-end anastomoses.

Chapter 50
Left Hemicolectomy

William E. Kelly, Jr.

PATIENT SELECTION

The general criteria for patient selection in laparoscopic colectomy parallel those for laparoscopic cholecystectomy. Surgeons who have not acquired much experience should restrict their procedures to thin, relatively healthy individuals with nonacute colonic pathologic conditions. Body habitus is an important consideration in patient selection for early procedures. A taller individual provides a larger peritoneal volume within which to work than does a shorter patient. Among patients of similar size, women are easier to operate upon than are men, because the female mesocolon contains less fatty tissue to impede dissection of the vessels and because these are less paracolic fat in women. The same considerations make obese patients less attractive surgical candidates than thin patients. The thickened omentum characteristic of obese patients also makes the dissection and mobilization of the splenic flexure considerably more difficult in these individuals. Finally, a history of multiple prior abdominal operations should alert the surgeon that extensive adhesiolysis might increase the difficulty of the operation and prolong operating room time.

As a surgeon's experience in laparoscopic colon surgery increases, body habitus becomes a less important concern. However, the extent of the colonic disease process continues to influence patient selection. Subacute diverticulitis or inflammatory bowel disease might result in local inflammation or scarring that could make dissection more difficult. A large diverticular mass of the left colon might increase operative risks as a result of local adhesion to the ureter. Acute diverticular bleeding is also a relative contraindication to laparoscopic surgery for the novice, because operative time is markedly prolonged by the laparoscopic technique. For the same reason, colonic perforation with peritonitis is an absolute contraindication to laparoscopic surgery for the inexperienced surgeon and remains a strong relative contraindication for the experienced surgeon. Colon obstruction markedly reduces exposure for laparoscopic surgery because of dilated proximal intestinal loops and also makes trocar insertion more hazardous. Large bulky neoplasms raise a relative contraindication to laparoscopic colectomy, since the incision must be large enough to readily accommodate removal of the lesion without crushing the tumor or contaminating the abdominal wall with malignant tissue. For this reason, various types of impermeable bags or sacs have been developed to remove malignant lesions through small incisions. The incision must, however, be large enough to accommodate the tumor. A bulky tumor may often require an incision large enough to perform a traditional open colon resection.

Comorbid medical illnesses affect patient

selection in much the same way that they affect traditional colon resection. These considerations are fully outlined in Chapter 9.

PREOPERATIVE EVALUATION

The time-honored principles of clinical evaluation of the patient by history and physical examination are of paramount importance in preparation for laparoscopic left hemicolectomy. Clinical indications for surgical intervention must be every bit as strict for laparoscopic surgery as they are for traditional operations. Having confirmed the indications for surgery, however, and having completed the traditional preoperative evaluation, the surgeon must address several considerations before laparoscopic colon resection can be scheduled.

Laparotomy by videolaparoscopy is primarily a visual and surface-oriented procedure. The ability to palpate deep structures and parenchymal lesions and to identify subtle masses in the colon is very limited. Therefore, an accurate preoperative colonoscopic evaluation is of critical importance to identify synchronous lesions and to chart their location accurately. If the laparoscopic surgeon does not perform the colonoscopy personally or if there is any question about the exact location of salient pathologic conditions after completion of the colonoscopy, then a barium enema should be performed. The proximal extent of diverticulosis cannot be accurately assessed laparoscopically. Small neoplasms and even relatively large polyps cannot be identified with confidence by laparoscopic technique. The surgeon must therefore be confident of the colonic pathologic condition preoperatively and must have a relatively precise plan for the anatomical resection that he or she will perform. Although a barium enema is often considered to be redundant and its results imprecise, it will frequently provide the surgeon with added certainty about the anatomical relationships of colonic pathologic conditions. The added cost of a barium enema will rapidly be made up in cost savings for operating time needed to confirm the location of a neoplasm or to resect extra colon to obtain an adequate margin for additional diverticular disease.

A more liberal use of computed tomographic (CT) scans should also be considered in the preoperative evaluation for laparoscopic colectomy. Since the liver cannot be accurately palpated, deep parenchymal liver metastases may be missed when operating for malignancy. This would have important prognostic significance and might indicate a more conservative operation. CT evaluation of a diverticular mass can often be helpful in predicting the degree of local inflammation, involvement of the left ureter, and involvement of adjacent structures, such as the bladder or small bowel. A less experienced laparoscopic surgeon should know these details in advance and factor them into the decision matrix for patient selection. Additional studies such as barium enema and CT scans should certainly not be considered standard in the preoperative evaluation for laparoscopic hemicolectomy. They should be used liberally, however, especially during a surgeon's early experience.

PREOPERATIVE PREPARATION

The osmotic fluid solutions have proven to be the most effective form of mechanical bowel preparation. In the absence of obstructive signs and symptoms, the patient is allowed to continue his or her normal diet until the day before surgery. On the morning of the first preoperative day, the patient initiates a clear liquid diet. After dinner, the patient takes one 10-mg tablet of metoclopramide. Beginning 1 hour later, the patient consumes two to three liters of GoLIGHTLY bowel preparation solution over a 2-hour interval. Two to 3 hours before surgery, the patient is given a Fleets enema to empty the distal colon of any residual fluid.

An oral antibiotic bowel preparation is routinely ordered. Neomycin and erythromycin base are given together in four doses at 3-hour intervals, beginning at 2:00 p.m. on the day prior to surgery. A single dose of a second generation cephalorsporin is given intravenously in the holding area preoperatively. If there is any unexpected contamination during the procedure, the intravenous antibiotic is continued at appropriate intervals for an additional 24 hours.

EQUIPMENT

A 10-mm 0-degree videolaparoscope is used throughout the procedure for the majority of left hemicolectomies. Occasionally, a 10-mm 30-degree laparoscope is useful to improve visualization during the mobilization of the splenic flexure. Although it is advisable to have a 30-degree laparoscope available, it is not often needed. A second laparoscope and light source may be helpful for transillumination of the mesocolon to assist in identification of the blood vessels. The 30-degree laparoscope can be used quite efficiently for that purpose.

Five trocars are used for standard port placement. Two 10-mm trocars are used for the retracting ports so that the first assistant can use either 5-mm atraumatic graspers or 10-mm ENDO BABCOCK* clamps. The 10-mm ports also permit alternative access points for the laparoscope. Three 12-mm trocars are used for the camera and dissecting ports to allow maximum flexibility for use of the ENDO GIA* stapler. Specifics of trocar placement and utilization are discussed below.

Various gripping devices are now available to fix the trocars within the abdominal wall and to help to prevent the trocars from sliding in and out during the extensive dissection required for left hemicolectomy. These devices help to prevent wasted time for reinsertion of the trocars and minimize trauma to the local tissues.

Atraumatic grasping forceps are critical to the safe execution of laparoscopic bowel surgery. Nondisposable Glassman and DeBakey forceps are available, but these can cause serosal injuries when traction is applied to bowel that is being fixed and held by these instruments. Disposable ENDO GRASP* forceps have proven to be the least traumatic forceps in our hands. The ENDO BABCOCK* forceps are slightly more traumatic, but are the most secure of the minimally traumatic bowel-grasping forceps.

Sharp, dependable scissors are also critical for laparoscopic bowel surgery. Laparoscopic scissors should be cautery-capable and must be reliably sharp every time. Up to the present time, the nondisposable scissors have been a disappointment, since they rapidly become dull with repeated use. Until durable scissors and less traumatic nondisposable graspers become available, the ENDO GRASP* forceps and disposable scissors appear to add a margin of safety and efficacy that fully justifies their expense.

Instruments for endoscopic suturing are among the most rapidly improving nondisposable laparoscopic devices. Diamond jaw needle holders are very important for use with curved needles. Knot-passing instruments are useful for passing individual ties and are helpful when the surgeon is not facile with intracorporeal knot tying. The use of a fisherman's knot for extracorporeal knot tying is somewhat more traumatic than individual knot passing and is not suitable for suturing delicate tissues.

The ENDO GIA* staplers have truly made laparoscopic colon surgery possible on a routine basis for properly trained laparoscopic surgeons. The 30-V cartridges reliably ligate and divide major blood vessels while the ENDO GIA* 3.5-mm cartridges divide the bowel without difficulty. Two or three applications of the 30-mm stapler are usually needed to divide the large intestine. By clamping and releasing the stapler, however, spasm is induced in the bowel wall, and the stapler can often be reapplied and fired across a somewhat smaller diameter of colon, requiring fewer applications (Fig. 50-1, A to C) With the advent of the 60-mm linear stapler, the division of larger segments of bowel and of longer lengths of mesocolon can now be accomplished more efficiently. The technique of intercorporeal anastomosis by a functional end-to-end technique has also been facilitated.

Multiple clip appliers are essential for the efficient progress of laparoscopic colon resection. Ligation of vessels of any significance requires the application of four clips before division. Single application clip appliers are too cumbersome and inefficient for this type of surgery. New ENDO CLIP* appliers offer the flexibility of varying clip lengths. Large clips permit ligation and division of bigger vessels than the traditional "medium-large" clips do.

Several fan-like retracting instruments are available that can be inserted as a cylinder and then adjusted to produce an "expanding fan" effect at the tip. Although these instruments are very important for vagotomy and for fundoplication, they are rarely needed for colon resection, except in obese individuals. Exposure is largely achieved by changing the position of the patient and sweeping the viscera away from the field of dissection, relying upon gravity to hold the bowel in place.

The technology of laparoscopic instrumentation is expanding at an incredible rate. As we have devised more and more complex surgical procedures, manufacturers have continued to supply us with instruments to facilitate our techniques. As the technology improves, so does the efficiency and safety of surgical procedures.

POSITIONING OF THE PATIENT

The patient is placed in the lithotomy position with the arms at the patient's side (Fig.

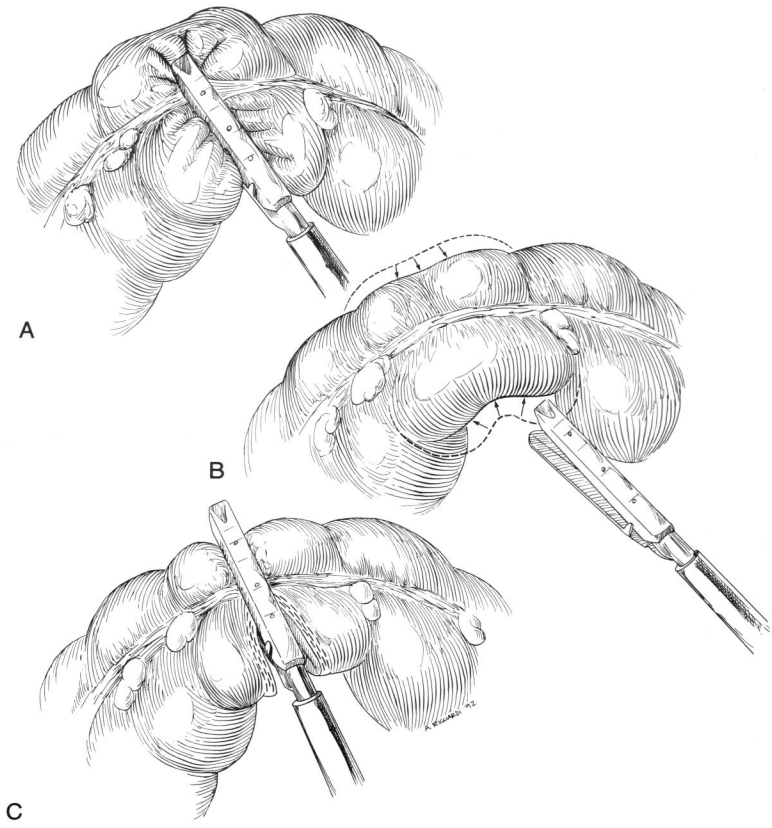

Figure 50-1.

50-2) The lithotomy position is chosen even if the preoperative evaluation indicates that the sigmoid colon may be spared. General endotracheal anesthesia is used, and a nasogastric tube is inserted for gastric decompression. A Foley catheter is inserted to evacuate the urinary bladder. If there is any question of ureteral involvement by a neoplasm or by an inflammatory mass, a left ureteral stent is inserted. A lighted ureteral stent can be particularly helpful in the obese patient when dissection in the area of the ureter is expected to be difficult. By dimming the light source of the videolaparoscope, the lighted stent can be readily seen, identifying the location of the ureter.

POSITIONING OF THE VIDEO EQUIPMENT

Two video monitors are used during left colectomy. At the beginning of the procedure, one monitor is positioned on each side of the patient (Fig. 50-2). The monitor to the patient's left begins at the patient's iliac crest. As the dissection moves toward the splenic flexure, the left side monitor is moved to the level of the patient's shoulder. This adjustment improves the surgeon's orientation as he or she proceeds with the dissection.

The assistant's monitor is positioned behind the surgeon. It is usually placed in a neutral position at the level of the patient's umbilicus. The camera operator begins the operation at the surgeon's left side, next to the patient's right shoulder. The scrub nurse is positioned between the patient's legs during most of the procedure.

TROCAR PLACEMENT

Typically, five trocars are used during the procedure (Fig. 50-3). Two 10-mm ports are inserted in the left midclavicular line, one just below the costal margin, and one just below the iliac crest. These ports provide access for atraumatic grasping forceps or for ENDO BABCOCK* clamps during most of the proce-

Left Hemicolectomy 551

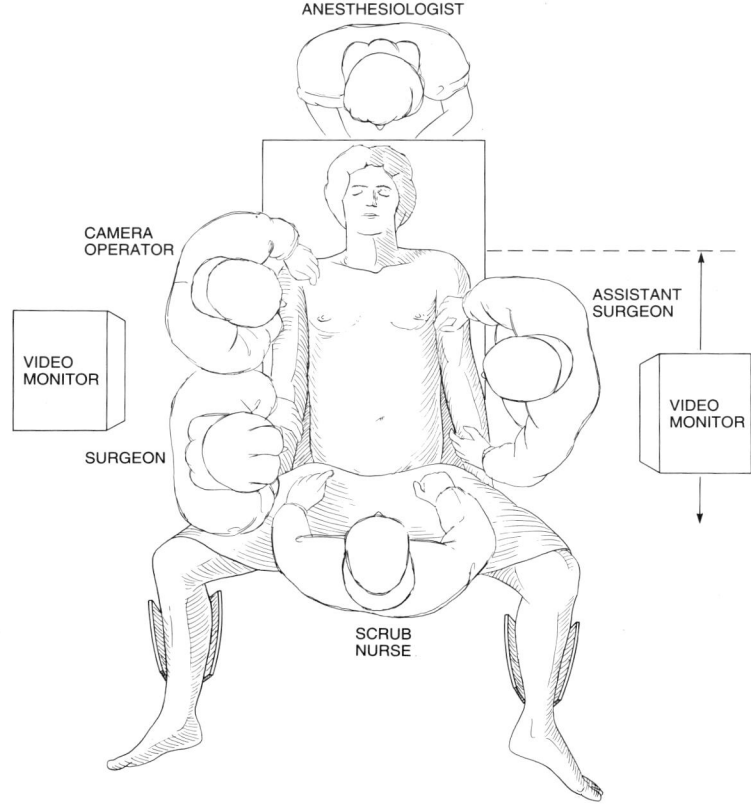

Figure 50-2.

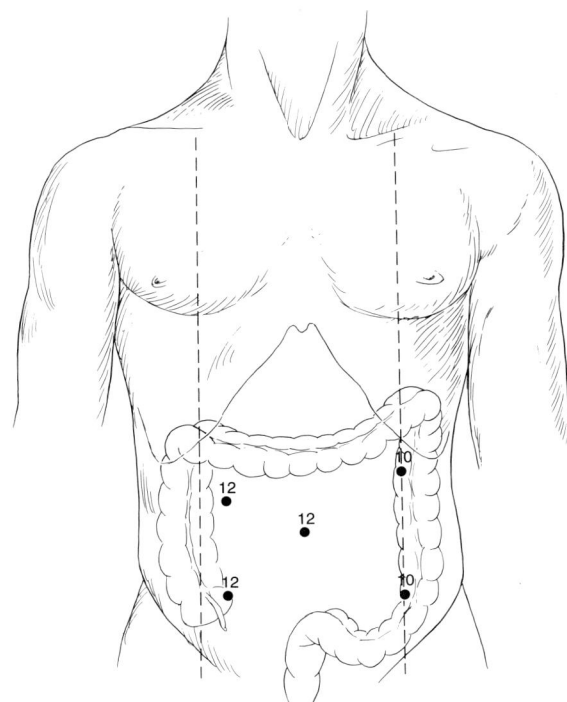

Figure 50-3.

dure. Three 12-mm ports are inserted, one at the umbilicus and two just medial to the right midclavicular line. The right-sided ports are positioned somewhat closer together than are the left-sided ports to permit the surgeon to use both hands in concert for two-handed dissecting technique. The videolaparoscope is positioned at the umbilical port during the majority of the procedure, but can be moved to the left lower quadrant or to the right upper quadrant port if the need arises to improve exposure. Any of the 12-mm ports can be used for application of the ENDO GIA* 30 stapler for transection of blood vessels or division of the bowel. When the ENDO GIA* 60 stapler is available, a 15-mm port may be substituted for the right lower quadrant trocar site.

The five-trocar distribution described here provides a flexible access to the left colon at all levels. The specific location of each port should be modified for each patient, following insertion of the laparoscope and exploration of the abdomen. As each surgeon gains experience in laparoscopic colectomy, the trocar placement will be modified to accommo-

552 Techniques of Laparoscopic Surgery

date individual styles of dissection. Several different approaches to port placement have already been described in other chapters.

METHODS OF EXPOSURE AND RETRACTION

Patient positioning and the force of gravity provide most of the exposure for laparoscopic colectomy. The patient is tilted 10 to 30 degrees downward to the right, during most of the procedure. The viscera can then be swept downward to the patient's right, and gravity will maintain the position of the small bowel. As the dissection progresses distally or proximally, the table is placed in the Trendelenburg or in the reverse Trendelenburg position, respectively. The colon is then retracted medially and posteriorly to provide exposure for mobilization along the lateral gutter or retracted laterally and upward to produce the exposure for dissection of the mesocolon.

METHODS OF DISSECTION

Most of the dissection is carried out sharply with scissors. Blunt dissection is used in the area of the ureter and to mobilize the descending mesocolon from the psoas and quadratus muscles and from Gerota's fascia. Most of the blunt dissection is performed with the back of the cautery scissors, or with a dissecting forceps to tease the tissue away from the ureter and gonadal vessels, while making judicious use of cautery. Some surgeons prefer to use laser energy to dissect through the mesocolon. The serosal surface of the mesocolon can be scored and incised with the noncontact laser, and the fatty tissue is then bluntly dissected free from the vessels using the suc-

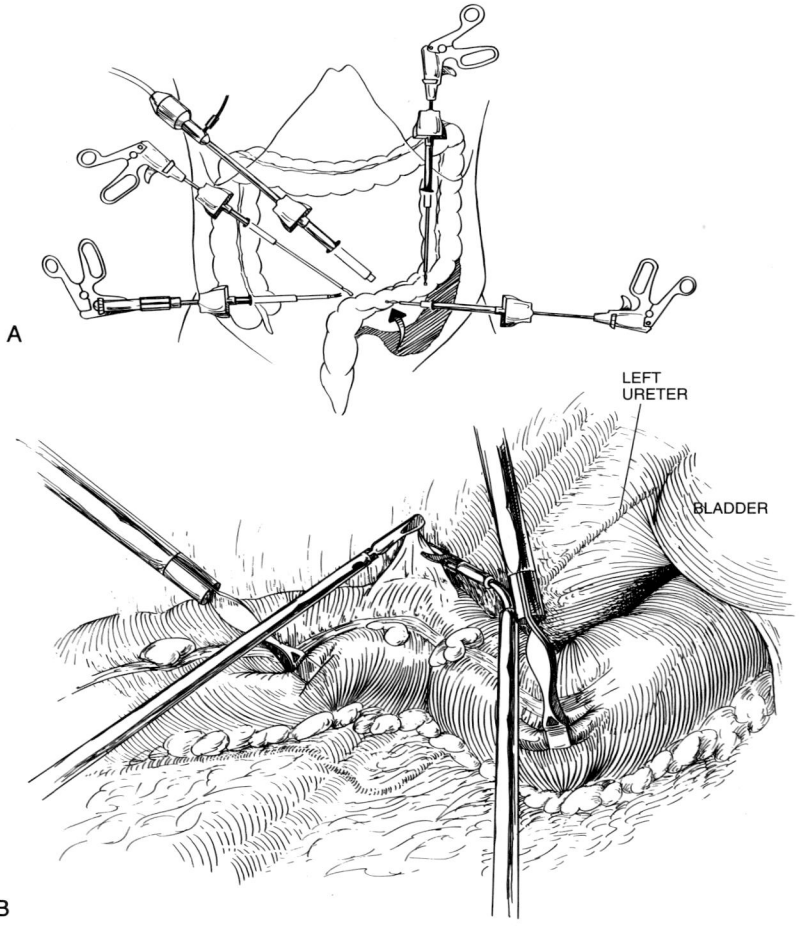

Figure 50-4.

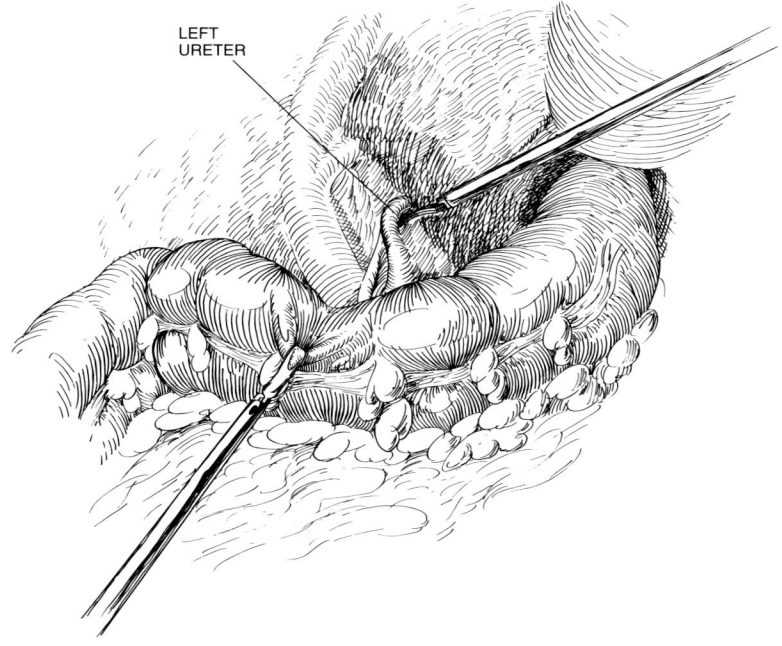

Figure 50-5.

tion-irrigation-laser probe. Alternatively, the cautery scissors can be used to score the mesocolon. The combined sharp and blunt dissection technique is particularly useful for obese patients and for male patients who tend to have thickened, fatty tissue surrounding the vessels of the mesocolon.

SPECIFIC DETAILS OF THE PROCEDURE

The patient is rotated 10 to 30 degrees to the right during most of the procedure. After the patient's abdomen is thoroughly explored, the table is rotated to the right and placed in a steep Trendelenburg position. The sigmoid colon is retracted medially using atraumatic grasping forceps or ENDO BABCOCK* clamps via the left upper quadrant and left lower quadrant ports. The sigmoid is then immobilized along the white line of Toldt using cautery scissors dissection with judicious application of cautery in the vicinity of the ureter. The videolaparoscope is positioned through the umbilical port and the surgeon operates through the two right-sided ports.

As the dissection develops, the left ureter is identified crossing the iliac artery (Fig. 50-4, A and B) The ureter is followed distally as the mobilization of the sigmoid continues toward the peritoneal reflection. The ureter must always be identified (Fig. 50-5). When an inflammatory mass is anticipated in the area of the ureter, it is advisable to pass a left ureteral stent preoperatively. The stent can usually be palpated with the dissecting forceps early in the course of the dissection to facilitate identification. A lighted stent can be even more helpful in difficult procedures. By dimming the laparoscopic light source, the light from the ureteral stent can readily be seen after the colon is reflected medially. Having completed the distal dissection, the surgeon then mobilizes the descending colon in the same fashion, progressing toward the splenic flexure. The table is changed to the reverse Trendelenburg position to improve exposure. The monitor on the patient's left is moved cephalad at this time to improve the surgeon's orientation. It is often helpful to change the position of the laparoscope to the left lower quadrant port and to retract from the right lower quadrant port while dissecting via the umbilical port as the proximal descending colon is mobilized (Fig. 50-6, A and B). The surgeon must be flexible in the use of the ports. The laparoscope port is often changed several times during the procedure to provide better visualization.

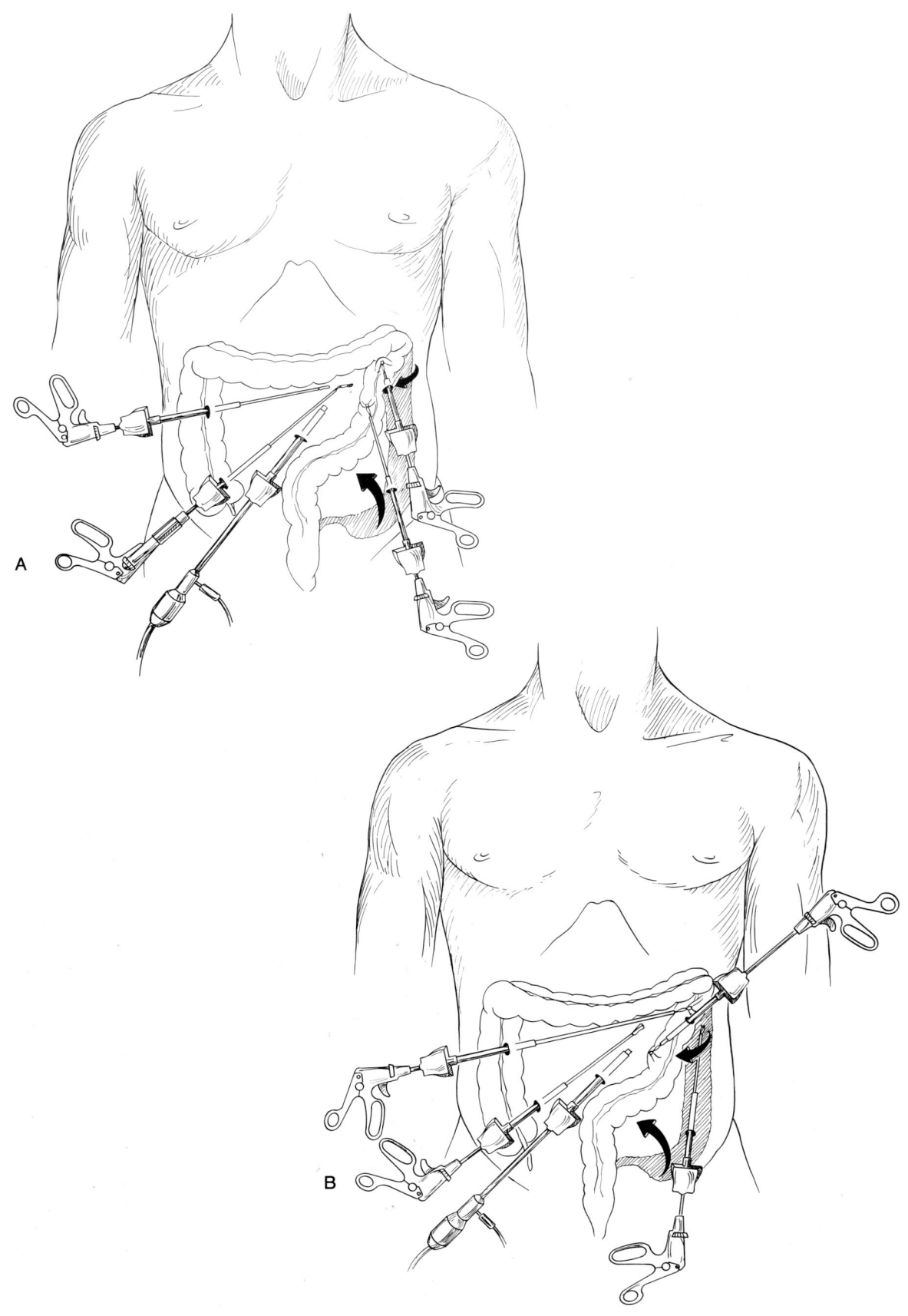

Figure 50-6.

Occasionally, an additional suprapubic port is inserted for the laparoscope to improve the exposure as the descending colon is mobilized. The suprapubic port is especially useful in obese patients.

As the splenic flexure is approached, attention is directed to the left transverse colon. The omentum is dissected free from the transverse colon in the avascular plane by cautery scissor dissection. The dissection begins well proximal to the anticipated level of transection of the colon and progresses in the direction of the lienocolic ligament. Unless a malignancy of the splenic flexure is expected, it is advisable to dissect close to the bowel as the splenic flexure is approached. The ENDO GIA* stapler is helpful in completing the dissection at the lienocolic ligament. In obese patients we have often used two or even three applications of the ENDO GIA* stapler in this area (Fig. 50-7). It is sometimes helpful to transfer the videolaparoscope to the right upper quadrant port as the splenic flexure is approached (Fig. 50-8).

For malignant lesions of the splenic flexure, a more radical resection of the gastrocolic omentum is carried out. In this case, the omentum is mobilized at the level planned for transection of the transverse colon. The gastrocolic omentum is then divided, progressing toward the greater curvature of the stomach. This dissection can be carried out in a relatively avascular plane. The omentum is then divided from right to left using cautery scissors dissection and endoscopic clips for hemostasis. In obese individuals, it is often safest to use the ENDO GIA* stapler liberally during this portion of the dissection to mini-

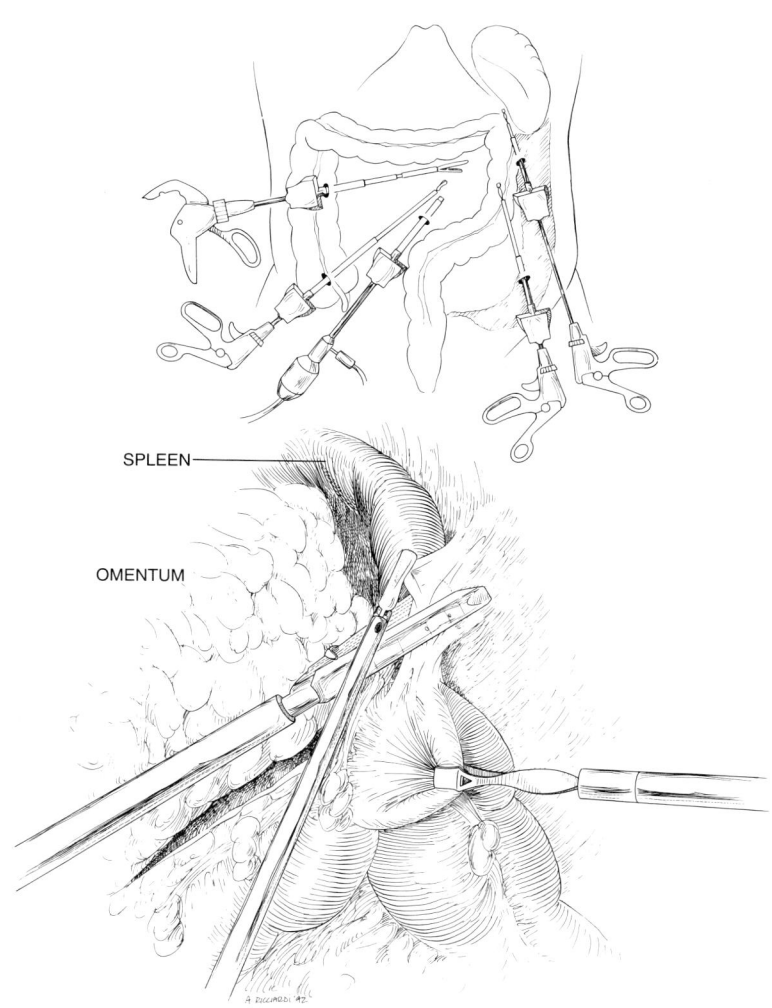

Figure 50-7.

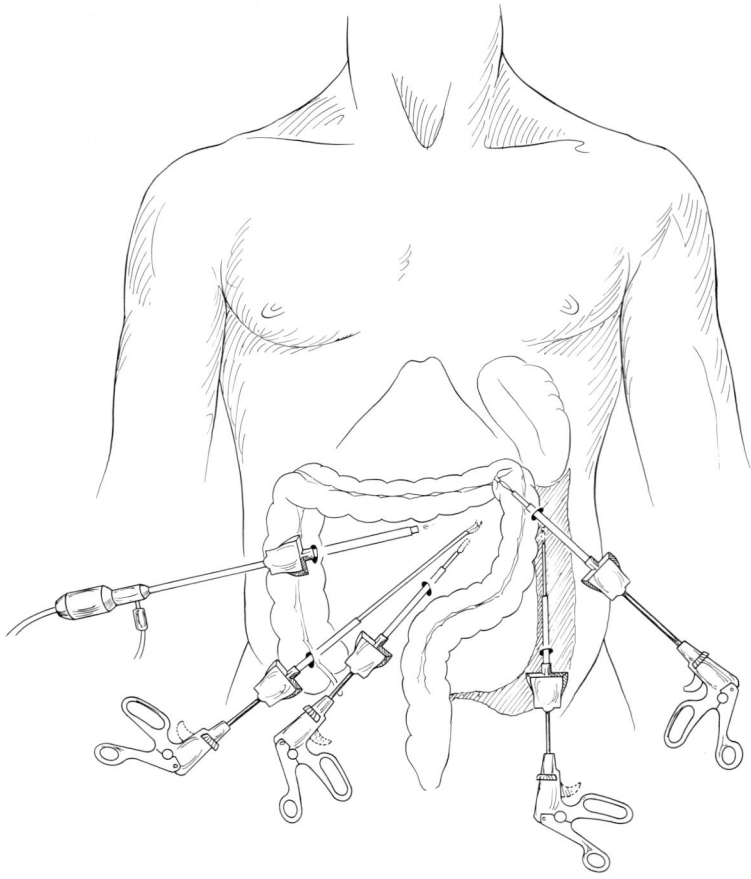

Figure 50-8.

mize bleeding. The vessels can be somewhat difficult to identify within the thickened omentum of an obese patient. The combined laser or sharp and blunt dissection technique is helpful in identifying the omental vessels.

After the splenic flexure is mobilized, the descending and left transverse colon is then reflected downward and to the right. The dissection continues on the posterior surface of the mesocolon, leaving the quadratus and psoas muscles and the left ureter exposed. The extent of this dissection depends upon the indication for surgery. In the case of a malignant lesion of the left colon, the origin of the left colic artery can be exposed, and the inferior mesenteric artery can be identified and isolated. The surgeon should have considerable experience with laparoscopic bowel surgery before proceeding with left hemicolectomy for a malignancy in this area.

At this point the transection of the mesocolon is initiated. The serosal surface of the mesocolon is scored along the intended line of dissection using either the laser or the cautery scissors. The vessels can then be dissected free from the fatty tissue and isolated. A second laparoscope and light source can be inserted via the left ports to transilluminate the major vessels. This technique is particularly useful in obese patients and in identifying the take-off of the left colic and the inferior mesenteric arteries.

The major vessels are ligated and divided using either the ENDO GIA* 30-V stapler or endoclips. The ENDO GIA* stapler has proven to be a safe and efficient instrument for division of major vessels, especially when the endoclips appear to be too short to completely ligate larger blood vessels. When endoclips are used, four clips should be applied, two proximally and two distally. When the vessels are divided, the tissue should be grasped on the arterial side as the ENDO GIA* stapler is released or as the scissors are applied. In this fashion, proximal control is assured in case bleeding results. Bleeding at the ENDO GIA* staple line is rare, but can occur. Bleeding through a doubly clipped vessel is also rare. If a bleeding point is encountered, however, the proper technique involves elevation and exposure of the vessel from behind with a grasping forceps. This technique presents the bleeding point and fixes it for prompt ligation by the ENDO CLIP* applier (Fig. 50-9). If necessary a SURGIETIE* or laparoscopic suture can be applied to further secure hemostasis.

An alternative method of transecting the mesocolon involves serial applications of the ENDO GIA* stapler without specifically identifying the vessels. This method can be somewhat faster than individual dissection and ligation of each vascular pedicle. It may offer some advantage for surgery in the obese patient. As the surgeon becomes experienced with laparoscopic bowel surgery, however, the time saving is reduced and the added cost for extra staple cartridges becomes difficult to justify on a routine basis.

After the division of the mesocolon is completed, the transverse colon is grasped and brought into approximation with the distal bowel to ensure that there is sufficient mobilization for a tension-free anastomosis (Fig. 50-10). The omentum is further dissected free from the right transverse colon if necessary. When a full left hemicolectomy with resection of the sigmoid colon is performed, the hepatic flexure may also have to be mobilized to gain sufficient length. The entire omentum is dissected free from the right transverse colon and the dissection is continued along the hepatic flexure. By staying close to the antimesenteric surface of the hepatic flexure, the hepatocolic ligament can be divided readily with cautery scissors dissection. Only a few endoscopic clips are needed if the dissection is directed adjacent to the colon.

COMPLETE HEMICOLECTOMY

If most of the sigmoid colon is to be resected, the anastomosis will be carried out using the Premium CEEA* stapling device. The transverse colon is brought up to the abdominal wall at a comfortable location in the left lower quadrant to identify the optimal site for exteriorization (Fig. 50-11). If possible, the exteriorizing incision should incorporate the left lower quadrant trocar site. The sigmoid colon is transected distally with the ENDO GIA* stapler via the right lower quadrant trocar with the videolaparoscope inserted through the umbilical port. Frequently, two applications of the 30-mm ENDO GIA* stapler are required. When the ENDO GIA* 60 stapler is available, a single application will routinely suffice. One helpful method for

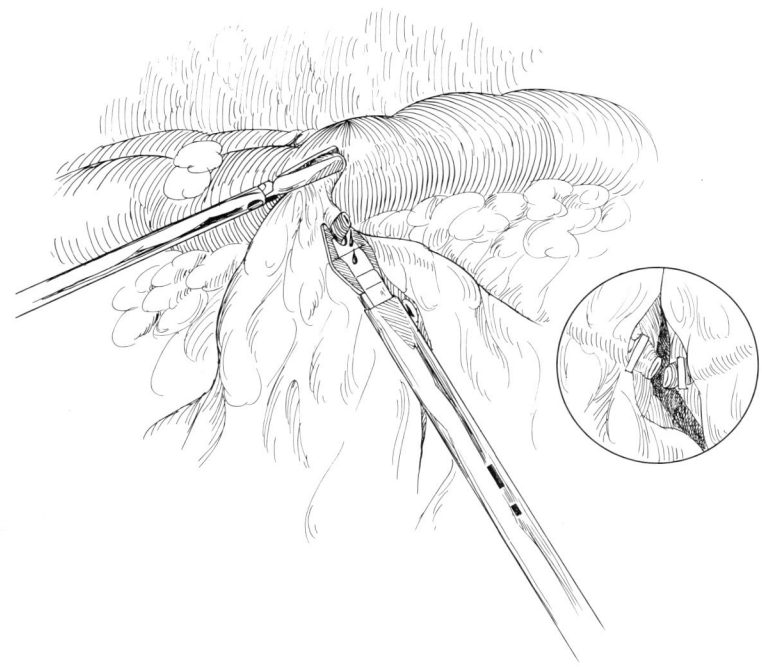

Figure 50-9.

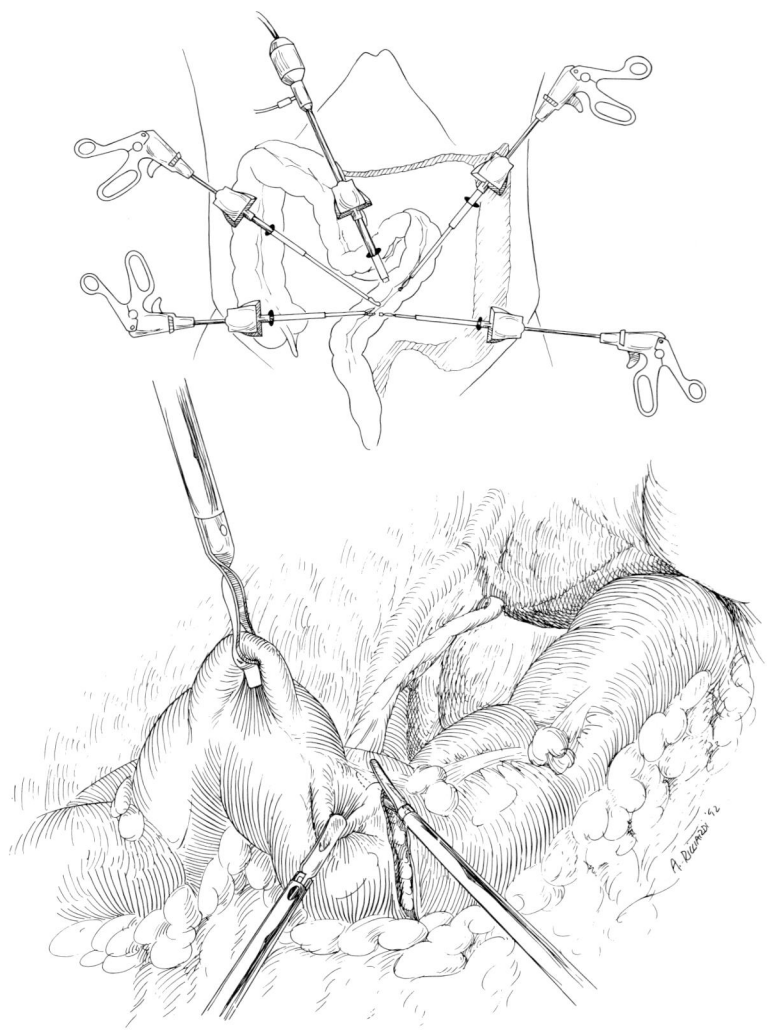

Figure 50-10.

reducing the number of applications of the ENDO GIA* is to clamp the stapler on the bowel at the transection site and to release it without firing. This maneuver is atraumatic and will not injure the bowel, but will produce spasm and thus contract the bowel and make the diameter to be divided smaller. Fewer cartridges are then needed to transect the bowel (Fig. 50-1).

The proximal cut end of the sigmoid is grasped on the antimesenteric surface with an ENDO BABCOCK* clamp via the right lower quadrant port (Fig. 50-12). The bowel is placed in the proper orientation to prevent torsion. A left lower quadrant incision is made, typically 4 to 7 cm in length, depending upon the size of the specimen. When possible, the incision begins along the lateral rectus border and extends laterally through the left lower quadrant trocar site. The external oblique aponeurosis is incised, and the oblique abdominus muscle layers are serially separated in the direction of the fibers. The peritoneum is incised, evacuating the pneumoperitoneum. The proximal end of the bowel is then exteriorized by advancing the ENDO BABCOCK* clamp through the incision. If there is a malignant lesion in the specimen, it is placed in a plastic bag before drawing it through the incision, to avoid seeding the abdominal wall with cancer cells.

At this point the bowel is divided and a purse-string suture is applied (Fig. 50-13A). The disposable purse-string device is applied

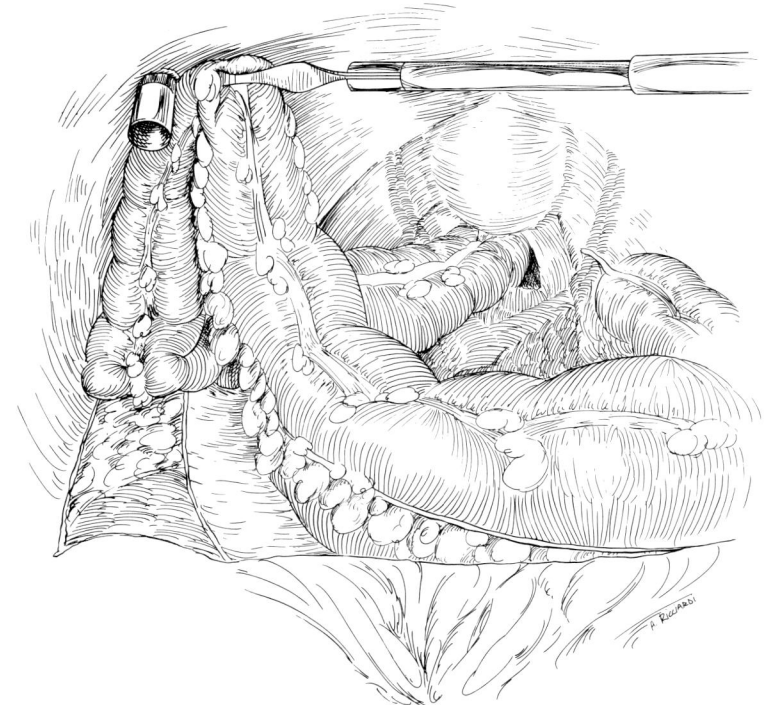

Figure 50-11.

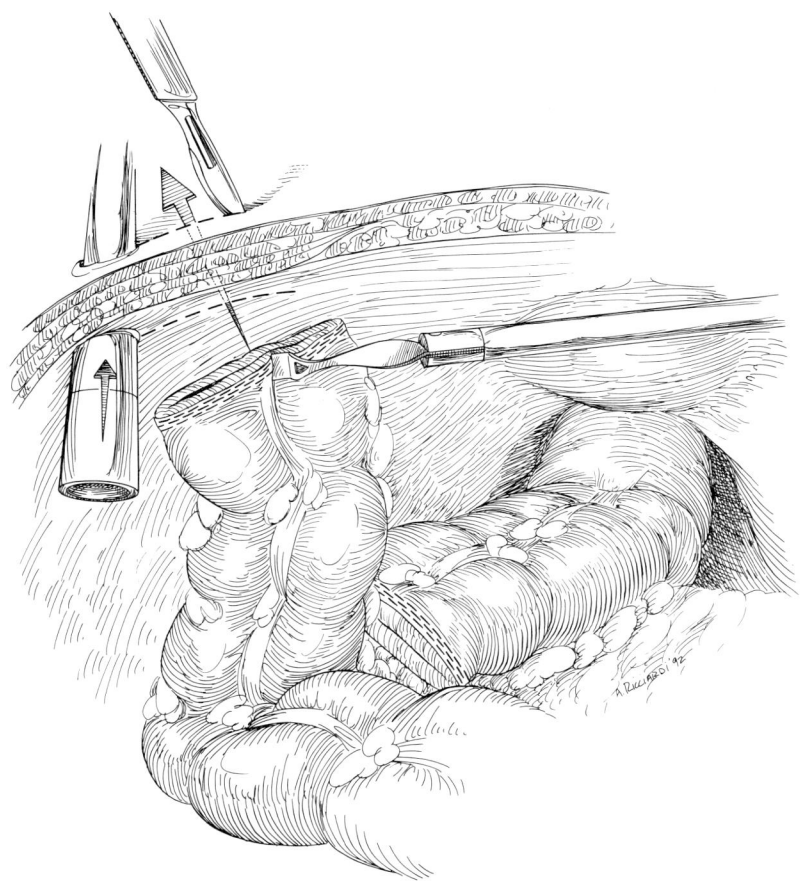

Figure 50-12.

559

to the skeletonized loop of colon at the level chosen for proximal transection. The instrument is fired, producing a circumferential row of staples, which hold the purse string along the serosal surface. The bowel is transected along the closed stapler and the specimen is sent for pathologic examination. If the purse-string device is not available, the bowel may be transected and a monofilament purse-string suture applied by hand.

The appropriate size of the circular stapling device is then chosen. The anvil is inserted into the proximal colon and the purse-string suture is tied (Fig. 50-13, *B* and *C*). The anvil and the proximal bowel are returned to the abdominal cavity. The peritoneum and external oblique aponeurosis are closed separately using running sutures. The pneumoperitoneum is reestablished with carbon dioxide. The patient is repositioned in the Trendelenburg position, right side down, and the distal staple line is exposed.

The rectosigmoid pouch is irrigated with Neosporin genitourinary irrigant by gravity through a three-way Foley catheter inserted per anum. This maneuver reduces the bacterial count and tests the pouch for possible leaks. The Premium CEEA* stapler is inserted transanally and advanced to the staple line. The CEEA* trocar is advanced through the staple line at the rectosigmoid (Fig. 50-14*A*). If the trocar cannot be lined up with the staple line, it can be brought out through the anterior surface of the bowel, leaving at least

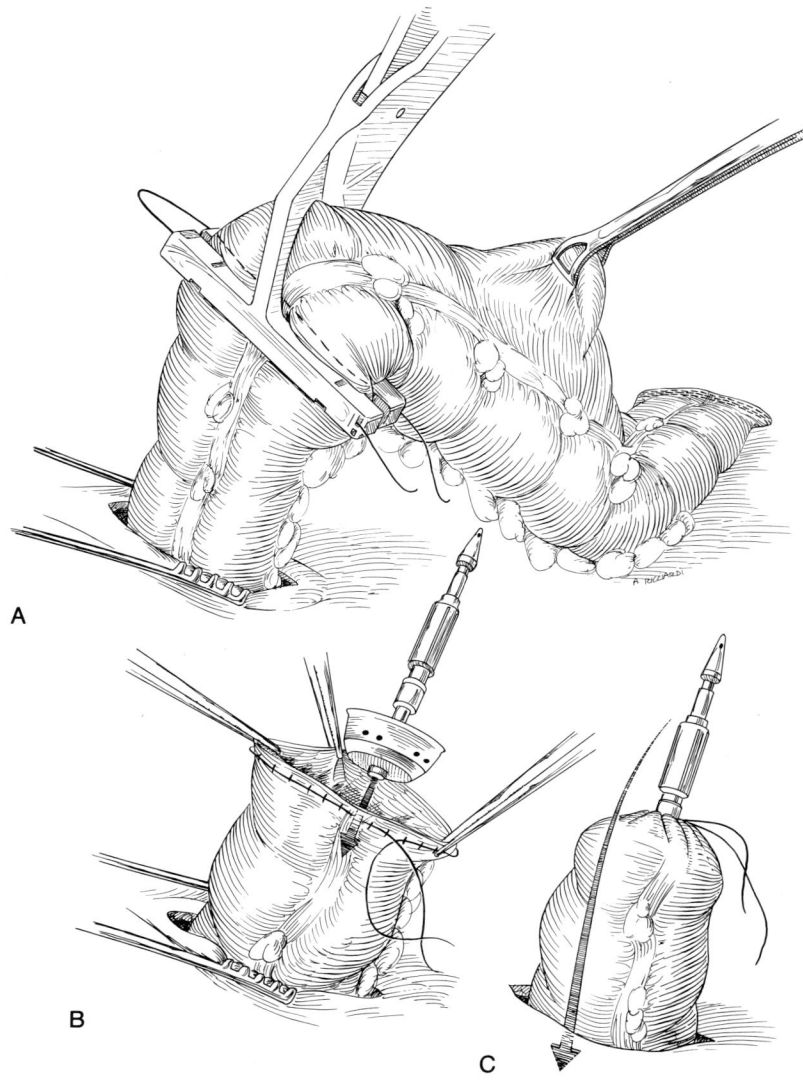

Figure 50-13.

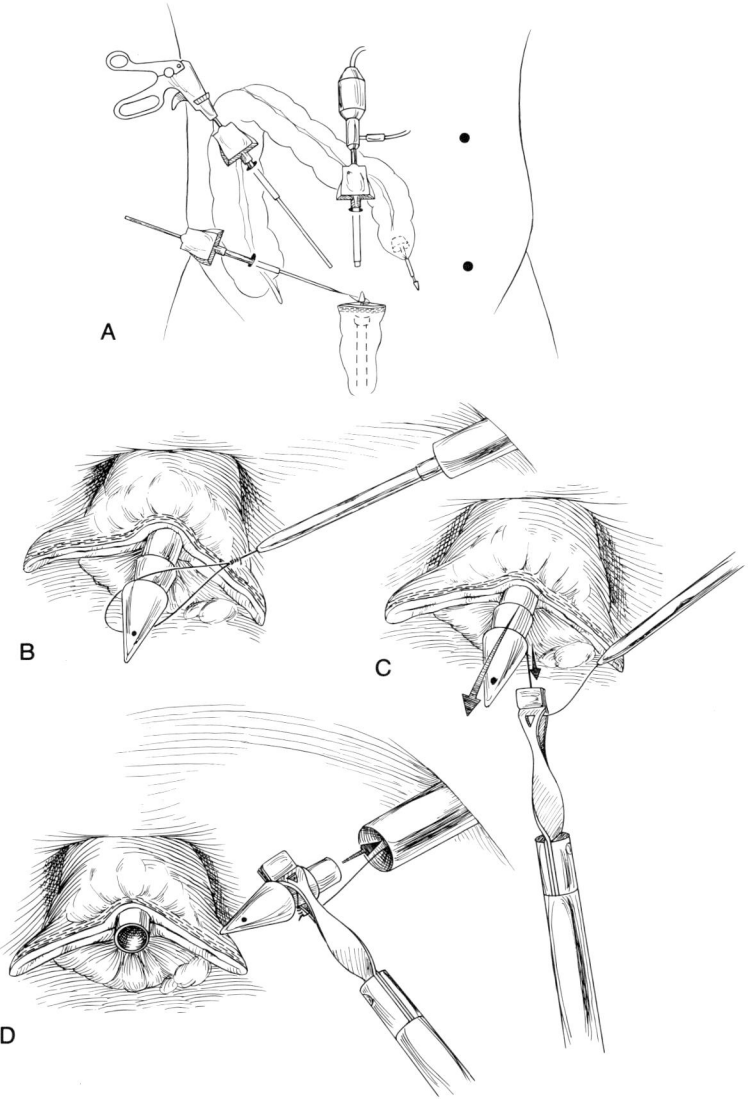

Figure 50-14.

1 cm between the linear staple line and the proposed circular staples.

The CEEA* trocar is encircled with a SURGITIE* via the right lower quadrant port (Fig. 50-14B). The trocar is dislodged by pulling on the SURGITIE* with an ENDO BABCOCK* clamp via the right upper quadrant port (Fig. 50-14C). The trocar itself is grasped and placed into the right lower quadrant port blunt end first (Fig. 50-14D) and is withdrawn from the abdomen by pulling the SURGITIE* out through the right lower quadrant port.

The post of the anvil is grasped with an ENDO BABCOCK* clamp through either the right upper quadrant or right lower quadrant port and is married to the CEEA* (Fig. 50-15). The CEEA* stapler is approximated and fired. The anvil is advanced three half turns and is withdrawn, along with the CEEA*, and removed from below. The CEEA* donuts are inspected for continuity. The anastomosis itself is inspected laparoscopically and is then tested.

To test the anastomosis, the pelvis is filled with irrigating solution to a level just covering the anastomosis. The three-way Foley catheter is reinserted through the anal canal, and the colon is compressed above the anastomosis. The rectum is inflated with air through

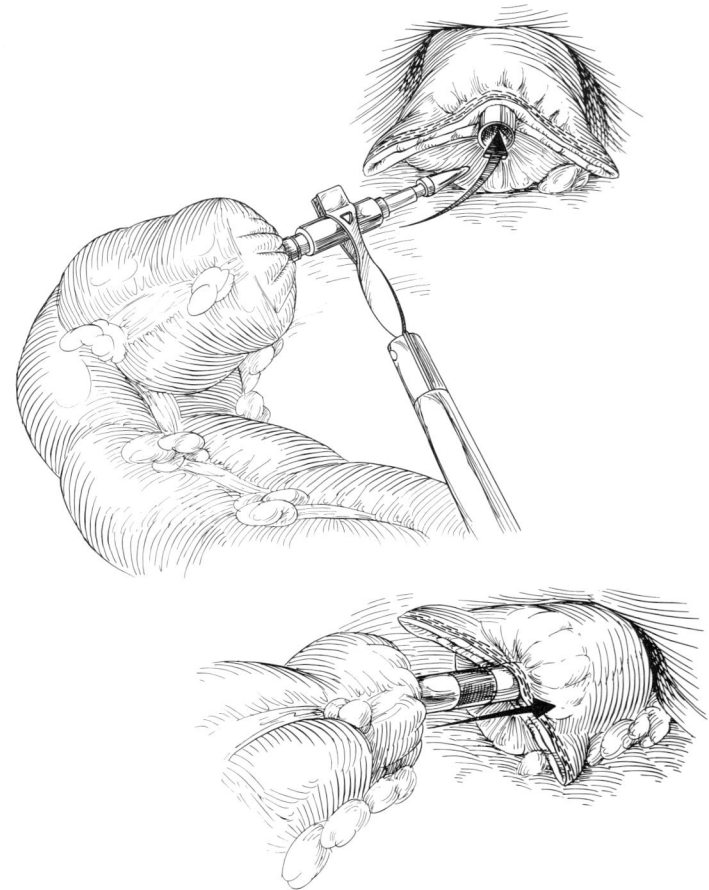

Figure 50-15.

the Foley catheter while the fluid is observed laparoscopically for bubbles. The absence of air bubbles confirms a satisfactory anastomosis.

The defect in the mesocolon is closed to prevent an internal hernia from forming (Fig. 50-16). The hernia stapler is preferred for approximating the mesocolon. If this device is not available, the defect can be closed with endosuture technique.

LEFT COLECTOMY SPARING THE SIGMOID COLON

If the sigmoid colon is to be spared, as in the case of a benign polyp of the splenic flexure or proximal descending colon, the anastomotic technique is substantially different. Following mobilization, the two points of the colon chosen for transection are held up against the abdominal wall to identify the optimal location for exteriorizing the bowel. When benign disease is present, the specimen is often sufficiently narrow that it can be brought out as a loop and resected both proximally and distally outside the abdomen. When a malignant or potentially malignant pathologic condition is present, however, the bowel should be divided at one point first and then exteriorized. In general, the incision can be kept smaller and trauma to the bowel wall can be minimized by dividing the colon at this point.

The transverse colon is divided with the ENDO GIA* stapler in the method described in the previous section. The two ends of the bowel are grasped on their antimesenteric surfaces with ENDO BABCOCK* clamps via the two right-sided ports. The orientation of the colon is checked to prevent torsion of the

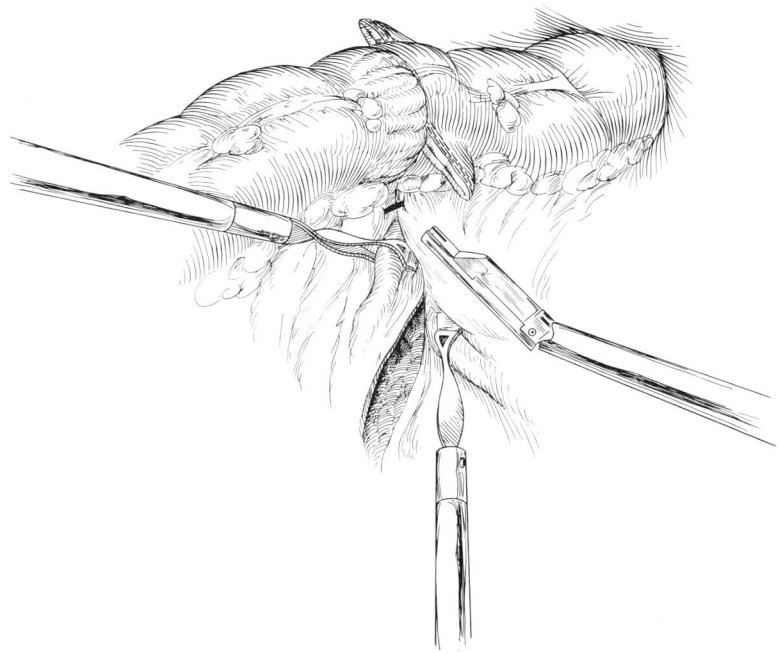

Figure 50-16.

loops prior to anastomosis. The small, transverse muscle splitting incision is made in the method described in the previous section. If the colon does not easily reach a lateral position, then a vertical incision can be made over the rectus muscle and the rectus fibers can be separated longitudinally. Alternatively, the umbilical incision can be extended and the rectus muscles retracted laterally if the sigmoid colon can reach this level without tension.

The distal transected end of the colon is exteriorized by advancing the right lower quadrant Babcock clamp through the incision. Once again, a malignant lesion is placed in a plastic bag before drawing it through the abdominal wall. The distal bowel is divided extracorporeally, and the specimen is sent for pathologic examination. The proximal end of the transverse colon is exteriorized by advancing the right upper quadrant Babcock clamp through the skin incision adjacent to the proximal end of the sigmoid colon. An extracorporeal anastomosis is carried out by either the stapled or sewn technique. The advantage of this procedure is that the surgeon can perform the type of anastomosis with which he or she feels most comfortable. It is recommended that surgeons begin their laparoscopic colectomy experience using the extracorporeal anastomosis technique, rather than an intracorporeal anastomosis.

The anastomosis is returned into the peritoneal cavity. The abdominal incision is closed with running sutures and the pneumoperitoneum is reestablished. The anastomosis is carefully inspected to ensure that the bowel has not been twisted during the course of exteriorization or during the anastomosis. The defect in the mesocolon is closed using either the hernia stapler or ENDO SUTURES*.

CLOSURE

At the conclusion of the procedure, care is taken to evacuate the pneumoperitoneum thoroughly. By evacuating the pneumoperitoneum, the likelihood of diaphragmatic irritation and resultant shoulder pain is minimized. The transverse, muscle-splitting incision has already been closed using running absorbable sutures. The 12-mm trocar incisions are closed at this time using interrupted 0-VICRYL* sutures on a UR-6 needle. This needle greatly facilitates suture placement through the narrow incisions. When possible, the fascia is also closed in this fashion at the 10-mm trocar sites.

POSTOPERATIVE MANAGEMENT

A nasogastric sump tube is left in place postoperatively usually until the morning of the second postoperative day. If excessive drainage is experienced, the nasogastric tube is left in place for an additional period of time. If the patient begins passing flatus prior to this time, the nasogastric tube is removed after a shorter interval. With this regimen, the average patient passes flatus on the second postoperative day. The average time for the patient's first bowel movement is 2½ days following surgery. Sips of clear liquids are ordered for the second postoperative day. The liquid diet is gradually advanced stepwise as the patient tolerates it. Typically, patients tolerate a liquid diet well by the third postoperative day.

The Foley catheter is left overnight following surgery and is removed on the morning of the first postoperative day. Antibiotics are not routinely administered after the patient leaves the operating room. A single dose of a second generation cephalosporin is administered in the holding area preoperatively. If unsuspected contamination is experienced during the operative procedure, the antibiotic is continued at appropriate intervals for 24 hours. If the pathologic specimen includes an inflammatory diverticular mass, intravenous antibiotics are continued for 48 hours postoperatively.

CRITERIA FOR PATIENT DISCHARGE

When patients are tolerating liquids well without nausea and are voiding without difficulty, they are eligible for discharge. They must be afebrile and tolerating adequate fluids by mouth to sustain a proper state of hydration. It is advisable that the patients be monitored in the hospital until they successfully move their bowels. Using these criteria, the average time for patient discharge has been the fourth postoperative day for patients under 80 years of age and the fifth postoperative day including all ages.

COMPLICATIONS SPECIFIC FOR THIS PROCEDURE

There have been no major complications with left hemicolectomy specific to the laparoscopic technique. The theoretical complications peculiar to laparoscopic surgery include unrecognized injury to the viscera caused by the restriction of laparoscopic exposure. Visceral or vascular injuries can also result from insertion of the Varess needle or trocars. Complications can result from the pneumoperitoneum, as noted in Chapter 9. Finally, injuries to the bowel can occur as a result of retraction, particularly if the proper atraumatic instruments are not used.

The early experience with laparoscopic cholecystectomy has been extremely positive. The authorities who have pioneered in this surgery have found that the infection rate is at or below that experienced with traditional surgery and that the overall complication rate is no higher. The safety and effectiveness of laparoscopic colectomy has been the direct result of the responsible approach taken by the surgeons who have developed the techniques of advanced laparoscopic general surgery. These surgeons have been careful to develop the procedures in animal models first and to be ready to convert to traditional laparotomy if the need arose. Conversion to open surgery is never a complication, but invariably represents sound surgical judgment. Surgeons must remain committed to the ideals of training, preparation, caution, self-assessment, and quality control if the early, encouraging experience of laparoscopic colon resection is to continue.

Further experience is needed with long term follow-up from multiple institutions to confirm the safety and efficacy of laparoscopic colon resection. Questions about cancer cure rates will certainly require long term follow-up with large numbers of patients. Surgeons are strongly encouraged to contribute their personal experience to centralized registries and to combined institution trials. Each individual institution must monitor ongoing experience with laparoscopic colon resection to ensure adequate quality control.

Chapter 51
Anterior Resection for Rectal Prolapse

Garth H. Ballantyne

Rectal prolapse has plagued mankind throughout history.[1] In the Old Testament, Jehoram, the son of Jehoshaphat, was punished for his "whoring" ways by a disease in which his "bowels [fell] out by reason of the sickness day by day."[2] Among the Greeks, Hippocrates advocated that when a rectal prolapse could not be easily reduced that "the patient hanging by the heeles be shaken, for so the gut by that shaking will returne to his place."[3] Other groups were also afflicted with this malady. Indeed, a Coptic mummy was found who had a rectal prolapse.[4] Various etiologies of rectal prolapse have been postulated. These include relaxation of the anal sphincter,[5] disfunction of the levator ani,[6] intussusception of the sigmoid colon into the rectum,[7,8] and a sliding hernia of the pouch of Douglas.[9] Surgeons have designed specific operations that correct each of these anatomic defects.

Treatment of rectal prolapse by anterior resection was first suggested by E. G. Muir.[10] This technique has been implemented by surgeons at the Mayo Clinic.[11,12] In this operation, the rectum is mobilized off of the sacrum down to the level of the coccyx. It is hoped that postoperative scarring of the presacral space will improve the fixation of the rectum and hinder recurrence of the prolapse. The lateral rectal ligaments are preserved. The sigmoid colon and part of the proximal rectum are resected. The anastomosis is constructed below the rectosigmoid junction in the proximal rectum above the anterior peritoneal reflection. Rates of recurrence of rectal prolapse following this procedure are less than 10 per cent with long term follow-up.

PATIENT SELECTION

Surgeons have designed a plethora of operative techniques for the repair of this affliction. These can be divided into perineal methods and abdominal procedures. The perineal techniques such as transanal proctectomy or Thirsch wire procedures have a low morbidity, but the recurrence rate is high. In contrast, the abdominal procedures such as Ripstein suspensions or anterior resections share the morbidity of major abdominal operations, but the recurrence rate is low. In view of this dichotomy, we have selected perineal operations for elderly debilitated patients tormented by rectal prolapse and abdominal approaches for more robust patients with a greater anticipated longevity.

Anterior resection offers distinct advantages for the treatment of rectal prolapse. The technique of this procedure is essentially the same as for other resections of the left colon for benign conditions. Consequently, the technique is familiar to most abdominal surgeons and, moreover, well practiced. The long term rates of recurrence of prolapse are as low as for other abdominal procedures. Furthermore, functional results are satisfactory. The major disadvantage of this operation, however, is the risk of anastomotic complications. We believe that this risk remains at an acceptably low rate if the anastomosis is constructed above the anterior peritoneal reflection.

PREOPERATIVE EVALUATION

Evaluation of patients is similar whether anterior resection is performed laparoscopically or with an open technique. Patients must be good candidates for general anesthesia. Since the patients treated laparoscopically will be subjected to a carbon dioxide pneumoperitoneum, their pulmonary and cardiac status must be evaluated carefully. A patient with chronic obstructive pulmonary disease who retains carbon dioxide or a patient with cardiac arrhythmias may not tolerate well the elevated partial pressure of carbon dioxide in the serum that will be generated by the pneumoperitoneum.

The colon of the patient is evaluated with colonoscopy or barium enema for evidence of occult neoplastic disease. Anal function is evaluated in patients who complain of incontinence.

PREOPERATIVE PREPARATION

The patients are admitted to the hospital on the night before the operation and are allowed nothing by mouth after midnight. They undergo a standard mechanical and antibiotic bowel preparation. Typically, the patients drink a gallon of a polyethelyene glycol-containing balanced electrolyte solution over a 3-hour period. Following this, they receive three doses of 1 g of neomycin and 1 g of erythromycin separated by 3-hour intervals. Broad spectrum antibiotics are also administered during the perioperative period.

EQUIPMENT

The following equipment is used:

1. Laparoscope: One 10-mm 0-degree telescope is needed. A second 10-mm 0-degree telescope or a 10-mm 30-degree telescope is helpful for transillumination of the mesentery.

2. Trocars: Five 10-mm trocars and one 12- or 15-mm trocars are required.
3. Instruments
   A. One disposable scissors
   B. One grasping instrument such as the ENDO DISSECT* (United States Surgical Corporation, Norwalk, CT)
   C. Two endoscopic Babcock clamps
   D. One reloadable endoscopic clip applier and clips
   E. ENDO GIA* 30 or ENDO GIA* 60 stapling device with blue (3.5-mm) cartridges
   F. One pre-tied endoscopic loop ligature
   G. One Premium CEEA* stapling device with a 31-mm cartridge, modified shaft, modified trocar, and low profile anvil
   H. One Automatic PURSTRING* (United States Surgical Corporation) device

POSITIONING OF THE PATIENT

The patient is placed in a supine position on an electric operating room table. The legs are supported with modified Lloyd-Davies stirrups. The thighs are as straight as possible, because flexed thighs impede the movement of the laparoscope and laparoscopic instruments. A nasogastric tube and urinary catheter are inserted in all patients, diminishing the risk of stomach and bladder injury during insertion of the trocars.

Positioning of the Video Equipment

The principal video monitor is stationed between the legs of the patient. The second monitor is placed on the left side of the patient. This second monitor proves helpful if mobilization of the descending colon is difficult.

Trocar Placement and Size Selection

Five 10-mm trocars are inserted at the initiation of the operation. The first 10-mm trocar is placed in the supraumbilical position (Fig. 51-1). Two are placed in the right lower quadrant and two in the left lower quadrant lateral to the rectus muscle. The caudad trocar in the right lower quadrant is replaced with a 12- or 15-mm trocar at the time of transection of the rectum with the ENDO GIA* 30 (United States Surgical Corporation) or ENDO

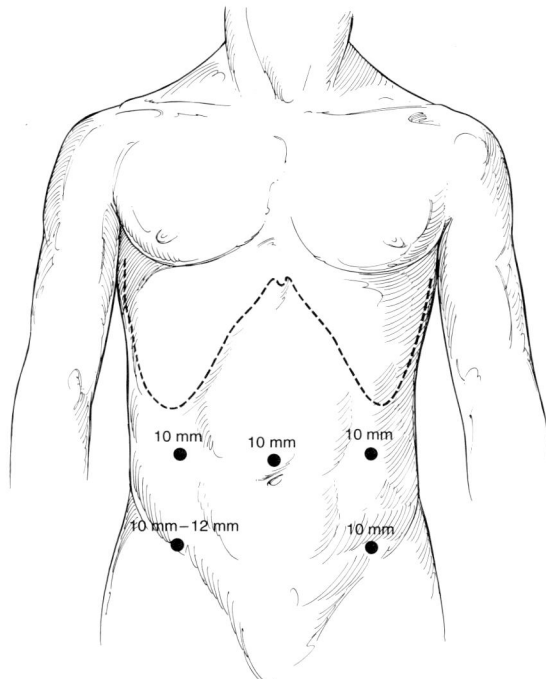

Figure 51-1.

GIA* 60 (United States Surgical Corporation) stapling device.

METHODS OF EXPOSURE AND RETRACTION

The patient is dropped into a deep Trendelenburg position. Once the critical angle is reached, the small bowel rolls out of the pelvis up toward the diaphragm. The left side of the pelvis and the left gutter are exposed by retraction of the rectosigmoid and sigmoid colon medially and anteriorly with two ENDO BABCOCK* clamps (United States Surgical Corporation), which are inserted through the right lower quadrant trocars.

Exposure of the presacral space is more difficult. Anterior and left lateral traction are applied to the proximal rectum and rectosigmoid with two ENDO BABCOCK* clamps, which are inserted through the left lower quadrant ports. Anterior displacement of the rectum is assisted by elevation with a dissecting instrument or laparoscopic retractor.

Exposure of the root of the sigmoid mesentery is problematic because of the extreme redundancy of the sigmoid colon in patients afflicted with rectal prolapse. The abdomen, despite the distention produced by the pneumoperitoneum, does not offer enough room for flattening out the entire sigmoid colon. The distal sigmoid vessels are exposed by lifting the rectosigmoid and distal sigmoid anteriorly and laterally with ENDO BABCOCK* clamps. In contrast, visualization of the proximal sigmoid vessels is tedious at best and consequently these vessels are divided extracorporeally.

METHODS OF DISSECTION

Mobilization of the rectum and sigmoid colon is readily accomplished with electrocautery scissors.

SPECIFIC DETAILS OF THE PROCEDURE

After induction of general endotracheal anesthesia, the abdomen is prepared and draped in a sterile fashion. The patient is dropped into a deep Trendelenburg position. The carbon dioxide pneumoperitoneum is established with a Veress needle in the supraumbilical site. The needle is replaced with a 10-mm trocar. The abdomen is inspected for evidence of bowel or vascular injury inflicted during insertion of the trocar. An additional four 10-mm trocars are inserted. The abdomen is explored for unsuspected disease.

The small bowel is grasped with ENDO BABCOCK* clamps and pulled out of the pelvis. The deep Trendelenburg position causes the small bowel to role away from the pelvis. The sigmoid colon is identified. The assistant stands on the right side of the patient. The rectosigmoid junction and distal sigmoid are retracted medially and anteriorly with the Babcock clamps by the assistant. The course of the common iliac vessels is identified. Often the pulsations of the iliac artery are discernible.

The surgeon stands on the left side of the patient, using the ENDO SHEARS* instrument in the dominant hand and a grasping instrument for countertraction in the nondominant hand. The posterior peritoneum is elevated off of the iliac vessels and incised. The incision of the retroperitoneum is first extended down into the pelvis and then up along the left gutter. The sigmoid mesentery is bluntly swept medially. Once the posterior periotoneum is cut, this blunt dissection is easily accomplished. The magnified video image broadcasted from the laparoscope conspicuously exposes the avascular planes in the retroperitoneum.

The left ureter is identified. In thin patients, the ureter is visible through the posterior peritoneum and easily protected. In other patients, identification of the ureter requires meticulous dissection. It is generally found, as in open operations, where it crosses the iliac vessels.

It is important to maintain a clear field of view throughout the operation. All tissues are divided with cautery. Clots of blood are troublesome because they clog aspiration devices and because the deep color absorbs light and darkens the laparoscopic video image. Clot formation is prevented by irrigation of the operative field with heparinized saline (3000 units/1000 ml of saline) before dissection is initiated. The heparin retards clot formation and allows aspiration of any blood in the operative field.

The rectum is mobilized off of the sacrum (Fig. 51-2). Postoperative scarring of this plane helps fix the rectum in place and retards the propensity for rectal prolapse to recur. This dissection is accomplished with the surgeon on the right side of the patient and the assistant on the left. The rectosigmoid and proximal rectum are elevated anteriorly and deflected laterally with two Endo Babcock clamps by the assistant. The surgeon visualizes the course of the right iliac vessels. The hard sacral promontory can often be identified by "palpation" with the laparoscopic scissors.

The visceral peritoneum over the sacral promontory is incised. The areolar plane between the fascia propria of the mesorectum and the retrorectal (Waldeyer's) fascia is identified. All vessels are cauterized in the presacral space. Even small amounts of blood stain the tissues and obscure the plane of dissection. The mesorectum is pushed bluntly off of the sacrum. The long shaft of the grasping instrument in the surgeon's nondominant hand assists with this maneuver. Other laparoscopic retractors can be substituted for this task.

Once the rectum is mobilized, the mesenteric dissection is accomplished. The inferior mesenteric and superior hemorrhoidal vessels are preserved. This ensures an excellent blood supply for the colorectal anastomosis. From the left side of the patient, the assistant grasps the rectosigmoid junction and the distal sigmoid colon. He or she attempts to flatten out the distal sigmoid mesentery while elevating it toward the anterior abdominal wall. The course of the inferior mesenteric artery is heralded by an arch-like fold visible at the base of the sigmoid mesentery.

The visceral peritoneum of the mesosigmoid is incised anteriorly to the inferior mesenteric vessels (Fig. 51-3). The individual sig-

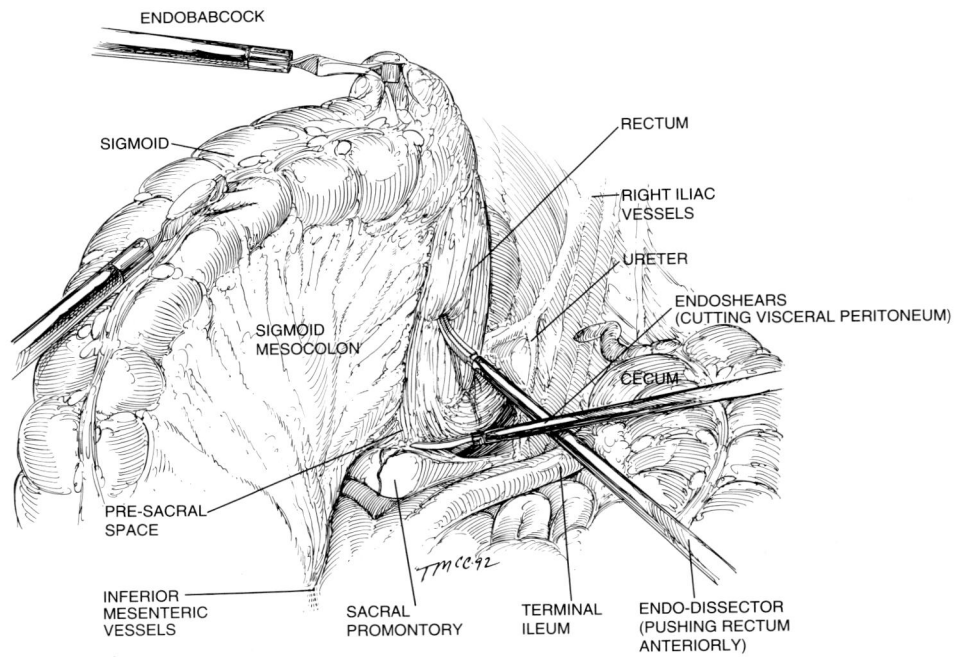

Figure 51-2.

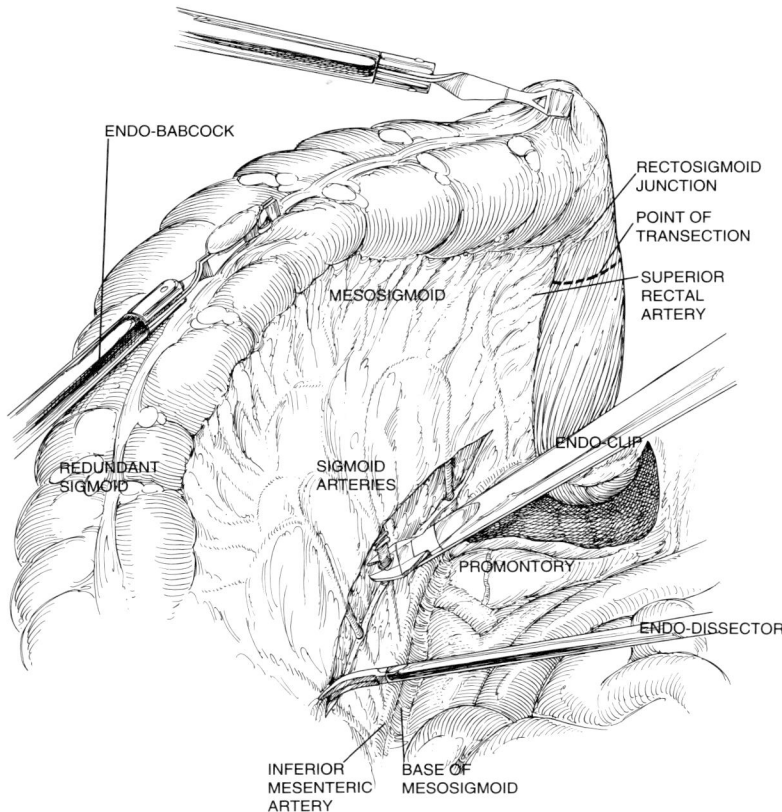

Figure 51-3.

moid branches are sharply and bluntly separated. This is most easily accomplished near the base of the mesosigmoid. Identification of these vessels can be assisted by transillumination of the sigmoid mesentery with a second laparoscope. The vessels are divided between clips. Each side of the vessel is clipped twice. Transection of vessels is continued distally until the selected point of distal transection of the rectum is reached.

Exposure of the more proximal sigmoid branches becomes increasingly difficult. Space limitations within the abdomen limit the ability to lay out the mesosigmoid for inspection. Consequently, division of these branches is more easily achieved extracorporeally. It is necessary to divide, however, enough of the sigmoid mesentery that the distal sigmoid can be easily delivered through an incision in the left lower quadrant (Fig. 51-4). Mobility of the distal sigmoid is checked by its elevation up to the abdominal wall at the planned site of incision.

The rectum is transected beyond the rectosigmoid junction in its proximal third (Fig. 51-5). The rectosigmoid junction is identified as the point of coalescence of the taenia with formation of a complete longitudinal layer of rectal muscle. The anastomosis is positioned above the anterior peritoneal reflection because of the lower risk of anastomotic dehiscence at this level. The caudad 10-mm trocar in the right lower quadrant is replaced with a 12- or 15-mm trocar. This position allows a perpendicular transection of the rectum with the laparoscopic stapling device. The rectum is transected and divided with multiple applications of the ENDO GIA* 30 or a single application of the ENDO GIA* 60 stapling device. The blue (3.5-mm) cartridge is used. The tips of the instrument are checked before firing. It is possible to pick up in the jaws of the stapling device unwanted structures such as the ureter.

The stapled closure of the specimen is grasped with a Babcock clamp, which is inserted through the caudad trocar in the left lower quadrant. The mobility of the specimen is again checked. The trocar is slid out of the abdominal wall over the shaft of the ENDO

570 Techniques of Laparoscopic Surgery

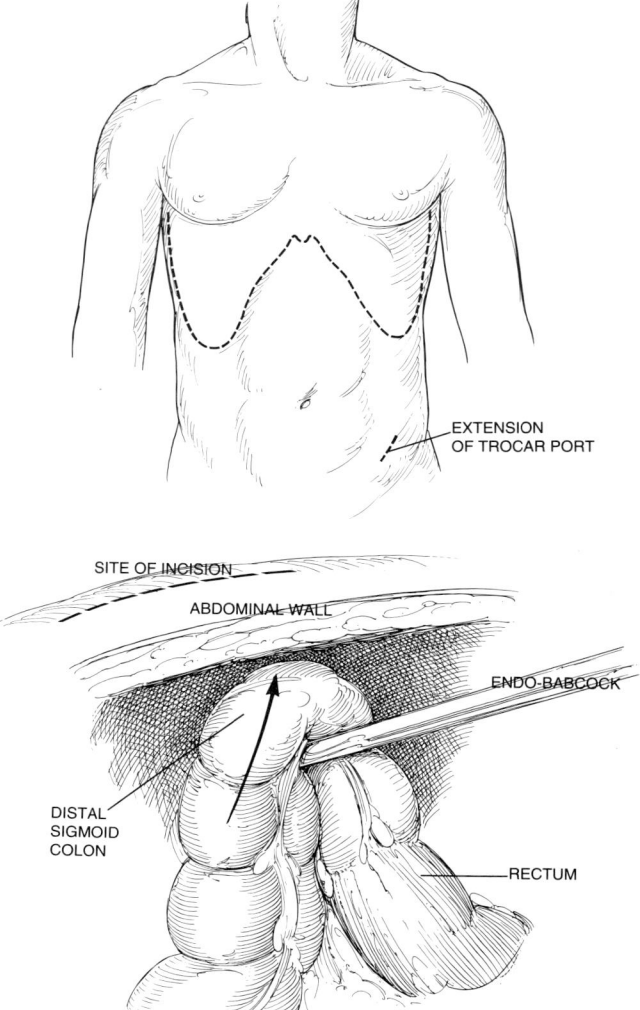

Figure 51-4.

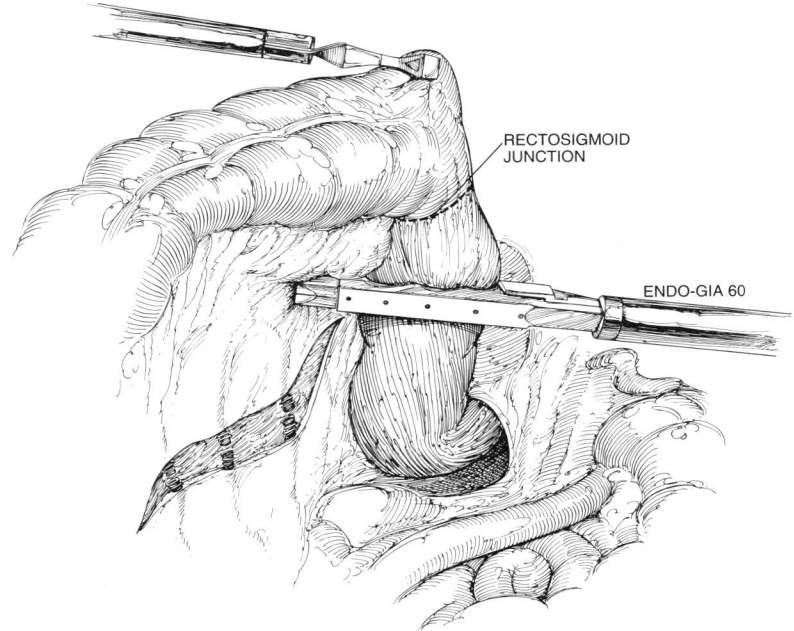

Figure 51-5.

BABCOCK* clamp (Fig. 51-6). The trocar site is extended as a transverse incision. A width of 1.5 inches is generally adequate. The distal end of the specimen is withdrawn from the abdomen out through this incision with the ENDO BABCOCK* clamp (Fig. 51-7). The pneumoperitoneum is deflated.

The remainder of the sigmoid branches are divided between clamps and ligated. The point of proximal transection is selected. The wall of the colon at this point is cleared of mesenteric fat for a distance of 1 inch. An Automatic PURSTRING* device is applied (Fig. 51-8). A crushing bowel clamp is placed on the specimen side. The colon is transected with curved Mayo scissors. The specimen is handed to a pathologist for gross inspection within the operating room.

The PURSTRING* device is opened. The edge of the colon is grasped with three Babcock clamps. The diameter of the colon is sized. Generally, a 31-mm cartridge can be used. The low profile anvil with modified shaft is inserted into the colon and tied into place with a purse-string suture. The end of the colon containing the anvil-shaft assembly is returned to the abdomen. It is carefully placed into the pelvis with the point of the shaft pointing toward the rectal stump.

The abdomen is liberally irrigated through the left lower quadrant incision. Any clot that has accumulated in the operative field is removed. The incision is closed with interrupted stitches of an absorbable suture. The pneumoperitoneum is re-inflated.

The anus is dilated to admit four fingers. The head of the Premium CEEA* stapling device is inserted through the anus and advanced up the rectum to the stapled closure. A suture is tied in a loop through the hole in the tip of the white trocar before the stapling device is inserted into the rectum. The white trocar is screwed through the staple line until the orange collar is visible (Fig. 51-9). A grasping instrument pushes against the rectal wall as the trocar is advanced. This helps to prevent a tear in the rectal wall.

The loop in the tip of the white trocar is held by a grasping instrument. An ENDO BABCOCK* pulls the trocar out of the head of the stapling device. The white trocar hangs vertically since the loop is away from its center of gravity. The white trocar is withdrawn through an anterior abdominal SURGIPORT*. When an older type of white trocar is used that does not have a hole in its tip, the white trocar is lassoed with a pre-tied endoscopic ligature. A Babcock clamp pulls the trocar out of the head of the stapling device. The suture is used to pull the trocar out through the 12-mm port. The Babcock clamp helps align the trocar with the axis of the trocar.

An ENDO BABCOCK* clamp is inserted

572 Techniques of Laparoscopic Surgery

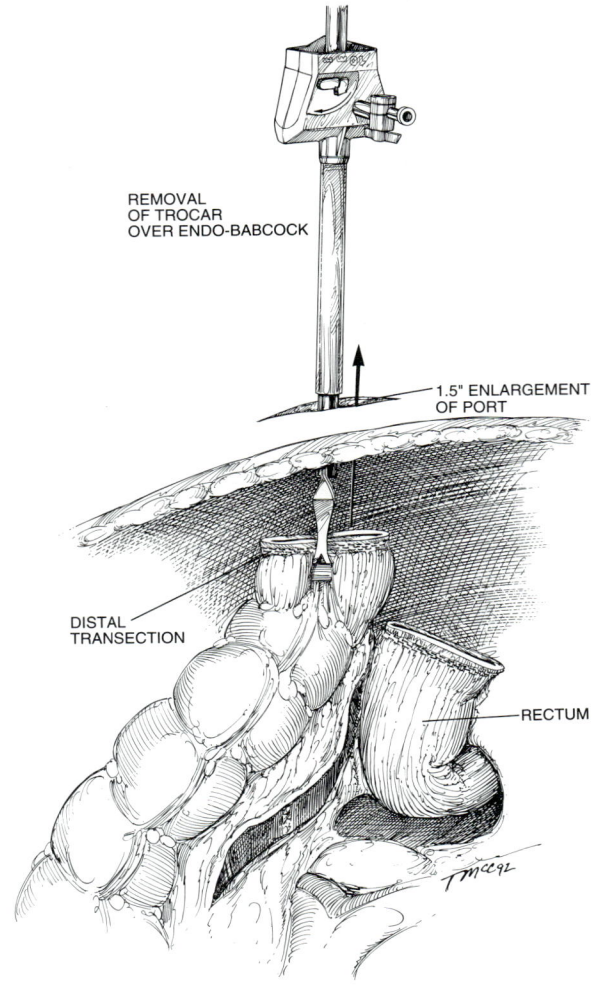

Figure 51-6.

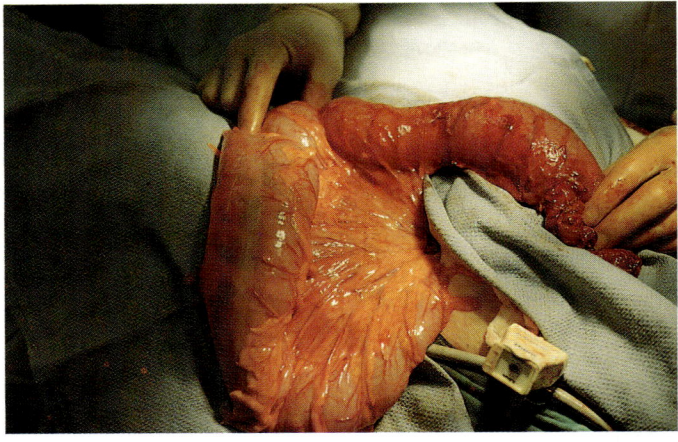

Figure 51-7.

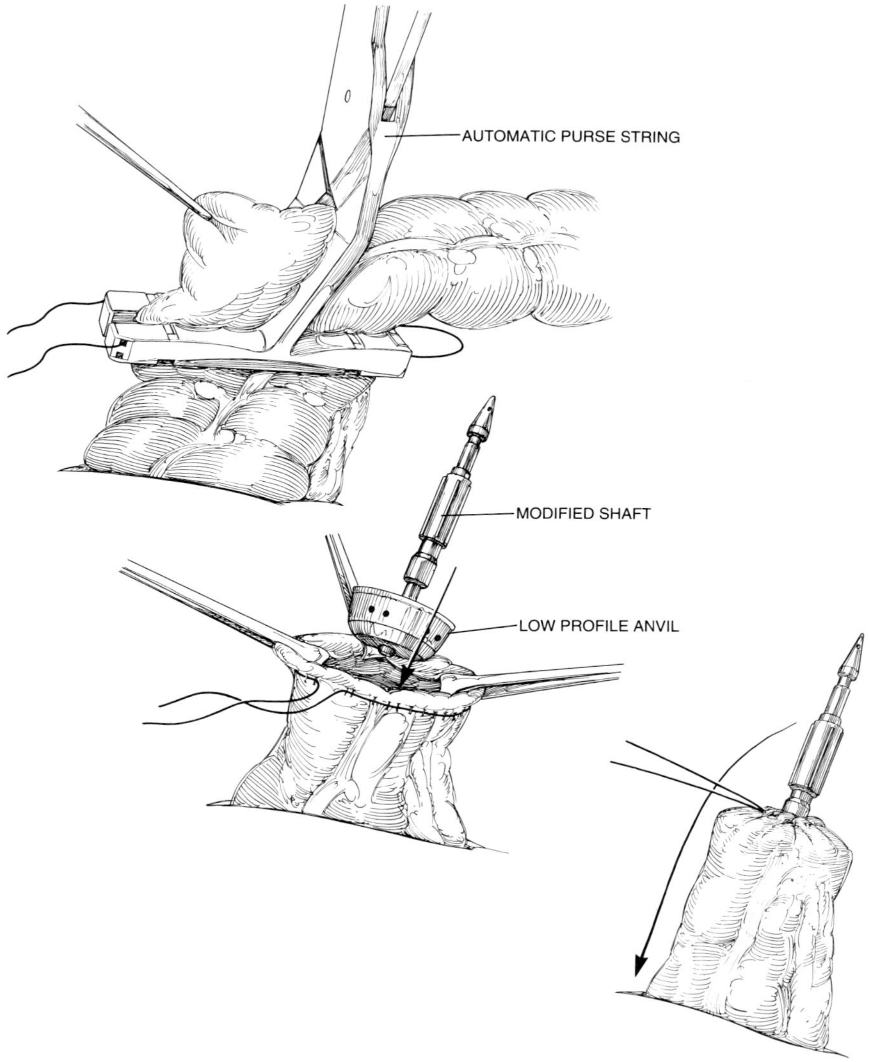

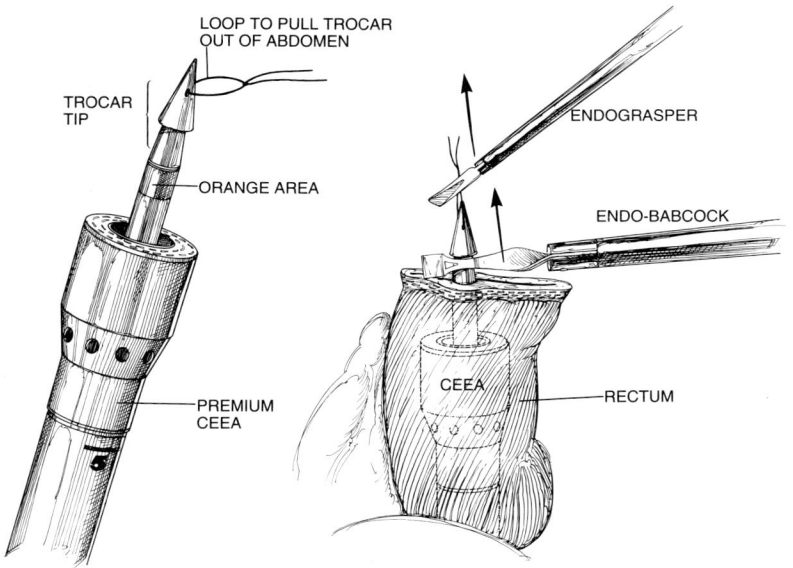

Figure 51-8.

Figure 51-9.

into the abdomen through the 12-mm trocar and used to grasp the modified shaft. The jaws of the Babcock clamp are locked into the groove of the shaft. It is important that the Babcock clamp be aligned perpendicularly to the long axis of the stapling device. The shaft is inserted into the orange collar of the cartridge of the CEEA* stapler. After docking the anvil-shaft assembly with the stapler, the taenia of the colon is traced back from the anastomosis to make sure that the colon is not twisted. Similarly, the mesentery of the colon is examined for evidence of a volvulus. The stapling device is screwed closed and fired. It is opened one full turn and withdrawn from the rectum. The anvil is opened, and the shaft is inspected for two intact donuts.

The pelvis is filled with warmed saline. A flexible or rigid sigmoidoscope is advanced through the anus up to the anastomosis. The staple line is scrutinized for hemostasis. The rectum is insufflated. The laparoscopic surgeon observes the pool of water in the pelvis for leakage of bubbles through the anastomosis. The saline is aspirated dry. The abdomen is checked for hemostasis.

CLOSURE

Drains can be inserted through a trocar and positioned near the anastomosis. The trocar is then withdrawn over the drain tubing. The trocars are removed one at a time. Each fascial defect is closed with interrupted stitches of an absorbable suture. The placement of the stitches is observed with the laparoscope. The pneumoperitoneum is deflated through the last trocar before it is extracted. The last fascial defect is closed. The skin edges are apposed with skin staples or Steri-Strips (3M Corporation, Minneapolis, MN). Band-Aids are applied over the wounds.

POSTOPERATIVE MANAGEMENT

The nasogastric tube is removed on the morning after the operation. The urinary catheter and pneumatic boots are not removed until the patient is able to move around. The patient is offered clear liquids on the first postoperative day. The intravenous line is removed. If fluids are tolerated, the diet is advanced to a regular diet. This is achieved sometimes on the second day but more commonly on the third.

CRITERIA FOR DISCHARGE

The patient is discharged when he or she can tolerate a regular diet. Also, the social conditions of the patient's domicile are assessed. A patient who lives with a supportive family and near the hospital may be discharged earlier than an elderly patient who lives alone. Generally, the patient should have had a bowel movement before discharge.

COMPLICATIONS SPECIFIC TO THIS PROCEDURE

Few of these procedures have been accomplished at present. Consequently, rates of anastomotic dehiscence remain undefined. Similarly, long term follow-up and rates of recurrence of rectal prolapse are unavailable.

REFERENCES

1. Ballantyne GH. The historical evolution of anatomic concepts of rectal prolapse. Semin Colon Rectal Surg 1991; 2:170–179.
2. Holy Bible (King James Version) II Chronicles 21:verses 1–16.
3. Pare A. Of particular tumors against nature. In Johnson T, trans. The Workes of That Famous Chirurgion Ambrose Parey Translated out of the Latine and Compared with the French. London, Tho. Cotes & R. Voung, 1634 (First English translation), Lib 8, C. XVIII. pp 313–314.
4. Moodie RL. Paleopathology. An Introduction to the Study of Ancient Evidence of Disease. Urbana, IL, University of Illinois Press, 1923, pp 400–401, Plate 78.
5. Mercuriale G (Hieronymus). De Morbis Puerorum. Tractatus Locupletissimi Variaque. Venetiis, Paulum Meietum Bibliopolam Patauinum, 1588, Liber I, C, X, pp 41–43.
6. Riolanus I. Methodus Medendi Tam Generalis Quam Particularis. Parisiis, Hadrianun Perier, 1598, pp 142–143.
7. Morgagni JB. The Seats and Causes of Diseases Investigated by Anatomy. (Alexander B, trans.) London, A Miller & T Cadell, 1769, Vol II, Letter 33 and 34, pp 110–163.
8. von Haller A. Pathological Observations, Chiefly from Dissections of Morbid Bodies. D Wilson & T Durham, 1756 (First English translation by the author), pp 53–55, 70.
9. Moschowitz AV. The pathogenesis, anatomy, and cure of prolapse of the rectum. Surg Gynecol Obstet 1912; 15:7–12. Reprinted in Dis Colon Rectum 1983; 26:553–565.
10. Muir EG. Rectal prolapse. Proc R Soc Med 1955; 48:33–44.
11. Schlinkert RT, Beart RW Jr, Wolff BG, et al. Anterior resection for complete rectal prolapse. Dis Colon Rectum 1985; 28:409–412.
12. Wolff BG, Dietzen CD. Abdominal resectional procedures for rectal prolapse. Semin Colon Rectal Surg 1991; 2:184–186.

Chapter 52
Low Anterior Resection

Patrick F. Leahy

Colorectal carcinoma is the second most common internal malignancy; only recently has this been surpassed by carcinoma of the lung. It is second only to carcinoma of the lung as a cause of death from carcinoma. In the United States it is estimated that there are approximately 155,000 new cases of colorectal carcinoma each year; this is estimated to be 15 per cent of all malignancies. Over the past 50 years there has been no decrease in the mortality rate from colorectal carcinoma in man and only a slight decrease in age-adjusted mortality rates for women in the United States and Canada.[1,2] However, the operative mortality rates have diminished because of better understanding of preoperative bowel preparation, antibiotic administration, and the availability of blood transfusions and better anaesthetic care and postoperative support.

PREOPERATIVE EVALUATION

Colonoscopy

The role of colonoscopy has assumed greater importance in the evaluation of colon disease. Colonoscopy now plays a major role in screening for colorectal carcinoma especially in high risk patients. With specific reference to its value in the assessment of patients with large bowel malignancy, colonoscopy has been recommended as a preoperative examination to detect the presence of synchronous neoplastic polyps or carcinomas. The necessity for perioperative and preoperative colonoscopy is still in contention, but growing evidence suggests that it plays an important role. The rationale for colonoscopy is that synchronous carcinoma exists in 2 to 7 per cent of patients. A group of surgeons concerned with the potential for implantation of malignant cells, exfoliated by preoperative colonoscopy, have opted for intraoperative palpation to detect synchronous carcinomas and postoperative colonoscopy to clear the colon of polyps.[3–5]

Radiology

Barium enema is the method by which the largest number of carcinomas of the colon are diagnosed. Various features are demonstrated such as the annular or napkin ring often seen in the left colon. The apple core defect is another feature of carcinoma. The air contrast barium enema has also been considered superior to the full column barium enema for detection of small polyps. For detection of the large constricting lesions the single contrast enema is superior to the double contrast enema.

Intravenous Pyelography

There is controversy as to whether an intravenous pyelogram is necessary preoperatively. Supporters suggest that it is helpful in advance to know whether the ureters or bladder are involved in the neoplastic process, whether two kidneys are present, or whether additional ureters may be present. One study has suggested that abnormalities are found in as many as 26 per cent of patients. Adversaries suggest that intravenous pyelography is not cost effective and not necessarily reliable in demonstrating the absence of disease involvement.

Ultrasound or Hepatic Scanning

Preoperative assessment of the liver by either ultrasonography or hepatic scanning may provide valuable information in considering the recommendations for the most appropriate management of patients with colorectal carcinoma.

Blood Markers

A tumor specific antigen was described by Gold and Freedman, and this heralded a new era in the assessment of the status of patients with colorectal carcinoma. Unfortunately, the carcinoembryonic antigen has not fulfilled its purpose as a simple blood test that would afford an early diagnosis of carcinoma of the colon.

PREOPERATIVE PREPARATION

Bowel Preparation

Preoperative bowel preparation has been the subject of considerable controversy. There is no question that the two elements of adequate mechanical preparation and antibiotic preparation are necessary. Mechanical cleansing may be accomplished by the use of vigorous laxatives along with repeated enemas until clearing. More recently the use of an oral lavage with a polyethylene glycol hypertonic electrolyte solution such as GoLYTELY or CoLYTE has become increasingly popular. The controversy as to whether oral or intravenous antibiotics or possibly both should be used continues. Antibiotics, when chosen, should be selected on the basis of gram-positive and gram-negative aerobic and anaerobic coverage. The timing of antibiotic administration is controversial, but it should be started preoperatively. The duration of antibiotic administration is also controversial, but the antibiotic is not necessary after the day of operation in all likelihood.

EQUIPMENT

The instruments needed for the Four-Puncture Technique are as follows:

1. One 12-mm trocar
2. Two 10-mm trocars and one 5-mm trocar
3. Two intestinal grasping devices and one Babcock clamp
4. Suture material for suspension of the intestine
5. Hand-shaped retractor
6. SURGIWIP*, disposable suture ligature and SURGITIE*
7. An ENDO GIA* stapling device
8. An ENDO CLIP* applier
9. Titanium clip applier

POSITIONING OF THE PATIENT

The patient is placed in a Trendelenberg lithotomy position. The patient's shoulders and arms are securely fastened to the operating table. A nasogastric tube and a urinary catheter are inserted.

POSITIONING OF THE VIDEO EQUIPMENT

The monitor of the video optical system is placed at the foot of the patient. Two monitors are preferable.

TROCAR PLACEMENT

A four-puncture technique is used (Fig. 52-1); the initial insertion is in the right upper quadrant. After creation of a pneumoperitoneum a 12-mm trocar is inserted into this area, carefully avoiding the liver, gallbladder, and colon. In the left upper quadrant a 5-mm trocar is inserted under direct vision. In the left lower quadrant a 10-mm trocar to accept the laparoscope is inserted. In the right lower quadrant a 12-mm trocar is inserted. This is to facilitate the entry of the ENDO GIA* stapling device.

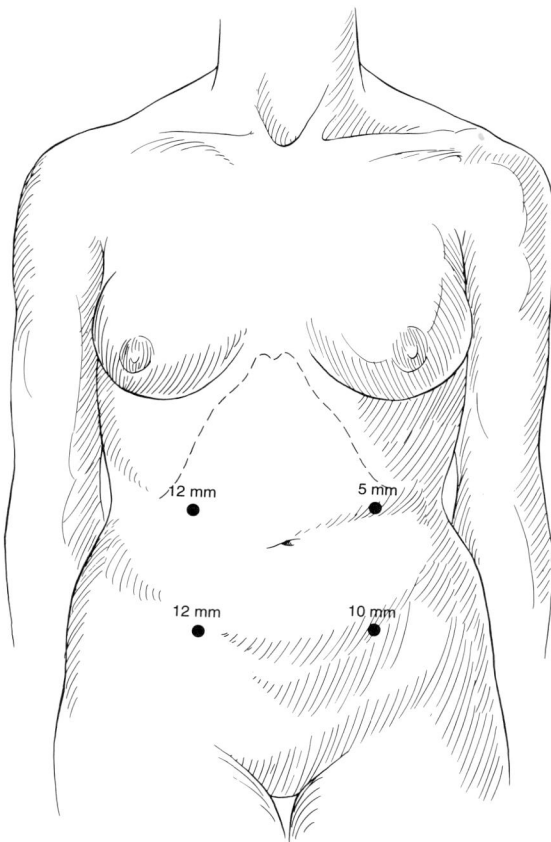

Figure 52-1.

PROCEDURE

Extensive examination and evaluation of the liver, colon, and pelvis are performed and the degree of the Trendelenberg position is increased. In a female patient it is imperative to suspend the uterus toward the anterior abdominal wall. This can be performed in two ways. One way is to place a suture one fingerbreadth above the pubis using a long Keith needle. This is inserted into the fundus of the uterus and then passed again to the anterior abdominal surface. By so doing the uterus is lightly suspended. Care is taken not to tighten the suture as this may cause extensive bleeding. Alternatively a suture may be passed around the fundus of the uterus; this can be clipped with an endoscopic clip and attached to the anterior abdominal wall.

If adhesions are present, they are divided and dissected; however, in some situations, if, for instance, the patient has had a previous appendectomy, it is often beneficial to leave the adhesions in place until the end of the operation. By so doing the intestine can be placed behind these adhesions, which form a shelf and thus prevent the small intestine from drifting into the pelvis and obscuring visualization and interfering with meticulous dissection. In a left hemicolectomy or left lower sigmoid colectomy, it is sometimes beneficial to rotate the table away from the area of dissection by approximately 15 degrees. A sigmoidoscope or colonoscope is placed through the rectum, and the lesion is identified in the rectosigmoid colon, by reducing the light intensity on the camera. This transillumination technique can be used to identify the lesion, which is then marked with an ENDO CLIP*. It is advisable to attach at least three endoscopic clips in case excessive mobilization may dislodge these clips.

Suspension of Intestine

A single suture is now inserted through the abdominal musculature into the parietal cavity, passed through the mesentery beneath the intestine, and then passed through to the surface of the anterior abdominal wall. This again is lightly clipped by a Mosquito clamp on the surface of the abdominal wall. It is important not to tighten the suture as it may transect the intestine. This allows elevation of the large bowel, thus freeing up the grasping devices for further manipulation of colon.

A grasping forceps is now inserted through the left upper quadrant 5-mm SURGIPORT* trocar (Fig. 52-2). A Babcock clamp is inserted through the right lower quadrant 12-mm SURGIPORT* trocar after the attachment of a 10-mm converter. The Babcock clamp is used to exert countertraction upon the intestine toward the right-hand side of the patient. Similarly the proximal aspect of the sigmoid colon is grasped by the first assistant using a 5-mm intestinal clamp. The lateral ligaments are identified. The surgeon replaces the 10-mm converter with a 5-mm converter and introduces either a laser fiber or an ENDO SHEARS* attached to low power monopolar electrocautery. It is advisable not to exceed Mark 4 on the monopolar electrocautery device. By a process of light coagulation followed by sharp dissection the lateral ligaments are divided. By carefully using the closed blades of the ENDO SHEARS* device the tissue is retracted entering the avascular plane. The common iliac and internal iliac vessels are visualized. The left ureter is identified as it traverses the iliac vasculature. This

578 Techniques of Laparoscopic Surgery

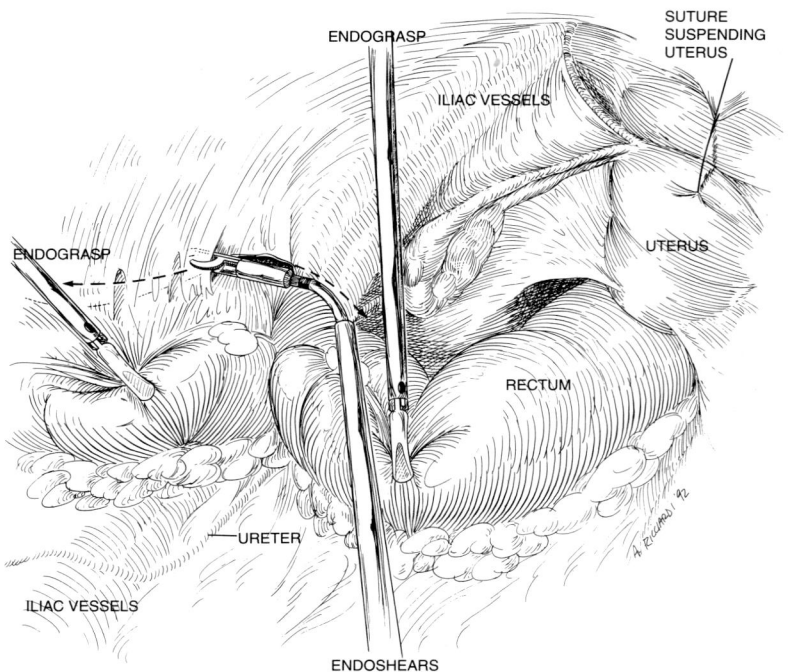

Figure 52-2.

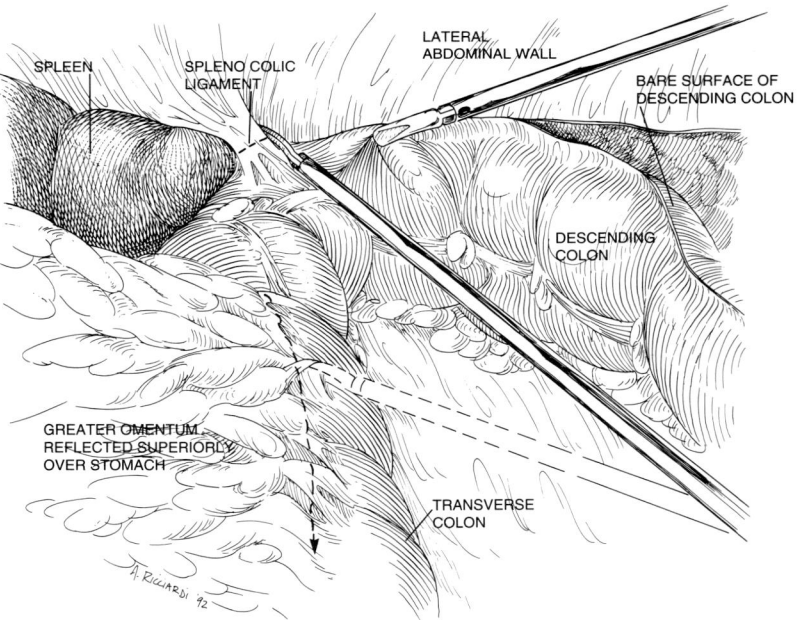

Figure 52-3.

dissection is continued in a cephalad direction and also toward the pelvis. Once the ureter has been identified the assistant surgeon now changes the grasping device to a more proximal position and again by exerting countertraction the intestine is displaced to the right of the patient. This affords tension on the peritoneal reflection in the left paracolic gutter. The surgeon continues to dissect along the paracolic gutter in a cephalad direction. It is important not to overdissect in this area as uncompromising bleeding may occur if one dissects into the area of the perinephric fat. As the dissection continues the colon, the mesentery and lymph nodes are swept toward the right-hand side of the patient, clearing away the mesentery and fatty tissue and lymph nodes from the underlying aorta and vena cava. At this stage attention is drawn to the splenic flexure (Fig. 52-3). The ligaments suspending the splenic flexure are divided. This step is imperative to avoid excessive tension upon the descending colon if an exteriorization of the colon is to be performed. The omentum is detached. Individual vessels can be skeletonized and ligated using a 9-mm endoscopic clip or a hand-suturing technique.

Attention is now drawn to the peritoneum on the right side of the mesentery (Fig. 52-4). The assistant surgeon grasps the proximal intestine and reflects the tissue toward the left-hand side of the patient, thus causing tension upon the peritoneum along the right side. This peritoneum is divided using either a laser or dissecting scissors. This division is continued vertically toward the pelvis and proximally toward the root of the mesentery. With careful meticulous dissection and blunt retraction the mesenteric fat is retracted from the underlying vessels. It is not always necessary to identify the ureter along the left side, but in patients with carcinoma in whom extensive resections are to be done it is preferable.

Transillumination of Mesenteric Arcade

A 10-mm telescope is now introduced into the left-hand side of the abdomen and placed

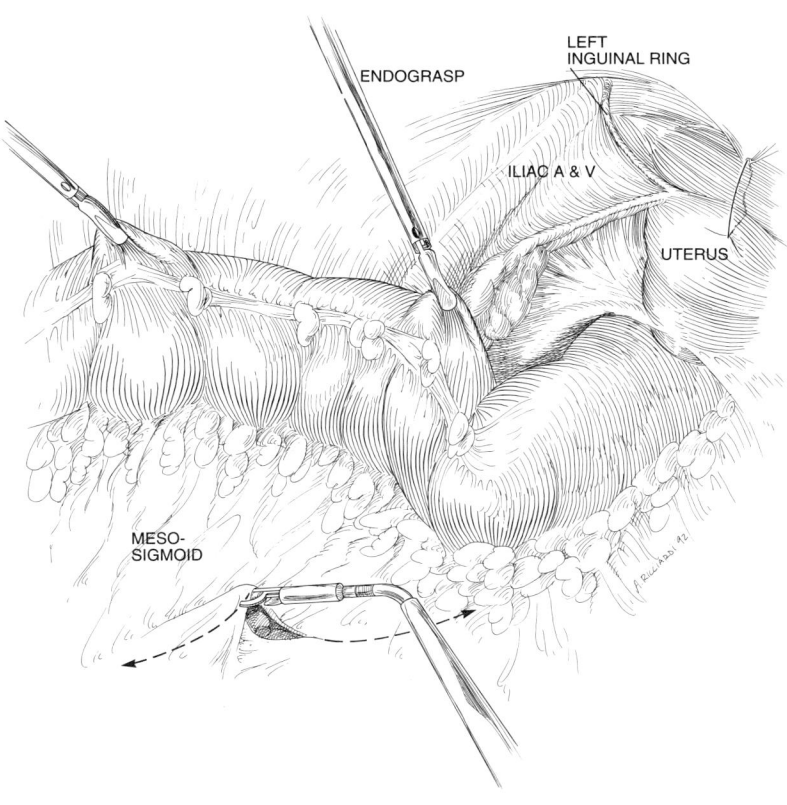

Figure 52-4.

adjacent to the mesentery. The intensity of the light source on the receptor camera is reduced. This allows transillumination of the mesenteric arcade. If the vessels do not transilluminate adequately then it is necessary to skeletonize the vessels by removing the excess fatty tissue so that the vessels can be more easily exposed by this transillumination technique. If this stage of the dissection is difficult, a Doppler probe can be inserted through a 5-mm port in the right lower quadrant to confirm the location of the mesenteric vasculature. Once the mesenteric vasculature is identified, the inferior mesenteric artery is carefully dissected free from other structures (Fig. 52-5). In patients with carcinoma this must be ligated flush with the aorta at the beginning of the procedure. To ligate this vessel a large endoscopic clip or an Abslok clip may be deployed or alternatively a hand-suturing technique using 30 chromic catgut or an ENDO GIA* stapler, may be used.

Extent of Resection

Once the inferior mesenteric artery has been transected the remainder of the mesenteric arcade must now be resected, bearing in mind that an extensive resection involves removal of all the lymph nodes for appropriate staging of the disease. If the vessels need to be ligated individually skeletonization of the mesenteric arcade is necessary. This involves removing the fatty tissue by combining sharp dissection with light electric coagulation and aspiration using a suction irrigation device. The creation of windows using this technique can be time consuming; this technique also has a higher susceptibility for hematoma formation. Alternatively after the ligation of the inferior mesenteric artery the ENDO GIA* stapling device can be used to transect the distal colon and the thickened mesentery. This step should not be done until an ENDO GAUGE* device has been applied to the mes-

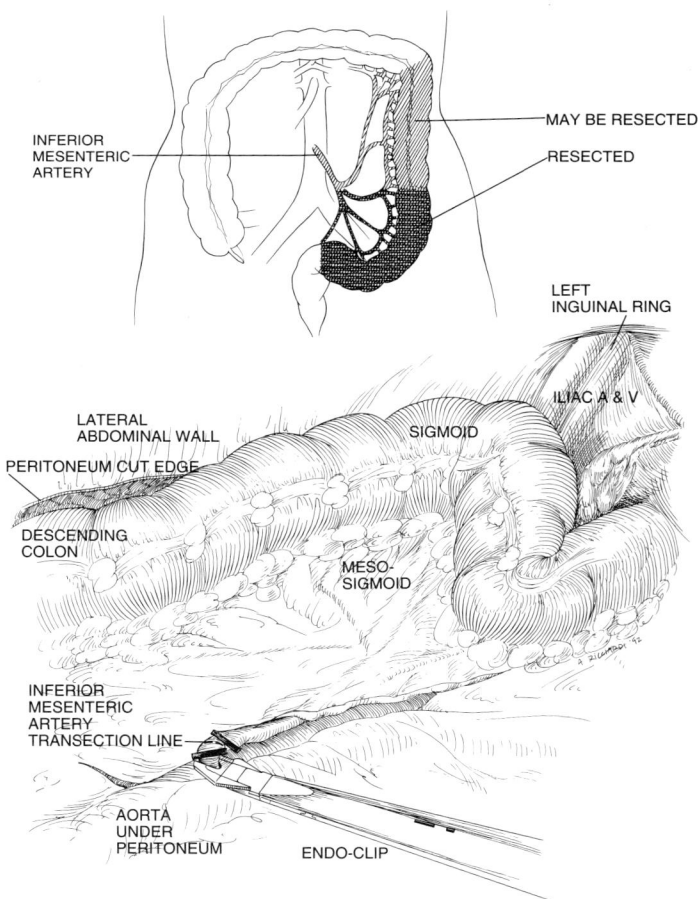

Figure 52-5.

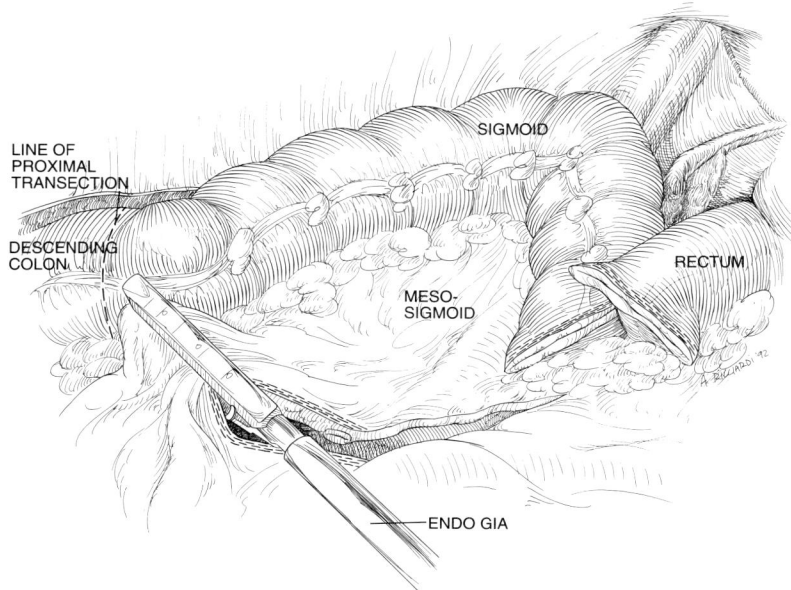

Figure 52-6.

entery to determine the thickness of the mesentery and to aid in the choice of the staple leg length. Either a 2.5-mm vascular cartridge will be used or a 3.5-mm staple leg length, which is the blue cartridge available in the disposable loading unit.

The sequential application of the ENDO GIA* stapling device is necessary for transections and ligation of the mesentery (Fig. 52-6). It is imperative that the ENDO GIA* stapling device be inserted into the V of the previously divided staple rows. It may be necessary to fire three to four lines of staples with the ENDO GIA*. The marginal artery is preserved. The intestine is transected at the proximal area and the specimen is placed in the pelvis prior to removal.

Carcinoma of the Colon

In patients with carcinoma, a double stapling technique is used whereby the proximal segment of the descending colon is transected in a similar fashion with the ENDO GIA* stapling device. This helps to reduce the theoretical possibility of sequestration of carcinoma cells in the proximal bowel. The immobilized and resected specimen of colon is placed in the pelvis to avoid its being obscured by the overlying loops of intestine. The proximal staple line is grasped by an atraumatic grasping forceps and brought to the left lower quadrant 10-mm port site. The skin incision is continued immediately to fashion an incision of 2.5 cm. The fascia is divided, and a muscle split incision is achieved. The incision must be of adequate size to allow the easy introduction of the anvil head and to remove the specimen. The mobilized segment of bowel is exteriorized, a PURSTRING* suture applier (United States Surgical Corporation) is applied to the proximal portion of bowel, and the jaws are closed. The excess intestine is excised, and a sizer is introduced into the bowel to determine which size anvil head will be used to fashion the anastomosis. The PURSTRING* device suture is snugly tightened with inversion of the intestine snugly on the shaft of the anvil. The anvil and intestine are reintroduced into the peritoneal cavity and placed in the pelvis. A purse-string prolene suture is applied to the peritoneum and fascia and the 10-mm trocar is introduced into this defect. The new pneumoperitoneum is recreated, and the distal resected specimen of intestine is grasped with a grasping forceps and brought to the left-sided incision site. The specimen is removed from the abdominal cavity; if there is serosal involvement an impermeable bag is introduced into the abdomen and the specimen is placed in this. After the tumor specimen is removed, the trocar is removed from the abdominal cavity and the fascia and skin are closed on the left lower quadrant.

A specially devised grasping forceps is introduced into the right lower quadrant to grasp the anvil of the stapling device. If this device is not available, an ENDO BABCOCK* is used. The shaft is placed adjacent to the rectal stump. The assistant surgeon now places the Premium CEEA* stapling device (United States Surgical Corporation) through the anus and advances the trocar 1 mm to the side of the staple line. After penetration of the rectal stump, the trocar is removed with a specially designed grasping forceps through the 12-mm port. Alternatively, the trocar is lasooed with a SURGITIE* and withdrawn through a port. The grasping device is reintroduced into the abdominal cavity to grasp the anvil shaft, and this is coupled to the locking mechanism on the circular stapler introduced through the rectum. The anvil is closed snugly as indicated by the stapling device. The safety mechanism is unlocked, and the staples are fired. The stapling mechanism is opened and twisted two turns and then removed from the rectum. Saline is insufflated into the abdominal cavity, and using a colonoscope air is insufflated into the rectum. This will determine if there are any leaks from the anastomotic line. Excellent visualization is achieved with the colonoscope which allows identification of any bleeding.

A drain is placed only in patients with inflammatory bowel disease or in whom excessive dissection was performed. A final inspection of the mesenteric defect and areas of dissection to determine whether there is any residual bleeding is performed and finally irrigation of the abdominal cavity is achieved using a pulsed irrigation system (Davol). The trocars are removed after decompression of the abdominal cavity, and the wounds are closed with a 30 Maxon subcuticular stitch. Steri-Strips are applied to the wound. The nasogastric tube is removed postoperatively.

REFERENCES

1. Gordon PH, Dalrymple S. The use of staples for reconstruction after colonic and rectal surgery. *In* Ravitch MM, Steichen FM, eds. Principles and Practice of Surgical Stapling. Chicago, Year Book Medical Publishers, 1987, pp 402–431.
2. Busuttil RW, Foglia RP, Longmire WP. Treatment of carcinoma of the sigmoid colon and upper rectum. A comparison of local segmental resection and left hemicolectomy. Arch Surg 1977; 112:920–923.
3. Russell A, Tong D, Dawson LE, et al. Adenocarcinoma of the proximal colon: Sites of initial dissemination and patterns of recurrence following surgery alone. Cancer 1984; 53:360–367.
4. Konishi F, Muto T, Kanazawa K, et al. Intraoperative irrigation and primary resection for obstructing lesions of the left colon. Int J Colorectal Dis 1988; 3:204–206.
5. Meijer S, Hoitsma HFW, van Loenhout RM. Intraoperative antegrade irrigation in complicated left-sided colonic cancer. J Surg Oncol 1989; 40:88–89.

Chapter 53
Drainage of a Diverticular Abscess

Anthony V. Coletta

PATIENT SELECTION

Standard approaches to patients with complicated diverticular disease not requiring immediate surgery include bowel rest, intravenous fluids, and antibiotics. Computed tomographic (CT) scans are often performed in this setting to identify peridiverticular abscess formation. Unilocular abscesses that can be accessed safely may be percutaneously drained in an effort to avoid emergency surgery (often requiring Hartmann resection). Patients whose abscesses are not responding to maximal medical therapy, however, and in whom CT scans do not identify abscess formation should be considered for laparoscopy in an attempt to identify and drain occult abscesses. In addition, patients in whom the CT scan demonstrates complicated, multilocular abscesses or abscesses not easily accessible percutaneously are candidates for laparoscopic exploration and drainage. Prior to therapeutic laparoscopy, these patients would have been considered for laparotomy with or without bowel resection along with abscess drainage and very often with the creation of a temporary (2 to 3 months) colostomy. Contraindications to the laparoscopic approach might include a severe bleeding diathesis or cardiovascular instability secondary to sepsis.

PREOPERATIVE EVALUATION

All patients give a thorough history and undergo a physical examination. Careful note is taken of prior operations. Routine laboratory studies are obtained. CT scans often not only identify peridiverticular abscess formation but also help to confirm the diagnosis of diverticulitis and identify potential involvement of surrounding organs. Barium enema and endoscopic examinations are avoided if possible in the face of acute diverticulitis.

PREOPERATIVE PREPARATION

Patients have generally had nothing by mouth upon admission into the hospital. Nasogastic suction is often helpful to lessen the distention of the viscera and thus improves laparoscopic visualization. Bowel preparation is not feasible in the setting of acute diverticulitis associated with abscess formation and should not be instituted solely because of the contemplated laparoscopic approach.

Broad spectrum antibiotic therapy is desirable and in these patients is instituted prior to any surgical approach and continued perioperatively.

EQUIPMENT

The following equipment is used:

1. Laparoscopes: 10-mm, 0-degree and 5-mm, 30-degree
2. Trocars: One 10-mm and two 5-mm
3. Instruments
   A. Two atraumatic bowel graspers
   B. One irrigation-suction instrument
   C. One Luken's trap on suction line
   D. One high pressure irrigation system
   E. Blunt tip monopolar cautery probe
   F. Monopolar scissors

POSITIONING OF THE PATIENT

Patients should be positioned in the dorsal lithotomy position with the legs well abducted but with the hips straight (not flexed) and on a level plain with the abdomen (Fig. 53-1). Easy access is necessary to the perineum for manipulation of the uterus or rectum if needed. Hips flexed in the lithotomy position often inhibit manipulation of laparoscopic instruments. The patient should be well secured on the operative table with arms at the side if possible. It is advisable to place padded shoulder braces to avoid slippage of the patient when in a steep Trendelenburg position.

A nasogastric tube should be placed if not placed preoperatively. A Foley catheter is also essential and should be secured in such a way that the circulating nurse can gain access to it to fill the bladder if necessary to delineate anatomic planes and check for bladder wall integrity if indicated.

POSITIONING OF THE VIDEO EQUIPMENT

Generally only one video monitor is necessary, and it should be placed at the foot of the table (Fig. 53-1). The video camera receiver, insufflator, and light source should be placed at the head of the table, usually to the patient's left side. Suction lines, cautery, and irrigation systems can be placed to the patient's right side. All lines should be secured to the surgical drapes in such a way that crossing of lines and tubes from one side of the table to the other is limited.

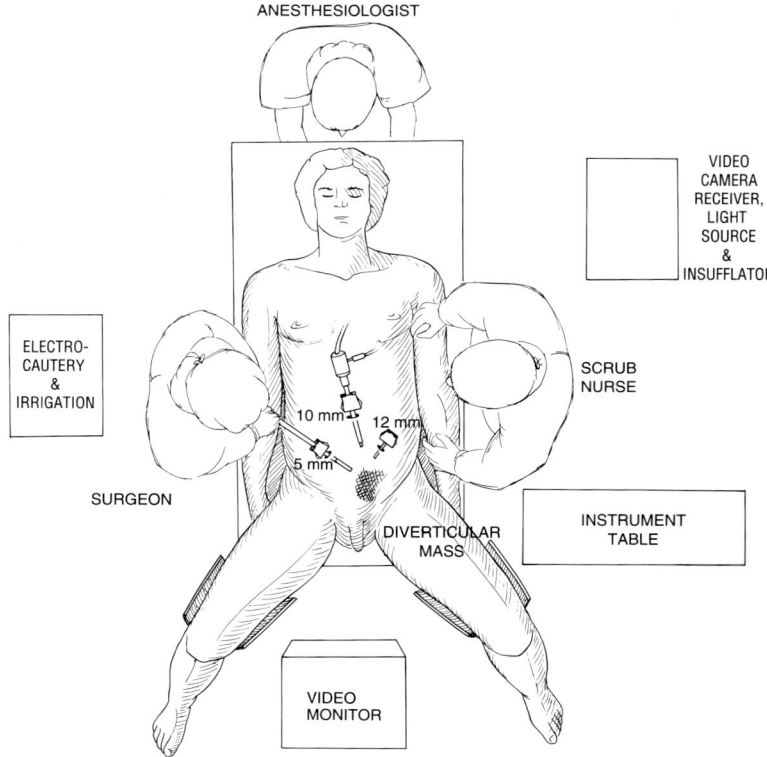

Figure 53-1.

TROCAR PLACEMENT AND SIZE SELECTION

A 10-mm umbilical trocar is placed for the laparoscope (Fig. 53-1). Two 5-mm trocars are placed in the right and left lower quadrants. Precise placement of these ports is determined following initial laparoscopic examination based upon the location of the inflammatory diverticular mass. Small size trocars are preferred to limit the size of abdominal wall incisions in the face of the suppurative intra-abdominal process.

METHODS OF EXPOSURE AND RETRACTION

It is essential to avoid inadvertent injury to inflamed bowel, which is often adherent to peridiverticular abscesses. Thus, methods of exposure should limit manipulation of viscera. As many abscesses will be located within the pelvis, visualization here is critical. This is greatly facilitated by a steep Trendelenburg position, allowing the gut to gently fall cephalad (Fig. 53-2). Further exposure can then be obtained by lifting the uterus anteriorly via a transvaginal uterine manipulator in women (Fig. 53-3). Lifting the posterior wall of the bladder anteriorly also helps to delineate pelvic tissue planes.

METHODS OF DISSECTION

Dissection of peridiverticular abscesses is essentially performed bluntly. Gentle use of bowel graspers to provide countertraction on loops of inflamed bowel avoids inadvertent bowel injury. Sharp dissection is usually limited to lysis of adhesions (Fig. 53-4).

A gentle and very effective manner in which to separate inflamed loops of bowel and identify diverticular abscesses is with the use of high pressure aquadissection (Fig. 53-5). Irrigation probes may be gently inserted into tissue planes. High pressure aquadissection is then instituted, and viscera will often separate along clean anatomic lines. Such high pressure irrigation is also useful in debriding inflammatory peel and debris away from the abscess and surrounding phlegmon.

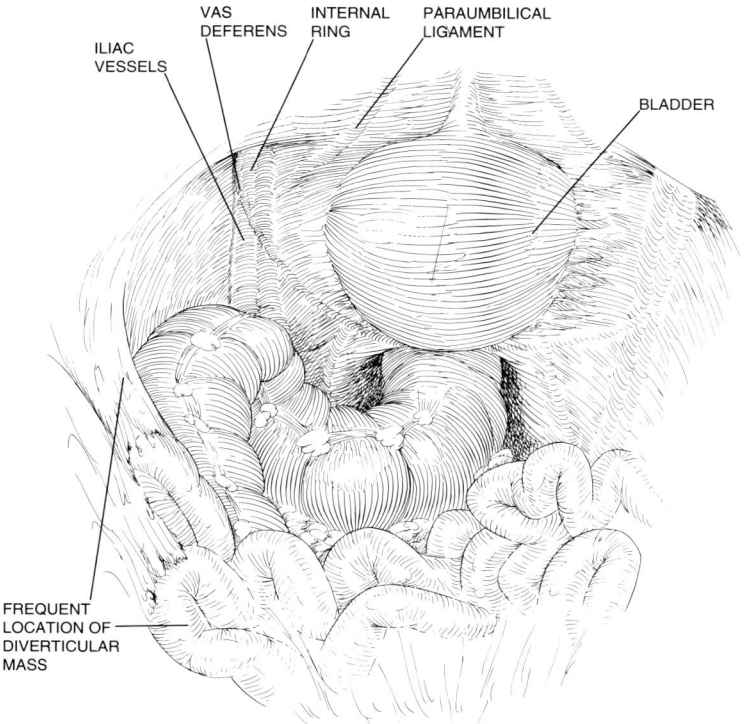

Figure 53-2.

586 Techniques of Laparoscopic Surgery

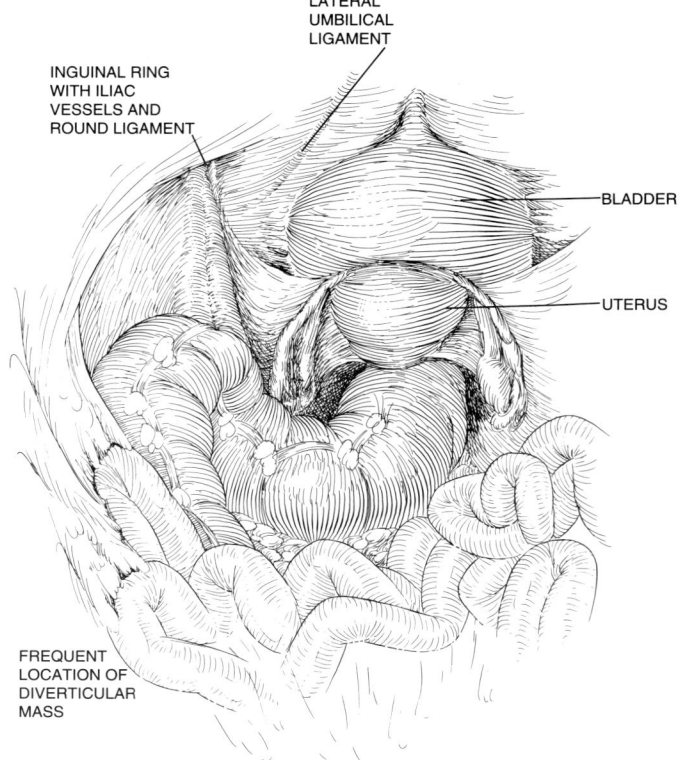

Figure 53-3.

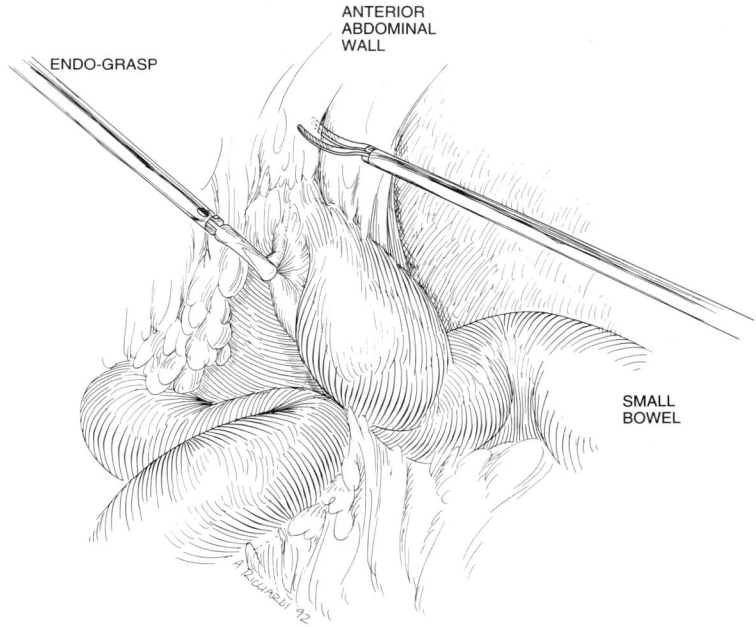

Figure 53-4.

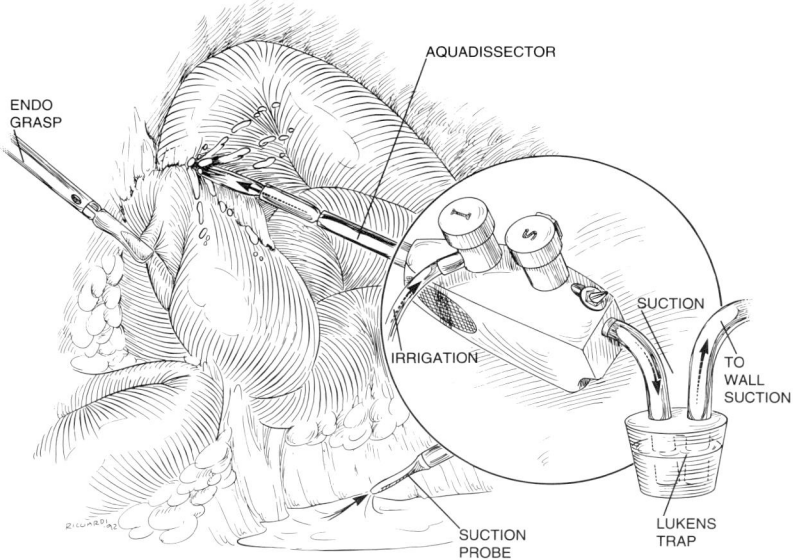

Figure 53-5.

SPECIFIC DETAILS OF THE PROCEDURE

Once the patient is properly positioned, general anesthesia is established and Foley catheter and nasogastric suction tubes are placed, the entire abdomen should be carefully palpated prior to preparation and draping. The size, shape, and location of inflammatory masses should be noted as these will have a direct impact on techniques of blind laparoscopy. If large midline masses are palpated in the region of the umbilicus, if distended, tympanitic loops of bowel are detected or if the patient has had prior lower abdominal surgery, open laparoscopy using the Hassan cannula is preferred to blind puncture.

A pneumoperitoneum is established with carbon dioxide at 15 mm Hg followed by the introduction of a 10-mm 0-degree laparoscope coupled with a video camera. A thorough laparoscopic examination is carried out. Free fluid is likely to be encountered and should be suctioned into a Luken's trap for culture. With the patient in the Trendelenberg position, note is taken of the location of inflammatory masses. Bowel may be noted to adhere to the anterior abdominal wall. Right and left lower quadrant ports (usually 5 mm) can then be placed. Bowel adherent to the abdominal wall can be sharply lysed using bowel graspers and sharp scissors. Landmarks should then be identified. The descending colon should be identified in the left gutter and followed caudad toward the sigmoid. The left paraumbilical ligament and internal ring should be noted as the vas deferens, spermatic vessels, and iliac artery and vein are in close proximity. The bladder and uterus are identified in the midline along with the adnexa in women. As dissection of the periverticular tissues is carried out, it is often useful to provide countertraction of tissues using a 5-mm blunt instrument via the left lower quadrant port while bluntly dissection with a suction irrigation probe via the right lower quadrant port is performed. Using the suction irrigation probe for this portion of the blunt dissection not only allows the use of aquadissection but also provides a source of immediate suction (and therefore culture with an in-line Luken's trap) as soon as any abscess is encountered, thus limiting the amount of peritoneal soilage.

As with open surgery, acutely inflamed tissue planes will often peel apart without force. Forceful dissection of more chronically inflamed tissues is not necessary and may be dangerous. Sharp dissection should be limited at this stage of the procedure. Once one or more abscess cavities have been identified and drained, it may be difficult to determine the end point of a dissection. In general, when these more chronically inflamed tissues are encountered, active dissection should be terminated.

An effort is then made to remove inflammatory exudate and peel that may serve as a continuing nidus of infection. High pressure (up to 200 mm Hg or more) hydrodissection is ideal for this purpose. Profuse irrigation is also carried out until the effluent is clear. An antibiotic may be added to the irrigant as with open surgery. The patient may be tilted head-up and head-down as well as side to side so that all dependent portions of the abdomen are well irrigated.

Finally, a drain should be placed in the abscess cavity (Fig. 53-6). A large, round Jackson-Pratt drain is ideal for this purpose and may be introduced into the abdomen through the left lower quadrant 5-mm port. Wetting the drain with saline helps it to glide through the port with ease. It can be grasped via the right lower quadrant port and placed into the abscess cavity. Prior to removal of the laparoscope, the abdomen should be desufflated while visualizing the drain to ensure that it does not dislodge as carbon dioxide is evacuated.

All port sights are then irrigated and closed via subcuticular closure. The drain is secured to the skin.

POSTOPERATIVE MANAGEMENT

It is advisable to continue nasogastric suction, intravenous fluids, and antibiotics as clinically indicated. An ileus may be encountered postoperatively in light of the inflammatory nature of the process. Antibiotic treatment should be adjusted according to results of cultures obtained operatively. The Foley catheter is often kept in place to assist with fluid management for several days. In general, all postoperative maneuvers are similar to those expected in any setting where an intra-abdominal abscess has been drained. A good response to the laparoscopic approach is heralded by an abatement of fever, pain, and leukocytosis over 48 to 72 hours. Persistent pain, fever, and sepsis mandates laparotomy. With improvement, consideration can be given to elective colectomy following proper evaluation. It would be anticipated that this

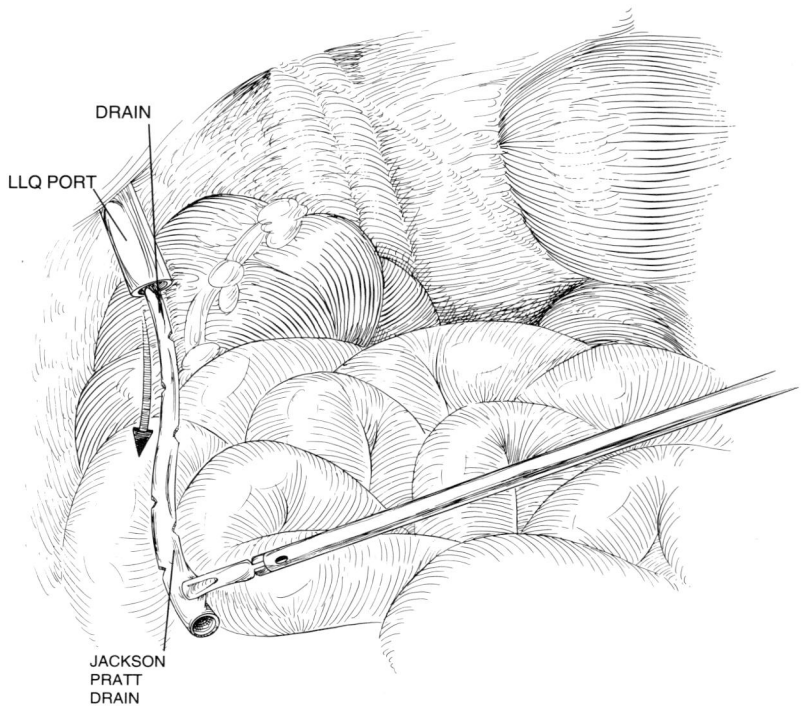

Figure 53-6.

could be performed as a one-stage procedure without colostomy formation.

CRITERIA FOR PATIENT DISCHARGE

Patients are considered for discharge when they are taking solid foods by mouth well and have been afebrile for 24 to 48 hours after completion of intravenous antibiotics (usually a 7- to 10-day course). Oral antibiotic treatment may be maintained after discharge if clinically indicated. If patients remain mildly to moderately symptomatic (abdominal pain, low grade fever, etc.), consideration may be given for further study (barium enema, flexible sigmoidoscopy), bowel preparation, and semielective resection of the diverticular segment prior to discharge. Otherwise, 6 to 8 weeks is a reasonable time interval prior to elective resection. If patients become completely asymptomatic and barium enema and flexible sigmoidoscopy do not show complicated disease (e.g., stricture, intra- or extramural tracking, or fistula), elective resection might be avoided altogether after careful counseling of the patient regarding the various options.

COMPLICATIONS SPECIFIC FOR THIS PROCEDURE

Because of the inflammatory nature of this process, which is often associated with mass formation, ileus, or obstruction and adhesions, closed laparoscopy may be particularly dangerous. The surgeon should not hesitate to convert to open laparoscopy techniques and should be familiar with these.

Bowel injury may occur with friable, inflamed tissues. Thorough inspection of all involved bowel is mandatory prior to completion of the procedure.

Vital structures may be adherent to inflamed, diverticular tissues. The iliac vessels and left ureter are particularly vulnerable to injury. Avoiding overaggressive sharp dissection and relying on gentle blunt dissection along with aquadissection are critical maneuvers.

Poorly controlled abscess drainage may result in diffuse contamination of the abdominal cavity by an otherwise localized process. Attention should be paid to the patient's position when the abscess is entered and if possible a level position should be maintained at this point. Dissection with the suction probe allows immediate evacuation of pus and limits this contamination.

Chapter 54
Closure of an Ileostomy

Garth H. Ballantyne

PATIENT SELECTION

On occasion, patients with inflammatory bowel disease require an emergency total abdominal colectomy with construction of a Brooke ileostomy. If the patient has chronic ulcerative colitis with relative rectal sparing or Crohn's colitis with sparing of the rectum, the rectum may be preserved and closed as a blind pouch.[1-10] Intestinal continuity is reestablished once the patient has recovered from the acute illness and has regained any weight that was lost during the affliction.

Laparoscopic closure of an ileostomy may be more difficult in some patients than in others. Laparoscopic techniques may be difficult to implement in patients with dense adhesions. Consequently, open techniques for closure might be more expeditious for patients in whom feculent peritonitis had developed or who have undergone multiple previous operations.

PREOPERATIVE EVALUATION

The evaluation of patients before laparoscopic closure of an ileostomy is the same as when closure is planned with traditional open techniques. Activity of the inflammatory bowel disease is assessed in the rectal pouch with rigid or flexible sigmoidoscopy. A minimally to moderately active disuse colitis is commonly encountered in the defunctionalized rectal stump and is not a contraindication for the reestablishment of intestinal continuity. The compliance of the rectal pouch is roughly gauged by air insufflation through the sigmoidoscope or more accurately as part of anal phsyiology studies using balloon catheters. Patients with a poorly expandable rectum because of chronic scarring of the rectal wall will suffer from poor functional results if an ileorectostomy is constructed. Anal sphincter function is measured with anal manometry. If the patient has poor compliance or inadequate sphincter function, an alternative procedure should be considered.

PREOPERATIVE PREPARATION

The patient takes nothing by mouth after midnight on the night before the operation. The patient is admitted on the night before surgery or the morning of the procedure. The patient receives several saline enemas which contain 1 g of neomycin. In addition, broad spectrum antibiotics are administered intravenously in the perioperative period.

EQUIPMENT

The following equipment is used:

1. Laparoscope: 10-mm 0-degree laparoscope
2. Trocars: Three 10-mm trocars

3. Instruments
   A. One ENDO DISSECT* instrument (United States Surgical Corporation, Norwalk, CT)
   B. One ENDO BABCOCK* instrument (United States Surgical Corporation)
   C. One ENDO SHEARS* instrument (only necessary if adhesions are encountered; United States Surgical Corporation)
   D. Premium CEEA* (United States Surgical Corporation) stapling device with modified shaft, modified trocar, and low profile anvil
   E. One Automatic PURSTRING* Device (United States Surgical Corporation)
   F. One SURGITIE* ligating loop (if modified trocar of CEEA* is not available; United States Surgical Corporation)
   G. One ENDO HERNIA* (United States Surgical Corporation) stapling device

POSITIONING OF THE PATIENT

The patient is placed in a supine position with legs supported on Lloyd-Davies stirrups. The thighs are straight because flexed thighs may limit the movement of the laparoscopic instruments or laparoscope. The calves are wrapped with pneumatic compression boots (Fig. 54-1).

A nasogastric tube and urinary catheter are inserted into all patients. This minimizes the risk of injury to the stomach and bladder during insertion of the trocars.

During mobilization of the ileostomy, the table remains flat. The patient is dropped into a deep Trendelenberg position while the anvil-shaft assembly is being docked into the cartridge of the Premium CEEA* stapling device.

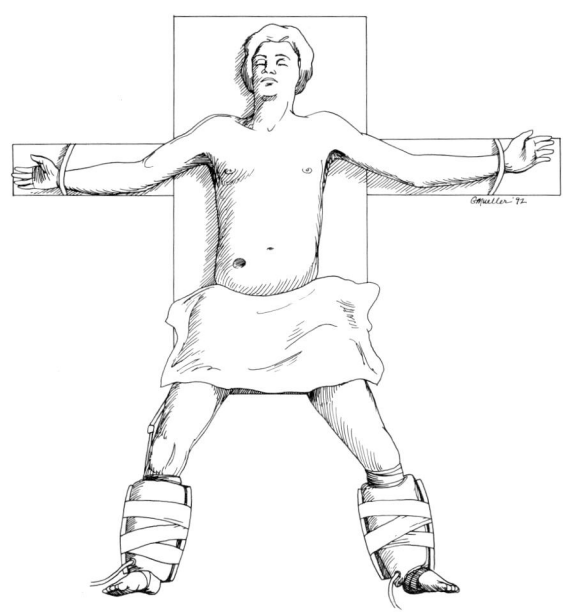

Figure 54-1.

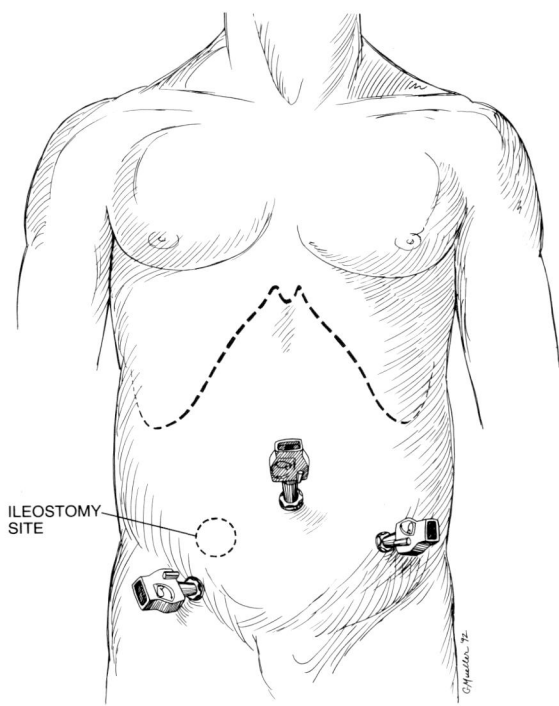

Figure 54-2.

POSITIONING OF THE VIDEO EQUIPMENT

Only one video monitor is generally required. It is best positioned between the legs of the patient. A second monitor sometimes proves helpful if adhesions are encountered in the upper abdomen. Under these circumstances, a second monitor stationed by the right shoulder of the patient may facilitate adhesiolysis.

TROCAR PLACEMENT AND SIZE SELECTION

Three trocars are required in this procedure (Fig. 54-2). A 10-mm trocar is placed in the right lower quadrant caudad to the ileostomy site after the ileostomy has been freed from the abdominal wall. A second 10-mm trocar is placed in the umbilicus. A third 10-mm trocar is inserted in the left lower quadrant lateral to the rectus sheath. The use of 10-mm trocars is required since ENDO BABCOCK* clamps are used to dock the anvil-shaft assembly into the cartridge of the circular stapling device.

Additional ports may be useful if adhesions are encountered. These are positioned based on the location of the adhesions.

METHODS OF EXPOSURE AND RETRACTION

The mobilization of the ileostomy is accomplished through the ileostomy site using traditional open surgical techniques. Lateral adhesions of the terminal ileum to the abdominal wall generated by efforts to close the lateral gutter of the ileostomy are particularly difficult to lyse laparoscopically. These are best exposed and divided under direct observation through the open ileostomy site.

Adhesions to the previous midline incision can also be visualized through the open stoma site. In most patients, these adhesions are readily swept off the incision bluntly with a finger or if they are more tenacious divided sharply with scissors or a cautery device.

If adhesions that cannot be lysed through the open ileostomy site are encountered, trocars are placed in the left upper quadrant and left lower quadrant lateral to the rectus sheath. Generally, the abdominal wall in the left upper quadrant is free of adhesions. This allows easy access with the laparoscope and the cautery scissors. Once the pneumoperitoneum is established, the distention of the abdominal wall generates traction on the adhesions. As a result, the avascular plane between the omentum or loops of bowel and the abdominal wall is conspicuously apparent.

Adhesions between the small bowel and the rectal stump can also be accessed through the open ileostomy site. These are bluntly or sharply divided.

The pelvis is exposed by placing the patient into a deep Trendelenburg position. This causes the small bowel to role back toward the diaphragm.

METHODS OF DISSECTION

Most of the dissection in this procedure is accomplished through the ileostomy site using either blunt or sharp dissection. Adhesions that are out of reach through the open stoma site are divided after establishment of the pneumoperitoneum with ENDO SHEARS*.

SPECIFIC DETAILS OF THE PROCEDURE

After induction of general endotracheal anesthesia, the nasogastric tube and urinary catheter are inserted. The abdomen is prepared and draped in a sterile fashion. A circular incision is made around the ileostomy and extended down to the fascia (Fig. 54-3). A small cuff of skin is left attached to the ileostomy. Adhesions between the ileostomy and abdominal wall are sharply incised. The abdominal cavity is entered along the lateral side of the stoma. Additional adhesions between the terminal ileum and the abdominal wall are divided under direct observation. It is particularly important to free any lateral attachments of the ileum to the right gutter. These are difficult to visualize through a centrally positioned laparoscope. Dissection is continued until sufficient mobility of the ileum is achieved to allow construction of a tension-free ileorectostomy.

The intussusception of the terminal ileum produced in the construction of the Brooke

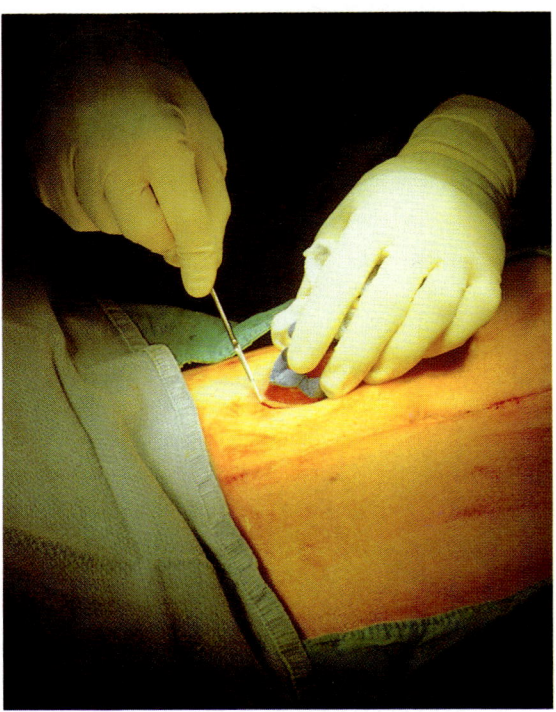

Figure 54-3.

ileostomy is reduced. The most distal several inches of the terminal ileum are excised if the bowel wall is unduly thickened. An Automatic PURSTRING* Device is applied at the selected level of transection of the ileum (Fig. 54-4). The diameter of the bowel is sized. Whenever possible I use a 31-mm cartridge for the Premium CEEA* circular stapling device. The anvil-shaft assembly of the stapling device is inserted into the terminal ileum. The low profile anvil is used since this is permanently secured to the shaft. During laparoscopic manipulations within the abdomen it is possible to inadvertently push the release button of the larger anvil separating the anvil from the shaft. Also, the modified shaft is selected since the additional groove generates a stronger purchase for the ENDO BABCOCK* clamp and facilitates docking of the anvil-shaft assembly into the cartridge of the CEEA*. The purse-string suture is tied around the modified shaft.

The terminal ileum is positioned in the pelvis of the patient through the open stoma site (Fig. 54-5). Care is taken to point the shaft directly toward the rectal pouch. The position of the patient should not be changed after the ileum is returned to the abdomen. Any movements of the patient may lead to displacement of the distal ileum under other loops of bowel.

Adhesions to the previous midline incision are lysed through the ileostomy wound. Any adhesions between loops of small bowel and the rectal stump can usually be reached through the ileostomy site and divided. The three 10-mm trocars are inserted under direct observation. A retractor such as a Deaver or a hand inserted through the wound elevates the abdominal wall during insertion of the trocars (Fig. 54-6). The fascial defect of the ileostomy is closed with interrupted sutures. The carbon dioxide pneumoperitoneum is insufflated through one of the trocars. The laparoscope is introduced into the abdomen.

The assistant surgeon now dilates the anus so that it admits four fingers. The rectal stump is irrigated with a diluted iodine solution. The head of the circular stapling device is advanced up the rectum. The progress of the cartridge of the instrument up the rectum is observed through the laparoscope. Often, the previous closure of the rectal stump is scarred down to the retroperitoneum. There is no advantage of freeing up this proximal end. This may prove to be a difficult and tedious dissection. Rather, the anastomosis is constructed through the anterior (antimesenteric) border of the proximal rectum.

The white trocar of the CEEA* stapling device is screwed out through the selected site for the anastomosis. The jaws of an ENDO BABCOCK* clamp are placed around the trocar as it penetrates the bowel wall. This countertraction helps to prevent a tear of the rectal wall. The trocar is advanced until the orange collar passes through the bowel wall (Fig. 54-7).

The white trocar is lassoed with a SURGITIE*. The trocar is pulled out of the orange collar either with a grasping instrument or by pulling on the suture (Fig. 54-8). The suture end is used to withdraw the white trocar into a 10-mm trocar. An ENDO BABCOCK* clamp aligns the axis of the white trocar with the axis of the 10-mm trocar. The white trocar may catch on the valve device of the 10-mm port. If this occurs, the 10-mm trocar is withdrawn, leaving the SURGIGRIP* device in place. The trocar tip is removed and the 10-mm trocar is reinserted through the SURGIGRIP* device.

A recent modification of the trocar tip of the Premium CEEA* stapling device allows an easier alternative technique for its retrieval. A hole has been drilled in the tip of the trocar. Before insertion of the stapling device into the rectum, a suture is tied in a loose loop through this hole. When the trocar is advanced through the rectal wall, this loop is pulled into the abdominal cavity. The loop is grasped between the jaws of a grasping instrument. Gravity aligns the trocar vertically so that it is easily pulled out through a 10-mm trocar.

The groove of the modified shaft of the anvil-shaft assembly is grasped with an ENDO BABCOCK* clamp (Fig. 54-9). This improves the mechanical advantage of the Babcock clamp and eases the docking of the

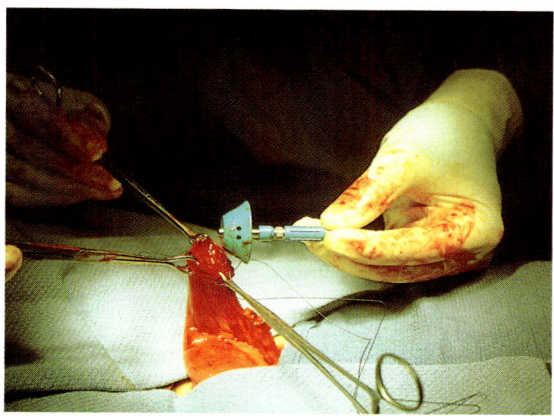

Figure 54-4.

594   Techniques of Laparoscopic Surgery

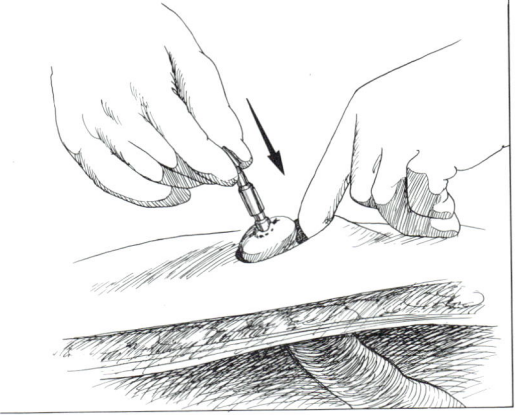

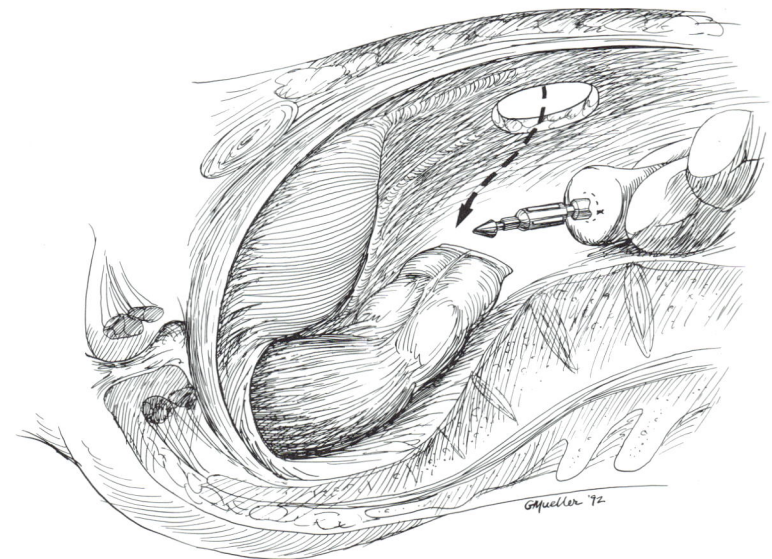

Figure 54-5.

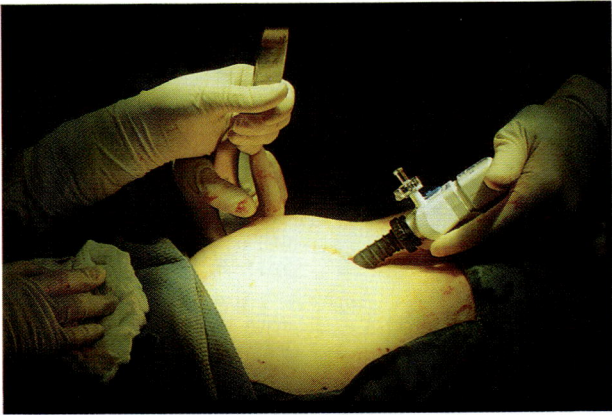

Figure 54-6.

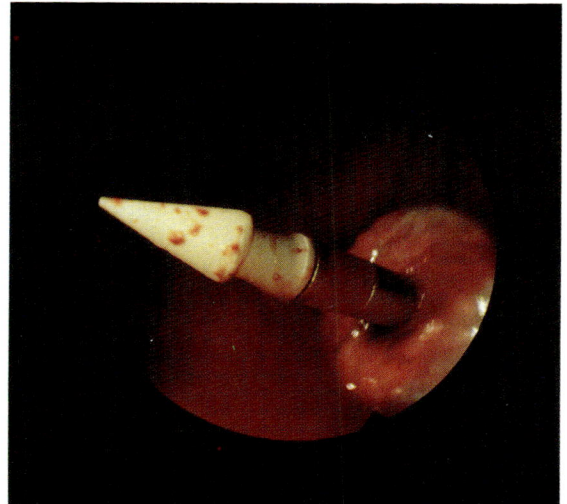

Figure 54-7.

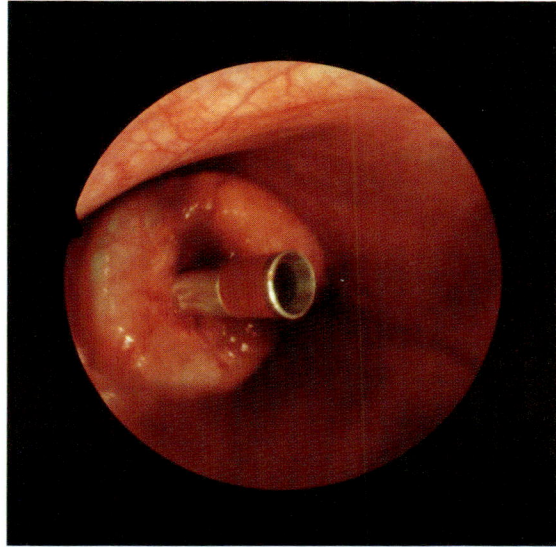

Figure 54-8.

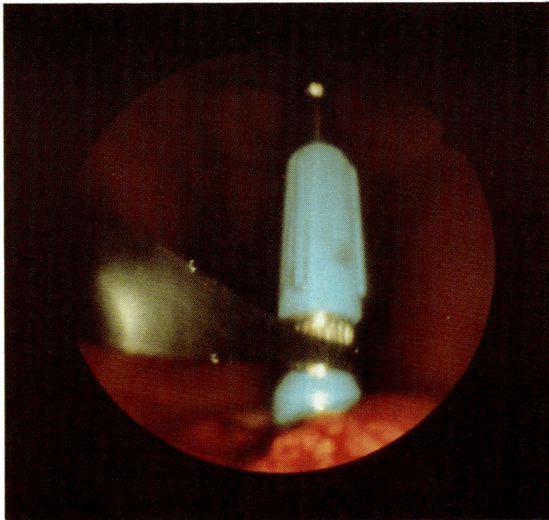

Figure 54-9.

shaft into the cartridge of the stapling device. The axis of the orange collar of the CEEA* device and the shaft must be aligned in all three dimensions. The shaft is snapped into the collar (Fig. 54-10A and B). The ileum is checked for any evidence of a volvulus. The ileal mesentery is traced down to its root. The circular stapling device is screwed closed and fired.

The Premium CEEA* stapling device is opened one full turn and removed. The stapling device is opened fully and checked for two complete donuts. The pelvis is filled with warmed saline. A flexible or rigid sigmoidoscope is inserted through the anus and advanced up to the anastomosis. The staple line is checked for hemostasis (Fig. 54-11). The rectum is insufflated. The light of the laparoscope is often visible through the wall of the bowel. The saline in the pelvis is observed for air bubbles.

CLOSURE

The saline in the pelvis is aspirated dry. The remaining defect in the mesentery can be closed with the ENDO HERNIA* stapler. Each staple is advanced halfway out. One tip of the exposed staple is used to latch onto the edge of the visceral peritoneum on one side of the mesenteric defect. This edge is pulled to the other, and the staple is then completely closed.

Drains, if desired, are inserted into the abdomen down one of the 10-mm trocars. The drain is positioned near the anastomosis. The trocar is removed leaving the tube of the drain in place.

The trocars are removed one at a time. The fascial defect of each is closed with interrupted absorbable sutures. The placement of these sutures is observed through the laparoscope. This ensures that stray loops of bowel are not snagged by the sutures. After all other trocar sites are closed, the laparoscope is removed from the last one. The pneumoperitoneum is slowly deflated through the last trocar, which is then re-

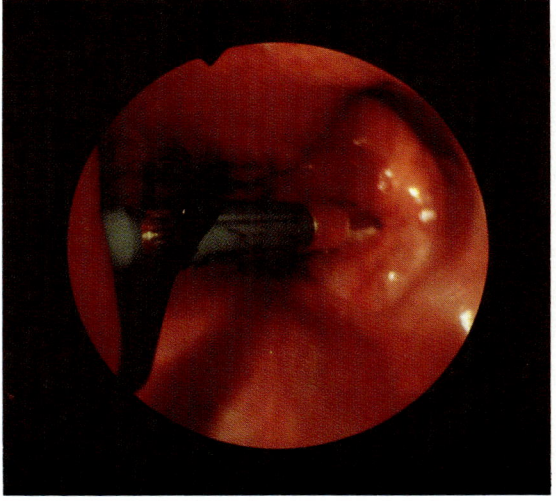

A

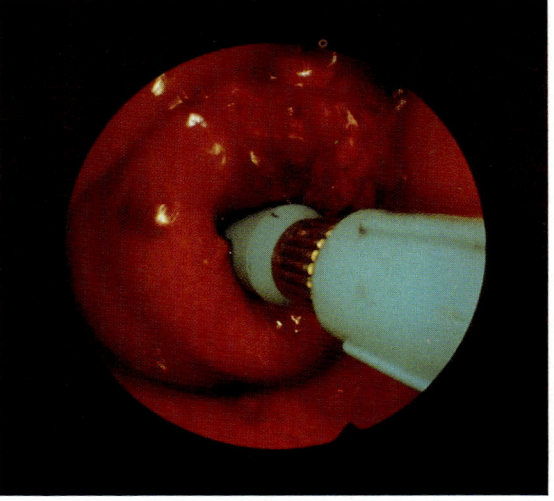

B

Figure 54-10.

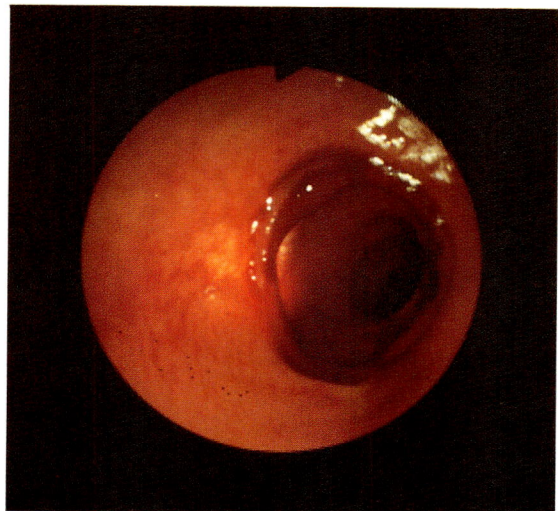

Figure 54-11.

moved. The last fascial defect is also closed with sutures. The skin edges of the trocar sites are apposed with skin staples or Steri-Strips (3M Corporation, Minneapolis, MN). Band-Aids cover the wounds.

POSTOPERATIVE MANAGEMENT

The nasogastric tube is removed in the operating room or on the first morning after the operation. The urinary catheter is removed when the patient is ambulating. Similarly, the pneumatic boots are not removed until the patient is up and walking.

The patient is allowed clear liquids by mouth on the morning after the operation. The intravenous line is removed when the patient is taking an adequate amount of liquids. If liquids are tolerated, the patient is given a regular diet on the second postoperative day. Often, however, the patient has little appetite until the third or fourth postoperative day.

CRITERIA FOR DISCHARGE

The patient may be discharged from the hospital when he or she is able to eat a regular diet. Hospitalization may be continued when social circumstances limit the availability of help at home. Similarly, patients who live near the hospital may be discharged sooner than patients who live farther away. It may not be necessary for the patient to have a bowel movement before discharge.

COMPLICATIONS SPECIFIC FOR THIS PROCEDURE

No specific complications have been identified for this laparoscopic procedure. As with all ileorectal anastomoses, the patient must be carefully followed for evidence of sepsis. The discharge of the patient should be delayed until after the seventh postoperative day if the patient cannot be followed closely at home or in a chronic care facility.

In patients with chronic ulcerative colitis, the remaining rectum must be carefully examined for evidence of dysplasia or malignancy. The risk of rectal cancer in patients with Crohn's disease may also be increased compared to the general population, but this risk remains incompletely defined.

REFERENCES

1. Aylett SO. Three hundred cases of diffuse ulcerative colitis treated by total colectomy and ileorectal anastomosis. Br Med J 1966; 1:1001.
2. Baker WN, Glass RE, Ritchie JK, Aylett SO. Cancer of the rectum following colectomy and ileorectal anastomosis for ulcerative colitis. Br J Surg 1978; 65:862–868.
3. Hawley PR. Ileorectal anastomosis. Br J Surg 1985; 72(Suppl):75–76.
4. Johnson WR, Hughes ESR, McDermott FT, Katrivessis H. The outcome of patients with ulcerative colitis managed by subtotal colectomy. Surg Gynecol Obstet 1986; 162:421–425.
5. Jones PF, Munro A, Ewen WB. Colectomy and ileorectal anastomosis for colitis: Report on a personal series, with a critical review. Br J Surg 1977; 64:615–623.
6. Khubchandani IT, Sandfort MR, Rosen L, Sheets JA, Stasik JJ, Rither RD. Current status of ileorectal anastomosis for inflammatory bowel disease. Dis Colon Rectum 1989; 32:400–402.
7. Leijonmarck CE, Löfberg R, Öst Å, Hellers G. Long-term results of ileorectal anastomosis in ulcerative colitis in Stockholm County. Dis Colon Rectum 1990; 33:195–200.
8. Oakley JR, et al. Complications and quality of life after ileorectal anastomosis for ulcerative colitis. Am J Surg 1985; 149:23–30.
9. Oakley JR. The fate of the rectal stump after subtotal colectomy for ulcerative colitis. Dis Colon Rectum 1985; 28:394–396.
10. Tonelli F, Bianchini F, Lodovici M, Valanzano R, Carderni G, Dolara P. Mucosal cell proliferation of the rectal stump in ulcerative colitis patients after ileorectal anastomosis. Dis Colon Rectum 1991; 34:385–390.

Chapter 55
Closure of a Hartmann's Colostomy

Anthony V. Coletta

PATIENT SELECTION

Hartmann resections, with removal of diseased bowel, oversewing of distal colon or rectum, and the creation of an end-colostomy are most often performed for acute diverticulitis, although obstruction of or trauma to the left colon is also an indication for the procedure. As the procedure is usually performed in acute settings, colostomy closure with reestablishment of gastrointestinal continuity is often delayed 2 to 3 months to allow infection or acute inflammation to subside. Closure of Hartmann's colostomy requires a second laparotomy with all its attendant morbidity and mortality, a 7- to 10-day hospital stay, and another 4 to 6 weeks for recovery. All such patients may be considered for laparoscopic colostomy closure. By avoiding a second laparotomy, a shorter hospitalization as well as a rapid return to normal activities would be an anticipated desirable outcome in these patients who have already undergone a prolonged recuperative period. Contraindications to laparoscopic closure include those for any laparoscopic procedure, i.e., severe cardiorespiratory disease or severe coagulopathy.

PREOPERATIVE EVALUATION

The time interval prior to consideration for laparoscopic colostomy closure following the initial Hartmann resection remains 2 to 3 months as with open colostomy closure.

The most important study preoperatively prior to laparoscopic colostomy closure is evaluating the distal colonic segment (Hartmann's pouch). Flexible fiberoptic sigmoidoscopy is best suited for this and in fact may be utilized intraoperatively to identify the full extent of the distal segment. Note should be taken of the length of the distal segment and whether or not it extends beyond the peritoneal reflection of the rectosigmoid (approximately 15 to 20 cm). A short rectal segment (less than 15 cm or below the peritoneal reflection) dictates that the procedure be done in the lithotomy position and that an intracorporeal stapled anastomosis will be required. Longer distal segments may be considered for extracorporeal anastomoses.

PREOPERATIVE PREPARATION

Preoperative preparation is identical to that for open colostomy closure. Full bowel preparation, both mechanical and antibiotic, should begin 2 to 3 days prior to the procedure. The patient begins to consume clear liquid diet 3 days prior to surgery. Two nights prior to surgery an oral cathartic is administered (e.g., 40 ml of Fleets Phospho-Soda). The day prior to surgery one Fleets enema is administered via the rectum, and the colostomy stoma is irrigated four times with 250 ml of a neomycin solution (1 g of neomycin in 1 liter of phosphate-buffered saline). If desired, oral antibiotics are also administered. Intravenous fluids are begun at 8 p.m. on the evening prior to the procedure, and a broad spectrum intravenous antibiotic is administered when the patient is taken to the operating room.

EQUIPMENT

The following instruments are used:

1. Laparoscopes: 10-mm 0-degree laparoscope and 5-mm 0- or 30-degree laparoscope
2. Trocars: Hassan cannula or 10-mm trocar, two 5-mm trocars, and one 12-mm trocar
3. Instruments
   A. Suction-irrigation probe
   B. Two atraumatic bowel graspers
   C. Laparoscopic Babcock forceps
   D. Laparoscopic "finger" retractor
   E. Fiberoptic sigmoidoscope
   F. End-to-end anastomotic stapler
   G. Surgical laparotomy tray
   H. Pre-knotted 0 chromic ties
   I. 10-mm ENDO CLIP* applier
   J. Monopolar scissors

POSITIONING OF THE PATIENT

In general, the dorsal lithotomy position with easy access to the perineum is preferred (Fig. 55-1). The legs should be abducted with the hips only minimally flexed. Flexed hips with the patient in the conventional dorsal lithotomy position can inhibit the movement of lower abdominal laparoscopic instrumentation. If possible, the arms should be well padded and kept at the patient's side. Shoulder pads anchored to the operative table should be used to prevent the patient from slipping when in a steep Trendelenberg position. As the patient may be in lithotomy stirrups for some time, the legs should be well padded, and sequential pneumatic compression boots are preferred (thigh-high).

A nasogastric tube should be placed following the induction of general anesthesia to keep the stomach well decompressed. At times the splenic flexure of the left colon may require mobilization and a distended stomach can interfere with this maneuver.

A Foley catheter is essential. It should be positioned so that circulating nurses may gain access to it to fill the bladder if neccesary to identify landmarks and ensure bladder wall integrity.

Although not essential, consideration should be given to placing ureteral stents following the induction of anesthesia. The pelvic dissection of a Hartmann's pouch may be difficult in light of prior inflammatory processes. Often the rectal stump is adherent to the left pelvic sidewall in the region of the iliac vessels and left ureter. A stent, as in open surgery, may make identification and protection of this ureter easier.

In women, a transvaginal uterine manipulator should be placed after pelvic examination to assist in pelvic exposure.

POSITIONING OF THE VIDEO EQUIPMENT

In general, only one video monitor is necessary. It should be positioned to the left of the patient at the foot of the table. The surgeon and camera assistant stand to the patient's right side. A second assistant, if necessary, stands to the patient's left. The scrub nurse is best positioned between the patient's legs. The camera receiver and light source as well as electrical energy sources and suction should be to the patient's right. Ideally, the insufflator is to the left of the patient where the surgeon can monitor intra-abdominal pressures and insufflation can be carried out through a lateral, grasping port.

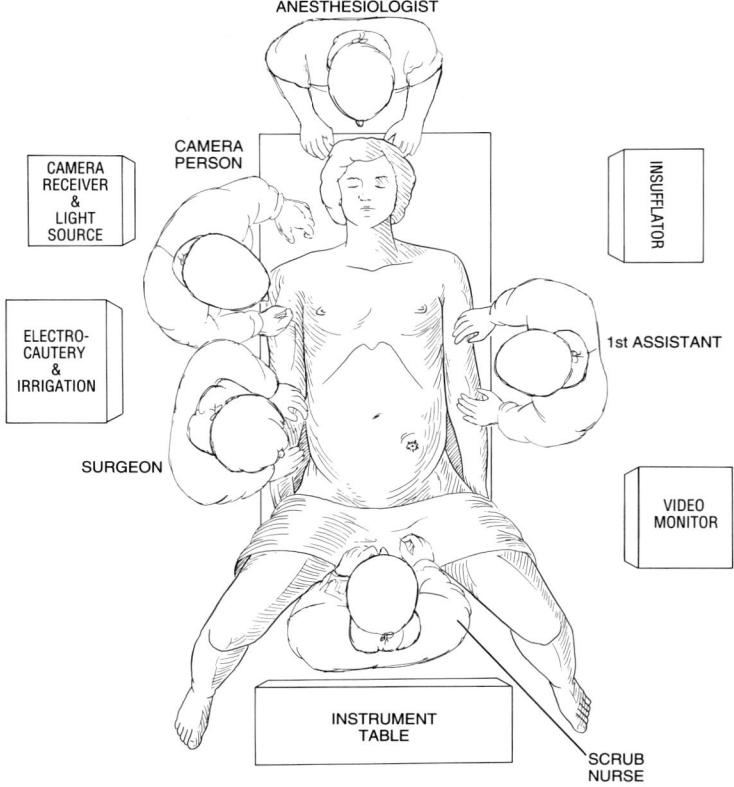

Figure 55-1.

TROCAR PLACEMENT AND SIZE SELECTION

Using the open laparoscopic technique, the Hassan cannula can be placed in the midline just above or below the umbilicus. This port is primarily used for the laparoscope (Fig. 55-2). Because extensive intra-abdominal adhesions are commonly encountered, primarily in the midline and left lower quadrant, the next port placed is often the right lower quadrant 12-mm port, lateral to the rectus sheath and in a plane just below the umbilicus. If the ENDO GIA* stapling device is used either for bowel or mesenteric resection, it is generally inserted via this port. Once adhesions are lysed and further exposure is obtained, two additional 5-mm ports are placed, usually suprapubically in the midline and in the left lower quadrant either above and lateral to the colostomy or just below it.

METHODS OF EXPOSURE AND RETRACTION

Initial exposure is obtained by lysing adhesions of bowel and omentum to the anterior abdominal wall. This can generally be carried out via the right lower quadrant 12-mm port initially with the placement of one of the two 5-mm ports when enough exposure is obtained to allow for additional countertraction and dissection. A steep Trendelenburg position is then essential for exposure of the pelvis and dissection of the rectal stump. In women the transvaginal uterine manipulator allows the uterus to be lifted anteriorly and to the patient's right. Multiple loops of small bowel are often adherent within the pelvis and must be dissected free to expose the rectal stump. A transanal rectal probe or a fiberoptic sigmoidoscope may assist in identification and exposure of the rectal stump (Fig.

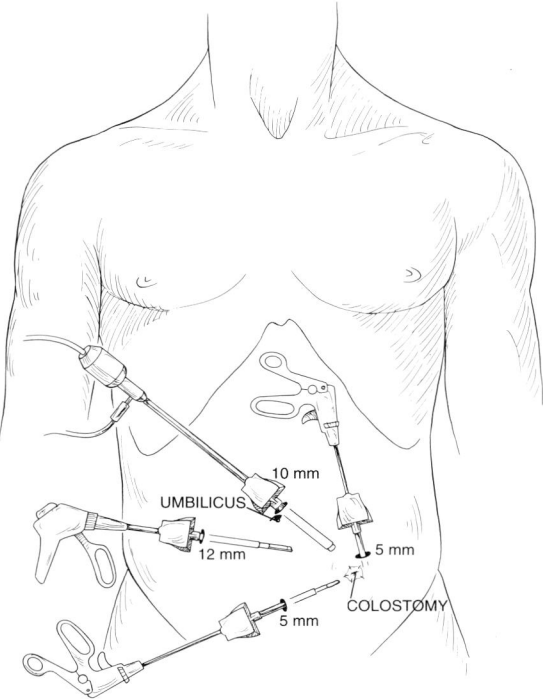

Figure 55-2.

55-3). Transillumination of the rectal wall with the fiberoptic scope may be possible if the rectal wall is not unduly thickened. Once the rectal stump has been identified, elevation of the bladder with a "finger" retractor placed via the right lower quadrant port greatly facilitates freeing the rectal stump prior to anastomosis (Fig. 55-4).

METHODS OF DISSECTION

Sharp adhesiolysis with and without the use of monopolar cautery is an essential element of the procedure. Often adhesions are matured in these patients to the point of being dense and thus will not separate freely simply with blunt dissection. Countertraction is essential to careful sharp dissection accomplished laparoscopically. Initially countertraction of adhesions to the anterior abdominal wall is provided simply via the draping of the viscera caused by the pneumoperitoneum. An avascular plane may be entered for this phase of the adhesiolyis, thus limiting the need for electrocautery. Aquadissection may be used as an adjunct here, by gently placing an irriga-

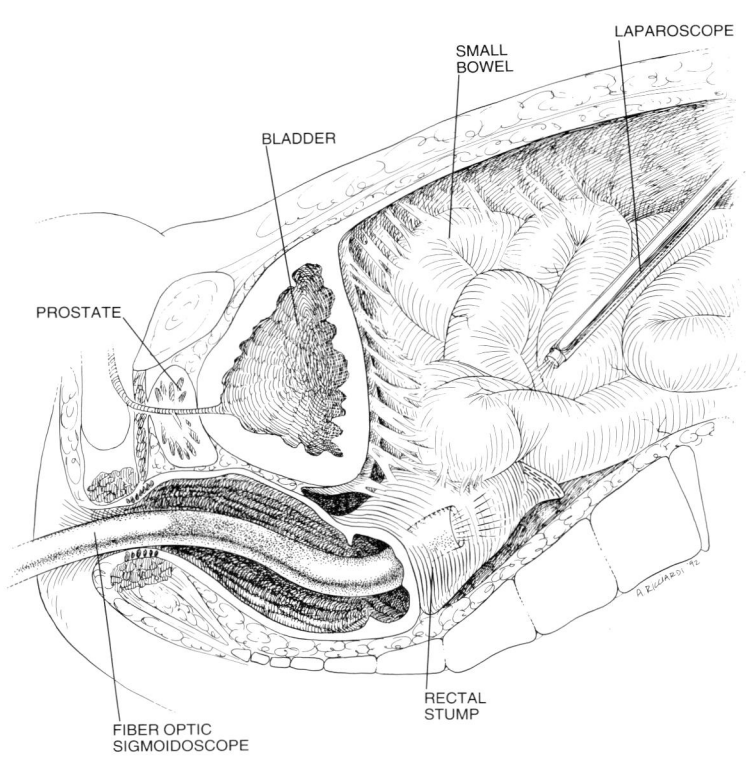

Figure 55-3.

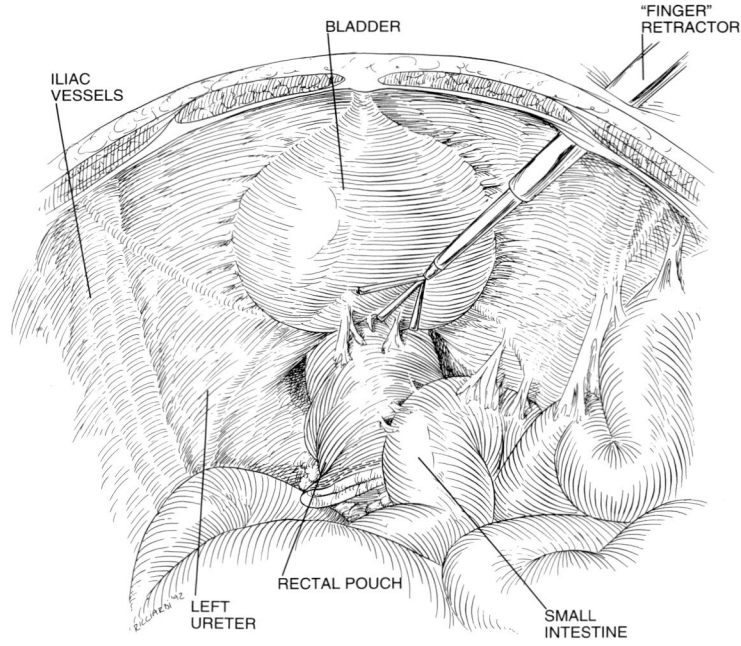

Figure 55-4.

tion probe between adhesions and the abdominal wall and initiation of high pressure flow to help separate adherent tissue planes.

SPECIFIC DETAILS OF THE PROCEDURE

Prior to beginning the procedure, the colostomy stoma should be oversewn with a 2-0 silk suture, inverting the skin edges to prevent fecal contamination as the procedure progresses. Establishing the pneumoperitoneum may be difficult in those patients who have had at least one prior laparotomy for inflammatory disease. Open laparoscopy is preferred although that approach may be difficult in the midline where adhesions predominate. Alternate insufflation sites may also be considered. Insufflation with the Veress needle in the ninth intercostal space, in the midaxillary line may provide a safe, alternate insufflation site. Open laparoscopy with the Hassan cannula can also be carried out in the right lower quadrant. Once a safe laparoscopic environment has been established, the fascia around the cannula may be secured with a purse-string suture and the Hassan cannula can be replaced with a 12-mm cannula.

Once adhesiolysis is complete and all trocars are placed, identification and dissection of the rectal stump in preparation for insertion of the end-to-end anastomosis (EEA) stapler and an intracorporeal anastomosis is begun. Identification of the rectal stump may be facilitated by transmural illumination via a flexible sigmoidoscope. Although circumferential dissection of the stump is not necessary in all patients, identification of the end point of the stump is critical to accurate placement of the end-to-end anastomosis. Prior to dissection of the end-colostomy, the proximal portion of the EEA stapler should be inserted, and it should be ascertained that the instrument is well approximated to the distal most portion of the rectal stump (Fig. 55-5).

At this point, laparoscopic mobilization of the descending colon colostomy is begun. Often this step is limited as the colostomy obscures clear visualization of the left paracolic gutter. Laparoscopic mobilization of bowel that might be adherent between the colostomy and the distal rectal stump is critical prior to open mobilization of the stoma and temporary loss of the pneumoperitoneum. In addition, an initial judgment must be made regarding the length of colon available for the coloproctostomy. If necessary and feasible, the splenic flexure and proximal left colon should be mobilized along the lateral peritoneal reflections prior to stoma excision.

After as much left colon dissection as is deemed necessary and safe has been carried

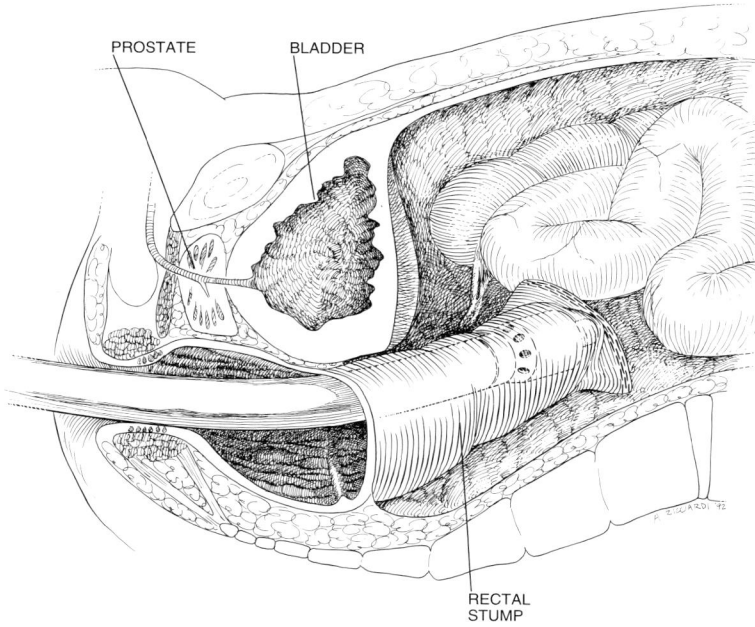

Figure 55-5.

out laparoscopically, conventional surgical techniques are then used to dissect the stoma free from the abdominal wall. Once the peritoneal cavity is entered, the pneumoperitoneum is lost, and the procedure is temporarily converted to open surgery. Via this approach, as much of the descending colon as can safely be mobilized without devascularization is brought out. The end stoma is excised from the proximal portion of bowel, the bowel is properly sized, and the anvil of the EEA stapler is inserted and purse-string sutures are applied. Prior to reinserting the descending colon into the abdomen and reestablishing the pneumoperitoneum, it is advisable that the sharp point of the EEA anvil be covered with an absorbable collagen material (e.g., Surgicel) secured with a chromic knot. This will prevent inadvertent bowel or vascular injury caused by the sharp trocar prior to return of laparoscopic visualization.

Once the proximal bowel is returned to the abdomen, the fascia is surgically reapproximated, and the pneumoperitoneum is reestablished. The chromic knot around the anvil may then be cut and the protective collagen hemostatic material removed. The EEA stapler is inserted transanally and the trocar is advanced through the distal end or anterior wall of the rectal stump (Fig. 55-6). The anastomosis is then carried out as with low anterior resection.

CLOSURE

If the Hassan cannula is used, the fascia should be reapproximated. The fascial opening surrounding the 12-mm port should also be closed. The skin is closed with subcuticular closure.

POSTOPERATIVE MANAGEMENT

The patient is given nothing by mouth until bowel function returns. Maintaining nasogastric suction is necessary only if postoperative distention ensues. With the return of bowel function, the diet is advanced as tolerated. The Foley catheter may be removed within 24 hours postoperatively. Antibiotics are continued for 24 hours as with open surgery.

CRITERIA FOR PATIENT DISCHARGE

Patients are discharged when they are taking solid foods well and normal bowel function has returned. This may be as early as 4 days postoperatively.

604 Techniques of Laparoscopic Surgery

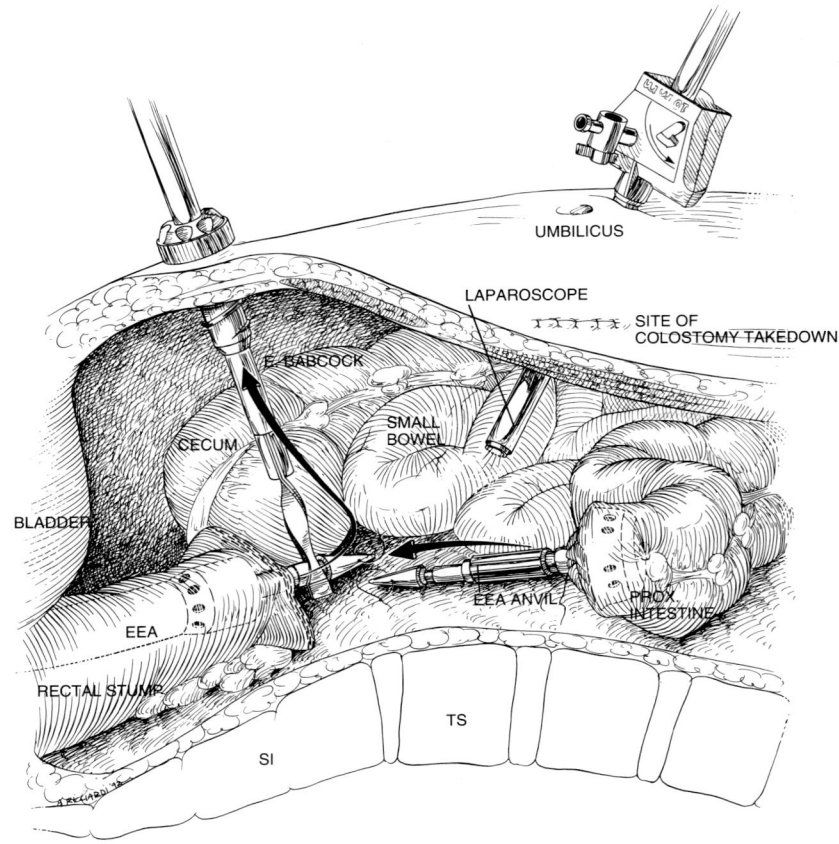

Figure 55-6.

COMPLICATIONS SPECIFIC FOR THIS PROCEDURE

Establishing a pneumoperitoneum may be difficult in these patients and visceral or vascular injury may be encountered. Open laparoscopy may minimize this complication.

If the location of the end-to-end anastomosis within the rectal stump is misjudged, inadvertent injury to the distal rectal wall or posterior bladder wall may ensue when the trocar is advanced. Insertion to its fullest extent along with palpation of the end of the instrument at the distal end of the rectal stump with a grasping instrument confirms proper placement.

It may be difficult to determine the amount of tension the stapled anastomosis is under once it is complete. Full mobilization of the left colon along with the splenic flexure minimizes this tension.

Chapter 56
Abdominal Perineal Resection

Garth H. Ballantyne

PATIENT SELECTION

Laparoscopically assisted abdominal perineal resection remains in an early period of development. Indeed, this procedure has been attempted in only a small number of patients. Consequently, useful criteria for patient selection are ill defined. As a general principle, however, indications for laparoscopically assisted abdominal perineal resection should be the same as for the traditional type of operation.

Patient selection will change as the experience of the individual surgeon broadens. During initial attempts with this procedure, the surgeon should select patients in whom this procedure can be more easily accomplished. The anterior pelvic dissection is more easily accomplished in women. Pneumoperitoneum is often difficult to establish in patients who have previously undergone abdominal operations. A previous hysterectomy may make the pelvic dissection particularly tedious. Extreme obesity obscures exposure of the pelvis and may make ligation of the mesentery difficult. Bulky lesions deep in the pelvis will shroud the pelvic dissection. Direct extension of the rectal cancer into contiguous organs is difficult to assess laparoscopically since the surgeon is unable to palpate these structures. Thus, a surgeon might best limit his early attempts at laparoscopically assisted abdominal perineal resection to patients who are thin, have relatively early distal rectal lesions, and have not previously undergone abdominal or gynecologic procedures.

PREOPERATIVE EVALUATION

The risk of operation for candidates for laparoscopic abdominal perineal resection is judged in the same manner as for standard operations. Three areas, however, require careful attention. The hypercarbia produced by the carbon dioxide pneumoperitoneum may lead to a respiratory acidosis in patients with limited respiratory reserve or fixed ventilatory capacity. Consequently, candidates for laparoscopic procedures should undergo pulmonary function testing. A baseline artery blood gas measurement may be helpful. Similarly, respiratory acidosis may precipitate cardiac arrhythmias in patients with arteriosclerotic coronary artery disease. Cardiograms are obtained in all patients. Extensive cardiac evaluations are pursued as warranted by history and other findings.

Locally advanced pelvic disease may hinder laparoscopically assisted resection of the rectal cancer. Preoperative staging of the rectal cancer may obviate such difficulties. A computed tomographic scan of the pelvis or intrarectal ultrasound may disclose direct extension of the rectal cancer into the prostate or vagina, trigone of the bladder, sacrum, or pelvic sidewalls. These findings do not preclude an attempt at laparoscopically assisted resection but will certainly facilitate decisions on the approach to resection of the lesion.

All patients are evaluated by an enterostomal therapist. The planned site of the stoma is selected and marked. Instruction in care of the stoma is begun before surgery.

PREOPERATIVE PREPARATION

The preoperative preparation for patients for whom laparoscopically assisted resection is planned is identical to that used for patients undergoing traditional abdominal perineal resections. The patient drinks 2 liters of GoLYTELY or NuLYTELY during a 3-hour period on the night before surgery. The patient receives an antibiotic bowel preparation such as neomycin and erythromycin or intravenous perioperative antibiotics.

EQUIPMENT

All instruments used in a traditional abdominal perineal resection should be available within the operating room. Hemorrhage or other complications may dictate rapid conversion to an open abdominal procedure. The table of instruments for the perineal dissection is set out in the same manner as for the standard operation.

Telescopes

The abdominal portion of the operation is accomplished with a 10-mm, 0-degree telescope. A second telescope for transillumination of the mesentery may prove helpful. A second telescope is also useful for observation of the tips of instruments as they are passed through the mesentery. In some patients, the pelvis may be better visualized through a 10-mm, 30-degree telescope. This angled telescope greatly facilitates mobilization of the splenic flexure when this proves necessary. In the future, flexible telescopes may improve exposure in all areas of the abdomen and pelvis.

Trocars and Ports

The number and sizes of trochars required for this procedure will vary from patient to patient. In general, six 10-mm ports are used. In addition, one 12-mm port is needed for transection of the bowel with the ENDO GIA* 30 stapling device or a 15-mm port for the ENDO GIA* 60.

Instruments

The number of laparoscopic instruments used in this procedure is small. These include:

1. One disposable scissors
2. One dissecting instrument such as the ENDO DISSECT* instrument
3. Two Babcock clamps
4. Two atraumatic bowel clamps
5. One needle driver
6. One suction device
7. One ENDO GIA* 30 stapling device with additional cartridges
8. One ENDO GIA* 60 stapling device with additional cartridges
9. One laparoscopic multifire clip applier

A new disposable scissors is the most important single instrument. Reusable scissors are inadequate because the edges dull too quickly.

POSITIONING OF THE PATIENT

The patient is placed in a supine position with the legs supported by Lloyd-Davies stirrups (Fig. 56-1). The legs are kept as straight as possible. Movement of the long handles on the laparoscopic instruments is limited by the legs if the hips are flexed. Almost all of the retraction of the bowel for exposure during the operation is achieved by varying the inclination and rotation of the table. Thus, it is essential that the table can be dropped into a deep Trendelenberg and a reverse Trendelenberg position as well as rotated to the left and right. An electric table facilitates these frequent changes in position.

A nasogastric tube and urinary catheter are inserted in all patients. These decrease the risk of injury during placement of the Veress needle and trocars. Ureteral catheters are helpful during a surgeon's early experience with this procedure. Illuminated catheters

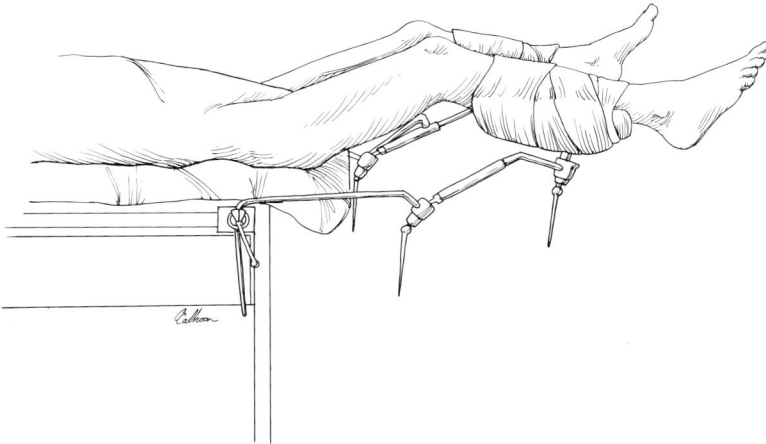

Figure 56-1.

greatly facilitate laparoscopic identification of the ureters.

POSITIONING OF THE VIDEO EQUIPMENT

Laparoscopic bowel surgery is a highly technical endeavor. The requisite equipment rapidly fills even the largest operating room. The equipment must be distributed within the room in a manner that facilitates the operation both in terms of movement of personnel within the room as well as comfort of the surgeon. The video monitors should be given the greatest priority in this regard. The primary video monitor is placed between the legs of the patient (Fig. 56-2). The surgeon and the assistant surgeon can comfortably view the pelvic dissection on this screen. A second monitor is positioned near the left shoulder of the patient. Mobilization of the descending colon and the splenic flexure, when necessary, is viewed on this screen. The video monitors should be easily moved. Often an adjustment of the screen as little as a foot in one direction or the other greatly increases the surgeon's comfort.

ESTABLISHMENT OF THE PNEUMOPERITONEUM

After induction of anesthesia, the abdomen and perineum are cleansed and draped in the same manner as used for standard abdominal perineal resection. The abdomen is draped widely so that trochars can be placed lateral to the rectus sheath. The patient is dropped into a deep Trendelenberg position. A small supraumbilical incision is made. A Veress needle is inserted into the abdominal cavity. Proper positioning of the needle is checked by rotation of the needle, injection and aspiration of saline, and observation of saline dropping rapidly down through the needle. If needle placement is unsatisfactory or if the patient has undergone previous abdominal operations, an open technique is used for trochar insertion. Insufflation of the abdominal cavity with carbon dioxide is commenced. Low intra-abdominal pressures (less than 10 mm Hg) should be initially observed. The regulator of the carbon dioxide insufflator is set at a pressure limit of 15 mm Hg or less. Carbon dioxide is pumped at a low rate for the first liter. Subsequently, a high flow rate is used. Once an adequate pneumoperitoneum is established, the Veress needle is removed. A 10-mm trochar is inserted into the abdomen through the supraumbilical incision. The abdomen is immediately inspected with a 10-mm 0-degree telescope for evidence of damage to bowel or other organs that may have occurred during insertion of the Veress needle or the supraumbilical trochar.

TROCAR PLACEMENT AND SIZE SELECTION

Sites of trocar placement are indicated in Figure 56-3. Placement of the umbilical trocar cephalad to the umbilicus allows a better angle for observation of the superior hemorrhoidal vessels at the level of the sacral promontory. Once the initial port is intro-

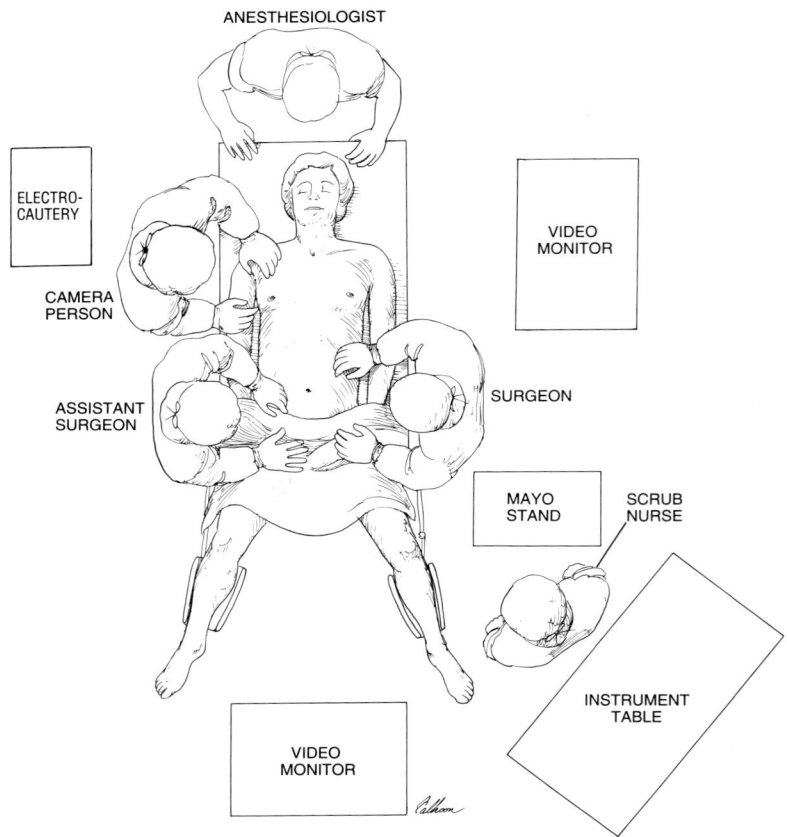

Figure 56-2.

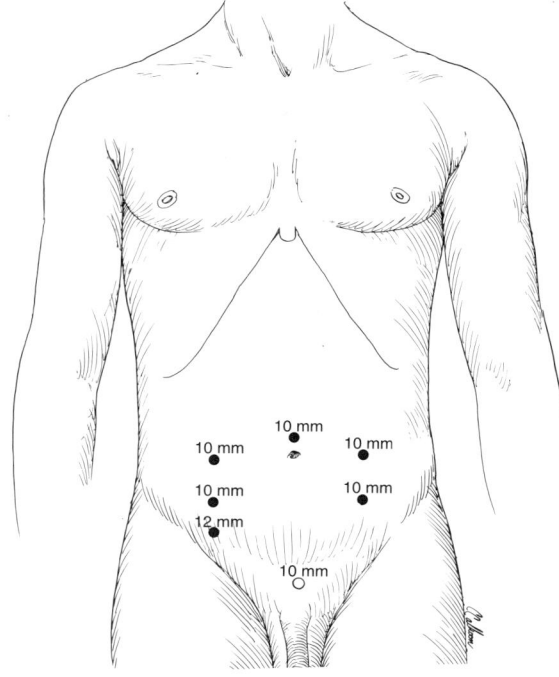

Figure 56-3.

duced, all others are introduced with direct visualization of the trocar tip as it enters the abdominal cavity. Two ports are placed lateral to the rectus sheath in the left and right lower quadrant. The surgeon and assistant surgeon, on opposite sides of the table, use two instruments each through these ports. The sixth port is placed at the level of the umbilicus lateral to the rectus sheath. The rectosigmoid when retracted out of the pelvis tends to cloak the telescope in the supraumbilical port. Consequently, the telescope is inserted through this sixth port during dissection of the right side of the pelvis and ligation of the superior hemorrhoidal vessels. This sixth port may not be necessary in some patients. Once the sigmoid is mobilized and the superior hemorrhoidal vessels are isolated, a port is picked for introduction of the stapling device. Typically, the caudad port on the right side is best situated for insertion of the stapling device. The 10-mm port is replaced by a 12-mm port for the ENDO GIA* 30 stapling device or a 15-mm port for the

ENDO GIA* 60 device. A suprapubic 10-mm port is useful in some patients. Many of the currently available laparoscopic instruments are too short to reach deeply into the pelvis. The suprapubic port adds to the functional length of the instruments.

METHODS OF EXPOSURE AND RETRACTION

Staging Laparoscopy

After placement of the trochars, the abdomen is explored. Placement of the patient in a reverse Trendelenberg position improves access and exposure to the liver (Fig. 56-4). The diaphragmatic surfaces of the liver are better visualized through a 10-mm 30-degree telescope. Superficial metastatic lesions are easily observed through the laparoscope (Fig. 56-4B and C). Laparoscopic ultrasound devices facilitate identification of lesions within the parenchyma of the liver.

The patient is returned to a deep Trendelenberg position. The omentum is grasped with atraumatic grasping forceps such as the ENDO GRASP* device and displaced cephalad. Unless adhesions limit movement of the omentum it is easily positioned above the transverse colon. The segments of small bowel are sequentially visualized by alternately grasping the bowel with the atraumatic instruments (Fig. 56-5). It is easier to identify the terminal ileum and to move proximally along the small bowel. It is well worth the effort at this point to free any adhesions that fix the small bowel in the pelvis or the sigmoid colon.

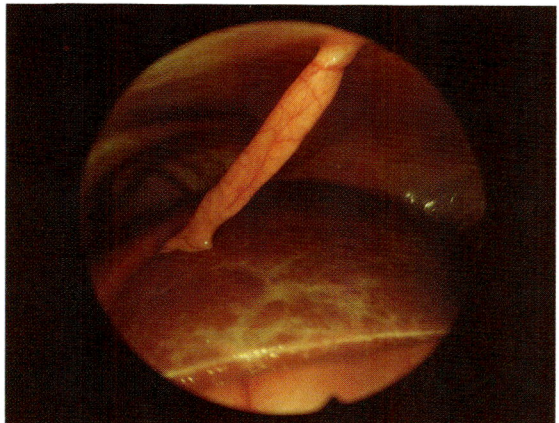

A

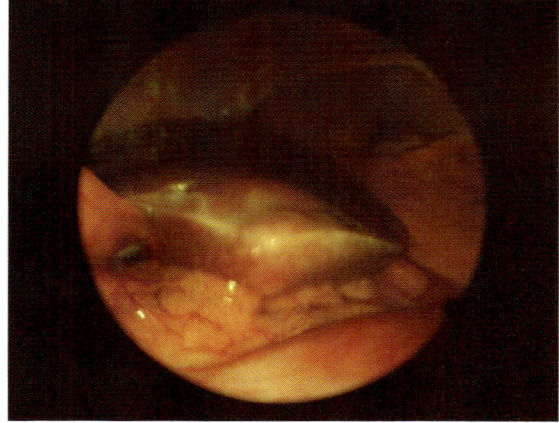

B

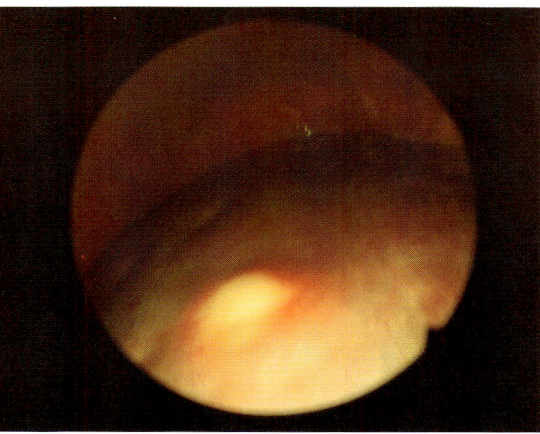

C

Figure 56-4.

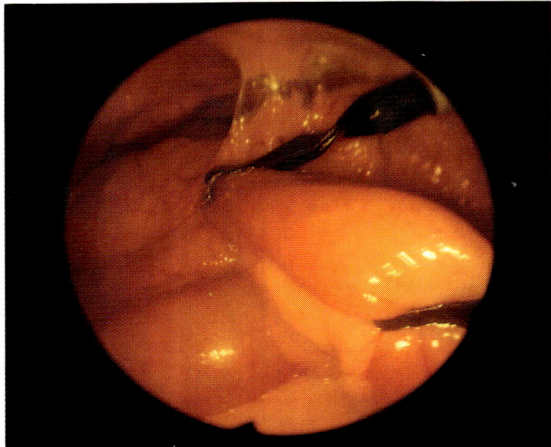

Figure 56-5.

Left Gutter and Left Pelvic Side Wall

The lateral fixation of the descending colon and sigmoid colon is easily exposed (Fig. 56-6). The patient is placed in a deep Trendelenberg position and the left shoulder is rotated up. The telescope is inserted through the supraumbilical port. The assistant on the right side of the patient retracts the sigmoid and descending colon medially and anteriorly with Babcock clamps. Traction on the colon moves the small bowel out of the way. Mobilization of the sigmoid is most easily observed on the monitor between the feet of the patient. Mobilization of the descending colon is better viewed on the monitor near the left shoulder of the patient.

Mesorectum and Right Pelvic Sidewall

These structures are exposed by positioning the patient in a deep Trendelenberg position and by rotation of the right shoulder up. The sigmoid and rectum are retracted to the left side and anteriorly with Babcock clamps. The small bowel is pulled out of the pelvis with atraumatic instruments and pushed cephalad (Fig. 56-7). If the angle of the table is adequate, the small bowel will roll up toward the transverse colon and remain out of sight. Sometimes the cecum and terminal ileum are fixed near the pelvic brim by congenital attachments or inflammatory adhesions. Under these circumstances, these points of fixation are divided. The mesentery of the terminal ileum and cecum is mobilized sufficiently so that the inclination of the table provides force for these structures to roll out of view. On occasion, the mesentery of the terminal ileum is so foreshortened or so fat that the inclination of the table does not provide sufficient exposure. The small bowel is then retracted cephalad with Babcock clamps or shielded out of the pelvis with fan-like retractors. The telescope is passed into the abdomen through the right lateral port at the level of the umbilicus. Dissection is observed on the monitor between the legs of the patient.

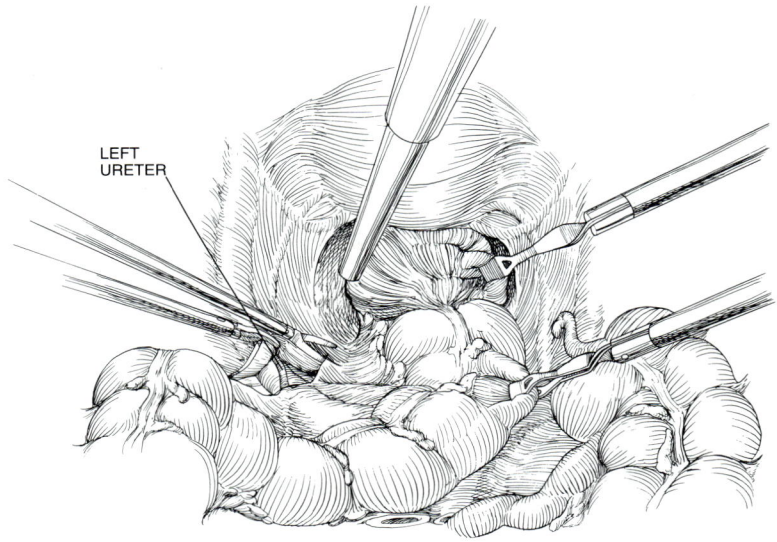

Figure 56-6.

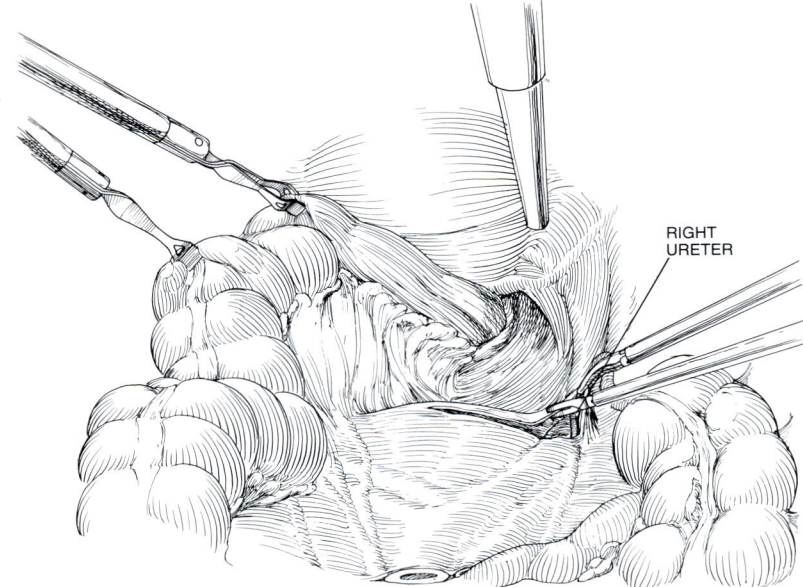

Figure 56-7.

High ligation of the inferior mesenteric artery requires a different orientation. The origin of the vessel is too near both the supraumbilical and cephalad right lateral ports for satisfactory visualization. The telescope is moved to the caudad right lower quadrant port. Rotation of the right shoulder down may better slide the small bowel away from the midline. The dissection is viewed on the monitor by the patient's left shoulder.

Presacral Space

Exposure of the presacral space requires anterior traction on the rectum and cephalad retraction on the rectosigmoid. Often this is easily accomplished with two Babcock clamps. This method, however, ties up both hands of the assistant. An alternative method is to suspend the rectum from the anterior abdominal wall with a suture. A long Kieth needle with a heavy suture such as 0 silk is passed through the abdominal wall just above the pubis (Fig. 56-8). Most of the suture is pulled into the abdomen. An ENDO DISSECT* instrument, which has been passed through the mesorectum near the rectal wall, is used to grasp the tip of the Kieth needle and pull it through the mesentery. The Kieth needle is passed back through the abdominal wall near its initial entry point. The suture is pulled tight and clamped. This pulls the rectum up against the anterior abdominal wall.

The mesorectum hangs below the rectum like a curtain. The superior hemorrhoidal vessels are retracted anteriorly away from the sacral promontory and concavity of the sacrum (Fig. 56-9). The surgeon supplements this retraction by pushing the mesorectum away from the sacrum with a blunt instrument. The dissection of the presacral space is viewed with a telescope passed into the abdomen through a right lateral port. Both the surgeon

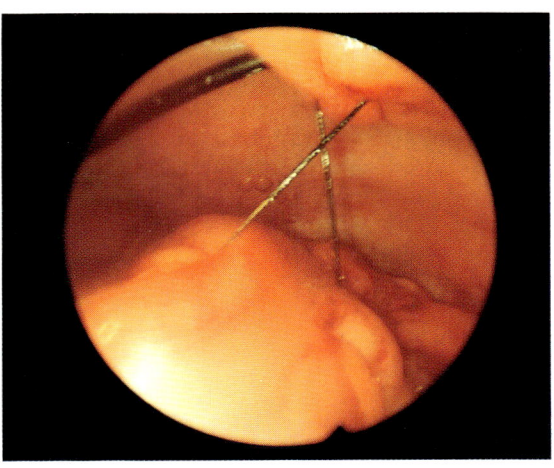

Figure 56-8.

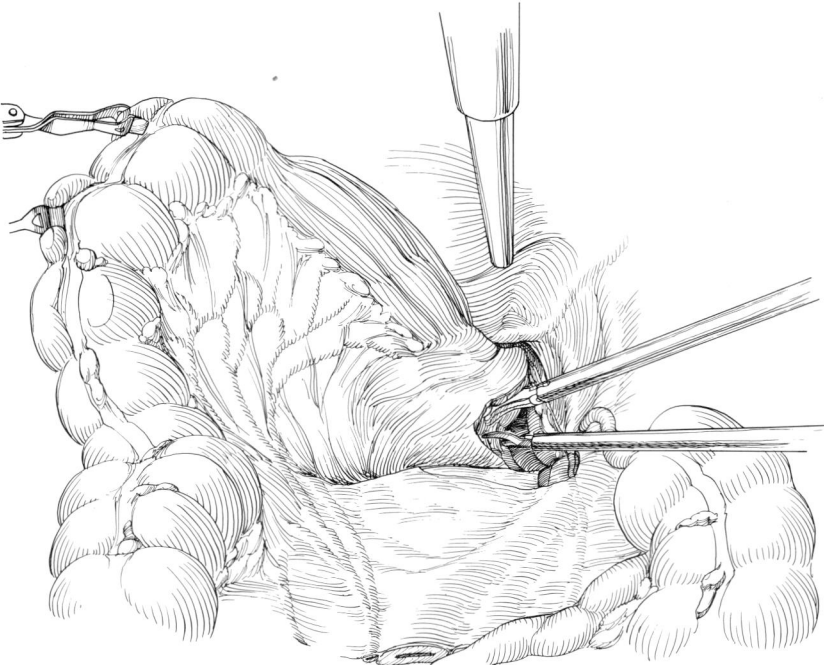

Figure 56-9.

and assistant face the monitor between the legs of the patient.

Anterior Pelvic Dissection

Exposure of the anterior pelvic dissection is difficult. In men, the patient is in a deep Trendelenberg position. Rotation first in one direction and then the other may be helpful. A finger or rigid proctoscope in the rectum can provide posterior traction on the rectum. This is aided by a Babcock clamp on the posterior cut edge of the parietal peritoneal reflection. Anterior countertraction, however, is difficult to obtain. A small hook-type retractor such as the ENDO MINI-RETRACT* instrument often achieves this goal. It may be necessary to place an additional suprapubic port to attain the correct angle of retraction. The telescope is introduced through the supraumbilical port. The dissection is watched on the monitor between the patient's legs.

In women, the task is somewhat simplified. Posterior retraction is achieved with a finger in the rectum. Excellent anterior retraction is maintained with a finger in the vagina. A Babcock clamp is placed on the posterior cut edge of the peritoneal reflection as in men. The uterus, however, often obscures the view of the anterior dissection between the rectum and vagina. The uterus is suspended from the abdominal wall with a suture. A Kieth needle is used as described previously for suspension of the rectum.

METHODS OF DISSECTION

Dissection is achieved with electrocautery scissors. Meticulous cauterization of even tiny vessels facilitates the operation since even small amounts of blood stain the tissues and obscure planes of dissection. Particularly during the pelvic dissection, the operative field should be frequently irrigated with heparinized (2000 to 3000 units/liter) saline and aspirated. This keeps the field clean and prevents clot formation. Clots are troublesome since they are difficult to remove, and they obstruct the lumen of the small caliber laparoscopic suction devices. The perineal dissection is accomplished by the technique to which the surgeon is accustomed.

Abdominal Perineal Resection

SPECIFIC DETAILS OF THE PROCEDURE

Mobilization of the Sigmoid

The patient is dropped into a deep Trendelenberg position. The left shoulder is rolled up. The 10-mm 0-degree telescope is inserted through the supraumbilical port. The dissection is followed on the video monitor between the patient's feet. The assistant surgeon grasps the rectosigmoid junction and apex of the sigmoid loop with two Babcock clamps from the right side of the table. The surgeon frees the sigmoid colon from its lateral attachments with electrocautery scissors and provides countertraction with a grasping instrument such as an ENDO DISSECT* instrument. Once the peritoneal reflection is incised along the white line of Toldt, the mesosigmoid is easily bluntly pushed toward the midline. The long shafts of the scissors and graspers accomplish this task. The lateral incision is extended over the pelvic brim down along the left wall of the pelvis to the midline in the anterior rectovesicle or rectovaginal pouch. The mesorectum is pushed medially by the surgeon. Even apparently avascular sheets of tissue are cut with cautery. Small amounts of blood stain the tissue planes and obfuscate structures.

Identification of the Left Ureter

The ureter is identified as soon as possible (Fig. 56-10). In thin patients, it may be visible through the transparent posterior parietal peritoneum. Otherwise it is pursued by the same techniques as commonly used in open procedures. If it is not identified where it crosses the common iliac artery, the descending colon is mobilized medially, and the ureter is sought in the retroperitoneum nearer to the kidney. Preoperative placement of illuminated ureteral stents facilitates localization of the ureter. When the intensity of the laparoscopic light source is turned down, the lighting of the stents becomes visible. Laparoscopic ultrasound devices might also prove helpful in verification of the location of the ureter.

Entering the Presacral Space

The table remains in a deep Trendelenberg position. The right shoulder is rolled up. The telescope remains in the supraumbilical port. The surgeon moves to the right side of the table. The assistant grasps the proximal rectum and distal sigmoid with two Babcock clamps. The surgeon pulls out with atraumatic bowel clamps any loops of small bowel that remain in the pelvis. If necessary, adhesions between the small bowel and sigmoid are incised. The surgeon applies countertraction to the retroperitoneum with a grasping instrument and incises with electrocautery scissors over the sacral promontory. The areolar tissue in the avascular presacral plane is found.

Dissection follows this areolar plane deep into the pelvis along the sacrum. The telescope dives down into the presacral space as the dissection advances (Fig. 56-11). The magnified views of the pelvic dissection represent the greatest dividend provided by a laparoscopic approach to this operation. The posterior peritoneum is incised down into the pelvis along the sidewall until the midline of the anterior rectovesicle or rectovaginal pouch is reached (Fig. 56-11). The right ureter is identified. If necessary for adequate exposure, the rectum is suspended from the abdominal wall with a suture as described previously. The arch of the inferior mesenteric artery and its extension as the superior hemorrhoidal artery are generally visible within the mesosigmoid and mesorectum anterior to the sacral promontory. Transillumination of the mesentery with a second telescope passed through one of the left lower quadrant ports clarifies the position of these vessels.

The primary telescope is moved to a right lateral port since retraction of the rectum out of the pelvis obstructs the view through the

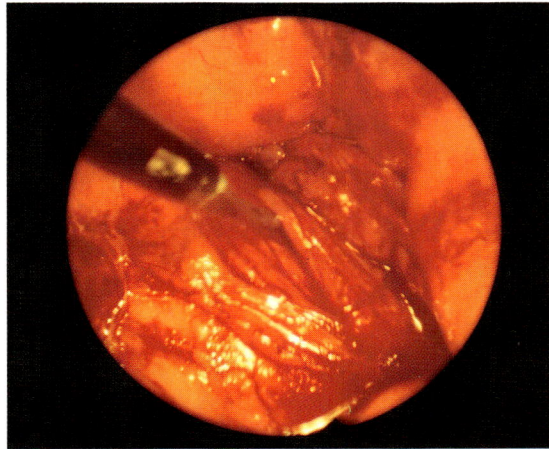

Figure 56-10.

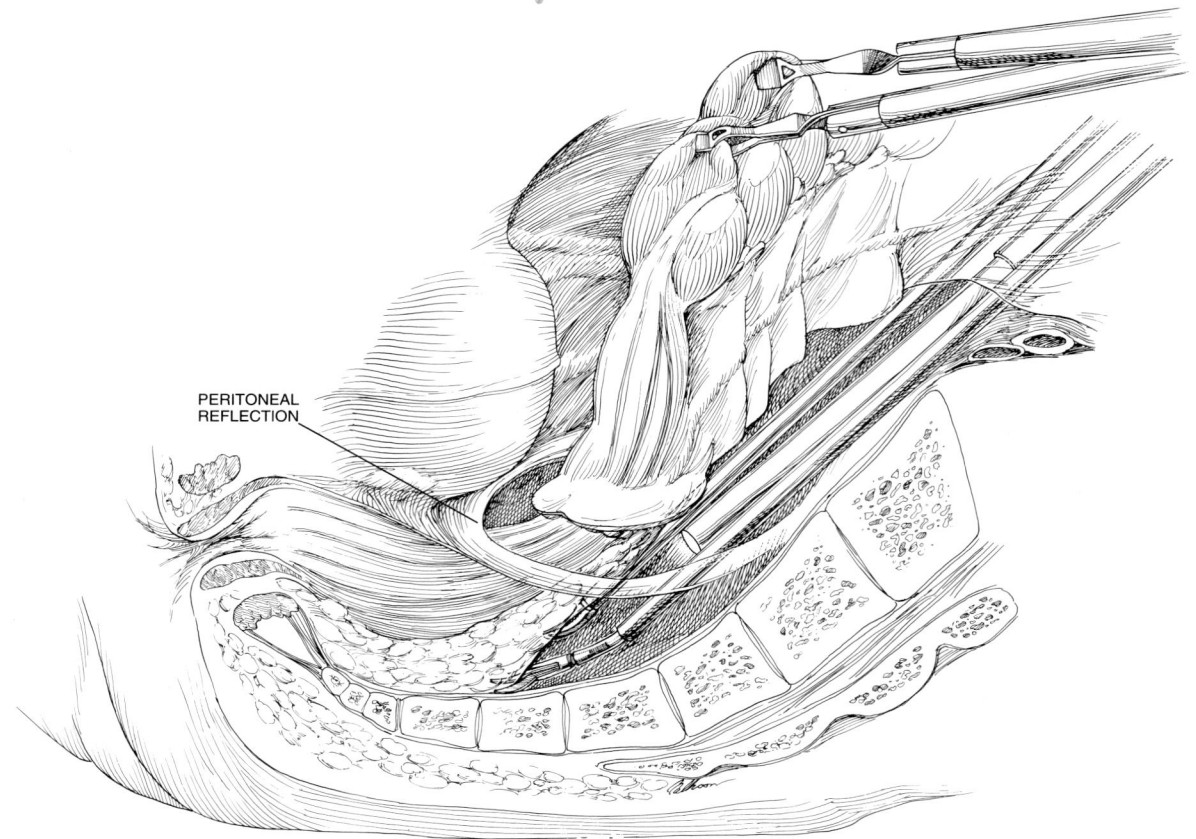

Figure 56-11.

supraumbilical port. The plane of dissection on the right side of the pelvis is connected with that of the left through the presacral space. The second telescope allows observation of the left ureter as the two planes are connected. Hemostasis is diligently maintained with the electrocautery scissors.

Ligation of the Superior Hemorrhoidal Vessels

Ligation of the blood supply of the rectum early in the procedure limits blood loss during the pelvic dissection. The superior hemorrhoidal vessels are isolated and skeletonized at the level of the sacral promontory (Fig. 56-12). Alternatively, the inferior mesenteric artery can be ligated near its origin if that is the custom of the operating surgeon. The 10-mm port in the right lower quadrant, which provides nearly perpendicular access to the superior hemorrhoidal vessels, is replaced with a 12-mm port. The thickness of the bundle of tissue is calibrated with the ENDO GAUGE* device. The appropriate size of cartridge is selected. The ENDO GIA* 30 stapling device is used to ligate and divide the vascular pedicle (Fig. 56-13). It places a total of six rows of staples, three on each side of the incision. Before the stapling device is fired, its tips are inspected with the second telescope to make sure that no extraneous tissue is included within its jaws. The location of the left ureter is confirmed.

In some patients, however, early division of the colon facilitates identification of the inferior mesenteric artery and superior hemorrhoidal vessels. In obese patients, adequate exposure of these vessels may be difficult. Once the colon is divided electrocautery dissection proceeds down the mesosigmoid to the root of its mesentery. The combination of freeing the mesosigmoid from over the sacral promontory and division of the mesosigmoid leaves the inferior mesenteric and superior hemorrhoidal vessels exposed at the apex of these two lines of dissection. When exposure

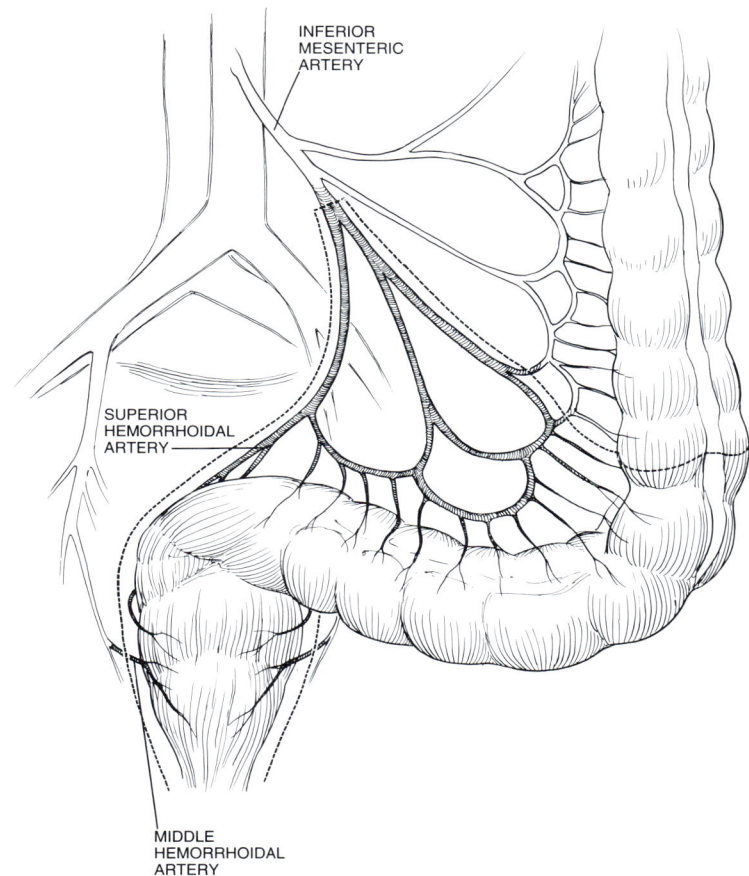

Figure 56-12.

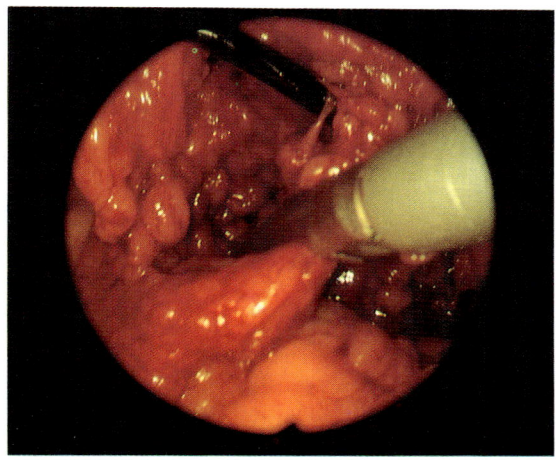

Figure 56-13.

of these vessels is unusually difficult, the perineal surgeon can run his or her hand up along the sacrum and elevate the vascular pedicle off of the sacral promontory. The laparoscopic surgeon then divides the vessels with the ENDO GIA* 30 stapling device.

Anterior Pelvic Dissection

The patient remains in a deep Trendelenburg position. The suture suspending the rectum from the abdominal wall is loosened. The primary telescope is inserted through the supraumbilical port. A finger in the rectum or a rigid sigmoidoscope applies posterior traction. The incisions in the peritoneum on the left and right side of the pelvis are connected anteriorly in the rectovesicle or rectovaginal pouch. The rectum is retracted toward the sacrum with a Babcock clamp attached to the posterior edge of the cut parietal peritoneum.

In men, the bladder is retracted anteriorly with an ENDO MINI-RETRACT* device. An additional suprapubic port provides a better angle of the mechanical effort for the retractor. The posterior wall of the bladder and vasa deferentia are retracted anteriorly (Fig. 56-14). Denonvilliers' fascia is incised. It is difficult to dissect this plane laparoscopically down to the level of the prostate because of difficulty with visualization with the telescope. If the plane is opened laparoscopically from above, the dissection can be completed by the perineal dissector.

In women, a finger in the vagina provides anterior retraction. The uterus is suspended from the abdominal wall with a suture. The tactile sensations of the two fingers inserted in the rectum and vagina can help direct the advance of dissection. If necessary, the perineal surgeon completes the anterior dissection.

Division of the Lateral Stalks

The table is in a deep Trendelenburg position. The patient's right shoulder is rolled up for dissection of the right side of the pelvis and the left shoulder is rotated up for the left side. The telescope obtains the best angle of view for the right sidewall dissection from a right lateral port and for the left dissection from the supraumbilical port (Fig. 56-15). The assistant retracts the rectum out of the pelvis and laterally with two Babcock clamps from the side of the table opposite to the surgeon. The lateral suspensory ligaments are divided under direct visualization with electrocautery scissors. Indeed, the magnification and closeup views, which are generated by the video system, project an image of the lateral stalks vastly more detailed than what is observed during an open operation. The inferior mesenteric vessels are divided between clips. The pelvic dissection proceeds easily down to about the middle of the rectum. Complete dissection down to the level of the pelvic floor from above is difficult early in one's experience with this technique. The perineal dissector can complete whatever part of the dissection is not accomplished by the laparoscopic surgeon. Moreover, a synchronous dissection by two teams will decrease the duration of the operation.

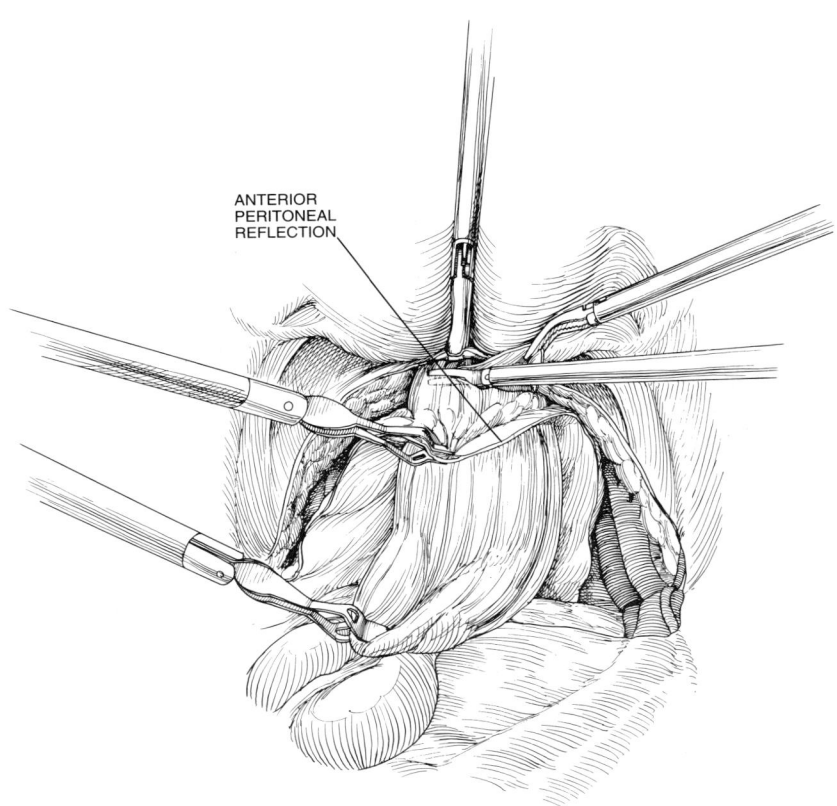

Figure 56-14.

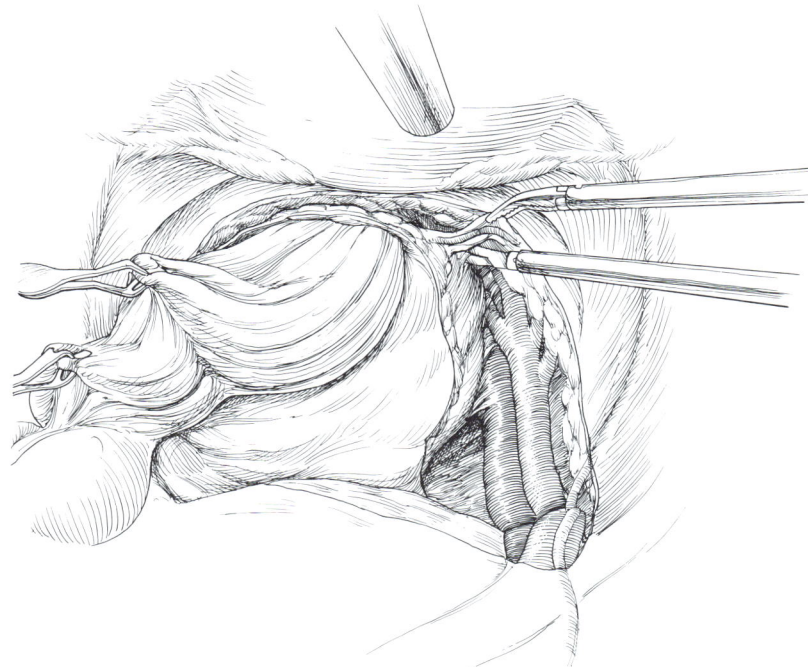

Figure 56-15.

Transection of Proximal Colon

Retraction of the rectum out of the pelvis is more easily accomplished while the colon and rectum remain in continuity. After division of the colon, the proximal end may obscure the pelvic dissection by sliding down into the pelvis. Transection of the colon is accomplished before initiation of the perineal dissection. Loss of gas through the perineal wound may compromise the pneumoperitoneum and interfer with exposure.

The patient remains in a deep Trendelenburg position. The small bowel is rolled away from the left colon by rolling up the left shoulder of the patient. The telescope is passed through a right lateral port. The second telescope is passed through a left lateral port. The surgeon, on the right side of the patient, views this maneuver on the monitor near the patient's left shoulder. The colon is grasped and elevated with two Babcock clamps placed proximally and distally to the selected point of transection (Figs. 56-16 and 56-17). The colon is aligned perpendicularly to the right lateral 12- or 15-mm port. It is not necessary to open a window in the mesentery before the bowel is divided. The thickness of the colonic wall is measured with the ENDO GAUGE* device. The proper cartridge is selected. The stapling device is applied to the bowel. The tips of the stapling device are observed with the secondary telescope. The stapler is fired, and the staple lines are inspected for hemostasis.

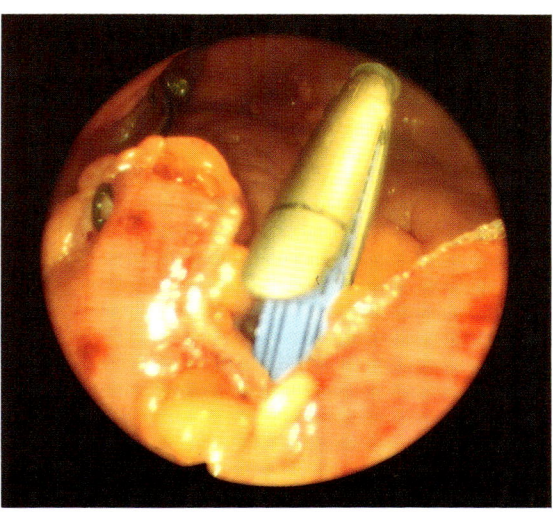

Figure 56-16.

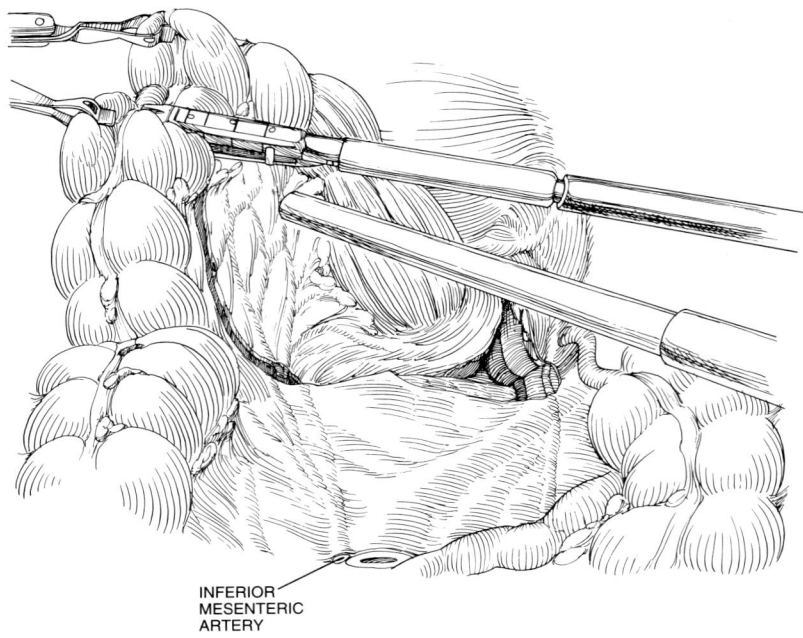

Figure 56-17.

Division of the Mesosigmoid

The mesosigmoid is divided either with the ENDO GIA* stapling device or electrocautery scissors and clips. The arcades of vessels near the colonic wall are most rapidly divided and ligated with the ENDO GIA* 30 device. It is then generally possible to follow a relatively avascular plane along the side of a sigmoid artery down to the root of the mesentery. When this avascular plane is not evident, one application of the ENDO GIA* 60 stapling device will usually divide and ligate most if not all of the mesosigmoid. The speed of this technique compensates for the expense of the stapling device. Alternatively, the mesentery is scored with the electrocautery scissors. Individual vessels are isolated, clipped, and divided. In thin patients this is rapidly accomplished, but in obese patients it may be tedious and time consuming.

Perineal Dissection

The perineal portion is approached in the same manner as with the traditional procedure. The anus is closed with a purse-string suture of 0 silk. An incision is made through the skin around the circumference of the anus. The edges of the perianal skin are grasped with Kocher clamps. The incision is extended down through the subcutaneous fat, through the ischiorectal fossa, to the level of the levators (Fig. 56-18). The inferior hemorrhoidal vessels are ligated and divided. The presacral space is entered anteriorly to the coccyx. The anococcygeal ligament is divided. A finger is slid into the presacral space. This finger slides along the superior aspect of the levator muscles freeing the mesorectum. The levators are pulled down with the finger and divided with electrocautery at the desired level.

After division of the anococcygeal ligament and the levators, the superficial transverse perineal muscle is divided (Fig. 56-19). The anterior surface of the rectum is freed in a plane at the posterior border of the deep transverse perineal muscle. The rectourethralis and puborectalis are divided.

Presacral Dissection

The perineal surgeon slides a hand with palm up behind the rectum into the presacral space. The hand easily advances cephalad along the sacrum in the avascular plane posterior to Waldeyer's fascia (Fig. 56-20). The perineal surgeon initially enters the laparoscopic plane of dissection posteriorly along

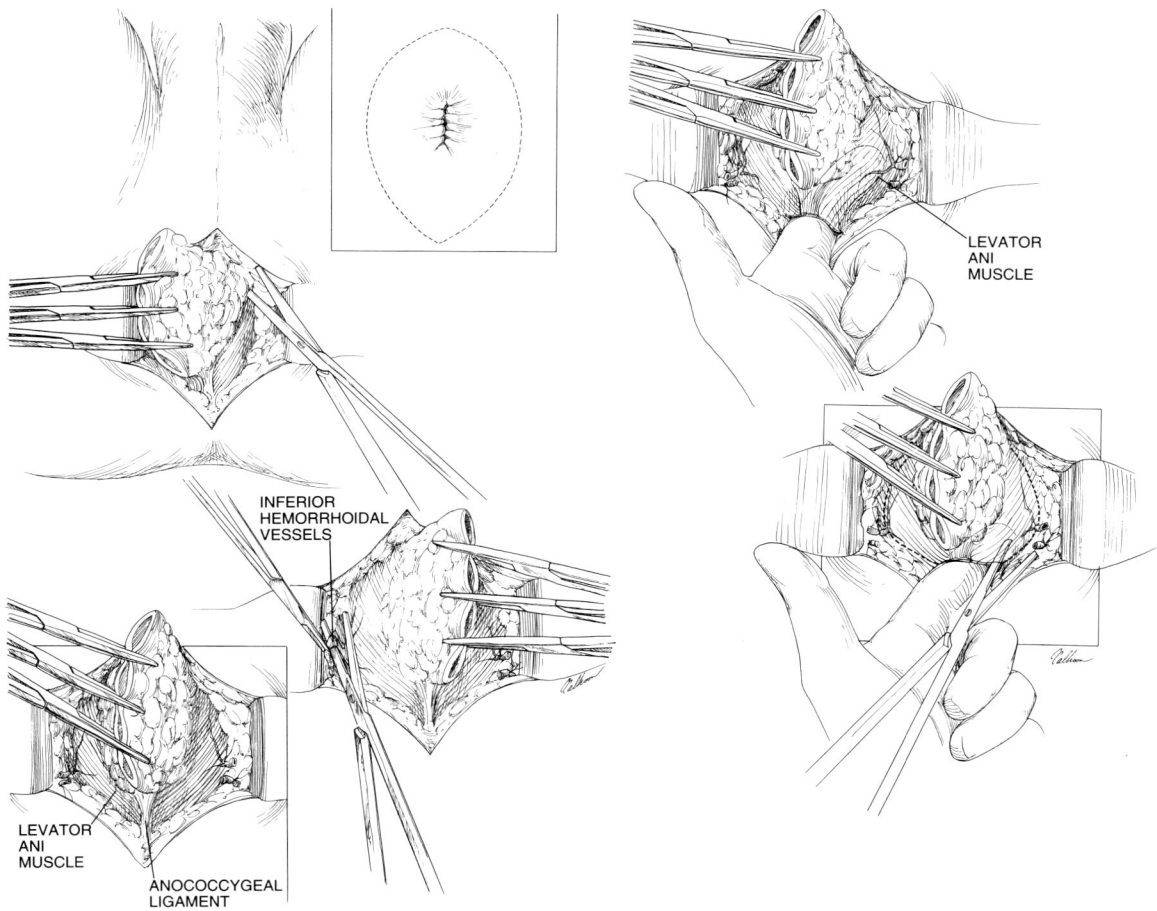

Figure 56-18.

the sacrum. This ensures that the ureters are not inadvertently injured. If Waldeyer's fascia has not been incised during the laparoscopic dissection, it is tented up by the fingers of the perineal surgeon. Under direct observation, Waldeyer's fascia is incised by the laparoscopic surgeon with electrocautery scissors. The bulk of the perineal surgeon's hand forms an airtight seal of the perineal wound and the pneumoperitoneum is maintained. This allows completion of the pelvic dissection with combined laparoscopic and blunt dissection. During combined dissection, the laparoscopic surgeon frequently checks the position of the ureters. Traction on the rectum may displace the ureters down into the pelvis where the perineal surgeon may inadvertently injure them. The preoperative placement of stents also minimizes the chance of injury since the perineal surgeon is then able to palpate these tubes and recognize the ureters. The hand of the perineal surgeon provides strong traction on the rectum and mesorectum. The remainder of the lateral suspensory ligaments are divided if exposure of these structures was previously inadequate. Similarly, the middle hemorrhoidal vessels may be more easily isolated with the hand of the perineal surgeon. Under direct observation, the laparoscopic surgeon applies clips to these vessels and then divides them with scissors.

Completion of the Anterior Dissection

Visualization of the anterior dissection is difficult with the laparoscope. This is more easily completed by the perineal surgeon. The peritoneal reflection in the rectovesicle or rectovaginal pouch, however, must first be incised by the laparoscopic surgeon. When possible Denonvilliers' fascia is also incised by the laparoscopic surgeon. After division of the lateral suspensory ligaments, the perineal

620 Techniques of Laparoscopic Surgery

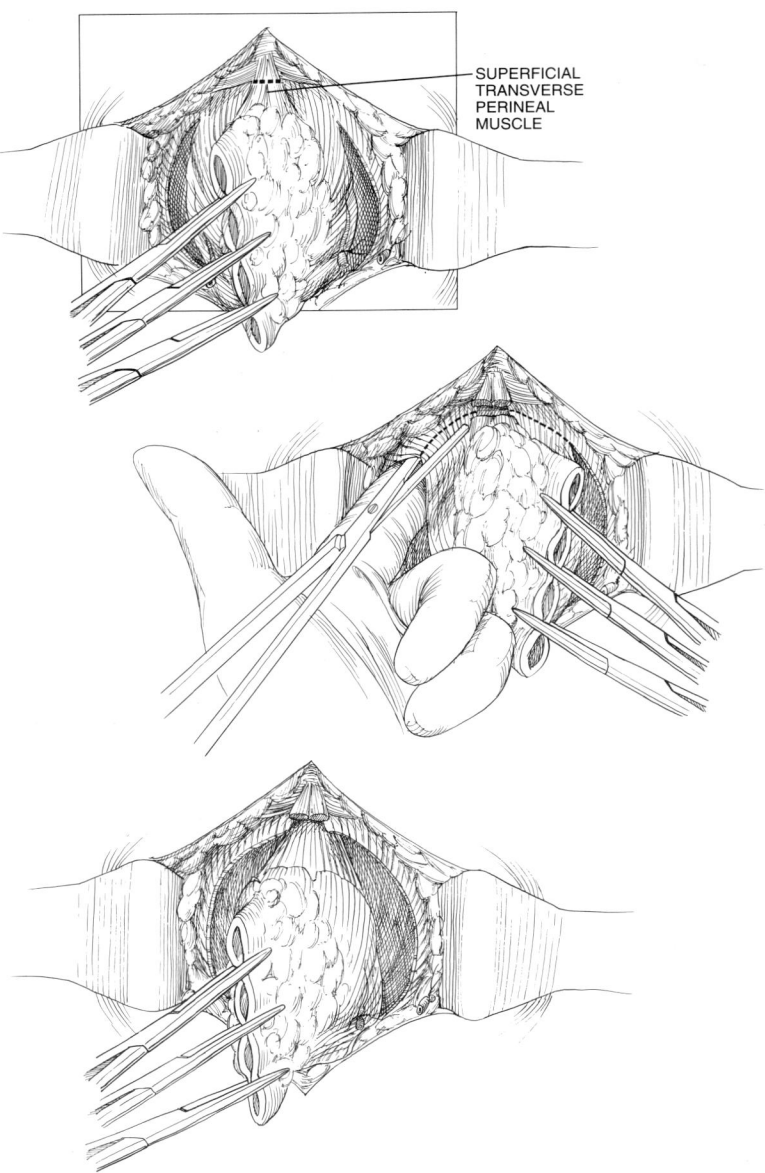

Figure 56-19.

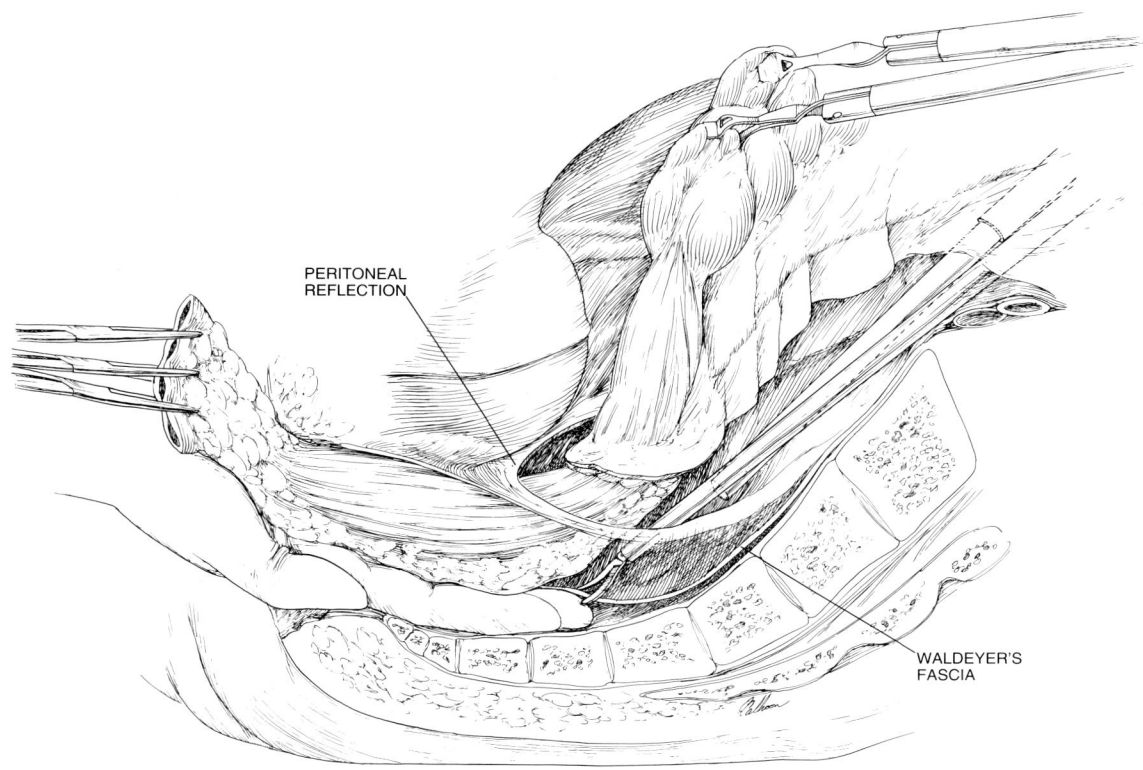

Figure 56-20.

surgeon slides a hand around to the front of the rectum. The laparoscopic surgeon retracts open the plane between the rectum and bladder or vagina with Babcock clamps or other grasping instruments. The fingers of the perineal surgeon bluntly slide down the anterior surface of the rectum.

Delivery of the Specimen

The staple line on the proximal end of the specimen is grasped with a Babcock clamp by the laparoscopic surgeon and placed into the hand of the perineal surgeon. The perineal surgeon's hand is withdrawn from the pelvis along the sacrum. The specimen is pulled out and left suspended by its attachments to the prostate in men or posterior wall of the vagina in women (Fig. 56-21). These remaining points of fixation are divided with cautery. The specimen is removed and opened within the operating room by a surgical pathologist. The margins of resection are inspected and the adequacy of resection judged.

During removal of the specimen, the pneumoperitoneum is lost through the perineal wound. The telescope must be withdrawn from the abdomen. The fiberoptic cables generate enough heat to burn the bowel wall or other abdominal organs if the tip of the telescope remains in contact with the organ for a prolonged amount of time.

CLOSURE

Perineal Wound

The pelvis is liberally irrigated with warmed saline through the perineal wound. Hemostasis is checked. The perineal wound is closed by traditional methods. Two flat suction drains are passed into the pelvis through two stab wounds in the skin and through the levators. The stab wounds are placed anterior to a line between the ischial tuberosities. The levators are apposed with interrupted sutures of 00 Dexon. The subcutaneous tissues are irrigated with an antibiotic-containing solution. The skin is closed with a continuous subcuticular suture of 0000 Dexon. A sterile dressing is applied.

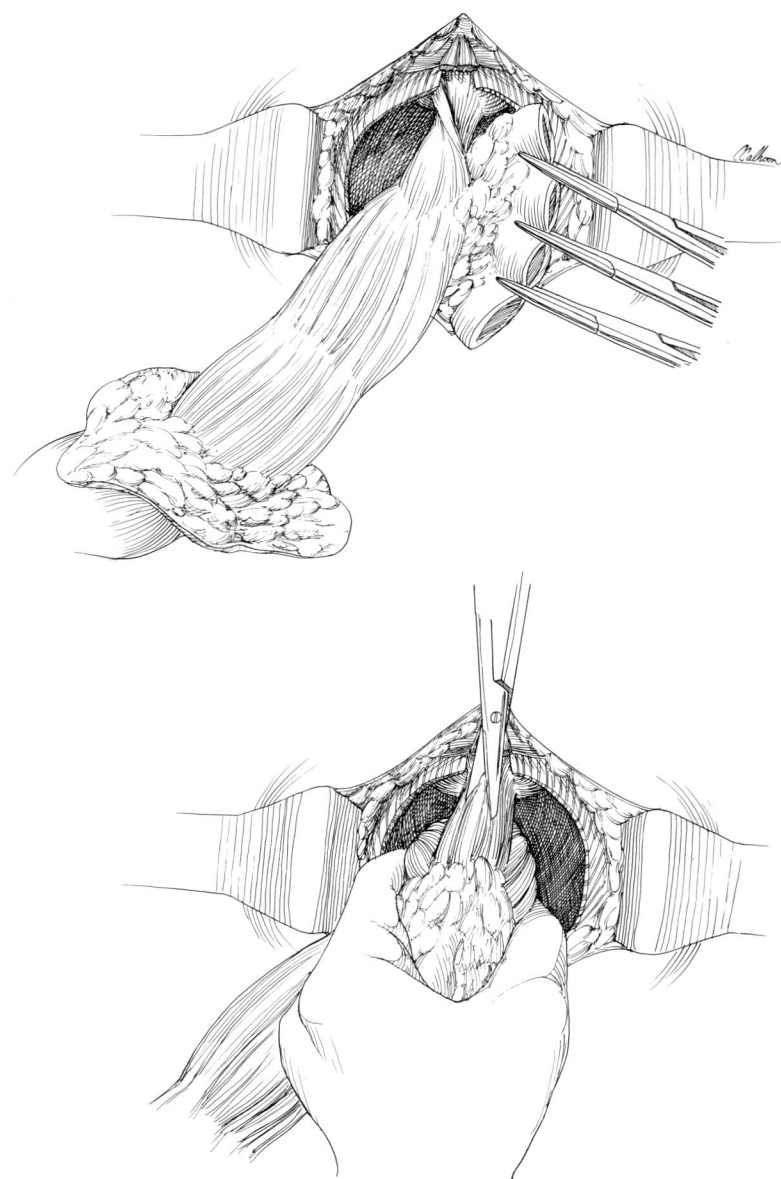

Figure 56-21.

Construction of the Colostomy

After the perineal wound is closed, the pneumoperitoneum is reestablished. The telescope is inserted through a right lateral port. The surgeon pushes against the previously marked stoma site with a finger. The indentation into the anterior abdominal wall produced by the finger is viewed on the video monitor. The stapled closure of the colon is grasped with a Babcock clamp and elevated toward the indentation caused by the finger (Fig. 56-22). The mobility of the colon is checked. If necessary more of the colon and mesosigmoid is freed from their retroperitoneal attachments.

The surgeon grabs the center of the colostomy site with a Kocher clamp. A disc of skin and subcutaneous fat is excised down to the level of the anterior rectus sheath. A cruciate

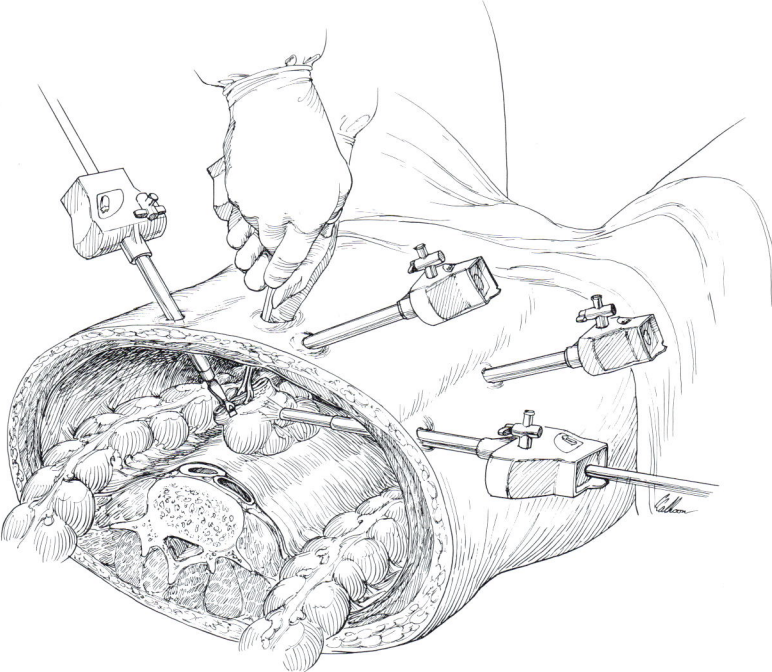

Figure 56-22.

incision is made in the anterior rectus sheath. A blunt clamp separates the fibers of the rectus muscle along the course of its fibers. A small stab wound is made through the posterior rectus sheath and anterior parietal peritoneum. The surgeon rapidly jabs a finger through this incision into the abdominal cavity. The finger seals the wound. The pneumoperitoneum is maintained. The surgeon introduces a Babcock clamp into the abdomen along the finger (Fig. 56-23). Under direct observation through the laparoscope, the stapled end of the colon is hoisted up to the stoma site. The surgeon clenches the staple line with the Babcock clamp. The mesentery of the colon is checked for tension and torsion. If necessary, remaining sigmoid branches are divided so that a tension-free colostomy is constructed. The colon is not pulled through the wound until the pneumoperitoneum is collapsed. Fixation of the colostomy prior to deflation may lead to excessive mobilization of the colon predisposing to prolapse of the stoma. Prior to extraction of the end of the colon, the ports are removed and fascial defects inflicted by ports 10-mm and larger are closed.

The incision in the posterior sheath is widened. The closed end of the colon is extracted. After all other wounds are closed, the staple line is excised. The colostomy is matured. Eight sutures of 000 chromic catgut fix the colostomy to the skin. Each stitch encompasses all layers of the edge of the colon and fixes the colon to the subcuticular layer of skin. There should be no tension on the colostomy. A stoma appliance covers the colostomy.

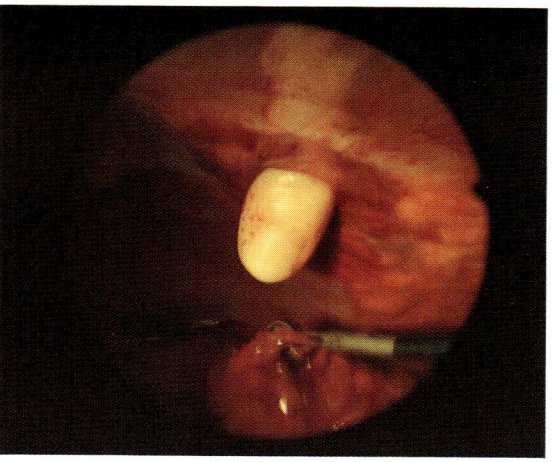

Figure 56-23.

Laparoscopy Wounds

The laparoscopy wounds are closed prior to maturation of the colostomy. After deflation of the pneumoperitoneum, the working ports are removed. The anterior fascia is closed with 00 Dexon in wounds generated by ports 10 mm in size or larger. The telescope is withdrawn. The last port is extracted. The skin edges of wounds created by smaller ports are apposed with Steri-Strips. The larger skin incisions are closed with continuous subcuticular sutures of 0000 Dexon. The wounds are covered with Band-Aids.

POSTOPERATIVE MANAGEMENT

Postoperative care of patients following laparoscopically assisted abdominal perineal resections is identical to that used for patients following traditional open operations. The nasogastric tube is removed following the operation or on the first morning after the operation. The urinary catheter is removed on the fifth postoperative day. The intravenous catheter is removed when the patient is taking adequate amounts of fluid orally. Subcutaneous heparin is administered while the patient remains in the hospital. The pelvic drains are pulled out when the volume of drainage subsides. The enterostomal therapist reinitiates patient education on stoma care early in the postoperative course. The patient is discharged as soon as he or she tolerates a regular diet and can care for the stoma.

Patients tend to progress more rapidly after laparoscopically assisted abdominal perineal resections than after traditional open operations. These patients do not suffer with pain associated with large abdominal incisions. Consequently, they tend to ambulate sooner after the operation and tolerate a diet earlier. The decreased pain and diminished requirement for narcotics may account for these differences in the postoperative course following laparoscopic operations.

COMPLICATIONS SPECIFIC FOR THIS PROCEDURE

Specific rates of complications following laparoscopically assisted abdominal perineal resection are not as yet established. It remains to be determined whether blood loss, fluid requirements, cardiovascular stress, and pulmonary compromise are diminished by the use of laparoscopic techniques. Since a large abdominal incision is avoided, wound complications should be decreased. The attenuated level of pain experienced by the patient may minimize the level of postoperative compromise of pulmonary function. In contrast, the rates of complications of the colostomy, perineal wound, and perineal sepsis are likely to remain unchanged.

Chapter 57
Herniorrhaphy

John D. Corbitt Jr.

Philip Mouret of Lyons, France, in 1987 was the first noted physician to remove a gallbladder laparoscopically.[1] This laparoscopic procedure was introduced in the United States in 1988. By 1992 it had gained widespread popularity and is now the accepted procedure of choice for removal of the diseased gallbladder.

Five hundred thousand cholecystectomies are performed each year in the United States, and an equal number of herniorrhaphies are also reported.[2] The enthusiastic response to laparoscopic cholecystectomy was not seen for the laparoscopic repair of the hernia, probably because cholecystectomy is a definitive procedure. Once the gallbladder has been removed successfully the patient is cured, and long-term follow-up is not necessary. Unfortunately, patients with herniorrhaphies must be followed on a long term basis to ascertain the efficacy of a repair.

A review of the literature indicates a significant recurrence rate with a groin approach using different types of repairs. The two exceptions to the high recurrence rate may be the Lichtenstein repair[3] and the preperitoneal approach described by Stoppa and Warlaumont.[4] Although these latter types of repairs are associated with a lower recurrence rate, they continue to have the disadvantage of the groin approach, using an incision in the inguinal area. The excellent results obtained with laparoscopic cholecystectomy, such as decreased pain, improved cosmesis, and a rapid return to normal activity, made it apparent that the laparoscopic herniorrhaphy should be considered. Although laparoscopic herniorrhaphy is in the early developmental stage, results would indicate that it is a viable, rewarding procedure with a low early recurrence rate.

HISTORICAL PERSPECTIVES OF HERNIA REPAIR

The classic inguinal herniorrhaphy was originally described by Bassini in 1884, since which time multiple modifications, such as the Shouldice, the McVay repair or the Ferguson repair, etc., have been attempted to improve the original herniorrhaphy. Despite modifications, these repairs still are associated with at least a 10 per cent recurrence rate. Despite being anatomically sound, most of the modifications of the Bassini repair place tension on the suture line. This tension is thought to contribute to the high recurrence rate. A significant reduction in the recurrence rate of all inguinal hernia repairs has been reported by Lichtenstein[3] using a prosthetic mesh to reconstruct the floor of the inguinal canal in a tension-free manner. For his most recent personal series of 1000 patients, he reports a recurrence rate approaching zero (personal communication). In a larger series of

7133 repairs on patients from nine different institutions, Lichtenstein in 1990 reported a recurrence rate of 0.28 per cent.[3] The follow-up on these patients was as long as 20 years. Stoppa and Warlaumont[4] and Nyhus et al.[5] have reported a preperitoneal approach to hernia repair, again using a prosthetic mesh to cover the floor of the inguinal canal. Their recurrence rate of 1.4 to 1.7 per cent (572 and 203 repairs), respectively, corresponds to the low recurrence rate reported by Lichtenstein. This repair is also considered a tension-free repair.

Another historical perspective of inguinal herniorrhaphy taken into consideration in the early development of laparoscopic herniorrhaphy was the work of Henry Marcy.[6,7] This American surgeon advocated that high ligation of the sac and closure of the internal ring were of paramount importance in preventing recurrence. Little was reported about the recurrence rate for this procedure, which was the first transabdominal approach to hernia repair. LaRoque modified Marcy's repair but still utilized a transabdominal approach.[8-10] He performed over 1700 of these procedures; however, LaRoque's follow-up was not published and his recurrence rate in this large series is unavailable.

Popp[11] in 1990 reported the first laparoscopic hernia repair in which a patient undergoing a myomectomy was found to have a hernia. This hernia was repaired with a piece of dehydrated dura mater secured to the floor with catgut ENDO SUTURES* tied extracorporeally over the internal ring. Ger[12,13] of New York also reported a series of 13 patients undergoing laparotomy for other reasons, who were noted to have hernias. In 12 of these patients hernias were repaired by using Michelle clips and a Kocher clamp to close the peritoneal opening of the hernia. In the 13th patient the hernia was closed laparoscopically using the "herniastat," an instrument developed by Ger. In this series, as well as a laboratory series using beagle dogs, the hernias were repaired leaving the distal sac in place. In Ger's patient series, a long term follow-up in excess of 5 years indicates that some patients died, but in those that continued to be followed hernias did not recur with this procedure, with the exception of one patient who had a recurrence following a repair of a direct inguinal hernia (personal communication). Hydroceles were not noted in any of the patients being followed, and the beagle dogs, which were used in the experimental phase of this procedure, were later sacrificed and found to have obliterated hernia sacs.

Leonard Schultz (personal communications)[14] of Minneapolis, Minnesota, began the first large series of laparoscopic herniorrhaphies in 1989 by placing a plug in the inguinal canal and a patch over the internal defect. Access was gained into the properitoneal area through an incision over the superior portion of the defect whether it was a direct or indirect hernia. Taking into consideration the work of Marcy and LaRoque, Corbitt[15] added high ligation of the sac in the indirect hernia and in those direct hernias containing a pseudosac. High ligation of the sac was originally accomplished using a pretied laparoscopic loop (ENDO LOOP*), and later the ENDO GIA* stapling device (United States Surgical Corporation). Both of these repairs took into consideration the work of Lichtenstein, Stoppa, and others, which resulted in a tension-free prosthetic repair. The patients were allowed to return to normal activity on the day following their hernia repair. Unfortunately, long term follow-up of those patients indicated a recurrence rate in excess of 20 per cent in both series (L. Schultz, personal communication). However, those patients who did not have an early recurrence and were examined over a 3-year period appeared to have an extremely good repair. Consequently, it seemed possible that a modification of this repair might result in an excellent laparoscopic approach with an acceptable recurrence rate.

Of greatest benefit in examining this series of early laparoscopic herniorrhaphies was the indication that an outpatient, pain-free repair could be performed, allowing the patient to return to normal activity rapidly. Equally significant was the absence of complications associated with all transinguinal approaches, such as wound infections, hematomas of the abdominal wall and testicles, injuries to the spermatic cord, ischemic orchitis, epididymitis paresthesia and neuralgias, and a prolonged, painful recovery period. In the early series, on a significant number of occasions, bilateral inguinal hernias were noted when only one hernia had been found preoperatively. Thus, it became clear that laparoscopy also offered improved diagnostic abilities because of the advantage of easy viewing of the unsuspected contralateral hernia.

LAPAROSCOPIC HERNIORRHAPHIES

After examination of the original laparoscopic plug, patch, and high ligation of the sac concept of hernia repair, it was evident from the high recurrence rate that this was not a satisfactory repair. Therefore, it was felt that a modification of this early concept of hernia repair should be examined in hopes of obtaining an ideal repair with less than a 1 per cent recurrence rate.

Intraperitoneal Approach

At the present time there are two major strategies for laparoscopic herniorrhaphy. The simplest approach is that of the "onlay" or intraperitoneal procedure. Fitzgibbons, Salerno et al.[16,17] originally worked in the laboratory, using onlay grafts in animals, which were later sacrificed to evaluate the procedure. In their clinical series they began using Marlex mesh as an onlay graft in both the direct and indirect inguinal hernias (personal communication). After early recurrence in some patients with the direct defects, they abandoned that procedure for the direct defect, but utilized the onlay procedure in the repair of the indirect inguinal hernia.

Toy and Smoot[18] and Spaw[19] are among other advocates of the intraperitoneal approach. In their procedure, Gor-Tex (polytetrafluoroethylene) is used as a prosthetic material and, at the present time, both direct and indirect hernias are being repaired with an intraperitoneal onlay graft with variations of the procedures.

The onlay procedure is performed by insufflating the abdomen to 15 mm Hg through an umbilical incision following which a laparoscope is introduced through this incision. With the use of two other ports, usually placed in a line at the level of the umbilicus but lateral to the rectus sheath, a graft is manipulated under direct vision over the hernia to be repaired. Depending upon the author describing the procedure: (1) the sac may either be left in place with the graft simply placed over the sac; (2) the sac may be reduced into the abdominal cavity with high ligation using either a pre-tied suture or the ENDO GIA* stapling device; or (3) a 360-degree circumferencial incision is made around the neck of the larger sacs leaving the distal sac in place, but exposing the preperitoneal area in this area of the inguinal floor only. The prosthetic material is then placed over the area of the defect and is stapled or sutured to the deep structures through the peritoneum. The peritoneum remains intact in the onlay repair, except as indicated previously. The size of the mesh varies depending upon the author's description of the procedure, but generally covers the area of the defect overlapping by 2 to 3 cm on all sides. In some instances, both the direct and indirect spaces are covered despite having only one or the other type of hernia present.

After a short term follow-up a high recurrence rate was noted (25 per cent) by Spaw, Toy and Smoot (personal communication) if a small graft was used and if it was attached only to the peritoneum. To decrease this unfavorable outcome a large graft which covers both the direct and indirect space has now replaced the smaller prosthesis in most "onlay" procedures. Many recurrences were noted in the medial aspect of the repair. Therefore, most surgeons using the intraperitoneal onlay method (IPOM) are now exposing Cooper's ligament and attaching the graft directly to this ligament or to the inguinal ligament medially. Use of the larger graft and exposure of the medial structures has reduced the recurrence rate of the IPOM repair to 2–5 per cent. The distal sacs of the indirect space hernias are now being left in place to avoid injury to the cord structures in this latter series.

The benefit of this procedure is that it may be done rapidly with little concern for the details of anatomy of the local area. It also avoids dissection of the preperitoneal structures, thus avoiding the complications associated with this part of the procedure. The disadvantages of this procedure are the exposure of the graft material to the intraabdominal contents, which may result in future adhesions and associated complications. Fitzgibbons[20] (personal communication) has suggested discontinuing the IPOM repair due to early postoperative complications associated with adhesions between the mesh and small intestines until these patients can be followed closely and further information becomes available. Other authors have not had this unfavorable experience (Toy, Smoot, Spaw, etc.). Nonetheless, this repair has only the stability of a prosthetic material being attached to deep structures in the areas to which it is sutured or stapled. In other areas it relies on the integrity of the peritoneum to hold the prosthetic mesh in place. How well the prosthetic material is attached to the underlying structures will determine whether the prosthetic material, along with the peritoneum, will slide back into a newly formed hernia defect, causing a prosthetic-lined recurrent hernia. Exposure of the medial structures (Cooper's ligament and the inguinal ligament) should drastically improve the onlay results.

This IPOM repair may be performed by capable laparoscopic surgeons without a great deal of additional training. The repair is simple to understand and has minimal complications associated with it. The recurrence rate with this new laparoscopic repair, however, remains to be determined.

Preperitoneal and Extraperitoneal Repair

The second and more tedious method of laparoscopic herniorrhaphy consists of a preperitoneal approach, which is advocated by this author,[21] M. Arregui,[22,23] J. Petlin (personal communication), and others. A method similar to the preperitoneal technique has been described by B. McKernan[24,25,26] (personal communication) and E. Phillips[27] (personal communication) and consists of an extraperitoneal approach to the same area.

To perform an extraperitoneal approach, the extraperitoneal area may be accessed by one of two methods. The first method, as described by McKernan, consists of placing a Hasson trocar into the umbilicus and the extraperitoneal area. The extraperitoneal space is then insufflated to 8 mm Hg pressure. The operating laparoscope is introduced through the Hasson cannula into this space, and dissection is performed by additional ports being placed under direct vision of the laparoscope, into the extraperitoneal space. Phillips, on the other hand, chooses to begin his approach by a standard intra-abdominal insufflation and initial placement of the laparoscope into the abdominal cavity. Under direct vision a Veress needle is placed into the extraperitoneal space which is insufflated with carbon dioxide to 8 mm Hg pressure. The scope is withdrawn and placed into the extraperitoneal space through the umbilical incision, and additional ports are put into place. With these additional ports the extraperitoneal dissection and the graft placement are carried out in a manner similar to that described later under the preperitoneal approach.

In most patients older than 50 years of age, both sides are repaired despite the absence of a hernia on the contralateral side. This is done because once the extraperitoneal space has been entered, it would be almost impossible to return to this area at a future date should a hernia occur on the then normal side.

Because of the difficulty of dissection in the area of the spermatic cord as will be described under the preperitoneal approach, an incision is made in the posterior graft to drape around the testicular vessels, the vas deferens, and iliac vessels. The same area of the inguinal floor, however, is covered by the graft and will further be described under preperitoneal repair. This graft is likewise tacked or sutured in place. This approach allows the graft to adhere to substantial structures in the preperitoneal space, and the abdominal contents are protected from the graft by the intact peritoneum covering the graft. Because of the difficulty in visualizing the structures in the preperitoneal space using the extraperitoneal approach, this method must be abandoned on occasions and would appear to be an extremely difficult procedure to teach the average laparoscopic surgeon. It can, however, be mastered by most surgeons with some time and effort. It is suggested that the transabdominal preperitoneal (TAPP) approach be mastered prior to the extraperitoneal approach.

It is the opinion of this author that the preperitoneal tension-free (TAPP) herniorrhaphy is the ideal laparoscopic procedure for repair of indirect, direct, and recurrent hernias at this time. One disadvantage of this approach is that complete understanding of the vital structures in the floor of the inguinal canal, as well as the iliac vessels is necessary. An additional disadvantage is that the surgeon has to dissect this area with the risk of invading these structures. It is a difficult procedure to learn initially, but after the surgeon becomes familiar with the anatomical structures, the repair may be done in a reasonable period of time (Fig. 57-1). The transabdominal preperitoneal laparoscopic herniorrhaphy has the advantage of direct visualization of all structures concerned. A portion of mesh covers the pelvic floor, which will include both the direct and indirect space, regardless of which type of hernia is present (Fig. 57-2). An additional advantage is the fact that the graft is attached in all areas to substantial fascial structures, including the transversalis fascia, iliopubic tract, or Cooper's ligament, with the expectation that these structures will firmly hold the graft in place. With this procedure, only the side containing the defect need be repaired and, should the patient develop a hernia on the contralateral side, it may be repaired in a similar manner at a future date. Therefore, disturbance of a normal inguinal floor is avoided.

Patient Selection

Laparoscopic tension-free preperitoneal inguinal herniorrhaphy can be performed in all the lack of postoperative pain despite repair of both sides. Physician referral and patient demand will soon produce a large number of laparoscopic herniorrhaphy requests from all patients.

Preoperative Evaluation

Patients should be evaluated for general anesthesia, although the use of epidural anesthesia is presently being investigated. Patients usually do better when the procedure is done under general anesthesia. If anesthesia is contraindicated, then an alternate repair should be considered.

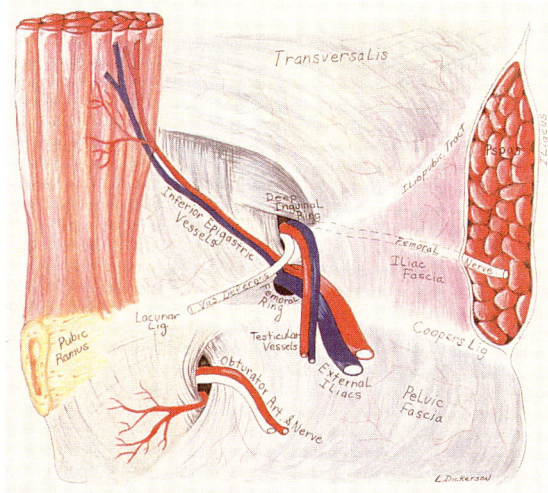

Figure 57-1. Schematic diagram of the pelvis indicating the important anatomical structures as well as the area of the direct and indirect hernia defect.

Preoperative Preparation

The patient should place a scopolamine patch on the postauricular area on the night prior to surgery. This, combined with 10 mg of Reglan given perioperatively has virtually eliminated postoperative nausea and vomiting. Routinely, a prophylactic long acting antibiotic is also administered preoperatively. This precaution is taken because of the use of a prosthetic mesh and may, in the future, be found to be unnecessary. However, at the present time most surgeons who perform this procedure deem it advisable. The patient is not shaved for this or other laparoscopic procedures, eliminating the uncomfortable regrowth of hair during the early postoperative phase. A protective barrier (Steri-Drape) is

patients with hernias regardless of size. These hernias include direct, indirect, and recurrent hernias (Fig. 57-3 through Fig. 57-7). (Femoral hernias may still be repaired with a modified plug and patch procedure, which will be described later but may also be repaired with the TAPP method.) Although all hernias may be repaired laparoscopically, the major indicators are the recurrent hernia (Fig. 57-8), because the anatomy is still preserved laparoscopically, and the bilateral hernia, because of

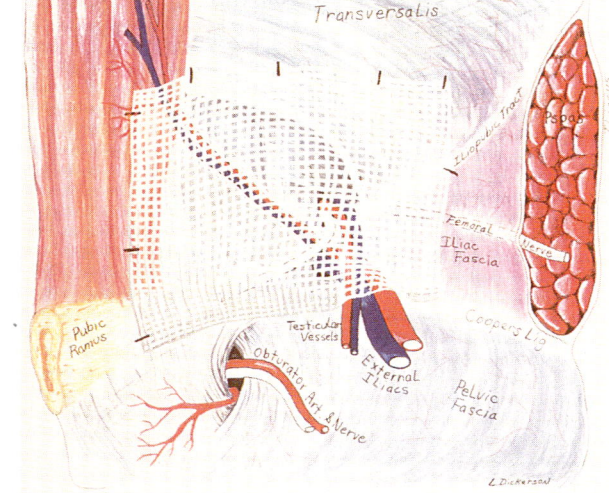

Figure 57-2. Proper mesh placement and peripheral staple placement. Additional staples may be placed in the body of the mesh as long as these staples are anterior to the iliopubic tract and do not compromise the important anatomical structures.

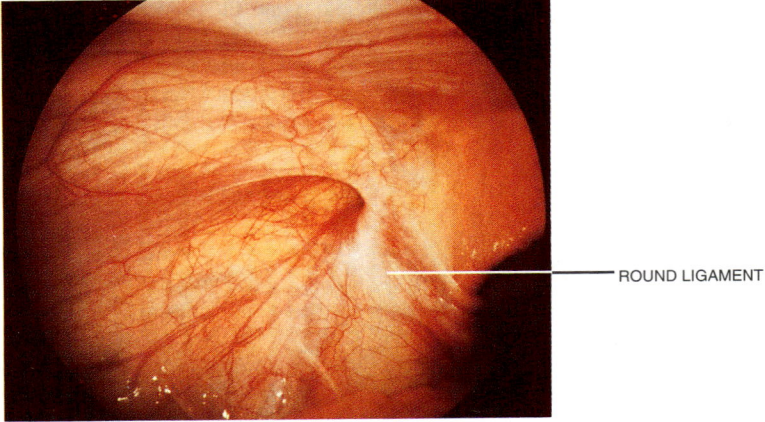

Figure 57-3. Left indirect inguinal hernia in a female.

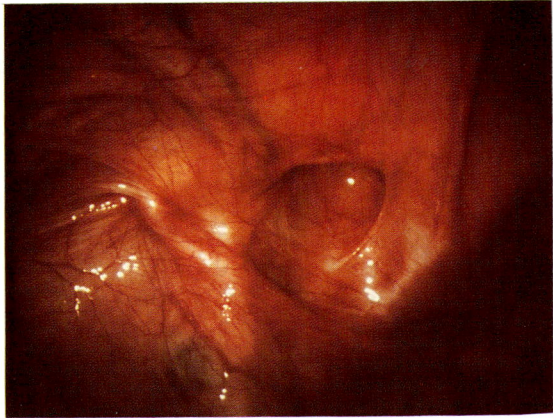

Figure 57-4. Left direct inguinal hernia.

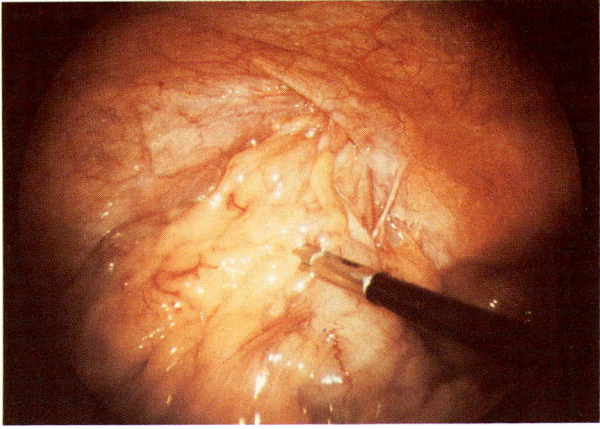

Figure 57-5. A sliding left inguinal hernia.

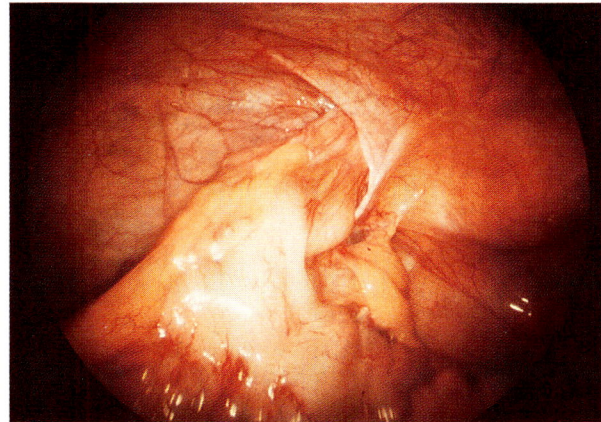

Figure 57-6. Reduction of sliding left inguinal hernia.

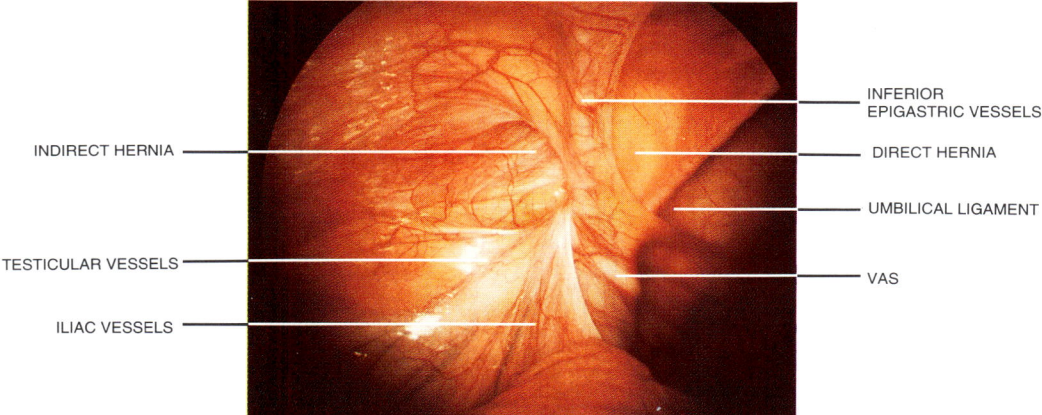

Figure 57-7. Left pantaloon hernia. Sac of the indirect component would be left in place. The direct sac would be reduced.

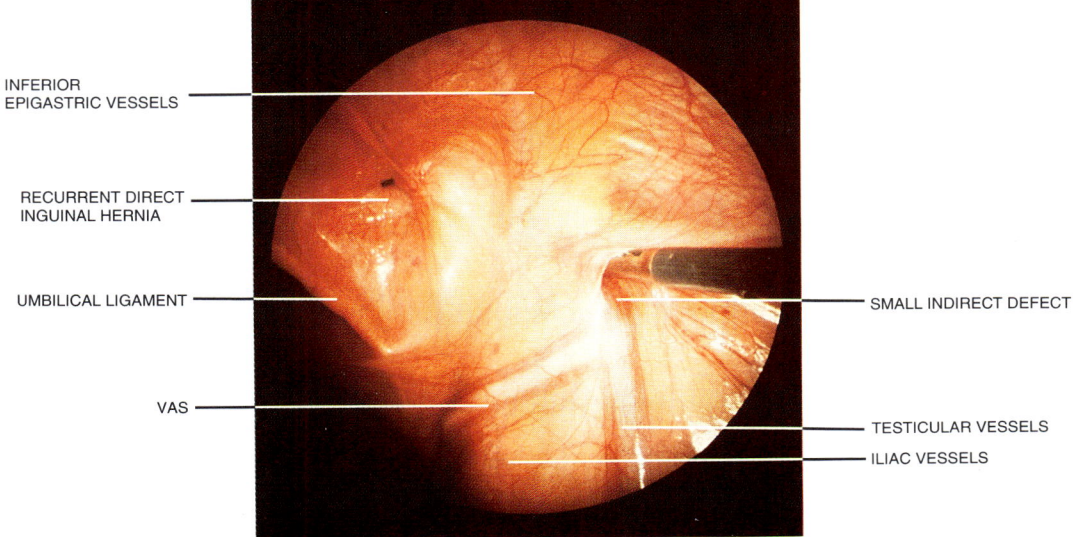

Figure 57-8. A recurrent direct inguinal hernia showing the preservation of the anatomy of the inguinal area.

used, however, in the draping process to isolate hair from the incisions.

Positioning of the Patient

At present, these laparoscopic herniorrhaphies are carried out with the patient placed in the Trendelenburg position. The patient may be rolled slightly to the right or left to further expose the area of the hernia, with rotation of the patient away from the hernia being repaired.

Trocar Placement and Size Selection

A 12-mm incision is made in the umbilicus, and an insufflation needle is used to insufflate the abdominal cavity to 15 mm Hg pressure. A 12-mm surgical port is then inserted through this incision. Through this port, a 10-mm laparoscope is inserted with a 0- or 30-degree lens, to observe the direct placement of additional ports (Fig. 57-9).

During the procedure use of the 30-degree lens has been found to be beneficial in some cases and will be of great benefit later when the stapling of the mesh is directly visualized. The 5-mm accessory ports are placed at the level of the umbilicus in a smaller patient or slightly inferior to the umbilicus in a larger patient to allow access to the pelvis for the dissecting instrument. The ports are placed lateral to the rectus sheath to avoid injury to the rectus muscle and postoperative hematoma. In cases where a 5-mm laparoscopic camera is not available, 10-mm ports may be substituted for the 5-mm ports and the same laparoscopic camera may be used throughout the procedure. However, it has been observed that use of 5-mm ports minimizes the patient's postoperative pain, lessens the chance of postoperative hematoma, and is extremely cosmetic. Meticulous care is taken in maintaining hemostasis during the pelvic dissection, so that the 5-mm camera will continue to allow adequate light and visualization of the areas concerned. The 10-mm laparoscope will be used during all dissection and placement of the graft. Only during stapling of the graft will the 5-mm laparoscope be utilized. The alternative secondary port placement for a surgeon performing a two-handed procedure is one port lateral to the rectus at the level of the umbilicus on the surgeon's side and the second in the midline between the umbilicus and pubis.

Methods of Exposure and Dissection

Regardless of the side on which the hernia appears, generally a right-handed surgeon will stand to the left of the patient and a left-handed surgeon to the right of the patient. A transverse incision is made in the peritoneum across the top of the hernia defect. If the incision is kept anterior to the defect, it can be made with little probability of damage to important structures. The only anterior structures that need to be protected are the inferior epigastric vessels. The transverse incision extends from the umbilical ligament medially, to the approximate area of the anterior superior iliac spine laterally. Although the dissection medially may extend beyond the umbilical ligament, the boundary of the peritoneal incision is found to be adequate if it is limited medially by the umbilical ligament (Fig. 57-10).

When the incision is extended laterally, palpation of dissecting instruments through

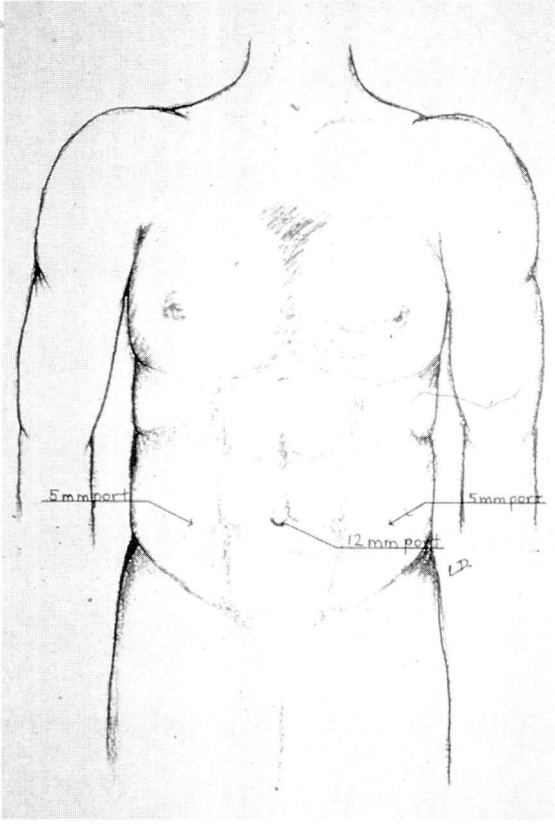

Figure 57-9. Port placement.

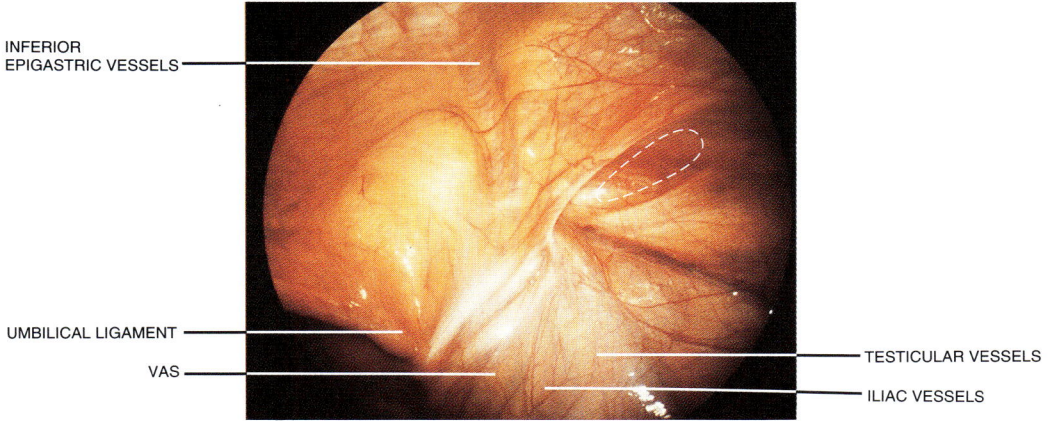

Figure 57-10. The right inguinal hernia showing important anatomical landmarks and the upper boundary of the transverse incision. The indirect sac in this hernia is amputated with a 360 degree circumferencial incision.

the anterior abdominal wall would indicate the extent of the incision. The tendency is for this incision to be extended far beyond the anterior superior spine and to gradually progress anteriorly rather than stay horizontal across the pelvis.

After the transverse incision is created, the posterior peritoneum is initially dissected to expose the entire floor of the pelvis. The anterior peritoneum is not dissected at this time because of its tendency to interfere with vision after it has been loosened from the anterior abdominal wall. Countertraction is placed on the posterior peritoneum, and a dissecting instrument (Kittner dissector) may be used to dissect the peritoneum free from all the structures in the pelvic floor or alternately traction and countertraction may be used to pull the perineum off of any structures that lie immediately under it. The most critical area of dissection is that which lies posterior to the iliopubic tract or inguinal ligament. This structure is the boundary of the posterior portion of the internal ring. It is more easily identified in the presence of an indirect hernia but still remains apparent when a hernia is not present. In the posterior portion of the indirect inguinal hernia or in the internal ring, the testicular vessels may be noted to run posteriorly and the vas deferens will tend to cross medially. Below these important structures, the iliac vessels are readily apparent through the laparoscope. It is this dissection and anatomical identification that are most important in the preperitoneal or extraperitoneal approach to hernia repair. These structures must be identified and carefully dissected during this stage and, during the latter portion of the repair, avoided when a stapling instrument is used to secure the mesh.

After the entire posterior portion of the inguinal floor has been identified, the anterior peritoneum may now be easily dissected. The inferior epigastric vessels are left attached to the abdominal wall and the peritoneum is easily removed from them. Again, this area consists of the only significant anterior structures to be avoided throughout the dissection.

In the original repairs, the fascia and the areolar tissue covering the floor of the pelvis in the preperitoneal area were left intact; however, at the present time all of this tissue is being removed to expose substantial fascia on which the graft will be placed. If a small lipoma is encountered, it may be left in place but a larger lipoma should be removed. When the initial transverse incision is made, as previously described, it may be placed across the superior aspect of the direct or small indirect hernia. However, if a large pseudosac is present in a direct defect or the patient has a large indirect inguinal hernia, a 360-degree circumferential incision is made inside the hernia defect to leave the distal sac in place. The great majority of the direct sacs are reduced with peritoneal dissection (Figs. 57-11 and 57-12). This 360-degree incision should not be made flush to the abdominal wall or there will be a hole in the peritoneum at the time the peritoneal tissue is reapproximated. Dissection of the distal sac, particularly with large indirect scrotal hernias, increases the chance of scrotal hematomas, injury to the cord structures or genito-femoral nerve, and

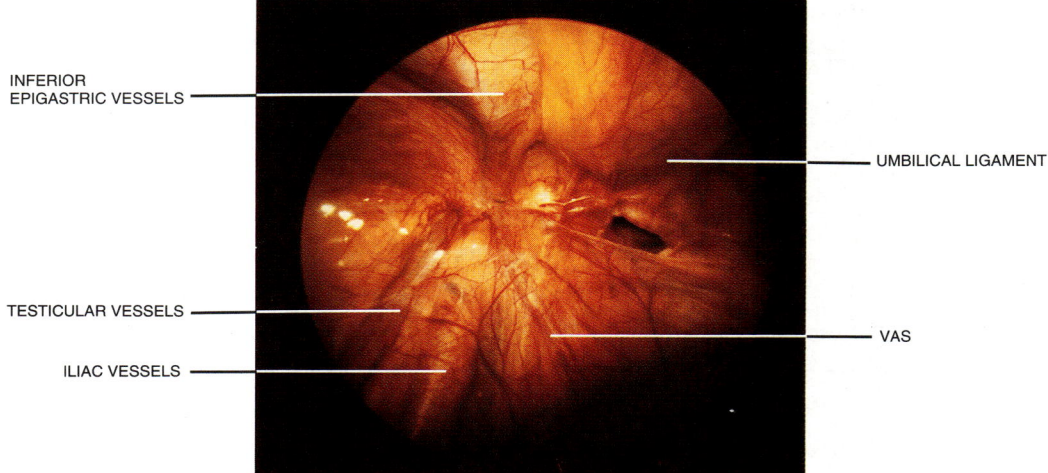

Figure 57-11. Left direct inguinal hernia.

confusion of the anatomical structures as the sac is reduced into the abdominal cavity. Leaving the distal sac in place will not cause a future hydrocele to occur. Smaller sacs may be reduced into the abdominal cavity and the procedure carried out as described previously.

Specific Details of the Procedure

After complete exposure of the entire inguinal floor, a prosthetic material may now be introduced into the abdominal cavity.

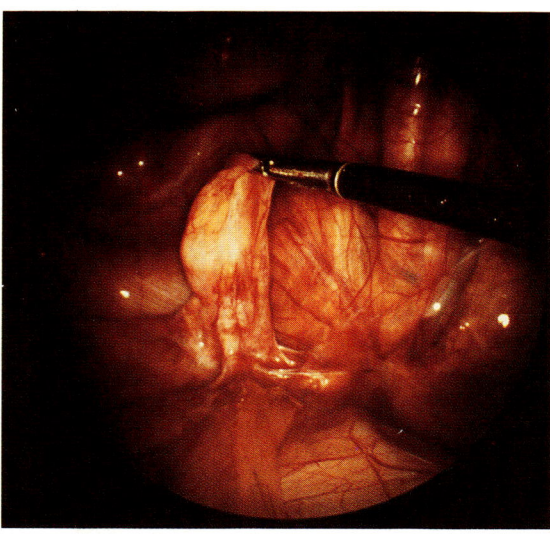

Figure 57-12. Reduction of the sac of a direct inguinal hernia.

Originally, Marlex was used for this procedure with excellent results; however, the present Marlex has a tendency to curl, making it somewhat difficult to lay onto the inguinal floor. A polypropylene mesh, SurgiPro, newly developed by United States Surgical, is now being used with excellent results. This mesh comes in a standard 3 by 5 inch size, which has been found to be the proper size mesh in over 90 per cent of patients. This larger piece of mesh should be used and may be adjusted in the smaller patient by increasing the area of dissection of the anterior and lateral peritoneal flap, if necessary. This mesh has the property of adhering to a moist surface, thus staying in place on the inguinal floor until it has been secured with staples. This adherence to the abdominal wall allows for easy adjustment into proper position.

Prior to insertion of this mesh, a plastic surgery marking pen is used to draw a horizontal line across the long axis of the mesh and vertical lines an inch from the margins on each end of the mesh. This "H" shaped diagram will allow the mesh to be positioned in a perfectly horizontal plane and at the time of stapling will allow exact identification of the location of important structures beneath the mesh, which need to be avoided. The graft is inserted into the abdominal cavity by removing the 10-mm camera and forcing the graft through the 12-mm port, which is pointed toward the pelvis. If SURGIPRO* mesh is used, it is not necessary to backload the mesh into a reducer prior to inserting it into the abdominal cavity.

After the mesh has been introduced into the pelvis, the 10-mm camera is then again placed into the 12-mm umbilical port, and the graft is positioned properly. If the secondary ports are 10-mm, the graft may be inserted through one of these ports and the laparoscope left in the umbilical port. The graft is allowed to cover the defect and extends from the area of the pubis medially to the area of the anterior superior iliac spine laterally. It extends from the transversalis fascia anteriorally down to and beyond the iliopubic tract or inguinal ligament posteriorly. The graft is allowed to drape over the iliac vessels, which is the only area in which the areolar tissue has been retained. Direct contact with these vessels is avoided by leaving this areolar tissue intact.

After the graft is positioned satisfactorily by the surgeon, the umbilical laparoscope is now removed and one of the 5-mm ports is used laterally for the camera. The 10-mm camera is replaced by a 5-mm angled laparoscope, which is inserted into the 5-mm port on the contralateral side of the hernia to observe and direct the placement of the staples into the graft. If 10-mm secondary ports are used, the 10-mm 0-degree lens may be replaced with a 30-degree laparoscope to have better access to the medial portion of the graft when it is being stapled to the pubic area. It is imperative that the staples are visualized when placing them directly into the graft to avoid injury to structures in the preperitoneal area. The "triangle of doom," consisting of the testicular vessels, vas deferens, and iliac vessels, must be visualized at all times. The autostapling devices now used to secure the graft are multifiring instruments capable of angulation.

The graft is usually secured by placing an anterior row of staples first. The surgeon's hand may be placed on the abdominal wall to allow counterpressure and easier seating of the staples into the anterior abdominal wall (Fig. 57-13). Using the stapler at 30–60 degrees will facilitate placement of these staples. A dissector is used through the secondary port on the side of the hernia to manipulate the graft and place it on tension when necessary, prior to putting additional staples in place. The ENDO* Universal 60° Stapler allows prepositioning of the staple, if necessary, and by placing one limb of the staple in the graft the stapler is used to move the graft into proper position prior to completing the firing of this staple. Two different staples are now manufactured. The 4.8-mm staple should be used when fixing the mesh to all fascia.

After placement of the anterior staples the lateral staples, or, if more convenient, the medial staples may be placed. The lateral staples extend over to the area of the anterior superior iliac spine. Medially, the staples are placed into the area of the pubic tubercle. In this area fixation of the mesh to the pubic tubercle and Cooper's ligament requires the use of the shorter, stronger 4.0-mm staple. The same staple gun may be used for both staples by changing the disposable loading unit (DLU) to the appropriate size staple.

With the graft secured on three sides, the posterior portion of the graft, which is the area of most concern, must be secured. The graft is tacked to the inguinal ligament (iliopubic tract) and to Cooper's ligament (Fig. 57-14). It is only necessary to place a few staples in the graft along this posterior boundary. Staples are not used posteriorly in the area of the iliac vessels, spermatic vessels, and vas deferens (triangle of doom). These are avoided throughout the procedure and injury to them represents the major concern with complications. A small vein and artery (the iliopubic vessels) consistently traverse Cooper's ligament and should also be

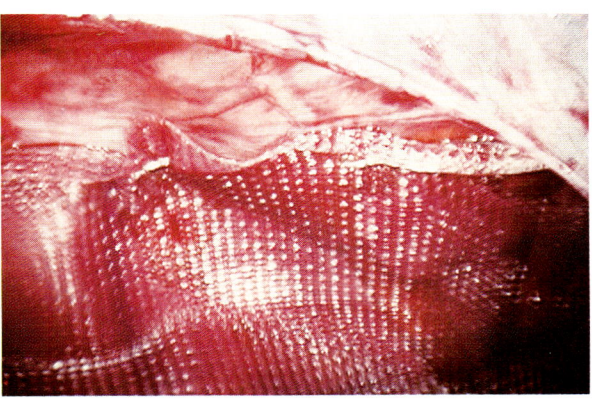

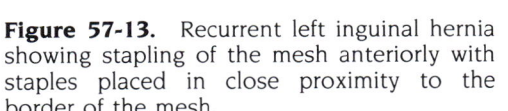

Figure 57-13. Recurrent left inguinal hernia showing stapling of the mesh anteriorly with staples placed in close proximity to the border of the mesh.

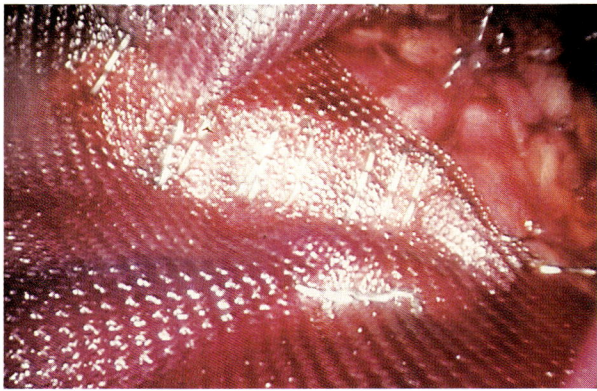

Figure 57-14. Multiple staples securing the mesh to Cooper's ligament.

avoided. This vein is of little significance other than being capable of producing a hematoma and obscuring the laparoscopic picture. Laterally no staples are placed below the iliopubic tract due to the possibility of injury to the lateral femoral cutaneous nerve. This important nerve runs posterior to the iliopubic tract but cannot be seen in most cases because it is superficial to the transversalis fascia. If necessary, the posterior lateral corner of the mesh may be held in place by stapling it to the soft areolar or fatty tissue in this area. This staple should not be placed into the fascia thus avoiding injury to the nerves in this area. The only structures of concern anteriorly are the inferior epigastric vessels, which are placed superficial to the graft. If these vessels interfere with placement of the graft, they may be divided, but it has been the author's experience that this is an unnecessary portion of the procedure and may cause additional complications. Fifteen to twenty staples are required to secure the graft in place. The staples only act to hold the prosthesis in place until it becomes firmly bound to the preperitoneal fascia. The graft will become extremely adherent to the preperitoneal surface in 24 to 48 hours.

Closure

After the graft has been secured as indicated, the intra-abdominal insufflator is reduced to 8 mm Hg with a corresponding evacuation of that amount of carbon dioxide from the abdominal cavity. This allows relaxation of the peritoneum, which will now be stapled with the same staples used to secure the mesh (Fig. 57-15). The peritoneum may be visualized at the time of removal of the remaining carbon dioxide to make sure no significant holes exist. The carbon dioxide and any irrigation fluid are completely evacuated from the abdominal cavity. The 12-mm umbilical incision is closed using a No. 1 PDS absorbable suture in the fascia. All skin incisions are closed with interrupted absorbable subcuticular sutures and Steri-Strips.

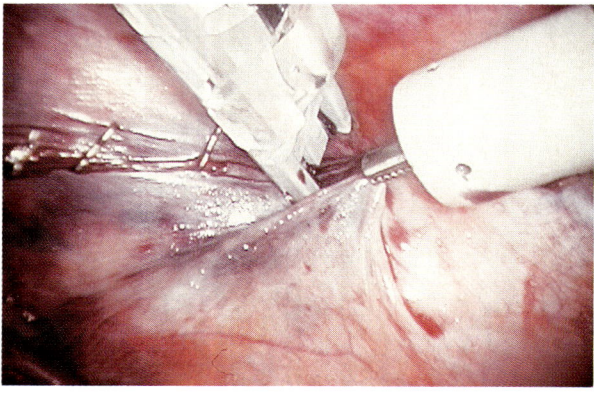

Figure 57-15. Closure of the peritoneum with placement of staples approximately 1-cm apart.

FEMORAL HERNIAS

Trocar Placement

Although much more infrequent, the femoral hernia is more easily repaired laparoscopically than direct, indirect, or recurrent hernias (Fig. 57-16). Femoral hernias are repaired by using the same port placement as previously described for other inguinal hernias and may be repaired using the procedure described previously so that all future hernias are avoided (direct and indirect).

Specific Details of the Procedure

If only the femoral hernia is to be repaired, the femoral hernia sac may be reduced into the abdominal cavity following which an incision is made in the anterior superior aspect of this sac. Care must be taken to avoid the femoral vessels. The loose areolar tissue is dissected from the area of the femoral hernia. The femoral hernia is then repaired using a modified plug and patch method. A small plug may be inserted in the area of the femoral hernia. This plug should be extremely small to avoid being palpable by the patient in the postoperative period. The plug is approximately 1 to 2 cm in length and is usually secured to the patch with a non-absorbable suture to prevent migration of this plug in the postoperative period. The "top hat" arrangement is placed into the femoral canal with the patch extending beyond the area of the femoral hernia. The plug and patch together are then secured to the inguinal ligament and Cooper's ligament with staples. A minimal amount of staples are required to secure this prothesis and must be placed under direct vision to avoid injury to the vascular structures in this area. Laterally the graft is allowed to drape over the iliac vessels. The area is then reperitonealized. The abdominal pressure is reduced to 8 mm Hg. This allows the peritoneum of the incised sac to come together and to be held permanently in place using the hernia stapler. This technique is similar to that described previously with the tension-free laparoscopic preperitoneal repair.

Postoperative Care

The patient who has undergone a transabdominal preperitoneal laparoscopic herniorrhaphy, (TAPP) is allowed to return to normal activity on the day following surgery. These patients have almost no pain and require less pain medication than the laparoscopic cholecystectomy patient. The patient is cautioned to limit lifting to 25 to 50 pounds during the first postoperative week. The patient is instructed to apply hydrogen peroxide to the wounds to avoid postoperative wound infections and is advised that if a bloated feeling occurs, he or she may take a laxative of his or her choice. No other care is required for this procedure.

Complications

Complications of all laparoscopic surgery are possible during the laparoscopic approach to hernia repair, and the patient should be advised of these during the informed consent. Complications of laparoscopic herniorrhaphy are rare, and major complications have not been seen at this time.

The complications of recurrent hernia repair remain unknown at this time; however, after a one- to three-year period of preperitoneal repairs, recurrences have been observed in fewer than 1 per cent of patients. A more frequent complication is that of scrotal emphysema particularly if an extraperitoneal repair is being done. With the patient under anesthesia at the termination of the procedure, the scrotal emphysema may be removed almost in its entirety by gentle compression of the scrotum. Preperitoneal hematomas may exist, but they have not been observed at this time to any significant degree.

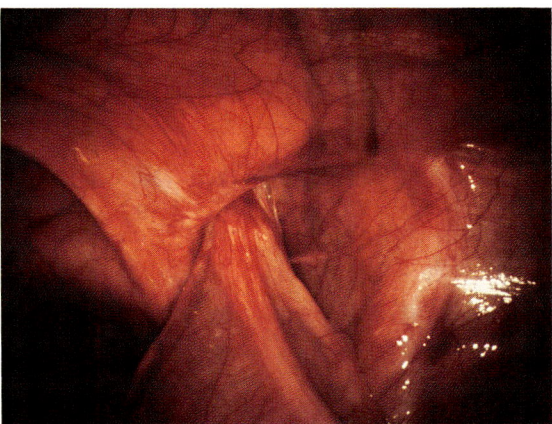

Figure 57-16. An incarcerated right femoral hernia.

Examination of the inguinal canal in some patients in the early postoperative period may reveal a bulge that is not increased with Valsalva's maneuver. This is thought to be a reaction to the graft or a small hematoma and usually resolves in 1 to 3 months.

Other complications of paresthesia along the distribution of the lateral cutaneous nerve of the thigh have been observed, but this is usually transient and will disappear in a 1- to 2-week period of time. This is thought to be caused by dissection laterally posterior to the iliopubic tract. If the paresthesia occurs several days after the repair, it will always be transient. If it occurs immediately following the repair, it may be due to staple placement posterior to the iliopubic tract through or into the lateral femoral cutaneous nerve and may take months to resolve with some persistent deficit. This complication is significant and is avoided by correct staple placement as indicated previously.

The most significant complications are related to injury to the iliac vessels, spermatic vessels, and vas deferens, which must be avoided during hernia repair. By careful identification of anatomical landmarks these structures can be avoided during dissection and placement of staples. This type of hemorrhagic complication will most likely result in conversion to open surgery during the procedure. Injuries to the epigastric vessels during port placement must be controlled as with other laparoscopic procedures and are avoided by staying lateral to the rectus muscle. If these vessels are injured during pelvic dissection, they will produce significant hemorrhage and must be controlled with ligation —not with electrosurgery.

Entrapment of a piece of small intestine through the peritoneum and into the inguinal space with obstruction has been reported in several patients. This was not directly observed by the author and, therefore, details are not known at this time. The intestine became incarcerated between the peritoneum and graft, requiring resection approximately 1 week postoperatively. To prevent this complication, the peritoneum must be completely closed without gaps between the staples. Bladder injuries are rare and are avoided by limiting the medial dissection to the boundary of the umbilical ligament (Fig. 57-17).

Conclusion

There have been a significant number of laparoscopic approaches to hernia repair, with an early recurrence rate of less than 1 per cent.[28,29] Laparoscopic herniorrhaphy is a viable procedure that at present is no longer considered to be investigational but rather developmental. The recurrence rate associated with laparoscopic hernia repair should soon become evident and establish this procedure as a standard of care. This procedure is initially more expensive and takes longer than hernia repair performed through a groin approach. However, the surgeon must keep in

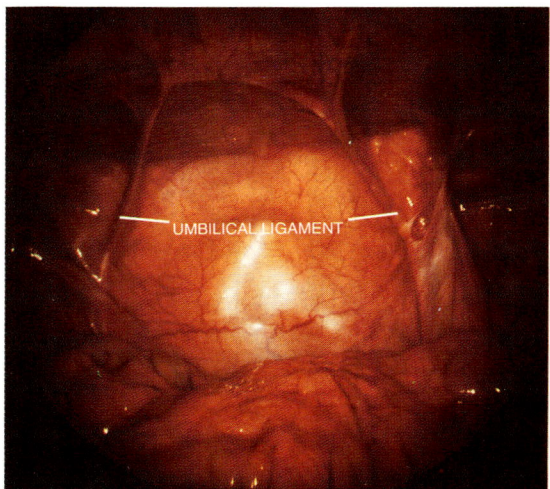

Figure 57-17. Pelvic view of the umbilical ligaments which indicate the medial boundary of dissection for herniorrhaphy.

mind that the primary obligation is to the patient and that a procedure resulting in a pain-free operation allowing rapid return to normal activity is a significant benefit and of primary importance to the hernia patient.

REFERENCES

1. Dubois F, Berthelot G, Levard H. Laparoscopic cholecystectomy: Historic perspective and person experience. Surg Laparosc Gastrosc, 1991; 1:52–57.
2. Selected data on hospital and use of services. In Polister P, Cunico E, eds. Socio-economic Factbook for Surgery, Chicago, American College of Surgeons, 1989, pp 25–42.
3. Lichtenstein IL. Scientific exhibit presented at the ASC meeting, San Francisco, Oct 1990.
4. Stoppa RE, Warlaumont CR. The preperitoneal approach and prosthetic repair of groin hernia. In Nyhus LM, Condon RE, eds. Hernia, 3rd ed. Philadelphia, JB Lippincott Co, 1989, Chap 10, pp 199–225.
5. Nyhus LM, Pollak R, Bombeck TC, Donahue PE. The preperitoneal approach and prosthetic buttress repair for recurrent hernia. Ann Surg 1988; 208:733–737.
6. Marcy HO. A new use of carbolized catgut ligatures. Boston Med Surg J 1871; 85:315–316.
7. Griffith CA. The Marcy repair of indirect inguinal hernias: 1870 to present. In Nyhus LM, Condon RE, eds. Hernia, 3rd ed. Philadelphia, JB Lippincott Co, 1989, Chap 5, pp 106–118.
8. Marcy HO. The cure of hernia. JAMA 1887; 8:589–592.
9. Marcy HO. Hernia. New York, Appleton Press, 1892.
10. LaRoque GP. The intra-abdominal method of removing inguinal and femoral hernia. Arch Surg 1932; 24:189–203.
11. Popp LW. Endoscopic patch repair of inguinal hernia in a female patient. Surg Endosc 1990; 4:12–20.
12. Ger R. The management of certain abdominal hernias by intra-abdominal closure of the neck. Ann R Coll Surg Engl 1982; 64:342–344.
13. Ger R, Monroe K, Duvivier R, Mishrick A. Management of indirect inguinal hernias by laparoscopic closure of the neck of the sac. Am J Surg 1990; 159:371–373.
14. Shultz L, Graber J, Pietrafitta J, Hickok D. Laser laparoscopic herniorrhaphy: A clinical trial preliminary results. J Laparoendo Surg 1990; 1:41.
15. Corbitt JD Jr. Laparoscopic herniorrhaphy. Surg Laparosc Endosc 1991; 1:23–25.
16. Salerno GM, Fitzgibbons RJ Jr, Filipi CJ. Surgical Laparoscopy, St Louis, Quality Medical Publishing Inc, 1991, Chap 14, pp 281–293.
17. Salerno GM, Fitzgibbons RJ Jr, Hart RO, Corbitt JD Jr, Filipi CJ. Laparoscopic Herniorrhaphy. In Zucker KA ed. Surgical Laparoscopic Update, St Louis, Quality Medical Publishing Inc, 1993, Chap 12, pp 373–394.
18. Toy FK, Smoot RJ Jr. Toy-Smoot laparoscopic hernioplasty, Surg Laparosc Endosc 1991; 1:151–155.
19. Spaw A. Laparoscopic hernia repair: The anatomic basis, J Laparoendosc Surg, 1991; 1:268–277.
20. Fitzgibbons RJ Jr, Annibali R, Litke B, Filipi C, Salerno A. A multicentered clinical trial on laparoscopic inguinal hernia repair: preliminary results. SAGES Scientific Session, 1993; 1:abstract 118.
21. Corbitt JD. Laparoscopic herniorrhaphy. In Reddick EJ, Saye WB, Corbitt JD eds. Atlas of Laparoscopic Surgery, New York, Raven Press, 1993, p 108.
22. Arregui M. Presentation at Advanced Laparoscopy Surgery, the International Experience, Indianapolis, IN, May 20–22, 1991.
23. Arregui M. Presentation at the International Minimal Access Surgery Symposium, Kansas City, MO, Nov 17–19, 1991.
24. McKernan JB, Laws HL. Laparoscopic preperitoneal prosthetic repair of inguinal hernias. Surgical Rounds 1992; 597–610.
25. McKernan JB. Personal communication. Laparoscopy in Focus. 1992.
26. McKernan JB, Laws HL. Laparoscopic repair of inguinal hernias using a totally extraperitoneal prosthetic approach. Surg Endosc 1993; 7(1):26–28.
27. Phillips EH, Carol BJ, Laparoscopic inguinal hernia repair. Gastrointes Endosc Clin N Am 1993; (in press).
28. 3rd World Congress of Endoscopic Surgery, Bordeaux, France, June 18–20, 1992.
29. The Forty-Third Surgical Forum, University of Southern California Medical Center, March 18–21, 1993.

Chapter 58
Iliopubic Tract Inguinal Hernia Repair with Inlay Buttress of Mesh

M. M. Gazayerli
M. E. Arregui
H. S. Helmy

Approximately 500,000 inguinal hernias are repaired each year in the United States.[1] This rivals the number of cholecystectomies performed annually and constitutes a large portion of the general surgeon's practice.

With the increase in minimally invasive surgery procedures, it has been estimated that the majority of cholecystectomies are now performed laparoscopically.[2] The success of this procedure does not necessarily suggest that laparoscopic inguinal hernia repair will gain wide acceptance.

The wide adoption of laparoscopic cholecystectomy can be credited to the fact that it is basically similar to the open operation that was first performed by Carl Yohann Langenbuch in Berlin in 1882. The laparoscopic adaptation of the traditional open procedure is familiar to all of us, but uses new instrumentation that causes less pain and morbidity.

The approach to laparoscopic inguinal hernia repair, in contrast, has been far less traditional. Many of the traditional operations for inguinal hernia repairs cannot be performed laparoscopically; however, a number of laparoscopic approaches to hernia repair have been developed (i.e., ring closure, plug, plug and small patch, plug and large patch, large piece of mesh placed intraperitoneally, large mesh placed preperitoneally, and iliopubic tract repair with inlay preperitoneal mesh).[3-10]

The theory behind some of these techniques has not been proven in open surgery. This raises the question: are surgeons justified in pursuing laparoscopic inguinal hernia repair when open repairs have recurrence rates of less than 10 per cent[11] and sometimes can be performed under local anesthesia as an outpatient procedure?

Although laparoscopic inguinal hernia repair, at this time, cannot be performed under local anesthesia, we feel that the laparoscopic approach can meet and exceed all the other criteria and offers the patient advantages not found with open surgery (i.e., reduced pain and morbidity, faster return to work, a repair that is more sound anatomically and that is minimally invasive).

We believe that there are only two traditional hernia repairs that can be performed laparoscopically: the Stoppa method,[12,13] known as the giant prosthetic reinforcement of the visceral sac (GPRVS), and the Nyhus, Condon, and Harkins method, known as preperitoneal or posterior approach and iliopubic tract repair (IPTR).[14-24]

The Stoppa repair is a preperitoneal repair advocated for use on all lower abdominal hernias. In open surgery, the method requires the insertion of a very large or giant piece of Dacron (polyester) mesh in the preperitoneal space to encase the entire lower abdomen. This procedure has been cited by many laparoscopic surgeons as the basis of their preperitoneal mesh repair.

It was Dr. Maurice Arregui[9] and Dr. Namir Katkhouda of Nice, France (personal communication) who first demonstrated that a wide dissection with suturing and stapling of a smaller piece of mesh than the Stoppa method can result in an effective cure of inguinal hernias. It was Dr. John D. Corbitt who first publicly abandoned the plug method and popularized the previously described laparoscopic adaptation of the Stoppa technique.

We (Gazayerli and Helmy) have adapted the Nyhus, Condon, and Harkins IPTR operation to the laparoscopic approach of hernia repair. We believe that the laparoscopic approach to this procedure is preferable to the open method because the large access incision is eliminated.

The laparoscopic IPTR is more difficult to learn than many other laparoscopic procedures. However, once one has mastered the suturing and tying techniques needed for this repair, other laparoscopic procedures can be approached with a greater degree of confidence.

If the surgeon is unfamiliar with IPTR, he or she should do a number of procedures by the open method to better grasp the anatomical structure of that area before approaching it laparoscopically.

PATIENT SELECTION

Laparoscopic IPTR can be performed in patients afflicted with any size of hernia defect. Among 113 patients referred to us for laparoscopic hernia repair, only 21 were advised against undergoing a laparoscopic approach.

The reasons for exclusion included multiple previous lower abdominal surgeries (1 patient), extreme obesity (4 patients), and concomitant cardiopulmonary conditions (16 patients). In the latter patients, it was felt that the added time of the surgery and the need for pneumoperitoneum made alternative methods of repair more suitable.

The preoperative evaluation of the candidates is similar to that for other laparoscopic procedures. Prior to surgery, patients are fed a regular diet. A broad spectrum, long acting cephalosporin is administered in the preoperative holding area. The patients are not given a preoperative bowel preparation.

EQUIPMENT

To perform laparoscopic inguinal hernia repair, we frequently use a 0-degree 10-mm laparoscope. A 30-degree 10-mm laparoscope, however, offers certain advantages, especially in port placement. More recently, a three-dimensional laparoscope made by American Surgical Technologies Corp. (Haverhill, MA) has been tested and offers distinct advantages, especially during needle grasping and manipulation. Based on this limited clinical test and the excellent needle handling and increased suturing facility, we believe that the three-dimensional laparoscope will facilitate the learning of laparoscopic IPTR and will one day become an essential part of the laparoscopic surgeon's armamentarium.

One 12-mm trocar and two 10-mm trocars are used during the procedure. A fourth 10-mm trocar is added if an abdominal retractor is used.

Additional instrumentation needed for the procedure includes: two double-action blunt graspers or dissectors, preferably long-jawed; one to three Gazayerli suture minders (Patent pending available from V. Mueller, Chicago, IL); the Gazayerli endoscopic retractor model 1[25]; a Thompson retractor; a Mediflex instrument holder (Islandia, NY) or other device to fix the retractor to the table frame; and if a first assistant is not available, the Flexbar camera holder.

To perform a laparoscopic IPTR with an inlay buttress of polypropylene mesh, the following instrumentation is very helpful: the Gazayerli knot-tying instrument or ligator[26] (patented, available from V. Mueller, Chicago, IL) (Fig. 58-1); a ROTICULATOR MULTIFIRE ENDO HERNIA* stapler (Patented, available from United States Surgical Corporation); an

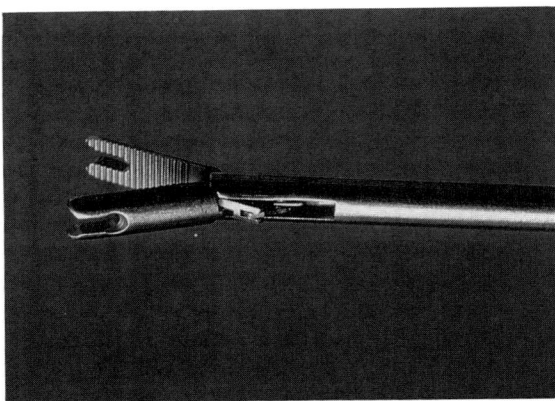

Figure 58-1.

ENDO CLIP* applier (Patented, available from United States Surgical Corporation); 30-inch 2-0 Ethibond suture on a non-removable tapered needle (e.g., X-411 on a tapered CT-2 needle or comparable suture material); and a racheted needle holder (V. Mueller-Jacoubek-Gazayerli needle holder).

We have found that the neodymium-yttrium-aluminum-garnet (Nd:YAG) laser greatly speeds up the dissection. If the laser is used, a laser fiber director, preferably combined with a right angle dissector, is useful (e.g., the Gazayerli laser fiber director and dissector available from Micro-France, Paris, France) (Fig. 58-2).

In addition, an 18-French Foley catheter with a 30-ml bag that can be passed through a 7.5 convertor can be used for preperitoneal sac dissection.[28]

PORT POSITIONS

For laparoscopic hernia repair, the patient is placed in a supine position at varying degrees of the Trendelenburg position. Elevation of the operative side of the table is rarely needed. A nasogastric tube and a Foley catheter are inserted after the anesthetic is administered. Ureteral stents are not used.

A single video monitor, placed at the foot of the table, or two video monitors, placed on either side of the patient's legs, can be used.

For treatment of unilateral hernias, the camera port is inserted in the umbilical scar or in the low epigastric area. The position of the umbilicus varies from person to person. If the scar is closer to the xiphisternum, the port can be inserted through the umbilicus. However, if it is low and closer to the symphysis pubis, the camera port should be placed above the scar in the low epigastric area.

The main operating port is placed contralateral to the hernia and as low as possible. Theoretically, the ideal port site for suture repair of a hernia with a nonrotatable (roticulating) needle holder would be in the upper thigh contralateral to the hernia, in order to have the jaws of the needle holder parallel to the hernia defect. Since this is not possible, the lowest possible point on the abdomen is chosen. This port should be a 12-mm trocar in order to introduce the MULTIFIRE ENDO HERNIA* stapler (Patented, available from United States Surgical Corporation, Norwalk, CT) toward the end of the procedure.

The assistant's port is placed on the same side as the hernia, between the midclavicular and anterior axillary lines, just below the costal margin. This allows adequate distance between the port site and the hernia defect to enable maneuvering of the instruments. The retractor port, if needed, is placed cephalad to the hernia defect, avoiding the inferior epigastric vessels. If the surgeon wants to operate with both hands, an extra port is placed between the contralateral and low epigastric ports.

For the treatment of bilateral hernias, the placement of the camera and main operating ports is unchanged. The assistant's port, however, is lowered as much as possible since suturing is technically more demanding. The retractor port is placed low in the midline, 1 to 2 inches above the symphysis pubis. This site may also be used when unilateral hernias are repaired to avoid injury to the inferior epigastric vessels. If a 12-mm port is not available, the hernia stapler can be intro-

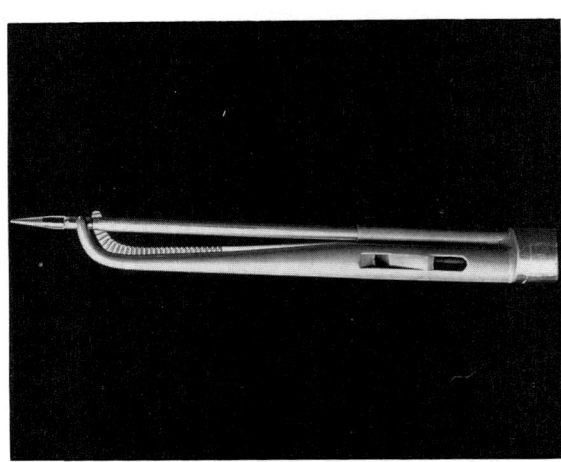

Figure 58-2.

duced through a 10-mm port by withdrawing the cannula and introducing the stapler directly through the incision.

For the treatment of a unilateral hernia, in which there is no experienced first assistant, the camera port is placed through the previously described assistant's port, high on the side of the hernia. Here a 30-degree laparoscope is very helpful. The surgeon manipulates the instruments through the contralateral and midline trocars.

METHODS OF DISSECTION

Once the trocars are in place and the abdomen is inspected, attention is directed to the hernia area (Fig. 58-3). The patient is placed in the Trendelenburg position, and adhesions are lysed.

The hernia sac is assessed, and the need for a Foley catheter to aid in the dissection is determined. In a direct hernia sac, it is very helpful to insert a 30-ml Foley catheter extraperitoneally and inflate it with 70 to 90 ml of saline prior to incising the peritoneum. This step is not useful in an indirect inguinal hernia sac dissection.

The peritoneum is then incised in a hockey stick fashion (Fig. 58-4) from the midline to a point just lateral to the internal ring. The lateral umbilical ligament and inferior epigastric vessels are clipped and ligated for better exposure (Fig. 58-5). The Nd:YAG laser or ENDO SHEARS* device (Patented, available from United States Surgical Corporation) with cautery are used to incise the peritoneum and make a flap extending down to the pubic ramus and Cooper's ligament. This is one of the few times when the laser is superior to

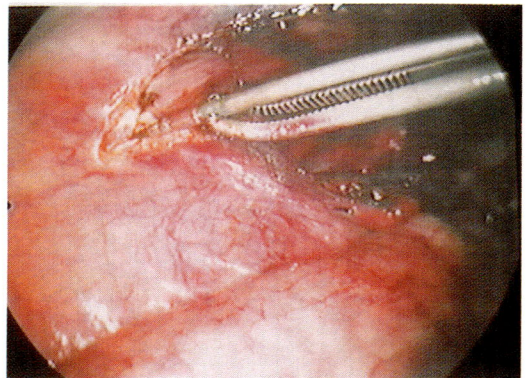

Figure 58-4.

cautery because it produces less charring of the areolar tissues and greatly facilitates the dissection of the flap.

If a large indirect inguinal hernia sac (possibly extending to the scrotum) is found, it is necessary to incise the peritoneum circumferentially around the neck of the sac. A decision is then made either to leave the distal sac in place or to dissect and remove it. The latter is accomplished by simple traction on the sac and blunt dissection of the areolar tissue. Removing a large sac will result in bruising of the external genitalia, and the patient should be so alerted prior to the procedure or immediately after the operation.

The need for an abdominal wall retractor is determined after the peritoneum and sac are dissected, just before beginning suturing. If the cephalad edge of the hernia defect, the transversalis fascia, is on a relatively horizontal plane in relation to the caudal edge, the iliopubic tract, then an abdominal wall retrac-

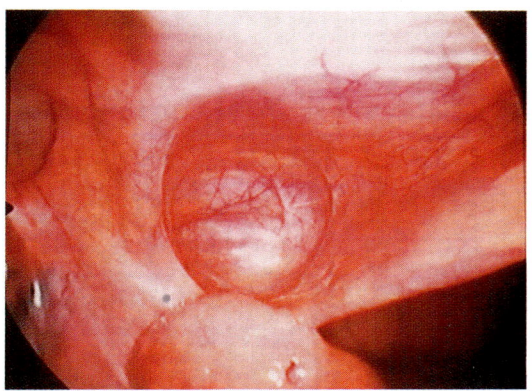

Figure 58-3.

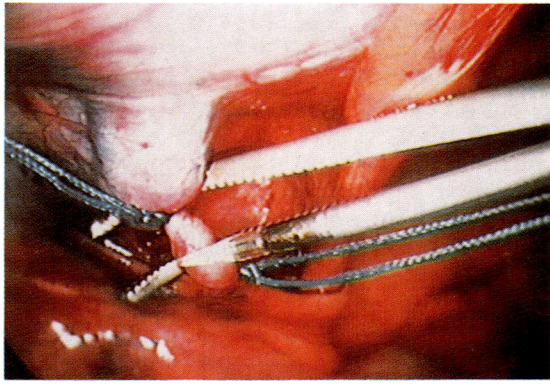

Figure 58-5.

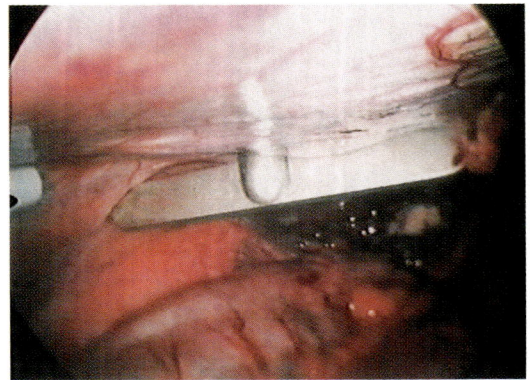

Figure 58-6.

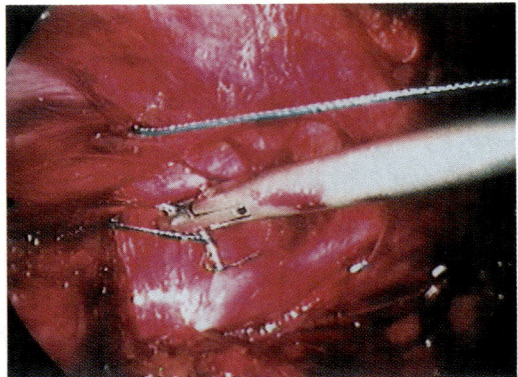

Figure 58-7.

tor is inserted (Fig. 58-6). The retractor is then fixed in place by means of a mechanical fixing device, e.g., a Thompson or Mediflex instrument holder.

IDENTIFYING THE LANDMARKS

Once the posterior wall of the inguinal canal has been dissected, one can identify the anatomical landmarks of that region. The vas deferens or round ligament will be seen reaching the internal ring from the 6:00 position. The cord structures and iliac vessels lie between the 3:00 and 6:00 positions in a right hernia, and the 6:00 and 9:00 positions in a left hernia. This area has been described by Corbitt as the "triangle of doom" and should be avoided in applying staples. Cooper's ligament is also identified.

More important, however, is the identification of the iliopubic tract, which is the inferior boundary of both a direct and indirect inguinal hernia. The superior boundary of both types of hernia is the transversalis fascia or its condensation, called the transversus abdominis arch.

In the indirect inguinal hernia, the iliopubic tract is also called the posterior crus, and the transversus abdominis arch becomes the anterior crus. The continuity of these structures is most apparent in a large indirect inguinal hernia. In these cases, the hernia stretches the internal ring medially and essentially eliminates the posterior wall of the inguinal canal. The looped inferior epigastric vessels around the medial edge of the sac are the only visible signs to indicate that it is a large indirect sac.

LAPAROSCOPIC ILIOPUBIC TRACT REPAIR

The actual hernia repair is started by introducing a 2-0 Ethibond suture on a non-pop-off needle and regrasping it with the needle holder through the 12-mm port. In the case of a direct inguinal hernia, the lateral most suture is placed first, just medial to the cord structures. A good "bite" of transversalis fascia and transversus abdominis arch is taken superiorly to approximate the edges to the iliopubic tract inferiorly (Figs. 58-7 and 58-8).

Once the most lateral suture is in place and tied using the Gazayerli ligator (Figs. 58-9 and 58-10), it is brought out through the operator's port for traction in order to facilitate the placement of the subsequent sutures (Figs. 58-11 and 58-12). Alternatively, for more control in suturing, the suture may be brought out through a suture minder. By placing the most lateral suture first, one re-

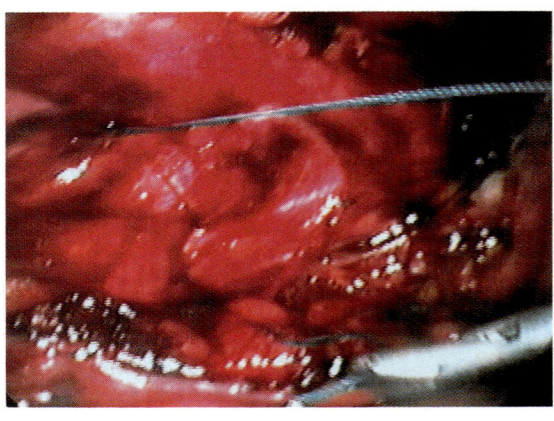

Figure 58-8.

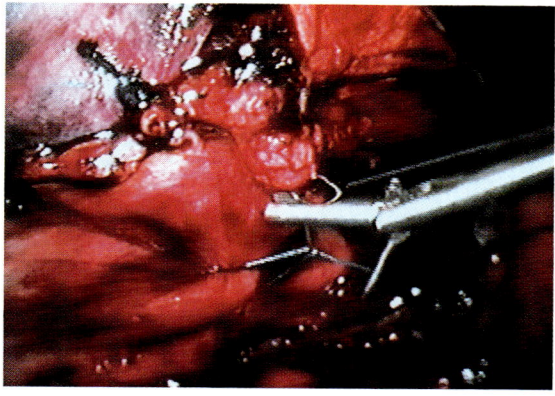

Figure 58-9.

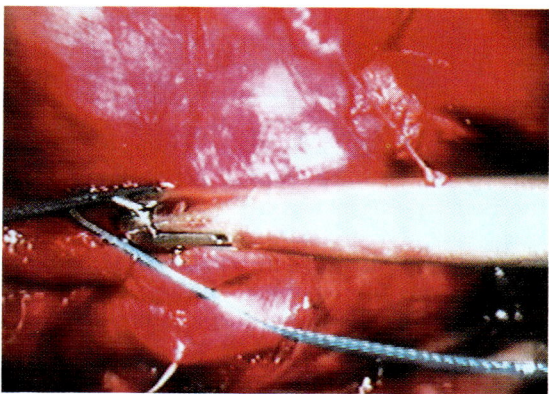

Figure 58-11.

duces the size of the hernia defect, and the two layers are approximated without tension. If tension is to be encountered, it is in this first suture.

Even though the abdomen is distended and the abdominal wall is often retracted, we have been able to approximate, without tension, these two structures in primary direct or indirect inguinal hernias of all sizes. In some types of recurrent inguinal hernias, however, the posterior inguinal wall is thickened and scarred so that it is impossible to approximate the edges of the hernia defect.

At first we were surprised to discover that some recurrent inguinal hernias have soft elastic tissue similar to that found in primary hernias. We then realized that in many anterior approach repairs, the transversus abdominis arch and iliopubic tract are never seen or sutured.

Suture repair of the transversalis fascia and transversus abdominis arch to the iliopubic tract proceeds medially. The most medially placed suture is in the iliopubic tract and Cooper's ligament, where these two transversalis fascia analogues meet at the pubic tubercle. One of the sutures of the repair, preferably the most medial, is left long for anchoring the polypropylene mesh.

After the sac is excised, the defect in an indirect inguinal hernia is found extending medially to the cord structures, superiorly to the anterior crus (transversalis fascia and transversus abdominis arch) and inferiorly to the posterior crus (iliopubic tract). The cord structures may be encircled with an 0 Ethibond ligature and displaced laterally by means of a Gazayerli suture minder. In this case the repair begins laterally and ends medially at the pubic tubercle or at the point where a sound posterior inguinal wall of transversalis fascia is encountered.

Alternatively, the cord may not be displaced laterally. In this case, the suture repair

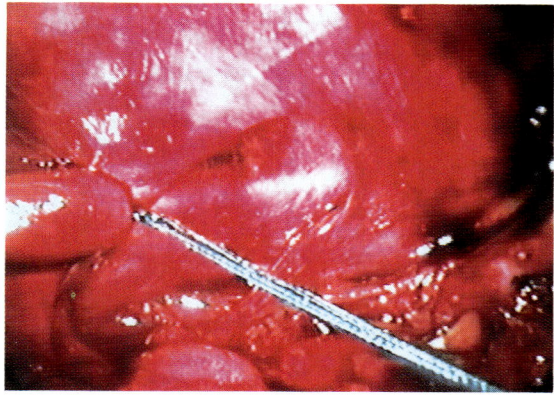

Figure 58-10.

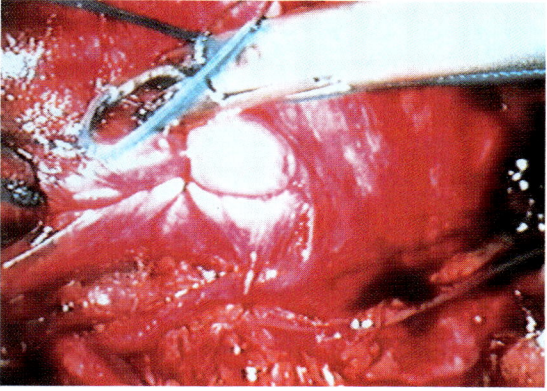

Figure 58-12.

is placed lateral to the cord structures, again approximating the anterior crus superiorly and the posterior crus inferiorly. The most medial of these sutures usually is placed first and left long for guiding and anchoring the polypropylene mesh.

After the suture repair is completed, a trimmed piece of polypropylene mesh is threaded outside the abdomen onto the suture. The mesh is then introduced through the port and guided to the posterior wall of the inguinal canal, where it is anchored. Staples are then used to secure the mesh superiorly, medially, and inferiorly (Figs. 58-13 and 58-14).

To avoid the iliac vessels, cord structures, and nerves, we do not staple the mesh lateral to the inferior epigastric vessels. The mesh is draped laterally over the internal ring area. Any excess mesh may be folded and stapled in a double layer. If the cord structures have been mobilized off the iliac vessels, the lateral part of the mesh is slit horizontally before introducing it, and an oval hole is made in the mesh. The mesh is then passed around the cord structures.

The peritoneum is then closed with staples or with a running purse-string suture of 2-0 material. We find suturing easier to do than stapling (Fig. 58-15).

At the conclusion of the repair, the skin incision is usually closed with 5-0 absorbable inverted subcuticular sutures. The deep fascia is closed by elevating it with skin hooks and approximating the edges with a 2-0 Vicryl suture. We find it useful to use a larger needle that has been bent into a V shape to facilitate this step. We have rarely found it necessary to close the deep fascia when using trocar sizes up to 10 mm. When 12 mm trocars are used it is essential that the deep fascia be closed to avoid incisional hernias.

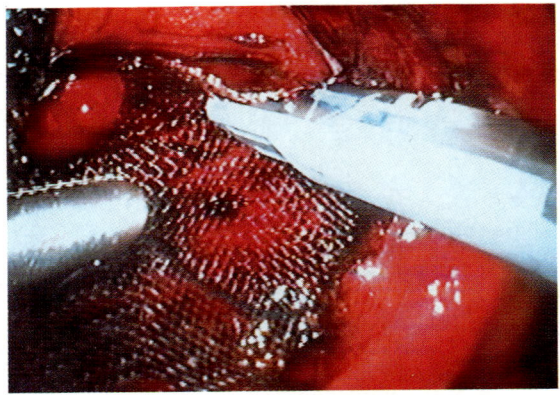

Figure 58-14.

ALTERNATIVE INSTRUMENTS AND SPECIAL TRICKS

We now carry our instruments from hospital to hospital, and even from continent to continent, to avoid using alternative instruments. However, when we first began performing laparoscopic inguinal repair we used more primitive instruments.

The Topol needle holder was the first advance in instrumentation that reduced the time it took to perform the procedure. This was replaced by the Codman racheted needle holder and more recently by the V. Mueller-Jacoubek-Gazayerli needle holder.

The Gazayerli ligator and endoscopic abdominal wall retractor were originally developed for hernia repair. The advantage of the

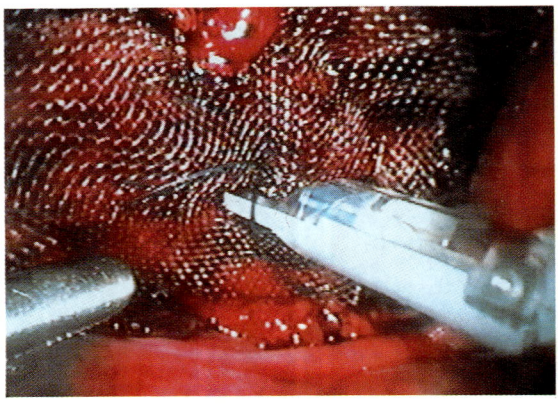

Figure 58-13.

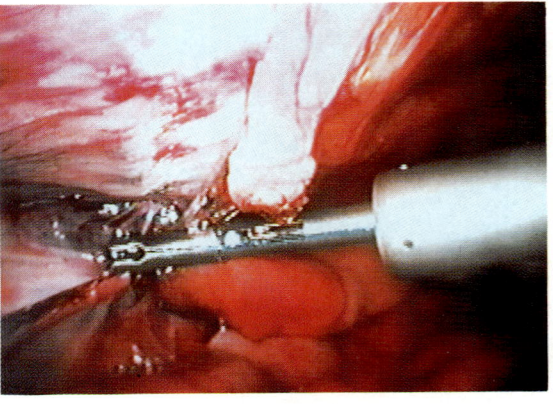

Figure 58-15.

ligator is that the sutures can be made expeditiously and placed squarely, while maintaining adequate tension to prevent slippage and loosening of the knots.[27]

To introduce the needle and suture, we thread the convertor on the shaft of the needle holder. We grasp the suture about 1.5 to 2 inches from the needle. The trailing end of the suture material is brought out alongside the needle holder shaft. The intra-abdominal trocar tip is then placed gently against the retroperitoneum or a loop of intestine to prevent loss of pneumoperitoneum. The trap-door valve on the trocar is then opened to introduce the needle partly down the shaft of the trocar. The convertor is then placed over the trocar to seal it. The intra-abdominal tip of the trocar is then elevated and the needle holder is advanced into the abdomen. A similar method is used to prevent loss of pneumoperitoneum during the introduction of the polypropylene mesh.

POSTOPERATIVE MANAGEMENT

At the conclusion of the procedure, the patient is taken to the recovery room where the nasogastric tube and Foley catheter are removed. Antibiotics are prescribed for 48 to 72 hours postoperatively, and the patient is encouraged to eat a normal diet as tolerated.

The patient is discharged when fully recovered from the anesthetic and tolerating oral intake. We encourage the patients to remain in the 23-hour unit until the following morning, but a number of patients have left the hospital on the day of the surgery.

RESULTS

We have repaired laparoscopically 102 hernias in 92 patients through March 1992. In the first 7 patients, we performed laparoscopic IPTR with no mesh. In these first patients, who have been followed for over 18 months, one hernia has recurred.

The next 48 patients were offered laparoscopic IPTR and a "plug" of mesh was placed in the inguinal canal as well as a preperitoneal inlay buttress of polypropylene mesh. These patients have been followed for 7 to 18 months, and no hernia has recurred. However, 5 of these 48 patients have complained of discomfort related to the inguinal canal plug. In 3 patients the complaints were severe enough to necessitate the removal of the plugs through a groin incision.

The plugs were found to be encased in areolar tissue and totally incapable of buttressing the anterior wall of the repair. We have also heard anecdotal reports of migration of these plugs into the anterior abdominal wall. We have stopped placing plugs in the inguinal canal and strongly recommend against doing so.

The subsequent 47 hernias were repaired by laparoscopic IPTR and preperitoneal inlay mesh when feasible, and no plugs were placed in the inguinal canal. These patients have been followed for over 3 months, and there have been no recurrences.

Of 34 direct hernias in this series, 26 had well defined anatomical structures, allowing the iliopubic tract repair with inlay buttress of mesh. The remaining eight patients had a generalized weakness that allowed no suture repair. In these cases, a Corbitt-Arregui-Katkhouda type of repair was performed.

There were 14 recurrent hernias: 1 was an indirect recurrent hernia, 6 resembled primary direct inguinal hernias, and 7 had scarred tissue with multiple defects. The 6 primary-resembling hernias were treated by the laparoscopic IPTR method with inlay mesh. For the 7 scarred hernias the defect edges could not be approximated, and they were treated by the Corbitt-Arregui-Katkhouda type of repair.

Thus of the 102 hernias upon which we have operated, 15 (8 direct hernias with generalized weakness and 7 scarred recurrent hernias) were not candidates for the Gazayerli-Helmy laparoscopic iliopubic tract repair with inlay buttress of polypropylene mesh.

As of mid-June 1993, over 250 patients have undergone laparoscopic repairs of inguinal hernias using, in most cases, the IPTR method. To date, no patient has developed a recurrence of an inguinal hernia. The only exception to this was one of the first 7 patients, who was discussed previously.

COMPLICATIONS SPECIFIC FOR THIS PROCEDURE

As with our experience with laparoscopic cholecystectomy, the advantages of laparoscopic inguinal hernia repair over open surgery include less postoperative pain and faster return to normal activities. However, complications do occur. Ecchymosis of the external genitalia is anticipated and described preoperatively to patients with large scrotal hernias.

In one early patient with Crohn's disease, a vesicocolic fistula was opened. This was repaired laparoscopically, and the bladder was drained with a Foley catheter for 10 days. Cystoscopy revealed complete healing.

In another patient, postoperative neuralgia of the inguinal area occurred and lasted for 2 weeks. This has prompted us to avoid using staples lateral to the inferior epigastric vessels.

Conclusion

The preperitoneal approach to inguinal hernial repair is not new. It was first introduced by Annandale[28] in 1876 and later revised by Cheattle[29] and Henry.[30] Nyhus, Condon, and Harkins[14] later improved on the Cheattle-Henry procedure by converting the vertical incision to a transverse incision.

We believe that laparoscopic IPTR, while essentially the same procedure as that of Nyhus, Condon, and Harkins,[14] further improves on the procedure by completely eliminating large access incisions. We believe that in both direct and indirect inguinal hernias the primary hernia defect is in the transversalis fascia and its analogues. Therefore, it is anatomically preferable to repair that defect than to artificially approximate structures that were never in close proximity to each other, as occurs in many anterior hernia repairs. The transversalis fascia is a large elastic layer that can be approximated with no tension. By adding the inlay buttress of the polypropylene mesh to a repaired posterior inguinal wall, one eliminates the bulge that is described when mesh is applied to the unrepaired defect. Since the abdomen is distended during laparoscopy it is impossible to rely on circumferential staples alone to eliminate the bulge.

In some recurrent inguinal hernias, as noted previously, the transversalis fascia is scarred and cannot be approximated to bridge the defect. In these patients it is sufficient to inlay a mesh patch and staple it to the edges of the defect after reducing the hernia sac and preperitoneal fat. The desmoplastic reaction of these recurrent hernias prevents bulging once the mesh is sutured or stapled in place.

Author's Note: One of the authors (M.E.A.), while endorsing the laparoscopic approach to inguinal hernia repairs, has his own preferred technique that does not include suturing of the transversalis fascia and transversus abdominis arch to the ileopublic tract.

REFERENCES

1. Selected data on hospitals and use of services. In Polister P, Cunico E, eds. Socio-Economic Factbook for Surgery, Chicago, American College of Surgeons, 1989, pp 25–42.
2. Conway D. Presentation at the Society of Laparoendoscopic Surgeons's Annual Meeting, Palm Beach, FL, 1992.
3. Ger R, Monroe K, Duvivier R, et al. Management of indirect inguinal hernias by closure of the neck of the sac. Am J Surg 1990; 159:371–373.
4. Schultz L, Graber J, Pietrafitta J, et al. Laser laparoscopic herniorrhaphy: A clinical trial preliminary results. J Laparoendosc Surg 1990; 1:41–45.
5. Corbitt J. Laparoscopic herniorrhaphy. Surg Laparosc Endosc 1991; 1:23–25.
6. Dion YM, Morin J. Laparoscopic inguinal herniorrhaphy. Can J Surg 1992; 35:209–212.
7. Seid AS, Deutsch H, Jacobson A. Laparoscopic herniorrhaphy. Surg Laparosc Endosc 1992; 2:59–60.
8. Salerno GM, Fitzgibbons RJ Jr, Filipi CJ. Laparoscopic inguinal hernia repair. In Zucker KA, ed. Surgical Laparoscopy. St Louis, Quality Medical Publishing, Inc., 1991, pp 281–293.
9. Arregui ME, Davis CD, Yucel O, et al. Laparoscopic mesh repair of inguinal hernia using a preperitoneal approach: A preliminary report. Surg Laparosc Endosc 1992; 2:53–58.
10. Gazayerli MM. Anatomical laparoscopic hernia repair of direct or indirect inguinal hernias using the transversalis fascia and iliopubic tract. Surg Laparosc Endosc 1992; 2:49–52.
11. Condon RE, Nyhus LM. Complications of groin hernias. In Nyhus LM, Condon RE, eds. Hernia, 3rd ed. Philadelphia, JB Lippincott, 1989, pp 106–118.
12. Stoppa RE, Rives JL, Warlaumont CR, et al. The use of Dacron in the repair of hernias of the groin. Surg Clin North Am 1984; 64:269–285.
13. Stoppa RE. The treatment of complicated incisional and groin hernias. World J Surg 1989; 13:545–554.
14. Nyhus LM, Condon RE, Harkins HN. Clinical experiences with preperitoneal hernia repair for all types of hernia of the groin; with particular emphasis to the importance of transversalis fascia analogues. Am J Surg 1960; 100:234–244.
15. Condon RE. Surgical anatomy of the transversus abdominis and transversalis fascia. Ann Surg 1971; 173:1–5.
16. Nyhus LM. An anatomic reappraisal of the posterior inguinal wall with special consideration of the iliopubic tract and its relation to groin hernias. Surg Clin North Am 1960; 44:1305–1313.
17. Nyhus LM. The preperitoneal approach and iliopubic tract repair of inguinal hernia. In Nyhus LM, Condon RE, eds. Hernia, 3rd ed. Philadelphia, JB Lippincott, 1989, pp 154–188.
18. Nyhus LM, Pollak R, Bombeck CT, et al. The preperitoneal approach and prosthetic buttress repair for recurrent hernia: The evolution of a technique. Ann Surg 1988; 733–737.

19. Nyhus LM, Klein MS, Rogers FB. Inguinal hernia. Curr Probl Surg 1991; 28:403-450.
20. Gaspar MR, Casberg MA. An appraisal of preperitoneal repair of inguinal hernia. Surg Gynecol Obstet 1971; 132:207-212.
21. Read RC. Preperitoneal herniorrhaphy: A historical review. World J Surg 1989; 13:545-554.
22. Lampe EW. Experience with preperitoneal hernioplasty. In Nyhus LM, Condon RE, eds. Hernia, 3rd ed. Philadelphia, JB Lippincott, 1989, pp 178-184.
23. Malanogoni MA, Condon RE. Preperitoneal repair of acute incarcerated and strangulated hernia of the groin. Surg Gynecol Obstet 1986; 162:65-67.
24. Greenburg AG, Saik RP, Peskin GW. Expanded indications for preperitoneal hernia repair: The high risk patient. Am J Surg 1979; 138:149-153.
25. Gazayerli MM. The Gazayerli endoscopic retractor, model one. Surg Laparosc Endosc 1991; 1:98-100.
26. Gazayerli MM. The Gazayerli knot tying instrument or ligator for use in diverse laparoscopic surgical procedures. Surg Laparosc Endosc 1991; 1:254-258.
27. Gazayerli MM, Helmy HS. The use of Foley catheters in laparoscopic surgery. In press.
28. Annandale T. Case in which a reducible oblique and direct inguinal and femoral hernia existed in the same side and were successfully treated by operation. Edinb Med J 1876; 21:1087.
29. Cheatle GL. An operation for the radical cure of inguinal and femoral hernia. Br Med J 1920; 2:68.
30. Henry AK. Operation for femoral hernia by a midline extraperitoneal approach with a preliminary note on the use of this route for reducible inguinal hernia. Lancet 1936; 230:531-533.

Chapter 59
Oophorectomy

Harry Reich

In 1980 Semm and Mettler reported 37 laparoscopic oophorectomies using a loop ligature and a tissue punch morcellator.[1] In 1985, Reich used bipolar electrosurgical desiccation to replace the ligature and culdotomy or umbilical extension incisions to eliminate the need to morcellate.[2-4]

PATIENT SELECTION

The indications for laparoscopic oophorectomy (or salpingo-oophorectomy) include pelvic pain secondary to ovarian adhesions from previous hysterectomy, pain from ovarian adhesions unresponsive to laparoscopic lysis, pelvic mass secondary to hydrosalpinx from pelvic inflammatory disease or previous surgery, and postmenopausal palpable ovary (PMPO). In women not desiring future fertility, oophorectomy should be considered for pain or a mass arising from ovarian endometrioma, hemorrhagic corpus luteum cyst, or dermoid cyst when the contralateral ovary is normal, especially if the lesion is on the left because the left ovary frequently heals adhered to the rectosigmoid. The acronym PMPO is used for the palpation of a postmenopausal ovary which, in a premenopausal woman, would be interpreted as normal size —3 to 4 cm in its largest dimension.[5] Such ovaries can almost always be removed intact through a culdotomy incision.[3,6-8] Women in families with two or more first degree relatives (mother or sister) with ovarian cancer may have a 50 per cent chance of developing this disease and should consider undergoing early prophylactic oophorectomy by age 35 if childbearing has been completed. Women without a family history of ovarian cancer have a 1 in 70 risk of developing this disease. Stage I ovarian cancer may be treated by laparoscopic oophorectomy, hysterectomy, omentectomy, and lymphadenectomy in selected cases.[9,10]

PREOPERATIVE EVALUATION

Endovaginal ultrasound is done to evaluate the ovaries in cases involving a pelvic mass, retrocervical nodules, or fibroid tumors. A CA 125 assay, which uses a monoclonal antibody that reacts to an antigen found in most nonmucinous ovarian cancers, is obtained. Intravenous pyelograms are rarely necessary preoperatively but are frequently ordered postoperatively if abdominal pain persists following surgery on or near the ureter.

PREOPERATIVE PREPARATION

Laparoscopy is performed prior to ovulation if possible. Norethindrone acetate, 10 mg daily, or depoleuprolide (Depo-Lupron),

3.75 mg intramuscularly once per month for 3 to 6 months, is often administered starting on the first day of menses until surgery to avoid operating on ovaries containing a corpus luteum. Patients are encouraged to hydrate and eat lightly for 24 hours before admission. Magnesium citrate and a Fleet enema are routinely administered the evening before surgery to evacuate the lower bowel. When extensive cul-de-sac involvement with endometriosis is suspected, either clinically or from another doctor's operative record, use of a mechanical bowel preparation is considered. Lower abdominal, pubic, and perineal hair is not shaved. Patients are encouraged to void when called to the operating room, and a Foley catheter is inserted only if the bladder is distended or a long operation is anticipated. Antibiotics are administered in all procedures lasting more than 2 hours.

EQUIPMENT

A suction-irrigator (aquadissector), special forceps, scissors, high flow insufflator, 30-degree tiltable operating room table, and an electrosurgical generator are indispensable tools for advanced surgical procedures. Five laparoscopes should be available: a 10-mm straight viewing laparoscope, a 10-mm operating laparoscope with a 5-mm operating channel, a 10-mm laser laparoscope with a 5-mm laser channel, a 12-mm laser laparoscope with a 7.2-mm laser channel, and a 5-mm straight viewing laparoscope for introduction through the 5-mm trocar sleeve. This author uses his right foot to activate the laser, his left foot for the bipolar electrosurgical pedal, and hand controls for unipolar electrodes. An average of 10 liters of Ringer's lactate irrigant is used per procedure; more than 40 liters have been used on occasion. Heparin is not added to the irrigating medium. High flow carbon dioxide (CO_2) insufflation up to 10 liters/min is used to compensate for the rapid loss of CO_2 during suctioning.

A Valtchev uterine mobilizer (Conkin Surgical Instruments, Toronto, Canada) is inserted to antevert the uterus and delineate the posterior vagina. Alternatively, a Cohen cannula or a curette may be inserted into the uterus (if present) for manipulation and tubal lavage.

Trocar sleeves are available in many sizes and shapes. For most instruments, 5.5-mm cannulas are adequate. Newer electrosurgical electrodes, which eliminate capacitance and insulation failures (Electroshield from Electroscope), will require 7/8-mm sleeves. Laparoscopic stapling is performed through 12/13-mm ports.

Trocar sleeves (5-mm) of a special design are used: short, self-retaining secondary to a screw grid around the external surface and without a trap (Richard Wolf, Apple Med).[11] These trocar sleeves facilitate efficient instrument exchanges and evacuation of tissue while allowing the introduction and removal of suture material. Once placed, their portal of exit stays fixed at the level of the anterior abdominal wall parietal peritoneum, permitting more room for instrument manipulation. United States Surgical Company disposable trocar sleeves with adjustable locking retention collars hold their position well for stapling. Their retention collars are used to prevent the umbilical 10-mm trocar sleeve from sliding out of the umbilicus.

POSITIONING OF THE PATIENT

All laparoscopic surgical procedures are done with the patient under general anesthesia and with endotracheal intubation and an orogastric tube. The patient is flat (0 degrees) until after the umbilical trocar sleeve has been inserted and then placed in a steep Trendelenburg position (20 to 30 degrees). The lithotomy position is obtained with Allen stirrups (Edgewater Medical Systems, Mayfield Heights, OH) or knee braces, which are adjusted to the individual patient before she is anesthetized. Anesthesia examination is always performed prior to preparing the patient.

POSITIONING OF THE VIDEO EQUIPMENT

The video monitor is opposite the surgeon. This arrangement is preferred, since only one monitor is necessary. The monitor is on the patient's right, the surgeon on her left, and the assistant between the patient's legs where the monitor can be viewed. Both surgeon and assistant have access to instrument tables beside or behind them, and a scrub nurse is not necessary, if a specially trained assistant is available. The circulating nurse tends the video recorder, irrigation supply, and laser.

This arrangement requires some hand-eye adjustment for the surgeon, since the monitor is rotated 90 degrees from the plane of surgery. However, it avoids neck and back strain from twisting to see a monitor placed between the patient's legs, especially if the surgeon operates with instruments in the left hand and laparoscope in the right. Hand-eye coordination (almost mirror image) is extremely difficult for the assistant, who often assumes a passive role of maintaining retraction or grasper positions achieved by the surgeon. Mirror image operating skills can be attained after extensive training and will greatly increase the efficiency of the surgical team.

TROCAR PLACEMENT AND SIZE SELECTION

For most pelvic procedures, the operative incisions are limited to three: 10-mm umbilical, 5-mm right lower quadrant, and 5-mm left lower quadrant. Three puncture sites in the anterior abdominal wall are sufficient for 90 per cent of laparoscopic procedures. Large puncture sites or incisions bordering on mini-laparotomy for tissue extraction should be replaced by an umbilical extension or a laparoscopic culdotomy approach.

The intraumbilical incision overlies the area where skin, deep fascia, and parietal peritoneum of the anterior abdominal wall meet, permitting little opportunity for the parietal peritoneum to tent away from the Veress needle. This vertical midline incision is made initially with a No. 15 blade (never a No. 11) on the inferior wall of the umbilical fossa extending to and just beyond its lowest point. In thin patients, this incision frequently traverses the deep fascia, but intraperitoneal injury is avoided by pulling the umbilicus onto the surgeon's forefinger, a maneuver that controls the incision's depth. Following CO_2 insufflation until the intra-abdominal pressure is more than 20 mm Hg, the trocar is seated vertically just inside the skin prior to a horizontal thrust. The result is a parietal peritoneal puncture directly beneath the umbilicus.

Placement of the lower quadrant trocar sleeves lateral to the deep epigastric vessels and just above the pubic hairline is preferred. These vessels, an artery flanked by two veins (venae comitantes), are located by direct inner laparoscopic inspection of the anterior abdominal wall. They are found lateral to the umbilical ligaments (obliterated umbilical artery) and cannot be found consistently by traditional transillumination. The left lower quadrant puncture is the major portal for operative manipulation. The right trocar sleeve is used for atraumatic grasping forceps to retract tissues as needed.

METHODS OF EXPOSURE AND RETRACTION

Prior to starting oophorectomy it is imperative that the surgeon visualize the course of the ureter. It crosses the external iliac artery near the bifurcation of the common iliac artery at the pelvic brim and is usually lower on the left, where its entrance into the pelvis is covered by the inverted V-shaped root of the sigmoid mesocolon. The peritoneum above the ureter can be opened with sharp scissors or CO_2 laser if visual identification through the peritoneum is difficult. Thereafter, the space can be further developed by flushing irrigant (lactated Ringer's solution) under pressure from an aquadissector into the space. Smooth grasping forceps are then opened parallel and perpendicular to the retroperitoneal structures until the ureter is identified and grasped. Scissors, laser, or aquadissector can then be used to further dissect the ureter throughout much of its course along the pelvic sidewall.

SPECIFIC DETAILS OF THE PROCEDURE

Oophorectomy

Prior to removal, the ovary must be released from all pelvic sidewall and bowel adhesions. Adhesions are divided and ovarian endometriomas are drained, if present (Figs. 59-1 and 59-2). The fallopian tube is grasped and pulled medially to stretch out the infundibulopelvic ligament containing the ovarian vessels. Kleppinger bipolar forceps are used to compress and desiccate the infundibulopelvic ligament, the broad ligament (mesovarium and mesosalpinx), the fallopian tube isthmus, and the utero-ovarian ligament (Figs. 59-3, 59-4, and 59-5).[3,4] These large blood vessels are compressed and bipolar cutting current is passed until complete desiccation is achieved, i.e., the current depletes tissue fluid and electrolytes until it ceases to flow between the forceps as determined by an ammeter or current flow meter (end point monitor: Electroscope EPM-1). In most cases, three contig-

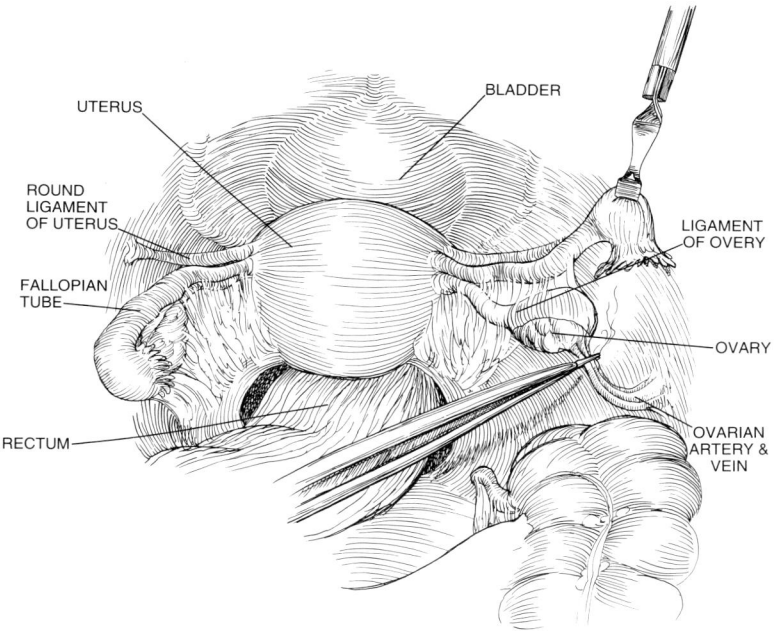

Figure 59-1.

uous areas are desiccated. Laparoscopic scissors are then used to divide the pedicle. In some cases the mesovarium alone can be desiccated and divided. Alternatively, the ENDO GIA* stapling device or suture may be applied.[12] Medial retraction with grasping forceps is helpful while the adnexa are being freed from the pelvic sidewall. The free ovary is then removed through the umbilicus or cul-de-sac.

Oophorectomy (Retroperitoneal Approach)

When the ovary or ovarian remnant is fused to or within the pelvic sidewall peritoneum, a retroperitoneal approach may be considered. Scissors or CO_2 laser is used to incise the peritoneum lateral to the infundibulopelvic ligament, progressing parallel to the tube and ovary up to the uterine end of the round ligament. With traction on the tube, ovary, or peritoneum, the retroperitoneal space is entered and its loose areolar tissue dissected with scissors or aquadissection. This dissection is continued downward until the ureter is identified. At this time, the ovarian vessels can be desiccated just caudad to where they cross over the iliac vessels. Following division of the infundibulopelvic ligament, it is placed on traction and the procedure continues caudad with division of the peritoneum just below its attachments to the ovary and lateral to its attachments to the rectosigmoid. Finally, the utero-ovarian ligament and proximal fallopian tube are desic-

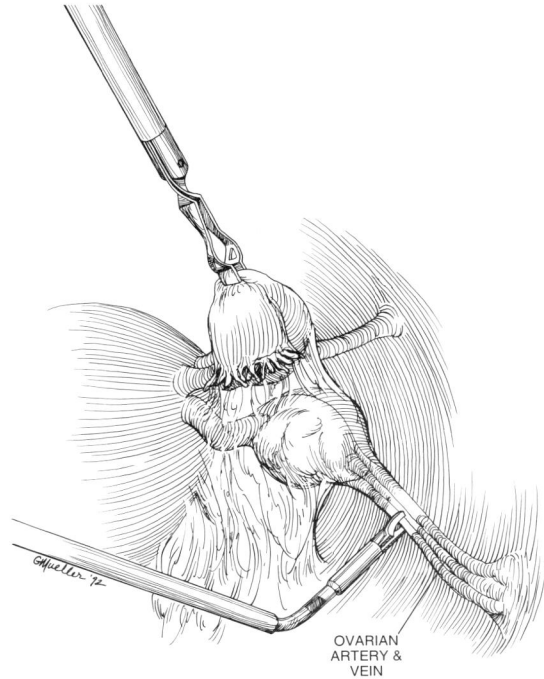

Figure 59-2.

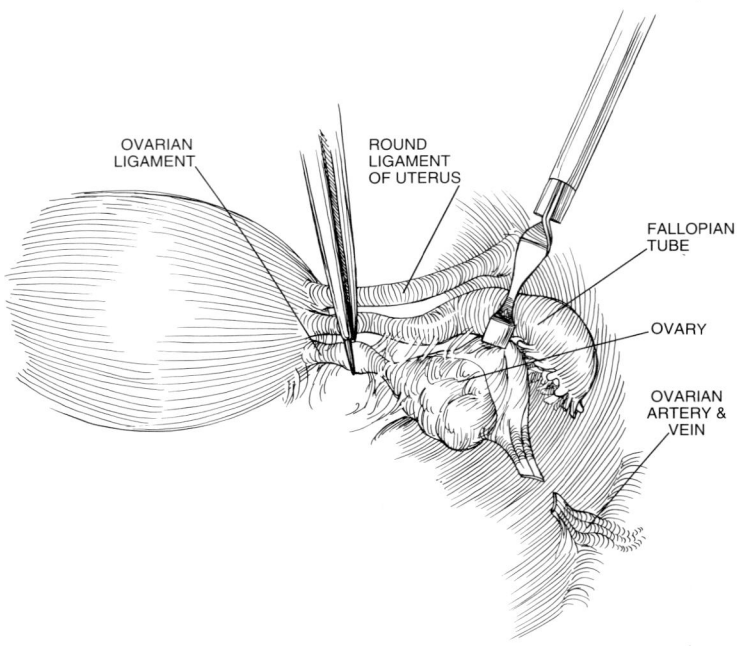

Figure 59-3.

cated and divided, freeing the specimen. Bipolar desiccation of this ligament is done most safely by inserting the forceps from the opposite side of the pelvis. The peritoneal sidewall defect is left alone.

Umbilical Extension (Fig. 59-6)

With decompressed ovaries (benign pathologic condition), the 11-mm umbilical incision can be enlarged, especially if the initial skin incision is vertically placed on the midline through the deepest part within the umbilicus. A 10-mm operating laparoscope with a 5-mm operating channel is used with a scissors in the operating channel. The tip of the laparoscope is placed 1 cm above the tip of the trocar sleeve, which is then carefully removed from the peritoneal cavity. Peritoneum first is visualized and incised downward in the midline with the scissors in the operating channel of the operating laparoscope. Next, deep fascia is identified and incised to add another 1 cm or more to the incision. Finally, the skin incision inside the umbilicus can be extended upward to incorporate the superior wall of the umbilical fossa. Compressible ovaries and cysts can be removed through this incision; this includes most benign cysts

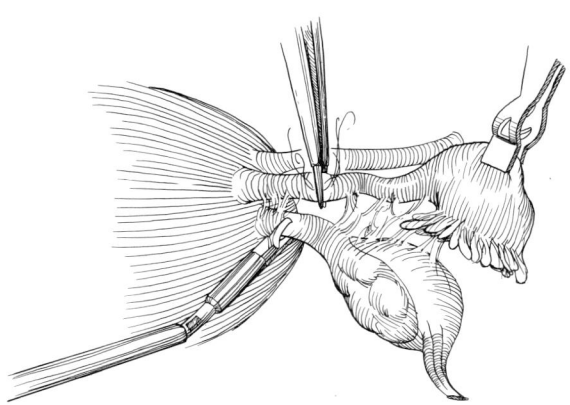

Figure 59-4.

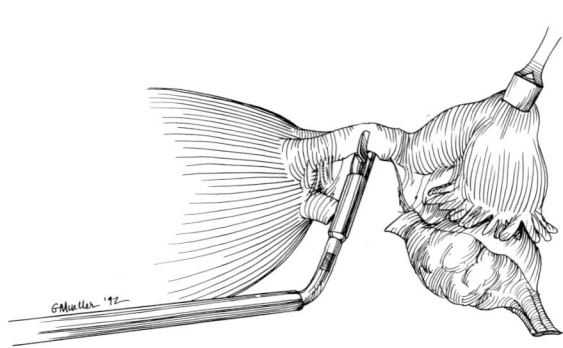

Figure 59-5.

Oophorectomy 655

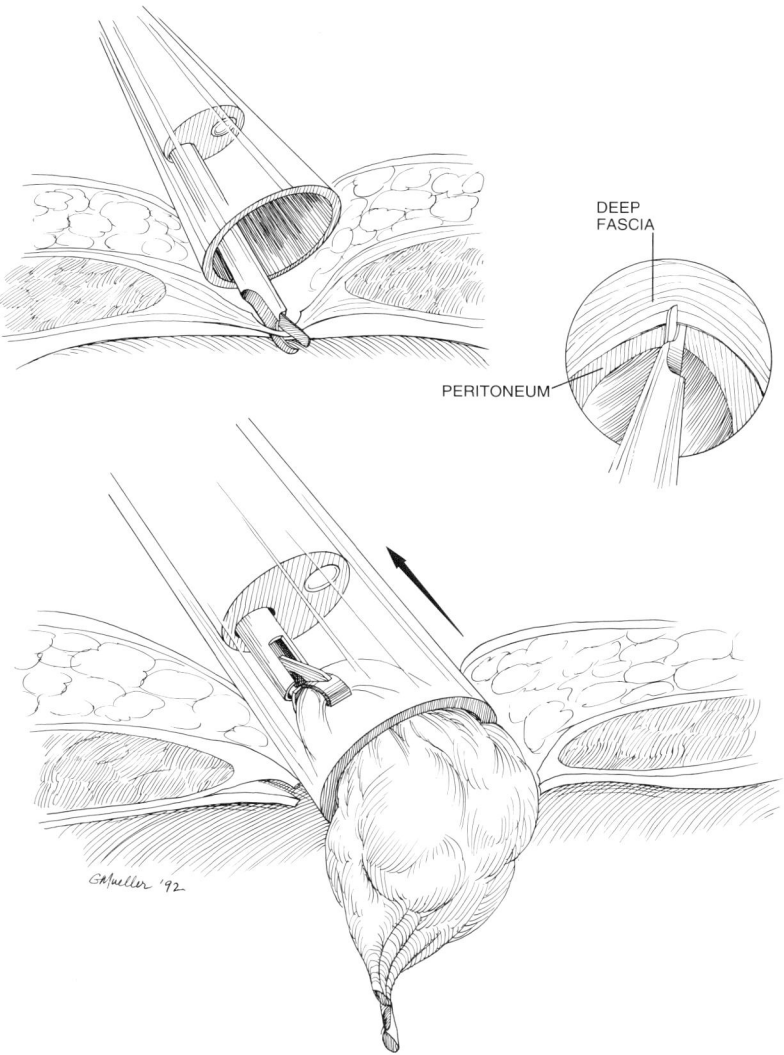

Figure 59-6.

and normal ovaries removed for adhesive disease. Five-millimeter biopsy forceps in the operating channel grasp the ovary, which is partially delivered into the tip of the umbilical trocar sleeve. The trocar sleeve and laparoscope are popped out of the umbilicus in one motion, after which the protruding tissue is grasped with hemostats or Kocher clamps and gently teased out of the peritoneal cavity. Alternatively a 5-mm laparoscope can be used for visualization through the 5-mm lower trocar sleeve, after which tissue to be removed is grasped with an 11-mm grasping forceps inserted through the umbilicus and extracted.

Laparoscopic Culdotomy (Figs. 59-7 and 59-8)

Solid and cystic ovaries of unknown pathologic condition separated intact from the pelvic sidewall are best removed through the cul-de-sac (Fig. 59-7). A posterior culdotomy incision using CO_2 laser or electrosurgery through the cul-de-sac of Douglas into the vagina is preferable to a colpotomy incision using scissors through the vagina and overlying peritoneum because complete hemostasis is obtained while making the culdotomy incision. Vaginal bleeding greater than 100 ml

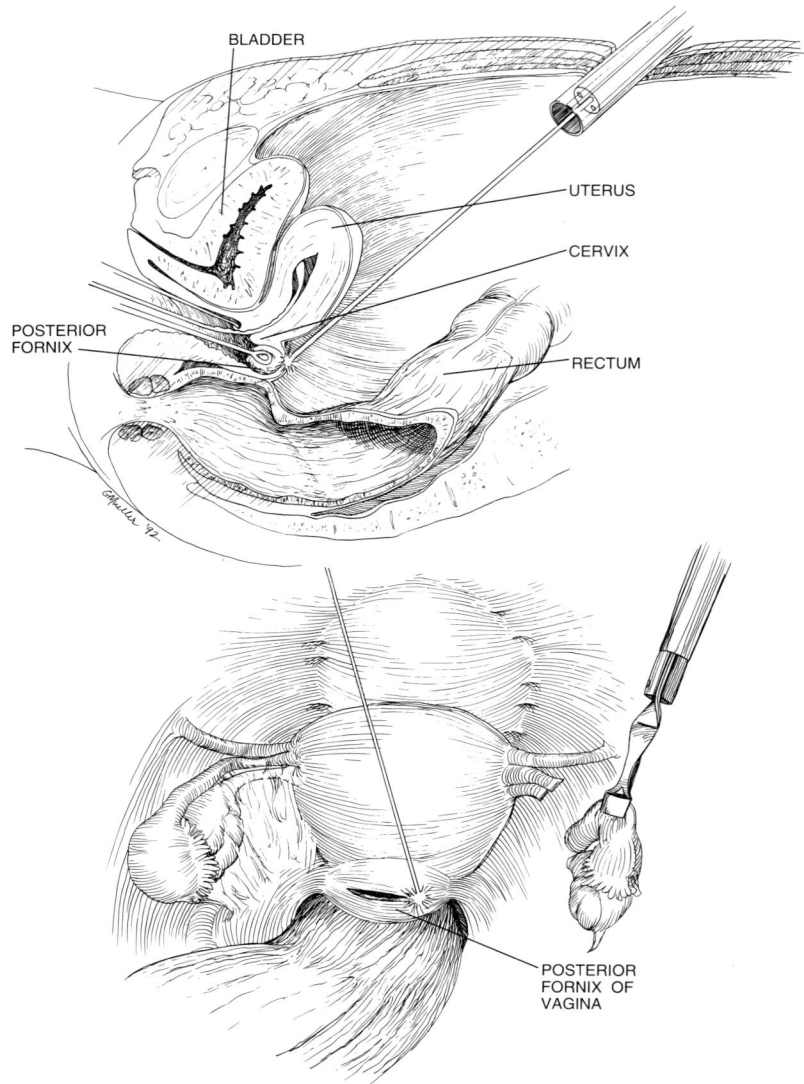

Figure 59-7.

is usual before all cuff bleeding is stopped after scissors colpotomy.

The anatomical relationship between the rectum and the posterior vagina must be confirmed before making the laparoscopic culdotomy incision to avoid cutting the rectum. A curette is placed in the uterus for elevation and anteversion. A wet sponge in a ring forceps is placed just behind the cervix to identify the posterior vaginal fornix by distending it. A rectal probe (Resnik Instruments, Skokie, IL) assures that the rectum is out of the way and aids in the dissection required should rectum cover the posterior vagina. Alternatively, a Valtchev uterine mobilizer can be inserted to antevert the uterus and delineate the posterior vagina. When this device is in the anteverted position, the cervix sits on a wide acorn making the cervicovaginal junction readily visible between the uterosacral ligaments when the cul-de-sac is inspected laparoscopically.

Before the rectal probe is removed, it may be necessary to reflect the rectum off the posterior vaginal fornix. This is performed using either cutting current through a spoon or angled spatula electrode or the laparoscopic CO_2 laser at 20 watts ultrapulse (Coherent, Palo Alto, CA). The peritoneum at the junction of the rectum and vagina is incised.

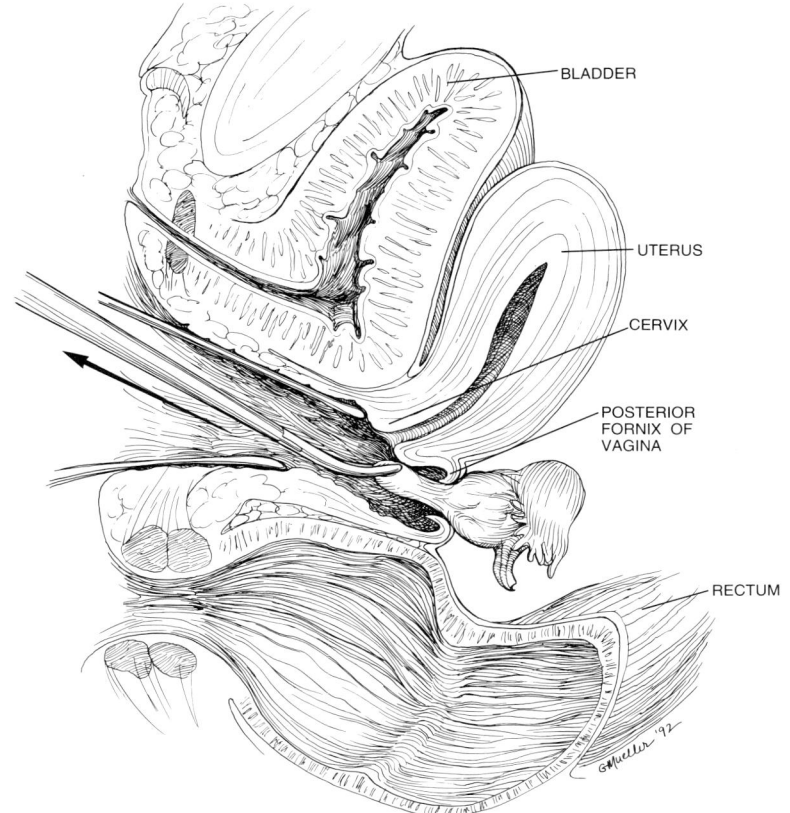

Figure 59-8.

The plane between rectum and vagina is developed using the aquadissector, and the rectum is pushed downward.

When it is clear that the rectum has been separated off the posterior vaginal wall or vaginal apex if the uterus has been removed, the upper vagina or posterior fornix is distended by the wet sponge on ring forceps. A transverse laparoscopic culdotomy incision is made with the knife electrode at 30 to 40 watts of blended current or the CO_2 laser with power set at 50 to 100 watts ultrapulse without the bleeding that accompanies a vaginal colpotomy incision made with scissors. The sponge in the posterior vagina rapidly comes into view. Some difficulty may be encountered maintaining adequate pneumoperitoneum once the vagina is entered, but the sponge in contact with the incision is usually adequate for this purpose. However, a sudden loss of pneumoperitoneum and field of view may create the potential danger of grasping bowel with a sharp forceps inserted through the vagina after losing sight of the lesion to be extracted. Following culdotomy, a sponge, pack, or 30-ml Foley balloon should be kept in close contact with the vaginal incision to avoid the loss of pneumoperitoneum and to facilitate the extraction of large masses. This loss of pneumoperitoneum can be minimized in some cases by manual labial apposition.

Laparoscopic biopsy forceps or ring forceps are inserted through the vagina and used to grasp the ovary or its attached tube and pull it out through the culdotomy incision (Fig. 59-8). Alternately, a 5-mm lower quadrant grasping forceps can be used to push the mass through the culdotomy incision. On occasion, the operator's fingers can be inserted into the peritoneal cavity to grasp the ovary.

For large cystic masses, a 14- to 18-gauge needle on a needle extension adapter (Crown Brothers, Decatur, GA) is directed through the vagina for cyst decompression. If a dermoid is present, the mass can be incised so that the thick cyst contents drain into the vagina until the mass is small enough to be pulled through the incision. Our most recent technique is to insert an impermeable sac (LapSac; Cook OB/GYN, Spencer, IN) intraperitoneally through the culdotomy incision. This 5 by 8 inch nylon bag has a polyurethane inner coating and a nylon drawstring. It is impermeable to water and dye. The ovary with intact cyst is placed in the bag which is closed by pulling its drawstring. The sac is delivered by the drawstring through the posterior vagina, the bag is opened, and the intact specimen is visually identified, decompressed, and removed.

Ovarian Remnant

Persistent pelvic pain following total abdominal hysterectomy with bilateral salpingo-oophorectomy may be secondary to an ovarian remnant, especially if the hysterectomy was performed for extensive ovarian adhesions and/or endometriosis.[13] In this author's experience with 12 patients treated laparoscopically, the ureter was contiguous with the ovarian remnant in all 12. Ten were left-sided and completely covered by the rectosigmoid in a retroperitoneal position. The two right-sided remnants were also retroperitoneal, with the rectosigmoid involved in one case.

Dissection on the left side should start well out of the pelvis where the descending colon meets the sigmoid colon. The lateral attachments of this junction in the paracolic gutter are divided and the descending colon/rectosigmoid junction reflected medially. Further dissection and reflection are necessary until the external iliac artery is exposed. Going along this large vessel, the ureter is identified and in most cases the ovarian vessel pedicle can be lifted just lateral to the ureter as it crosses the external iliac artery. Both are followed into the deep pelvis with careful dissection. The rectosigmoid is carefully reflected from the deeper ureter and the ovarian vessel pedicle which lies above until the ovarian remnant can be identified. Once the rectosigmoid is completely detached from the sidewall, ureteral dissection proceeds deeper into the pelvis, just beyond all attachments to the remnant. Thereafter the ovarian vessel pedicle is desiccated with bipolar forceps, divided, and put on medial traction to further expose the lateral limits of the ovary attached to retroperitoneal structures, usually the superior vesicle and obturator vessels. Dissection continues until the ovary is completely freed from the pelvic sidewall. Bleeding from neovascularization is controlled with the microbipolar forceps, usually underwater. The ovarian remnant is removed from the peritoneal cavity through the umbilical incision.

CLOSURE

At the close of each operation, an underwater examination is used to confirm complete hemostasis on the pelvic sidewall and the rectosigmoid in stages; this detects bleeding from vessels and viscera tamponaded during the procedure by the increased intraperitoneal pressure of the CO_2 pneumoperitoneum. The CO_2 pneumoperitoneum is displaced with 2 to 5 liters of Ringer's lactate solution, and the peritoneal cavity is vigorously irrigated and suctioned with this solution until the effluent is clear of blood products, usually after 10 to 20 liters. Underwater inspection of the pelvis is performed to detect and control any further bleeding using the Vancaillie microbipolar forceps (Storz) to coagulate through the electrolyte solution.

First, complete hemostasis is established with the patient in the Trendelenburg position. Next, complete hemostasis is secured through underwater examination with the patient supine and in the reverse Trendelenburg position using underwater microbipolar coagulation. Finally, complete hemostasis is documented with all instruments removed, including the uterine manipulator.

To visualize the pelvis with the patient supine, the 10-mm straight laparoscope and the aquadissector are manipulated together into the deep cul-de-sac beneath floating bowel and omentum, and this area is alternately irrigated and suctioned until the effluent is clear both in the pelvis and the upper abdomen. During this copious irrigation procedure, clear fluid is deposited into the pelvis and circulates into the upper abdomen, displacing upper abdominal bloody fluid, which is suctioned after flowing back into the pelvis.

A final copious lavage with Ringer's lactate solution is undertaken, and all clot is isolated, usually in the pararectosigmoid gutters, and aspirated; at least 2 liters of lactated Ringer's solution are left in the peritoneal cavity to displace CO_2 and to prevent fibrin adherences from forming by separating raw operated-upon surfaces during the initial stages of reperitonealization. No other antiadhesive agents are used. No drains, antibiotic solutions, or heparin is used. The lactated Ringer's solution is absorbed in 2 to 3 days.[14]

The umbilical incision is closed with a single 4-0 Vicryl suture opposing deep fascia and skin dermis. The knot is buried beneath the fascia.

The culdotomy incision is closed from below or laparoscopically with interrupted, figure of eight, or running 0 Vicryl suture. Vaginal suturing is aided by the use of a lateral vaginal retractor used to spread the lateral vagina adjacent to the culdotomy incision (Euro-Med, Redmond, WA; Simpson/Basye, Wilmington, DE). This device is self-retaining with a thumb-ratchet release that keeps it open and in place. Vaginal suturing can be difficult as the vaginal incision frequently becomes edematous during the procedure making exposure inadequate. Thus, the surgeon may elect to close the culdotomy incision from above using 1-3 curved needle sutures (Vicryl on a CT-2 needle) tied extracorporeally with the Clarke knot pusher.[12]

POSTOPERATIVE MANAGEMENT

After stabilization in the recovery room, the patient is transferred to the short stay unit. Diet is advanced as tolerated. Anaprox DS is used for pain. Vistaril, 50 mg intramuscularly, is used for nausea and vomiting.

The Foley catheter is removed when the patient is alert and aware of the catheter, and bethanechol chloride (Urecholine), 25 mg orally, is then given. If no antibiotic was administered in the operating room, Septra DS is given before discharge. If spontaneous voiding of approximately 250 ml does not occur within 4 hours of catheter removal, a straight catheter is inserted and 50 mg of bethanechol chloride is administered. Should voiding in good quantities not occur over the next 3 hours, the patient is admitted overnight with a Foley catheter in place to be removed in the morning.

Following voiding, the patient is usually discharged with Anaprox DS as the only pain medication. Because of the large amount of Ringer's lactate irrigant left in the peritoneal cavity, fluid commonly oozes from patients' lower quadrant 5-mm incision sites, which have been covered with Collodion without suture. This oozing of fluid ceases within 24 hours, but many patients are discharged with Chux nonwoven disposable underpads or a towel inside their undergarments.

CRITERIA FOR PATIENT DISCHARGE

In most cases the decision for discharge is made by the patient and her family. If she is awake and alert with minimal discomfort, she may leave the hospital for home or a nearby hotel room on the day of the procedure. In 75 per cent of cases, patients undergoing laparoscopic oophorectomy will be discharged the same day.

COMPLICATIONS SPECIFIC FOR THIS PROCEDURE

Bipolar desiccation of ovarian and uteroovarian vessels has been a safe method of ligation in this author's experience. Postoperative pain is less than following suture ligation as electrosurgical desiccation eliminates later distal ischemic necrosis. There have been no late bleeding episodes in over 400 oophorectomies performed in this manner.

While culdotomy surgery offers an opportunity for invasion by organisms already present in the genital tract, the use of an electrosurgical or laser incision, aspiration of all blood clots, and copious irrigation with over 2 liters of irrigant left in the peritoneal cavity at the close of the procedure eliminates the environment necessary for proliferation of these organisms. Pelvic cellulitis and postoperative sepsis with laparoscopic culdotomy using these techniques have not been reported.

REFERENCES

1. Semm K, Mettler L. Technical progress in pelvic surgery via operative laparoscopy. Am J Obstet Gynecol 1980; 138:121–127.
2. Reich H, McGlynn F. Laparoscopic oophorectomy and salpingo-oophorectomy in the treatment of benign tuboovarian disease. J Reprod Med 1986; 31:609.
3. Reich H. Laparoscopic oophorectomy and salpingo-oophorectomy in the treatment of benign tubo-ovarian disease. Int J Fertil 1987; 32:233–236.
4. Reich H. Laparoscopic oophorectomy without ligature or morcellation. Contemp Obstet Gynecol 1989; 9:34–46.
5. Barber HR, Graber EA. The PMPO syndrome (postmenopausal palpable ovary syndrome). Obstet Gynecol, 1971; 38:921–923.
6. Levine RL. Pelviscopic surgery in women over 40. J Reprod Med 1990; 35:597–600.
7. Parker WH, Berek JS. Management of selected cystic adnexal masses in postmenopausal women by operative laparoscopy: A pilot study. Am J Obstet Gynecol 1990; 163:1574–1577.

8. Mann W, Reich H. Laparoscopic adnexectomy in postmenopausal women. J Reprod Med 1992; 37:254–256.
9. Reich H, McGlynn F, Wilkie W. Laparoscopic management of Stage I ovarian cancer. J Reprod Med 1990; 35:601–605.
10. Reich H, McGlynn F, Wilkie W. Laparoscopic management of stage I ovarian cancer. Obstet Gynecol Surv 1990; 45:772–773.
11. Reich H, McGlynn F. Short self-retaining trocar sleeves. Am J Obstet Gynecol 1990; 162:453–454.
12. Reich H, Clarke HC, Sekel L. A simple method for ligating in operative laparoscopy with straight and curved needles. Obstet Gynecol 1992; 79:143–147.
13. Price FV, Edwards R, Buchsbaum HJ. Ovarian remnant syndrome: Difficulties in diagnosis and management. Obstet Gynecol Surv 1990; 45:151–156.
14. Rose BI, MacNeill C, Larrain R, Kopreski MM. Abdominal instillation of high-molecular-weight dextran or lactated Ringer's solution after laparoscopic surgery: A randomized comparison of the effect on weight change. J Reprod Med 1991; 36:537–539.

Chapter 60
Pelvic Lymphadenectomy

Dudley Seth Danoff
Alex Gershman

Pelvic lymphadenectomy has gained widespread acceptance as the *final* staging procedure in the definitive treatment of prostatic cancer. The standard open procedure of bilateral pelvic lymphadenectomy, which routinely precedes radical prostate cancer surgery, has both a significant morbidity and considerable negative economic impact associated with abdominal incision and lengthy hospitalization and convalescence. The introduction of new instrumentation has made laparoscopic pelvic lymphadenectomy not only feasible but a standard part of clinical practice for many urologists. The development of laparoscopic pelvic lymphadenectomy techniques and instrumentation suggests that open lymphadenectomy is unnecessary. Laparoscopic lymphadenectomy is an extremely useful cost-effective staging procedure when combined with perineal prostatectomy or transperineal radioactive implants in the treatment of prostatic carcinoma. The veritable explosion in the number of operable carcinomas of the prostate being diagnosed at an early stage by virtue of the widespread use of prostate-specific antigen (PSA) screening makes it essential for all urologists to learn this technique. The use of pelvic computed tomography (CT), transrectal magnetic resonance imaging, (MRI) and elevated PSA to evaluate the status of the obturator and iliac lymph nodes is unreliable, when compared to laparoscopic pelvic lymphadenectomy. Although the learning curve may be steep initially, the urologist's prior experience with the cystoscope gives a clear edge in learning laparoscopic techniques, applying many of the same principles used in transurethral surgery.

PATIENT SELECTION

Prostatic carcinoma has been diagnosed in all patients after having undergone transrectal ultrasonically guided prostate biopsy. In general, those patients who are suspected of having positive nodes are ideal candidates for laparoscopic pelvic lymphadenectomy. This is usually determined by elevation in the PSA value, a suspicious MRI or CT scan, a high Gleason grade of the biopsy specimen, multifocal prostatic disease, a suspicious lesion noted on the transrectal ultrasound, or a bone scan suggestive of metastatic disease.

Those patients with either a significantly elevated prostatic acid phosphatase or bone scan and confirmatory skeletal survey that are unequivocally positive for metastatic bone disease are not considered candidates for radical prostatectomy and therefore would not undergo staging laparoscopic pelvic lymphadenectomy in our series. In our experience, identification of metastatic obturator or pelvic lymph nodes by pelvic CT scan or MRI is not reliable. Consequently, laparoscopic pelvic lymphadenectomy is undertaken prior to radical prostatectomy to ensure a tissue diagnosis. We have encountered a significant number of patients in whom both the PSA and acid phosphatase were normal and the transrectal MRI or pelvic CT disclosed normal appearing lymph nodes and yet nonetheless positive lymph nodes were found at exploration. Consequently, bilateral laparoscopic pelvic lymphadenectomy for us is the final and definitive staging procedure for prostatic neoplasm.

PREOPERATIVE EVALUATION

All patients who are suspected of having prostate cancer are initially screened with a digital rectal examination, transrectal prostate ultrasound, and serum prostate acid phosphatase and PSA tests. Then, an ultrasonically guided transrectal prostate biopsy is done. If the pathologist reports adenocarcinoma of the prostate, the patient's disease is further staged with either a pelvic CT scan or, preferably, a transrectal MRI. We have found that the use of the transrectal probe with MRI has allowed us improved visualization of the obturator area and has increased our ability to detect the possibility of positive lymph nodes. It is well known that the findings of positive nodes drastically alters the survival of patients with prostate cancer. The finding of positive nodes should direct the treating physician to an alternate form of therapy. If metastatic disease is identified, we do not proceed with radical prostatectomy and laparoscopic lymphadenectomy has spared the patient an incisional procedure.

PREOPERATIVE PREPARATION

Patients are admitted to the hospital on the evening prior to surgery. Patients are prepared for laparoscopic pelvic lymphadenectomy in the same manner as they would be prepared to undergo radical prostatic surgery, with the assumption that the lymph nodes will be negative. If positive lymph nodes are identified by frozen section at the time of the laparoscopic procedure, the radial surgery is abandoned, and the patient is discharged from the hospital either on the same day or the following day. Routine preoperative laboratory studies include chest x-ray, electrocardiogram, complete blood count including platelet count, basic chemistry panel, prothrombin time, partial thromboplastin time, and template bleeding time. On the evening before surgery, the patient is given a liquid diet. An intravenous infusion of 5 per cent dextrose in 0.25 normal saline is started. The patient is given intravenous antibiotics. We use a second generation cephaloridine, which provides broad spectrum and gram-negative coverage. The patient is started on a mechanical and chemical bowel preparation which includes:

1. A clear liquid dinner.
2. GoLYTELY, 2 to 3 liters by mouth, which is the essence of the mechanical preparation.
3. Neomycin base with erythromycin base, 1 g by mouth. We start this on the afternoon prior to the contemplated surgery, giving one dose at 2:00 p.m., a second dose at 4:00 p.m., and a third dose at 8:00 p.m. If the patient is admitted later in the afternoon we change the hour of the doses accordingly so that the first dose is given at hour 0, the second dose is given at hour 2, and the third dose is given at hour 6. Both the neomycin base and erythromycin base are given together.
4. A tap water enema on the morning of surgery.

We feel that this bowel preparation is very important, even though the possibility of rectal or intestinal injury is remote. Should bowel injury occur, we feel comfortable enough with this bowel preparation to proceed with a primary closure instead of a diverting colostomy. Also, a mechanically cleansed bowel makes retraction and movement of these intraperitoneal structures out of the pelvis easier during the laparoscopic procedure.

EQUIPMENT

In order to perform adequate laparoscopic pelvic lymphadenectomy, five major types of capital equipment are necessary as a functional unit.

1. Insufflators. A high flow carbon dioxide (CO_2) peritoneal insufflator must be capable of delivering flow rates of at least 8 to 10 liters/min. The high flow feature is very important in case the pneumoperitoneum is lost during the procedure. Automatic pressure control is essential to prevent overinsufflation and maintain constant pressure while instruments are being loaded and unloaded through the trocars invariably with some

loss of the pneumoperitoneum. Ideally, laparoscopy for pelvic lymphadenectomy is carried out at a pressure of 15 to 16 mm Hg. We specifically request that at least two CO_2 tanks of 300-liter capacity each be readily available and connected to the field by a minimum of 4 m of tubing, so that the tanks are well away from the field and other video equipment (Fig. 60-1).

2. Suction-irrigation systems. There are a number of such suction/irrigation devices available. Both the suction tubing and saline irrigation must be set up prior to insufflating the abdomen because they must be readily available in case of bleeding during the laparoscopic dissection.

3. Videoendoscopy systems (Fig. 60-2). A "chip camera" is used to reproduce high resolution video images on two video monitors placed on either side of the table, so that the surgeon and the assistant each are looking at their own monitors across the table as they face the patient. This arrangement dramatically facilitates eye-hand coordination between the surgeon and the assistant. Cameras that attach directly to the laparoscope are preferable to those that require additional coupling. A zoom feature on the camera is essential, especially when working deep in the pelvis. Be sure, when selecting the camera, that the zoom controls do not interfere with the focusing adjustment. A sharp, clear, and in focus image is absolutely essential for doing this kind of surgery successfully. Video monitors (Fig. 60-3) placed on either side of the operating table should be at least 13 inches diagonally with at least 400 lines of horizontal resolution. The use of two monitors facilitates the procedure and allows the remaining people on the operating team to

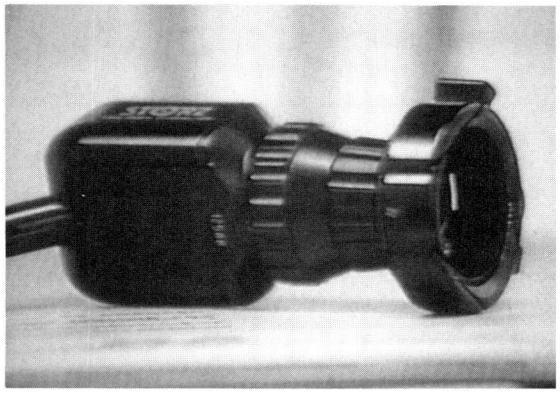

Figure 60-2.

have a constant view of the laparoscopic appearance of the surgical field. The success of pelvic lymphadenectomy is limited by the clarity of the images projected onto the monitor screen and the highest standard of equipment is therefore necessary to achieve this goal. Especially during the learning curve, all laparoscopic pelvic lymphadenectomies should be recorded on videotape. These tapes can be used for later review and familiarization with the anatomical structures necessary to carry out successful laparoscopic pelvic lymphadenectomy.

We use a laparoscope with a 0-degree lens, which provides an image of what is directly in front of the camera. The urologist is familiar with this image from the use of the urethrotome or resectoscope. A 30-degree lens

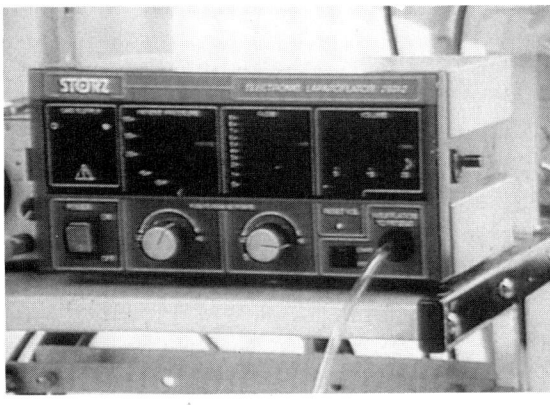

Figure 60-1.

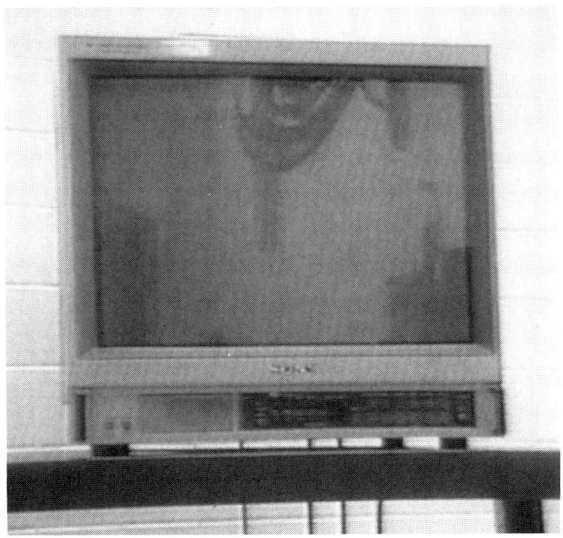

Figure 60-3.

may also be used, but for pelvic work the 0-degree lens is most useful. The lens system has a depth of field that ranges from 1 mm to 10 cm. The distal tip of the laparoscope is kept between 1 and 2 cm from the actual operative field, and at this range the picture and image are sharp and clear.

A video printer can also be added to the system and allows the surgeon to produce a photograph from the video image, which can be placed as a permanent part of the patient's record and used in educating other physicians on the remarkable access to the pelvis gained through the laparoscope.

4. Endoscopic light sources (Fig. 60-4). A 300-watt xenon endoscopic light source is ideally suited for pelvic lymphadenectomy through the laparoscope.

5. Electrosurgical unit.

6. Lasers (optional). We have not found lasers to offer any advantage in the performance of bilateral pelvic lymphadenectomy over monopolar electocautery. However, two types of lasers are applicable to laparoscopic pelvic lymphadenectomy. Both the neodymium-yttrium-aluminum-garnet (Nd:YAG) and the krypton:Nd:YAG lasers are used. If the urologist feels comfortable with use of the YAG laser, then it can be used for pelvic lymphadenectomy. As laser technology advances and specialized tips made of sapphire or hardened quartz or other heat-resistant optically transparent materials develop, and if the smoke problem can be resolved, then lasers may prove to be an excellent adjunct in the performance of laparoscopic pelvic lymph node dissection.

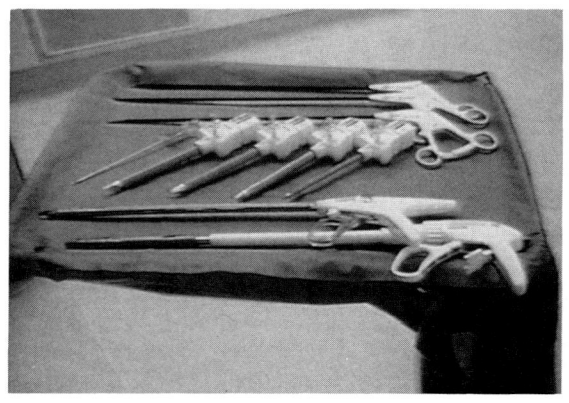

Figure 60-5.

INSTRUMENTATION (Fig. 60-5)

A Veress needle is used to create the pneumoperitoneum. Its spring-loaded obturator advances in front of the needle and this safety feature prevents perforation of intraabdominal organs. The Veress needle is placed infra- or subumbilically, as the abdominal wall is elevated. To confirm the correct placement of the needle, it is first aspirated with a syringe and then 5 to 10 ml of normal saline are injected and should flow smoothly and drain into the abdomen. Once proper placement of the Veress needle is ensured, the tubing from the insufflator is attached, and a pneumoperitoneum is created gradually to 15 to 16 mm Hg. If this is not the case, the needle must be removed.

Five trocars are used: one 11-mm SURGIPORT* trocar, two 10-mm SURGIPORT* trocars, and two 5-mm SURGIPORT* trocars. Their placement will be described later in the chapter. In addition, two SURGIPORT* 10.5-mm convertor-reducers are needed along with two SURGIPORT* 5.5-mm convertor-reducers.

One ENDO SHEARS* device is required as well as one medium and one large ENDO CLIP* applier. One endoscopic vein retractor and one endoscopic Kittner should be in the setup. Several types of endoscopic graspers and dissectors must also be available for use. The purpose of the 5.5-mm convertor-reducer is to prevent escape of the pneumoperitoneum when a 5-mm instrument is used through a 10- or 11-mm trocar. Prior to the use of this instrument, the reducer or gasket must be placed to provide a tight seal around the smaller diameter of the working instrument as it passes

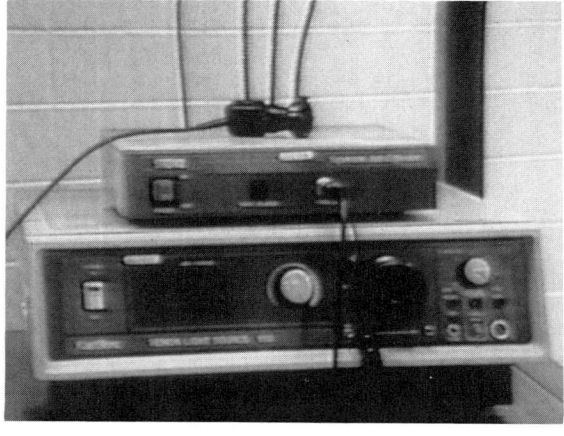

Figure 60-4.

through the larger diameter of the trocar. The endoscopic vein retractors are used through the 10-mm trocar and function exactly as in open surgery.

ENDO CLIP* appliers, both medium and large, are placed through the 10-mm trocar and are used for vessel, vas deferens, and lymphatic ligation. The ENDO CLIP* applier has a 360-degree rotational head and is extremely useful in the pelvis.

The ENDO SHEARS* with monopolar cautery attached also has full rotational capability. This is the most useful and versatile of all of the laparoscopic instruments. It is used as a cutting instrument, blunt dissector, spreader, and cauterizer. A variety of grasping forceps are also used, usually being placed through the 5-mm trocar or through the 10-mm trocar with an appropriate reducer.

POSITIONING OF THE PATIENT

The patient is placed supine (Fig. 60-6). The foot of the table is lowered and the legs are placed down as far as they will go. The table is then tilted into the maximum Trendelenburg position. With the legs down, the patient does not slip to the head of the table with this extreme position. In addition, the table is tilted a full 30 degrees away from the side that is being dissected. If the node dissection is begun on the right side, the patient is placed in the maximum Trendelenburg position and then the table tilted 30 degrees to the left. This causes all of the intraperitoneal contents to fall *away* from the right pelvic side wall. Similarly, the iliac artery, vein, inguinal ring, and obturator area become accessible without having to retract bowel. It is always necessary to securely tape the patient to the table to prevent slippage. Shoulder braces, pillows, and straps are also useful.

A Foley catheter is placed prior to creating a pneumoperitoneum and the bladder is drained and completely decompressed. The bowel preparation results in complete decompression of the colon and small intestines for maximal exposure. No nasogastric tube is used. The ureters are not stented or catheterized. In addition, the arms of the patient are placed at the patient's side and rolled under a towel. A small sandbag or rolled towel is placed under the patient's lumbar spine so that the normal lordotic curve of the pelvis is neutralized.

POSITIONING OF THE VIDEO EQUIPMENT AND OPERATING ROOM SETUP

The surgeon and assistant are placed on opposite sides of the table (Fig. 60-7). Each has his or her own video monitor placed conveniently so that it is viewed across the table. The light source, camera control, and suction and irrigation apparatus are placed at some distance from the table so as not to interfere with movement of either surgeon or assistant. The tubing from the suction and irrigation apparatus must be long enough to be comfortably secured on the operative field and yet not interfere with the movement of the instruments through the trocars. The electrosurgical unit is placed at the foot of the table, well away from the operative field.

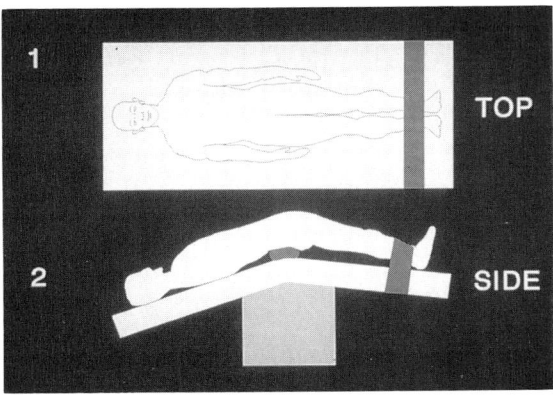

Figure 60-6.

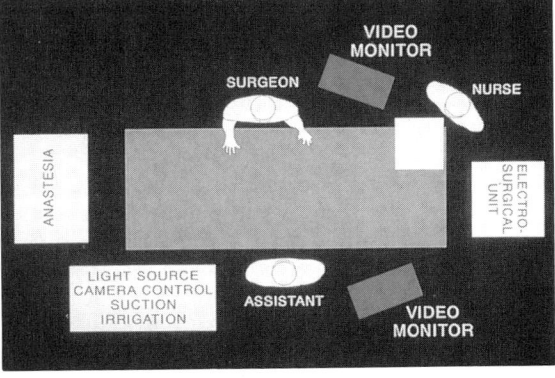

Figure 60-7.

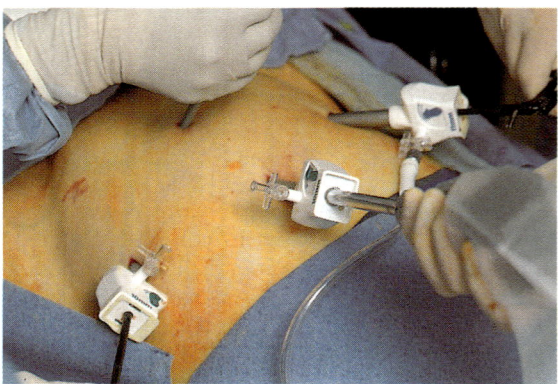

Figure 60-8.

TROCAR PLACEMENT AND SIZE SELECTION

The size and selection of trocars have evolved since we first started to do bilateral pelvic lymphadectomies through the laparoscope. Initially, four ports were utilized: one for the camera in the subumbilical region, a second in the midline approximately 2 cm above the symphysis pubis, and two additional trocars just anterior and medial to each iliac crest (Fig. 60-8). Once experienced, the laparoscopy technician can be trained to hold and direct the camera. This allows usage of five ports, including two working ports for the surgeon and two for the assistant. The midsuprapubic port is deleted. The infraumbilical port is kept for the camera and two working ports are placed on each side of the patient. The first port is placed somewhat medial and above the anterior iliac crest and then a second port is placed 2 cm above an imaginary line drawn between the port holding the camera and the port just medial to the anterior iliac crest. Two similar ports are placed on the opposite side (Fig. 60-9).

The surgeon and the assistant can each work through two ports, and this works best when the surgeon uses the ENDO SHEARS* device with coagulation through the port closest to the anterior iliac crest on the side *opposite* to the lymphatic chain being dissected. The assistant retracts through the ports opposite the surgeon. For example, if the right iliac nodes are being dissected, the surgeon stands on the left side of the table and uses the ENDO SHEARS* device and a grasper through the two ports in proximity to the left iliac crest. The assistant is standing on the right side of the patient, retracting with two grasping forceps through the ports in proximity to the right anterior iliac crest (Fig. 60-10).

A 10-mm trocar is placed in the subumbilical region, and this will be used for the video equipment. The trocars placed closest to each anterior iliac crest are one 10-mm and one 11-mm trocar. A 10-mm cannula will be inserted through the 11-mm trocar to remove the nodal tissue once dissected. The two trocars superior to the iliac crest are 5 mm each and are used mostly for grasping, dissecting with the ENDO SHEARS* device and coagulation. A Kittner can also be placed through the 5-mm ports.

METHODS OF EXPOSURE AND RETRACTION

The patient's preoperative bowel preparation, which has mechanically cleansed and decompressed all of the bowel and intestinal structures, will allow easy mobilizing of all the intestinal structures out of the pelvis. In addition, the extreme Trendelenburg position and 30-degree tilt, either right or left, also enhance retraction of the peritoneal contents out of the field of vision. A Kittner can be placed through one of the 5-mm trocars for further blunt retraction. The endoscopic vein retractor on the iliac vein, artery, or obturator nerve can be placed through one of the 10-mm trocars. No further retraction is usually needed.

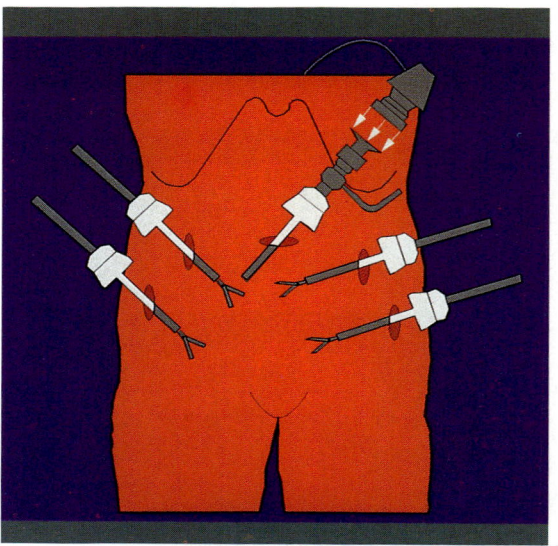

Figure 60-9.

Pelvic Lymphadenectomy   667

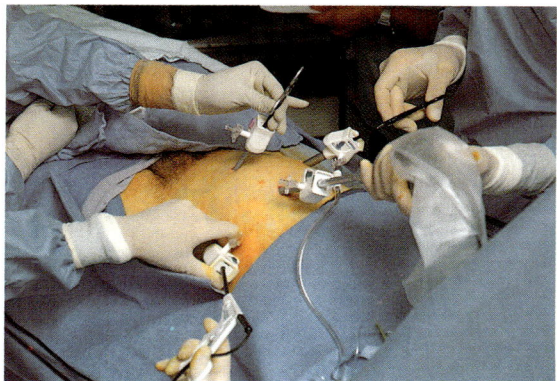

Figure 60-10.

With the camera positioned in the midline, both the right and left operative fields can be visualized (Fig. 60-11).

METHODS OF DISSECTION AND SPECIFIC DETAILS OF THE PROCEDURE

Once the abdomen and pelvis have been explored with the laparoscope, the side of interest is dissected first. If the lesion is right-sided, the nodal dissection is begun on the right side and vice versa. For purposes of this chapter, we will begin with the description of the right nodal chain (Fig. 60-12).

The landmarks are outlined (Fig. 60-13): the umbilical ligament in yellow; the vas deferens crossing over the umbilical ligament and the iliac artery in blue; and the outline of the external iliac artery in red. The spermatic vessels can be visualized at the extreme right of the field. The dissection is started by incising the peritoneal reflection just lateral to the

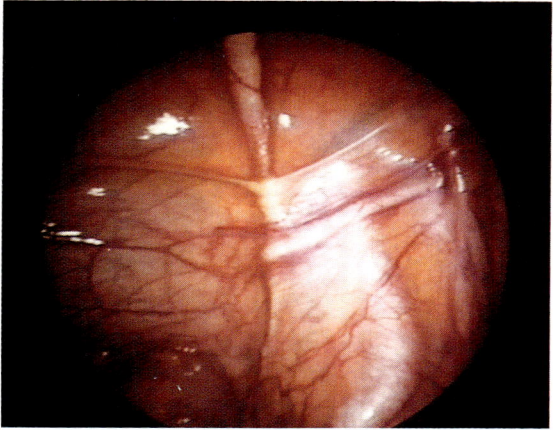

Figure 60-12.

umbilical ligament. The surgeon, who is standing on the left of the patient, first grasps the umbilical ligament with a toothed-rigid grasping forceps (Fig. 60-14). Through the opposite port contiguous to the right anterior iliac crest and with the ENDO SHEARS* device, the peritoneum is incised along the dotted line (Fig. 60-14) using a combination of blunt and sharp dissection and electrocautery. The key is to try to extend the line of dissection as far anteriorly as possible until the undersurface of the symphysis pubis at Cooper's ligament is exposed. This is an important landmark. The dissection is then carried down over the vas deferens and curves laterally across the base of the external iliac artery just below its bifurcation with the internal iliac artery. At this point, the vas deferens is grasped and using curved ENDO SHEARS*

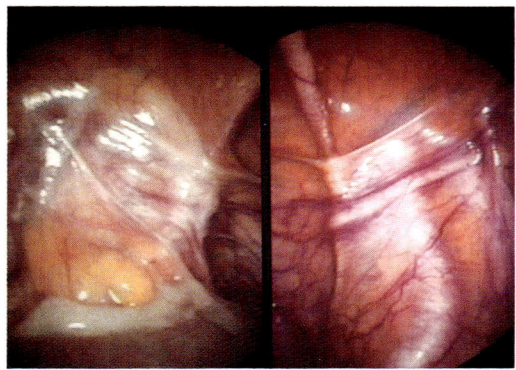

Figure 60-11.

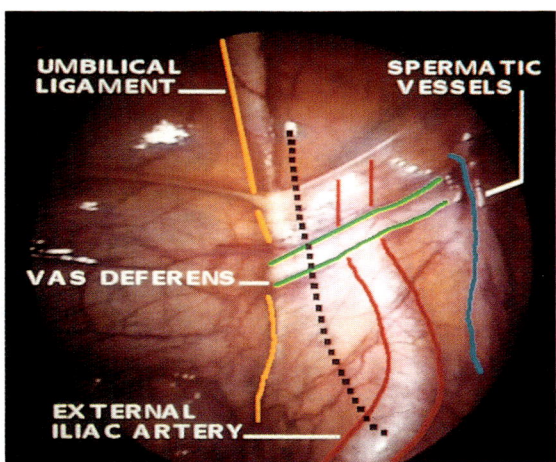

Figure 60-13.

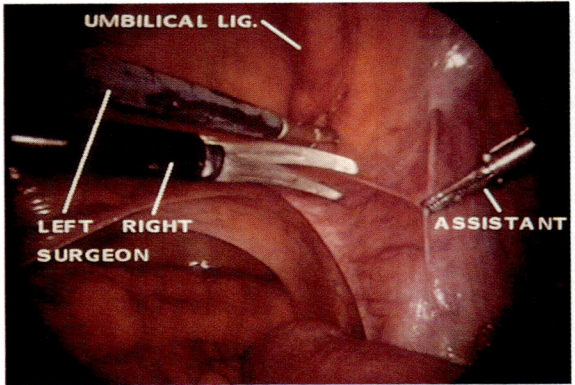

Figure 60-14.

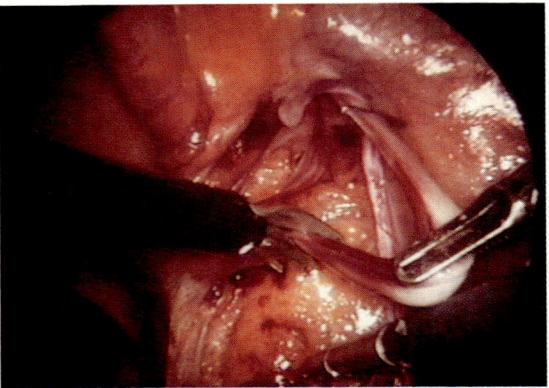

Figure 60-16.

device is freed from the surrounding structures (Fig. 60-15). It is elevated and the surgeon places an ENDO CLIP* applier through the 10-mm trocar and clips it, and it is taken and removed through one of 10-mm ports (Fig. 60-16). The surgeon then grasps the medial portion of the cut vas deferens and the assistant grasps the lateral portion and they retract in opposite directions. This opens the space medial to the iliac artery and vein and lateral to the umbilical ligament. This is the area of interest and where most of the significant obturator and iliac lymph nodes are found (Fig. 60-17 and 60-18).

The dissection of the lymph nodes is started as close to Cooper's ligament as possible (Fig. 60-19). The lymph chain is separated from the area of Cooper's ligament by sharp and blunt dissection. An ENDO CLIP* applier, placed through a 10-mm trocar, is used to begin the dissection. Sometimes, the circumflex iliac vein is encountered at this point

and care must be taken not to injure it or considerable bleeding will ensue (Fig. 60-20). The lymphatic chain is then grasped by the surgeon, using an atraumatic grasper, and with the other hand, the ENDO SHEARS* device is used to tease the nodal package free. With some practice, the chain can be removed intact. At the same time, an endoscopic vein retractor holds the iliac vein laterally. At this point, the obturator nerve is encountered, as it enters the obturator fossa. With the umbilical ligament retracted medially, the nodal chain being dissected cephalad, and the obturator nerve or iliac vein being retracted laterally, the nodal package is exposed and delivered.

A key maneuver is to cleanly expose the pubic bone at the apex of the dissection (Fig. 60-21). By establishing this landmark, the nodal chain can be grasped and brought medial to the obturator nerve and iliac vessels (Fig. 60-22). We have found a "Russian-type"

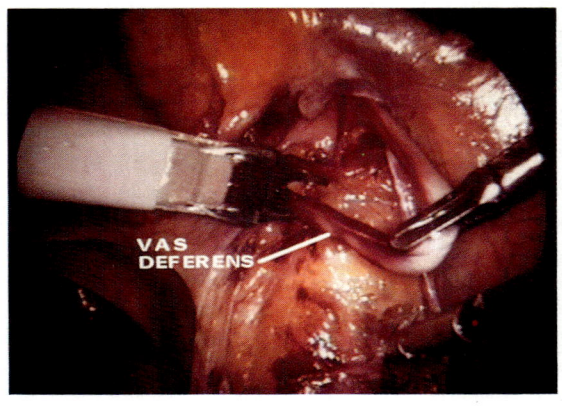

Figure 60-15.

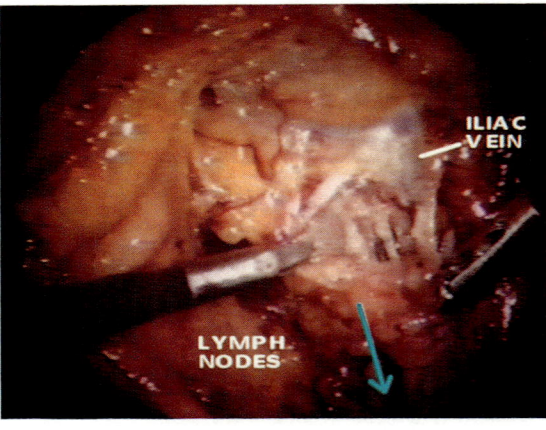

Figure 60-17.

Pelvic Lymphadenectomy   669

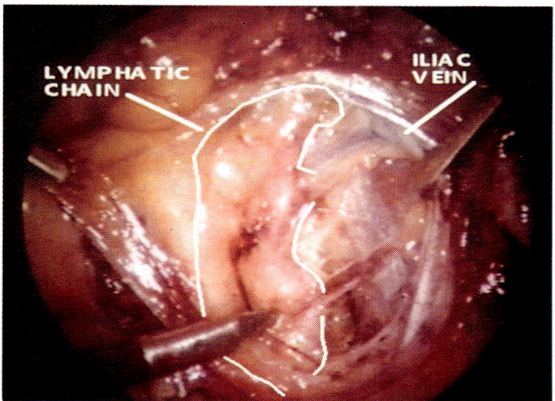

Figure 60-18.

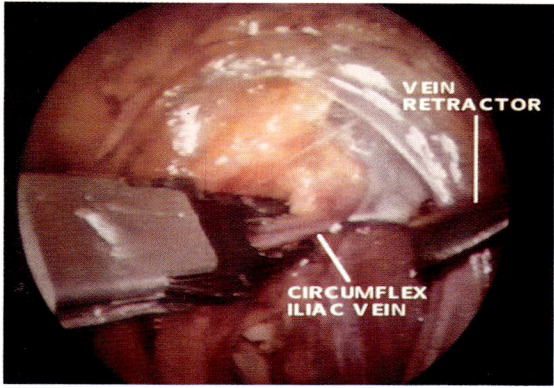

Figure 60-20.

pickup used by the surgeon through either port to be a most useful instrument. With this instrument, a teasing technique is used to bring the nodal tissue from around the obturator nerve. This technique separates the nodal tissue from some of the adherent fat, without injuring any vascular structures or traumatizing the obturator nerve (Fig. 60-23). Lymphocele has not been a problem because the opening in the peritoneum is not closed and any accumulated lymphatic fluid is absorbed back into the peritoneal cavity.

Should any part of the lymph chain being retracted cephalad and dissected come free, these nodal structures are placed conveniently in the pelvis, so that all of the nodes for each side are removed at the same time through one trocar in a single maneuver (Fig. 60-24). Smoke from the electrocautery is usually dissipated throughout the peritoneal cavity once the pneumoperitoneum is created and is not problematic.

Once the dissection is complete (Fig. 60-25) and the nodes removed, meticulous inspection is made of the area to be certain that there is perfect hemostasis. Should there be any signs of bleeding, a suction-irrigator is placed through one of the 10-mm trocars. Major bleeding has not been encountered thus far in our series.

Dissection on the left side is universally more difficult than that on the right because bowel adhesions are usually attached to the umbilical ligament. These can be lysed quickly and expeditiously. We have observed that the CO_2 used to create the pneumoperitoneum literally dissects and defines the avascular planes. This makes lysis even easier through the laparoscope than it is in open surgery.

The dissection is carried along the descending sigmoid colon, which is retracted cephalad, as it adheres to the area overlying the umbilical ligament and vas deferens (Fig.

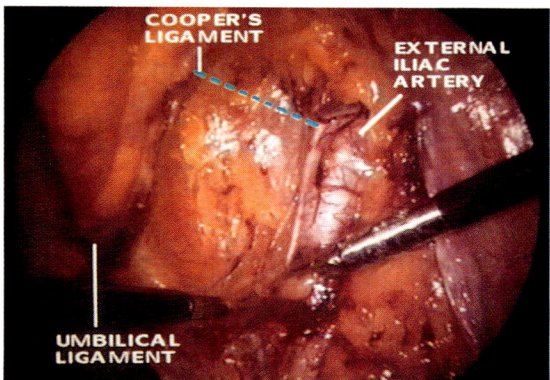

Figure 60-19.

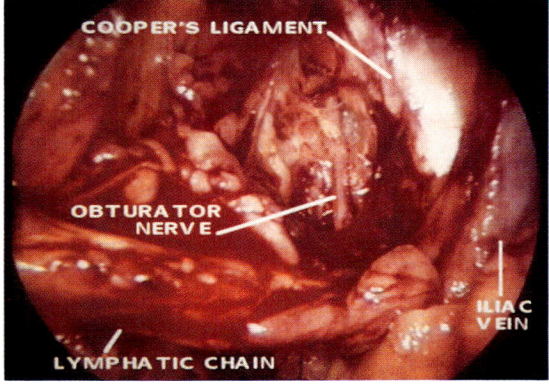

Figure 60-21.

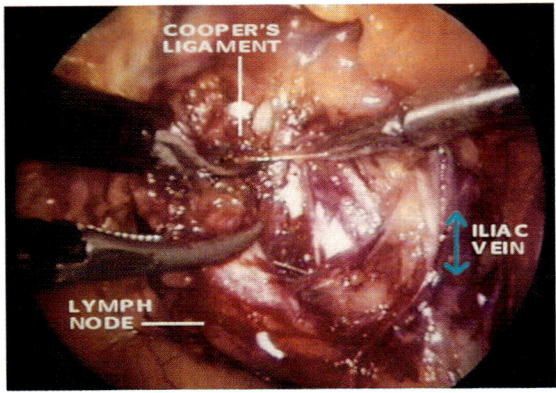

Figure 60-22.

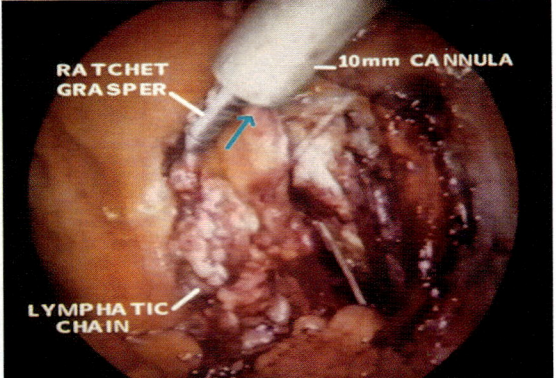

Figure 60-24.

60-26). The dissection of these adhesions can proceed rapidly and safely. Once this is done, the vas deferens will appear underlying the adhesions, similar to its appearance on the right side (Fig. 60-27). The left umbilical ligament is then grasped medially by the surgeon, who in this case is standing on the right side of the table, and is retracted. The assistant, standing on the left side of the table, will pick up the vas deferens and retract it laterally. The vas is completely dissected free of the surrounding structures and a clip is applied to each end of the vas, which is then taken. With exactly the same technique as on the right side, each end of the vas is pulled in opposite directions to open the field of interest medial to the left iliac artery and vein and lateral to the umbilical ligament. Once the bowel adhesions are lysed, the operative field is exactly the same as on the right side.

On several occasions in our early experience, we encountered positive nodes which appeared to be entrapping the obturator nerve (Fig. 60-28). In the first several cases we struggled heroically in attempting to remove these obviously positive nodes from around the obturator nerve. We realized, however, that a positive lymph node would justify termination of the procedure. Consequently, we introduced an extra long biopsy needle, placed directly through the abdominal wall under the visual control of the laparoscope. We used this merely to sample the involved node by taking several cores of tissue for pathologic examinations. On two occasions, we were able to make a diagnosis of metastatic carcinoma based on this small sample of tissue without actually removing the positive node.

In summary, the key to the successful removal of the obturator lymph nodes is that

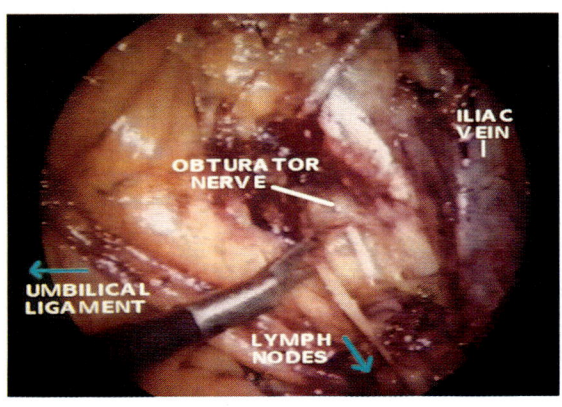

Figure 60-23.

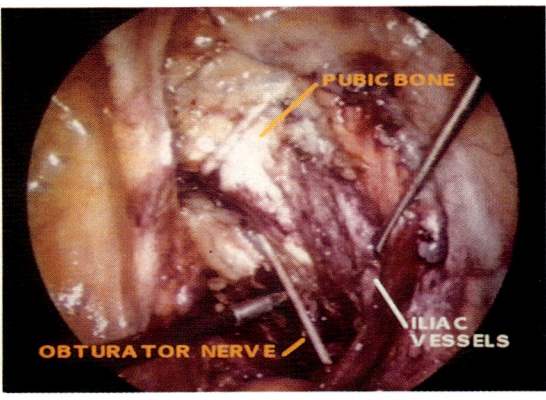

Figure 60-25.

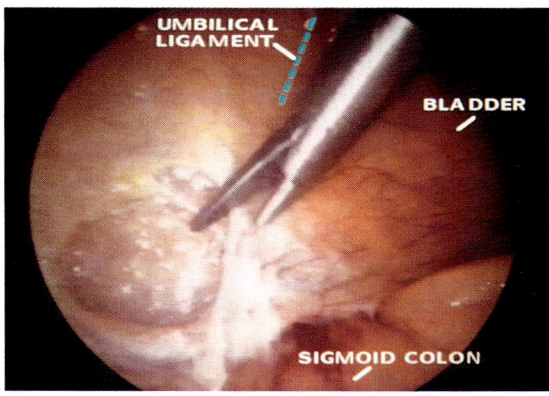

Figure 60-26.

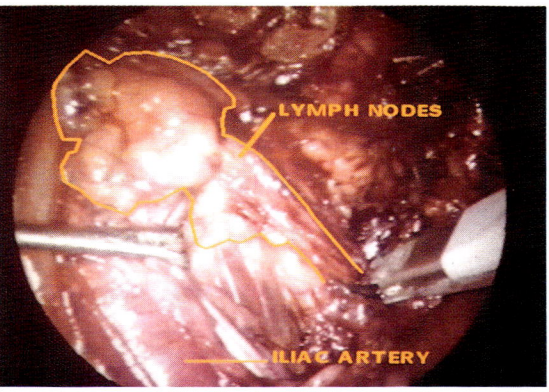

Figure 60-28.

the incision in the peritoneal reflection must be made just lateral to the umbilical ligament and it must be carried caudad to Cooper's ligament. It is very important to *start* the node dissection at Cooper's ligament in order to remove the entire chain expeditiously. Other important points to remember are: to use the extreme Trendelenburg and tilting position, to use a mechanical bowel preparation to ensure maximum decompression of all bowel and small intestine, to keep the patient's hands tucked in at his side to ensure maximum movement for the surgeon and assistant toward the patient's head for good angulation in the pelvis, and to be sure that the surgeon is working from the side of the table *opposite* to the pelvic lymph nodes being dissected in order to obtain maximal mechanical advantage. Regarding instrument use, the current development of instrumentation for pelvic lymphadenectomy through the laparoscope is explosive. There are endless numbers of graspers and forceps being designed, and the surgeon and assistant must select instruments suited to their personal taste and surgical style. In general, toothed forceps work best for grasping the nodal tissue and smooth instruments must be used around the obturator nerve and iliac vessels.

CLOSURE

Prior to closure, the camera is angled to visualize the withdrawal of all trocars. Occasionally there is bleeding from the puncture site, which only becomes apparent *after* the trocar is removed. Should bleeding be seen at a trocar site, it is coagulated either intraperitoneally or from the outside by grasping the vessel and utilizing the Bovie coagulator. It is also important to inject Marcaine at the trocar site to decrease postoperative discomfort. The camera site should be the last of the trocars to be removed. The abdomen is then decompressed. Occasionally, a pneumoscrotum is created. This is easily decompressed by applying manual pressure before removing the last cannula. Pneumoscrotum has not been problematic in our experience, although to the uninitiated the size of the pneumoscrotum can be impressive before decompression. We make no special effort to close the small openings in the peritoneum or the fascia. Skin clips are applied to these small abdominal wounds, and we have had no problem with hernia to date. A Band-Aid is then placed over the puncture sites.

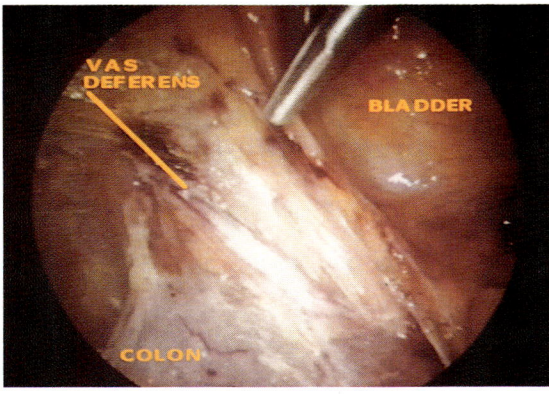

Figure 60-27.

POSTOPERATIVE MANAGEMENT

In spite of opening the peritoneum at both the right and the left iliac fossa and then extensively dissecting the iliac artery, vein and obturator nerve, as well as taking the vas deferens on each side, the postoperative course for these patients is truly remarkable for its paucity of problems. No nasogastric tube is necessary. The pain is surprisingly minimal and rarely requires parenteral analgesia. Postoperative ileus is rare, and the patient can often tolerate fluids and solid foods by mouth once recovered from the effects of the anesthesia. Initially, we were very cautious in giving the patient nothing by mouth, at least on the day of surgery, but time and time again were badgered by patients on the evening of the operation because they were "hungry." As soon as bowel sounds are apparent, the patient is fed a regular diet. Postoperatively intravenous fluids are maintained until intake by mouth is adequate. Intravenous antibiotics are usually continued for 24 hours. A Foley catheter is left in place overnight or until the patient is fully ambulatory.

CRITERIA FOR PATIENT DISCHARGE

Patients are usually discharged on the first postoperative day, although some patients (later in our series), were discharged on the same day of the procedure. It is surprising how stable and pain-free these patients are in spite of the extensive bilateral laparoscopic pelvic surgical dissection. Criteria for discharge include: no pain, no fever, voiding easily without a Foley catheter, ability to tolerate food by mouth, and no abdominal tenderness or drainage from the trocar sites. As a rule, patients are not given oral analgesics or antibiotics on discharge. They are not restricted from resuming full regular exercise as they wish. They are asked to return to the office in 7 to 10 days for the abdominal clips to be removed from the puncture wounds.

It should be noted that when laparoscopic pelvic lymph-adenectomy is done at the same time as either radical prostatectomy or cystectomy, then discharge plans and postoperative management are dictated by the more complex and extensive open surgery. In general, no special criteria are added because the patient has undergone concurrent laparoscopic pelvic lymph node dissection.

COMPLICATIONS SPECIFIC FOR LAPAROSCOPIC PELVIC LYMPHADENECTOMY

This procedure has been remarkably complication free. Intraoperative morbidity has been nil. Average blood loss for laparoscopic pelvic lymphadenectomies done by us was less than 100 ml. Although a back table is always set up for open laparotomy, this has not been used in any of our patients. There have been no major vessel injuries nor injury to the obturator nerve. There have been no bowel perforations or injuries. It has not been necessary to abandon any procedures because of prior operations or inability to lyse adhesions. Two procedures had to be terminated prematurely because of failure of the optical equipment to function adequately. In addition, one patient had a transient obturator nerve palsy which resolved within 48 hours. Adequate nodal tissue was recovered for pathologic examination in all patients. In one patient, grossly suspicious nodal tissue was removed and examined by frozen section and reported as negative.

We proceeded with radical retropubic prostatectomy. When the final reports on the sections of the nodes removed originally at laparoscopy were received, there were several microscopic foci of metastatic nodal involvement, which were not originally recognized. There is always the potential problem that nodal tissue sampled and reported as negative at the time of laparoscopy may subsequently be found positive for tumor after further pathologic study. If a surgeon does proceed to a radical operation under the same anesthesia as the laparoscopy, then the risk of occasionally missing microscopic nodal involvement exists. The risk-benefit ratio of doing the pelvic lymphadenectomy laparoscopically on one occasion, removing and sampling the nodes, and then allowing the pathologist to proceed with a full and complete examination under ideal conditions, is weighed against the patient undergoing two anesthesia episodes, assuming the nodes are negative.

There have been no lymphoceles or chronic lymphedema of either the scrotum or the lower extremities. There have been no hernias. Our longest follow-up to date is approximately 2 years. There have been no thromboembolic episodes, attributable in part to early ambulation made easier by essentially no incisional discomfort. In addition, the surgical procedure accomplished laparoscopically rarely exceeds one hour, avoiding venous stasis.

Conclusion

Laparoscopic pelvic lymphadenectomy as the final and ultimate staging procedure in the definitive treatment of both prostatic cancer and bladder cancer provides nodal tissue adequate to or superior to that provided in an open procedure. The question of whether laparoscopic pelvic lymph node dissection is better than the standard treatment can be argued by the fact that there is no large incision, and there is clearly minimal disfigurement, decreased postoperative pain, decreased morbidity, shortened hospitalization and convalescence, lower cost, and ultimately, accurate node sampling. Laparoscopic pelvic lymph node dissection is clearly the modality of the future and it is incumbent upon all urologists and those dealing with the treatment and diagnosis of prostate and bladder cancer to become proficient in this technique. Progress in medicine is notable not just by looking at change, but measuring change in terms of improvement. As Sir H. Ogilvie stated:

Advancement means progress to something better not necessarily progress to something new.

Other indications and uses for laparoscopic surgery in urologic procedures include bladder suspension, nephrectomy, total or partial cystectomy, urinary diversion, radical prostatectomy, retroperitoneal lymph node dissection, ureteral injury repair and the treatment of varicoceles, undescended testicles, inguinal hernias, and vesicostomies. The procedures at this time that can be done by laparoscopic surgical techniques are limited only by the surgeon's imagination and the availability of appropriate instruments and retraction apparatus to do the job. As this chapter is written, laparoscopy in urology is in its infancy and short of organ transplantation, we predict that virtually no open urologic surgery will exist within the next several years.

Section VIII
Postdoctoral Training for Laparoscopic Surgery

Chapter 61
Setting up and Running Courses

Joris Bannenberg
Dirk Meijer

The introduction of the rapidly expanding field of laparoscopic surgery has created for surgeons the need to become familiar with its techniques and perspectives. Hands-on training courses can be an efficient means of achieving a minimum level of manual dexterity and the necessary insight for the performance of laparoscopic surgery in a safe manner. For those not familiar with the organization of these courses, we report on our experiences with the laparoscopic training courses that we have organized at the University of Amsterdam.

WHY TEACH COURSES?

Benefits for the patient but also pressure from the patient, insurance companies, and instrument manufacturers, and the doctor's own ego force surgeons to become familiar with laparoscopic procedures/minimal invasive techniques. These procedures differ enormously from the standard surgical technique. They require extensive and adequate training for their safe performance.

The Society of American Gastrointestinal Endoscopic Surgeons (SAGES) was the first to recommend criteria for credentialing surgeons performing laparoscopic procedures.[1] Other societies such as the Society for Surgery of the Alimentary Tract (SSAT) and the European Association for Endoscopic Surgery (EAES) followed with similar guidelines. These recommendations include *minimum* requirements for training for those without formal education in laparoscopic techniques.

In Europe, a general system of credentialing and granting privileges by hospital boards is not known. Training in laparoscopic procedures is totally the European surgeon's own responsibility. At this time, the demand for clinical operations has not been met with a sufficient number of trained surgeons. Moreover, the demand is only likely to increase because of the obvious advantages of laparoscopic procedures for the patients and because of the rapid extension of the field. Until laparoscopic surgery training has found its place within formal resident training, there will be a demand for specialized training courses. Hands-on training courses can be a very efficient means of transferring the working knowledge of the experienced laparoscopic surgeon to the novice wanting training. The setting of these courses can generate a critical mass in which peer learning takes place.

At the time of the chaotic introduction of laparoscopic cholecystectomy, the lack of training facilities led to situations (in the United States as well as in Europe) in which major complications and even deaths were reported. Because of the different structure of medical welfare and the scarce availability of laparoscopic equipment, the general adaptation to this technique has only recently started in Europe. In Eastern Europe (or Middle Europe as some like to call it) laparoscopic surgery is only at its dawning.

We are convinced that a course without extensive training with animals is inadequate. The use of an animal laboratory provides direct operative experience by mimicking conditions similar to the actual clinical situation. In contrast to that clinical situation, it exemplifies in a better way the complex situations, complications, and complication handling of laparoscopic surgery. Protocols for laparoscopic procedures in humans should be followed during animal training procedures. All use of animals in training settings requires approval of animal ethics commissions and has to be performed according to legal regulations. To guarantee the quality of hands-on training courses and to minimize the use of animals, it is important that these training courses are authorized by the professional societies involved in endoscopic surgery. Both the EAES and the SAGES have issued recommendations for basic minimum requirements for laparoscopic training courses.

WHAT TO EXPECT FROM COURSES

Hands-on training courses must provide the opportunity for the attendees to become familiar with the laparoscopic technique. In addition, these courses should reveal to the surgeon his or her own capabilities in the application of laparoscopic techniques. Moreover, the surgeon must gain insight into his or her own limitations with these techniques.

Each course must offer a theoretical session. Subjects that should be covered in these formal presentations include the principles of general laparoscopy, basic information on the variety of available instruments and equipment, and its functioning, a step by step demonstration of the procedure, thorough explanations on how to avoid pitfalls and how to manage complications. No program is complete without a presentation of clinical results.

Hands-on practice should provide enough time to study the different steps involved in the particular procedure. Each small group of course attendees is supervised by a clinically experienced instructor with qualified teaching capabilities. Training sessions allow enough time for demonstrations and an opportunity to practice the specific procedure. It is also important to allot time to demonstrate pitfalls of the procedure and for the exchange of seemingly small details concerning the procedure. These details can make a world of difference in the actual clinical situation. Throughout the course, attendees should interact directly with the experienced clinical instructors.

No training in laparoscopic general surgery is complete without clinical experiences. Although observation of live procedures may be informative, it cannot replace the experience of assisting. Providing clinical experiences may be beyond the scope of a hands-on training course but should be offered to all participants. Experience can be acquired in the clinic of the organizing hospital where the course attendee can assist with laparoscopic procedures in humans. Furthermore, it is important that the course attendee is guided by an experienced laparoscopic surgeon when undertaking his or her first procedures.

In contrast to the United States, it is not customary in Europe to videotape the whole laparoscopic procedure. Thus, the opportunity for screening of the laparoscopic technique used by an instructor or proctoring is not possible.

In the next section an overview of the basic requirements for setting up laparoscopic courses is presented.

COURSE ORGANIZATION

The general organization of the course consists of the following parts:

1. Course objectives, target groups, and the program.
2. Course Facilities.
3. Faculty.
4. Course administration, marketing, and finance.

Course Objectives, Target Groups, and the Program

The objectives for courses in laparoscopic surgery are partly determined by the rules of SAGES and EAES, as described earlier. These rules state that a course should, at the minimum, contain introductory lectures, inanimate training, and animal training in the laboratory. For a course to be recognized by one of these organizations, it is important that these rules be strictly followed, so the student can be officially certified.

There are two types of courses: introductory courses and applied (or advanced) courses. The introductory courses expose the surgeon to the basics of laparoscopic surgery and teach, in general, a single standard technique (e.g., cholecystectomy, pelvic lymph node dissection). The objective of the applied or advanced courses is to train already experienced laparoscopic surgeons in a specific technique (e.g., herniorrhaphy, vagotomy, bowel resection).

Both types of courses are taught according to the above-mentioned standard items.

TARGET GROUPS

The target groups are general surgeons, cardiac-thoracic surgeons, urologists, and gynaecologists.

OBJECTIVES

The main objectives of a laparoscopy course are to teach:

1. The safe operation of the optical and electrical equipment required for laparoscopic surgery.
2. The pathophysiology of pneumoperitoneum.
3. The selection of appropriate patients for laparoscopic surgery.
4. The fundamental techniques of laparoscopic surgery.
5. The safe performance of standard operations.
6. Prevention of complications of laparoscopic surgery.

Additional objectives of an applied or advanced course depend on the subject of the course.

COURSE PROGRAM

A good basic course should contain the following lectures.

Introductory Lecture. In this introduction all necessary information needed to safely perform laparoscopy is provided. It is always advisable to keep this part very basic. Too much unnecessary information is confusing. As the quality of this lecture is closely related to the didactic gifts of the faculty, careful selection is obligatory.

Introduction to Laparoscopic Surgery. In this section the objectives and the course program are explained. A short historical introduction with emphasis on the development of the subject of that particular course is given. It is also wise to give information about the several societies devoted to laparoscopic surgery and about some of the journals for laparoscopic surgery. Subscription forms should be available.

It is also advisable to mention the value of checklists of instruments, the value of video recording of procedures, and the importance of controlled prospective clinical trials.

Instrumentation and Basics of Laparoscopic Surgery. One of the central lectures is devoted to the instrumentation required for laparoscopic surgery. In this lecture the basic instruments and techniques are explained.

Check-list. Because incomplete instrumentation is hazardous for patients undergoing laparoscopic surgery, the value of a checklist of the necessary instruments for each particular laparoscopic intervention should be explained. This is especially necessary in clinics where performance of laparoscopic surgery has just started, and the operating room staff are not familiar with it yet. The checklist should be attached onto the monitor before the procedure starts. It is then the responsibility of the surgeon to check if all items are available.

Minimum Conditions for Laparoscopy. The minimum requisite conditions for laparoscopy procedures, such as light source, capacity of the insufflator, quality of the camera, coagulation, and suction should be stated. Complications arising from incomplete, wrong, or malfunctioning equipment have to be mentioned. Instruments should always be divided into disposable and nondisposable. The function of the trocars, the risks of introduction and the groups at risk for complications during introduction (e.g. patients suspected to have adhesions or obese patients), and the use of Hasson trocars for the open technique should be explained. The use of electrocautery, monopolor versus bipolar, laser, and argon beamer and the physical basics of these techniques should be taught.

Basic Techniques

1. Indications and contraindications. It is very important to mention the indications for laparoscopic procedures and the close relation to the level of experience of the surgeon. It is advisable to emphasize what type of patient should be chosen to undergo a laparoscopic procedure. No less important are the contraindications. The absolute contraindications and relative contraindications for laparoscopic surgery should be mentioned.
2. Preoperative preparation. This must include informed consent; including letting the patient know that there is a possibility that conversion to the open procedure may be necessary.
3. Anesthesia.
4. Establishing and maintaining pneumoperitoneum. How to do an open and closed technique properly and how to avoid complications (e.g., trocars, carbon dioxide) are covered.
5. Golden rule. Do not hesitate to convert to the open procedure.
6. Basic-technique operation. The most common and simple operative technique is taught in the hands-on part of the course. Presentation of the operative technique should be clear and straightforward and supported with educational videotapes and slides. It is important to keep the lecture as basic as possible and explain the critical parts of the procedure, only mentioning the alternatives. A thorough explanation of all alternatives will be confusing.

Complications. It is essential for the student to understand which serious mistakes can be made, and more important, how to avoid these. It is important to discourage heroic interventions, and to emphasize how to perform procedures safely.

Inanimate Laboratory: Laparoscopic Training Boxes. The students are instructed in the operation of the optical and electrical equipment required for laparoscopic surgery on real equipment. They are shown how to "troubleshoot" common problems in the operation of this sophisticated equipment. The fundamental techniques of laparoscopic surgery will be demonstrated by experienced laparoscopic surgeons on inanimate materials shaped like human organs (Figs. 61-1 and 61-2). The students in the course will then practice these techniques under conditions that simulate laparoscopic surgery. The Laparoscopic Training Box is a model of the human abdomen, which blocks direct visualization of the inanimate practice materials. The students introduce laparoscopic surgical instruments through the simulated abdominal wall of the Laparoscopic Training Box and view the simulated organs on the monitor of the videolaparoscope. They then practice the fundamental techniques of laparoscopic surgery using the actual instruments under simulated conditions on inanimate objects. The number of surgeons is limited to a maximum of two per Laparoscopic Training Box. Depending on the type of course, the instructor

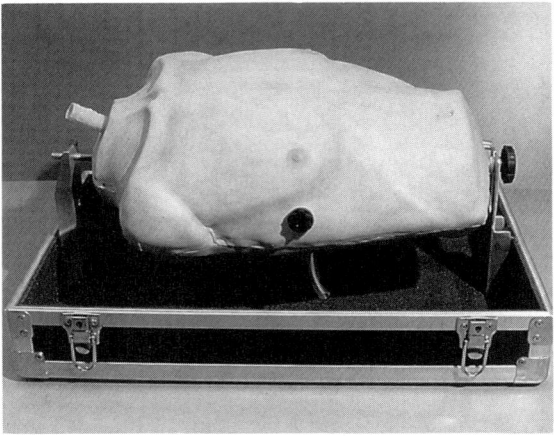

Figure 61-1. Laparoscopic Training Box used for training surgeons in laparoscopic procedures.

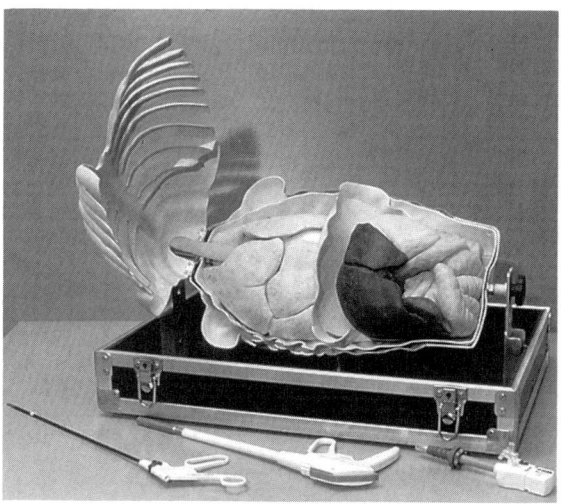

Figure 61-2. The Laparoscopic Training Box utilizes simulated organs on which one can learn new procedures.

can handle one or two inanimate practice stations at the same time.

Animal Laboratory. Experienced laparoscopic surgeons will demonstrate safe surgical techniques and methods of safely performing operations on live animals. The students of the course then practice these techniques and operations on live animals. The experienced surgeons will observe the students in these endeavors and offer pointers and correct errors of technique.

The number of students per animal varies per course type; the maximum is usually three students and one instructor per station. The students rotate so they will be the operating surgeon, the first assistant, or the cameraman. After each procedure the students will rotate to their next position. The instructor is responsible for overseeing that every student gets about the same operation time.

Evaluation and Certification. The evaluation is the most important instrument used to judge the quality of every part of the course, including the lecturers and the participating industry. A detailed evaluation form must be filled in by every participant at the end of the course. In the evaluation form the students can score every item so that statistical analysis and improvement of the course are eventually possible.

At the end of the course, the student receives the course certification, which is approved by SAGES (United States) or by EAES (Europe).

Course Facilities

Organizing courses depends on suitable accommodations, which must include the following facilities.

ROOM FOR INTRODUCTORY LECTURES

The introductory lectures can be held in a standard auditorium equipped with modern audiovisual equipment, including a slide projector, overhead projector, and video equipment. The latter is very important because most operations are recorded on videotape. Because the instructors may come from different countries, which may use different systems (PAL/NTSC or SECAM) or different videotapes (VHS or U-Matic), multisystem monitors and videoplayers have to be available.

INANIMATE LABORATORY

The inanimate laboratory training does not require extended laboratory facilities. This training can be performed either in a simple classroom or in an animal laboratory. A table on which the Laparoscopic Training Box and the laparoscopic equipment can be placed is the only need.

ANIMAL LABORATORY

The animal laboratory is central to the success of the training course (see Appendix 1). The laboratory should be equipped with one or more training stations. Every station requires at least an operation table that can be put in different positions, complete anesthesia equipment including mechanical ventilation, electrocautery with connections for laparoscopy instruments, suction/irrigation systems and, of course, a complete set of laparoscopy equipment. Electrocardiogram registration, an extra monitor, an argon beamer, laser, and diagnostic equipment, such as echocardiographic equipment, are optional. In the laboratory the help of biotechnicians is necessary. One biotechnician is, in general, able to monitor a maximum of two stations.

Faculty

GENERAL

The quality of the faculty determines the quality of the course. The ideal faculty member should be an experienced clinical surgeon who is also a skilled teacher. The latter means that the instructor must be patient enough to teach. The faculty should be selected according to the above-mentioned requirements. A good indicator of the quality of selection is the course evaluation.

INSTRUCTION OF THE FACULTY

The responsibilities of each instructor must be individually enumerated. The faculty should be given a detailed schedule, the contents of which are amplified at a faculty meeting that precedes the course. To avoid repetition, it is strongly advised that the content of every lecture is reviewed beforehand. Also instructors should be informed of the evaluation before the start of the course.

MODERATOR

Every session, including the laboratory sessions, must have a moderating instructor. The task of the moderator is keep the introductory lectures on schedule and to explain what is required in the laboratory sessions (e.g., type of procedure).

Course Administration, Marketing, and Finance

No course will be perfect in its first run. We believe that full time professional medical and administrative staff for course organization is a must. The course administration is responsible for all matters concerning registration, correspondence, follow-up and implementation of the outcome of the evaluation, marketing, finance, and industrial participation. Although the subjects of marketing and finance are beyond the limits of this chapter, a few remarks are necessary, as these vary from country to country. In the United States laparoscopic courses tend to be very commercial and highly priced. In Europe, courses are organized more academically, which means that the prices are, in general, lower. Eventually one must realize that the price of a course is determined, on one hand, by the fees paid to the faculty and, on the other hand, by the sponsoring of industries.

If an industry sponsors the course, a basic condition is that the course must not be hampered by commercial restrictions or commitments. All instruments and equipment having sound technical or significant advantages for a certain procedure should be demonstrated regardless of the manufacturer.

FUTURE OF LAPAROSCOPIC SURGERY COURSES

More and different laparoscopic procedures will be performed in the future. As more clinical data become available, the uses of laparoscopic surgery will be determined. The ongoing development of technical equipment will facilitate new procedures and initiate more indications. Surgical research centers will play an important role in this development. As laparoscopic surgery becomes normal in general surgery training programs, the need for these courses will be less necessary. The remaining courses will change character: basic techniques and knowledge of instrument handling will be replaced by more technical explanations and demonstrations of a particular procedure. Not only will hands-on training in the animal laboratory be provided, live demonstrations with intensive communication between the trainees and the chief surgeon will become part of the courses. When courses are organized under the authorization of societies such as the SAGES and the EAES the didactic quality will improve and become standarized.

As in open surgery, each new procedure requires minimum training. Every hospital will send one of their surgeons to seek training to become adept with a new laparoscopic technique. Knowledge and skills will then be passed on to other staff members and residents. The quality of laparoscopic surgery in a hospital will be as good as the quality of the instructor in that hospital.

Summary

In our experience hands-on courses for laparoscopic surgery are still the most effective and efficient means to transfer the working knowledge of experienced laparoscopic surgeons to novice laparoscopists. High quality courses can only be guaranteed when these courses are organized as part of an on-going program, because the fast development of laparoscopic techniques necessitates continuous updating. Full time medical and administrative staff support is needed both for the unbiased presentations of the procedures and for course evaluation afterward, which should influence the structure and contents of subsequent courses.

Laparoscopic surgery courses should offer the following:

1. A sound and unbiased factual basis and enough insight into the dynamics to be able to follow and understand the future developments.
2. Enough interaction with the instructors to acquire the working knowledge desired by every participant.
3. Enough opportunity for manual dexterity to evolve.
4. Instructors with ample clinical experience and good teaching capacities.
5. Written course material, which provides concise information on all the key issues, itemized by these key points.

6. Organizers who maintain a broad understanding of the evolving field of laparoscopic surgery. They should also have enrolled in courses themselves as participants.

7. Evaluation in detail, with changes based on these comments implemented in the next course.

8. Easy access for participants to course organizers for postcourse support, e.g., to discuss further practical questions.

REFERENCE

1. Society of American Gastrointestinal Endoscopic Surgeons. Granting of priviliges for laparoscopic (peritoneoscopic) general surgery. Los Angeles: Society of American Gastrointestinal Endoscopic Surgeons, 1991.

APPENDIX 1: ANIMAL LABORATORY

Laboratory Animals

A number of laboratory animals are suitable for laparoscopic surgery training. The most ideal and cost-effective animal is the pig, which is suitable for almost all intra-abdominal applications. The use of dogs is only recommended for thoracic surgery, as the porcine thorax is far from ideal and very different from that in the human. In some gynecology courses, rabbits are used because of the easy accessible cloaca-uterus complex.

The specifications for an animal laboratory for most courses are listed below.

Laparoscopic Cholecystectomy

Animal:	Pig
Weight:	20–35 Kg
Anaesthesia:	Mechanical ventilation
Position of table:	Anti-Trendelenburg
Position of the laparoscopic equipment:	Top
Position of animal:	Back on table
Position of trocars:	See Figure 61-3

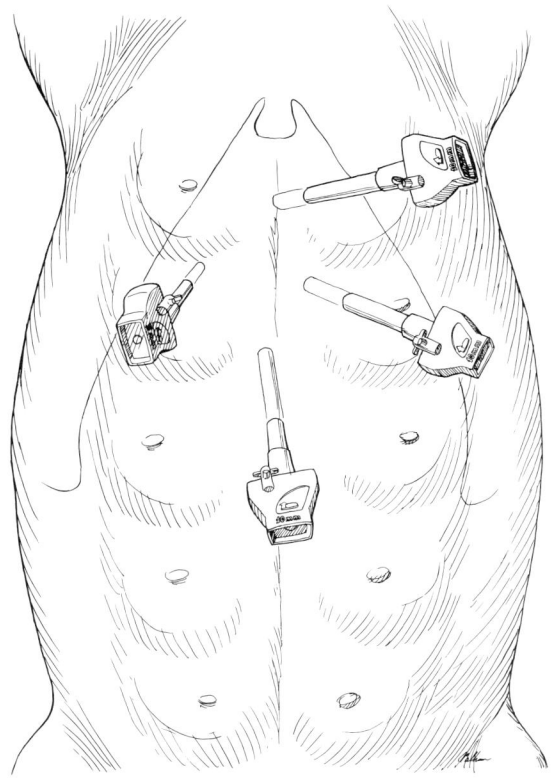

Figure 61-3. Position of trocars for laparoscopic cholecystectomy in a porcine model.

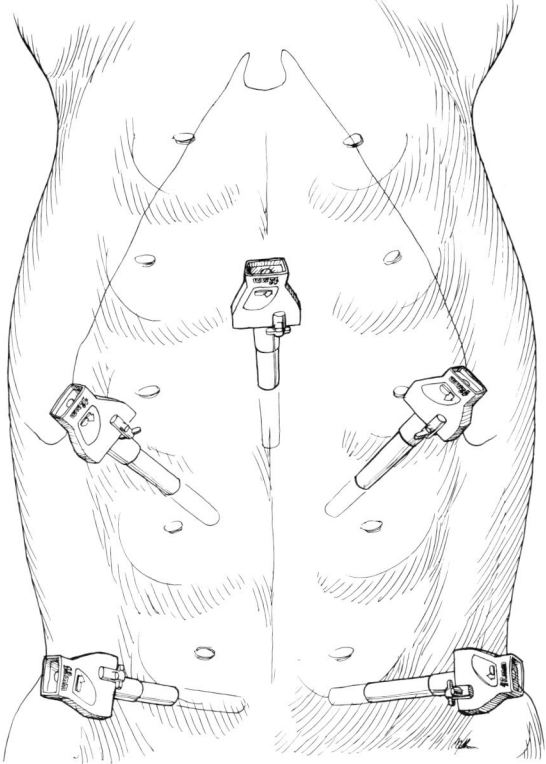

Figure 61-4. Position of trocars for advanced laparoscopic procedures in a porcine model.

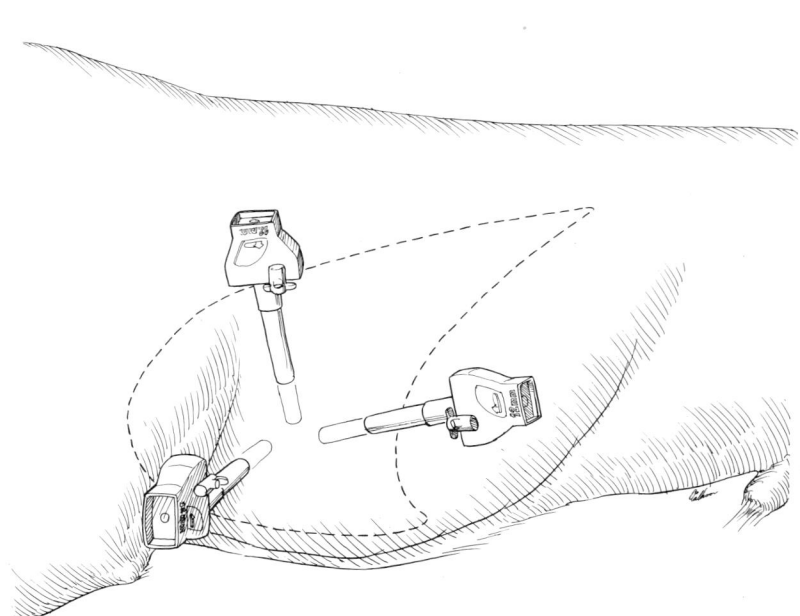

Figure 61-5. Position of trocars for thoracoscopy in a canine model.

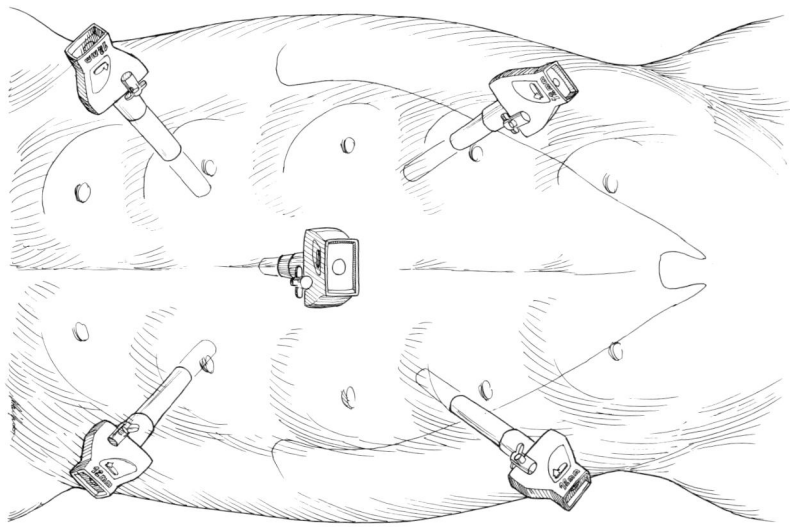

Figure 61-6. Position of trocars for laparoscopic urology and laparoscopic gynecology procedures in a porcine model.

Advanced Laparoscopic Procedures

Animal: Pig
Weight: 20–35 Kg
Anesthesia: Mechanical ventilation
Position of table: Depends on procedure
Position of the laparoscopic equipment: Depends on procedure
Position of animal: Back on table
Position of trocars: See Figure 61-4

Thoracoscopy

Animal: Dog
Weight: 20–30 kg
Anesthesia: Right-sided Mechanical ventilation
Position of table: Horizontal
Position of the laparoscopic equipment: Top
Position of animal: Right side down
Position of trocars: See Figure 61-5

Urology

Animal: Pig
Weight: 20–35 kg
Anesthesia: Mechanical ventilation
Position of table: Trendelenburg
Position of the laparoscopic equipment: Bottom
Position of animal: Back on table
Position of trocars: See Figure 61-6

Gynaecology

Animal: Pig
Weight: 20–35 kg
Anaesthesia: Mechanical ventilation
Position of table: Trendelenburg
Position of the laparoscopic equipment: Bottom
Position of animal: Back on table
Position of trocars: See Figure 61-6

Chapter 62
Hospital Credentialing

Kenneth A. Forde

In this chapter we will discuss the issues involved in the credentialing process for laparoscopic surgery, the evaluation of the process, and valuable existing guidelines.

Hospital credentialing in current parlance refers to the granting of clinical privileges by hospitals' "credentials committees." This is an obvious misnomer in that "credentials," in the strict sense, refers to documentation of training or experience. Nevertheless, the process by which a physician has been permitted to perform procedures or care for patients in general (the granting of privileges) has been the responsibility of the local hospital's credentials committee. This process, as noted by Dent,[1] "was designed to insure that patients receive skillful care by competent practitioners." During the years the process has been based on a combination of: (a) accreditation requirements, (b) guidelines of professional societies, (c) modifications to fit the peculiar needs of a specific institution, and (d) local or regional custom.

Whereas heretofore local hospital credentials committees dealt with physicians seeking privileges in their own traditional specialty (for example, radiology, gastroenterology, medicine, or surgery), the rapid development of medical technology shared by more than one subspecialty and the evolution of imaging and display modalities have made the process of credentialing more difficult. The interventional cardiologist, interventional radiologist, endoscopic surgeon, imaging physician, and other new categories of physicians seeking privileges have increased the complexity of credentialing. Some institutions do not have enough experienced members in the disciplines involved to act as "local experts" or consultants to credentials committees. Issues of infringement on traditional referral and practice patterns frequently cause too many conflicts to allow a smooth process. Issues of turf, economic gain or loss, and professional jealousy often make the process overly confrontational, vindictive, and sometimes litiginous.

Among the elements involved with hospital credentialing for laparoscopic surgery are: professional societies, groups of surgeons and some physicians who have been traditionally involved in diagnostic and operative laparoscopy (including general surgeons, gynecologists, and some gastroenterologists), hospital credentials committee members, regulatory agencies, third party payers, surgical program directors, postgraduate course directors, instrument and equipment makers, hospital associations,[2] hospital administrators and their legal counsel, and the general public. Another current problem is the fact that most postgraduate laparoscopy courses to date have used laparoscopic cholecystectomy as the training model, which is inappropriate for the colorectal, thoracic, urologic, or other subspecialty surgeon.

Surgeons have traditionally been able to introduce new procedures by a gradual process. Sometimes this initially occurred in the animal laboratory, at times through working clinically with others at their own or other institutions, and most commonly at teaching institutions with eventual wider utilization if a procedure appeared to be safe and successful. *Laparoscopic surgery* has not had the luxury of this evolution. In a few short years it has been embraced by a significant percentage of surgeons in many specialties (general surgery, gynecologic surgery, colorectal surgery, urology, thoracic surgery, and others) and in one major area—cholecystectomy—it has rapidly become the "usual and customary." Adding to the confusion in all this is the valid question: If a procedure can be done safely by a well trained individual, is that enough justification for the granting of privileges? What if the procedure is thought by some to be inappropriate or inferior to current approaches? While this is a critical question and is of paramount importance to those cynical about some of the laparoscopic surgical procedures being developed, it is definitely not in the purview of credentials committees. Some specialty societies (for example, the Society of American Gastrointestinal Endoscopic Surgeons and the American Society for Gastrointestinal Endoscopy) have been concerned enough about this issue to prepare and present guidelines on clinical practice, reviewing the literature and attempting to conduct follow-up studies and obtain end results. Those responsible for quality assurance in individual institutions must also address this issue. It goes hand in hand with the granting of privileges to perform procedures.

The Committee on Surgical Practice in Hospitals of the American College of Surgeons has identified hospital credentialing as a problem area and has recommended that the College consider development of a strong statement on the credentialling of surgeons for the performance of procedures.[3]

Hospitals throughout the country have suddenly been deluged with requests for privileges to perform this "new surgery." Obviously, even if the surgeon has spent a lifetime, for example, in biliary tract surgery, the approach to the gallbladder through a different route, utilizing different technology and requiring additional skills, of necessity requires additional training and experience. How the surgeon acquires these and how he or she is "credentialed" is an important consideration.

The gynecologists, who for many years performed diagnostic and operative laparoscopy in their specialty, are involved in this process in several ways. At some institutions they may be the instructors of general surgeons who wish to become involved in laparoscopic surgery. Some gynecologists themselves wish to extend their laparoscopic expertise to areas traditionally managed by general or colorectal or urologic surgeons and so conflicts arise at local institutions. Some gastroenterologists, many with training and expertise in diagnostic laparoscopy, have had a long involvement in fiberoptic and videoendoscopy and see a possible challenge in or advantage to involvement in more operative laparoscopy. The following policy statement was endorsed by the governing board of the ASGE[4]:

Laparoscopic cholecystectomy is a complex surgical procedure which should be performed only by surgeons with training in both traditional and laparoscopic methods of biliary surgery. The first assistant is also critical to the performance of the procedure and must be a physician or surgical assistant with special training in laparoscopic techniques

This statement highlights the concerns of that group about patient safety on the one hand (the need for the laparoscopic cholecystectomist to be first a biliary tract surgeon) and the turf issue on the other, by making sure that the operating team is composed of members generic to the realm of laparoscopy. Will there be a movement to credential surgical assistants? What about surgical trainees (residents and fellows)?

The first organization to address this issue of hospital credentialing for laparoscopic procedures in a formal fashion was SAGES. In a 1989 policy statement this national organization of endoscopic surgeons declared[5]:

Laparoscopic cholecystectomy is currently an investigational procedure. It is the opinion of the Society of American Gastrointestinal Endoscopic Surgeons that for optimal quality patient care this procedure should be performed only by surgeons who are qualified to perform open cholecystectomy. Only such surgeons possess the skill to perform biliary tract surgical procedures; only such surgeons are able to determine the best method of cholecystectomy and only such surgeons can treat complications subsequent to Laparoscopic Cholecystectomy

Thus SAGES emphasized patient safety and the need for the endoscopic surgeon to be first trained in traditional surgical techniques to recognize and recover from anticipated pitfalls in this nascent discipline of laparoscopic surgery.

Eight months later, the American College of Surgeons of the United States and Canada, representing not only general surgeons but including specialties such as urology, gynecology, thoracic surgery, colon and rectal surgery, orthopedic surgery, and others, issued a policy statement, essentially echoing the SAGES document.[6] As the field of laparoscopic surgery began to spread beyond the gallbladder, it was recognized that broader guidelines would need to be developed. SAGES has provided further guidelines that could be used by hospital credentials committees.[7] These guidelines emphasize where responsibility lies for the credentialing of surgeons in particular, pathways to competence in the broad field of laparoscopic surgery, and elements felt necessary for adequate training. The stated purpose of the document was to

outline principles and provide practical suggestions to assist hospital credentialing committees in their task of granting privileges to perform laparoscopic surgery. In conjunction with the standard JCAHO [Joint Commission on Accreditation of Healthcare Organizations] guidelines for granting hospital privileges, implementation of these methods should help hospital staffs insure that laparoscopic surgery is performed only by individuals with appropriate competency, thus assuring high quality patient care and proper procedure utilization.

As the SAGES document points out (and this is supported by JCAHO standards), it is the responsibility of the chief of the clinical department to recommend individual surgeons for privileges in laparoscopic general surgery as for other procedures performed by members of the department. With regard to training and determination of competence the SAGES guidelines suggested[8]:

A. formal fellowship or residency training in general surgery (as the basic requirement) and
B. the following methods of determination of competence in laparoscopic surgery:
   1. completion of a surgical residency or fellowship program which incorporates structured experience in laparoscopic surgery, with such competence documented by the instructor or instructors,
   2. for those in whose training programs this was not possible (but who have had experience), proficiency in laparoscopic surgical procedures and clinical judgment equivalent to that obtained in a residency or fellowship program with documentation and demonstrated competence,
   3. for those without residency training which included laparoscopic surgery and for those without documented prior experience as in (2), the basic requirements for training are described as follows:
      a. completion of a general surgical residency,
      b. privileged in diagnostic laparoscopy,
      c. training in laparoscopic general surgery by an experienced laparoscopic surgeon or through completion of a university- or academic society-sponsored, recognized didactic course which included clinical experience and hands-on laboratory practice, as well as,
      d. experience as first assistant
      e. proctoring
      f. monitoring of laparoscopic performance

The fourth element was that the applicant's laparoscopic training director confirm the student's experience and the explanation that a residency program of 5 years of general surgery involving, as it does, cognitive experience in anatomy, physiology, and pathology combined with progressive development of visual and psychomotor skills contains important elements for surgeons in particular. The training director's opinion was felt to be superior to any specific number of procedures done or courses attended.

As proctoring is more commonly employed definitions become increasingly necessary. Satara[9] and Reed[10] have recently pointed out the issues involved and offer help in clarifying the proctor's role and responsibilities.

The Society for Surgery of the Alimentary Tract (SSAT) has issued its own guidelines for laparoscopic cholecystectomy specifically[11] and they include: the requirements (1) that general surgeons with competence to perform open cholecystectomy and manage complications be the basic group given privileges, (2) that they have expertise through experience or training in the performance of laparoscopy, and (3) that they have had supervised laparoscopic cholecystectomy experience including animal laboratory work.

With these promulgated guidelines available, how is the issue to be addressed at the individual hospital? The JCAHO requires that the "medical staff" assume overall responsibility for clinical privileges and establish hospital-specific mechanisms for the granting and renewal or revision of clinical privileges.[12] "Clinical privileges" are defined as: "permission to provide medical or other patient care services in the granting institution within well-defined limits, based on the individual's professional license and his/her experience, competence, ability and judgment." There are requirements that there be "a mechanism to assure that all individuals with clinical privileges provide services within the scope of privileges granted." *Each clinical department* is expected, according to the JCAHO, "to develop its own criteria for recommending such privileges."

During the year 1990 to 1991 this issue was a topic discussed by representatives of the American Board of Surgery, the American Hospital Association, and the JCAHO, resulting in a consensus statement on Certification and Hospital Credentialing to be presented to the American Board of Medical Specialties.[3] With the goal of the best possible patient care, the purpose of this document (like all other such guidelines) was to provide hospital credentialing bodies with insight into the relationship between postgraduate education, certification, and credentialing. The document reiterated the charge to credentialing committees, namely "assuring the medical staff and health care consumer that a physician can safely perform the requested privileges." Careful reading of these guidelines reveals amplification and corroboration of the guidelines offered by the various specialty societies. They point out the need for credentialing committees to "augment the information provided by certification with documentation of specific experience (especially for requested procedures) and by clinical observation of new applicants by appropriate senior members of the medical staff and, prior to credentialing individuals for procedures, "the physician must demonstrate thorough familiarity with the disease process which the procedure proposes to address, as evidenced by appropriate education and training." The document further advises "the physician must be prepared to manage the complications of the procedure. . . ." For laparoscopic surgery, this therefore means that the requirement is for an approved surgical residency training and certification in the particular area in which laparoscopic surgery is to be performed. For example, general and colorectal surgeons would need adequate prior training and certification in colectomy in order to perform laparoscopic colectomy.

Although this is an evolving area, hospital credentialing bodies do have considerable consensus upon which they can draw in establishing guidelines for granting privileges to surgeons if the focus is patient safety and if the yardsticks remain adequate surgical background training and proficiency in surgical management of diseases in both the traditional and newer techniques. In 1990 Dent, at a postgraduate course of the American College of Surgeons,[1] presented the criteria used by the Abington Memorial Hospital for granting of Clinical Privileges in Laparoscopic Cholecystectomy. At this institution, in addition to considering the SAGES and SSAT guidelines, they felt that observation of the procedure in humans needed to be supplemented with assisting in the procedure prior to becoming the primary surgeon. SAGES has also recently adopted this position.[8] At Abington Memorial proctoring is mandatory. It is pointed out (and we think this a most important point) that the proctor need not be privileged in laparoscopic cholecystectomy but only in biliary tract operations, since with televised procedures ". . . an experienced biliary tract surgeon should be able to determine the skill of the laparoscopic surgeon without necessarily being skilled in laparoscopy."

Because of the system of reporting incidents and adverse outcomes, the New York State Department of Health has accumulated a disturbing list of complications and deaths related to laparoscopic cholecystectomy when compared with recent morbidity statistics for open cholecystectomy.[13,14] As a result of this, in consultation with a national panel of surgeons, this agency has recommended credentialing guidelines similar to but more specific than the SAGES guidelines. The panel found that the major problem was with the granting of privileges to individuals who learned to perform laparoscopic cholecystectomy outside of a residency training program and for those individuals the New York State Department of Health is recommending as the primary mechanism for the delineation of privileges:

1. Certification (or eligibility) by the American Board of Surgery.
2. Credentialing in open cholecystectomy, common bile duct exploration, and liver procedures.
3. Completion of a "practicum," with ele-

ments of didactic course work, inanimate laboratory, animal laboratory, objective testing, and certification.

4. Assistance at laparoscopic surgery (minimum number 5 to 10 procedures).

5. A form of proctoring (performance under direct supervision of a surgeon already priveleged) (minimum number 10 to 15 procedures).

We have attempted to trace the evolution and consensus among responsible groups in this rapidly developing area of "endosurgery." Laparoscopic and other endoscopic surgical techniques are a permanent part of the surgeon's armamentarium for the foreseeable future. All who have seriously addressed this issue are concerned not only with the maintenance of acquired technical ability but also the acquisition of new skills and feel[1,2,15] that recertification should be based on review of experience and results in accordance with quality assurance mechanisms in place at the individual institution. While laparoscopic cholecystectomy is clearly in the lead, other laparoscopic surgical procedures (and procedures using similar technology in other body cavities) have been subsequently developed, and many more will undoubtedly follow. In keeping with current surgical tradition, additional training in other procedures will probably be by a combination of postgraduate course or other didactic program, coupled with observation and assisting colleagues.[1] However, as with other clinical privileges, the surgeon, monitored by the clinical chief of service and the credentials committee, should recognize when and how such additional formal training is necessary.

REFERENCES

1. Dent TL. Clinical privileges for laparoscopic general surgery. Am J Surg 1991; 161:399–403.
2. IQA² Continuous Performance Improvement through Integrated Quality Assessment. Hospital Association of New York State, 1991.
3. Carrico CJ. Ten specialty boards report goals and achievements. American Board of Surgery Bulletin. Am Coll Surg 1991; 76:50–54.
4. ASGE Newsletter. Manchester, MA, American Society for Gastrointestinal Endoscopy, Jan 1992; p 3.
5. Statement on laparoscopic cholecystectomy issued by the Society of American Gastrointestinal Endoscopic Surgeons (SAGES), Los Angeles, Oct 18, 1989.
6. Statement on laparoscopic cholecystectomy. Bull Am Coll Surg 1990; 75:22.
7. SAGES: Granting of privileges for laparoscopic general surgery. Am J Surg 1991; 161:324–325.
8. SAGES Guidelines: Guidelines for granting of privileges for laparoscopic (peritoneoscopic) general surgery. Surg Endosc 1993; 7:67–68.
9. Satara RM. Proctors, preceptors, and laparoscopic surgery. Editorial. Surg Endosc 1993; 7:283–284.
10. Reed WP. Proctors, preceptors, and laparoscopic surgery. Editorial. Surg Endosc 1993; 7:284.
11. Tompkins RK. Laparoscopic cholecystectomy—Threat or opportunity? Am J Surg 1990; 125:1245.
12. The 1992 Joint Commission Accreditation Manual for Hospitals. Oakbrook Terrace, IL, Joint Commission on Accreditation of Healthcare Organizations, 1991.
13. Laparoscopic Surgery. New York State Department of Health Memorandum, Series 92-20, June 12, 1992.
14. Nenner RP, Imperato PJ, Alcorn CM: Serious complications of laparoscopic cholecystectomy in New York State. N Y State J Med 1992; 92:179–181.
15. Greene FL. Training, credentialling and privileging for minimally invasive surgery. Probl Gen Surg 1991; 8:502–506.

Index

Note: Page numbers in *italics* refer to illustrations; page numbers followed by t refer to tables.

A

Abdomen, acute, 327–330
  adjunctive techniques for decision-making with, 327
  contraindications to laparoscopy in, 329t
  diagnostic laparoscopy in, 328–329, 329t
  laparoscopic surgery for, 329–330
Abdominal pain, 85, 324
Abdominal perineal resection, 605–624
  closure after, 621–624
  complications of, 614
  dissection methods for, 612
  equipment for, 606
  exposure methods for, in anterior pelvic dissection, 612
    of left gutter and left pelvic side wall, 610
    of mesorectum and right pelvic side wall, 610–611
    of presacral space, 611–612
    staging laparoscopy and, 609, *609–610*
  patient positioning for, 606–607
  patient selection for, 605
  pneumoperitoneum for, 607
  postoperative management of, 624
  preoperative evaluation for, 605–606
  preoperative preparation for, 606
  procedural details for, 613–621
    in anterior pelvic dissection, 615–616
    in completion of anterior dissection, 619, 621
    in delivery of specimen, 621, *622*
    in division of lateral stalks, 616, *616–617*
    in division of mesosigmoid, 618
    in entering presacral space, 613–614
    in identification of left ureter, 613

Abdominal perineal resection *(Continued)*
    in ligation of superior hemorrhoidal vessels, 614–615
    in mobilization of sigmoid, 613
    in perineal dissection, 618, *619–620*
    in presacral dissection, 618–619, *621*
    in transection of proximal colon, 617, *617–618*
  retraction methods for, in anterior pelvic dissection, 612
    of left gutter and left pelvic side wall, 610
    of mesorectum and right pelvic side wall, 610–611
    of presacral space, 611–612
    staging laparoscopy and, 609, *609–610*
  trocar placement and size selection for, 607–609
  video equipment positioning for, 607, *608*
Abdominal wall injuries, 84–85
Abdominoperineal resection (APR), versus low anterior resection for rectal cancer, 250
Abscess(es), diverticular, drainage of, 583–589. See also *Diverticular abscess drainage.*
  splenic, 158
Achalasia, cardiomyotomy for, 400–404. See also *Cardiomyotomy.*
Acid production, suppression of, in peptic ulcer disease, complications of, 147
Acid production, suppression of, in peptic ulcer disease, 142
Acidosis, respiratory, from carbon dioxide pneumoperitoneum, 64
  in laparoscopic cholecystectomy, 50
Adhesions, lysis of, 484–498. See also *Bandolysis.*

Adnexal torsion, 371, 372
Anal encirclement, for rectal prolapse, 293
Anastomosis, 125–134
  of colon, intracorporeal, 127–133
    double-stapled technique for, 131, 132
    hand-sewn purse-string suture for, 131, 132
    triple-stapling technique for, 131, 132, 133
Anemia, hemolytic, 154–155
Anesthesia, 42–58
  complications related to, 78–80, 79t
Aneurysm, splenic artery, 158
Anismus, constipation in, 296
Anterior resection, for rectal prolapse, 293–294
Antireflux procedures, laparoscopic, operating room configuration for, 39–40
Antrectomy, laparoscopic, 442–443
  with Billroth II anastomosis, 444–447
    closure for, 446–447
    equipment for, 444–445
    patient positioning for, 445
    patient selection for, 444
    postoperative management of, 447
    preoperative evaluation for, 444
    preoperative preparation for, 444
    procedural details for, 445–446
    trocar placement and sizes for, 445
    video equipment positioning for, 445
Aponeurosis, 334
Appendectomy, 215–220, 499–506
  advantages claimed for, 220
  closure following, 504–505
  complications of, 89t, 89–90, 505–506
  contraindications to, 220
  conversion rate of, 219
  exposure methods for, 501–502
  fecal fistula complicating, 219
  hospital stay following, 219
  in children, 219–220
  operating room configuration for, 36–38
  patient positioning for, 500
  patient selection for, 500
  postoperative management of, 505
  pregnancy and, 219
  preoperative evaluation for, 500
  preoperative preparation for, 500
  procedural details for, 502, 502–504, 504, 505
  results of, 216t
  stump leakage complicating, 219
  technique of, 217–219

Appendectomy (Continued)
  traditional open, 215–216
    results of, 216t
    versus laparoscopic, 217
  trocar placement and size selection for, 501
  versus traditional open, 217
  video equipment positioning for, 500–501
Appendicitis, acute, appendectomy for, 215–220
  differential diagnosis of, 500t
  laparoscopic diagnosis and treatment of, in pregnant patient, 73–74
Arginine vasopressin (AVP) release, by pneumoperitoneum, 64–65
Arrhythmias, cardiac, anesthesia-related, 79
Artery(ies), cystic, management of, in emergency cholecystectomy, 191–193
  inferior mesenteric, high ligation of, for colorectal cancer, 249
  splenic, aneurysm of, 158
Aspiration, anesthesia-related, 79–80
Astler and Coller's system, for colorectal cancer staging, 270–271
Australian clinico-pathology system, for colorectal cancer staging, 272
Autoimmune hemolytic anemia, idiopathic, 155

B

Bandolysis, 484–498
  adhesions in, avoiding reoccurrence of, 486–487
  complementary, 495
  definition of, 484
  dissection in, 484–485
  experience with, from second look operation, 497–498
  exposure methods for, 491–492
  for exposure, 495
  justification of, 487–488
  laser cut in, 486
  monopolar electrosurgery in, 485–486
  patient positioning for, 492–495
  patient selection for, 489
  postoperative management of, 496
  preoperative preparation for, 491

Bandolysis *(Continued)*
  procedural details for, 495–496
  procedures for, 489–491
  result of, 497
  retraction methods for, 491–492
  section with scissors in, 485
  stapling section in, 486
  symptoms treated by, 489–491
  technique of, 484–486
    acquisition of, 496–497
  therapeutic, 495–496
  trocar placement for, 492, 492–493
Bile duct, common. See *Common bile duct.*
  injury to, 88
Bile leaks, 88
Biliary system, 173–212
  acute cholecystitis in, 183–197. See also *Cholecystitis, acute.*
  cholecystectomy on, 175–182. See also *Cholecystectomy laparoscopic.*
  injury to, 87
Bismuth compounds, for peptic ulcer disease, 142
Bladder, anatomy of, 368
  endometriosis involving, 385, *389*
  injury to, 87
Bleeding. See *Hemorrhage.*
Blood markers, 576
Blood supply, to colon, 234, *235*, *236*
  to rectum, 236–237
Blood vessels, control of, 121–123
  injury to, 86–87
    management of, 105, *105*
  spread of colorectal cancer through, 240–241
Bowel. See also *Colon; Rectum.*
  endometriosis involving, 385, *388*
  injury to, complicating laparoscopic cholecystectomy, 87–88
  perforated, management of, 104–105, *105*
  pneumoperitoneum and, 65
  small. See *Small bowel.*

C

Camera, charged coupled device, 4–6
  competitive profiles of, 18t
  video, exposure and, 115

Cancer, colorectal, 233–259. See also *Colorectal cancer.*
  of colon, recurrence of, 257–258
    surgical management of, 242–245, *243*, *245*
  of esophagus, esophagogastrectomy for, 397–399
  of liver, 322–323
  of ovary, 376–378
  of pancreas, 167–169
  of prostate. See *Prostate cancer.*
  of rectum. See *Rectum, cancer of.*
  of spleen, 157
  of stomach, 321–323
Cannula, 7–10
Carbon dioxide, exogenous, complications of laparoscopic cholecystectomy involving, 52–53
  for insufflation, 81
  for insufflator, 6
  for pneumoperitoneum, 62
  in pregnant patient, 70–71
Carcinoma(s), 167–169. See also *Cancer.*
  epithelial origin of, classification and, 267–268
Cardiac arrest, anesthesia-related, 79
Cardiac arrhythmia, anesthesia-related, 79
Cardiac output, changes in, from pneumoperitoneum in laparoscopic cholecystectomy, 49–50
  pneumoperitoneum and, 64
Cardiomyotomy, 400–404
  closure of, 404
  complications of, 404
  discharge criteria for, 404
  dissection methods for, 401–403
  equipment for, 401
  exposure methods for, 401
  patient positioning for, 401
  patient selection for, 400
  postoperative management of, 404
  preoperative evaluation for, 400
  preoperative preparation for, 401
  procedural details for, 403–404
  retraction methods for, 401, *402*
  trocar placement for, 401, *402*
  trocar size selection for, 401
  video equipment positioning for, 401
Cardiovascular system, anesthesia-related complications of, 78–79
  changes in, associated with Trendelenburg position, 48
  pneumoperitoneum creation and, 49–50

Cecal volvulus, 312–315
  cecopexy for, results of, 315t
  cecostomy for, results of, 315t
  detorsion of, results of, 314t
  diagnosis of, 313–314
  laparoscopic surgery for, 315
  resection for, results of, 315t
  treatment of, 314–315
Charged coupled device (CCD) camera, 4–6
Children, appendectomy in, 219–220
Cholangiography, intraoperative, in emergency cholecystectomy, 190
  laparoscopic, in stone management, 205
Cholecystectomy, laparoscopic, 175–182, 448–455
  anesthetic management of, 53–56, 54t
    agents for, 54–56
    technique for, 53–54
  closure after, 453
  common bile duct stones and, 455
  complications of, 47t, 47–53, 87–89, 88t, 454–455
    from exogenous carbon dioxide, 52–53
    from pneumoperitoneum creation, 49t, 49–52
    from reverse Trendelenburg position, 53
    from Trendelenburg position, 47–49, 48t
    from trocar insertion, 47, 47t
  contraindications to, 45, 45t, 178t
  controversies over, 181–182
  conversion of, to open cholecystectomy, indications for, 45, 46t, 47, 177–178
  development of, 175–177
  discharge criteria for, 453
  dissection methods for, 451
  electrocautery for, 31
  emergency, 183–197
    bleeding complicating, 193–194
    cannula placement for, 184–185
    cystic artery management in, 192
    cystic duct dissection in, 191–193
    decompression of gallbladder in, 185–186
    dissection in, 189–190
    dissection in from liver bed, 193–195
    drainage catheter placement in, 195
    gallbladder extraction in, 195–196

Cholecystectomy (Continued)
    intraoperative cholangiography in, 190
    pneumoperitoneum in, 184
    postoperative care in, 196
    retraction for, 186–187
    stone removal in, 188, 188–189, 190–191
    tears of gallbladder during, 187–189
  exposure methods for, 450–451
  in pregnant patient, 74–75
  indications for, 45t, 177–178
  injury from, 179–181
  monitoring during, 56
  open cholecystectomy compared with, 44t
  operating room configuration for, 36, 37
  patient positioning for, 450
  patient selection for, 449
  postoperative management of, 453
  preoperative evaluation for, 449–450
  preoperative preparation for, 450
  procedural details for, 451–453, 452–454
  retraction methods for, 450–451
  surgical technique for, 44–45
  traditional open cholecystectomy compared with, 42–44
  trocar placement and size selection for, 450
  open, adverse event rate for, 43t
Cholecystitis, acute, definition of, 83–84
  management of, 183–197, 197t
  operative technique for, 184–197
  preoperative preparation in, 183–184
Choledochoscopy, cystic duct, 455
Choledochotomy, direct laparoscopic, 206–207, 208
Cigarette smoking, ulcer healing and, 141
Cimetidine, for peptic ulcer disease, complications of, 147
Circulatory system, effects of pneumoperitoneum on, 64
Clips, metal, in blood vessel control, 122, 122
Coagulation, electrocautery, 27–28
Colectomy, laparoscopic, complications of, 91
  right, 522–525
    closure after, 525
    complications of, 525

Colectomy *(Continued)*
  discharge criteria for, 525
  dissection methods for, 524
  equipment for, 522
  patient positioning for, 524
  patient selection for, 522
  postoperative management of, 525
  preoperative evaluation for, 522
  procedural details for, 524
  trocar placement and size selection for, 523, *524*
  video equipment positioning for, 523
 sigmoid, 244–245, *245*
  for sigmoid volvulus, 307
Colitis cystica profunda, with rectal prolapse, 292
Colomyotomy, for colonic diverticulitis, 226
Colon, abnormal transit in, in intractable constipation, 298–299
 anastomosis of, intracorporeal, 127–133
 carcinoma of, recurrence of, 257–258
  surgical management of, 242
 descending, carcinoma of, surgical management of, 243–244, *244*
 disorders(s) of, 290–299
  diverticular, 223–227. See also *Diverticular disease, colonic.*
  intractable constipation as, 294–299
  rectal prolapse as, 290–294. See also *Constipation, intractable.*
 dysmotility of, constipation from, 295–296
 laparoscopic surgery on, indications for, 131t
 left, blood supply of, *235*, 236
  lymphatic drainage of, 236, *236*
 microscopic anatomy of, 238, *238*
 polyps in, polypectomy for, 509–518. See also *Polypectomy, for colonic polyps.*
 resection of, and anastomosis of, 125–134
  operating room configuration for, 38–39
 right, blood supply of, 234, *235*
  carcinoma of, surgical management of, 243
  lymphatic drainage of, 234, *236*
 sigmoid, blood supply of, *235*, 236–237
  carcinoma of, surgical management of, 244–245, *245*
  lymphatic drainage of, 236, *236*

Colon *(Continued)*
  volvulus of, 301–312. See also *Sigmoid volvulus.*
 surgery of, complications of, 251–257
 surgical anatomy of, 234, *235–236*, 236–238
 transverse, blood supply of, *235*, 236
  carcinoma of, surgical management of, 243, *243*
  lymphatic drainage of, 236, *236*
  volvulus of, 315
 volvulus of, 301–316
Colonoscopic polypectomy, laparoscopically assisted, 509
 procedural details for, 513–514, *515*
Colonoscopy, preoperative, for low anterior resection, 575
Colopexy, for sigmoid volvulus, 307
Colorectal cancer, 233–259
 Broders' classification of, 267
 detection of, radioimmune, 277–280
  scanning in, devices for, gamma, hand-held, 278–280
   limitations of, 278
   techniques of, 277–278
 distribution of, by site, 238–239
 evaluation of, 273–280
  computed tomography in, 274
  digital rectal examination in, 273–274
  ultrasonography in, 275–277
 laparoscopic resection of, role of, 259
 low anterior resection for, 575–582. See also *Low anterior resection.*
 spread of, intramural, curative versus palliative resection and, 248t
  lymphatic, 239–240
  ovarian, 241
  patterns of, 239–241
  vascular, 240–241
  within bowel wall, 239
 staging of, 266–281
  Astler and Coller's system for, 270–271
  Australian clinico-pathology system for, 272
  Dukes' system for, 268–269
  future directions of, 273
  future of, 280–281
  Gabriel, Dukes, and Bussey's system for, 269
  Gunderson and Sosin's system for, 271–272
  history of, 266–273

Colorectal cancer *(Continued)*
    Kirklin, Dockerty, and Waugh's system for, 270
    Lockhart-Mummery system for, 268
    methods of, using multivariate statistical analysis, 273
    Simpson and Mayo's system for, 270
    TNM system for, 272t, 272–273
    Turnbull, Kyle, Watson, and Spratt's system for, 271
  surgical management of, 241–245
    complication(s) of, 251–257
      anastomotic, 253–254, 256–257
      intestinal obstruction as, 255–256
      intraoperative, 251–253
      postoperative, 253–257
      pulmonary, 257
      urinary tract, 252, 254
      vascular, 252–253
      wound problems as, 254–255
  surgical technique for, 245–247
Colostomy, construction of, after abdominal perineal resection, 622–623
  Hartmann's, closure of, 598–604. See also *Hartmann's colostomy, closure of.*
Colotomy and polypectomy, laparoscopic, 509
  procedural details for, 515–518
  laparoscopically assisted, 509
    procedural details for, 515, *516*
Common bile duct, exploration of, 456–466
  direct laparoscopic approach to, closure after, 463, *465*
    discharge criteria for, 466
    postoperative management of, 466
    procedural details of, 463, *464*
  dissection methods for, 459
  equipment for, 458–459
  exposure methods for, 459
  patient positioning for, 459
  patient selection for, 456–457
  preoperative evaluation of, 457
  preoperative preparation for, 457–458
  retraction methods for, 459
  transcystic duct approach to, 459–463
    closure after, 462
    direct laparoscopic approach to, 463, *464–465*, 466
    postoperative management of, 462–463
    procedural details for, 439–462
  trocar placement and size selection for, 459

Common bile duct *(Continued)*
  video equipment positioning for, 459
  stones in, removal of, 455
Composite video, 18
Computed tomography (CT), in colorectal cancer evaluation, 274
Constipation, in rectal prolapse, 292
  intractable, 294–299
    current approach to, 299
    evaluation of, 297–299
    extracolonic causes of, 296t
    from colonic dysmotility, 295–296
    from disordered defection, 296–297
    functional causes of, 296t
    in adult Hirschsprung's disease, 297
    in anismus, 296
    in descending perineum syndrome, 296–297
    in disturbed rectal sensation, 297
    in rectal prolapse, 297
    in rectocele, 297
    management of, 297–299
    patient assessment in, 295
Credentialing, hospital, 686–690
Cryptorchidism, 358–361
  location of testes in, 359t
Cul-de-sac, posterior, endometriosis involving, 385, *390–392*
Currents, blended, in electrosurgery, 28
  solid state versus vacuum tube generated, in electrosurgery, 28–29
Cyst(s), ovarian, 375–376
  paraovarian, 371
  splenic, 158
Cystic artery, management of, in emergency cholecystectomy, 191–193
Cystic duct, dissection of, in emergency cholecystectomy, 191–193
  stones in, removal of, 190–191
Cystic duct choledochoscopy, 455

D

Davol Arthro-Flo irrigation system, 10
Defecation, disordered, constipation from, 296–297
Descending perineum syndrome, constipation in, 296–297
Diagnostic laparoscopy, 319–325
  in abdominal pain, 324
  in acute abdomen, 329

Diagnostic laparoscopy (Continued)
   in trauma, 323–324
   indications for, 312–323, 320t
   operating room configuration for, 40
   technique of, 319–321
Digital rectal examination, 273–274
Dissecting instruments, 10–12
Dissection techniques, 119–121
Diverticular abscess drainage, 583–589
   complications of, 589
   discharge criteria for, 589
   dissection methods for, 585, *586–587*
   equipment for, 584
   exposure methods for, 585, *585–586*
   patient positioning for, 584
   patient selection for, 583
   postoperative management of, 588–589
   preoperative evaluation of, 583
   preoperative preparation for, 583
   procedural details for, 587–588, *588*
   retraction methods for, 585
   trocar placement and size selection for, 585
   video equipment positioning for, 584
Diverticular disease, 222–230
   colonic, 223–227
      anatomy of, 223
      complications of, 224
      etiology of, 223
      location of, 224
      pathogenesis of, 223
   jejunal-ileal, 227–229
Diverticulitis, 232
   colonic, colomyotomy for, 226
      CT-guided percutaneous drainage for, 226
      Hartmann's procedure for, 225
      one stage resection for, 227
      recurrent, extent of resection and, 224–227
Diverticulum, ileal, 229
   Meckel's, 229–230
Documentation, video tape for, 15–16
Drainage, of diverticular abscess, 583–589. See also *Diverticular abscess drainage*.
   percutaneous, CT-guided, for colonic diverticulitis, 226
Dukes' system, for colorectal cancer staging, 268–269
Dundee internal slip knot, 112, *112*
Duodenal ulcer, perforation of, management of, 145–146
   standard operations for, results of, 143t
   surgical management of, 143

E

Ectopic pregnancy, 371–372
   laparoscopic evaluation of, 72–73
Ectopic spleen, 158
Electrical injury, 85
Electrocautery, applications of, 29–30
   coagulation by, 27–28
   cutting by, 27
   devices for, adaptation of, 30
      monopolar, 30
         versus bipolar, 29
   experimental studies on, 31
   for advanced gastrointestinal procedures, 31–32
   in endoscopic surgery, 26
   in laparoscopic cholecystectomy, 31
   safety of, 30–31
   technique of, cautions in, 32
Electrosurgery, blended currents in, 28
   frequency of current in, 26–27
   fulguration in, 28
   historical background of, 22–26
   physics of, 26–32
   solid state versus vacuum tube generated currents in, 28–29
Elliptocytosis, hereditary, 155
Embolism, gas, 86–87
   from pneumoperitoneum, 62–63
   management of, 105
Emphysema, subcutaneous, in extraperitoneal insufflation, 82
   management of, 105
Endobronchial intubation, Trendelenburg position and, 48–49
Endocrine tumors, pancreatic, 169t
Endometriosis, 373–375, 379–392
   diagnosis of, 381, *381–382*
   etiology of, 379, *380*, 381
   treatment of, 381, 383–385, *386–387*, *388–392*
      outcome of, 385, 387
      pregnancy outcome after, 384t
Endoscopic imaging, basic principles of, 16
Endoscopic sphincterotomy, for stone removal, 199–201
   preoperative, for duct clearance, 201, *202*
Endoscopic surgery, electrocautery in, 26
Endoscopic techniques, percutaneous, for stone removal, 198–199
Epidural anesthesia, for outpatient laparoscopy, 54

Equipment, 3–14
  failures of, complications from, 85
  for operating room, 35–36
  video, exposure and, 115
Esophagogastrectomy, 397–399
Esophagus, carcinoma of, esophagogastrectomy for, 397–399
  staging of, 321
Excision, local, for rectal cancer, 251
Exposure, 114–118
  laparoscope for, 115
  pneumoperitoneum for, 115
  port placement for, 115–117
  position of patient for, 117
  techniques for grasper and retractor use in, 117–118
  video equipment for, 115
Extraperitoneal insufflation, 82–83

F

Fallopian tubes, anatomy of, 367
  disorders of, 369–371
Fascia, 334
  pelvic, 237–238
Fecal fistula, complicating appendectomy, 219
Feeding gastrostomy tube, 470–471
Feeding jejunostomy, 467–470
  closure after, 470
  equipment for, 468
  exposure methods for, 468–469
  patient positioning for, 468
  patient selection for, 467–468
  postoperative management of, 470
  procedural details for, 469–470
  retraction methods for, 468–469
  Roux-en-Y, 471
  trocar placement and size selection for, 468
  tube placement in, 467–468
  video equipment positioning for, 468
Felty's syndrome, 157–158
Femoral hernias, repair of, 637–638
Fentanyl, perioperative administration of, 55
Fetal physiology, pneumoperitoneum and, 72t
Fistula, fecal, complicating appendectomy, 219

Fulguration, in electrosurgery, 28
Fundoplication, Nissen, 430–439. See also *Nissen fundoplication.*

G

Gabriel, Dukes, and Bussey's system, for colorectal cancer staging, 269
Gallbladder, decompression of, in emergency cholecystectomy, 185–186
  disease of, laparoscopic cholecystectomy for, 42–58. See also *Cholecystectomy, laparoscopic.*
  dissection of, from liver bed in emergency cholecystectomy, 193–195
    in emergency cholecystectomy, 189–190
  extraction of, in emergency cholecystectomy, 195–196
  removal of, 448–455. See also *Cholecystectomy, laparoscopic.*
  tears in, in emergency cholecystectomy, 187–189
Gallstones. See also *Stones.*
  cholecystectomy for, 175–182. See also *Cholecystectomy, laparoscopic.*
  extraction of, 188, *188–189*
  surgical treatment of, history of, 177t
Gamma scanning devices, hand-held, 278–280
Gas embolism, 86–87
  from pneumoperitoneum, 62–63
  management of, 105
Gas leak, at trocar site, management of, 101, 103
Gastrectomy, distal, for peptic ulcer disease, 150
Gastric. See also *Stomach.*
Gastric outlet obstruction, complicating peptic ulcers, 146–147
Gastrinoma, 169t
Gastrointestinal procedures, advanced, electrocautery for, 31–32
Gastrointestinal tract, injury to, as complication, 85–86
  lower, surgery of, 213
    appendectomy as, 215–220. See also *Appendectomy.*
    for diverticular disease, 222–230. See also *Diverticular disease.*

Gastrointestinal tract *(Continued)*
  surgery on, complications of, 91
Gastrostomy tube, feeding, 470–471
Gaucher's disease, 158
General anesthesia, for laparoscopic cholecystectomy, 53
Genitourinary tract injury, 87
Glucogonoma, 169t
Graspers, use of, 117–118
Gunderson and Sosin's system, for colorectal cancer staging, 271–272
Gynecologic disorder(s), adnexal torsion as, 371, *372*
  anatomy in, normal, 366–368
  endometriosis as, 373–375, 379–392. See also *Endometriosis.*
  functional cysts as, 375–376
  ovarian masses as, 375
  ovarian neoplasms as, 376–378
  paraovarian cysts as, 371
  tubal disorders as, 369–371
  uterine masses as, 368–369

H

H_2-receptor antagonists, for peptic ulcer disease, 142
  complications of, 147
Hairy cell leukemia, 157
Halothane, for laparoscopic cholecystectomy, complications of, 50
Hartmann's colostomy, closure of, 598–604
  complications of, 604
  discharge criteria for, 603
  dissection methods for, 601–602
  equipment for, 599
  exposure methods for, 600–601, *601*
  patient positioning for, 599, *600*
  patient selection for, 598
  postoperative management of, 603
  preoperative evaluation for, 598–599
  preoperative preparation for, 599
  procedural details for, 602–603, *603–604*
  retraction methods for, 600–601, *602*
  trocar placement and size selection for, 600, *601*
  video equipment positioning for, 599
Hartmann's procedure, for colonic diverticulitis, 225

Hartmann's procedure *(Continued)*
  for sigmoid volvulus, 307
Hasson trocar, 10
Heart. See *Cardiac* entries.
Helicobacter pylori infection, peptic ulcer disease and, 140
Helium, for pneumoperitoneum, 62
Hemicolectomy, complete, 557–558, *559–560,* 560–562, *561–563*
  left, 547–564
    closure after, 563
    complications of, 564
    discharge criteria for, 564
    dissection methods for, 552–553
    equipment for, 548–549, *550*
    exposure methods for, 552
    patient positioning for, 549–550, *551*
    patient selection for, 547–548
    postoperative management of, 564
    preoperative evaluation of, 548
    preoperative preparation for, 548
    procedural details for, 553, *554–555,* 555–557, *556–558*
    retraction methods for, 552
    sparing sigmoid colon, 562–563
    trocar placement for, 550–552
    video equipment positioning for, 550, *551*
  right, with extracorporeal anastomosis, 536–546
    closure after, 544–545
    complications of, 546
    discharge criteria for, 546
    dissection methods for, 539
    equipment for, 537
    exposure methods for, 538–539
    patient positioning for, 537
    patient selection for, 536–537
    postoperative management of, 546
    preoperative evaluation for, 537
    preoperative preparation for, 537
    procedural details for, 539–540, *541–542,* 542–544, *543–545*
    retraction methods for, 538–539
    trocar placement and size selection for, 537–538
    video equipment positioning for, 537, *538*
  with intracorporeal anastomosis, 526–535
    closure after, 534
    equipment for, 527
    patient positioning for, 527–528

Hemicolectomy (Continued)
    patient selection for, 526
    postoperative management of, 534
    preoperative evaluation for, 526–527
    preoperative preparation for, 527
    procedural details for, 529, 530–531, 531–533, 532–533
    trocar placement and sizes for, 528, 529
    video equipment positioning for, 528
Hemicolectomy, left, 243, 244
Hemolytic anemias, 154–155
Hemorrhage, 86
    abdominal wall, 84
    complicating emergency cholecystectomy, 193–194
    complicating peptic ulcers, 144–145
    from trocar site, 103
Hemostasis, electrocautery for, 29–30
Hereditary elliptocytosis, 155
Hereditary spherocytosis, 154–155
Hernia(s), abdominal wall, 85
    femoral, repair of, 637–638
    inguinal, iliopubic tract, repair of, with inlay buttress mesh, 640–648. See also *Iliopubic tract inguinal hernia repair with inlay buttress mesh.*
    inguinofemoral, 332–344. See also *Inguinofemoral hernia.*
    repair of. See *Herniorrhaphy.*
Herniorrhaphy, 625–639
    closure after, 636
    complications of, 90
    dissection methods for, 632–634
    exposure methods for, 632–634
    extraperitoneal approach to, 628
    for femoral hernias, 637–638
    historical perspectives of, 625–626
    intraperitoneal approach to, 627–628
    operating room configuration for, 38
    patient positioning for, 632
    patient selection for, 628–629, 630–631
    preoperative evaluation for, 629
    preoperative preparation for, 629, 632
    preperitoneal approach to, 628, 629
    procedural details for, 634–636
    trocar placement and size selection for, 632
Hirschsprung's disease, constipation in, 297
Hodgkin's disease, 157

Hospital credentialing, 686–690
Hypercarbia, from carbon dioxide pneumoperitoneum, 63–64
    from halothane anesthesia, 50, 52–53
Hypersplenism, 156–157
Hypotension, anesthesia-related, 79
Hypoventilation, pneumoperitoneum-induced, in laparoscopic cholecystectomy, 50
Hypoxemia, during laparoscopic cholecystectomy, 50–51, 51t

I

Ileostomy, 590–597
    closure after, 596–597
    complications of, 597
    discharge criteria for, 597
    dissection methods for, 592
    equipment for, 590–591
    exposure methods for, 592
    patient positioning for, 591
    patient selection for, 590
    postoperative management of, 597
    preoperative evaluation for, 590
    preoperative preparation for, 590
    procedural details for, 592, 592–593, 593, 594–596, 596, 597
    retraction methods for, 592
    trocar placement and size selection for, 591–592
    video equipment positioning for, 591
Ileum, diverticular disease of, 227–229
Ileus, postoperative, pneumoperitoneum and, 66
Iliopubic tract inguinal hernia repair, with inlay buttress mesh, 640–648
    alternative instruments and special tricks for, 646–647
    complications of, 647–648
    dissection methods for, 643–644
    equipment for, 641–642
    landmark identification in, 644
    laparoscopic iliopubic tract repair in, 644–646
    patient selection for, 641
    port positions for, 642–643
    postoperative management of, 647
    results of, 647
Image, laparoscopic, creation of, 16–19

Imaging, 15–21
  endoscopic, basic principles of, 16
  for documentation, 15–16
Imaging system, 3–7
  charged coupled device camera in, 4–6
  image sensor in, 4–6
  laparoscope in, 3–4
  light service in, 6
Incontinence, fecal, 292
Infections, superficial wound, of abdominal wall, 84–85
Inferior mesenteric artery, high ligation of, for colorectal cancer, 249
Inguinal hernia, iliopubic tract, repair of, with inlay buttress mesh, 640–648. See also *Iliopubic tract inguinal hernia repair, with inlay buttress mesh.*
Inguinofemoral hernia, anatomy of, 333–334
  etiology of, 332–333
  laparoendoscopic surgery for, 333
  laparoscopic repair of, 335–336, 337–339, 340, 341–344
    preperitoneal approach to, 335
      for direct hernia, 340, 341–342
      for femoral hernia, 340, 343–344
      for indirect hernia, 336, 337–340, 340
    preperitoneal mesh in, 336
    prosthetic material in, 335
  treatment of, 333–335
Instruments, complications caused by, 80, 85–87
  dissecting, 10–12
  for abdominal perineal resection, 606
  for colon resection and anastomosis, 125–127
  for thoracoscopy, 346t
  ligation, 12–13
  manipulating, 10–12
  suturing, 12–13
Insufflation, aberrant pressure patterns during, 100t
  agents for, choice of, 81
  extraperitoneal, 82–83
  mesenteric, 82
  omental, 82–83
  preperitoneal, 82
Insufflator, 6–7
Insulinoma, 169t
Intestinal intussusception, 290–291
Intestinal obstruction, 284–288
  classification of, etiolgical, 285t

Intestinal obstruction *(Continued)*
  clinical features of, 284–285
  mechanical, pathophysiology of, 285–286
  operative findings in, 286–288
Intrapulmonary shunting, during laparoscopic cholecystectomy, 51
Intravenous pyelography, 576
Intubation, endobronchial, Trendelenburg position and, 48–49
Intussusception, intestinal, 290–291
Irrigator, 10
Islet cell neoplasms, 169–170

J

Jejunostomy, feeding, 467–470. See also *Feeding jejunostomy.*
Jejunum, diverticular disease of, 227–229

K

Kidneys, pneumoperitoneum and, 65
Kirklin, Dockerty, and Waugh's system, for colorectal cancer staging, 270
Knot tying, laparoscopic, 109, *110–111*, 111–113, *112*

L

Laparoendoscopic surgery, for inguinofemoral hernias, 333
Laparoscope, 3–4
  exposure and, 115
Laparoscopic hand-held gamma detection probe, 279–280
Laparoscopic image, creation of, 16–19
Laparoscopy, complications of, 77–91, 78t
  contraindications to, 81t
  diagnostic, 319–325. See also under specific technique, e.g., *Cholecystectomy, laparoscopic; Diagnostic laparoscopy.*
  open, complications of, 84

Leiomyomas, 368–369
Leukemias, 157
Ligament(s), definition of, 334
  uterine, 366
Ligation instruments, 12–13
Ligation techniques, 107–113
  in laparoscopic vs. open surgery, 107–108
Light sources, for endoscopic imaging, 16, 17t
  high intensity, 6
Lighting, operating room, 35
Lithotripsy, mechanical, 203, 204
Liver, malignancies in, staging of, 322–323
  metastases of colorectal cancer to, intraoperative ultrasound detection of, 277
  pneumoperitoneum and, 65
  scanning of, preoperative, 576
Local anesthesia, for laparoscopic gynecologic procedures, 53–54
Lockhart-Mummery staging system, for rectal cancer, 268
Low anterior resection (LAR), 575–582
  equipment for, 576
  patient positioning for, 576
  preoperative evaluation for, 575–576
  preoperative preparation for, 576
  procedure for, 577, 578, 579–581, 579–582
    extent of resection in, 580–581, 581
    for carcinoma of colon, 581–582
    suspension of intestine in, 577, 578, 579, 579
    transillumination of mesenteric arcade in, 579–580, 580
  trocar placement for, 576, 577
  versus abdominoperineal resection, for rectal cancer, 250
  video equipment positioning for, 576
Lung(s), complications of, anesthesia-related, 79–80
  edema of, anesthesia-related, 80
  pneumoperitoneum and, 63–64
Lymph nodes, pelvic, dissection of, 351–355
  metastases to, incidence of, tumor grade and clinical stage and, 352, 352t, 353t
  resection margins for, in prostate cancer, 354
  status of, noninvasive detection of, 352–353

Lymphadenectomy, pelvic. See *Pelvic lymphadenectomy.*
Lymphatic drainage, of colon, 234, 236, 236
  of rectum, 236, 236–237
Lymphatic extension, of colorectal cancer, 239–240
Lymphatics, pelvic, anatomy of, 353–354
Lymphomas, 157
  staging of, 323
Lysis, of adhesions, 484–498. See also *Bandolysis.*

M

Manipulating instruments, 10–12
Maryland Dissector, 30
Meckel's diverticulum, 229–230
Media, recording, alternative, 20–21
Mesenteric artery, inferior, high ligation of, for colorectal cancer, 249
Mesenteric insufflation, 83
Mesorectum, distal, resection of, for rectal cancer, 250
Metaplasia, myeloid, 157
Metastasis, to pelvic lymph nodes, incidence of, tumor grade and clinical stage and, 352, 352t, 353t
Microsurgical square knot, tying, 109, 111, 111–112
Monitors, 19
  use of, complications and, 80
Morbidity, 77–78
Mortality, 77–78
Multivariate statistical analysis, methods of colorectal staging system using, 273
Myeloid metaplasia, 157

N

Narcotics, perioperative administration of, for laparoscopic cholecystectomy, 55
Needle(s), for suturing, 108
  Veress. See *Veress needle.*
Neoplasms. See also *Cancer.*
  islet cell, 169–170
Nephrectomy, laparoscopic, 361

Neuroendocrine tumors, of pancreas, 169–170
Nezhat-Dorsey hydrodissection pump, 10
Nissen fundoplication, 430–439
    closure of, 435
    complications of, 91
    discharge criteria for, 436
    equipment for, 432
    exposure method for, 433
    laparoscopic, complications of, 91
    patient evaluation for, 431–432
    patient positioning for, 432
    patient selection for, 431
    postoperative management of, 435–436, 439
    procedural details for, 433–435, 433–438
    retraction method for, 433
    trocar placement for, 432–433
Nitrous oxide, for insufflation, 81
    for laparoscopic cholecystectomy, 55–56
"No-touch" technique, for colorectal cancer, evaluation of, 246
Nonsteroidal anti-inflammatory agents (NSAIDs), peptic ulcer disease due to, 140

O

Obstetric disorder(s), anatomy in, normal, 366–368
    ectopic pregnancy as, 371–372
Omental insufflation, 82–83
Omeprazole, for peptic ulcer disease, 142
    complications of, 147
Oophorectomy, 650–659
    closure after, 658–659
    complications of, 659
    discharge criteria for, 659
    equipment for, 651
    exposure methods for, 652
    for laparoscopic culdotomy, 655–658
    patient positioning for, 651
    patient selection for, 650
    postoperative management of, 659
    preoperative evaluation for, 650
    preoperative preparation for, 650
    procedural details for, 652–658
        in ovarian remnant, 658
        in retroperitoneal approach, 653–654
        in umbilical extension, 654–655

Oophorectomy (Continued)
    prophylactic, for colorectal cancer, 247
    retraction methods for, 652
    trocar placement and size selection for, 652
    video equipment positioning for, 651–652
Open laparoscopy, complications of, 84
Operating room, configuration of, 34–41
    for diagnostic and staging laparoscopy, 40
    for laparoscope cholecystectomy, 36, 37
    for laparoscopic antireflux procedures, 39–40
    for laparoscopic appendectomy, 36–38
    for laparoscopic colon resection, 38–39
    for laparoscopic herniorrhaphy, 38
    for laparoscopic small bowel resection, 38
    for laparoscopic vagotomy, 39–40
    for operative thoracoscopy, 40
    equipment for, 35–36
    lighting in, 35
    table in, 34–35
Ovary(ies), anatomy of, 367
    cysts of, functional, 375–376
    endometriosis involving, 385, 386–387
    masses in, 375, 375t
    metastasis of colorectal cancer to, 241
    neoplasms of, 376–378
        classification of, 377t
        diagnostic characteristics of, 376t

P

Pain, abdominal, diagnostic laparoscopy in, 324
    postoperative, 85
Pancreas, carcinoma of, 167–169, 169t
    staging of, 322
    diseases of, 165–171
        laparoscopic approaches to, applications of, 166t, 167–171
        for islet cell neoplasms, 169–170
        for pancreatic carcinoma, 167–169
        historical issues on, 165–166
        infragastric approach to, 167
        supragastric approach to, 166–167

Pancreas (Continued)
    technical aspects of, 166–167
    endocrine tumors of, clinical features of, 169t
Pancreatitis, acute, 170–171
    chronic, 171
Paraovarian cysts, 371
Paul-Mikulicz resection, for sigmoid volvulus, 307
Pelvic fascia, 237–238
Pelvic floor, dysfunction of, intractable constipation with, 299
    evaluation of, in intractable constipation, 297–298
    normal function of, intractable constipation with, 298–299
Pelvic inflammatory disease (PID), 369–371
Pelvic lymph nodes, dissection of, 351–355
    metastases to, tumor grade and clinical stage in, 352, 352t, 353t
    resection margins for, in prostate cancer, 354
    status of, noninvasive detection of, 352–353
Pelvic lymphadenectomy, 661–673
    closure after, 671
    complications of, 672
    discharge criteria for, 672
    dissection methods for, 667–671
    equipment for, 662–664
    exposure methods for, 666–667
    for other genitourinary malignancies, 354–355
    in staging and prognosis of prostate cancer, 351–352
    instrumentation for, 664–665
    laparoscopic, technique of, 355–356
    operating room setup for, 665
    patient positioning for, 665
    patient selection for, 661–662
    postoperative management of, 671–672
    preoperative evaluation for, 662
    preoperative preparation for, 662
    procedural details for, 667–671
    retraction methods for, 666–667
    trocar placement and size selection for, 666, 666–667
    video equipment positioning for, 665
Pelvic lymphatics, anatomy of, 353–354
Peptic ulcer disease, 137–151

Peptic ulcer disease (Continued)
    bleeding from, recurrent, predicting, 145t
    classification of, 138, 139
    clinical course of, 138–142
    epidemiology of, 138
    gastric outlet obstruction complicating, 146–147
    highly selective vagotomy for, 150
    laparoscopic treatment of, 420–428
    management of, 142–150
        complications/side effects of, 147–148
        costs of, 148
        for acute complications, 144–147
        laparoscopic approaches to, 148–150
        medical, 142
        surgical, 143–144
    pathogenesis of, 138–141
    pathophysiology of, 138–141
    perforation complicating, 145–146
    surgical options for, 405–406
    symptomatic, natural history of, 141–142
    truncal vagotomy for, 149–150
    vagotomy for, 405–419. See also *Vagotomy.*
Percutaneous drainage, CT-guided, for colonic diverticulitis, 226
Percutaneous endoscopic techniques, for common bile duct stone removal, 198–199
Perforation, of peptic ulcers, management of, 145–146
Perineal rectosigmoidectomy, for rectal prolapse, 293
Perineal resection, abdominal, 605–624. See also *Abdominal perineal resection.*
Peritoneal cavity, trocar not entering, management of, 103–104, 104
Peritoneal inflammation, pneumoperitoneum and, 66
Photography, still, 19–20
Pixels, in image creation, 17–18
Pneumomediastinum, anesthesia-related, 80
Pneumoperitoneum, carbon dioxide, in pregnant patient, 70–71
    circulatory effects of, 64
    complications of, 81–85
    creation of, complications of laparoscopic cholecystectomy involving, 49t, 49–52

Pneumoperitoneum (Continued)
   technique for, 98–101
  exposure and, 115
  fetal physiology and, 72t
  gas embolism from, 62–63
  gas for, selection of, 62
  hazards of, future research on, 65
  historical notes on, 62
  maternal physiology and, 72t
  pathophysiology of, 61–66
  peritoneal inflammation and, 66
  postoperative ileus and, 66
  vasopressin release by, 64–65
  venous return and, 65–66
  ventilatory effects of, 63–64
Pneumothorax, anesthesia-related, 80
  tension, during laparoscopic cholecystectomy, 51
Polypectomy, 508–521
  colonoscopic, laparoscopically assisted, 509
  for colonic polyps, closure after, 518
    colonoscopic, laparoscopically assisted, procedural details for, 513–514, 515
    dissection methods for, 512–513
    equipment for, 510
    exposure methods for, 512
    laparoscopic colotomy and, procedural details for, 515–518
    laparoscopically assisted colotomy and, procedural details for, 515, 516
    patient evaluation for, 509
    patient positioning for, 510
    postoperative management of, 518
    preoperative preparation for, 509
    procedural details for, 513–518
      for exploration of abdomen, 513
      for localization of polyp, 513, 513–514
    retraction methods for, 512
    trocar placement for, 510, 512
    video equipment placement for, 510, 511
  for rectal polyps, 518–521
    complications of, 521
    discharge criteria for, 521
    equipment for, 519
    patient positioning for, 519
    patient selection for, 518–519
    preoperative evaluation for, 519
    preoperative preparation for, 519

Polypectomy (Continued)
    procedural details for, 519–521
  laparoscopic colotomy and, 509
  laparoscopically assisted colotomy and, 509
  patient selection for, 509
Port(s), for abdominal perineal resection, 606
  placement of, 115–117
    for colon resection and anastomosis, 126, 128
Positioning, of patient, exposure and, 117
  for colon resection and anastomosis, 126, 127
Postdoctoral training, 675–690
  animal laboratory for, 683, 683–684, 685
  courses in, administration of, 682
    expectations for, 678
    facilities for, 681
    faculty for, 681–682
    financing of, 682
    future of, 682
    marketing of, 682
    objectives of, 679
    organization of, 678–681
    program for, 679–681
    reasons for teaching, 677–678
    target groups for, 679
  hospital credentialing and, 686–690
Pregnancy outcome after surgery for endometriosis, 384t
Pregnant patient, laparoscopy in, 69–75
  for appendicitis, 73–74, 219
  for cholecystectomy, 74–75
  for ectopic pregnancy, 72–73, 371–372
  future prospects for, 75
  safety considerations for, 69–72
  technical considerations for, 69–72
Premedication, for laparoscopic cholecystectomy, 54
Preperitoneal insufflation, 82
Prostaglandin E analogues, for peptic ulcer disease, 142
Prostate cancer, pelvic lymph nodes in, resection margins for, 354
  staging and prognosis of, 351–352
  tumor grade and clinical stage of, incidence of pelvic metastases and, 352, 352t, 353t
Purpura, 156
Pyelography, intravenous, preoperative, for low anterior resection, 576

R

Radiology, preoperative, for low anterior resection, 575
Recorders, video, 20
Recording media, alternative, 20–21
Rectocele, constipation in, 297
Rectopexy, sling, for rectal prolapse, 294
Rectosigmoidectomy, perineal, for rectal prolapse, 293
Rectum, blood supply of, 235, 236–237
  cancer of, 248–251
    operation for, choice of, 247–248
    recurrence of, 258–259
    resectability of, determination of, 247
    spread of, 267
    spread of, Miles on, 267
    surgical management of, 247–251
      abdominoperineal versus low anterior resection in, 250
      factors determining, 250
      level of lesion and, 248
      level of vascular and lymphatic ligation and, 249
      local excision in, 251
      margins of resection and, 248–250
      radical, failure of, 250–251
      resection of distal mesorectum in, 250
  lymphatic drainage of, 236, 236–237
  microscopic anatomy of, 238, 238
  polyps of, polypectomy for, 518–521. See also *Polypectomy, for rectal polyps.*
  prolapse of, 290–294
    anterior resection for, 565–574
      closure after, 574
      complications of, 574
      discharge criteria for, 574
      dissection methods for, 567
      equipment for, 566
      exposure methods for, 567
      patient positioning for, 566
      patient selection for, 565–566
      postoperative management of, 574
      preoperative evaluation of, 566
      preoperative preparation for, 566
      procedural details for, 567–569, 568–571, 571, 572–573, 574
      retraction methods for, 567
      trocar placement and size selection for, 566–567

Rectum (Continued)
      video equipment positioning for, 566
    clinical features of, 291–292
    complete, 291
      anatomic abnormalities associated with, 291t
      etiology and diagnosis of, 291
    current approach to, 294
    definitions of, 290–291
    differential diagnosis of, 292
    mucosal, 290
    occult, 290–291
    surgical therapy for, 293t, 293–294
    symptoms of, 292
    syndromes related to, 292
  sensation in, disturbed, constipation in, 297
  surgery of, complications of, 251–257
  surgical anatomy of, 234, 235–236, 236–238
Resection, laparoscopic, for sigmoid volvulus, with end-to-end anastomosis, 311–312, 313
  with side-to-side and end-to-end anastomosis, 307–311
  of colon, instrumentation for, 125–127
    operating room configuration for, 38–39
  of small bowel, operating room configuration for, 38
Respiratory acidosis, from carbon dioxide pneumoperitoneum, 64
  in laparoscopic cholecystectomy, 50
Respiratory system, anesthesia-related complications of, 79
  pneumoperitoneum creation and, 50–52
  Trendelenburg position and, 48
Retractors, use of, 117–118
RGB video, 18–19
Roeder external slip knot, tying, 108, 109
Roux-en-Y feeding jejunostomy, 471

S

Safety, of electrocautery, 30–31
  of laparoscopy, in pregnant patient, 69–72
Salpingitis, 369–371
  clinical diagnostic criteria for, 369t

Salpingo-oophorectomy, 650–659. See also *Oophorectomy*.
Sarcoidosis, 158
Sensor, in video camera, 16–17
Seromyotomy, anterior fundic, right truncal vagotomy with, 420–426. See also *Truncal vagotomy, right, with anterior fundic seromyotomy*.
anterior lesser curve, for peptic ulcer disease, 150
Shunting, intrapulmonary, during laparoscopic cholecystectomy, 51
Sickle cell disease, 155
Sigmoid colectomy, for sigmoid volvulus, 307
Sigmoid colon, blood supply of, 235, 236
carcinoma of, surgical management of, 244–245, 245
lymphatic drainage of, 236, 236
Sigmoid volvulus, 301–312
diagnosis of, 303
etiology of, 301–303
treatment of, 303–312
colopexy in, 307
definitive, rationale for, 303, 304t, 305–306
Hartmann's procedure in, 307
laparoscopic surgery in, 306–312, 313
with end-to-end anastomosis, 311–312, 313
with side-to-side functional end-to-end anastomosis, 307–311
Paul-Mikulicz resection in, 307
resuscitation in, 303
sigmoid colectomy in, 307
sigmoidoscopic reduction in, 306
surgical, 306–312
Signal output, from camera, 18
Simpson and Mayo's system, for colorectal cancer staging, 270
Sling rectopexy, for rectal prolapse, 294
Small bowel, injury of, 86
resection of, 473–483
closure after, 482
complications of, 483
discharge criteria for, 483
dissection methods for, 475, 476
equipment for, 474
exposure methods for, 475
laparoscopic, operating room configuration for, 38
patient positioning for, 474
patient selection for, 473

Small bowel (*Continued*)
postoperative management of, 482
preoperative evaluation for, 473
preoperative preparation for, 473–474
procedural details for, 475, 477, 477–478, 479, 479–481, 481–482
retraction methods for, 475, 476
trocar placement and size selection for, 474–475
video equipment positioning for, 474
Smoking, ulcer healing and, 141
Solid state currents, versus vacuum tube generated currents in electrosurgery, 28–29
Spherocytosis, hereditary, 154–155
Sphincterotomy, endoscopic, for common bile duct removal, 199–200
preoperative, for duct clearance, 201, 202
Spleen, abscess of, 158
cysts of, 158
disorder(s) of, hemolytic anemias as, 154–155
hypersplenism as, 156–157
neoplastic, 157
purpura as, 156
ectopic, 158
salvage of, after trauma, 161–162
surgery on, 154–162
trauma to, 159
tumors of, 158
Splenectomy, historic review of, 154
laparoscopic technique of, 159–162
Splenic artery aneurysm, 158
Splenic flexure, volvulus of, 316
Staging, laparoscopic, operating room configuration for, 40
Staplers, 13–14
Staples, in blood vessel control, 122, 122–123
Stapling instruments, 127, 128, 129
Stomach, malignancies in, staging of, 321–323
outlet obstruction of, 146–147
resection of, 441–443
for peptic ulcer disease, 150
ulcers of, perforation of, 145–146
perforation of, management of, 146
surgical management of, 144
Stones, in common bile duct, 198–209
difficult removal of, 201–203, 202–203
intransigent, 204–205
management of, 205–207

Stones (Continued)
    direct laparoscopic choledochotomy in, 206–207, *208*
    laparoscopic cholangiography in, 205
    laparoscopic exploration in, 205–209
    nonsurgical, 198–201
    removal of, 455
        endoscopic sphincterotomy for, 199–201
        intracorporeal electrohydraulic lithotripsy in, 203–204, *204*
        mechanical lithotripsy in, 203, *204*
        percutaneous endoscopic techniques for, 198–199
  in distal cystic duct, removal of, 190–191
  in gallbladder. See *Gallstones.*
Stump, appendiceal, leakage from, 219
Subcutaneous emphysema, in extraperitoneal insufflation, 82
  management of, 105
Sucralfate, for peptic ulcer disease, 142
Surgiwand Tip system, 30
Suturing, laparoscopic, 108–109
Suturing instruments, 12–13
S-video, 18, 20

T

Table, operating room, 34–35
Tackers, 13–14
Telescopes, for abdominal perineal resection, 606
Tension pneumothorax, during laparoscopic cholecystectomy, 51
Testes, undescended, 358–361
  location of, 359t
Thalassemia, 155
Thermal injury, of small bowel, 86
Thoracoscopy, 345–349
  applications of, 345–346
  diagnostic, 345–346
  instrumentation recommended for, 346t
  operative, operating room configuration for, 40
  technique of, 346–349
  therapeutic, 346

Thrombocytopenic purpura, 156
Tissue approximation techniques, 107–113
  in laparoscopic versus open surgery, 107–108
TNM system, for colorectal cancer staging, 272t, 272–273
Traction/countertraction, in laparoscopic dissection, 120
Training, postdoctoral, 675–690
Transverse colon, volvulus of, 315
Trauma, diagnosis of, laparoscopy in, 323–324
  splenic, 159
Trendelenburg position, complications of laparoscopic cholecystectomy involving, 47–49, 48t
  reverse, in laparoscopic cholecystectomy, 53
Trocar, 7–10
  for abdominal perineal resection, 606
  injuries from, 83–84
  insertion techniques for, closed and open, 97–106
    complications of laparoscopic cholecystectomy involving, 47, 47t
    creating pneumoperitoneum in, 98–101
    detailed, 98–106
    for additional trocars, 101, *103*, *104*
    for first trocar, 101, *102*
    historical background on, 97–98
    pitfalls of, 101, 103–105
  not entering peritoneal cavity, management of, 103–104, *104*
  placement of, in pregnant patient, 69–70
  removal of, 106
Truncal vagotomy, 420–428
  bilateral, and pyloric dilatation with balloon, 427, 427–428
  for peptic ulcer disease, 149–150
  right, with anterior fundic seromyotomy, 420–426
    anterior fundic seromyotomy in, 423–426
    complications of, 426
    dissection techniques for, 422
    equipment for, 421
    parietal closure in, 426
    patient positioning for, 421, 422
    patient selection for, 420
    pneumoperitoneum in, 422

Truncal vagotomy *(Continued)*
    postoperative care in, 426
    preoperative care in, 421
    preoperative evaluation for, 420–421
    results of, 426
    technique of, 422–423, *424*
    trocar placement for, 421–422
    video equipment positioning for, 421
    with anterior highly selective vagotomy, 427–428
Tumors, splenic, 158
Turnbull, Kyle, Watson, and Spratt's system, for colorectal cancer staging, 271

U

Ulcer(s), duodenal, perforation of, management of, 145–146
    surgical management of, 143
  gastric, perforation of, management of, 146
    surgical management of, 144
  peptic, 137–151. See also *Peptic ulcer disease.*
  solitary rectal, with rectal prolapse, 292
Ultrasonography, for colonic cancers, 276
  for rectal cancer, 275–276
  in colorectal cancer evaluation, 275–277
  in preoperative evaluation for low anterior resection, 576
  intraoperative, in hepatic metastases detection, 277
  laparoscopic, in colorectal cancer evaluation, 277, *278*
  three-dimensional, for colorectal cancer, 277
Ultrasound probes, endoscopic, for colorectal cancer, 276–277
Ureter, anatomy of, 367–368
  injury to, complicating laparoscopic, 87
Urologic disorder(s), 351–362
  cryptorchidism as, 358–361
  laparoscopic nephrectomy for, 361
  laparoscopy for, complications of, 362
  pelvic lymphadenectomy for, 351–356. See also *Pelvic lymphadenectomy.*

Urologic disorder(s) *(Continued)*
  varicocele as, 356–358
Urologic procedures, laparoscopic, complications of, 90–91
Uterus, anatomy of, 366
  masses in, 368–369

V

Vacuum tube generated currents, versus solid state currents, in electrosurgery, 28–29
Vagotomy, 405–419
  anterior highly selective, right truncal vagotomy with, 427–428
  closure in, 414–415
  complications of, 91, 415
  discussion of, 415–418
  evolving techniques in, 415–418
  for peptic ulcer disease, 149–150
  initial assessment in, 408
  insufflation and, 408
  operating room configuration for, 39–40
  patient positioning for, 407
  patient preparation for, 407
  patient selection for, 406
  posterior vagus nerve identification and division in, 409–414
  postoperative management of, 415
  preoperative evaluation for, 406
  retraction of left lobe of liver in, 409
  trocar placement for, 407–408
  truncal, 420–428. See also *Truncal vagotomy.*
Varicocele, 356–358
Vascular injury, 86–87
  management of, 105, *105*
Vasopressin release, by pneumoperitoneum, 64–65
Venous return, pneumoperitoneum and, 65–66
Ventilation, effects of pneumoperitoneum on, 63–64
Veress needle, 7, *8*
  injuries from, 83–84
  placement of, in pregnant patient, 69–70
VHS video, 20
Video printers, 20–21

Video recorders, 20
Video tape, for documentation, 15–16
Vipoma, 169t
Visick system, in ulcer treatment evaluation, 147
Volvulus, cecal, 312–315. See also *Cecal volvulus.*

Volvulus *(Continued)*
  of colon, 301–316
  of transverse colon, 315
  sigmoid, 301–312. See also *Sigmoid volvulus.*
  splenic flexure, 316

ISBN 0-7216-6648-5

90071